Miller's Nursing for Wellness in Older Adults

Miller's Nursing for *Wellness* in Older Adults

CANADIAN EDITION

Sandra P. Hirst, RN, PhD, GNC(c)

Associate Professor, Faculty of Nursing
University of Calgary
Calgary, Alberta, Canada

Annette M. Lane, RN, PhD

Associate Professor, Faculty of Nursing
Center for Nursing and Health Studies Athabasca University
Athabasca, Alberta, Canada

Carol A. Miller, MSN, RN-BC, AHN-BC

Gerontological Clinical Nurse Specialist and Nurse Care Manager
Care & Counseling
Cleveland, Ohio

Clinical Faculty
Frances Payne Bolton School of Nursing
Case Western Reserve University
Cleveland, Ohio

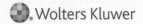. Wolters Kluwer

Philadelphia • Baltimore • New York • London
Buenos Aires • Hong Kong • Sydney • Tokyo

Executive Acquisitions Editor: Patrick Barbera
Product Development Editor: Shana Murph
Editorial Assistant: Dan Reilly
Design Coordinator: Holly Reid McLaughlin
Art Director, Illustration: Jennifer Clements
Manufacturing Coordinator: Karin Duffield
Prepress Vendor: S4Carlisle Publishing Services

Canadian Edition

9 8 7 6 5 4 3 2 1

Printed in China

Library of Congress Cataloging-in-Publication Data
Hirst, Sandra P., 1951- , author.
Miller's nursing for wellness in older adults / Sandra P. Hirst, Annette M. Lane, Carol A. Miller. -- Canadian edition.
   p. ; cm.
  Nursing for wellness in older adults
  Based on: Nursing for wellness in older adults / Carol A. Miller. 7th ed. 2015.
  Includes bibliographical references and index.
  ISBN 978-1-4511-9391-6— ISBN 1-4511-9391-2
  I. Lane, Annette M., 1962- , author.   II. Miller, Carol A., author.   III. Miller, Carol A. Nursing for wellness in older adults. Based on (work):   IV. Title.   V. Title: Nursing for wellness in older adults.
  [DNLM: 1. Geriatric Nursing—Canada.   2. Aged—psychology—Canada.   3. Health Promotion—Canada.   4. Nursing Theory—Canada.   WY 152]
  RC954
  618.97'0231—dc23
                                                                                    2014040804

Dedications

To Martin, Robbie Burns once said "And I will love thee still, my dear,
Till all the seas gang dry." Sandra P. Hirst

To my parents, Gysbert and Jeannette de Bruyn, who lived well and with courage
despite progressing dementia in their later years. Annette M. Lane

Contributors & Reviewers

CONTRIBUTORS

Marlette B. Reed, BEd, MA
Chaplain and Consultant
Calgary, Alberta

Georgia Anetzberger, PhD, ACSW
Assistant Professor, Health Care Administration
Cleveland State University and Case Western
Reserve University
Cleveland, Ohio
Sacramento, California

A Student's Perspective Contributors

*These features were contributed by students from
the following programs:*

Brigham Young University
Provo, Utah

Western Michigan University
Kalamazoo, Michigan

Angelo State University
San Angelo, Texas

REVIEWERS

Beryl Cable-Williams, PhD, RN
Faculty
Trent/Fleming School of Nursing
Trent University
Peterborough, Ontario, Canada

Deborah Fischer, MSN, RN
Faculty
Irene Ransom Bradley School of Nursing
Pittsburg State University
Pittsburg, Kansas

Nancy Fleming, MAEd, HBSCN, RN
Professor
Lakehead University & Confederation College
Collaborative BScN Nursing Program
Thunder Bay, Ontario, Canada

Marian George, EdD
Nursing Educator
Red Deer College
Red Deer, Alberta, Canada

Sandra Gordon, MN, BN, GNC(c)
Assistant Chair and Associate Professor
Mount Royal University School of Nursing
Calgary, Alberta, Canada

Rae Harwood, EdD, RN
Instructor
College of Nursing, Faculty of Health Sciences
University of Manitoba
Winnipeg, Manitoba, Canada

Beverley Jones, MScN, MPA
Professor
School of Nursing
St. Clair College
Windsor, Ontario, Canada

Susan C. Maloney, PhD, FNP-BC
Assistant Professor
Edinboro University
Edinboro, Pennsylvania

Mitzi G. Mitchell, PhD, DNS, MN, MHSc, BScN, BA, RN, GNC(c)
Professor
Seneca College of Applied Arts & Technology
King City, Ontario, Canada

Christina Murray, PhD, MN, BScN, BA, RN
Assistant Professor
School of Nursing
University of Prince Edward Island
Charlottetown, Prince Edward Island, Canada

Verna Pangman, MEd, MN, RN
Faculty of Nursing
Helen Glass Centre for Nursing
University of Manitoba
Winnipeg, Manitoba, Canada

Cynthia Ploutz, MS, FNP-BC
Assistant Professor of Nursing
Hartwick College
Oneonta, New York

Jocelyn Rempel, MN, RN, GNC(c)
Associate Professor
School of Nursing
Faculty of Health and Community Studies
Mount Royal College
Calgary, Alberta, Canada

Deborah A. Vandewater, MN, RN
Professor
St. Francis Xavier University
Distance Nursing Program
Antigonish, Nova Scotia, Canada

Kevin Y. Woo, PhD, RN, FAPWCA
Assistant Professor
School of Nursing
Queen's University
Kingston, Ontario, Canada

Preface

Why is a Canadian textbook in gerontological nursing so important and needed at this time? It seems like a rhetorical question as many settings in which nurses work—medical units, outpatient clinics, community-based day programs, psychiatric units and continuing care settings—all involve contact with older adults. This question is not intended to be rhetorical, but truly reflective. As professional nurses, we need to know the clients that we work with; however, *know* is an amazing word and covers a wide diversity of knowledge and skills. This knowledge and skills needs to be applied to a population that demonstrates tremendous heterogeneity in ages, life stages, health and illness, and cultures and beliefs. This textbook was adapted for the Canadian audience; its focus is on the older Canadian and the professional Canadian-based nurse. This Canadian approach enables students and registered nurses to acquire fundamental knowledge about the health issues faced by older Canadians and the resources that this country can offer us to provide quality nursing care.

In every chapter of this textbook, you will see that Canadian content and resources abound. This was clearly one of our intents. We want to showcase and share many of the best practices that were developed and are being used in this country. In addition, we specifically added an evidence-informed nursing practice box that illustrates some of the research being done in this country. This is research that provides you and us, as Canadian nurses, with the evidence to inform our nursing practice. Evidence-informed practice is an expectation of the Canadian Nurses Association and all provincial/territorial jurisdictions.

I (Sandra P. Hirst) remember the first conference on gerontological nursing held in Victoria, British Columbia, in 1983, although we did not even call it our first—that came the following year in Winnipeg, Manitoba. The organizers expected about a hundred or so participants, but they had over three hundred. I felt so proud and thrilled that I had colleagues who talked the same language that I did, who valued working with older adults as I did—but to my naïve surprise at the time, not all of them worked in continuing care settings or in acute care hospitals. I remember too, in 1999, when gerontological certification was first awarded by the Canadian Nurses Association—another key point in our history.

For Annette and I, aging and gerontological nursing is an ongoing process and privilege. We have worked with older adults for most of our nursing careers. The stories that we hear and share with them have enriched our nursing practice, and we are so appreciative to them.

Annette and I are truly honoured to have been asked to adapt Miller's work. We would like to express our appreciation to Carol for the strong foundation that she laid for us when we adapted this book for the Canadian nursing audience. We believe that wellness is a lifespan experience and that nurses facilitate this journey. But more importantly, we are proud to be Canadian gerontological nurses.

Sandra P. Hirst, RN, PhD, GNC(c),
and Annette M. Lane, RN, PhD

ORGANIZATION

Miller's Nursing for Wellness in Older Adults, Canadian Edition, has 29 chapters, organized into five parts. Chapters in Parts 1 and 2 introduce topics relevant to aging, wellness, diversity, older adults and the role of nurses in promoting wellness in older adults. Chapters in Parts 3 and 4 are organized around the Functional Consequences Theory of Gerontological Nursing, so each facet of physiologic or psychosocial function is presented according to age-related changes, risk factors, functional consequences, nursing assessment, nursing diagnosis, wellness outcomes, nursing interventions and evaluation of nursing care. The three chapters in Part 5 help nurses provide holistic care for older adults during illness.

The intent of Part 1 (Chapters 1 through 4), Older Adults and Wellness, is to help nurses apply a wellness philosophy to their care of older adults. Chapters 1 and 2 integrate the concepts of wellness and aging and provide an overview of characteristics and diversity of older adults, with emphasis on the uniqueness of each older adult. Chapter 3 explicates the Functional Consequences Theory, which is applied throughout this book as a framework for wellness-oriented nursing care of older adults. Chapter 4 provides an overview of theories that are pertinent to aging well.

Part 2 (Chapters 5 through 10), Nursing Considerations for Older Adults, introduces gerontological nursing as a subspecialty within nursing and addresses the unique challenges of caring for older adults. Chapter 5 discusses nursing care of older adults as a specialization and as a responsibility for all nurses. This chapter also addresses health promotion with emphasis on ways in which nurses can apply evidence-based guidelines to help older adults develop health-promoting behaviours. Chapter 6 helps nurses identify the many types of community-based services and health care programs that address the complex needs of older adults. This section also covers the multifaceted topics of assessment, medications, and legal and ethical concerns because nurses address these aspects of care with the majority of the older adults for whom they provide care. The important topic of elder abuse and neglect is addressed in this section, with emphasis on the roles of nurses in preventing, identifying and addressing this serious—and all too common—issue.

Part 3 (Chapters 11 through 15), Promoting Wellness in Psychosocial Function, extensively reviews cognitive and psychosocial function and provides guidelines for a comprehensive nursing assessment of psychosocial function, with emphasis on healthy older adults. In addition, this part covers delirium, dementia and depression, which are three of the most commonly occurring pathologic conditions that have serious psychosocial consequences for older adults.

Part 4 (Chapters 16 through 26), Promoting Wellness in Physical Function, includes chapters that address each of the following specific aspects of functioning in older adults: hearing, vision, digestion and nutrition, urinary function, cardiovascular function, respiratory function, mobility and safety, integument, sleep and rest, thermoregulation and sexual function. Selected common pathologic conditions are also addressed in these chapters when these conditions affect a particular aspect of functioning in older adults.

Part 5 (Chapters 27 through 29), Promoting Wellness in All Stages of Health and Illness, has been added to address topics of caring for older adults during illness and when they are experiencing pain or are at the end of life.

NEW AND SPECIAL FEATURES

Special features from past editions have been retained in this edition, and several new features have been added.

Pedagogical Features

- **Learning Objectives** help the reader identify important chapter content and focus his or her reading.
- **Key Terms** listed at the beginning of the chapter and bolded in the text highlight important vocabulary.
- **Theory Illustrations** at the beginning of each chapter on specific aspects of functioning present an overview of the Functional Consequences Theory in the context of the nursing process.
- **Icons** identify the five major components of the Functional Consequences Theory:

   Age-related changes

   Risk factors

   Functional consequences

   Nursing assessment

   Nursing interventions

- **Online Learning Activities** direct readers to websites that provide enhanced information related to the topic, including resources, access to articles and evidence-based guidelines.

Canadian Evidence-Informed Nursing Practice Research Boxes

- **Unfolding Case Studies** provide real-life examples of the cumulative effects of age-related changes and risk factors, beginning in young-old adulthood and continuing through all the stages of later adulthood. **Thinking Points** after each segment of the case assist the student in applying the content of the chapter to the case example. Many chapters include a concluding case study with a sample **Nursing Care Plan**.
- **Chapter Highlights** facilitate review of the material.
- **Critical Thinking Exercises,** at the end of each chapter, help readers to gain insight and develop problem-solving skills through purposeful, goal-directed thinking.
- **References** give readers additional information about the most up-to-date research that supports evidence-based practice.

Practice-Oriented Features

- **QSEN** examples provide application of Knowledge, Skills and Attitudes for care plans related to unfolding case examples.
- **Evidence-Based Practice** boxes are included in clinically oriented chapters to summarize guidelines for research-based care of older adults.
- **Wellness Opportunities** are sprinkled throughout the clinically oriented chapters to draw attention to ways in which nurses can promote wellness during the usual course of their care activities.
- **A Student's Perspective** provides reality-based stories written by nursing students that illustrate the application of wellness concepts in clinical practice.
- **Cultural Considerations** boxes help the reader to appreciate cultural differences that may influence his or her approach to a patient, resident or client.
- **Diversity Notes** give brief information about differences among specific groups (e.g., men and women, whites and First Nations).
- **Assessment Boxes** provide the reader with specific approaches for nursing assessment. Commonly used assessment tools are described (and, in many cases, illustrated).
- **Interventions Boxes** provide succinct guides for nursing interventions, with a strong focus on health promotion. Guides for "best practices" in nursing interventions are given.

Many of the interventions boxes can be used as tools for teaching older adults and their caregivers about how to improve functional abilities. Interventions boxes that double as teaching tools can be downloaded from the Point at http://thepoint.lww.com/miller6e.

TEACHING AND LEARNING PACKAGE

Instructor Resources

Tools to assist you with teaching your course are available upon adoption of this book at http://thePoint.lww.com/Miller6e. Many of these tools are also included on the Instructor's Resource DVD-ROM.

- An **E-Book** allows access to the book's full text and images online.
- The **Test Generator** lets you generate new tests from a bank of NCLEX-style questions to help you assess your students' understanding of the course material.
- **PowerPoint Presentations** provide an easy way for you to integrate the textbook with your students' classroom experience, either via slide shows or handouts. Multiple-choice and True/False questions are integrated into the presentations to promote class participation and allow you to use i-clicker technology.
- A sample **Syllabus** provides guidance for structuring your course.

- An **Image Bank** contains illustrations from the book in formats suitable for printing and incorporating into PowerPoint presentations and Internet sites.
- **Journal Articles**, corresponding to book chapters, offer access to current research available in Lippincott Williams & Wilkins journals.
- Access to all student resources.

Student Resources

Students can also visit at http://thePoint.lww.com/miller6e and access the following tools and resources using the codes printed in the front of their textbooks:

- An **E-Book** allows access to the book's full text and images online.
- **Journal Articles**, corresponding to book chapters to offer access to current research available in Lippincott Williams & Wilkins journals.
- Internet **Resources**, include links to clinical tools, evidence-based practice and health education materials.
- Plus **NCLEX alternate-item format tutorial, a Spanish–English audio glossary, Learning Objectives** and **Interventions Boxes** from the textbook.

Sandra P. Hirst, RN, PhD, GNC(c)
Annette M. Lane, RN, PhD
Carol A. Miller, MSN, RN-BC, AHN-BC

Acknowledgments

We would first like to thank Carol Miller for allowing us to adapt her book. We would also like to acknowledge some of the stops along our journey of gerontological nursing practice. Each stop has been a teachable moment for us, an encounter with an older adult or a family member that encouraged us to continue learning and refining our knowledge and skills and returning these to practice. We believe that we give quality nursing care but we have the stops along our journey that have helped us both achieve this outcome.

We appreciate the staff at Wolters Kluwer | Lippincott Williams & Wilkins, who first approached us with Canadianizing the text. They helped us move from idea to fruition, and we are so grateful.

Contents

part **4**

Promoting Wellness in Physical Function 305

chapter **16**

Hearing 306

chapter **17**

Vision 328

part 5

Promoting Wellness in All Stages of Health and Illness 555

chapter 27
Caring for Older Adults During Illness 556

chapter 28
Caring for Older Adults Experiencing Pain 571

Assessment, Intervention and Evidence-Based Practice Boxes

E·B·P EVIDENCE-BASED PRACTICE BOXES

part **1**

Older Adults and Wellness

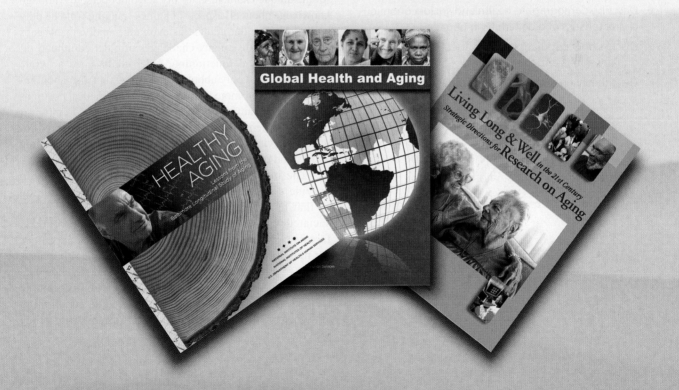

Seeing Older Adults Through the Eyes of Wellness

Despite the common perception that older adulthood involves an extended period of declining health and functioning, conceptualizations of aging are broadening. Currently, most gerontologists and many older adults themselves view aging as a complex process that includes both losses and gains. This perspective is consistent with the broadening base of knowledge about ways in which older adults can achieve what gerontologists call "healthy aging" or "successful aging." It is also consistent with a bio-psycho-social-emotional-spiritual perspective on aging, which addresses all aspects of aging with particular attention to increasing diversity of older adults as a group and respect for the unique characteristics of each older person. Although knowledge about all aspects of aging—ranging from healthy aging to frail older adults—is evolving rapidly, many gaps still exist. Because many challenges of older adulthood involve health and functioning, older adults need accurate information, not only about normal aging, but also about interventions to promote wellness. Nurses are in ideal positions to teach older adults about health and aging and empower them to implement problem-solving strategies directed toward achieving and maintaining a high level of functioning and a good quality of life.

The intent of this gerontological nursing text is to provide comprehensive and research-based information so that nurses can distinguish between the changes associated with normal aging and those that result from risk factors. In addition, the text provides tools and guides for nursing assessment, interventions and health education in relation to all aspects of physical and psychosocial functioning. Nurses can use this information to promote wellness—which includes improved health, functioning and quality of life—for the older adults for whom they provide care.

This chapter provides an overview of concepts related to wellness and aging and presents information about myths and realities. It also presents information about older adults in Canada in terms of demographic, health and socioeconomic characteristics. Last, it presents a brief overview of aging worldwide to provide a broader perspective.

THE RELATIONSHIP BETWEEN WELLNESS AND AGING

If asked to define wellness and aging, most people associate wellness with peak achievement in younger adulthood, and they associate aging with declining health that eventually leads to death. Although somewhat accurate with regard to biologic aging, this description of wellness does not address well-being of the body, mind and spirit. Similarly, many definitions of human aging focus narrowly on physical health and functioning rather than holistically—and accurately—on humans as complex bio-psycho-social-spiritual individuals. Thus, the apparent disconnect between definitions of wellness and aging results not only from misunderstandings about aging, but also from a narrow focus on physical health and functioning.

Promoting wellness in older adults is an ideal; however, nurses may not believe it is achievable in practice because of barriers such as the following:

- Older adults may be pessimistic about their ability to improve their health and functioning.
- Survival needs and a multitude of health problems may take precedence over the "luxury" of being able to focus on wellness and quality of life.
- Despite the increasing emphasis on wellness and health promotion, health care environments focus more on treating disease than on preventing illness and addressing whole-person needs.
- Often older adults and health care providers mistakenly attribute symptoms to aging rather than identify and address the contributing factors that are reversible and treatable.
- Health care providers may not believe that older adults are capable of learning and implementing health-promoting behaviours that are inherent in wellness-oriented care.
- Because many of these barriers arise from myths, misperceptions and lack of knowledge, accurate information about older adults and the relationship between aging and wellness is an indispensable tool for addressing these barriers.

Wellness and Older Adults

The concept of wellness came to public attention a half century ago when Halbert L. Dunn, MD, PhD, retired from his formal public health career and became a "lecturer and consultant in high-level wellness work" (Dunn, 1961, p. 244). Dunn believed that education at all points in a person's life was the key to high-level wellness, and he developed a series of radio talks with the theme "High-Level Wellness for Man and Society." He defined high-level wellness as an "integrated method of functioning that is oriented toward maximizing each person's potential, while maintaining a continuum of balance and purposeful direction within the person's environment" (Dunn, 1961, pp. 4–5). In one radio program, Dunn addressed stereotypes about aging and emphasized that "healthy maturity" is characterized not only by physical decline, but also by wisdom. Moreover, he discussed the relationship between mind, body and spirit and stressed the importance of older adults having a purpose in life, communicating with others, maintaining personal dignity and contributing to society (Dunn, 1961).

Even before addressing aging in his public education series, Dunn had published an article in *Geriatrics* while he was chief of the National Office of Vital Statistics in the United States. In the article, he advised all health care workers to foster a sense of value and dignity for older adults by directing interventions toward improved health and functioning (Dunn, 1958). Dunn (1958) described the role of health care professionals with regard to older adults as follows:

> *The later years of life will come to be more widely regarded as years of opportunity for older people and for society if, in addition to prevention, care, and various health-related activities, direct attention is devoted to the promotion of high-level wellness. This will require a major reorientation.* (p. 51)

Wellness and Nursing Care of Older Adults

Nurses have many opportunities to promote wellness for older adults through actions that are integral to holistic nursing. A major focus of a "wellness approach" to older adult health care is addressing the body–mind–spirit interconnectedness of each older adult as a unique and respected individual. This requires that nurses assess each older adult in the full context of his or her personal history and current situation. Based on this holistic assessment, nurses identify realistic wellness outcomes and plan interventions directed toward improved health, functioning and quality of life. This approach may seem challenging—or even impossible—for older adults who are seriously or terminally ill or for those who have overwhelming chronic conditions. Even when caring for someone who is seriously ill or dying, however, nurses can implement interventions directed toward improved physical comfort and psychological and spiritual growth. Some nursing actions that promote wellness for older adults are as follows:

- Addressing the body–mind–spirit interrelatedness of each older adult.
- Identifying and challenging ageist attitudes (including their own), especially those that interfere with optimal health care.
- Assessing each older adult from a whole-person perspective.
- Incorporating wellness nursing diagnoses as a routine part of care.
- Planning for wellness outcomes, which are directed toward improved health, functioning and quality of life.

- Using nursing interventions to address conditions that interfere with optimal functioning (including lack of accurate information about aging).
- Recognizing each older adult's potential for improved health and functioning as well as psychological and spiritual growth.
- Teaching about self-care behaviours to improve health and functioning (or teaching caregivers of dependent older adults).
- Promoting wellness for caregivers and other people who provide care for older adults (including self-care for nurses).

McMahon and Fleury (2012) published a concept analysis of wellness related to nursing care of older adults and stated,

> Wellness coexists across all functional and health statuses.... In its current state of development within geriatric nursing, wellness has the potential to provide geriatric nurses with tools to foster being well and living values among older adults by addressing their strengths and promoting growth while simultaneously addressing their changing and diverse needs. (p. 49)

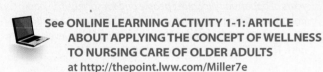

See **ONLINE LEARNING ACTIVITY 1-1: ARTICLE ABOUT APPLYING THE CONCEPT OF WELLNESS TO NURSING CARE OF OLDER ADULTS** at http://thepoint.lww.com/Miller7e

Definitions of Aging

Gerontologists and lay people define aging from many perspectives. Objectively, **aging** is a universal process that begins at birth; in this context, it applies equally to young and old people. Subjectively, however, aging is typically associated with being "old" or reaching "older adulthood," and people define aging in terms of personal meaning and experience. Children usually do not view themselves as aging, but they delight in announcing how old they are, and they anticipate birthdays with great enthusiasm. They view their birthdays as positive events that will permit them to enjoy additional opportunities and responsibilities. Adolescents, likewise, view aging as the mechanism that allows them to participate legally in important activities, such as driving and voting. In contrast, adults tend to view "old age" as something to be avoided and they are likely to define the onset of older adulthood as a decade beyond their current age.

The term **subjective age** (also referred to as *feel* age or **age identity**) describes a person's perception of his or her age. Subjective aging experiences are multidimensional, with perceptions of physical and social-cognitive functioning having a strong influence (Miche et al., 2014). Nurses often observe this phenomenon when they hear people whose chronologic age is 75 years, 80 years or older refer to "old people" as if they were a group older than and distinct from themselves. Studies show that many older adults feel significantly younger than their chronological age and that this perception helps them maintain a positive view of themselves

(Weiss & Freund, 2012; Weiss & Lang, 2012). Studies also indicate that self-perception of feeling younger can positively influence an older adult's health, functioning and sense of well-being (Low et al., 2013; Stephan et al., 2013). **Perceived age**, defined as other people's estimation of someone's age, is another aspect of aging that gerontologists are studying. For example, a recent study of same-sex twins aged 70 years and above found that those who were perceived as chronologically older had shorter life expectancy, even after adjusting for other factors (Christensen et al., 2009).

Objectively, people define **chronologic age** as the length of time that has passed since birth. North American culture is particularly fascinated by numbers, quantities and relative values that can be measured. Among the questions frequently asked and answered are *How much? How far? How often?* and *How old?* Our fascination with age is particularly evident in media newspaper articles, which invariably state the age of the subjects, regardless of the relevance of age to the topic. In addition to being easily measured, another advantage of chronologic age is that it serves as an objective basis for social organization. For example, societies establish chronologic age criteria for certain activities, such as education, voting, driving, marriage, employment, alcohol consumption, military service and the collection of retirement benefits. To participate legally in these activities, people must provide documentation of a certain chronologic age.

Sixty-five years of age became the marker for old age in Canada, due to government initiatives. In 1965, the eligibility age for the existing Old Age Security plan in Canada was reduced from 70 years of age to 65 years (through one-year gradations). In 1965, the Canada Pension Plan and Quebec Pension Plan were introduced and they came into effect in 1966 (Human Resources Development Canada, n.d.). With the linkage of retirement benefits to 65 years, this age became correlated to old age.

During the 1960s, gerontologists also viewed 65 years of age as an acceptable chronologic criterion for aging processes. In recent decades, however, gerontologists agree that aging is too complex to be defined only by one's birth date. From both scientific and humanistic perspectives, a person's chronologic age is relatively insignificant because there is no biologic measurement that applies to everyone at a specific age. Consequently, gerontologists have commonly divided older adulthood into subgroups, such as young-old, middle-old, old-old and oldest-old. As one of the first gerontologists to challenge the original criterion stated,

> We have used sixty-five as the economic marker, then as the social and psychological marker, of old age. A set of stereotypes has grown up that older persons are sick, poor, enfeebled, isolated, and desolated. While these stereotypes have been greatly overdrawn even for the old-old, they have become uncritically attached to the whole group over sixty-five. (Neugarten, 1978, pp. 47–48)

The trend in gerontology to divide old age into chronologic subcategories is an improvement over the categorization of all people older than 65 years as one homogeneous group, but it has the disadvantage of creating additional stereotypes and age biases. For example, if a chronologically old-old person needs a complicated or expensive medical treatment to maintain or potentially improve his or her health status, such treatment may be discouraged based on advanced age. Currently, geriatricians emphasize that decisions about preventive care and treatment of disease should consider all factors that affect the person's health, functioning and quality of life.

For health care providers whose practice focuses on older adults, as well as for many older adults, the important indicators of age are physiologic health, psychological well-being, socioeconomic factors and the ability to function and participate in desirable activities. On the basis of this understanding of aging, gerontologists have used the term functional age for several decades. This concept is associated with a shift in emphasis from chronologic factors to such factors as whether individuals can contribute to society and experience personal quality of life. Functional age is a concept that is used worldwide, but its definition varies according to different cultural contexts. For example, industrialized societies may associate functional age with self-sufficiency and physiologic function, whereas other cultures might associate it more closely with social or psychological function than with physiologic function.

One advantage of functional definitions of age over chronologic definitions is that the former are associated with higher levels of well-being and with more positive attitudes about aging. From a holistic perspective, the concept of functional age provides a more rational basis for care than the measurement of how many years have passed since the person was born. Thus, the question *How functional?* is more relevant than *How old?* Even more relevant for promoting wellness in older adults are questions such as the following:

- How well do you feel?
- What goals do you have for improving your level of wellness?
- Is there anything that you would like to do that you cannot do?
- What goals do you have for improving your quality of life?

In this text, the term *older adult* applies to individuals experiencing the cumulative effects of age-related changes and risk factors that affect their health and functioning. As will be discussed in Chapter 3, a person does not automatically reach "old age" at a particular point in time. Rather, from a holistic perspective, this conceptualization addresses all aspects of bio-psycho-social-spiritual health and functioning, as discussed in the next section.

Descriptions of Successful Aging

Since the early 1960s, gerontologists have focused on identifying the most agreed-upon components of successful aging and determining how many older adults can be categorized as such. A widely recognized model, which is based on the large-scale longitudinal studies of the MacArthur Research Network on Successful Aging, identified three components of successful aging: an active engagement with life, high cognitive and physical function, and low probability of disease and disability (Rowe & Kahn, 1997). In 2013, several gerontologists commented on differing views of successful aging (Flatt et al., 2013). They stated,

> *The ideas that one can "succeed" at aging, and that some strategies and interventions might increase that success, has reached a position of near-ubiquity within gerontology today—despite the distinctly varied interpretations of the meanings and applications of "successful" aging.* (p. 944)

Currently, there is emphasis on optimal physical, mental, emotional, spiritual and social well-being and quality of life as essential components of successful aging. According to this broad perspective, successful aging encompasses the experiences of older adults who apply adaptive processes to preserve their well-being and transcend limitations associated with diseases and functional limitations (Woods et al., 2012). In one Canadian study, older adults with chronic illnesses noted how drawing on personal resources and engagement in meaningful leisure activities that exercised their minds or bodies strengthened their sense of well-being, despite the limitations imposed by their illnesses (Hutchinson & Nimrod, 2012).

Gerontologists are also emphasizing that the concept of successful aging can be applied to people who have overcome disabilities and disease, in which case the term *aging successfully* is used (Morley, 2009). To illustrate this concept, Morley cited the following examples of well-known people who have aged successfully:

- Grandma Moses (Anna Maria Robertson) became a famous painter after arthritis interfered with her ability to make quilts.
- Monet developed the painting technique known as modern impressionism after his eyesight was clouded by cataracts.
- Renoir painted with a clenched fist after he developed arthritis.
- Pablo Casals played his cello each day in his 90s.
- Maurice Ravel composed the famous *Bolero* after he was affected with dementia.

A Student's Perspective

My interview with Mr. H. was an enlightening experience. I was able to learn a great deal about the time period in which this man grew up. Also, it was eye opening to see how healthy a man of 84 years could be. His health reinforced what we are learning. He does have a chronic illness, diabetes (like 80% of those aged 65+), but he is still independent and free of any noticeable cognitive impairments. He can still drive and get around, which also defeats a lot of ageist attitudes. Negative attitudes that I have heard about elders were defeated by this man. Reading about aging in a book is one thing, but actually interacting with elders and learning firsthand is much more influential. Mr. H. really taught me not to hold ageist attitudes.

Jordan S.

A recent study of older adults with late-life disability supports the perspective that aging successfully has a subjective component that involves using adaptation and coping strategies to "align their perception of successful aging with their experiences" (Romo et al., 2013).

ATTITUDES TOWARD AGING

Images of and attitudes toward aging arise from long-term patterns of falsely attributing pathologic conditions and undesirable characteristics to normal aging. In reality, many older adults function independently and report high levels of satisfaction with their health and quality of life, even with their high prevalence of chronic conditions. Historically, societal attitudes toward aging have ranged from respect and veneration to fear of aging and idealization of youth. As indicated in Figure 1-1, the pendulum is slowly swinging again toward positive attitudes toward aging and older adulthood. This shift is attributable to the increasing emphasis on successful aging and the emergence of accurate information about the difference between aging and disease. Despite this focus on successful aging, however, care of older adults continues to be influenced by long-standing negative attitudes toward aging that are held by society, as well as health care professionals. Thus, an important part of gerontological nursing is to recognize the effects of ageism and address attitudes that can interfere with holistic care of older adults.

Ageism

The term *ageism* was coined by Robert Butler in 1968 and was first used in a publication, *The Gerontologist*, the next year (Butler, 1969). With the 1975 publication of Butler's Pulitzer Prize-winning book *Why Survive? Being Old in America*, ageism became an accepted new word in the English language (Butler, 1975). Butler defined ageism as "the prejudices and stereotypes that are applied to older people sheerly on the basis of their age. . . . Ageism, like racism and sexism, is a way of pigeonholing people and not allowing them to be individuals with unique ways of living their lives" (Butler et al., 1991, p. 243). It is widely recognized that in contrast to the social categories related to gender or race, only age encompasses the category that every living person potentially joins (North & Fiske, 2012).

A review of ageism among younger and older adults proposed that younger adults develop ageist attitudes to protect themselves from death anxiety, whereas older adults develop ageist attitudes because of negative stereotypes about their own group (Bodner, 2009). Another study found that among groups of older adults between the ages of 68 and 98, participants aged 81 to 98 held more ageist stereotypes and reported more avoidance of older adults than those aged 63 to 73 (Bodner et al., 2012). Common manifestations of ageism include negative stereotypes of social isolation, psychological rigidity, asexual behaviour, lack of creativity, physical and mental decline, and economic and familial burden. For example, a review of 262 articles published in the *Economist* between 1997 and

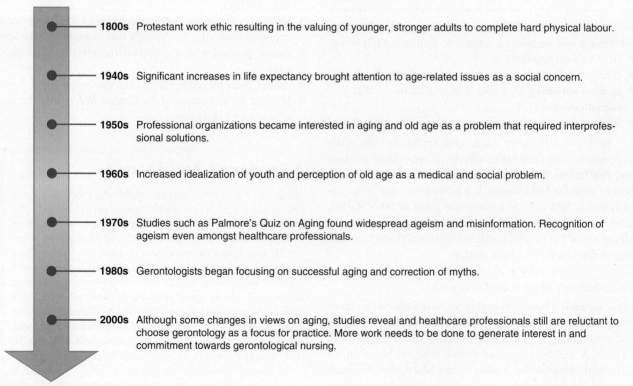

1800s Protestant work ethic resulting in the valuing of younger, stronger adults to complete hard physical labour.

1940s Significant increases in life expectancy brought attention to age-related issues as a social concern.

1950s Professional organizations became interested in aging and old age as a problem that required interprofessional solutions.

1960s Increased idealization of youth and perception of old age as a medical and social problem.

1970s Studies such as Palmore's Quiz on Aging found widespread ageism and misinformation. Recognition of ageism even amongst healthcare professionals.

1980s Gerontologists began focusing on successful aging and correction of myths.

2000s Although some changes in views on aging, studies reveal and healthcare professionals still are reluctant to choose gerontology as a focus for practice. More work needs to be done to generate interest in and commitment towards gerontological nursing.

FIGURE 1-1 Historical trends in views on aging in Canada

2008 found that 64% portrayed an ageist view of older people being a burden on society (Martin et al., 2009).

In the late 1960s, Erdman Palmore and other researchers concluded that between 1950 and 1970, the effects of ageism diminished more slowly than those of racism (Palmore, 2005). On the basis of his research, Palmore developed two versions of a 25-item Facts on Aging Quiz, as indirect measures of ageism. These quizzes have been used in hundreds of studies and classrooms and consistently show more negative bias than positive bias toward older adults (Palmore, 2005). Palmore later developed the Ageism Survey, a 20-item ageism review, to directly measure older adults' experiences of ageism (Fig. 1-2). Studies using this survey in Canada and the United States indicate that most respondents in both countries frequently experienced ageism (Palmore, 2005). For example, one study of 247 community-dwelling adults between the ages of 60 and 92 years found that 84% of the participants said they had experienced at least one type of ageism, with the most common forms being jokes and greeting cards that poked fun at older people (McGuire et al., 2008).

Although ageism is not unique to Canada, it does not exist in all cultures. In North America, ageism has developed and grown as a result of dominant cultural beliefs and trends, such as the glorification of youth, the perception of the individual as autonomous and the equating of human worth with economic worth. Contrasting cultural perspectives on independence versus interdependence is another factor that can account for differences in attitudes about aging (Plath,

2009). For example, Levy and Leifheit-Limson (2009) found that older adults in the United States and Japan were likely to make age attributions, but these were associated with worse functional health only among the Americans. This difference was attributed to the Japanese acceptance of interdependence, which is rooted in the Confucian precept that adult children should respect and support parents. A potentially positive outcome of the increasing cultural diversity in Canada and the United States is that the dominant cultural values that foster ageism may be challenged by cultural values of other groups. Box 1-1 identifies cultural perspectives on elders and family caregiving relationships.

Effects of Ageism

In recent years, gerontologists have identified some of the specific effects of negative attitudes and stereotypes on older adults. A review of studies found the following serious negative consequences of ageism (North & Fiske, 2012):

- In medical care: older people often receive less aggressive treatment for common ailments, which are dismissed as a natural part of aging.
- In the workplace: older job applicants are rated less positively than younger ones, even when they are similarly qualified and despite considerable research showing that job performance does not decrease in older adults.
- In nursing homes and home settings: elder abuse and neglect is underreported.
- In media: older adults are underrepresented and stereotyped.

The Ageism Survey

Please put a number in the blank that shows how often you have experienced that event: Never = 0; Once = 1; More than once = 2. ("Age" means older age.)

_____ 1. I was told a joke that pokes fun at old people.

_____ 2. I was sent a birthday card that pokes fun at old people.

_____ 3. I was ignored or not taken seriously because of my age.

_____ 4. I was called an insulting name related to my age.

_____ 5. I was partronized or "talked down to" because of my age.

_____ 6. I was refused rental housing because of my age.

_____ 7. I had difficulty getting a loan because of my age.

_____ 8. I was denied a position of leadership because of my age.

_____ 9. I was rejected as unattractive because of my age.

_____ 10. I was treated with less dignity and respect because of my age.

_____ 11. A waiter or waitress ignored me because of my age.

_____ 12. A doctor or nurse assumed my ailments were caused by my age.

_____ 13. I was denied medical treatment because of my age.

_____ 14. I was denied employment because of my age.

_____ 15. I was denied promotion because of my age.

_____ 16. Someone assumed I could not hear well because of my age.

_____ 17. Someone assumed I could not understand because of my age.

_____ 18. Someone told me, " You're too old for that."

_____ 19. My house was vandalized because of my age.

_____ 20. I was victimized by a criminal because of my age.

Please write in your age: _____

Please check: Male _____ Female _____

What is the highest grade in school that you completed? _____

Survey © Copyright 2000 by Erdman Palmore.

FIGURE 1-2 The Ageism Survey is being used to measure the prevalence and identify types of ageism. (Used with permission from Palmore, E. [2000]. *The ageism survey* [6th ed.]. Durham, NC: Duke Centre for the Study of Aging.)

Box 1-1 Cultural Considerations: Cultural Perspectives on Elders and Family Caregiving Relationships

Aboriginals (Canadian)

- Elder status is characterized by health status and roles as counsellors, teachers or grandparents.
- Grandparents often care for grandchildren, who then are expected to care for the elders; grandmother may be called mother.

Chinese

- Traditional Chinese values place family and society above the individual.
- Elders are highly respected and honoured.
- Multigenerational households are common.

Filipinos

- Respect for elders is a cornerstone of Filipino values, demonstrated by deference in verbal and nonverbal communication.
- Children (especially the oldest daughter) are expected to care for parents to repay their debt of gratitude (*utang na loob*).

Indians

- Older Indians who live in multigenerational housing often act as the "head" of the household.
- Older adults play a significant role in raising grandchildren.

Japanese

- Elders are highly respected and those who are able help in caring for children and grandchildren.
- Elders commonly maintain separate households; when they need help, the eldest son's family is expected to care for them at home.

Koreans

- Caring for elderly kin is a family duty that is associated with respect for elders and family bonds inherent in Confucianism.
- Grandparents frequently provide care for grandchildren; elders are welcome to live with family during times of need.

Vietnamese

- The more one respects the elderly, the greater one's chance is of reaching old age.
- Young adults are expected to assume full responsibility for caring for elders at home.

Source: Lipson, J. G., & Dibble, L. (2005). *Culture and clinical care.* San Francisco, CA: UCSF Nursing Press.

One study found that women, but not men, associated older-age identities with pessimistic outlooks about their own cognitive aging (Schafer & Shippee, 2010).

Another outcome of ageism is aging anxiety. This anxiety is experienced by people of all ages as fears and worries about detrimental effects associated with older adulthood (e.g., social losses, financial insecurity, changes in appearance and declines in health and functioning). One study found that aging anxiety about loss of attractiveness was higher among women who were younger, white, employed, heterosexual, separated or divorced, and less financially independent (Barrett & Robbins, 2008). Aging anxiety is reinforced by negative stereotypes of older adults and the associated fear that these problems are likely to occur in one's own later life. In contrast, people who have accurate information about aging and positive experiences with older adults are less likely to have aging anxiety.

One aspect of ageism that is particularly relevant to providing care for older adults is related to age attribution, which is the tendency to attribute problems to the aging process rather than to pathologic and potentially treatable conditions. For example, the phrase *senior moment* has been used since the mid-1990s to describe a lapse in memory. Because age attribution can have the effect of a self-fulfilling prophecy, health care professionals need to be cognizant of messages they give to older adults. Negative effects of age attribution include worse physical functioning, delayed treatment for health problems and an increased risk of mortality (Levy et al., 2009). One study found that exposure to images associated with healthy aging had a more positive effect on older adults, as compared with younger adults (Lineweaver et al., 2009).

When older adults or health care professionals falsely attribute symptoms of pathologic conditions to normal aging, they are likely to overlook treatable conditions, and significant harm can result from this negligence. An important responsibility of gerontological nurses is to be knowledgeable about the differences between age-related changes and pathologic conditions, so appropriate nursing interventions can be initiated. An essential first step in planning interventions, especially health-promotion interventions, is to identify those factors that are not inherent consequences of aging. Throughout this text, emphasis is placed on differentiating between age-related changes, which cannot be modified, and those factors that can be addressed through interventions. Chapter 3 describes a nursing model for this approach to promoting wellness for older adults.

Another consequence of ageism is the emergence of the anti-aging movement, which has been promoted by the American Academy of Anti-Aging Medicine since the early 1990s. The anti-aging movement views aging as a process that can be stopped and the lifespan as something that can be extended for up to 200 years. Anti-aging interventions include exercise and lifestyle modifications, but there also is strong emphasis on dietary supplements and other products that have not been proved effective. While the anti-aging movement is more prominent in the United States than in Canada, the emphasis on appearing younger through routes such as dietary supplements and youth enhancement mechanisms (injections, surgeries, etc.) are very much present. A main criticism is that the anti-aging movement is directed more toward selling products than toward the advancement of sound scientific evidence. One gerontologist concluded that anti-aging concepts are based on an understanding of aging as a bodily failure, which can be counteracted only when scientists no longer hold ageist preconceptions that are embedded in a wider ageist culture (Vincent, 2008).

Addressing Attitudes of Nurses

Negative attitudes about aging that are held by health care workers can negatively affect the care older adults receive.

Box 1-2 Evidence-Informed Nursing Practice

Background: Research generally confirms that nursing students do not choose gerontology as a career preference after graduation. However, there is some evidence that suggests that attitudes toward working with older adults is improving.

Questions: What are novice and experienced nursing students' attitudes toward working with older adults, as well as children? Do these attitudes change in their willingness to care when nursing students become advanced? And, do advanced nursing students demonstrate changes in their willingness to care across the academic year?

Methods: Within this study, nursing students from a baccalaureate program in Eastern Canada were assessed for willingness to care for children and older adults twice. The sample included 114 novice nursing and 56 advanced nursing students. Novice nursing students and advanced nursing students were tested at the beginning of the academic year and again at the end of the year. Students were asked to rate their willingness to work with both populations on a Likert-like scale (1–7 with 1 indicating "not willing at all").

Results: Novice nurses became less positive about nursing all age groups by the end of the first year (not just caring for older adults). Additionally, advanced nursing students revealed some negative attitudes toward caring for both children and older adults. Despite these findings, the researchers concluded that the students were relatively positive about caring for older adults, particularly when they compared their results with previous studies. Furthermore, they noted that the advanced nursing students were much more positive in their attitudes toward working with older adults than were novice nursing students.

Implications: The researchers concluded that nurse educators should attempt to address negative stereotypes about aging in novice nursing students by providing them with positive clinical experiences, such as working with healthy older adults who reside in the community. They suggested that advanced nursing students may need to learn (through positive role models, for example) that caring for older adults can be intellectually challenging and requires sophisticated nursing skills.

Gould, O. N., & MacLennan, A. (2012). Career preferences of nursing students. *Canadian Journal on Aging, 31*(4), 471–482.

A Student's Perspective

I personally have aging anxiety. After working at an assisted-living facility for the past year and a half, I have seen some pretty tragic and depressing events happen in the lives of these residents. Many of these residents tell me they do not know why God has kept them around this long. But listening to the stories of others has given me hope. I found it very encouraging to see the elderly people taking classes and enjoying the discussions they were a part of. I would imagine that it would be tempting to give up when the mental or physical functioning is not what it used to be, but some of the people gave me hope for aging. They make me want to be a stronger person even now at the age of 19 years. They seem to have so much passion and intensity to their lives. Not only can they serve to encourage people in their younger years to continually embrace life, but I hope other elderly people can be encouraged that they do not have to let go of their dreams just because they are aging. You can age successfully as these people have by living life to its fullest and persevering to keep your individuality and talents alive.

Jessica S.

experiences that are integral to their self-identities. Nurses have daily opportunities to learn about aging and older adulthood simply by listening to the older adults for whom they provide care. In addition, nurses can equip themselves with accurate information about the older adult population. Accurate information may be the most effective antidote to negative attitudes resulting from misunderstandings or myths. The next sections address myths about aging by providing an accurate snapshot of older adults in Canada.

DEBUNKING MYTHS: UNDERSTANDING REALITIES ABOUT OLDER ADULTS IN CANADA

As a consequence of ageism and negative attitudes about aging, many myths and negative stereotypes about older adults have been perpetuated, especially with regards to aspects of health and functioning. These myths and stereotypes can be particularly detrimental when health care providers lack accurate information on which to base their decisions or actions about older adults because misconceptions lead to suboptimal goals for care. At best, older adults do not experience the benefits of wellness-focused care; at worst, they experience unnecessary decline.

This chapter provides information about characteristics of the older adult population, and Chapter 2 extends this overview by addressing cultural diversity of older adults. Chapters in Part 3 of this book address aspects of functioning that can be significantly affected by myths and misunderstandings about aging. Table 1-1 lists some of the myths and misperceptions about aging that are commonly held by older adults and health care professionals. The related realities about each aspect of health and functioning are also identified, along with a reference to the chapter that provides accurate information to dispel the myths.

Although studies have found that nurses and nursing students hold negative attitudes about caring for older adults, these attitudes are slowly improving because of a broader base of evidence-based information in nursing education (Baumbusch et al., 2012; Eymard & Douglas, 2012; see Box 1-2). Nurses and all health care workers are likely to be influenced not only by ageism in society but also by their own experiences in health care, which often are with those older adults who are the most impaired and in need of interventions. It is important, therefore, that health care workers in all clinical settings recognize that many older adults are healthy and functional and strive toward improved levels of wellness and functioning.

Attitudes are changed through education, but changing attitudes requires first recognizing their existence. Because ageism is subtle but pervasive in Canadian society, nurses first need to become aware of the attitudes they hold toward older adults. The first critical thinking exercise at the end of this chapter suggests ways of becoming aware of one's own attitudes about older adults. Another way of improving negative attitudes about older adults is to listen carefully to older adults as they talk about beliefs, values, hopes and

TABLE 1-1 Myths and Realities of Aging

Myth	Reality
Older adulthood is something to be dreaded because it represents disability and death.	Most older adults live independently, have high levels of self-reported health and are aging successfully. *(Chapter 1)*
People consider themselves "old" on their 65th birthday.	People usually feel old on the basis of their health and function rather than their chronologic age. *(Chapter 1)*
Gerontologists have discovered that, by the age of 75 years, people are quite homogeneous as a group.	The more gerontologists learn about aging, the more they realize that, with increased age, people become more diverse and individuals become less like their age peers. *(Chapters 1, 2 and 4)*
Ageism is a natural part of all societies.	Ageism is more common in industrialized societies and is highly influenced by stereotypes and cultural values. *(Chapter 1)*
Gerontologists have recently discovered a theory that explains biologic aging.	Theories about biologic aging continue to evolve, and there is little agreement on any one theory. *(Chapter 4)*
In today's society, families no longer care for older people.	In Canada, 80% of the care of older adults is provided by their families. *(Chapter 1)*
As people grow older, it is natural for them to want to withdraw from society.	Because older people are unique individuals, each of them responds differently to society. *(Chapter 4)*
By the age of 70 years, an individual's psychological growth is complete.	People never lose their capacity for psychological growth. *(Chapters 4 and 12)*
Increased disability in older people is attributable to age-related changes alone.	Although age-related changes increase one's vulnerability to functional impairments, the disabilities are attributable to risk factors, such as diseases and adverse medication effects. *(Chapter 3)*
Health-promotion efforts are not beneficial to older adults who have two or more chronic conditions.	Research has debunked the myths that prevention is not effective after onset of chronic illness. *(Chapter 5)*
About 20% of people aged 65 years and older live permanently in nursing homes.	About 5% of older adults live in a nursing home at any time. *(Chapters 1 and 6)*
Widowhood and other life events have been found to have a consistently negative impact on older people.	No one life event affects all older people negatively. The most important consideration governing the impact of an event is its unique meaning for the individual. *(Chapter 12)*
In old age, there is an inevitable decline in all intellectual abilities.	A few areas of cognitive ability decline in healthy older adults but other areas show improvement. *(Chapter 11)*
Older adults cannot learn complex new skills.	Older adults are capable of learning new things, but the speed with which they process information slows down with age. *(Chapter 11)*
Constipation develops primarily because of age-related changes.	Constipation is attributable primarily to risk factors, such as restricted activity and poor dietary habits. *(Chapter 18)*
Urinary incontinence is a normal consequence of aging that is best managed by using incontinence products.	In most cases, underlying causes of urinary incontinence can be ddressed and a variety of self-care methods can be initiated. *(Chapter 19)*
Skin wrinkles can be prevented by using oils and lotions.	The best way to prevent skin wrinkles is to avoid exposure to ultraviolet light. *(Chapter 23)*
Older people are less sexually active primarily because they lose the ability to enjoy sex.	Declines in sexual activity in older people are primarily because of risk factors, such as diseases, adverse medication effects, and loss of partner. *(Chapter 26)*
Health care professionals readily recognize adverse medication effects in older adults.	Adverse medication effects are often overlooked in older adults because they are mistakenly attributed to aging or pathologic conditions. *(Chapter 8)*
Some degree of "senility" is normal in very old people.	"Senility" is an inaccurate term used to refer to dementing conditions, which are always caused by pathologic changes. *(Chapter 14)*
Most old people are depressed and should be allowed to withdraw from society.	About one third of older people exhibit depressive symptoms; however, depression is a very treatable condition at any age. *(Chapter 15)*

The characteristics of the older adult population in Canada summarized in this chapter are based on census data and other reliable sources; however, this information can only reflect trends and grouped data. The intent is to provide an overview of population demographics and characteristics of older adults that are most pertinent to holistically caring for older adults. Nurses need to keep in mind that older adults are a highly diverse group and this general information does not necessarily apply to every older individual.

Demographics of Aging

Discussions of current demographic trends in Canada inevitably focus on the so-called **baby boomers**, which is the very large group of people born between 1946 and 1964. Baby boomers began turning 65 in 2011, and as a group they are bringing about major demographic changes. Based on chronologic age, baby boomers will be identified as the "newcomers" of older adulthood until the subsequent generation begins turning 65 in 2029, when the first baby boomers will be 83 years old. Although baby boomers were all born during one 18-year period, this period was characterized by dramatic changes in socioeconomic and political trends. As with other socially labelled groups, the baby boomer generation is extremely heterogeneous, and each person in this group has a unique life story. The influence of this and other population trends, such as greater cultural diversity (see Chapter 2) and increased life expectancy (see Chapter 4), is reflected in the statistics summarized in Box 1-3 and Figure 1-3.

Health Characteristics

A major focus of health characteristics of older adults is on chronic conditions and levels of functioning. During the past few decades, the prevalence of disability among older adults has been gradually decreasing, and a notable percentage of older adults report very good to excellent health, as illustrated in Figure 1-4. At the same time, many older adults live with chronic health conditions, as illustrated in Figure 1-5. Thus, a major focus of health care is on interventions to prevent and

---

Box 1-3 Stats in Brief: Changing Demographics of Aging in Canada

Median Age

- 1956   27.2 years
- 2006   38.8 years
- 2056 (projection)   46.9 years

Average Life Expectancy at Age 65 Years

- 1921   13.3 years (13.6 for women, 13 for men)
- 1971   15.7 years (17.6 for women, 13.8 for men)
- 2007/2009   20.2 years (21.6 for women, 18.5 for men)

Actual and Projected Percentage of People Aged 65+ Years

- 1920s–1930s   5%
- 2005   13.1%
- 2036   24.5%

Actual and Estimated Percentage of People Aged 85+ Years

- 1981   0.8%
- 2011   2%
- 2041   5.8%

Approximate or Estimated Number of Centenarians

- 2001   3,795
- 2011   5,825
- 2036   Up to 20,300

Sources: Statistics Canada. (2007). *Some facts about the demographic and ethnocultural composition of the population.* Retrieved from www.statcan.gc.ca/pub/91-003-x/2007001/4129904-eng.htm

Statistics Canada. (2007). *A portrait of seniors in Canada, 2006.* Retrieved from http://www.statcan.gc.ca/pub/89-519-x/89-519-x2006001-eng.pdf

Statistics Canada. (2013). *National Seniors' day . . . by the number.* Retrieved from http://www42.statcan.gc.ca/smr08/2013/smr08_178_2013-eng.htm

Election Canada. (2012). *Canadian seniors: A demographic profile.* Retrieved from http://www.elections.ca/content.aspx?section=res&dir=rec/part/sen&document=index&lang=e

Statistics Canada. (2012). *Life expectancy at birth and age 65, by sex, by province and territory.* Retrieved from http://www.statcan.gc.ca/tables-tableaux/sum-som/l01/cst01/health72a-eng.htm

Statistics Canada. (2013). *Remaining life expectancy of women and men at age 65, Canada, 1921–2007.* Retrieved from http://www.statcan.gc.ca/pub/89-503-x/2010001/article/11441/tbl/tbl002-eng.htm

---

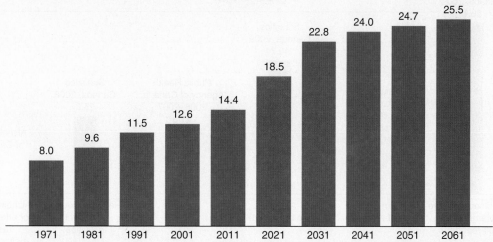

Population 65 years and over, Canada, Historical (1971–2011) and projected (2012–2061) (percentage)

1971	1981	1991	2001	2011	2021	2031	2041	2051	2061
8.0	9.6	11.5	12.6	14.4	18.5	22.8	24.0	24.7	25.5

FIGURE 1-3 Actual and projected total population of Canada, 1971 to 2011 and projected population (2012–2061). (Statistics Canada. [2011]. *Canadians in context.* Retrieved from www4.hrsdc.gc.ca/3ndic.1t.4r@eng.jsp?iid=33)

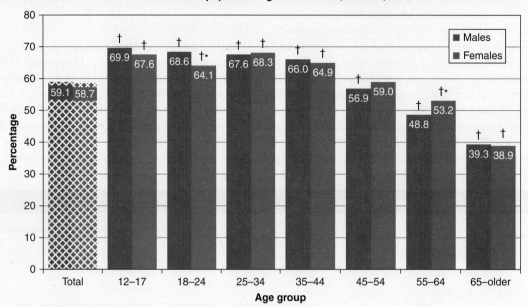

Percentage reporting excellent or very good health, by age group and sex, household population aged 12 or older, Canada, 2008

* *Significantly different from estimate for males (p < 0.05)*
† *Significantly different from overall estimate for same sex (p < 0.05)*

FIGURE 1-4 Percentage of people aged 65+ reporting excellent or very good health, by age group and sex, household population aged 12 or older, Canada, 2008. (Canadian Community Health Survey, 2008. Retrieved from http://statcan.gc.ca/pub/82-229-x/2009001/status/phx-eng.htm)

manage chronic diseases so older adults can maintain optimal levels of functioning, as discussed in detail in Chapters 5 and 6. In recent years, increasing attention has been paid to the negative consequences of health disparities among groups of Canadian Aboriginal peoples and other minorities, as discussed in more detail in Chapter 2. See Chapter 4 for more information on life expectancy and race.

Socioeconomic Characteristics

Socioeconomic characteristics that are most strongly correlated with healthy aging are poverty and lower educational level.

Higher levels of education and income are linked with longer life expectancy and better ratings of self-reported health. This is particularly the case for women (Labonte et al., 2010).

Although census data predict gradual and continuing increases in level of education for older adults—with associated better health and higher incomes—many older adults will remain socioeconomically disadvantaged. For instance, according to the 2010 Healthy Populations report, Canadians living in Newfoundland have higher levels of diabetes and lower life expectancies than those living in other regions of Canada (Labonte et al., 2010). Newfoundland and Labrador

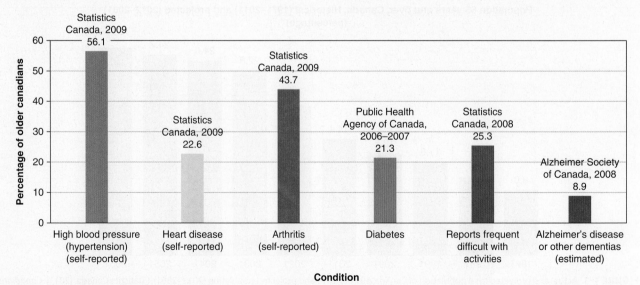

FIGURE 1-5 Chronic conditions among Canadian seniors (65 years of age and older). (Adapted from Public Health Agency of Canada. [2010]. *The Chief Public Health Officer's Report on the state of public health in Canada.* Retrieved from http://www.phac-aspc.gc.ca/cphorsphc-respcacsp/2010/fr-rc/cphorsphc-respcacsp-06-eng.php)

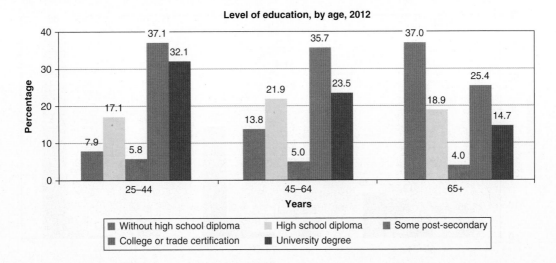

Level of education, by age, 2012

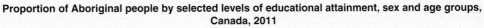

FIGURE 1-6A Educational levels of Canadian adults by age groups, 2012. (Employment and Social Development Canada. [2014]. *Indicators of well-being in Canada: Learning-education attainment.* Retrieved from http://www4.hrsdc.gc.ca/.3ndic.1t.4r@-eng.jsp?iid=29)

also have the lowest percentage of individuals below 65 who are university educated, and of those who have university educations, Newfoundland and Labrador also have low employment rates for the university educated and the lowest percentage of employed individuals with less than high school education (Statistics Canada, 2012a). In this example, lower levels of education are correlated with poorer health and lower life expectancy. Figures 1-6A and 1-6B illustrate educational levels of older Canadians.

In recent decades, the overall poverty rate for older adults has been declining, but this does not mean that all older people are economically better off today than they were

40 years ago. For example, economic conditions of older adults vary considerably as indicated below:

● Older Canadian women are almost twice as likely to live in poverty than are older men (6% compared with 3.3%; Library of Parliament, 2009).
● Poverty rates for individuals above the age of 75 are higher than those for individuals below 75, particularly among women (Conference Board of Canada, 2014).
● Rates of poverty are much higher among Aboriginal Canadians than non-Aboriginal individuals. For instance, not only is the average income of a non-Aboriginal Canadian significantly higher than an Aboriginal individual,

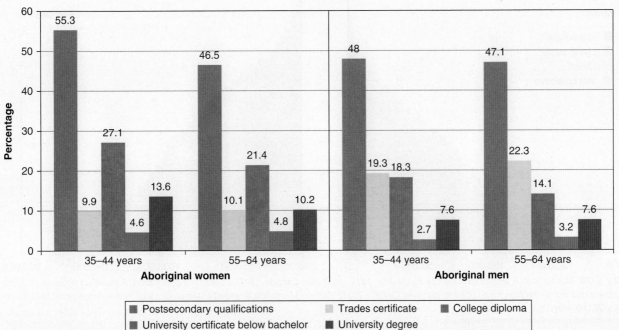

Proportion of Aboriginal people by selected levels of educational attainment, sex and age groups, Canada, 2011

FIGURE 1-6B Educational attainment by Aboriginal peoples in Canada. (Statistics Canada. [2013]. *The educational attainment of Aboriginal people in Canada.* Retrieved from http://www12.statcan.gc.ca/nhs-enm/2011/as-sa/99-012-x/99-012-x2011003_3-eng.cfm)

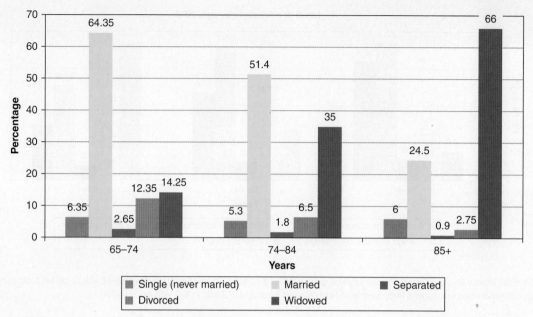

FIGURE 1-7A Marital status by age in Canada. (Statistics Canada. [2012b]. *2011 Census of Canada: Families, households and marital status (Catalogue no. 98-312-XCB2011041).* Ottawa, ON: Author. Percentages calculated from Census numbers—percentages rounded up to the nearest decimal point.)

but also, Statistics Canada data from 2006 suggest that Aboriginal individuals are four times more likely than non-Aboriginals to live in crowded dwellings (Library of Parliament, 2009).

- Recent immigrants to Canada have a much higher rate of low income than other Canadians. According to the 2006 Canadian census, racialized (individuals from visible minorities) communities had double the rate of low income than did non-racialized individuals. In some racialized communities, the percentage of those living in poverty are very high. For instance, according to Statistics Canada, 40% of Koreans were living in poverty in 2006 (Government of Canada, 2013).

Marital status affects other aspects of older adults' lives in many ways, including economic resources, living arrangements and availability of a caregiver for those who are dependent. Marital status varies significantly by sex and age, as illustrated in Figures 1-7A and 1-7B. Box 1-4 summarizes statistics about socioeconomic characteristics of older adults in Canada.

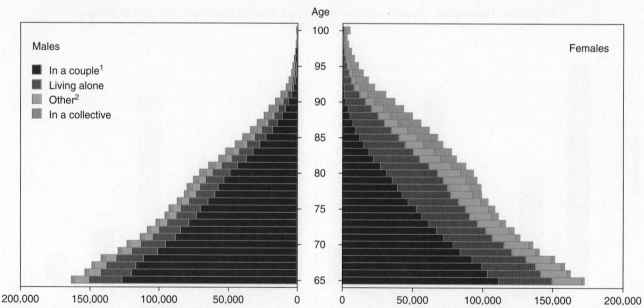

FIGURE 1-7B Marital status adults 65+ by sex in Canada, 2011. (Statistics Canada. [2011]. *Census of population, Population pyramid by living arrangement and sex for the population aged 65 and over, Canada, 2011.* Retrieved from http://www12.statcan.gc.ca/census-recensement/2011/as-sa/98-312-x/2011003/fig/fig3_4-1-eng.cfm)

1. Includes married couples and common-law spouses
2. Includes older adults who are living with relatives or nonrelatives or adult children who are living with an elderly parent

Box 1-4 Stats in Brief: Socioeconomic Characteristics of People Aged 65+ Years in Canada

Education	No High School Certificate	High School (Without Postsecondary Certificate)	Postsecondary Certification
• 2012	37%	18.9%	40.1%
Low Income Cut-Off (LICO)	**1995**	**2007**	**2010**
• Below LICO	10%	4.8%	5.2%
Marital Status	**Men**	**Women**	
• Married or common-law	72.1%	43.8%	

Sources: Employment and Social Development Canada. (2012). *Indicators of well-being: Learning-educational attainment.* Retrieved from http://www4.hrsdc.gc.ca/.3ndic.1t.4r@-eng.jsp?iid=29

Statistics Canada. (2012). *Low income in Canada: A multi-line and multi-index perspective* (Catalogue no. 75F0002M-001). Retrieved from http://www.statcan.gc.ca/pub/75f0002m/75f0002m2012001-eng.pdf

Statistics Canada. (2011). *Living arrangements of seniors.* Retrieved from http://www12.statcan.gc.ca/census-recensement/2011/as-sa/98-312-x/98-312-x2011003_4-eng.pdf

Living Arrangements of Older Adults

Living arrangements for older adults are influenced by such factors as health, marital status, family relationships and socioeconomic conditions, as indicated in the 2011 enumeration conducted by Statistics Canada (2012b):

● Just more than 56% of Canadian older adults live as part of a couple (married or common law). Just more than 70% of men and approximately 44% of women lived as a couple in 2011. By the time older adults reach 85 years of age and older, however, only about 24% lived with a spouse or partner.

Figure 1-8 provides additional details about living arrangements of older Canadians.

The statistic that is most relevant for nurses is that, overall, about 92% of the older adult population lives in independent housing settings in the community, with the remaining 8% divided between nursing facilities and settings that provide some assistance with daily needs (e.g., assisted living;

Statistics Canada, 2012b). Many older adults who live in independent settings receive significant levels of assistance from family members as discussed in the following sections on caregiving. Many also receive significant levels of support from the broad range of community-based services and agencies that increasingly are available (discussed in Chapter 6).

Older adults also have an increasingly wide range of housing options that address the needs of the growing number of older adults who require daily assistance but not full-time care. For example, assisted-living residences (sometimes equated with designated living facilities) are now available in many areas of the country. Although the services provided by these facilities vary widely, basic services generally include a single residential unit, at least one daily meal and 24-hour availability of assistance. People who live in assisted-living facilities usually need help with three or more daily activities, and these services are provided either as part of the care agreement or through other arrangements.

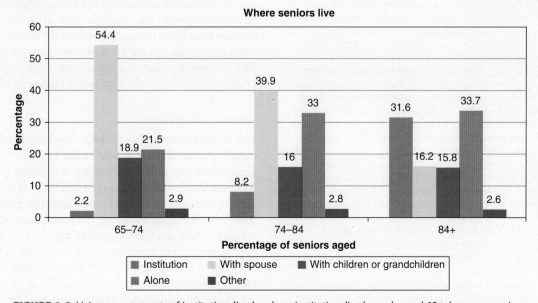

FIGURE 1-8 Living arrangements of institutionalized and noninstitutionalized people aged 65+ by age groupings in Canada. (Elections Canada. [2012]. *Canadian seniors: A demographic profile.* Retrieved from http://www.elections.ca/content.aspx?section=res&dir=rec/part/sen&document=index&lang=e)

Because the range of housing options and community-based services is rapidly increasing, decisions about staying in one's own home or moving to another type of living facility are becoming more complex. Although terms, such as *continuing care* and *aging in place*, have been widely used in recent decades, definitions vary significantly. For example, some aging-in-place or continuing-care programs require that residents move to a new location within a larger group of facilities when their needs change. Because these moves require that older adults adjust to new staff and a different environment, they can be as disruptive as a move that is not defined as continuing care.

Although nurses may not be familiar with all the housing options in their communities, at a minimum, they need to know about the various types of facilities that are commonly available. Moreover, nurses are responsible for suggesting referrals to social service agencies and seniors' centres so that older adults and their families can find additional information. Box 1-5 describes various housing options for older adults that are available in a number of parts of Canada.

Assisted-Living Facilities

Many older adults receive a wide range of health care services in assisted-living facilities and continuing-care

Box 1-5 Housing Options for Older Adults

Homecare Suite or In-Law Suite: A fully functional and accessible modular apartment built as an addition, remodelled in basements or installed in attached garages

Shared Housing: A house or apartment shared by two or more unrelated people, with each occupant having a private or semi-private bedroom. Occupants share expenses and responsibilities.

Retirement Community: A specially designed residential development occupied by self-sufficient older adults. Recreational programs and support services are usually available.

Cohousing Communities: Cohousing communities are new to Canada. Within the last several years, groups in various Canadian provinces have begun to talk about starting these communities. Cohousing communities are residential developments of 15 to 25 individually owned houses and commonly owned land and buildings designed to encourage community interaction. These communities typically emphasize individual privacy, resident involvement in planning and collaborative community management. Intergenerational cohousing communities began in the United States in the 1990s, and in recent years, some communities have been developed for adults older than 50 or 55 years as senior cohousing communities.

Life-Care or Continuing-Care Retirement Community: A residential complex designed to provide a wide range of services and accommodations to meet each resident's needs as they change. The development includes independent housing, congregate housing, assisted living and nursing home care.

Congregate Housing: Individual apartments within a specially designed, multi-unit dwelling. Supportive services typically include meals, laundry, housekeeping, limited transportation, and social and recreational activities.

Assisted-Living Facility: A residential facility with individual apartments, which typically consists of one to three rooms and a bathroom, and shared space for meals and social activities. Services, licensing, regulation and funding are similar to those described for foster care homes.

retirement communities. Although assisted-living facilities developed during the 1980s as settings for independent living, some of these facilities have evolved to provide levels of care similar to that provided in nursing homes. Initially these facilities were based on a "social model," but in recent years, there has been an increasing shift toward addressing the needs of older adults with complex medical needs in assisted-living facilities (McNabney et al., 2014). Because of this trend, some assisted-living facilities are integrally associated with and physically connected to nursing homes and provide a high level of care for residents who no longer can live semi-independently. Another recent development is that some assisted-living facilities provide specialized dementia care, as discussed in Chapter 6. End-of-life care is another issue being addressed in assisted-living facilities because residents express the desire to die at home. Because of this, some older Canadians may receive palliative care services while residing in assisted-living facilities.

See **ONLINE LEARNING ACTIVITY 1-2:**
ADDITIONAL INFORMATION ABOUT OLDER ADULTS IN CANADA
at http://thepoint.lww.com/Miller7e

OLDER ADULTS AS GIVERS AND RECIPIENTS OF CARE

Major demographic trends in Canada have brought about important changes in many aspects of family and societal relationships in recent decades. Trends toward improved health and increased longevity for older adults have occurred in parallel with trends toward increased diversity of family constellations among all generations. Concurrent with these trends, the prevalence of dementia and other chronic conditions that lead to functional decline has led to increased demands for family caregiving. On the other side of the coin, societal changes have led to increased demands for grandparents to assume roles of caregiving for dependent younger generations. This section discusses implications of these shifting demographics in relation to their influence on care of older adults.

Family Caregivers

The increasing numbers of middle-aged adults who simultaneously juggle the demands of caring for older and younger generations are referred to as the **sandwich generation**. Responsibilities of middle-aged adults with parents who depend on them for care (i.e., the sandwich generation) are described demographically by the parent support ratio. According to the Canadian Caregiver Coalition (2014), there are approximately 4 to 5 million family caregivers in Canada. At least half of family caregivers are providing care to parents or parents-in-law and over one quarter (28%) of all family caregivers are providing care to both parents and children (Sinha, 2013). Additionally, the numbers of middle-aged caregivers (45 years of age and older) has increased significantly between 2007 and 2012. Between these years, the number of middle-aged family caregivers increased by 760,000, or 20% (Sinha, 2013). Demographics such as these have influenced patterns of family caregiving, particularly for women. The mid-1980s, for example, marked the beginning of an era in which the average woman in North America spent more time caring for her parents than for her children. Despite the emphasis on women as caregivers for older adults, it is important to recognize that about one quarter of caregivers are men. However, studies show that female caregivers are more likely to provide a higher level of care than are male caregivers (defined as helping with at least two activities of daily living and providing more than 40 hours of care per week; Sinha, 2013).

Since the preindustrial period, nuclear family living arrangements have been predominant in North America and Western Europe. Typically, younger family members establish separate households after marriage, and older family members attempt to maintain independent households for as long as possible. For much of Canadian history, the "ideal" relationship between older and younger generations in families has been to be far enough away to preserve independent lifestyles, but close enough for social support and emotional connectedness. Moreover, this kind of family relationship provides for meeting occasional caregiving needs of family members while allowing for the maintenance of differing lifestyles for both younger and older generations. These family relationships are based on the principle of reciprocity across generations, characterized by mutual assistance and extensive exchanges among kin. The current trend in Canada is that caregiving needs of elders are met primarily by spouses and secondarily by adult children, especially daughters and unmarried children.

In recent years, increased rates of divorce and remarriage among younger generations have resulted in the proliferation of varieties of blended families across several generations. In addition, increased rates of remarriage among older adults who are widowed or divorced have led to increasing numbers of later-life blended families. One consequence of these trends is that family dynamics can become quite complex, particularly when adult stepchildren assume new roles as caregivers or decision makers for dependent older adults. For example, adult children may share caregiving and decision-making responsibilities regarding their impaired parent with a parent's spouse whom they hardly know. Similarly, adult children may assist their parent with caregiving or decision making about a stepparent whom they are just getting to know. In addition, concerns among members of blended families regarding assets and financial resources often complicate decisions about caregiving responsibilities and plans for care.

Expectations and attitudes about caregiving practices also have changed due to societal trends that affect relationships between older adults and their families. In the early 1900s, for example, the tradition of deep involvement in generational assistance, reinforced by strong family and ethnic values, was dominant in Canadian culture. By the mid-1960s, trends were shifting toward individualistic values and lifestyles, due in part to the proliferation of public support and

services for older Canadians. Another major influence has been the increasing numbers of women who have careers independent of their roles in families, which can lead to conflict between the younger generation of adult children and older family members who expect care. Even with complex and evolving social and demographic trends in Canada, studies consistently show that about 80% of care for dependent older adults is provided by family members and other "informal" sources. The term **informal caregiver** refers to the provision of assistance to a family member or friend in a nonprofessional and unpaid role to support the person in a community setting. Spousal and filial responsibilities are traditions that have directed family caregiving in Canada for more than a century, and this continues even though the specific dynamics of the care are changing. Box 1-1 summarizes some cultural perspectives related to older adults and family caregiving.

Multigenerational families are now the norm with 10% of older people having at least one child who is also older than 65 years, 25% of people aged 58 to 59 years having at least one living parent, and about half of young children having all grandparents alive. Implications of these demographic trends for older adults are discussed in the following sections.

Grandparents Raising Grandchildren

Skipped-generation households were first counted in 2001 in the Canadian census (Statistics Canada, 2012c). These households are ones in which there are children younger than 18 years living with a grandparent without parents present. Households in which children are being raised by both their parents and grandparents are called three-generation, shared-care households (or multigenerational households). Studies of children's living arrangements and grandparent caregivers provide the following data about grandparents raising grandchildren in Canada:

- Between the years of 1991 and 2001, there was a 20% increase in the number of skipped-generation households containing children 18 years of age or younger and one or more grandparents (Fuller-Thomson, 2005).
- According to the 2011 Canadian census (2012d), just more than 30,000 children 14 years of age and younger lived in skipped-generation families (with one or more grandparents and no parents).
- Of these 30,000 children, 57.8% of these grandchildren lived with both of their grandparents, while the remaining 42.2% lived with just one grandparent (Statistics Canada, 2012d).
- Geographically, the greatest percentages of skipped-generation households in 2011 were located in Nunavut (2.2%), the Northwest Territories (1.8%) and Saskatchewan (1.4%) (Statistics Canada, 2012d).
- Grandparents raising grandchildren alone are most likely to be female, Aboriginal and unemployed (Fuller-Thomson, 2005; Statistics Canada, 2013).

Although the overall percentage of older adults and children in these situations is small and the numbers of grandparents/grandchildren in these situations are relatively stable within Canada, there still are implications for children, grandparents and society. Common reasons for grandparent custody include child abuse, teen pregnancy, parental abuse of drugs or alcohol, and death, disability, mental illness or incarceration of adult parents. Some studies have found positive effects of becoming a custodial grandparent; however, more studies have documented negative effects (Namkung, 2010). Rewards of grandparent caregiving include role enhancement, sense of purpose in life, motivation to keep physically active, close relationships with younger generations, and satisfaction with maintaining family well-being. Negative consequences include significant stresses, role overload, social isolation, detrimental effects on health and increased likelihood of being poor. Specifically, studies have found that custodial grandparents were more likely to report more functional limitations, poorer self-rated health, increased prevalence of chronic disease, more depressive symptoms and lower levels of life satisfaction than were noncaregivers (Namkung, 2010).

OLDER ADULTS IN THE WORLD

This chapter has presented characteristics of older adults in Canada that are pertinent to gerontological nursing, but it would be incomplete without a brief perspective on global aspects of aging because the world's population is now aging at an unprecedented rate. Declines in fertility rates and improvements in health and life expectancy that occurred during the 20th century are resulting in significant increases in the number and proportion of older adults in most of the world. Even more significantly, projections for 2050 indicate continued increases in all groups of older adults, compared with much lower increases in younger age groups, as illustrated in Figure 1-9.

Much of the information about global aging discusses differences between *developed* countries and *developing* countries because of significantly different conditions that

Box 1-6 Stats in Brief: Global Aging	
Population Changes: People Aged 65 + Worldwide	
• 2008	7%
• 2040	14%
World Population Aged 65 + Living in Developing Countries	
• 2008	62%
• 2040	76%
Projected Increase in World Population Between 2008 and 2040	
• Age 80+	233%
• Age 65+	160%
• All ages	33%
Countries With Highest Proportion of People Aged 65 +	
• Japan	21.6%
• Italy	20.0%
• Germany	20.0%
• Greece	19.1%
Source: U.S. Census Bureau, An Aging World, 2009.	

affect population aging in these two types of countries. Organizations, such as census bureaus, the United Nations and the World Health Organization, use these terms to differentiate between countries according to level of development. Although there are no universally accepted standards for classifying countries as more or less developed, commonly used criteria include life expectancy, literacy rate and per capita income. The United Nations classifies Japan, Australia, New Zealand and all nations in Europe and North America as developed nations, and all other nations of the world as developing nations. World population trends show that the most developed nations have the highest percentages of older adults and the highest median age and some may have more grandparents than young children by 2050. However, many of the developing countries are experiencing more recent and rapid declines in fertility rates, so the proportion of older adults in developing countries is expected to increase significantly during the next decades (Kinsella & He, 2009). Box 1-6 summarizes demographic information about global aging.

Chapter Highlights

The Relationship Between Wellness and Aging

• Since the late 1950s, health care professionals have recognized the importance of incorporating wellness goals in their care of older adults; however, there are many conceptual and practical barriers.

• Barriers to promoting wellness in older adults include older adults' negative attitudes about being able to improve, the existence of more serious or pressing health concerns, the focus of health care environments on disease treatment rather than prevention or health promotion, the false attribution of symptoms of pathologic

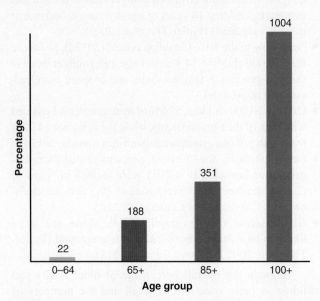

FIGURE 1-9 Percentage change in the world's population by age: 2010–2050.

conditions to normal aging processes, and the belief that older adults are not capable of learning and implementing health-promoting behaviours inherent in wellness-oriented care.

- Rather than having a narrow focus on physical health and functioning, wellness-focused nursing considers the older adult's physical, mental, social and spiritual well-being.
- Definitions of aging can be understood in terms of subjective age, perceived age, chronologic age or functional age. Concepts related to functional age are most appropriate in wellness-oriented nursing care.
- The current emphasis on successful aging involves optimal physical, mental, emotional, spiritual and social well-being and quality of life.

Attitudes Toward Aging

- Negative images of aging and ageism are pervasive in modern societies (Fig. 1-1) and can have a negative impact on care provided to older adults, especially when health care providers—including nurses—base their care on myths and inaccurate information.
- Ageism is pervasive in Canadian and American societies and is associated with negative consequences on older adults.
- Nurses need to identify myths about older adults (Fig. 1-2), examine attitudes toward aging (including their own) and use accurate information as an antidote so they can provide wellness-oriented care for older adults (Table 1-1).
- Cultural perspectives have a significant influence on attitudes about aging, older adults and family caregiving relationships (Box 1-1).

Debunking Myths: Understanding Realities About Older Adults in Canada

- The older adult population in Canada has been increasing and will continue to increase at a rapid pace (Fig. 1-3).
- Despite a high prevalence of chronic illnesses, most older adults report good to excellent health (Figs. 1-4 and 1-5).
- Socioeconomic characteristics and living arrangements of older adults vary significantly among subgroups (Boxes 1-3, 1-4, Figs. 1-6A and 1-6B, 1-7A and 1-7B, 1-8).
- Older adults have a number of choices of community-based housing options (Box 1-5).

Older Adults as Givers and Recipients of Care

- The current trend in Canada is that caregiving needs of elders are met primarily by spouses and secondarily by adult children, especially daughters and unmarried children.
- Older adults may be responsible for raising grandchildren in skipped-generation households.
- Declines in fertility rates and improvements in health and life expectancy have led to an aging population worldwide (Box 1-6 and Fig. 1-9).

Older Adults in the World

- Populations in both developed and developing countries is aging (Box 1-6 and Fig. 1-9).

Critical Thinking Exercises

1. Increase your awareness of attitudes toward aging and older adults through the following exercises:
   - During the next 2 weeks, as you go about your usual activities, keep a small notebook handy and jot down examples of images of older adults that you see or hear in the following media: newspapers, magazines, the Internet, television, greeting cards and social conversations. Note whether the images convey a neutral, positive or negative image.
   - During the next 2 weeks, pay attention to your thoughts and conversations about older adults and identify the perceptions you hold, the terms you use and the images you convey.
   - Rephrase each of the 20 questions in the Ageism Survey (Fig. 1-2) and ask yourself how often you have done any of those activities in the past few months (e.g., "How often did I tell a joke that pokes fun at old people?").
   - Ask an older relative, friend or acquaintance to fill out the Ageism Survey and discuss his or her experiences.
2. Carefully review the cultural perspectives on elders and family caregiving relationships (Box 1-1) and think about how you have formed your attitudes about aging.
3. Review the myths and realities of aging listed in Table 1-1 and think about times in your personal or professional experiences when you might have "bought into" a myth.
4. On the Internet, use the key words about types of housing options in Box 1-5 to find information about residential settings for older adults in your community. Consider which of these are most appropriate for independent older adults who are interested in social contacts and which would be most appropriate for older adults who have cognitive or functional limitations.

 For more information about the topics discussed in this chapter, be sure to check out the interactive Online Learning Activities and other helpful resources at http://thepoint.lww.com/Miller7e

REFERENCES

Barrett, A. E., & Robbins, C. (2008). The multiple sources of women's aging anxiety and their relationship with psychological distress. *Journal of Aging and Health, 20*(1), 32–65.

Baumbusch, J., Dahlke, S., & Phinney, A. (2012). Nursing students' knowledge and beliefs about care of older adults in a shifting context of nursing education. *Journal of Advances in Nursing, 68*(11), 2550–2558.

Bodner, E. (2009). On the origins of ageism among older and younger adults. *International Psychogeriatrics, 21*(6), 1003–1014.

Bodner, E., Bergman, Y. S., & Cohen-Fridel, S. (2012). Different dimensions of ageist attitudes among men and women: A multigenerational perspective. *International Psychogeriatrics, 24*(6), 895–901.

Butler, R. N. (1969). Ageism: Another form of bigotry. *The Gerontologist, 9*, 243–246.

Butler, R. N. (1975). *Why survive? Being old in America.* New York, NY: Harper & Row.

Butler, R. N., Lewis, M. I., & Sunderland, T. (1991). *Aging and mental health* (4th ed.). New York, NY: Merrill/Macmillan.

Canadian Caregiver Coalition. (2014). *Caregiver facts*. Retrieved from http://www.ccc-ccan.ca

Conference Board of Canada. (2014). *Elderly poverty*. Retrieved from www.conferenceboard.ca/hcp/details/society/elderly-poverty.aspx

Christensen, K., Thinggaard, M., McGue, M., et al. (2009). Perceived age as clinically useful biomarker of ageing: Cohort study. *British Medical Journal, 339*, b5262. doi:10.1036/bmj.b5256

Dunn, H. L. (1958). Significance of levels of wellness in aging. *Geriatrics, 13*(1), 51–57.

Dunn, H. L. (1961). *High-level wellness*. Arlington, VA: R.W. Beatty.

Eymard, A. S., & Douglas, D. H. (2012). Ageism among health care providers and interventions to improve their attitudes toward older adults: An integrative review. *Journal of Gerontological Nursing, 38*(5), 26–35.

Flatt, M. A., Settersten, R. A., Jr., Ponsaran, R., et al. (2013). Are "Anti-Aging Medicine" and "Successful Aging" two sides of the same coin? Views of anti-aging practitioners. *The Journals of Gerontology: Psychological Sciences and Social Sciences, 68*(6), 944–955.

Fuller-Thomson, E. (2005). *Grandparents raising grandchildren in Canada: A profile of skipped-generation families* (SEDAP Research Paper No. 132). Retrieved from http://socserv.mcmaster.ca/sedap/p/sedap132.pdf

Government of Canada. (2013). Poverty profile: *A snapshot of racialized poverty in Canada*. Retrieved from http://www.esdc.gc.ca/eng/community/reports/poverty_profile/snapshot.shtml

Human Resources Development Canada. (n.d.). *Reducing poverty, 1952–1967: The history of Canada's Public Pension*. Retrieved from www.historymuseum.ca/cmc/exhibitions/hist/pensions/cpp-a52-wcr_e.shtml

Hutchinson, S. L., & Nimrod, G. (2012). Leisure as a resource for successful aging by older adults with chronic health conditions. *International Journal of Aging and Human Development, 74*(1), 41–65.

Kinsella, K., & He, W. (2009). *An aging world: 2008* (U.S. Census Bureau, International Population Reports, P95/09-1). Washington, DC: Government Printing Office.

Kreider, R. M. (2008). *Living arrangements of children: 2004* (U.S. Census Bureau, Current Population Reports, P70/s114). Washington, DC: Government Printing Office.

Labonte, R., Muhajarine, N., Winquist, B., et al. (2010). *Healthy population—A report of the Canadian Index of Wellbeing*. Retrieved from https://uwaterloo.ca/canadian-index-wellbeing/sites/ca.canadian-index-wellbeing/files/upload/files/HealthyPopulation_DomainReport.sflb_pdf

Levy, B. R., & Leifheit-Limson, E. (2009). The stereotype-matching effect: Greater influence on functioning when age stereotypes correspond to outcomes. *Psychology and Aging, 24*(1), 230–233.

Levy, B. R., Ashman, O., & Slade, M. D. (2009). Age attributions and aging health: Contrast between the United States and Japan. *The Journal of Gerontology: Psychological Sciences and Social Sciences, 64*(3), 335–338.

Library of Parliament. (2009). *A statistical profile of poverty in Canada*. Ottawa, ON: Government of Canada.

Lineweaver, T. T., Berger, A. K., & Hertzog, C. (2009). Expectations about memory change across the life span are impacted by aging stereotypes. *Psychology and Aging, 24*(1), 169–176.

Low, G., Molzahn, A. E., & Schopflocher, D. (2013). Attitudes to aging mediate the relationship between older peoples' subjective health and quality of life in 20 countries. *Health and Quality of Life Outcomes, 11*, 146. doi:10.1186/1477-7525-11-146

Martin, R., Williams, C., & O'Neill, D. (2009). Retrospective analysis of attitudes to ageing in the economist: Apocalyptic demography for opinion formers? *British Medical Journal, 339*, b4914. doi:10.1136/bmj.b4914

McGuire, S. L., Klein, D. A., & Chen, S. L. (2008). Ageism revisited: A study measuring ageism in East Tennessee, USA. *Nursing and Health Sciences, 10*(1), 11–16.

McMahon, S., & Fleury, J. (2012). Wellness in older adults: A concept analysis. *Nursing Forum, 47*(1), 39–49.

McNabney, M. K., Onyike, C., Johnston, D., et al. (2014). The impact of complex chronic diseases on care utilization among assisted-living residents. *Geriatric Nursing, 35*(1), 26–30.

Miche, M., Wahl, H. W., Diehl, M., et al. (2014). Natural occurrence of subjective aging experiences in community-dwelling older adults. *Journals of Gerontology: Psychological Sciences and Social Sciences, 69*(2), 174–187.

Morley, J. E. (2009). Successful aging or aging successfully. *Journal of the American Medical Directors Association, 10*(2), 85–86.

Namkung, E. H. (2010). *Grandparents raising grandchildren: Ethnic and household differences in health and service use*. Paper presented at the Society for Social Work and Research 14th Annual Conference, New Orleans, LA.

Neugarten, B. L. (1978). The rise of the young-old. In R. Gross, B. Gross, & S. Seidman (Eds.), *The new old: Struggling for decent aging* (pp. 47–49). Garden City, NY: Anchor Press/Doubleday.

North, M. S., & Fiske, S. T. (2012). An inconvenienced youth? Ageism and its potential intergenerational roots. *Psychology Bulletin, 138*(5), 982–997. doi:10.1037/a0027843

Palmore, E. (2005). Three decades of research on ageism. *Generations, 29*(3), 87–90.

Plath, D. (2009). International policy perspectives on independence in old age. *Journal of Aging and Social Policy, 21*(2), 209–223.

Romo, R. D., Wallhagen, M. I., Yourman, L., et al. (2013). Perceptions of successful aging among diverse elders with late-life disability. *The Gerontologist, 53*(6), 939–949.

Rowe, J. W., & Kahn, R. L. (1997). Successful aging. *The Gerontologist, 37*, 433–440.

Schafer, M. H., & Shippee, T. P. (2010). Age identity, gender, and perceptions of decline: Does feeling older lead to pessimistic dispositions about cognitive aging? *Journals of Gerontology Series B, 65*(1), 91–96.

Sinha, M. (2013). *Portrait of caregivers, Catalogue 89-652-x*. Ottawa, ON: Statistics Canada.

Statistics Canada. (2012a). *Educational attainment and employment: Canada in an international context* (Catalogue no. 81-599-x, Issue no. 008). Ottawa, ON: Government of Canada.

Statistics Canada. (2012b). *Living arrangements of seniors: Families, households and marital status, structural type of dwelling and collectives, 2011 census of population*. Retrieved from www12.statcan.gc.ca/census-recensement/2011/as-sa/98-312-x/98-312-x2011003_4-eng.pdf

Statistics Canada. (2012c). *Fifty years of families in Canada: 1961–2011* (Catalogue no. 98-312-X2011003). Ottawa, ON: Government of Canada.

Statistics Canada. (2012d). *Portraits of families and living arrangements in Canada*. Retrieved from http://www12.statcan.gc.ca/census-recensement/2011/as-sa/98-312-x/98-312-x2011001-eng.pdf

Statistics Canada. (2013). *Aboriginal peoples in Canada: First Nations people, Métis and Inuit* (National Household Survey, 2011, Catalogue no. 99-011-X2011001). Ottawa, ON: Author.

Stephan, Y., Chalabaev, A., Kotter-Gruhn, D., et al. (2013). "Feeling younger, being stronger": An experimental study of subjective age and physical functioning among older adults. *The Journals of Gerontology: Psychological Sciences and Social Sciences, 68*(1), 1–7.

Vincent, J. A. (2008). The cultural construction old age as a biological phenomenon: Science and anti-aging technologies. *Journal of Aging Studies, 22*(2008), 331–339.

Weiss, D., & Freund, A. M. (2012). Still young at heart: Negative age-related information motivates distancing from same-aged people. *Psychology and Aging, 27*(1), 173–180.

Weiss, D., & Lang, F. R. (2012). "They" are old but "I" feel younger: Age-group dissociation as a self-protective strategy in old age. *Psychology and Aging, 27*(1), 153–163.

Woods, N. F., Cochrane, B. B., LaCroix, A. Z., et al. (2012). Toward a positive aging phenotype for older women: Observations from the Women's Health Initiative. *The Journals of Gerontology: Biological Sciences and Medical Sciences, 67*(11), 1191–1196.

chapter 2

Addressing Diversity of Older Adults

LEARNING OBJECTIVES

After reading this chapter, you will be able to:

1. Discuss the importance of providing linguistically and culturally competent care for older adults.
2. Perform a cultural self-assessment.
3. Describe three major health belief systems that influence cultural perspectives on health and wellness.
4. Describe health disparities that affect older adults of different cultural groups.
5. Identify sources of information that nurses can use to improve their cultural competence.
6. Describe characteristics of the cultural groups of older adults in Canada.

KEY POINTS

cultural competence   health belief system

cultural self-assessment   health disparities

ethnogeriatrics   linguistic competence

The increasing diversity of all age groups in Canada affects almost every facet of health care as cultural background significantly influences values, communication, health beliefs and health-related behaviours, and many other aspects of daily life. It is imperative to recognize that seven or more decades of cultural influences significantly affect health beliefs and behaviours of older adults, as well as their relationships with health care providers and their receptivity to interventions. Although it is beyond the scope of this text to discuss all the implications related to cultural diversity

of older adults, this chapter provides overviews of diverse groups of older adults in Canada. It also addresses the topic of health disparities because differences are closely related to cultural diversity and are especially pertinent to health promotion for older adults. As with any information related to cultural diversity, it is imperative to recognize that, at best, the overviews provide basic statistics about particular groups. Each group comprises many individuals, and each individual has some characteristics that are common to the group and many that are not. Because overviews do not apply to individuals within the group, nurses need to avoid stereotypes and generalizations as they care for individual older adults.

CULTURAL DIVERSITY IN CANADA

As discussed in Chapter 1, remarkable changes have occurred in the demographic characteristics of all countries because of increased life expectancy among most groups and decreased fertility rates among many groups. At the same time that the trend toward population aging has been occurring worldwide, a trend toward increasing diversity by race and ethnicity has been occurring in Canada, notably, the substantial increase in Asian and Middle East individuals immigrating to this country. Historically, the largest percentage of immigrants came from Europe (Statistics Canada, 2013a). While Europeans still immigrate to Canada, the largest number of immigrants to arrive between 2006 and 2011 came from the Philippines, followed by those arriving from China and India (Statistics Canada, 2013a). Additionally, 19.1% of the Canadian population self-identified as being part of a visible minority group; of those who self-identified as having come from a visible minority, just more than 65% immigrated to Canada and almost 31% were born in this country. As of 2011, the three largest visible minority groups within Canada were South

Asians, Chinese and Black Canadians (Statistics Canada, 2013a). Because of low birth rates, projections indicate that by mid-21st century, most of the population growth in Canada will come from immigration (Statistics Canada, 2012). Information about the increasing diversity of the older adult population is provided in the sections of this chapter on overviews of cultural groups.

The increasing diversity that is characteristic of the general Canadian population is also reflected in the health care workforce and is especially noticeable in nursing staff, including nursing assistants, who provide care for older adults in community and long-term care settings. In urban home care settings, care is often provided by caregivers who have recently come to Canada and have not learned to speak English or French fluently, or who speak one of our official languages with accents unfamiliar to older adults. In these situations, communication barriers between care providers and care recipients are a challenge that needs to be addressed. Thus, it is important to recognize that cultural diversity in health care settings encompasses a wide range of situations, and each situation requires a high degree of cultural competence on the part of the health care provider.

CULTURAL COMPETENCE

During the 1950s, transcultural nursing (i.e., the provision of nursing care across cultural boundaries) focused on the comparative study of different cultural groups. Although transcultural nursing is an important specialization, the demographic trend toward ever-expanding diversity requires that *all* health care professionals are culturally competent. Every nurse–client encounter involves some degree of cultural differences because of the distinctive values and characteristics of each individual. Even when two people have ostensibly similar cultural backgrounds, each one experiences and expresses cultural factors in a unique way. Consequently, nurses, nursing organizations and faculties of nursing are among the groups that are taking action to ensure the provision of culturally competent care. In adopting the Registered Nurses of Ontario's (RNAO, 2007) definition of cultural competence, the Canadian Nurses Association (CNA, 2010) stated,

> ... *cultural competence is the application of knowledge, skills, attitudes or personal attributes required by nurses to maximize respectful relationships with diverse populations of clients and co-workers. ... cultural competence enables them to work effectively in cross-cultural situations.* (p.1)

Cultural competence is essential for improving the health of individuals from various ethnic backgrounds, as well as to eliminate **health disparities** between cultural groups (Engebretson & Headley, 2009; Maddalena, 2009). Within Canada, some organizations such as the Canadian

Association on Gerontology and the federal government's National Seniors Council are emphasizing the need to address cultural diversity in the aging population. The term **ethnogeriatrics**, which is defined as the component of geriatrics that integrates the influence of race, ethnicity and culture on health and well-being of older adults, has been introduced into health care practice to promote ethnoculturally appropriate care while avoiding stereotyping (American Geriatrics Society, 2006).

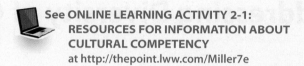

See **ONLINE LEARNING ACTIVITY 2-1: RESOURCES FOR INFORMATION ABOUT CULTURAL COMPETENCY** at http://thepoint.lww.com/Miller7e

Performing a Cultural Self-Assessment

Nursing texts emphasize that individual **cultural competence** is an ongoing process, rather than an end point, in which the nurse continuously strives to work effectively within the cultural context of the individual, family or community (Andrews, 2012a). This process is often described as a progression from judgmental attitudes and practices to positive approaches. For example, Purnell (2013) described a continuum that begins with being *unconsciously incompetent*, which is being unaware that one is lacking knowledge about another culture. When the person becomes aware of this knowledge gap, he or she is *consciously incompetent* and takes actions to learn about the cultural group. The next stage of being *consciously competent* involves learning about the other culture, verifying generalizations and providing culturally specific interventions. In the final stage, the care provider is *unconsciously competent* and automatically provides culturally congruent care to clients of diverse cultures.

Although health care professionals rarely achieve high levels of cultural competency in relation to a broad spectrum of different ethnic/cultural groups, they are expected to achieve cultural competency in relation to the specific cultural groups for whom they provide care. Moreover, they are expected to be nonjudgmental and avoid stereotyping by recognizing the extent to which cultural views and practices influence their own attitudes and perceptions, as well as the care they provide. This can be achieved through a **cultural self-assessment**, which is an awareness-raising tool for gaining insight into the health-related values, beliefs, attitudes and practices that one holds (Andrews, 2012a). Box 2-1 describes a cultural self-assessment that is particularly applicable for nurses caring for older adults. It is important to recognize that people can internalize social stigma and prejudices that apply to members of one's own groups. Thus, the self-assessment includes questions to increase one's awareness of internalized stigma.

Box 2-1 Cultural Self-Assessment for Nurses Working With Older Adults

What Self-Identity Influences My Worldview?

- With what sociocultural and religious groups do I most closely identify?
- What does it mean to belong to these groups?
- Is there any stigma associated with any of these groups?
- What negative and positive images are associated with these groups?
- What do I like and dislike about these groups and my sociocultural identity?

How Has My Cultural Background Influenced Me?

- How has (does) the society in which I grew up (currently live in) influence(d) the dominant values that I now hold?
- What is my perception of concepts such as time, work, leisure, health, family and relationships?
- How do my perceptions differ from those of people who come from different cultural backgrounds?

What Is My Attitude Toward People, Especially Older Adults Who:

- Are immigrants?
- Have difficulty with the English language?
- Have difficulty communicating?
- Have a cultural background different from my own?
- Look or act like the stereotype of people who are gay, lesbian or transgender?

What Are My Attitudes About and Experiences With Health Practices That Differ From My Own?

- Do (did) members of my family have health care practices that differ(ed) from conventional Western medicine practices (e.g., herbs, poultices, folk remedies)?
- Do (did) they consult with folk, indigenous, religious or spiritual healers?
- How do I feel about alternative or complementary health care practices for myself and for older adults?

How Well Do I Communicate and Understand?

- What do I do and how do I feel when I have difficulty understanding people whose accents and primary language are different from my own?
- What have I learned about myself because of this self-assessment?

A Student's Perspective

After completing the cultural assessment, I learned that I do not have a thorough grasp on my own culture. We learned in class that nurses must be aware and knowledgeable about their own culture before they can relate to their clients. I have not gotten that one under wraps yet. I do not know, for example, what religious group that I best fit in with. I know that it is necessary to firmly understand your own beliefs and background before you can help a client be comfortable with theirs, yet I obviously

do not! Doing the cultural assessment does make me aware of biases. I do feel uncomfortable thinking about immigrants, in that, I do not know who I define as immigrants or where I believe they come from. I also tend to imagine "we are all the same," when in reality all cultures are very different in positive ways, and to generalize is to say that the things that make cultures different are unimportant, when that is not true.

It is definitely the time to answer these questions about culture. Not only is it important for me to identify with my culture, but I also need help in developing an understanding of other people's cultures. Doing this assessment is only the first step; I must continue to question what I believe, where I come from, and who I relate to. Then I can help my clients.

Erin H.

Linguistic Competence in Care of Older Adults

Linguistic competence, which refers to health care services that are respectful of and responsive to a person's linguistic needs, is one small part of cultural competence. This concept is important for gerontological nurses because they frequently work with older adults whose primary language differs from their own. Immigrants who come to Canada as adults may be particularly disadvantaged because they may not have the same opportunities to learn English as do school-age children. The challenge of communicating with people who do not speak the same language or dialect is magnified when the person also has dementia or sensory impairments, as is often the case in long-term care settings.

Nurses need to be aware of interpreter resources that should be accessible to all health care settings. For example, the Language Line Services offers immediate telephone interpretation services for subscribers. In situations where no interpreters are available, nurses can obtain immediate fee-based telephone interpretation services from Language Line Services by calling 1-800-752-6096. Box 2-2 summarizes guidelines for using interpreters in health care settings with older adults.

 Box 2-2 Guidelines for Using Interpreters

Before the Interaction

- Whenever possible, use the services of a professional interpreter. Avoid using visitors or staff from auxiliary services unless permission to do so has been obtained from both the older adult and the interpreter.
- Given that there are more than 140 languages spoken in North America, be certain that the correct language and dialect have been identified before arranging for an interpreter. For example, does the person speak Cantonese or Mandarin Chinese?
- If an interpreter for the primary language is unavailable, determine whether the older adult speaks other languages. For example, many older adults from Vietnam and some African nations are also fluent in French.

(continued)

Box 2-2 *(continued)*

- Be aware of age, gender and socioeconomic class considerations in selecting an interpreter. In general, it is best to use an interpreter who is the same gender and of the same approximate age and socioeconomic class as the older adult.
- Organize your thoughts and plan ahead to ensure that the most important topics are covered.
- Allow sufficient time for the interaction and expect that it will take longer than an interaction with an older adult for whom English is the primary language.

During the Interaction

- Review the importance of confidentiality.
- Talk to the older adult, not the interpreter.
- Talk about only one topic at a time.
- Use short sentences and simple vocabulary.
- Use the active voice. Avoid vague modifiers.
- Avoid professional jargon, idioms and slang.
- Be aware that many words do not translate into another language. For instance, the English word *depression* has no equivalent in many Asian and other languages.

CULTURAL PERSPECTIVES ON WELLNESS

As discussed in Chapter 1, nurses have numerous opportunities to promote wellness for older adults, even under the most challenging of circumstances, through holistic nursing interventions to improve physical comfort and psychological and spiritual growth. To achieve this, nurses need to have a good understanding of the meaning of health and wellness to each older adult. Nurses can explore this with older adults by asking questions such as "What does it mean to you to be healthy?" or "How do you achieve wellness in your life?" If appropriate, nurses can explore this topic from the perspective of cultural diversity with a question such as "I'm interested in knowing more about how Chinese people view wellness. Can you tell me your thoughts about this?"

Health care practices and beliefs of individuals are strongly influenced by the **health belief system** (defined as the health-related attitudes, beliefs and practices) of one's cultural group. Andrews (2012b) described three major health belief systems that underpin health beliefs and health-related behaviours of individuals, as summarized in Box 2-3. It is important to recognize that many people integrate beliefs from two or all of these paradigms, but some people are firmly entrenched in one health belief system. Nurses need to be aware of the health beliefs that influence their clients, so they can adapt their interventions accordingly. For example, people who adhere to the holistic paradigm described in Box 2-3 may view their condition as an imbalance between "hot" and "cold" energies and request a particular food or herbal remedy for restoring balance.

Box 2-3 Cultural Considerations: Major Health Belief Systems

Magico-Religious Paradigm

- Supernatural forces dominate the fate of the world, and all those in it depend on the actions of supernatural forces (e.g., God, gods).
- Origins of illness include sorcery, breach of a taboo, intrusion of a disease object, intrusion of a disease-causing spirit and loss of soul.
- Illness is initiated by a supernatural agent with or without justification, or by a person who practises sorcery or engages the services of sorcerers.
- *Health is* a gift or reward given as a sign of God's blessing and goodwill.
- Health and illness belong first to the community and then to the individual, so there is a strong sense of community.
- These beliefs are common among Black Canadians (Caribbean), African Canadians and Middle Eastern groups.

Holistic Paradigm

- Forces of nature must be kept in balance or harmony.
- Human life is only one aspect of nature and a part of the general order of the universe.
- The whole person is viewed in the context of the total environment.
- Disease is caused by an imbalance or disharmony between the human, geophysical and metaphysical forces of the universe.
- Illness is not an intruding agent but is a natural part of life's rhythmic course; health and illness are both natural parts of a continuum.
- Diseases of civilization (e.g., unemployment, discrimination, ghettos, suicide) are just as much illnesses as are biomedical diseases.
- *Health* and *healing* reflect the quality of wholeness associated with healthy functioning and well-being.
- These beliefs are common among Asian, First Nations peoples, and British and European Canadians.

Scientific (Biomedical) Paradigm

- Life is controlled by a series of physical and biochemical processes that can be studied and manipulated by humans.
- Principles of determinism: a cause-and-effect relationship exists for all natural phenomena.
- Principles of mechanism: life processes can be controlled through mechanical, genetic and other engineered interventions.
- Principles of reductionism: all life can be reduced or divided into smaller parts (e.g., the mind and body are two distinct entities).
- Disease is a breakdown of the human machine as a result of stress, internal damages, or external trauma or invasion.
- *Health* is the absence of disease.
- These beliefs are common among most Western cultures, including Canada.

Source: Andrews, M. M. (2012b). The influence of cultural and health belief systems on health care practices. In M. M. Andrews & J. S. Boyle (Eds.), *Transcultural concepts in nursing care* (pp. 73–88). Philadelphia, PA: Lippincott, Williams & Wilkins.

A Student's Perspective

I came from a highly educated, Christian, Caucasian family, and this affects how I see the world both consciously and unconsciously. Education is a very important part of my life. My Christian upbringing makes me value honesty, justice, compassion and forgiveness. I was raised to have an open mind and not judge people until I got to know them. I think that has been the most important idea that I live my life around.

One thing I learned was how I see everyone who was not born in Canada and those who do not speak English as immigrants. I get very frustrated when I don't understand people because of their heavy accent or inability to speak English. Because one of my grandmothers used plenty of home remedies, I was exposed to alternative medicine from an early age. I think it is important to take into consideration other's beliefs and incorporate them as best as you can into their care. I am sure I will continue to discover my true values and beliefs as I grow in nursing. I think it is a good idea to keep reviewing my own cultural beliefs so that I become aware of them and how they affect my practice.

Sarah L.

HEALTH DISPARITIES

In recent years, there has been increasing awareness of major health disparities among racial and ethnic minorities. **Health disparities** are defined as significant differences with regard to the rates of disease incidence, prevalence, morbidity, mortality or life expectancy between one population and another. The most widely identified health disparities affecting older adults are listed in Cultural Considerations Box 2-4. There is, however, relatively little research conducted on health disparities between visible minority groups and the larger Canadian population (Rodney & Copeland, 2009). Often, the focus of research studies involves how immigrants from visible minorities use health care services, especially screening (e.g., Pap tests for cervical cancer or mammography), the access barriers they face in service utilization and their health beliefs. Perhaps it has been assumed that the findings of research studies conducted on ethnic groups within their

Box 2-4 Cultural Considerations: Major Health Disparities Affecting Older Adults

South Asians as Compared With Canadian Population Overall:

Higher rates of heart disease and hypertension, especially for women (Long, 2010)
Higher rates of diabetes (Chiu et al., 2010)
Strokes experienced earlier (Chiu et al., 2010)

Chinese as Compared With Canadian Population Overall:

More episodes of depression (Lai, 2004; Long, 2010)

Black Canadians as Compared With Canadian Population Overall:

Higher rates of diabetes (Chiu et al., 2010)
Earlier diagnosis of diabetes (Chiu et al., 2010)
Higher rates of hypertension (Chiu et al., 2010; Veenstra, 2012)
Males experience stroke earlier (Chiu et al., 2010).

Aboriginal Canadians as Compared With Canadian Population Overall:

Higher rates of diabetes (Johnson et al., 2009)
Greater consequences from tuberculosis (Health Canada, 2012)
Substantial increase in cancer rates among Inuit, in particular, lung cancer (Circumpolar Inuit Cancer Review Working Group, 2008)

country of origin can be applied to those who have moved to Canada. While it may be possible to make some comparisons between the health care systems, for example, between Canada and the Philippines and their influence upon how cultural groups access health services, it does not speak to health discrepancies. Furthermore, as Canada has a universal health care system and is considered multicultural, some may erroneously assume that there are few health disparities (Rodney & Copeland, 2009). However, research conducted with visible minorities within Canada suggests that this assumption is incorrect; inequities in health and health care access exist.

One factor that contributes to health disparities, especially for preventable diseases, is the fact that health-promotion materials and programs typically are developed for Caucasians, and this approach may not be effective for people of other cultural backgrounds. However, progress has been made in recent years in identifying evidence-based approaches to disease prevention and health promotion for specific diverse groups.

There is a healthy immigration effect in Canada, such that immigrants are more likely to have better health profiles than the Canadian-born population (Newbold, 2009). Yet, it is also known that the health of older immigrants may decline years after immigration to Canada. Kim and colleagues (2013) examined the trajectory of health for new immigrants to Canada over a 4-year period, including Chinese individuals. At the time of immigration, health was rated as being very good. However, shortly after immigration, health began to deteriorate. Chinese men revealed poor health over time at a much greater rate than did their European counterparts. Chinese women showed even greater declines in health than did Chinese men. The researchers concluded that unemployment, minimal income, difficulties in acquiring English-language skills and discrimination contributed to their declining health (Kim et al., 2013). This holds true for a number of visible minority groups.

OVERVIEW OF CULTURAL GROUPS OF OLDER ADULTS IN CANADA

To provide culturally competent care, nurses need to learn about the cultural groups in their patient populations. Although the study of aging in Canada has focused almost exclusively on Caucasian individuals, researchers are increasingly addressing interrelationships among race, ethnicity, aging and health. Furthermore, researchers are beginning to address age-related concerns of other diverse groups, such as rural, homeless and incarcerated older adults. Even today, terminology used in reference to subgroups is inconsistent, and definitions of specific groups may vary. Current terminology includes the following:

● *Aboriginal*—The term "Aboriginal" is a collective term for indigenous peoples in North America (Health Canada, 2003). Canada uses the term "Aboriginal" to cover registered and non-registered First Nations, Métis and Inuit people (Health Canada, 2003). The term "**Indigenous**" is also used to refer to these three groups of Aboriginal people.

- *Indian*—A term that was used to refer to all indigenous people in Canada who were not Métis or Inuit. Within Canada, this word has largely been replaced by the term "First Nations" (Health Canada, 2003).
- *First Nations*—This term replaced the word "Indian" in the 1970s and is commonly used; there is no legal definition for it (Health Canada, 2003).
- *Inuit*—This term refers to Aboriginal individuals living in Arctic Canada, including Nunavut, the Northwest Territories, and northern Quebec and Labrador (Health Canada, 2003). Within Canada, Inuit has replaced the word "Eskimo."
- *Métis*—A group of Aboriginal people that descend from a mixed First Nations and European ancestry (Health Canada, 2003).
- *Visible Minority*—According to the Employment Equity Act (http://laws-lois.justice.go.ca), visible minorities refer to individuals who are non-Caucasian in race or non-white in colour, and who are not Aboriginals. Individuals who are considered visible minorities include South Asians, Chinese, Blacks, Southeast Asian, Filipinos, Latin Americans, Arabs, West Asians, Japanese and Koreans (Statistics Canada, 2009b).
- *South Asian Canadians*—The South Asian grouping include individuals who have come from Bangladesh, India, Pakistan, Sri Lanka and Nepal (Surood & Lai, 2010).
- *Black Canadians*—The term Black Canadians refers to individuals who have emigrated from Caribbean countries, such as Trinidad or Jamaica. It can also describe African Canadians, those who have come to Canada from Africa. However, this term can signify Black individuals whose families have resided for centuries in Nova Scotia and came as escaped slaves from the United States in the 1700s (Beagan & Chapman, 2012).

Although progress is being made in research related to ethnic and racial diversity of older Canadians, many subgroups continue to be combined together. Thus, it is important to realize that conclusions from studies may not apply to all the subgroups when they are grouped as a collective. Furthermore, many immigrants from the aforementioned subgroups, such as those coming from China, initially experience very good health when coming to Canada. However, their health advantages disappear over time due to the acculturation stresses and changes in diet and other living circumstances (Kim et al., 2013).

Information about the largest minority groups of older adults within Canada is presented in the following sections. These studies are conducted on minorities living within Canada, and, as noted earlier, the amount of research is limited. Nevertheless, nurses can use this information to learn about the cultural traditions of patient populations, keeping in mind, however, that they should not generalize or stereotype

on the basis of an individual's race or ethnicity. More research using larger sample sizes needs to be conducted with visible minority groups in Canada.

Canadian Aboriginals

As stated earlier in this chapter, formally recognized Canadian Aboriginals include First Nations (61%), Métis (32%) and Inuits (4%) (percentages are approximated; Statistics Canada, 2013b). These recognized groups gave up land titles to the Canadian government to receive separate tracts of land (reserves), specific rights (e.g., hunting and fishing), as well as social welfare benefits. Other smaller bands of Aboriginals have not signed treaties with the government (e.g., Cherokee, M'kmaq, Lubicon) and hence are not officially recognized by the Canadian government (Schub & Pravikoff, 2014).

The Aboriginal population is growing much faster than the general population in Canada (Statistics Canada, 2013b). The Aboriginal population is younger than the non-Aboriginal population in Canada, in part due to higher birth rates and shorter life expectancy (Statistics Canada, 2013b). Adults 65 years of age and older comprise only 5.9% of the Aboriginal population, as compared to non-Aboriginal older adults comprising 14.2% of the general population (Statistics Canada, 2013b).

A number of social problems affect the health of Canada's Aboriginal peoples. For instance, Aboriginals experience higher rates of unemployment, poor housing, violence, crime, incarceration and substance abuse (Schub & Pravikoff, 2014). In addition to the health issues mentioned in Cultural Considerations Box 2-4, Aboriginals have higher rates of risky health behaviours, such as smoking and binge drinking (this is particularly problematic among the Inuit; McDonald & Trenholm, 2010). They often do not consume the recommended 5 servings of vegetables and fruit per day (as per Canada Food Guide; Quadir & Akhtar-Danesh, 2010). In 2008, the rate of HIV was 3.6 times higher in the Aboriginal population than in the general Canadian population (Public Health Agency of Canada, 2010). Finally, the rates of suicide and self-injury are very high among Aboriginal individuals, particularly among adolescents (Adelson, 2005).

Many older Aboriginal Canadians experienced the trauma of residential schools. In the late 19th century, the Canadian government believed it was its responsibility to educate and care for Aboriginal people. It believed that Aboriginals should learn English and adopt Canadian customs and the Christian faith. It was hoped that they would pass their adopted lifestyle onto their children and native traditions would diminish within a few generations. So young Aboriginal children were placed into residential schools. Throughout their school years, they lived in substandard conditions and experienced physical, emotional and sexual abuse. They were in residential school 10 months a year, away from their parents, and had few opportunities to see examples of normal family life. Their letters to their parents were written in English, which most parents could not read. When the students returned to the reserve, they often found they did not belong. They did not have the skills to help their parents with traditional hunting and fishing and became ashamed of their native heritage (Aboriginal and Northern Affairs Canada).

South Asian Canadians

South Asians are the largest visible minority in Canada (Statistics Canada, 2011a) and immigrated from Bangladesh, India, Pakistan, Sri Lanka and Nepal. They may follow different faiths, such as Sikh, Hindu and Muslim (Bedi et al., 2008). Genetics, culture and faith may affect how South Asian Canadians respond to illness. South Asians experience more cardiovascular problems than do other ethnic groups, due in part to physiological differences, such as smaller coronary arteries and greater plasma lipids (Prayaga, 2007). However, they may not follow through with cardiac rehabilitation (Galdas et al., 2011), due in part to culture and religious reasons. For instance, South Asian Canadian women of Sikh faith may be challenged to comply with rehabilitation due to a lack of understanding about what cardiac disease entails, a faith paradigm that embraces fate or destiny as well as difficulty in adhering to a heart-healthy diet (King et al., 2006). Sikh South Asian Canadian males reported factors that affected their ability to manage cardiac disease, including decreased physical activity in Canada, an inability to speak English or French (with health care providers), a lack of understanding about what cardiac illness involves, as well as their Sikh beliefs about illness being part of God's plan (Bedi et al., 2008).

Besides experiencing challenges in following treatment regimens for cardiac disease, South Asians may be less likely to have screening tests, such as Pap smears, than the overall Canadian population (Amankwah et al., 2009). Older South Asians report the following barriers to accessing health services, including culture and language differences, lengthy waiting lists, inconvenient office hours and not having transportation (Lai & Surood, 2010). While South Asians believe that herbal medications have less side effects than western ones (Surood & Lai, 2010), they are not averse to utilizing western treatments.

Southeast Asians

Immigrants from Southeast Asia include those from Brunei, Burma (Myanmar), Cambodia, Indonesia, Laos, Malaysia, Philippines, Singapore, Thailand and Vietnam (ASEAN, n.d.). Of these countries, Canada is home to a number of individuals from the Philippines, Vietnam, Cambodia and a small number from Laos. Vietnamese, Laotian and Cambodian refugees came to Canada in large numbers between 1978 and 1982 (Dorais, 2000) to escape war and political unrest. While most of the immigrants came after 1979, there were some who came to study in Canada before 1975. Also, there were professionals who had come from Vietnam in 1975 and 1976 to escape the Communist takeover. In 1979, Canada agreed to take refugees from these countries. During 1979 and 1980, Canada received over 60,000 refugees from Vietnam, Cambodia and Laos. In the following few years,

the Canadian government accepted many more immigrants from these countries, in an effort to support family reunification. These immigrants were sponsored by relatives already in Canada (Dorais, 2000).

Examining health disparities within the Southeast Asian population is difficult as many studies lump Asians from various countries together under the title Asian, despite the fact that individuals come from very different regions with different ethnicities, culture and dietary habits (Carolan, 2013). There are limited Canadian studies examining immigrants from the Southeast Asia. As such, we need to access studies from various countries, such as the United States or Britain, but recognize that the findings may not always apply (e.g., differences in health care systems).

That being said, there are some notable health disparities between immigrants from Southeast Asia as compared with white Canadians. For instance, individuals from Southeast Asian countries have significantly higher rates of Hepatitis B infection. The rate of Hepatitis B is between 5% and 10% in Southeastern Asia (Grytdal et al., 2009; WHO Fact Sheet, 2012). Additionally, according to one study, Filipino women in the United States have higher rates of type 2 diabetes than do white Americans (Araneta et al., 2002). Within the United States, women of Vietnamese origins have higher rates of cervical cancer than do women of other ethnicities. Historically, they were less likely to undergo Pap screening for cervical cancer. With this understanding, education was targeted to a Vietnamese community in a large American city. In examining the impact of the educational efforts, researchers concluded that the disparities in cervical cancer screening is decreasing (Taylor et al., 2009).

In relation to accessing health services, Southeast Asians are less likely to use mental health services than the overall Canadian population (Tiwari & Wang, 2008). However, in comparison with the general Canadian population, individuals of Southeast Asian descent (including Filipino) were more likely to access influenza vaccinations (Quach et al., 2012).

Older Vietnamese and Cambodian immigrants living in North America may experience poorer health than do some of their counterparts from other Asian countries. For example, studies from the United States have shown that older Vietnamese Americans may experience higher rates of disability and poorer health than do their Asian counterparts (Fuller-Thomson et al., 2011; Mui & Kang, 2006), but still may experience less disability than do white Americans (Fuller-Thomson et al., 2011). Similarly, Cambodian older adults may experience poor physical and mental health in comparison with their Asian and American counterparts (Marshall et al., 2005; Wong et al., 2011). The poor health status has been attributed to the war trauma experienced before immigrating to America (Marshall et al., 2005).

Chinese Canadians

Up until 2006, Chinese Canadians made up the largest visible minority in Canada. It is believed that the Chinese first immigrated to Canada (British Columbia) in 1858 upon hearing that gold had been found in the Fraser Valley. In the early 1880s, approximately 15,000 Chinese were enlisted to complete the last part of the Canadian Pacific Railway in British Columbia. The Chinese Immigration Act (also known as the Chinese Exclusion Act) almost banned the immigration of Chinese to Canada (Radio Canada International, 2013). In 1947, the Act was rescinded and Chinese Canadians were granted the right to vote. In 1997, with Hong Kong handed back to the Chinese, immigration of Chinese to Canada rapidly grew (Radio Canada International, 2013).

Research on Chinese Canadians suggests that aging Chinese individuals experience good health. For instance, Chow (2010) interviewed 147 Chinese seniors in a western Canadian city about their health. Chow concluded that the majority of them described their health as being good or very good. However, some studies indicate that older Chinese adults may experience some degree of mental illness. In one study, almost 25% of older Chinese adults interviewed revealed experiencing at least mild symptoms of depression, related in part to cultural barriers (Lai, 2004).

Black Canadians

Black Canadian immigrants may be from Caribbean countries (e.g., Trinidad, Jamaica) or from Africa (largely from Algeria, Morocco, Ethiopia and Nigeria; Government of Canada, 2012). These individuals tend to be more recent immigrants to this country. However, there are Black individuals who have resided for centuries in Nova Scotia from ancestors who came as slaves from Africa in the 1700s (Beagan & Chapman, 2012). Within Nova Scotia, particularly in Halifax, Black Africans comprise the largest visible minority.

In addition to the health problems noted in Cultural Considerations Box 2-4, such as hypertension, HIV/AIDS is disproportionately higher in Canadians from Caribbean and African countries (Gardezi et al., 2008). Furthermore, culture may play a role in the admission of mental health problems. For instance, even when feeling depressed, African Canadian women may be reluctant to talk about depression (Etowa et al., 2007). In one study, Black women living in rural areas of Nova Scotia felt reluctant to go to hospital due to a fear of discrimination (Etowa et al., 2007). While discrimination may discourage African Canadians from accessing health services, the relationship between disease and discrimination is not as clear. For example, in one study (Veenstra, 2012), telephone interviews were conducted with 706 adults living in Toronto and 838 adults living in Vancouver to examine the relationship between racial identity and hypertension. It was found that Black Canadians had a much higher rate of hypertension than did Canadians of other ethnicities. It was determined that lower educational level played a stronger role in hypertension risk than did perceived discrimination. Discrimination alone was not believed to be related to hypertension. As such, more research needs to examine the health experiences of Black Canadians.

Case Study

Mrs. A. is an 81-year-old Black Canadian who lives with her daughter, Mildred, and teenage great-grandson in a two-bedroom apartment in a large metropolitan area of Ontario. Mildred works as a nursing assistant in a nearby nursing home and often works double shifts. Mrs. A. was born in Jamaica and lived there until 20 years ago when her husband died, and she moved in with her daughter (who lived alone at the time). Seven years later, Mildred took on responsibility for raising her infant grandson, who is now 13 years old. Mrs. A. has glaucoma, arthritis and hypertension, and she had a stroke several years ago. She admits to having "a little problem" with her memory, but Mildred says, "She remembers what she wants to remember." Mrs. A. takes an over-the-counter analgesic as needed for her arthritis and has two prescription medications for hypertension. She also uses prescription eye drops twice daily. Mrs. A. has her blood pressure checked by the parish nurse about once monthly; she sees a doctor and nurse practitioner at a neighbourhood clinic for checkups about twice yearly. The parish nurse often tells her that her blood pressure is "a little on the high side" and encourages her to see her doctor, but Mrs. A. has difficulty getting appointments because she depends on Mildred to take her there. Mrs. A. is about 20 kg overweight and she walks very slowly. When she is out of the house, Mildred provides a supportive hand to assist her with steadiness and mobility. Mildred shops for groceries, but Mrs. A. prepares most meals for the family.

THINKING POINTS

- How might Mrs. A.'s living arrangements influence her health and functioning, both positively and negatively?
- What factors are likely to influence the kind of health care Mrs. A. receives?
- If you were the parish nurse, what actions would you take to decrease health risks and promote quality of life for Mrs. A.?
- What additional resources could be used to improve Mrs. A.'s situation?

See **ONLINE LEARNING ACTIVITY 2-2: RESOURCES FOR INFORMATION ABOUT BLACK CANADIANS AND THEIR HISTORY** at http://thepoint.lww.com/Miller7e

See **ONLINE LEARNING ACTIVITY 2-3: RESOURCES FOR INFORMATION ABOUT CHINESE AND ASIAN OLDER ADULTS RESIDING IN CANADA AND THEIR HISTORY** at http://thepoint.lww.com/Miller7e

See **ONLINE LEARNING ACTIVITY 2-4: RESOURCES FOR INFORMATION ABOUT CANADIAN ABORIGINAL PEOPLES AND THEIR HISTORY** at http://thepoint.lww.com/Miller7e

Case Study

Mrs. C. is a 76-year-old Chinese Canadian widow who lives in an apartment in the Chinatown section of Vancouver. She has lived within the same 2-km radius since her parents brought her to Vancouver from Mainland China when she was 9 years old. All three of her children are married; two live about an hour away, and the other one lives on the East Coast. Although she can speak and read English, Mrs. C. prefers to use her native Chinese dialect, and all of her reading materials are in Chinese. She completed a high-school education in Chinatown and married a Chinese immigrant when she was 19 years old. She served as her husband's primary caregiver after he developed lung cancer several years ago until his death last year.

Mrs. C. is enrolled in the On Lok Senior Health Program, a health-maintenance organization that provides a wide range of health and social services. She attends a daily meal program and sees the nurse at the centre for blood pressure checks every month. She has hypertension, arthritis and coronary artery disease. Mrs. C. sees a local herbalist every few weeks to obtain the herbal medicines that will keep her yin and yang energies in balance, and she chooses foods according to their yin and yang characteristics. She periodically has acupuncture treatments when her arthritis bothers her. Although Mrs. C. believes she can control her heart problem and high blood pressure with herbs and diet, she takes her two medications as prescribed because the nurse at the On Lok clinic has emphasized that these pills are essential for keeping her energy in balance.

Mrs. C. recently had a stroke and received medical treatment and rehabilitation services. She is being discharged to her apartment with a referral to the On Lok home care services for skilled nursing and speech, physical and occupational therapies. Discharge orders also include the need to instruct Mrs. C. in a low-sodium diet. In addition to having some aphasia and left-sided paralysis, Mrs. C. has some residual memory impairment from the stroke. Before discharge from the rehabilitation program, she said she would not need any home care assistance because she expected that her daughter and daughter-in-law would take turns coming over every day and that they would take care of her. You are the nurse assigned to do the initial assessment and your visit is scheduled for the day after discharge, when the daughter-in-law will be there. Although you have been a home care nurse for several years, you have recently moved to Vancouver and you began working for On Lok 2 weeks ago.

THINKING POINTS

- What cultural factors might influence Mrs. C.'s acceptance of you, as the skilled care nurse, and of home care services in general?
- What would you do to gain cultural competence to work more effectively with Mrs. C. and other patients in the On Lok health care program?
- What are your specific health care concerns for Mrs. C., and what strategies would you use to develop an effective and acceptable care plan?

Case Study

Mrs. I. is an 72-year-old Plains Cree who lives with her daughter and son-in-law. In accordance with Cree traditions, Mrs. I. believes that health is closely linked with being in harmony with the environment, family members and supernatural forces. She regularly attends native healing ceremonies and protects her family and herself from sickness through songs, stories, rituals and prayers. Mrs. I. has had diabetes and hypertension for several years and is about 20 kg more than her ideal weight. She receives medical care at the Cree First Nations Healing Centre, where you are the nurse. During a recent visit, you found Mrs. I.'s blood pressure was 164/98 mm Hg; her random blood sugar level as measured on the glucometer was 9.9 mmol/L. You know from previous visits that Mrs. I. does not want to take any prescription medications because she thinks they are not in harmony with spiritual forces. When you explain that both her blood sugar and blood pressure are high, she promises you that she will ask the healer at the sweat lodge for healing. You know from your experience with the Cree First Nations Healing Centre that sweat lodge practices may include fasting for healing.

THINKING POINTS

- What cultural factors are likely to influence Mrs. I.'s understanding of diabetes and hypertension?
- How would you use metaphors and cultural knowledge to help Mrs. I. understand her diabetes and hypertension?
- What questions would you ask Mrs. I. to identify teaching strategies and other interventions that might be successful with regards to her diabetes and hypertension?
- What strategies are likely to be successful in implementing dietary and lifestyle interventions for Mrs. I.?
- What steps would you take to improve your cultural competence in working with Mrs. I.?

OLDER ADULTS IN OTHER DIVERSE GROUPS

It is important to recognize that the concept of cultural competence applies even to one's own group because individuals within groups have unique combinations of characteristics. Another consideration is that many culturally based characteristics are subtle, not noticed or even purposefully hidden (e.g., sexual orientation, religious affiliations). Thus, nurses need to learn about groups of older adults that may be less visible and smaller in numbers but with unique needs. In recent years, gerontologists are identifying the needs of some of these groups, such as those considered rural or homeless. Other groups, such as those who are discriminated against because of sexual orientation or gender identity, are advocating on their own behalf to identify and address their unique needs. Information about some of these groups is discussed in this section, and nurses are encouraged to use the resources listed in Online Learning Activity 2-5 to learn more about these and other groups. Again, as with all aspects of cultural diversity, what is known about a group of people does not necessarily apply to individuals within that group.

Older Adults in Rural and Remote Areas

As noted in the *Rural and Small Town Canada Analysis Bulletin* (Statistics Canada, 2008a), the definition of rural includes the population outside of settlements of 1,000 or more persons with a population density of 400 or more individuals per square kilometre. Within Canada, the rural population is growing; however, much of the growth occurs near metropolitan areas. Depending upon how rural is defined (there are different definitions), between 19% and 30% of Canadians were living in rural regions in 2006 (Statistics Canada, 2008a). A greater percentage of older Canadians live in rural areas as compared with urban centres; 15% are in rural Canada compared with 13% in urban areas (Statistics Canada, 2008b). Most immigrants live in large urban centres. This means that only a small proportion of immigrants reside in rural Canada. For example, in 2006 the immigrant population in rural and small towns ranged from 0.9% in Newfoundland and Labrador to 12% in British Columbia (Statistics Canada, 2009a). While relatively few immigrants settle in rural areas and small towns in Canada, there are a few exceptions. Some new immigrants who arrived in Canada between 2001 and 2006 settled in areas around Winkler and Steinbach, Manitoba, as well as Fort McMurray, Alberta (Statistics Canada, 2009a).

Although significant local differences exist among rural areas, researchers have identified some common characteristics and needs. Populations in rural regions, including older adults, tend to be more impoverished and less educated and have poorer health outcomes than their urban counterparts. Rural women may be less likely to acknowledge health problems due to a desire for self-sufficiency and resilience and thus attempt to reduce their dependency on formal health care services (Keating, 2008; Wanless et al., 2010). In addition, rural older adults have more limited transportation options and less access to services, including meal and social programs, because of isolation. Using the Canadian Community Health Survey 2.1, McDonald and Conde (2010) examined determinants of various measures of health services use by Canadians aged 55 or older across a range of urban and rural areas of residence. Findings indicated that older residents in rural areas made fewer visits to a general practitioner, to a specialist and to a dentist compared with urban residents.

Geographical location is a determinant of health. One of the challenges in meeting the health care needs of older Canadians who reside in rural and remote areas is that these communities have declining populations, and it is difficult to develop and maintain an effective health care system for them. Acute care hospitals, for example, may be located several hours away, and rehabilitation and specialist services may be lacking. Older adults living in remote and rural Canada are disadvantaged when compared with those living in urban centres.

Homeless Older Adults

The category of "older homeless" typically extends downward to the age of 50 to 55 years because homeless people have significant health problems and other characteristics, such as appearing much older, which are typically associated with older chronologic age. Increased homelessness among older adults is associated with increased poverty rates and declining availability of affordable housing. Homeless people 65 years old and older are entitled to Medicare and social security benefits, but they may have difficulty accessing funding if they do not have a permanent address. Characteristics of homeless older adults include significantly higher mortality rates, higher levels of disability, longer length of homelessness and higher overall rates of chronic illnesses and mental illness than younger homeless adults or older adults who are not homeless (Bonin et al., 2010; Joyce & Limbos, 2009). Since the mid-1980s, social service and health care providers have recognized the need to provide rehabilitative services to address health, social and behavioural problems of homeless older adults, in addition to addressing their basic needs for food and shelter. However, homeless older adults are difficult to reach with health care services. They may be transient, using different drop-in centres or living from week to week in low-rate hotel rooms. Because of their life experiences of poverty, mental illness and homelessness, some of these older adults may have difficulty adjusting to long-term care facilities.

Lesbian, Gay, Bisexual and Older Adults

According to a 2009 Canadian Community Health Survey, 2% of Canadians 18 to 59 years of age identify as lesbian, gay or bisexual (Statistics Canada, 2011b). Not surprisingly, this group of older adults has been called "the invisible elderly" (Jablonski et al., 2013). That being said, nurses are increasingly recognizing the need to identify and address the unique needs of these diverse groups (Hardacker et al., 2013; Jablonski et al., 2013). The acronym LGBT is an umbrella term that includes three groups whose sexual orientation is not heterosexual (lesbian, gay or bisexual) and several groups whose gender identity and/or gender expression differs from the sex they were assigned at birth (e.g., transgender, cross-dressers). Although sexual orientation and gender identity are distinct entities, these subgroups share a common bond of being viewed outside the norms of sexual expression and identity and they all experience similar societal stigma, isolation, stereotypes and prejudices. Compared with ethnicity and race, the needs of older LGBT people are a less studied area of diversity in aging. Donahue and McDonald (2005) cited a major methodological concern with the existing literature on the needs of older LGBT people, specifically that samples are often recruited through clinical settings or single gay-friendly events with little representation from lower-income groups or visible minorities.

Despite the relatively small numbers and invisibility of LGBT older adults, there is growing recognition of the unique barriers, challenges and inequalities that this group faces. Major progress has been made to address these concerns, and Canada is learning from the experiences of its southern neighbour—the United States. The National Gay and Lesbian Task Force published a 165-page report, *Outing Age 2010* (Grant, 2010), to promulgate research about critical concerns of LGBT older adults and make recommendations related to key issues, such as health, housing, caregiving, discrimination and access to services.

Although there is great diversity among LGBT older adults, one issue they have in common is their experience of various levels and types of stigma. Even this common experience, however, has been shaped by vastly different sociopolitical forces. For example, cohorts of LGBT adults older than 70 years entered into young adulthood at a time when nonheterosexual orientation was considered a crime or a mental illness. Detrimental effects of stigmatization—which for some has included the experience of violence—include fear, anxiety, chronic stress, social isolation and avoidance of needed services and entitlements (LGBT Movement Advancement Project, 2010). Many LGBT people experience their sexual orientation along a continuum, and they do not necessarily live as either heterosexual or gay/lesbian during their entire adult lives. Thus, it is important to recognize that older LGBT individuals vary widely in the length of time they have identified themselves as such.

Some LGBT individuals have biologic, adopted or step children, grandchildren or great-grandchildren. In the past, very few had close relationships with their families. Anecdotal evidence, as well as a few case studies, suggests that some gay and lesbian adults who are estranged from their families provide a source of support for many older adults (Allen, 2005). Other LGBT older adults have no biologic family—or have been rejected by their families—but they have strong bonds with their "family of choice." This extended network of family and friends often become the caregivers for older LGBT adults who need assistance; however, all people involved in these situations face social, economic and legal challenges that do not affect heterosexuals. Older LGBT adults vary greatly in their intimate relationships, and many have had or continue to have monogamous committed partnerships. Relatively few are able to have a legally recognized marriage, and these marriages are not recognized at the federal level. An important aspect of providing culturally competent care for LGBT older adults is using gender-neutral terminology in reference to intimate or partner relationships (as discussed in Chapter 26).

Although some LGBT older adults, especially couples in committed long-term relationships, live very comfortably, LGBT older adults as a group are poorer and less financially secure than other older adults. Many older LGBT adults have limited income and assets because discrimination limited their job opportunities. Only rarely are LGBT partners able to obtain financial benefits that are similar to those of legally married couples, and this has a negative impact on retirement income, assets and access to health care. One study found that older lesbian couples are twice as likely to be poor in comparison with heterosexual couples (Goldberg, 2009). The most significant health disparities that affect older LGBT adults include poorer overall health, lack of access to care, and higher prevalence of cancer, depression, HIV/AIDS, chronic disease and disability, and risky behaviours (e.g., smoking, drug and alcohol abuse; LGBT Movement Advancement Project, 2010). Among older gays and lesbians, but especially for older men, access to services may be restricted due to HIV/AIDS. Furlotte and colleagues (2012) reported on the lack of housing options for older adults living with AIDS in Ottawa (see Box 2-5).

Box 2-5 Evidence-Informed Nursing Practice

Background: There is little Canadian research examining the housing challenges faced by older adults with HIV/AIDS.

Question: What are the experiences of older adults with HIV/AIDS in finding housing with Ottawa, Canada?

Method: The researchers conducted semistructured interviews with 11 individuals—50 years of age and older—who had HIV/AIDS. The sample was composed of 2 women and 9 men, ranging from 52 to 67 years of age. Of the 11 participants, 8 had been aware of their HIV-positive status for more than 10 years. Research participants reported living in various kinds of housing situations, such as renting an apartment, owning a home, living with family members or being homeless. Interviews were recorded and examined for themes.

Findings: Several major themes emerged from the data analysis. First, participants were concerned about access to retirement and long-term care facilities; they worried about whether or not they would be accepted in these facilities and if they would receive appropriate care. Second, participants spoke about the need for subsidized housing for aging individuals with HIV/AIDS. Third, participants who were currently homeless or who had been homeless in the past spoke about the unhealthiness of shelters for those with HIV/AIDS.

Implications for Nursing Practice: Nurses should be aware of the growing need for housing for aging adults with HIV/AIDS. Nurses can advocate on behalf of these vulnerable older adults.

Furlotte, C., Schwartz, K., Koornstra, J. J., et al. (2012). "Got a room for me?" Housing experiences of older adults living with HIV/AIDS in Ottawa. *Canadian Journal on Aging, 31*(1), 37–48.

Older Adults With Intellectual Disabilities

Older adults with intellectual disabilities are a relatively new, emerging grouping of aging individuals. In the past, these individuals rarely lived until older age; however, individuals with moderate to severe disability are now commonly living into their late 50s or even into their 60s (Hirst et al., 2013). The term *intellectual disability* is used to describe individuals who have significant limitations in intellectual functioning, as well as in conceptual, social and practical behavioural skills; these difficulties begin before 18 years of age (Schalock et al., 2010). Typically, this term is used for individuals who have disorders such as cerebral palsy (Patja et al., 2001) and Down syndrome (Sherman et al., 2007).

Individuals with intellectual disabilities are often considered "older" when they reach about 45 years of age or older. This is because pre-existing neurological and physical impairments result in signs of aging that are not usually seen in the general population until 20 or 30 years later (Thomas et al., 2010). For instance, there is a higher prevalence of Alzheimer's disease among those with Down syndrome, and this often occurs when individuals are in their 40s. In one Dutch study, the incidence of dementia was 16.8% among 506 individuals with Down syndrome 45 years of age and older (Coppus et al., 2006).

There are a number of challenges faced by older adults with intellectual disabilities. Some of these challenges revolve around their limited knowledge about health and negative past experiences with health care. For example, aging individuals with intellectual disabilities may have little understanding about the changes they experience as a result of aging. Furthermore, they may have difficulties communicating changes in their bodies or pain or sensations that are different from usual for them. If they have had unpleasant experiences with health care providers in the past, they may be fearful, resistant and uncommunicative with a physician or nurse when needing care (Hirst et al., 2013). As such, older adults with intellectual disabilities should receive education about their health, as well as regular preventative screening, such as eye exams or screening for prostate or breast cancers. Reciprocally, health care professionals require education on how to best communicate with these aging individuals.

In addition to the importance of education for older adults with intellectual disabilities and their health care providers, there is a need for appropriate housing for this aging cohort. Some of these aging individuals may have resided in group homes for decades, and yet if they are now experiencing dementia, staff within group homes may not know how to manage symptoms of dementia, such as delusions, hallucinations or agitation. Similarly, if aging individuals with intellectual disabilities are placed in nursing homes, staff may be uncertain in how to relate to individuals with Down syndrome. In addition to instruction about dementia for staff within group homes, as well as education about intellectual disabilities for staff in nursing homes, research needs to be conducted on what types of environments are most suited for the care of aging individuals with intellectual disabilities (Lane et al., 2013).

 See **ONLINE LEARNING ACTIVITY 2-5: RESOURCES FOR INFORMATION ABOUT AGING CANADIANS WHO ARE HOMELESS, HAVE INTELLECTUAL DISABILITIES OR IDENTIFY AS LGBT** at http://thepoint.lww.com/Miller7e

Chapter Highlights

Cultural Diversity in Canada

- One out of every five Canadians belongs to a visible minority group, largely due to the country's growing South Asian population.
  1. Chinese is the most common language spoken at home after English and French.
  2. Most immigrants live in metropolitan areas.
- Gerontologists are identifying health care needs of many diverse subgroups of older adults by characteristics such as race/ethnicity, socioeconomic factors, rural residency, homelessness, intellectual disabilities and self-identification as LGBT.

Cultural Competence

- All nurses are expected to develop cultural competence by assessing their own attitudes (Box 2-2) and learning about culturally diverse groups (Box 2-6).
- All health care providers need to be linguistically competent and to use resources to address needs of patients who are not proficient in English (Box 2-3).

Cultural Perspectives on Wellness

- Nurses need to explore what health and wellness mean to individual older adults.
- Definitions of health and wellness are rooted in the three major health belief systems (Box 2-4).

Health Disparities

- Members of racial or ethnic groups experience many health disparities, and these have significant implications for older adults (Box 2-4).

Overview of Cultural Groups of Older Adults in Canada

- Racial and ethnic groups recognized as being the largest include Aboriginals, South Asian Canadians, Chinese Canadians and Black Canadians.
- Nurses can develop cultural competence by educating themselves about the cultural traditions of the older adults in their geographic areas.
- Characteristics of some of these groups are summarized, but it is important to recognize that the larger groups are composed of many subgroups and there is great diversity within these groups.

Older Adults in Other Diverse Groups

- Researchers and nonprofit organizations are identifying and addressing the unique needs of other diverse groups,

---

Box 2-6   Examples of Health Disparities Affecting Older Adults, Based on National Data and Reviews of Studies

Life Expectancy and Levels of Functional Impairment

- First Nations and Inuit peoples in Canada have a life expectancy of 5 to 10 years less than Canadians as a whole (Heart & Stroke Foundation, 2012).
- Aboriginal peoples in Canada have higher rates of disability than do non-Aboriginal Canadians (Durst et al., 2006).

Disparities Related to Preventive Care

- South Asian immigrant women have lower rates of accessing mammography than the general Canadian population (Ahmad et al., 2013).
- Older South Asian immigrants may fail to seek health services due to barriers such as lack of knowledge, complicated procedures to use services, professionals not speaking language of immigrants and lack of finances (to buy nutritious foods or appropriate housing; Lai & Surood, 2013).
- Canadians with low income, including older adults, are less likely to access dental care due to costs (Wallace & MacEntee, 2012).
- Canadian Aboriginal women are less likely to seek screening for breast and cervical cancers (Schub & Pravikoff, 2014).

Disparities Related to Chronic Diseases

- Immigrants from Latin American countries to Canada are one of the highest risk urban populations for diabetes (Otero et al., 2011).
- Individuals of South Asian descent in Canada experience coronary artery disease at younger ages and at higher rates than those of European or Chinese descent (Galdas et al., 2012).
- Aboriginal Canadians have very high rates of diabetes; there has been a 150% increase in type 2 diabetes over the past two decades (Schub & Pravikoff, 2014).
- First Nations' individuals have a greater risk for chronic renal failure and end-stage renal disease than do other Canadians (Schub & Pravikoff, 2014).

Leading Causes of Death by Race and Hispanic Origin (Ng—Statistics Canada, 2011)

- Immigrants to Canada generally have lower rates of age-standardized mortality rates, believed due to the "healthy immigration effect." However, women living in Toronto and Montreal who emigrated from India, and women who came from the United Kingdom and resided in Vancouver had similar age-standardized mortality rates as Canadian-born women in these cities.
- When cause of death examined, women from India living in Toronto and Montreal had higher rates of circulatory disease and women coming from the United Kingdom had higher rates of circulatory disease and cancer (Ng—Statistics Canada, 2011).

Disparities Related to Nursing Home Use and Care

- There are few Aboriginal nursing homes in Canada (on and off the reserve; Beatty & Berdahl, 2011).
- Although Asian and South Asian communities have promoted the idea of families caring for their older members, there are nursing homes geared to specific ethnic backgrounds in Canada. For instance, in Toronto, there are nursing homes for aging Chinese individuals.
- Influencing factors: Increased use of more preferred settings (e.g., assisted living), which are less accessible to those with lower incomes.

---

including rural, homeless, LGBT older adults, as well as those with intellectual disabilities.

Critical Thinking Exercises

1. Complete the cultural self-assessment in Box 2-2, and think about how you are similar to and differ from the many cultural groups to which you belong.
2. Reflect on your encounters during the past few weeks with people who differ from you culturally. Make a list of the obvious differences and another list of differences that you may not have recognized but most likely existed (e.g., you most likely interacted with someone who was LGBT). Ask yourself how accepting and nonjudgmental you feel about these people.
3. Identify one culturally diverse group that you are likely to work with in your current geographic area. Contact local agencies and organizations that serve these groups and find out what services they offer; ask about unique health care issues affecting these particular groups.
4. Use Online Learning Activities 2-5 to find information about the history of various cultures that might inform your understanding of the cultures you may work with in the future. How might that information assist you in your work with older adults?
5. Think of the various settings in which you work with older adults and describe what you would do or whom you would call if you needed to communicate with a patient who did not speak English.

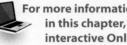 **For more information about the topics discussed in this chapter, be sure to check out the interactive Online Learning Activities and other helpful resources at http://thepoint.lww.com/Miller7e**

REFERENCES

Aboriginal Affairs and Northern Development Canada. *Indian Residential Schools*. Retrieved from http://www.aadnc-aandc.gc.ca/eng/110010001 5576/1100100015577(n.d.)

Adelson, N. (2005). The embodiment of inequity: Health disparities in Aboriginal Canada. *Canadian Journal of Public Health*, 96(2), S45–S61.

Ahmad, F., Jandu, B., Albagli, A., et al. (2013). Exploring ways to overcome barriers to mammography uptake and retention among South Asian immigrant women. *Health and Social Care*, 21(1), 88–97. doi:10.1111/j.1365-2524.2012.01090.x

Allen, K. (2005). Gay and lesbian elders. In M. Johnson (Ed.), *The Cambridge handbook of age and ageing* (pp. 482–489). New York, NY: Cambridge University Press.

Amankwah, E., Ngwakongnwi, E., & Quan, H. (2009). Why visible minority women in Canada do not participate in cervical cancer screening. *Ethnicity & Health*, 14(4), 337–349.

American Geriatrics Society. (2006). *Position statement on ethnogeriatrics*. Retrieved from http://americangeriatrics.org/Products/Positionpapers/ethno_committeePF.shtml

Andrews, M. M. (2012a). Culturally competent nursing care. In M. M. Andrews & J. S. Boyle (Eds.), *Transcultural concepts in nursing care* (6th ed., pp. 17–37). Philadelphia, PA: Lippincott Williams & Wilkins.

Andrews, M. M. (2012b). The influence of cultural and health belief systems on health care practices. In M. M. Andrews & J. S. Boyle (Eds.), *Transcultural concepts in nursing care* (6th ed., pp. 73–88). Philadelphia, PA: Lippincott Williams & Wilkins.

Araneta, M. R., Wingard, D. L., & Barrett-Connor, E. (2002). Type 2 diabetes and metabolic syndrome in Filipina-American women: A high-risk nonobese population. *Diabetes Care, 25*(3), 494–499.

Association of South East Asian Nations. Retrieved from http://www.asean.org

Beagan, B. L., & Chapman, G. E. (2012). Meanings of food, eating and health among African Nova Scotians: 'Certain things aren't meant for Black folk'. *Ethnicity & Health, 17*(5), 513–529.

Beatty, B. B., & Berdahl, L. (2011). Health care and Aboriginal seniors in urban Canada: Helping a neglected class. *The International Indigenous Policy Journal, 2*(1). Retrieved from http://ir.lib.uwo.ca/iipj/vol2/iss1/10/

Bedi, H., LeBlanc, P., McGregor, L., et al. (2008). Older immigrant Sikh men's perspective of the challenges of managing coronary heart disease risk. *Journal of Men's Health, 5*, 218–226.

Bonin, J. P., Fourner, L., Blais, R., et al. (2010). Health and mental health care utilization by clients of resources for homeless persons in Quebec City and Montreal, Canada: A 5-year follow-up study. *Health and Mental Health Care Utilization, 37*, 95–110.

Canadian Nurses Association. (2010). *Position statement: Promoting cultural competence in nursing.* Retrieved from http://www.cna-aiic.ca/~/media/cna/page-content/pdf-en/6%20-%20ps114_cultural_competence_2010_e.pdf

Carolan, M. (2013). Gestational diabetes mellitus among women born in South East Asia: A review of the evidence. *Midwifery, 29*(9), 1019–1026. doi:10.1016/j.midw.2012.09.003

Chiu, M., Austin, P. C., Manuel, D. G., et al. (2010). Comparison of cardiovascular risk profiles among ethnic groups using population health surveys between 1996 and 2007. *Canadian Medical Association Journal, 182*(8), E301–E310. doi:10.1503/cmaj.091676

Chow, H. P. (2010). Growing old in Canada: Physical and psychological well-being among elderly Chinese immigrants. *Ethnicity & Health, 15*(1), 61–72.

Circumpolar Inuit Cancer Review Working Group. (2008). Cancer among the circumpolar Inuit, 1989-2003. II. Patterns and trends. *International Journal of Circumpolar Health, 67*(5), 408–420.

Coppus, A., Evenhuis, H., Verberne, G. J., et al. (2006). Dementia and mortality in person's with Down's syndrome. *Journal of Developmental Disability Research, 50*, 768–777.

Donahue, P., & McDonald, L. (2005). Gay and lesbian aging: Current perspectives and future directions for social work practice and research. *Families in Society, 86*, 359–366.

Dorais, L. J. (2000). *The Cambodians, Laotians and Vietnamese in Canada* (Canada's ethnic group series, Booklet No. 38). Ottawa, ON: The Canadian Historical Association.

Durst, D., South, S., & Bluechardt, M. (2006). Urban First Nations people with disability speak out. *Journal of Aboriginal Health, 3*(1), 34–43.

Engebretson, J. C., & Headley, J. A. (2009). Cultural diversity and care. In B. M. Dossey, L. Keegan, & C. E. Guzetta (Eds.), *Holistic nursing: A handbook for practice* (5th ed., pp. 573–597). Boston, MA: Jones and Bartlett.

Etowa, J., Keddy, B., Egbeyemi, J., et al. (2007). Depression: The 'invisible grey fog' influencing the midlife health of African Canadian women. *International Journal of Mental Health Nursing, 16*, 203–213. doi:10.1111/j.1447-0349.2007.00469.x

Etowa, J., Wiens, J., Bernard, W., et al. (2007). Determinants of black women's health in rural and remote communities. *Canadian Journal of Nursing Research, 39*(3), 56–76.

Fuller-Thomson, E., Brennenstuhl, S., & Hurd, M. (2011). Comparison of disability rates among older adults in aggregated and separate Asian American/Pacific Islander subpopulations. *American Journal of Public Health, 101*(1), 94–100.

Furlotte, C., Schwartz, K., Koornstra, J. J., et al. (2012). Got a room for me? Housing experiences of older adults living with HIV/AIDS in Ottawa. *Canadian Journal on Aging, 31*(1), 37–48.

Galdas, P. M., Oliffe, J. L., Wong, S. T., et al. (2012). Canadian Punjabi Sikh men's experiences of lifestyle changes following myocardial infarction: Cultural connections. *Ethnicity & Health, 17*(3), 253–266.

Galdas, P. M., Ratner, P. A., & Oliffe, J. L. (2011). A narrative review of South Asian patients' experiences of cardiac rehabilitation. *Journal of Clinical Nursing, 21*, 149–159. doi:10.1111/j.1365-2702.2011.03754.x

Gardezi, G., Calzavara, L., Husbands, W., et al. (2009). Experiences of and responses to HIV among African and Caribbean communities in Toronto, Canada. *AIDS Care, 20*(6), 718–725.

Goldberg, N. G. (2009). *The impact of inequality for same-sex partners in employer-sponsored retirement plans.* Los Angeles, CA: University of California School of Law, The Williams Institute.

Government of Canada. (2012). *Facts and figures 2011—Immigration overview: Permanent and temporary residents.* Retrieved from http://www.cic.gc.ca/english/resources/statistics/facts2011/permanent/10.asp

Grant, J. M. (2010). *Outing age: Public policy issues affecting lesbian, gay, bisexual and transgender elders.* Washington, DC: National Gay and Lesbian Task Force.

Grytdal, S. P., Liao, Y., Chen, R., et al. (2009). Hepatitis B testing and vaccination among Vietnamese- and Cambodian-Americans. *Journal of Community Health, 34*, 173–180. doi:10.1007/s10900-008-9141-5

Hardacker, C. T., Rubinstein, B., Hotton, A., et al. (2013). Adding silver to the rainbow: The development of the nurses' health education about LGBT elders cultural competency curriculum. *Journal of Nursing Management, 22*(2), 257–266. doi:10.1111/jonm.12125

Health Canada. (2003). Closing the gaps in Aboriginal health. *Health Policy Research, 5*, 1–16.

Heart and Stroke Foundation. (2012). *First Nations, Inuit, and Metis resources.* Retrieved from www.heartandstroke.com

Hirst, S. P., Lane, A. M., & Seneviratne, C. C. (2013). Growing old with a developmental disability. *Indian Journal of Gerontology, 27*(1), 38–54.

Jablonski, R. A., Vance, D. E., & Beattie, E. (2013). The invisible elderly: Lesbian, gay, bisexual, and transgender older adults. *Journal of Gerontological Nursing, 39*(11), 46–52.

Johnson, J. A., Vermeulen, S. U., Toth, E. L., et al. (2009). Increasing incidence and prevalence of diabetes among Status Aboriginal population in urban and rural Alberta, 1995–2006. *Canadian Journal of Public Health, 100*(3), 231–236.

Joyce, D. P., & Limbos, M. (2009). Identification of cognitive impairment and mental illness in elderly homeless men. *Canadian Family Physician, 55*, 1110–1117.

Keating, N. (Ed.). (2008). *Rural ageing: A good place to grow old?* London, England: Policy Press.

Kim, I. H., Carrasco, C., Muntaner, C., et al. (2013). Ethnicity and post migration health trajectory in new immigrants to Canada. *American Journal of Public Health, 103*(4), e96–e104. doi:10.2105/AJPH.2012.301185

King, K. M., LeBlanc, P., Sanguins, J., et al. (2006). Gender-based challenges faced by older Sikh women as immigrants: Recognizing and acting on the risk of coronary artery disease. *Canadian Journal of Nursing Research, 38*(1), 16–40.

Lai, D. (2004). Impact of culture on depressive symptoms of elderly Chinese immigrants. *Canadian Journal of Psychiatry, 49*(12), 820–827.

Lai, D., & Surood, S. (2010). Types and factor structure of barriers to utilization of health services among aging South Asians in Calgary, Canada. *Canadian Journal on Aging, 29*(2), 249–258.

Lai, D., & Surood, S. (2013). Effect of service barriers on health status of aging South Asian immigrants in Calgary, Canada. *Health & Social Work, 38*(1), 41–50.

Lane, A. M., Hirst, S. P., & Reed, M. B. (2013). *Older adults: Understanding and facilitating transitions.* Dubuque, IA: Kendall Hunt.

LGBT Movement Advancement Project. (2010). Retrieved from http://www.lgbtmap.org/lgbt-movement-overview/2010-national-lgbt-movement-report

Long, P. M. (2010). *Improving health care system responses to chronic disease among British Columbia's immigrant, refugee, and corrections population: A review of current findings and opportunities for change.* Retrieved from http://www.phsa.ca/NR/rdonlyres/0E0E5401-E596-4D8B-96C9-3923D577A9B5/0/ReducingHealthInequitiesLitReviewExecutiveSummaryMarch2010.pdf

Maddalena, V. (2009). Cultural competence and holistic practice, implications for nursing education practice and research. *Holistic Nursing Practice, 23*(3), 153–157.

Marshall, G. N., Schell, T. L., Elliott, M. N., et al. (2005). Mental health of Cambodian refugees 2 decades after resettlement in the United States. *Journal of the American Medical Association, 294*(5), 571–579. doi:10.1001/jama.294.5.571

McDonald, J. T., & Conde, H. (2010). Does geography matter? The health service use and unmet health care needs of older Canadians [Special issue]. *Canadian Journal on Aging, 29*(1), 23–37.

McDonald, J. T., & Trenholm, R. (2010). Cancer-related health behaviours and health service use among Inuit and other residents of Canada's north. *Social Science & Medicine, 70*, 1396–1403.

Minister of Public Works and Government Services, Canada. Health Canada. (2012). *First Nations & Inuit health: Tuberculosis.* Retrieved from http://www.hc-sc.gc.ca/fniah-spnia/diseases-maladies/tuberculos/index-eng.php

Mui, A. C., & Kang, S. Y. (2006). Acculturation stress and depression among Asian immigrant elders. *Social Work, 51*(3), 243–255.

Newbold, B. (2009). Health status and Canada's immigrant population: Evidence from LSIC. *Ethnicity and Health, 14*, 315–336.

Ng, E. (2011). *The healthy immigrant effect and mortality rates. Statistics Canada.* Retrieved from www.statcan.gc.ca/pub/82-003-x/2011004/article/11588-eng.pdf

Otero, L., Fong, M., Papineau, D., et al. (2011). Testing a prediabetes screening approach for a Latin American population in Vancouver, Canada. *Journal of Nursing and Healthcare of Chronic Illness, 3*, 329–338. doi:10.1111/j.1752-9824.2011.01110.x

Patja, K., Molso, P., & Livanainen, M. (2001). Cause specific mortality of people with intellectual disabilities in a population-based, 35-year follow-up study. *Journal of Developmental Disability Research, 45*, 30–40.

Prayaga, S. (2007). Asian Indians and coronary artery disease risk. *American Journal of Medicine, 120*(3), e15.

Public Health Agency of Canada. (2010). *Population-specific HIV/AIDS status report: Aboriginal peoples.* Ottawa, ON: Author.

Purnell, L. D. (2013). *Transcultural health care: A culturally competent approach.* Philadelphia, PA: F. A. Davis.

Quach, S., Hamid, J. S., Pereira, J. A., et al. (2012). Influenza vaccination coverage across ethnic groups in Canada. *Canadian Medical Association Journal, 184*(15), 1673–1681.

Quadir, T., & Akhtar-Danesh, N. (2010). Fruit and vegetable intake in Canadian ethnic populations. *Canadian Journal of Dietetic Practice and Research, 71*(1), 11–16.

Radio Canada International. (2013). *Asian Heritage Month—Chinese Canadian history.* Retrieved from http://www.rcinet.ca/patrimoineasiatique/en/le-mois-du-patrimoine-asiatique-au-canada/limmigration

Registered Nurses Association of Ontario. (2007). *Diversity in health care: Developing cultural competence.* Retrieved from http://rnao.ca/sites/rnao-ca/files/Embracing_Cultural_Diversity_in_Health_Care-Developing_Cultural_Competence.pdf

Rodney, P., & Copeland, E. (2009). The health status of Black Canadians: Do aggregated racial and ethnic variables hide health disparities. *Journal of Health Care for the Poor and Underserved, 20*(3), 817–823.

Schalock, R. L., Borthwick-Duffy, S. A., Bradley, V. J., et al. (2010). *Intellectual disability: Diagnosis, classification, and systems of support* (11th ed.). Washington, DC: American Association on Intellectual & Developmental Disabilities.

Schub, T., & Pravikoff, D. (2014, April 25). Aboriginal people living in Canada: Providing culturally competent care. *CINAHL Nursing Guide, Evidence-Based Care Sheet,* 1–2.

Sherman, S. L., Allen, E. G., Bean, L. H., et al. (2007). Epidemiology of Down syndrome. *Mental Retardation and Developmental Disabilities Research Reviews, 13*, 221–227.

Statistics Canada. (2008a). *Rural and small town Canada—Analysis bulletin. Structure and change in Canada's rural demography: An update to 2006 (Catalogue No. 21-006-x).* Ottawa, ON: Author.

Statistics Canada. (2008b). *Rural and small town Canada analysis bulletin: Seniors in rural Canada—Key findings.* Retrieved from http://www.statcan.gc.ca/pub/21-006-x/2007008/findings-resultats-eng.htm

Statistics Canada. (2009a). *Rural and small town Canada—Analysis bulletin. Immigrants in rural Canada: 2006 (Catalogue no. 21-006-x).* Ottawa, ON: Author.

Statistics Canada. (2009b). *Visible minority of person.* Retrieved from http://www.statcan.gc.ca/concepts/definitions/minority-minorite1-eng.htm

Statistics Canada. (2011a). *Immigration and ethnocultural diversity in Canada: National household survey (Catalogue No. 99-010-X2011001).* Ottawa, ON: Author.

Statistics Canada. (2011b). *Gay Pride by the numbers.* Retrieved from www42.statcan.gc.ca/smr08/2011/smr08_158_2011-eng.htm

Statistics Canada. (2012). *Population growth in Canada: From 1851 to 2061—Population and dwelling counts, 2011 census (Catalogue No. 98-310-X2011003).* Ottawa, ON: Author.

Statistics Canada. (2013a). *Immigration and ethnocultural diversity in Canada—National Household Survey, 2011 (Catalogue No. 99-010-X2011001).* Ottawa, ON: Author.

Statistics Canada. (2013b). *Aboriginal peoples in Canada: First nations people, Métis and Inuit, The National Household Survey, 2011 (Catalogue No. 99-011-X2011001).* Ottawa, ON: Author.

Surood, S., & Lai, D. (2010). Impact of culture on use of western health services by older South Asian Canadians. *Canadian Journal of Public Health, 101*(2), 176–180.

Taylor, V. M., Yasui, Y., Nguyen, T. T., et al. (2009). Pap smear receipt among Vietnamese immigrants: The importance of health care factors. *Ethnicity & Health, 14*(6), 575–589.

Thomas, E., Strax, T. E., Luciano, L., et al. (2010). Aging and a developmental disability. *Physical Rehabilitation Clinics of North America, 21*, 419–427.

Tiwari, S. K., & Wang, J. (2008). Ethnic differences in mental health service use among white, Chinese, South Asian and South East Asian populations living in Canada. *Social Psychiatry and Psychiatric Epidemiology, 43*, 866–871.

Veenstra, G. (2012). Expressed racial identity and hypertension in a telephone survey sample from Toronto and Vancouver, Canada: Do socioeconomic status, perceived discrimination and psychosocial stress explain the relatively high risk of hypertension for Black Canadians? *International Journal for Equity in Health, 11*, 1–10. Retrieved from http://www.equityhealthj.com/content/11/1/58

Wallace, B. B., & MacEntee, M. I. (2012). Access to dental care for low-income adults: Perceptions of affordability, availability and acceptability. *Journal of Community Health, 37*, 32–39. doi:10.1007/s10900-011-9412-4

Wanless, D., Mitchell, B. A., & Wister, A. (2010). Social determinants of health for older women in Canada: Does rural-urban residency matter? *Canadian Journal on Aging, 29*, 233–247.

Wong, E. C., Schell, T. L., Marshall, G.N., et al. (2011). The unusually poor physical health status of Cambodian refugees 2 decades after resettlement. *Journal of Immigrant & Minority Health, 13*(5), 876–882.

World Health Organization. (2012). *Hepatitis fact sheets.* Retrieved from http://who.int/topics/hepatitis/factsheets/en/index.html

Applying a Nursing Model for Promoting Wellness in Older Adults

As discussed in Chapter 1, myths about aging are insidious and pervasive in society and form the foundation of ageism, which has serious detrimental effects on older adults. Nurses are influenced not only by societal myths and ageist attitudes but also by their experiences with older adults in health care settings, which often reinforce the perception that older adults are frail, confused, depressed and dependent. These attitudes can lead to a sense of pessimism—or even hopelessness—regarding caring for older adults. Fortunately, knowledge can be an effective antidote to ageism, and the theoretical base of information about aging has expanded exponentially during the past half-century (as discussed in Chapter 4). Research-based information enables health care providers to differentiate between age-related changes that are inevitable and risk factors that can be addressed or even prevented. Chapters in this book provide research-based information about age-related changes and risk factors affecting a particular aspect of functioning, with emphasis on the changes and risks that nurses can address. Nurses can apply this information to promote wellness for older adults by identifying ways of improving functioning and quality of life.

Theories about aging and older adults attempt to answer questions about why and how people age, and they provide a basis for identifying the risk factors that health care providers can address. However, they do not address *nursing* care of older adults, as does a *nursing theory* that explains relationships among the core concepts of person, nursing, health and environment. Discipline-specific nursing theories guide nursing care and are essential to promoting wellness for older adults. A recent review of literature identified major gaps in evidence-based information to help nurses intentionally promote wellness (Strout, 2012). The **Functional Consequences Theory for Promoting Wellness in Older Adults**, which is delineated in this chapter and used throughout this text, provides a framework that nurses can use to promote wellness and improve functioning and quality of life for older adults.

A NURSING THEORY FOR WELLNESS-FOCUSED CARE OF OLDER ADULTS

During the 1980s, Miller proposed a model for gerontological nursing, which was the organizational framework for the first edition of the book *Nursing care of older adults: Theory and practice* (Miller, 1990). Since its inception, this model has emphasized the significant role of nurses in using health education interventions to promote optimal health, functioning and quality of life for older adults. In the fifth and sixth editions, some terminology was revised to reflect current emphasis on adding life to years in conjunction with adding years to life. Thus, the model is now called the Functional Consequences Theory for Promoting Wellness in Older Adults. In addition, the updated model reflects and incorporates the evolving understanding of wellness as an integral aspect of health care. Nurses are among the health care professionals who have increasingly emphasized the need to incorporate wellness-oriented goals into their care plans. The Functional Consequences Theory can be used to achieve these goals in all aspects of nursing care for older adults because it addresses essential questions, such as *What is unique about promoting wellness for older adults?* and *How can nurses address unique wellness needs of older adults?*

The purpose of nursing theories is to describe, explain, predict or prescribe nursing care based on scientific evidence. Since the time of Florence Nightingale, nurses have developed theories that address the relationships among the domains of person, nursing, health and environment. The Functional Consequences Theory is based on a combination of research on aging and health and Miller's four decades of providing nursing care for older adults. It also draws on theories that emphasize concepts related to wellness, health promotion and holistic nursing. In this text, up-to-date and evidence-based information about specific aspects of functioning is applied to nursing care of older adults in the framework of the Functional Consequences Theory. The basic premises of the Functional Consequences Theory are as follows:

- Holistic nursing care addresses the body–mind–spirit interconnectedness of each older adult and recognizes that wellness encompasses more than physiologic functioning.
- Although age-related changes are inevitable, most problems affecting older adults are related to risk factors.
- Older adults experience positive or negative functional consequences because of a combination of age-related changes and additional risk factors.
- Interventions can be directed toward alleviating or modifying the negative functional consequences of risk factors.
- Nurses can promote wellness in older adults through health promotion interventions and other nursing actions that address the negative functional consequences.
- Nursing interventions result in positive functional consequences, also called wellness outcomes, which enable older people to function at their highest level despite the presence of age-related changes and risk factors.

This theoretical framework, shown in Figure 3-1, can be illustrated by the following example. Because of age-related visual changes, older adults experience an increased sensitivity to glare and have difficulty seeing clearly when they face bright lights or when lights reflect off shiny surfaces. For instance, it is difficult to see clearly when driving toward the sunlight or reading shopping mall maps that are enclosed in glass cases. In addition to this age-related change, older adults are likely to have disease-related conditions, such as cataracts, that further interfere with their visual abilities. In addition, environmental factors, such as bright lights, highly polished floors and white or glossy paint, can intensify glare. These age-related changes and risk factors can interfere with vision to the extent that older adults stop performing activities or perform them unsafely.

To counteract these functional consequences, the older person or a nurse can initiate any of the following interventions, which are discussed in Chapter 17:

- Wearing sunglasses and using glare-reducing glasses (self-care).
- Addressing environmental conditions by using adequate nonglare lighting (self-care).
- Obtaining periodic evaluations from an ophthalmologist (self-care).
- Teaching about the use of sunglasses and glare-reducing glasses (nursing action).
- Teaching about and facilitating environmental modifications (nursing action).
- Taking actions to avoid glare (e.g., not standing in front of a bright window when talking with an older adult) (nursing action).
- Teaching older adults about the importance of having their eyes evaluated at least annually for treatable conditions (nursing action).

Wellness outcomes resulting from these interventions include improved safety, function and quality of life (Box 3-1).

CONCEPTS UNDERLYING THE FUNCTIONAL CONSEQUENCES THEORY

The Functional Consequences Theory draws from theories that are pertinent to aging, older adults and holistic nursing. The nursing domain concepts of person, environment, health and nursing are linked together specifically in relation to older adults. Before discussing these domain concepts, however, the concepts of functional consequences, age-related changes and risk factors are explained. Box 3-2 summarizes the key concepts in the Functional Consequences Theory for Promoting Wellness in Older Adults.

Functional Consequences

Functional consequences are the observable effects of actions, risk factors and age-related changes that influence the quality of life or day-to-day activities of older adults. Actions include, but are not limited to, purposeful interventions initiated by either older adults or nurses and other caregivers. Risk factors can originate in the environment or arise from physiologic and psychosocial influences. Functional consequences are negative when they interfere with a person's

A Nursing Model for Promoting Wellness in Older Adults

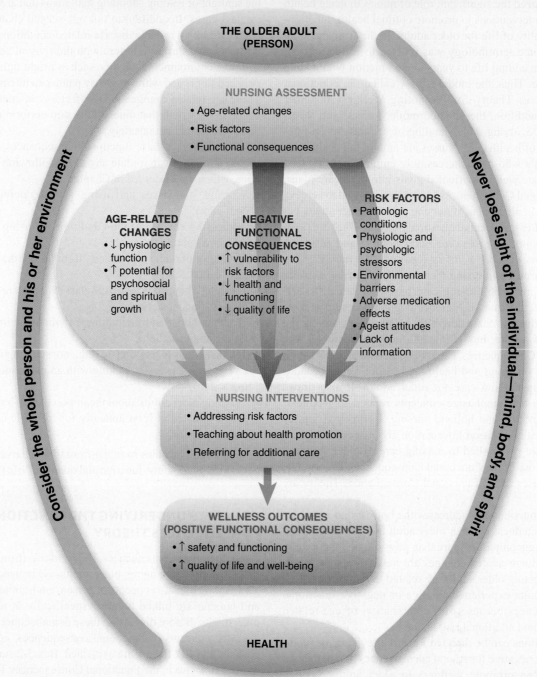

FIGURE 3-1 The Functional Consequences Theory for Promoting Wellness in Older Adults. Age-related changes and risk factors combine to cause negative functional consequences. Nurses holistically assess older adults and initiate interventions to counteract or minimize negative functional consequences. Nursing actions result in wellness outcomes.

level of function or quality of life or increase a person's dependency. Conversely, they are positive when they facilitate the highest level of performance and the least amount of dependency.

Negative functional consequences typically occur because of a combination of age-related changes and risk factors, as illustrated in the example of impaired visual

performance. They may also be caused by interventions, in which case the interventions become risk factors. For example, constipation resulting from the use of an analgesic medication is an example of a negative functional consequence caused by an intervention. In this case, the medication is both an intervention for pain and a risk factor for impaired bowel function.

Box 3-1   Evidence-Informed Nursing Practice

Background: Frail older adults represent 75% of home care users. In this setting, there are numerous opportunities to promote health for older adults, but they are often missed.

Question: What is the effectiveness of nurse-led multicomponent health promotion and disease prevention interventions?

Method: Three randomized controlled trials that included 498 community-residing frail older adults using home care services in Southern Ontario were conducted. Older adults either received usual home care services (e.g., coordinating services, referrals, consultations) or were enrolled in a multicomponent program (e.g., monthly home visits, enhanced assessment, follow-up from an interprofessional team). Across the studies, the same strategy was used to measure the change in health-related quality of life and the cost of service use.

Findings: Nurse-led multicomponent interventions for frail older adults provided greater improvements in quality of life than did usual home care services.

Implications for Nursing Practice: Nurses need to consider multicomponent interventions when providing care in the home setting.

Markle-Reid, M., Browne, G., & Gafni, A. (2013). Nurse-led health promotion interventions improve quality of life in frail older home care clients: Lessons learned from three randomized trials in Ontario, Canada. *Journal of Evaluation in Clinical Practice, 19*, 118–131.

Box 3-2   Concepts in the Functional Consequences Theory for Promoting Wellness in Older Adults

Functional Consequences: Observable effects of actions, risk factors and age-related changes that influence the quality of life or day-to-day activities of older adults. The effects relate to all levels of functioning, including body, mind and spirit.
- *Negative Functional Consequences*: Those that interfere with the older adult's functioning or quality of life.
- *Positive Functional Consequences*: Those that facilitate the highest level of functioning, the least dependency and the best quality of life. When positive functional consequences are the result of nursing interventions, they are called wellness outcomes.

Age-Related Changes: Inevitable, progressive and irreversible changes that occur during later adulthood and are independent of extrinsic or pathologic conditions. On the physiologic level, these changes are typically degenerative; however, on psychological and spiritual levels, they include potential for growth.

Risk Factors: Conditions that increase the vulnerability of older adults to negative functional consequences. Common sources of risk factors include diseases, environment, lifestyle, support systems, psychosocial circumstances, adverse medication effects and attitudes based on lack of knowledge.

Older Adult (Person): A complex and unique individual whose functioning and well-being are influenced by the acquisition of age-related changes and risk factors. When risk factors cause the older adult to be dependent on others for daily needs, his or her caregivers are considered an integral focus of nursing care.

Nursing: The focus of nursing care is to minimize the negative effects of age-related changes and risk factors and to promote wellness outcomes. Goals are achieved through the nursing process, with particular emphasis on health promotion and other nursing interventions that address the negative functional consequences.

Health: The ability of older adults to function at their highest capacity, despite the presence of age-related changes and risk factors. It is not limited to physiologic function and encompasses psychosocial and spiritual functions. Thus, it addresses well-being and quality of life as defined by each older adult.

Environment: External conditions, including caregivers, that influence the body, mind, spirit and functioning of older adults. Environmental conditions are risk factors when they interfere with function, and they are interventions when they enhance function.

Positive functional consequences can result from automatic actions or purposeful interventions. Often, older adults bring about positive functional consequences when they compensate for age-related changes with or without conscious intent. For example, an older person might increase the amount of light for reading or begin using sunglasses without realizing that these actions are compensating for age-related changes. At other times, older adults initiate interventions in response to a recognized need. In the example cited earlier, improved function would likely result from purposeful interventions, such as cataract surgery or environmental modifications. In a few instances, positive functional consequences are caused directly by age-related changes. For example, a woman may view the postmenopausal inability to become pregnant as a positive effect of aging. Consequently, sexual relationships may become more satisfying in later adulthood. Similarly, positive functional consequences, such as increased wisdom and maturity, can result from psychological growth in older adulthood. In the context of the nursing process, positive functional consequences are called wellness outcomes because they result from purposeful nursing interventions.

The concept of functional consequences draws on concepts and research regarding functional assessment, which focuses on a person's ability to perform activities of daily living that affect survival and quality of life, as discussed in Chapter 7. From a research perspective, functional assessment provides a framework for research and a method for planning health services for dependent people. From a clinical perspective, health care practitioners view the multidimensional functional assessment as an important component in the care of older people. Evidence-based tools are widely available for assessing specific aspects of functioning and activities of daily living, and there is strong support for using these tools in clinical settings. Although the Functional Consequences Theory draws on concepts related to functional assessment, its scope is much broader. The Functional Consequences Theory differs from functional assessment in the following ways:

- It distinguishes between age-related changes that increase a person's vulnerability and risk factors that affect function and quality of life.
- It focuses on functional consequences that can be addressed through nursing interventions.
- It focuses on assessment of conditions that affect functioning, rather than on identification of a person's functional level.
- It leads to interventions that address negative functional consequences.
- It leads to wellness outcomes, such as improved functioning and quality of life.

Many standardized and easy-to-use assessment tools are available for use in clinical settings, and those that are most pertinent to nursing care of older adults are cited in clinically-oriented chapters of this book. In addition, all clinically-oriented chapters contain comprehensive assessment and intervention boxes that apply evidence-based information to a wellness-oriented approach to nursing care of older adults (see list in the front matter of this book).

Age-Related Changes and Risk Factors

A unique challenge of caring for older adults is the need to differentiate between age-related changes and risk factors, because the interventions for age-related changes differ from those for risk factors. Age-related changes cannot be reversed or altered, but it is possible to compensate for their effects so that wellness outcomes are achieved. By contrast, risk factors can be modified or eliminated to improve functioning and quality of life for older adults.

In the Functional Consequences Theory, **age-related changes** are the inherent physiologic processes that increase the vulnerability of older people to the detrimental effects of risk factors. From a body–mind–spirit perspective, however, age-related changes are not limited to physiologic aspects but include potential for increased cognitive, emotional and spiritual development. Thus, nurses holistically focus on the whole person by identifying age-related changes that can be strengthened to improve the older adult's ability to adapt to physiologic decline. For example, nurses can work with older adults to strengthen their coping skills, as discussed in Chapter 12. In addition, nurses have many opportunities to build on the wisdom of older adults, especially their "everyday problem-solving" skills (as discussed in Chapter 11) by teaching about interventions to address risk factors.

A Student's Perspective

Most older adults live outside nursing homes and are actively involved in maintaining their independence and functional abilities as much as possible. Having worked in an acute care setting for many years, it is very easy for me to assume that all older adults have many underlying chronic diseases and do very little to comply with their medical therapies. It does help to separate what is part of the aging process from what is part of a chronic condition, since problems resulting from chronic conditions may be receptive to medical and nursing interventions.

Darris C.

The definition of age-related changes in the context of the Functional Consequences Theory draws primarily on research on aging. Biologic theories can help differentiate between age-related and disease-related processes; usually, however, there is some overlap among these processes, as discussed in Chapter 4. In addition to biologic theories of aging, other theories about aging and older adulthood can shed light on age-related changes that contribute to the ability of older adults to respond to the challenges of aging. Clinically-oriented chapters in this book discuss research on age-related changes pertinent to specific aspects of functioning.

Risk factors are the conditions that are likely to occur in older adults and have a significant detrimental effect on their health and functioning. Risk factors commonly arise from environments, acute and chronic conditions, psychosocial conditions or adverse medication effects. Although many risk factors also occur in younger adults, they are more likely to have serious functional consequences in older adults because of the following characteristics:

- They are cumulative and progressive (e.g., long-term effects of smoking, obesity, inadequate exercise or poor dietary habits).
- The effects are exacerbated by age-related changes (e.g., effects of arthritis are exacerbated by diminished muscle strength).
- The effects may be mistakenly viewed as age-related changes rather than reversible and treatable conditions (e.g., mental changes from adverse medication effects may be attributed to normal aging or dementia).
- They would not have negative functional consequences in a younger person (e.g., glare or background noise would not affect the vision or hearing of someone who is not experiencing age-related sensory changes).

Researchers and health care providers commonly address risk factors in relation to prevention and treatment of medical conditions. For example, evidence-based practice guidelines for pharmacologic or surgical treatments often weigh the probable risks versus benefits. Similarly, studies focus on identifying risk factors for developing conditions, such as heart disease, so that these risks can be addressed through health promotion interventions. Further, in some countries, such as the United States, Australia and Canada, chronic disease models are being implemented. For instance, the Ontario Chronic Disease Prevention and Management Framework involves changes to the health care system, as well as professional and peer support for individuals living with chronic diseases. Within such a framework, individuals are encouraged to work in close collaboration with an inter-professional team. Older adults with chronic diseases have access to education, skills training to manage their illnesses, behaviour modification programs to address problematic behaviours (such as smoking), as well as counselling.

Nurses incorporate the concept of risk factors in many aspects of the nursing process. For example, many nursing diagnoses, interventions and outcomes address risk control, risk identification or risk detection. According to NANDA-I, a risk nursing diagnosis is "a clinical judgment about human experiences/responses to health conditions/life processes that have a high probability of developing in a vulnerable individual, family, group, or community" (Herdman, 2012, p. 96).

A major focus of nursing is to identify risk factors that can be addressed through health promotion interventions. For example, from a holistic perspective, nurses routinely assess for risks associated with stress, smoking, obesity, poor nutrition and inadequate physical activity. A unique aspect of caring for older adults is the need to assess for risk factors associated with myths or ageist attitudes that can affect interventions. For example, if urinary incontinence is mistakenly attributed to "normal" aging, then the older adult will not receive appropriate evaluation and interventions. Environmental risks are also particularly pertinent to older adults because additional risk factors, such as sensory, mobility or cognitive impairments, can compromise their safety and functioning. Identification of risk factors is an integral aspect of the Functional Consequences Theory because nurses have numerous opportunities for promoting wellness by identifying and addressing the many modifiable factors that affect functioning and quality of life for older adults.

Person

In the Functional Consequences Theory, the concept of **person** applies specifically to older adults. Because the holistic approach of the theory views each **older adult** as a complex and unique individual whose functioning and well-being are influenced by many internal and external factors, older adults are not defined simply according to chronologic criteria. From this perspective, an older adult is characterized by the acquisition of physiologic and psychosocial characteristics that are associated with increasing maturity. Physiologic characteristics include slowing down of physiologic processes, compromised ability to respond to physiologic stress and increased vulnerability to pathologic conditions and other risk factors. Psychosocial characteristics include an increased potential for psychosocial strengths, such as wisdom and creativity, and the potential for advanced levels of personal and spiritual growth.

Because aging is a complex and gradual process involving all aspects of body, mind and spirit, a person does not suddenly become an older adult at a particular chronologic age. Rather, people who live long enough recognize at some point that they have reached a stage of life that society categorizes as older adulthood. When they reach this point, they may or may not identify with social labels, such as elder, senior or older adult. Although this concept has the distinct disadvantage of being difficult to measure, it has the advantage of accurately reflecting the realities of older adulthood as a continuum within the life-course continuum. Because people become more heterogeneous rather than homogeneous as they age, any definition of the older adult must, by its nature, be broad. In the context of the Functional Consequences Theory, an individual is an older adult when he or she manifests several or many functional consequences attributable to age-related changes alone or to age-related changes in combination with risk factors. Stated simply, the accumulation of age-related functional consequences defines someone as an older adult. Moreover, because aging involves many gradual, interacting and cumulative processes, each older adult experiences his or her own unique continuum. This concept is applied in the progressive case examples in chapters of Parts 3 and 4 of this book, which illustrate the progression of one person from young–old to old–old as he or she is affected by functional consequences pertinent to a particular aspect of functioning.

The older adult is further conceptualized in the context of his or her relationships with others because a person is not an isolated entity but a dynamic being who continually influences and is influenced by the environment and other people. This context is particularly important for older adults, because the more functionally impaired a person is, the more important are supporting resources and environmental factors. When functional consequences accumulate to the extent that the older adult depends on others for daily needs, nurses broaden their focus to include caregivers during nursing assessments and interventions. Even for older adults who do not rely on others for assistance, it is important to address the needs of older adults in the context of their relationships because older people have a long history of interpersonal relationships that influence their health behaviours and well-being.

Although no characteristics are universally applicable to all older adults, all are affected by the cumulative effects of aging and all are vulnerable to the effects of risk factors. Thus, it is imperative to be knowledgeable about the facts and myths about normal aging so that nursing care can address negative functional consequences. The Functional Consequences Theory emphasizes the importance of identifying and respecting the unique characteristics of each older adult that affect his or her functioning and well-being.

Nursing

The conceptualization of **nursing** in the Functional Consequences Theory draws on nursing theories, including those of the following long-established theorists, as described in Box 3-3.

An additional aspect of the Functional Consequences Theory is its emphasis on person-centred care, which focuses on older adults as the centre of their own care. The individualized needs of older adults are addressed, and there is a sharing of power and responsibility. Nurses involve older adults in decision-making because they recognize that older adults are experts in their own health. Thus, it is essential that nurses get to know the person, which can be achieved

---

Box 3-3 Nursing Theories That Support the Conceptualization of Nursing in the Functional Consequences Theory

Florence Nightingale: Nurses foster an environment conducive to healing and health promotion.

Virginia Henderson: Nurses provide assistance with daily activities to help patients/clients gain independence as rapidly as possible.

Imogene King: Nurse and client interact to achieve a specific health-related goal.

Jean Watson: Nursing consists of knowledge, thought, values, philosophy, commitment and action with passion in human care transactions.

Martha Rogers: Nurses promote person–environment interactions for unitary human beings.

Margaret Newman: Nursing is the act of assisting people to use their power to evolve toward higher levels of consciousness.

through nursing assessments, as discussed in all clinically-oriented chapters of this book.

Health

The Functional Consequences Theory defines **health** as the ability of older adults to function at their highest capacity, despite the presence of age-related changes and risk factors. It encompasses psychosocial as well as physiologic functions, including well-being and quality of life as defined by each older adult. In this model, health is individually determined on the basis of the functional capacities that are perceived as important by that person. For example, one person might define the desired level of function as a capacity for intimate relationships, whereas another might define it as being able to perform aerobic exercise for half an hour daily. Definitions of health by major nursing theorists that are consistent with the conceptualization of health in the Functional Consequences Theory are summarized in Box 3-4.

Wellness is a closely related concept (defined in Chapter 1) that is used throughout this book in reference to outcomes that address the person's highest potential for well-being. In recent years, nurse researchers have focused on identifying components of wellness in relation to care of older adults. A concept analysis of wellness in older adults by McMahon and Fleury (2012) concluded that scholars agree that wellness is not dependent on states of health or illness. They synthesized a collective description of wellness as it relates to older adults as "a purposeful process of individual growth, integration of experience, and meaningful connection with others, reflecting personally valued goals and strengths, and resulting in being well and living values" (McMahon & Fleury, 2012, p. 48). This evidence-based conclusion is consistent with the concept of health in the Functional Consequences Theory as it is applied in this text. It is also consistent with the *Nursing Call to Action* report of the Canadian Nurses Association (CNA, 2012) that nurses intentionally promote wellness and disease prevention and improve health care outcomes throughout the life span and with the principles advocated by the federal government (Health Canada, 2013, 2014) national organizations such as the Canadian Mental Health Association (2012), Canadian Nurses Association (2010) and the Community Health Nurses of Canada (2012).

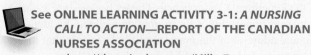 See **ONLINE LEARNING ACTIVITY 3-1:** *A NURSING CALL TO ACTION*—REPORT OF THE CANADIAN NURSES ASSOCIATION at http://thepoint.lww.com/Miller7e

Environment

In the Functional Consequences Theory, **environment** is a broad concept that includes all aspects of the setting in which the care is provided; for dependent older adults, the environment also includes their caregivers. Some aspects of the conceptualization may seem to be contradictory because the environment can be a source of both negative functional consequences and wellness outcomes. For example, the environment is a risk factor when it interferes with functioning (e.g., glare or poor lighting), but it also can facilitate wellness outcomes when it is used to improve functioning (e.g., grab bars, or bright and nonglare lighting). Box 3-5 summarizes some nursing conceptualizations of environment that are pertinent to the Functional Consequences Theory.

Since the 1970s, gerontologists have studied the influence of the environment on functioning of older adults. For example, the Person–Environment Fit Theory (discussed in Chapter 4) focuses on the interrelationship between the individual person and his or her environment. This theory has been used in studies of the effects of environments (e.g., homes, neighbourhoods) on many aspects of functioning and quality of life for older adults and people with mobility limitations (Greenfield, 2012; Rosenberg et al., 2013). Some of the questions that are addressed by gerontologists, as well as nurses, include the following:

- How does the environment affect the older adult's level of functioning?

Box 3-4 Definitions of Health That Support the Conceptualization of Health in the Functional Consequences Theory

Florence Nightingale: To be well, but to be able to use well every power we have.
Imogene King: A dynamic life experience involving continuous adjustment to stressors through optimum use of one's resources to achieve maximum potential for daily living.
Calista Roy: A state and process of being and becoming integrated and whole.
Jean Watson: Unity and harmony within the mind, body and soul; congruence between the self as perceived and the self as experienced.
Margaret Newman: Expanding consciousness; evolving pattern of the whole of life.
Rosemarie Parse: A way of being in the world; the living of day-to-day ways of being.
Madeleine Leininger: A state of well-being that is culturally constituted, defined, valued and practised by individuals or groups that enables them to function in their daily lives.

Box 3-5 Definitions of Environment from Nursing Theories That Are Pertinent to the Functional Consequences Theory

Florence Nightingale: A healthy environment is essential for healing and includes specific aspects such as noise level, cleanliness and nutritious food.
Madeleine Leininger: The totality of an event, situation or particular experience that gives meaning to human expressions, interpretations and social interactions, in particular physical, ecologic, sociopolitical and cultural settings.
Imogene King: The background for human interactions, which is both internal and external to the individual.
Margaret Newman: All internal and external factors of influences that surround the client or system.
Calista Roy: All conditions, circumstances and influences that surround and affect the development and behaviour of humans.

- How does the environment affect the older adult's quality of life?
- Is the environment comfortable for the older adult?
- Is the environment a source of risks that interfere with functioning and well-being of the older adults; for example, does it increase the risk of falls?
- How can the environment be adapted to improve functioning for the older adult?

Throughout this text, the Functional Consequences Theory provides a framework for addressing questions such as these as an integral part of the nursing assessment and interventions for specific aspects of functioning.

A Student's Perspective

Today I cared for L.C., who has had two previous cerebrovascular accidents, with the second one leading to left-sided hemiplegia. As I was caring for her, I noticed a few things in her room that may have significance for her. First, I noted that she had poles both by her bed and in the bathroom; both were bolted to the ceiling and the floor. These poles made it easier for L.C. to stand on her own with little assistance from anyone else. I feel that these make her more independent and help her use the strong side of her body. L.C. also had a divided box, with different kinds of tea in each section. I feel that this is significant to her because she is able to have the type of tea she likes whenever she wants it. It allows her to make choices each day and provides one of the comforts of "home." A third item was a triangle pillow that she sleeps on rather than a regular one. This is significant because it allows her to breathe better in the night or whenever she is sleeping. Because L.C. has chronic obstructive pulmonary disease, it is hard for her to breathe.

Kelly Z.

APPLYING THE THEORY TO PROMOTE WELLNESS IN OLDER ADULTS

In the context of the Functional Consequences Theory, nurses direct their care toward addressing risk factors and promoting wellness outcomes for older adults. The focus and goals of this type of care vary in different settings. For acute care, the focus is on treatment of pathologic conditions that create serious risks; goals include helping vulnerable older adults recover from illness and maintain or improve their level of functioning. For long-term care, the focus is on addressing multiple risk factors that interfere with functional abilities; goals include improved functioning and quality of life. The Functional Consequences Theory is particularly pertinent in rehabilitation settings, where the focus is on preventing negative functional consequences and promoting wellness outcomes (Gouveia et al., 2011). For home and community settings, the focus is on short- and long-term interventions aimed at age-related changes and risk factors; goals include improving or preventing declines in functioning and addressing quality-of-life concerns. In all settings, nurses can incorporate wellness outcomes to address each older adult's personal aspirations toward well-being of body, mind and spirit. Examples of these wellness outcomes are delineated in all clinically-oriented chapters of this book.

Nurses apply the nursing process to assess age-related changes and risk factors, identify nursing diagnoses, plan wellness outcomes, implement nursing interventions to achieve wellness outcomes and evaluate the effectiveness of their interventions. A major focus of nursing care is on educating older adults and caregivers of dependent older adults about interventions that will eliminate risk factors or minimize their effects. The educational aspects are particularly important when older adults are influenced by myths and misunderstandings about age-related changes. For example, nurses can provide information about the difference between normal aging changes and risk factors to an older person who believes that functional impairments are a necessary consequence of old age, and identify ways of minimizing the effects of risk factors and compensating for the effects of age-related changes.

The Register Theory of Generative Quality of Life for the Elderly is a middle-range theory developed by nurses that is pertinent to the concepts in the Functional Consequences Theory. According to this model, quality of life for older adults is synonymous with connectedness, and a goal of nursing care is to establish patient-centred connections that can result in generative older adults who establish or sustain a variety of connections in response to the daily forces and processes they encounter (Register & Herman, 2006, 2010). Register and Herman (2006) cited the following examples of generative nursing interventions to address specific aspects of quality of life for older adults:

- *Metaphysical connectedness*: teaching about guided imagery, journaling activities and activities that increase self-esteem and a sense of optimism.
- *Spiritual connectedness*: arranging transportation to local church services or making referrals to faith-based groups.
- *Biologic connectedness*: facilitating participation in congregate meals, doing group exercises to music.
- *Connectedness to others*: providing comfort touch, encouraging participation in social and educational activities.
- *Environmental connectedness*: encouraging and facilitating activities in nature, referring for transportation resources.
- *Connectedness to society*: providing information about supporting resources, helping older adults develop contingency plans for emergencies.

Providing nursing care for older adults is both challenging and rewarding, despite the common perception that it is futile and discouraging. Although nursing care of older adults is often associated with limited goals, a holistic perspective focuses on the potential of every person to experience wellness by achieving higher levels of psychological or spiritual functioning. Even older adults who have dementia, and other progressive conditions that can profoundly affect psychological function, may have potential for spiritual growth in ways that are not always observable or measurable.

The Functional Consequences Theory helps nurses see older adults as more than an accumulation of age-related physiologic changes and pathologic conditions leading to diminished functioning. Thus, it provides a framework for promoting wellness because it addresses the whole-person needs of the older adult and his or her relationships with self, others and the environment. It reminds nurses to identify strengths and potentials in relation not only to physical aspects of functioning but also to psychological and spiritual well-being. Moreover, it leads to nursing interventions directed toward achieving wellness outcomes, such as improved quality of life for older adults.

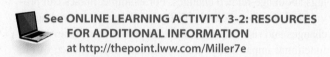

See ONLINE LEARNING ACTIVITY 3-2: RESOURCES FOR ADDITIONAL INFORMATION
at http://thepoint.lww.com/Miller7e

Chapter Highlights

A Nursing Theory for Wellness-Focused Care of Older Adults (Fig. 3-1)

- The Functional Consequences Theory explains the unique relationships among the concepts of person, health, nursing and environment in the context of promoting wellness for older adults.

Concepts Underlying the Functional Consequences Theory (Boxes 3-2 through 3-5)

- Combinations of age-related changes and risk factors increase the vulnerability of older people to negative functional consequences, which interfere with the person's level of functioning or quality of life.
- Nurses assess the age-related changes, risk factors and functional consequences, with particular emphasis on identifying the factors that can be addressed through nursing interventions.
- Wellness outcomes enable older adults to function at their highest level despite age-related changes and risk factors.

Applying the Theory to Promote Wellness in Older Adults

- Nurses can incorporate wellness outcomes to address each older adult's personal aspirations for well-being of body, mind and spirit.
- Nurses educate older adults and caregivers about interventions to minimize risk factors or their effects.
- Providing nursing care for older adults is rewarding when approached from a holistic perspective that sees opportunities for wellness in physical, psychological and spiritual aspects of function.

Critical Thinking Exercises

Bring to your mind a vivid image of an older friend, relative or patient who is at least 80 years old, and apply the following questions to one obvious functional consequence (e.g., impaired mobility). Develop an opportunity to talk with that person about what you have learned about the Functional Consequences Theory for Promoting Wellness in Older Adults, and use Figure 3-1 as a basis for discussion.

1. What age-related changes and risk factors interact to contribute to this functional consequence?
2. What environmental conditions either improve or interfere with the affected aspect of functioning?
3. How can you use your nursing knowledge to improve health and quality of life in relation to that aspect of functioning?

For more information about the topics discussed in this chapter, be sure to check out the interactive Online Learning Activities and other helpful resources
at http://thepoint.lww.com/Miller7e

REFERENCES

Canadian Mental Health Association. (2012). *Women and health care.* Retrieved from http://www.cmha.ca/public-policy/policy-statements/

Canadian Nurses Association. (2010). *Social justice: A means to an end, an end in itself.* Retrieved from http://cna-aiic.ca/~/media/cna/page-content/pdf-en/social_justice_2010_e.pdf

Canadian Nurses Association. (2012). *A nursing call to action.* Retrieved from http://www.cna-aiic.ca/~/media/cna/files/en/nec_report_e.pdf

Community Health Nurses of Canada. (2012). *Public health nursing: Primary prevention of chronic disease.* Retrieved from http://www.chnc.ca/documents/2012MayCHNCCDPReport.pdf

Gouveia, B. R., Jardim, H., & Martins, M. M. (2011). Foundation of gerontological rehabilitation nursing: Applicability of the Functional Consequences Theory. *Referencia, 1*(4 Suppl.), 475.

Greenfield, E. A. (2012). Using ecological frameworks to advance a field of research, practice, *and policy on aging-in-place initiatives. The Gerontologist, 52*(1), 1–12.

Health Canada. (2013). *Healthy living.* Retrieved from http://www.hc-sc.gc.ca/hl-vs/index-eng.php

Health Canada. (2014). *First Nations and Inuit Health.* Retrieved from http://www.hc-sc.gc.ca/fniah-spnia/index-eng.php

Herdman, T. H. (Ed.). (2012). *NANDA international nursing diagnoses: Definitions and classification 2012–2014.* Oxford, England: Wiley-Blackwell.

McMahon, S., & Fleury, J. (2012). Wellness in older adults: A concept analysis. *Nursing Forum, 47*(1), 39–50.

Miller, C. A. (1990). *Nursing care of older adults: Theory and practice.* Glenview, IL: Scott, Foresman/Little, Brown Higher Education.

Register, M. E., & Herman, J. (2006). A middle range theory for generative quality of life for the elderly. *Advances in Nursing Science, 29,* 340–350.

Register, M. E., & Herman, J. (2010). Quality of life revisited: The concept of connectedness in older adults. *Advances in Nursing Science, 33*(1), 53–63.

Rosenberg, D. E., Huang, D. L., Simonovich, S. D., et al. (2013). Outdoor built environment barriers and facilitators to activity among midlife and older adults with mobility disabilities. *The Gerontologist, 53*(2), 268–279.

Strout, K. (2012). Wellness promotion and the Institute of Medicine's Future of Nursing Report. *Holistic Nursing Practice, 26*(3), 129–136.

chapter 4

Theoretical Perspectives on Aging Well

LEARNING OBJECTIVES

After reading this chapter, you will be able to:

1. Describe theoretical perspectives on the relationships among aging, disease, health and quality of life.

2. Discuss pertinent concepts from biologic theories of aging and their relevance to nursing care of older adults.

3. Discuss pertinent concepts from sociocultural theories of aging and their relevance to nursing care of older adults.

4. Discuss pertinent concepts from psychological theories of aging and their relevance to nursing care of older adults.

KEY POINTS

active life expectancy

activity theory

age stratification theory

caloric restriction theory

compression of morbidity

cross-linkage theory

disengagement theory

free radical theory

gerotranscendence

human needs theory

immunosenescence theories

life expectancy

life span

person–environment fit theory

program theory

rectangularization of the curve

selection, optimization and compensation

senescence

socioemotional selectivity theory

strength and vulnerability integration theory

subculture theory

wear-and-tear theory

People have always looked for answers to universal questions, such as *How long can we live? Why do we age?* and *How can we prevent the unwanted effects of aging?* Since early times, scientists and philosophers have tried to answer these questions from various perspectives, such as biologic, sociologic and psychological theories. As knowledge about unique and variable aspects of aging expanded, it became evident that aging is multidimensional and requires a multidisciplinary approach. Now, a dominant question is *How can we live both long and well?* and the concept of **aging well** is prominent in studies. Fernandez-Ballesteros and colleagues (2013) analysed terminology in studies related to aging well and described the following commonly used definitions:

- Healthy aging: no illness and preserved functioning in activities of daily living
- Active aging: high physical and cognitive functioning and positive affect and control
- Productive aging: social participation and engagement
- Successful aging: the full concept of aging well

This chapter discusses theoretical perspectives pertinent to aging well and applies this information to nursing care of older adults.

HOW CAN WE LIVE LONG AND WELL?

Questions about how long we can live are addressed by measuring life span, life expectancy, and morbidity and mortality rates. The more important questions about how we can live both long and well are addressed by exploring the relationships among aging, health and disease, as is the current focus of gerontological research. For the past several decades, gerontological research has increasingly focused on identifying ways to delay the effects of aging and maintain high levels of functioning and quality of life. This more optimistic approach is attributable to the large group of adults who are currently turning 65—the so-called baby boomers—who view themselves as aging better than the way previous generations aged or are aging (Madden & Cloyes, 2012). Gerontologists have not discovered answers to the questions *What is usual or normal aging?* and *What differentiates healthy aging from pathologic aging?* However, they are intensely investigating this complex topic. For example, within the 21st century, there has been a notable increase in the number of research projects investigating "health span" in Canada.

Life Span and Life Expectancy

Two measures that gerontologists use to address questions about how long we can live are life span and life expectancy. **Life span,** defined as the maximum survival potential for a member of a species, is relatively stable as evident by the barely perceptible extensions that occur over the evolutionary time scale. Human life span is about 110 to 115 years, with only 1 of 5 million people living beyond 110 years in industrialized nations and far fewer in less developed countries (Andersen et al., 2012). Jeanne Calment lived for 122 years and 165 days and is verified to be the longest living human.

Life expectancy is the predictable length of time that one is expected to live from a specific point in time, such as birth or age 65. In contrast to the relatively stable time frame for life span, life expectancy at birth has increased from 59 years of age for men and 61 years of age for women in 1920 to approximately 79 years of age for men and 82 years of age for women in 2012 (Statistics Canada, 2012a). Another way of looking at this is by recognizing that during the past century humans have gained more years of average life expectancy at birth than in the last 10,000 years (Caruso et al., 2012). The dramatic increase in life expectancy at birth is due largely to improved infant and child mortality and control of communicable disease. This is illustrated by the following statistics: in 1900, about 40% of babies born in Western countries were expected to live past age 65; today 88% of babies born in those same countries will live beyond age 65 (Caruso et al., 2012). It is important to recognize that life expectancies vary, not only between developed and developing nations, but also by gender, racial characteristics and socioeconomic situations (i.e., homeless older adults compared with those with financial resources) in Canada.

Life expectancy has been extended not only at birth, but also during middle and later adulthood. For example, many more Canadians are living to age 65 years and beyond; in the past several decades, the proportion of the population of individuals 65 years of age and older increased from 9% to 14% (PHAC, 2010). The life expectancy beyond 65 years of age has also increased; Canadians living until 65 years of age in 2009 could expect to live another 20.2 years (Statistics Canada, 2012b). And, according to the national census, there were 5,825 centenarians in Canada in 2011; this has increased from 3,795 centenarians in 2001. In 2011, of those individuals who lived to 100 years of age,

approximately 60% could expect to reach 101 years (Statistics Canada, 2012c). Gerontologists estimate that between 1994 and 2012, the estimated prevalence of centenarians in developed nations doubled from 1 in 10,000 to 1 in 5,000, (Sebastiani & Perls, 2012). Because of these changes in life expectancy trends, centenarians are now the fastest growing demographic group worldwide, with projections that their numbers will more than quintuple between 2005 and 2030 (Willcox et al., 2010).

Rectangularization of the Curve and Compression of Morbidity

Despite the remarkable changes, life expectancy at birth will be limited to about 90 years because major causes of death—represented by mortality rates—cannot be eliminated (Carnes et al., 2013). Mortality rates are graphically represented in a survivorship curve, which illustrates the changes occurring in death rates over different periods of time (Fig. 4-1a and b). The vertical axis designates the percentage of survivors, whereas the horizontal axis represents the age of survivorship. Since the 1980s, the rate of increase in average longevity has continued to rise, but the pace of increase has slowed down. This change in pace has resulted in the squaring of the human survival curve, meaning that life expectancy has not been prolonged as significantly after age 75 or 80 years. This **rectangularization of the curve** is attributed to changes in survival caused by various significant factors occurring at different points in time (Fig. 4-2).

The first major change, during the age of pestilence and famine, resulted from improved housing and sanitation, and the second major change was brought about by the advent of immunization programs and other advances in public health practices during the age of pandemics. The third major change, which occurred between 1960 and 1980, is attributable to biomedical breakthroughs, such as organ transplants, heart–lung machines and cancer treatments. Recently, gerontologists identified a fourth stage—the age of delayed degenerative diseases—characterized by the later onset of death from diseases that cause disability and chronic illness. Although it is clear that increased life expectancy involves a longer time in chronic illness, it is less clear whether this is necessarily associated with a longer time in a state of disability. Thus, the focus of geriatric research and practice shifted from an emphasis on disease processes per se to an emphasis on the functional losses that are of key importance to older people.

James Fries, a physician, first brought attention to this concern in an article on the **compression of morbidity,** in which he argued that the onset of significant illness could be postponed, but that one's life expectancy could not be extended to the same extent. Consequently, disease, disability and functional decline are "compressed" into a period averaging 3 to 5 years before death. Fries and a colleague emphasized that preventive approaches must be directed toward preserving health by postponing the onset of chronic

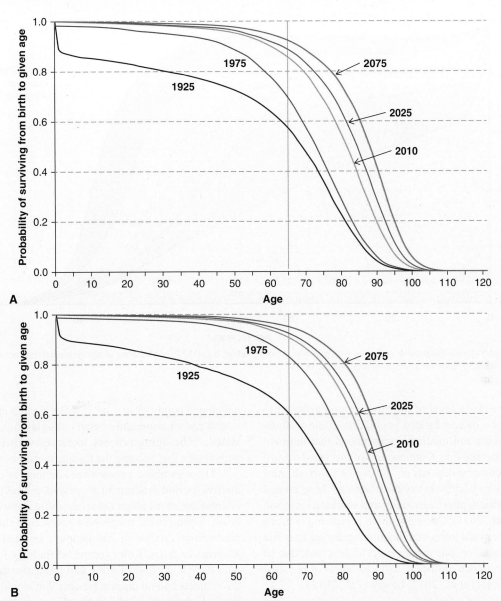

FIGURE 4-1 Survival curves at birth. A. (Males) and B. (Females) (based on period life tables). (Office of the Superintendent of Financial Institutions, Mortality Projections for Social Security Programs in Canada, April 2014, http://www.osfi-bsif.gc.ca/eng/oca-bac/as-ea/Pages/mpsspc.aspx)

illnesses (Fries & Crapo, 1981). Results of population studies and ongoing longitudinal studies that began in 1984 and 1986 support this theory, confirming that health-promotion interventions, such as exercise and risk-reduction behaviours, can postpone disability by 10 to 16 years compared with control or high-risk groups (Fries, 2012).

Active Life Expectancy

Spurred partly by Fries' compression of morbidity hypothesis, gerontologists developed the concept of **active life expectancy**, which is measured on a continuum ranging from inability to perform activities of daily living to full independent functioning, as an indicator of quality of life during later adulthood. Gerontologists emphasize that the goal of science, medicine and gerontology should be the

extension of healthy lifespan through research on health-promotion interventions rather than disease-oriented mechanisms (Carnes & Witten, 2013; Rattan, 2013).

Since the 1980s, gerontologists have analysed longitudinal data about functional disability (i.e., loss of various self-maintenance functions) in Canada and other developed countries as a reliable measure of health status and quality-of-life issues. Most, but not all, studies indicate that younger cohorts of older adults (i.e., those people turning 65 more recently) are living longer with less disability (Manton et al., 2008; Hung et al., 2011). One analysis of data concluded that more recent cohorts are likely to experience a decade free of disability, with increased disability being associated with stroke, arthritis, diabetes and hip fracture (Taylor & Lynch, 2011).

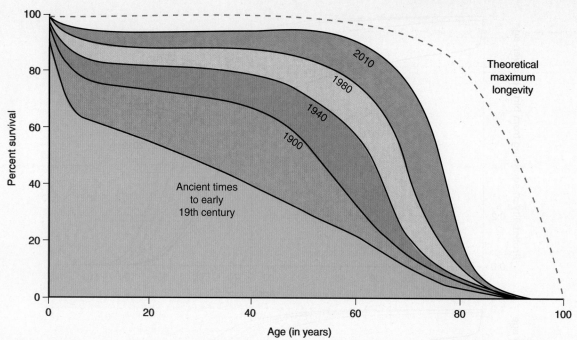

FIGURE 4-2 Human survivorship curve. (Adapted with permission from Strehler, B. L. [1975]. Implications of aging research for society. *Proceedings of the Federation of American Societies for Experimental Biology, 34,* 6.)

Improvements in level of functioning are attributed to factors such as a more educated population of older adults and environments and medical interventions that improve function and accessibility. Continuation of this trend toward improved functioning depends on the degree to which individuals engage in healthy behaviours, such as those related to weight, nutrition, physical activity and smoking cessation (Wolinsky et al., 2011). Currently, there is growing concern that this trend toward improved functioning during later life will not continue, or that it may even be reversed, due to increasing prevalence of obesity and low levels of physical activity (Antonucci et al., 2012; Lowry et al., 2012).

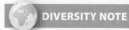

DIVERSITY NOTE

In 2006/2007, 20% of Canadian seniors (non–First Nations) reported having diabetes. This is starkly different from the 35% of older First Nations seniors living on the reserve who have diabetes (according to a 2002/2003 report; Public Health Agency of Canada, 2010).

Relationships Among Aging, Disease and Death

Whether or not age-associated diseases are inevitable is an important question related to living both long and well. The noted gerontologist Leonard Hayflick described the complex relationship between aging and disease as analogous to the "weak links" in automobiles. According to his analogy, both humans and particular makes and models of cars are characterized by weak links that increase the probability of component failure. For cheap cars, the "mean time to failure" is 4 or 5 years; for Canadians born today, it is about 81 years (Statistics Canada, 2012a). The weakest links for people in

developed countries are the vascular system and the cells in which cancer commonly occurs. As Hayflick (2001–2002) stated, "The aging process increases vulnerability to the pathologies that become the leading causes of death." (p. 21)

Theories about **senescence**, defined as the postreproductive period leading to increased probability of death, address questions about the relationships between aging and death. Kohn (1982) proposed a senescence theory based on postmortem studies of 200 people who died at the age of 85 years or older. Kohn compared findings from autopsies with the listed cause of death and found that at least 26% of the subjects had no disease process that would be a cause of death. Kohn concluded that had the same degree of disease occurred in middle-aged people, the condition would not have been fatal. Thus, he concluded that aging itself was the actual cause of death in a large fraction of the aged population (Kohn, 1982). Kohn further suggested that when death in older people cannot be ascribed to a disease process that would cause death in middle-aged people, the cause of death should be listed on the death certificate as senescence.

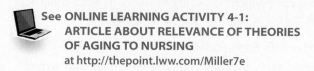

See **ONLINE LEARNING ACTIVITY 4-1: ARTICLE ABOUT RELEVANCE OF THEORIES OF AGING TO NURSING** at http://thepoint.lww.com/Miller7e

Studies of Older Adults Who Are Healthy and Long Lived

Studies of long-lived people who are healthy and functional explore the most important question of all: *How can we live a life that is not only long but also functional, productive and satisfying?* This question is particularly relevant to the growing attention to adding quality, not just quantity, to life. The first study of "extreme longevity" was the Okinawa Centenarian Study, which began in 1975, and since then more than a dozen major longitudinal studies have been ongoing worldwide for a decade or more (Willcox et al., 2010). As these studies progressed, they also included "exceptional survivors" or "supercentenarians," defined as the oldest-old population who are 110 years or older. For example, the New England Centenarian Study in the United States currently has the largest sample in the world, with about 107 supercentenarians and about 1,600 centenarians as study participants in 2014 (New England Centenarian Study, 2014). People who survive to 100 years and older are a heterogeneous group with a wide range of health and socioeconomic characteristics. Most centenarians experience good health and relatively good functioning until their mid-90s or later because they have escaped the common pathologies, such as stroke, cancer and myocardial infarction (Andersen et al., 2012; Vacante et al., 2012). Common health characteristics of the New England Centenarian Study (2014) include the following:

- Lean or healthy body mass index
- No history of smoking
- High levels of cognitive functioning
- Better than average ability to handle stress
- Family history of exceptional longevity

Variables commonly identified as predictors of healthy longevity include nutritional patterns with a high intake of plant-based foods (i.e., fruits, vegetables, nuts), high levels of physical activity and strong social networks (Davinelli et al., 2012). Psychosocial variables found in centenarians include maintaining strong interest, feeling satisfied with life and being resilient in the face of stress (Hutnik et al., 2012; see Box 4-1).

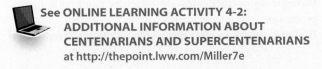

See ONLINE LEARNING ACTIVITY 4-2: ADDITIONAL INFORMATION ABOUT CENTENARIANS AND SUPERCENTENARIANS at http://thepoint.lww.com/Miller7e

HOW DO WE EXPLAIN BIOLOGIC AGING?

Biologic theories of aging address questions about the basic aging processes that affect all living organisms. These theories answer questions, such as *How do cells age?* and *What triggers the process of aging?* Biologic aging is the gradual and progressive decline in physiologic functioning that occurs throughout adulthood and ends in death. It is important to recognize that each biologic theory of aging attempts to explain a specific aspect of aging from a particular perspective. As such, each theory provides a narrow lens through which biologic aging can be viewed, but they do not provide a broad vision.

Box 4-1 Evidence-Informed Nursing Practice

Background: A number of studies focusing on centenarians are quantitative, looking at specific factors that contributed to longevity. There are fewer studies that qualitatively examine the perspectives and lived experiences of centenarians.

Question: What characteristics do centenarians view as important to their longevity?

Method: Researchers from the University of Waterloo (Canada) and Cologne (Germany) utilized secondary data (interview data or recorded video available on the Internet) to examine why centenarians believed they had lived so long. Interviews/videos from 19 English-speaking centenarians (ages 100–115 years; 14 men and 5 women) were used.

Findings: The researchers identified four themes from the data: lifestyle choices, community and environment, attitude toward life, and goal setting and attainment. They found that centenarians made lifestyle choices that were generally healthy and engaged regularly in activities. These individuals stressed the importance of being connected to others and having spirituality or faith as an active part of their lives. Furthermore, they lived in a purposeful manner, in that they volunteered or continued to work.

Implications for Nursing Practice: In working with older adults, it is important to help individuals examine what brings meaning to their lives and encourage them to make connection with others, to express themselves spiritually and to find and engage in meaningful activities.

Freeman, S., Garcia, J., & Marston, H. R. (2013). Centenarian self-perceptions of factors responsible for attainment of extended health and longevity. *Educational Gerontology*, 39, 717–728. doi:10.1080/03601277.2012.750981

Overview of and Conclusions About Biologic Theories

Biologic theories provide insight into the inevitable consequences of normal aging as well as the increased susceptibility of older adults to diseases. In addition, these theories attempt to identify the factors that can predict long as well as healthy lives. Hundreds of biologic theories of aging have been proposed during the past several centuries, and, although some have been disproved, others continue to provide groundwork for gerontologists today. Table 4-1 summarizes some commonly cited theories of aging that have laid the groundwork for studies of biologic aging.

Much of the current research on biologic aging has evolved since the 1990s as an outcome of major advances in genetic science. Studies of twins and families confirm that genetic factors account for about 25% of a person's life expectancy, with environmental factors during the prenatal time and early life accounting for another 25% of variability and life circumstances during adulthood accounting for the other 50% (Caruso et al., 2012; Melzer et al., 2013). Current studies indicate that the genetic effect on longevity is due to modest effects of many genes interacting, with some genes increasing one's susceptibility to age-related disease and early death and other genes slowing the aging process and leading to a longer life (Murabito et al., 2012).

TABLE 4-1 Biologic Theories of Aging

Theory	Description
Wear-and-tear theory	A human body is like a machine: It functions well for a certain time and broken parts can be fixed or replaced, but eventually it stops working because of accumulated effects of wear and tear. Longevity is affected by the genetic components, as well as by the care provided. For humans, the wearing-out process is exacerbated by harmful factors, such as stress, disease, smoking, poor diet and alcohol abuse.
Free radical theory	Free radicals are ionized oxygen molecules that are highly unstable because they have an extra electron. They are waste products of metabolism and they can damage cells. Healthy bodies have protective mechanisms that can remove and repair damaged cells; however, these mechanisms become less effective with increased age and cellular damage becomes cumulative.
Immunosenescence theories	Immunosenescence, which is an age-related decline of the immune system, increases the susceptibility of older people to diseases, such as cancer and infections. The immune system may even attack healthy cells, leading to autoimmune conditions, such as rheumatoid arthritis.
Cross-linkage theory	Biochemical processes create linkages, or connections, between structures that normally are separated. This causes a buildup of collagen-like substances that leads to failure of tissues and organs.
Program theory	The life span of each animal species is predetermined by a genetic program, which allows for a maximum of about 110 years in humans. Abnormal cells, such as cancer cells, are not subject to this predictable program and can proliferate an indefinite number of times.
Caloric restriction theory	Numerous animal studies have found that reducing caloric intake by 30% to 40% without causing malnutrition results in enhanced ability to protect cells, increased resistance to stress and overall longer and healthier life expectancy. However, to date, this research has not been applied to humans.

Since the early 2000s, when the Human Genome Project mapped the location of each human gene, gerontologists have access to a wealth of data that is improving our understanding of genetic factors that influence aging. In particular, gerontologists are applying information from the Human Genome Project to address questions about the relationship between health, diseases and long life. For example, Bloss and colleagues (2011) proposed the following explanations about the relationship between longevity and genetic factors:

1. An individual does not possess disease-predisposing genetic variations, and therefore does not develop life-threatening diseases to the same extent as others.
2. A person lives in a health-enhancing environment and/or engages in healthy behaviours.
3. An individual possesses disease-predisposing genetic variations or lives in an unhealthy environment, but also possesses "protective" genetic variations that mitigate detrimental effects.
4. A person has a combination of these factors.

Recent studies of genome sequences indicate that centenarians would be in the third category, that is, they have genetic variants associated with increased risk for age-related disease (e.g., stroke, cancer, heart disease) but they also have high numbers of genetic variants associated with longevity (Sebastiani et al., 2012, 2013).

In conclusion, all biologic theories of aging recognize that aging is a multidimensional process that is directly influenced by many interacting factors. Moreover, because of the great variability among people—which increases with aging—no single theory can explain the complex phenomenon of aging, which involves many processes and mechanisms. Although no one theory can explain biologic aging, these theories lead to the following conclusions:

- Biologic aging affects all living organisms.
- Biologic aging is natural, inevitable, irreversible and progressive with time.
- The course of aging varies from individual to individual.
- The rate of aging for different organs and tissues varies within individuals.
- Biologic aging is an intrinsic process that is independent of external factors but is strongly influenced by nonbiologic factors.
- Biologic aging processes are different from pathologic processes.
- Biologic aging increases one's vulnerability to disease.

Relevance to Nurses

A primary role of nurses is to help older adults identify and address the modifiable factors that can lead to diseases, disability and death as well as those health-promoting factors that can contribute to a longer and healthier life. Thus, nurses need to understand not only the relationship between aging and disease but also what "causes" healthy aging and longevity. Biologic theories of aging shed light on the differences between age-related changes and the risk factors that affect the health and functioning of older adults. Nurses then can use this knowledge to implement interventions that promote wellness and a higher level of functioning.

Biologic theories of aging are also applicable to attitudes of health care professionals about aging. If, for example, health care providers hold the perspective of "what do

Case Study

Imagine that you are 72 years old and your mother and father are 96 and 95 years old, respectively, and they live in an assisted-living apartment. You have a brother who died last year at the age of 70 and you have a sister who is 69 years old. You have two children, three grandchildren and two great-grandchildren. Your mother is moderately obese and has osteoarthritis, hypertension, glaucoma and type 2 diabetes. Functionally, she uses a walker, needs help with getting in and out of the bathtub, and has some trouble reading but can still see well enough to watch television and get around familiar environments. Your father has hypertension, osteoarthritis and a recent diagnosis of prostate cancer. Functionally, he is independent in his basic activities of daily living but is quite hearing impaired. Both of your parents have some memory impairment, but the support services at the facility where they live address their needs for meals, medication administration and reminders about getting to activities.

THINKING POINTS

- Using the concepts of rectangularization of the curve and compression of morbidity, what would you expect the health, functioning and life expectancy to be for each of the five generations in your family?
- Pick the biologic theory of aging that you think is most applicable for your family and use it to explain to your great-grandchildren why their great-great-grandparents are still living.
- Choose a theory about the relationships among age, disease and death or a theory about active life expectancy and functional health, and use it to respond to your mother's statement, "I'm 96 years old—what does it matter if I follow a diabetic diet? If the sugar hasn't killed me so far, then eating two doughnuts this morning isn't going to kill me. It's old age that will take me, not my diet."
- Pick a theory about the relationships among age, disease and death or a theory about active life expectancy and functional health, and use it to respond to your father's declaration that "Of course, I have prostate cancer! I'm 95 years old!"
- What perspectives on aging would you want your father's primary care provider to use in addressing your father's prostate cancer?

you expect, you're old," reversible disease conditions may go untreated. Similarly, if health care providers subscribe to the theory that aging is an ultimately fatal disease, their attitude may reflect a hopelessness that pervades their care for older patients. Biologic theories of aging can be used to point out that such fatalistic perspectives are outdated. Nurses can base their care on a holistic perspective and use studies of healthy and functional oldest-old people to identify health-promotion interventions that will improve quality of life for older adults. Nurses often are in positions to serve as teachers and advocates for older adults whose care might be based on outdated or narrow approaches that incorrectly equate aging and disease. The functional consequences theory for promoting wellness in older adults (discussed in Chapter 3) provides a framework for a holistic approach that identifies the risk factors and addresses those that are modifiable in older adults. This text addresses each aspect of functioning from this perspective, with emphasis on those factors that nurses can address through health-promotion interventions.

Biologic theories highlight the need for health-promotion interventions to prevent disease conditions and minimize the negative effects of aging. However, these theories do not address the significant influence of nursing, medical and psychosocial interventions that can improve a person's functioning and life expectancy. From a broader perspective, aging is more than an unrelenting progression of cellular deterioration. Survival to old age is an accomplishment that denotes strong will and the ability to adapt. As emphasized throughout this book, older adulthood is a dynamic part of the life span continuum and has the potential to be a very rewarding part of the life cycle, during which one experiences personal growth and self-understanding, fulfilment of potential and the ability to establish clear priorities. These aspects of aging are addressed in the following sections, which describe sociocultural and psychological theories of aging.

A Student's Perspective

One thing I feel I did well during my first week of providing patient care was seeing my patient for the person that she is and not just as a set of problems that needed caring for. I can understand how difficult it may be in today's health care settings to stop for a minute and really "see" the patient. When I cared for Mrs. S., I was able to look past the wrinkles and white hair and see the spunky spirit that she really is. It is easy to just categorize someone in your mind as old, senile or dependent. One very important lesson that I will take with me for the rest of my career is that you cannot categorize someone because everyone is so different. It's amazing what you can discover if you actually take the time to see people for who they truly are. Taking care of a person holistically means taking care of them physically, psychologically, and spiritually as well.

Sarah L.

SOCIOCULTURAL PERSPECTIVES ON AGING

Sociocultural theories of aging attempt to explain the interrelationship between older adults and the societies and environments in which they live. Early sociocultural theories viewed older adults in the context of societal problems, but more recent theories explore the complex interrelationship between older people and their personal, cultural, physical, political and socioeconomic environments. The following sections present a sampling of the widely recognized sociocultural theories of aging.

Disengagement Theory

Disengagement theory, the first sociologic theory of aging, proposed that society and older people engage in a mutually beneficial process of reciprocal withdrawal to maintain social equilibrium (Cumming & Henry, 1961). This process occurs systematically and inevitably and is governed by society's needs, which override individual needs. Moreover, older people desire this withdrawal and are happy when it occurs. As the number, nature and diversity of the older person's social contacts diminish, disengagement becomes a circular process that further limits opportunities for interaction. This theory challenged traditional beliefs about the relationship between a person and society and stimulated much discussion and controversy, but it is no longer viewed as credible.

Activity Theory

During the early 1970s, social gerontologists built upon the work of Havighurst and Albrecht (1953), which emphasized the relationship between successful aging and keeping active, and proposed the **activity theory**. The activity theory postulates that older people remain socially and psychologically fit if they remain actively engaged in life. For example, one's self-concept is affirmed through activities associated with various roles, and the loss of roles in old age negatively affects life satisfaction. Support for this theory comes from many studies finding that volunteer activities and altruistic attitudes improve life satisfaction, positive affect and quality of life for older adults (Cattan et al., 2011; Kahana et al., 2013). This theory underlies many current theories about successful aging, which recognize that later life can be a time of engagement, contribution and well-being (Johnson & Mutchler, 2013).

Subculture and Age Stratification Theories

The **subculture theory**, first proposed by Rose in the early 1960s, states that old people, as a group, have their own norms, expectations, beliefs and habits; therefore, they have their own subculture (Rose, 1965). The theory also maintains that older people are less well integrated into the larger society and interact more among themselves, compared with people from other age groups. Moreover, the theory

> ## A Student's Perspective
>
> *I think that over the past few weeks, I have really been able to see that it doesn't matter if a person is 90 or 50 or 5, he or she has a story, a family, a life. He or she has values and friends and things that are important to him or her. I think that this is what I will take away from this experience the most. I will try to remember in my nursing career that each patient has a story and that I will be a better nurse if I take the time to find out that story and connect with my patients, no matter what age they are.*
>
> *Erika B.*

holds that the formation of an aged subculture is primarily a response to the loss of status resulting from old age, which is so negatively defined in Canada that people do not want to be viewed as old. In the aged subculture, individual status is based on health and mobility, rather than on the occupational, educational or economic achievements that were previously important. Rose (1965) envisioned that one outcome of the aged subculture would be the development of an aging group consciousness that would serve to improve the self-image of older people and change the negative cultural definition of aging.

Because the aged subculture has millions of members in Canada, it constitutes a minority group that can organize and make public demands. A group such as CARP is evidence of the social importance of the aged subgroup. When considered along with the activity theory, the subculture theory supports the perspective that there is a strong relationship between peer-group participation and the adjustment process of aging.

The **age stratification theory**, first proposed by Riley et al. (1972), addresses the interdependencies between age as an element of the social structure and the aging of people and cohorts as a social process. This theory emphasizes the following concepts:

- People pass through society in cohorts that are aging socially, biologically and psychologically.
- New cohorts are continually being born, and each experiences a unique sense of history.
- A society can be divided into various strata according to age and roles.
- Society itself is continually changing, as are the people and their roles in each age stratum.
- A dynamic interplay exists between individual aging and social change.
- Aging people and the larger society are thus constantly influencing each other and changing both the cohorts and the society.

Based on this theory, older adults will always be viewed as an "out-group" that is subject to ageist attitudes—despite the fact that ageism is one form of discrimination that allows the "nonold" to discriminate against their "future selves" (Jonson, 2013).

Person–Environment Fit Theory

The **person–environment fit theory** considers the interrelationships between personal competence and the environment (Lawton, 1982). According to this theory, personal competence involves the following factors, which collectively contribute to a person's functional ability: ego strength, motor skills, biologic health, cognitive capacity and sensory–perceptual capacity. The environment is viewed in terms of its potential for eliciting a behavioural response from the person. Lawton asserted that for each person's level of competence, there is a level of environmental demand, or environmental press, which is most advantageous to that person's function. People who function at relatively lower levels of competence can tolerate only low levels of environmental press, whereas people who function at higher levels of competence can tolerate increased environmental demands. An often-quoted correlate is that the more impaired the person, the greater the impact of the environment. This theory is often used in planning appropriate environments for older adults with disabilities.

Emerging Sociocultural Theories

A current focus of sociocultural theories is on issues that are associated with the increasing diversity in Canada; as of 2011, 19.1% of the population was comprised by visible minorities, such as South Asians and Chinese (Statistics Canada, 2013), as compared with 50 years ago when immigrants largely came from Europe and there were relatively few visible minorities (Li, 2000). For example, in response to the increasing numbers of minorities, in many nations there is much current focus on cultural influences in various aspects of caregiving (Knight & Losada, 2011). Another currently emerging focus is on identifying sociocultural factors, such as inequities in social and economic resources that contribute to the racial and ethnic disparities in health among older adults (Keith, 2014). Current theories also address questions about the effects of education and other sociocultural factors that affect mortality and longevity differences across racial and ethnic groups (Hummer et al., 2014); for instance, there are a number of Canadian studies examining the healthy immigrant effect, whereby immigrants who come to Canada have much better health than the general population, but whose health declines over time (Islam, 2013). A third evolving trend is the development of feminist gerontology, which examines aging from perspectives specific to the experiences of older women. These types of theories address gender inequalities with regard to caregiving roles, diseases (e.g., cardiovascular disease) and economic status (Meyer & Parker, 2011).

Relevance of Sociocultural Theories of Aging to Nurses

Sociocultural theories of aging help nurses view older adults in relation to society and environments. Thus, these perspectives contribute to a better understanding of influences, such as culture, family, education, community, ascribed roles,

Case Study

Imagine that you are 87 years old and have been retired for 10 years. Create an image of yourself at that age, making sure that you incorporate some changes that are likely to occur as you grow older. Describe the people who are an active part of your relationships during a typical month. Describe the activities you would engage in during a typical week for each of the following aspects of your life: leisure activity, physical activity, intellectual stimulation, emotional growth, social interaction and spiritual nurturing. Are you active in any volunteer organizations? What would your health and functioning be and where would you be living? Based on the image of yourself at 87 years old that you just created, answer the following questions:

THINKING POINTS

- How could you apply either the activity theory or the disengagement theory to your life, as it compares with your life at your present age?
- Would any of the concepts in the subculture or age stratification theories explain your activities and relationships?
- How would the person–environment fit theory explain the relationship between you and your environment?

cohort effects, home and living setting, and personal and political economics. These theories remind health care practitioners that there are patterns of similar responses among cohorts, but within those larger patterns, each person is unique. Some older people achieve their identity in a subculture, others may define successful aging in relation to their activities and still others may find new roles in society.

Sociocultural perspectives encourage nurses to consider not only the cultural needs of individual older adults, but also the role of culture in shaping societal attitudes about aging. Feminist-based theories provide a broad and holistic understanding of the needs of older adults as well as their families and caregivers. Information about diverse aspects of aging, such as cultural or gender differences, are discussed throughout this book, and pertinent information gleaned from studies appears in the Diversity Notes. Theories about person–environment interactions are stimulating interest in broadening the environments of institutional settings to include pets and intergenerational activities.

In addition, these theories emphasize the importance of assessing both environmental and psychosocial factors that influence the functioning of an older person. Concepts from the person–environment fit theory help nurses appreciate the importance of environmental adaptations as interventions to improve functional status, especially when working with dependent older adults. Lawton's theory also suggests that when an older person has difficulty, coping interventions can be directed toward improving personal competency or decreasing environmental demands, or both. Some of the risk factors discussed throughout this book identify environmental factors that interfere with the health and functioning of older adults. Similarly, many of the nursing interventions discussed in this book identify ways of modifying the environment to improve the functioning of older adults.

PSYCHOLOGICAL PERSPECTIVES ON AGING

Psychological theories of aging focus on the psychological factors that affect health, longevity and quality of life. These theories are especially relevant to psychosocial aspects of aging because they address variables such as learning, memory, emotions, intelligence and motivation. The following sections review some of the major psychological theories of aging. In addition, relevant psychological theories about cognitive function, stress and coping, and depression are discussed in Chapters 11, 12 and 15, respectively.

Human Needs Theory

Maslow's hierarchy of needs framework forms the basis of the **human needs theory**, one of the psychological theories that gerontologists use to address the concepts of motivation and human needs. According to Maslow's (1954) theory, the five categories of basic human needs, ordered from lowest to highest, are physiologic needs, safety and security needs, love and belongingness, self-esteem and self-actualization. The attainment of lower-level needs takes priority over higher-level needs; self-actualization can occur only when lower-level needs are met to some degree. People continually move between the levels but always strive toward higher levels. This theory is particularly applicable to older adults because Maslow describes self-actualized people as fully mature humans who possess such desirable traits as autonomy, creativity, independence and positive interpersonal relationships.

Life-Course and Personality Development Theories

Two closely related types of psychological theories of aging are personality development theory, which identify personality types as predictive forces of successful or unsuccessful aging, and life-course theory, which address old age within the context of the life cycle. Carl Jung's (1960) personality development theory categorizes personalities as either extroverted, and thus oriented toward the external world, or introverted, and therefore oriented toward subjective experiences. A balance between the two orientations, both of which are present to some degree in all people, is essential for mental health. Jung further theorized that people tend to be more extroverted in their younger years because of the nature of the demands and responsibilities associated with family and social roles. As these demands change and diminish, beginning around the age of 40 years, people become more introverted. Jung (1954) described later adulthood as a period of taking stock, a time during which a person looks backward rather than forward and is responsible for devoting serious attention to self. Successful aging, according to Jung's theory, depends on accepting one's diminishing capacity and increasing number of losses.

Erik Erikson's (1963) original theory about the eight stages of life has been used widely in relation to older adulthood. Erikson defined the stages of life as trust versus mistrust, autonomy versus shame and doubt, initiative versus guilt, industry versus inferiority, identity versus identity diffusion, intimacy versus self-absorption, generativity versus stagnation, and ego integrity versus despair. Each of these stages presents the person with certain conflicting tendencies that must be balanced before he or she can move successfully from that stage. As in other life-course theories, how one stage is mastered lays the groundwork for successful or unsuccessful mastery of the next stage. In works published between 1950 and 1966, Erikson emphasized the life course from childhood to young adulthood; in later publications, however, he reconsidered the meaning of these stages. In 1982, when he was 80 years old, Erikson described the task of old age as balancing the search for integrity and wholeness with a sense of despair. He believed that the successful accomplishment of this task, achieved primarily through life-review activities, would result in wisdom. Erikson's conceptualization of continuing development throughout adulthood is cited as "seminal" work underlying current gerontological research (Kivnick & Wells, 2013).

Peck (1968) expanded Erikson's original theory and divided the eighth stage—ego integrity versus despair—into additional stages occurring during middle age and old age. The stages described by Peck as specific to old age are ego differentiation versus work-role preoccupation, body transcendence versus body preoccupation, and ego transcendence versus ego preoccupation.

Some life-course theories concentrate on middle or later adulthood and address tasks of late life such as the following:

- Adjusting to decreasing physical strength and health
- Coping with physical changes of aging
- Adjusting to retirement and reduced income
- Adjusting to the death of a spouse
- Redirecting energy to new roles and activities, such as retirement, widowhood and grandparenting
- Establishing an explicit association with one's age group
- Adapting to social roles in a flexible way
- Establishing satisfactory physical living arrangements
- Accepting one's own life
- Developing a point of view about death

A current focus of life-course theories is on "human potential stages," with emphasis on the "ever extant potential for growth that occurred not in spite of old age but because of it" (Agronin, 2013).

Psychological Theories of Successful Aging

Psychological theories of aging address questions, such as *How is emotional well-being maintained during older adulthood? Does psychological well-being differ in younger and older adults?* and, perhaps most importantly, *How do people define and achieve "successful aging?"*

Many studies found an "unexpected positive relationship between aging and happiness"—a phenomenon that is referred to as "the paradox of well-being" because ageist stereotypes portray older adulthood as a time of loss and sadness (Carstensen et al., 2011; Gana et al., 2013). Four psychological theories of aging that help explain this finding are selection, optimization and compensation; socioemotional selectivity; gerotranscendence; and strength and vulnerability integration.

The theory of **selection, optimization and compensation** has been proposed to explain successful aging on the basis of a dynamic model of development as a continuous process of specialization and loss (Zarit, 2009). According to this theory, older adults *select* certain goals and tasks while disengaging from other goals; they *optimize* necessary resources to achieve these goals; and they *compensate* by establishing new resources to substitute for lowered or lost abilities and skills (Rohr & Lang, 2009). Morley (2009) described some of the following examples of well-known people who illustrate this theory:

- Former prime minister of Canada, Pierre Elliott Trudeau, worked as a lawyer after leading Canada up until his death at 80 years of age, despite having Parkinson's disease and prostate cancer.
- Grandma Moses became a famous painter of miniatures after arthritis limited her ability to make quilts.
- Monet invented modern impressionism when his eyesight was clouded by cataracts.
- Renoir held his paintbrush in his clenched fist after he developed arthritis.
- Maurice Ravel composed his famous *Bolero* after he developed dementia.

Researchers have used this theory extensively to explain aspects of aging well, such as coping with stress, managing careers and recovering from stroke (Donnellan & O'Neill, 2014; Unson & Richardson, 2013).

The **socioemotional selectivity theory** has been proposed to explain emotional well-being during older adulthood. This theory proposes that in contrast to younger adults, who view time as unconstrained, older adults recognize that their time is limited, so they focus on emotional goals rather than on knowledge-seeking goals (Kryla-Lighthall & Mather, 2009). Studies using this theory found that, when compared with younger adults, older adults found more meaning in life because they had less time in which to fulfil their goals (Hicks et al., 2012). Another study supporting both the socioemotional selectivity theory and the selection, optimization and compensation theory found that older adults reported more goals focused on the present, emotions,

generativity and prevention of loss and fewer goals focusing on the future or knowledge acquisition (Penningroth & Scott, 2012).

The theory of **gerotranscendence** was proposed in the early 1990s by Lars Tornstam (1994) and has become widely recognized in Sweden and other Scandinavian countries. This theory proposes that human aging is a process of shifting from a rational and materialistic metaperspective to a more cosmic and transcendent vision. This shift includes the following aspects (Tornstam, 1996):

- Decreased self-centredness
- Less concern with body and material things
- Decreased fear of death
- Discovery of hidden aspects of self
- Increased altruism
- Increased time spent in meditation and solitude
- Decreased interest in superfluous social interaction
- Urge to abandon roles
- Increased understanding of moral ambiguity
- Increased feelings of cosmic union with the universe
- Increased feelings of affinity with past and coming generations
- A redefinition of one's perception of time, space and objects

Recent studies based on this theory indicate that gerotranscendence (i.e., a shift from a materialistic and rational vision to a more cosmic and transcendent one) may explain successful aging, or psychological well-being, to counteract negative influence of functional decline in people who are 90 years and older (Gondo et al., 2013). A longitudinal study found that gerotranscendence was higher among older adults who experienced more negative life events (Read et al., 2014).

The **strength and vulnerability integration theory** posits that older adults experience age-related gains, as well as losses in emotion-related processes, but overall they maintain a relatively positive level of emotional experience (Charles, 2011). Strengths of older adults include improved abilities to (1) direct emotional attention away from negative stimuli, (2) appraise situations and (3) remember experiences more positively. Age-related vulnerabilities are defined as diminished physiologic ability to respond to high levels of stress. This theory is relatively new, but one study found that it is a useful model for understanding age-related patterns in emotional experiences of people diagnosed with colorectal cancer (Hart & Charles, 2013).

Relevance of Psychological Theories of Aging to Nurses

In caring for older adults, nurses can use psychological theories of aging as a framework for addressing certain issues, such as response to losses and continued emotional development. Maslow's hierarchy of needs framework is useful for conceptualizing the nature of interventions in institutional or home settings. For instance, if older adults are

A Student's Perspective

My comfort level at the nursing home increases each and every week, and I find myself enjoying my time there more and more. Today there was a children's program in the dining room for all the residents. It was very cute. The kids were great, and most of the residents expressed true appreciation and enjoyment while the kids visited. For instance, my patient Mr. B. was chatting with a young boy and his mother. As the boy got more and more involved in the conversation, Mr. B.'s attitude changed completely; he became so happy and engaged with the young boy. I had seen Mr. B. smile a couple of times before, but not to the extent of how he smiled and laughed with the little one. After the boy left, Mr. B. told me that the boy reminded him of his own grandson, whom he doesn't get to see very much. I think it brought Mr. B. joy and a sense of comfort because he felt like he was with his family. Personally, I was quite touched. Sometimes, everyone gets so caught up in current tasks or problems, when really at the end of the day it comes down to making people smile and helping them to enjoy life to the best of one's abilities.

Caitlin B.

unable to purchase food, they are unlikely to feel secure. Likewise, if older adults feel insecure about being able to meet their shelter needs, they are unlikely to have a sense of trust. Older adults who have already met their lower-level

Case Study

Imagine, again, that you are 87 years old and add the following information to the description of yourself that you created for the discussion of sociocultural theories. Describe your personality, including, but not limited to, the following characteristics: emotional stability, adjustments to losses, contentedness with life, optimism versus pessimism, engagement in activities versus withdrawal from activities, and feelings of self-efficacy versus feelings of powerlessness. Describe your beliefs about your gender-specific roles (i.e., those aspects of roles that are defined by you being a woman or a man). Based on this image of yourself at 87 years of age, answer the following questions:

THINKING POINTS

- Where do you think you would be in Maslow's or Erikson's stages and how would you have moved between the levels in the past decades?
- What aspects of your lifestyle at 87 years of age could be explained by the continuity theory?
- How would any concepts in the personality development theories apply to you?
- Based on your own experiences, how has your perception of your role as a woman or man changed over time?

needs, however, can be encouraged to focus on higher-level achievements such as self-actualization.

In addition, psychological theories imply that devoting some time and energy to life review and self-understanding can be beneficial for older adults. Nurses can facilitate this process by asking sensitive questions and by listening attentively to older adults as they share information about their past. Reminiscence is a positive experience that is essential for continued psychological development, and it can be promoted by nurses either on an individual or group basis.

Life-course models can help nurses identify those areas of personality that are likely to change and those that are more likely to remain stable. Nurses have used lifespan theories to develop a multidisciplinary theory of thriving (Haight et al., 2002). This model proposes that thriving is achieved when there is concordance between the person and the human and nonhuman environment, that is, when these three elements are mutually engaged, supportive and harmonious. In contrast, failure to thrive is the result of discordance among these three elements, causing a failure of engagement and mutual support and disharmony (Haight et al., 2002). In addition to these implications, nurses consider implications regarding specific aspects, such as cognitive function and coping responses (see Chapters 11 and 12), in the context of psychological theories of aging.

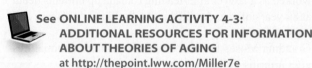

See ONLINE LEARNING ACTIVITY 4-3:
ADDITIONAL RESOURCES FOR INFORMATION ABOUT THEORIES OF AGING
at http://thepoint.lww.com/Miller7e

A HOLISTIC PERSPECTIVE ON AGING AND WELLNESS

From a holistic perspective—the one that is most pertinent to promoting wellness—it is necessary to consider the body–mind–spirit interconnectedness of each older adult for whom nurses provide care. Thus, questions about how we can live long and well must be answered in the context of the interplay among the many factors that influence health and aging. This requires an integrated perspective on aging, an avoidance of stereotypes and a commitment to identifying the factors that most directly affect—both negatively and positively—health and quality of life for each unique older adult. Current theories point to the following determinants of living long and well:

- Inherit good genes.
- Avoid oxidative damage (e.g., from tobacco, environmental conditions).
- Protect from oxidative damage with antioxidants from natural sources (e.g., fruits and vegetables).

- Maintain optimal weight.
- Engage in physical exercise.
- Engage in meaningful social interactions.
- Develop close personal relationships.
- Maintain a sense of spiritual connectedness.
- Reject ageist stereotypes.

The functional consequences theory for promoting wellness that was presented in Chapter 3 provides a nursing framework for addressing the factors that affect the health and functioning of older adults. Although it is beyond the scope of any nursing book to address all aspects of body–mind–spirit interconnectedness, nurses can use the functional consequences perspective, in conjunction with information from theories discussed in this chapter, to help older adults answer their own questions about aging. When older adults express resignation in the "What-do-you-expect-you're-old?" outlook, nurses can rephrase that viewpoint and ask "So, what *do* you expect because you are older?" or "What *will* you expect when you are older?" Nurses can challenge ageist stereotypes and approach the question from a holistic perspective that acknowledges the interconnectedness among one's body, mind and spirit. From this point of view, nurses can emphasize that even though some degenerative changes affect one's body with increasing age, one's mind and spirit can continue to thrive and even improve.

Because self-responsibility is an essential component of wellness, nurses can ask older adults to identify for themselves those factors that most significantly influence their health and functioning and can focus care on those aspects that are within the scope of nursing. Nurses also need to avoid communicating ageist stereotypes, which requires that we examine our own attitudes about aging and make sure that our nursing care of older adults is based on accurate, theory-based information. Nurses can check their attitudes about their own aging and periodically ask, *What do I expect (or wish) for my own wellness when I am older tomorrow? . . . a week from now? . . . a month from now? . . . a year? . . . 10 years? . . . 20 years?* Even more important, ask, *What am I doing today that will affect how well I am aging tomorrow? . . . 10 years from now?* If we acknowledge that no matter what else is happening, we are aging biologically, we are likely to pay careful attention to health-related behaviours that affect how well we age. Likewise, if we approach our care of older adults holistically, we will be able to identify interventions that promote wellness of body, mind and spirit.

Chapter Highlights

How Can We Live Long and Well? (Fig. 4-1)

- Gerontologists develop theories to answer questions about how and why we age. From a holistic perspective, the most important question is *How can we live a life that is both long and healthy?* Nurses address this question by promoting wellness and facilitating optimal level of functioning for older adults.

- The rectangularization of the curve illustrates the changes in survivorship and life expectancy that have been occurring in developed countries.
- The compression of morbidity describes the phenomenon of postponing disability until the last years before death.
- Studies of people who are healthy and long lived provide insights into characteristics of healthy aging.

How Do We Explain Biologic Aging? (Table 4-1)

- Biologic theories of aging address questions about inevitable consequences of normal aging.
- Examples of biologic theories of aging are wear and tear, free radical, immunosenescence, cross-linkage, program and caloric restriction.
- Nurses can apply information about biologic theories of aging to teach older adults about health-promotion interventions.

Sociocultural Perspectives on Aging

- Sociocultural theories of aging attempt to explain how a society influences its old people and how old people influence their society.
- Sociocultural theories include disengagement, activity, subculture, age stratification and person–environment fit theories.
- Nurses can apply information from sociocultural theories to holistically address the multidimensional needs of older adults.

Psychological Perspectives on Aging

- Psychological theories of aging provide a framework for addressing certain psychosocial issues that are common among older adults (e.g., responses to losses and continued emotional development).
- Maslow's human needs theories and theories of Jung, Erikson and Peck underlie many psychological theories of aging.
- Gerontologists are especially interested in theories of successful aging, such as selection, optimization and compensation; socioemotional selectivity; gerotranscendence; and strength and vulnerability integration.
- Psychological theories of aging help nurses address the psychosocial needs of older adults.

A Holistic Perspective on Aging and Wellness

- Nurses can use theories of aging developed by other disciplines in conjunction with the functional consequences theory (see Chapter 3) to develop and implement a holistic approach to promoting wellness in older adults.

Critical Thinking Exercises

You are assessing an 87-year-old woman who is being admitted to the hospital with congestive heart failure for the third time in the past 2 years. She does not have any cognitive impairment, and she lives alone in her own home. When you ask her why she came to the hospital, she states, "I'm 87 years old, you know. Isn't that a good enough reason to be sick? Don't you think you'll be in the hospital when you're my age?"

1. How do you respond to her?
2. What additional assessment information would you want?
3. What health teaching would you think about incorporating into your care plan?

For more information about topics discussed in this chapter, be sure to check out the interactive Online Learning Activities and other helpful resources at http://thepoint.lww.com/Miller7e

REFERENCES

Agronin, M. E. (2013). From Cicero to Cohen: Developmental theories of aging, from antiquity to the present. *Gerontologist, 54*(1), 30–39. doi:10:10.1093/geront/gnt032

Andersen, S. L., Sebastiani, P., Dworkis, D. A., et al. (2012). Health span approximates life span among many supercentenarians: Compression of morbidity at the approximate limit of life span. *Journals of Gerontology: Biological Sciences and Medical Sciences, 67*(4), 395–405.

Antonucci, T. C., Ashton-Miller, J. A., Brant, J., et al. (2012). The right to move: A multidisciplinary lifespan conceptual framework. *Current Gerontology and Geriatrics Research, 2012* [Article ID 873937]. doi:10.1155/2012/873937

Bloss, C. S., Pawlikowska, L., & Schork, N. J. (2011). Contemporary human genetic strategies in aging research. *Ageing Research Review, 10*(2), 191–200.

Carnes, B. A., & Witten, T. M. (2013). How long must humans live? *Journals of Gerontology: Biological Sciences and Medical Sciences, 69*(8), 965–970. doi:10.1093/gerona/glt164

Carnes, B. A., Olshansky, S. J., & Hayflick, L. (2013). Can human biology allow most of us to become centenarians? *Journals of Gerontology: Biological Sciences and Medical Sciences, 68*(2), 136–142.

Carstensen, L. L., Turan, B., Scheibe, S., et al. (2011). Emotional experience improves with age: Evidence based on over 10 years of experience sampling. *Psychology of Aging, 26*(1), 21–33.

Caruso, C., Passarino, G., Puca, A., et al. (2012). "Positive biology": The centenarian lesson. *Immunity & Ageing, 9*(1), 5. Retrieved from http://www.immunityageing.com/content/9/1/5

Cattan, M., Hogg, E., & Hardill, I. (2011). Improving quality of life in ageing populations: What can volunteering do? *Maturitas, 70*(4), 428–432.

Charles, S. T. (2011). Emotional experience and regulation in later life. In K. W. Schaie & S. L. Willis (Eds.), *Handbook of the psychology of aging* (7th ed., pp. 295–310). New York, NY: Elsevier.

Cumming, E., & Henry, W. (1961). *Growing old: The process of disengagement.* New York, NY: Basic Books.

Davinelli, S., Willcox, C., & Scapagnini, G. (2012). Extending healthy ageing: Nutrient sensitive pathway and centenarian population. *Immunity Ageing, 9,* 9. Retrieved from http://www.immunityageing.com/content/9/1/9

Donnellan, C., & O'Neill, D. (2014). Baltes' SOC model of successful ageing as a potential framework for stroke rehabilitation. *Disability and Rehabilitation, 36*(5), 424–429. doi:10.3109/09638288.2013.793412

Erikson, E. H. (1963). *Childhood and society* (2nd ed.). New York, NY: W. W. Norton.

Fernandez-Ballesteros, R., Molina, M.-A., Schettini, R., et al. (2013). The semantic network of aging well. *Annual Review of Gerontology and Geriatrics, 33,* 79–107.

Fries, J. F. (2012). The theory and practice of active aging. *Current Gerontology and Geriatrics Research, 2012* [Article ID 420637]. doi:10.1133/2012/420637

Fries, J. F., & Crapo, L. M. (1981). *Vitality and aging: Implications of the rectangularization of the curve.* San Francisco, CA: W. H. Freeman.

Gana, K., Bailly, N., Saada, Y., et al. (2013). Does life satisfaction change in old age: Results from an 8-year longitudinal study. *Journals of Gerontology: Psychological Sciences and Social Sciences, 68*(4), 540–552.

Gondo, Y., Nakagawa, T., & Masui, Y. (2013). A new concept of successful aging in the oldest old. *Annual Review of Gerontology and Geriatrics, 33,* 109–132.

Haight, B. K., Barba B. E., Tesh, A. S., et al. (2002). Thriving: A life span theory. *Journal of Gerontological Nursing, 28*(3), 14–22.

Hart, S. L., & Charles, S. T. (2013). Age-related patterns in negative affect and appraisals about colorectal cancer over time. *Health Psychology, 32*(3), 302–310.

Havighurst, R. J., & Albrecht, R. (1953). *Older people.* New York, NY: Longmans, Green.

Hayflick, L. (2001–2002). Anti-aging medicine hype, hope, and reality. *Generations, 20,* 20–26.

Hicks, J. A., Trent, J., Davis, W. E., et al. (2012). Positive affect, meaning in life, and future time perspective: An application of socioemotional selectivity theory. *Psychology and Aging, 27*(1), 181–189.

Hummer, R. A., Melvin, J. E., Sheehan, C. M., et al. (2014). Race/ethnicity, morality, and longevity. In K. E. Whitfield & T. A. Baker (Eds.), *Handbook of minority aging* (pp. 11–129). New York, NY: Springer.

Hung, W. W., Ross, J. S., Boockvar, S., et al. (2011). Recent trends in chronic disease, impairment and disability among older adults in the United States. *BioMed Central Geriatrics, 11,* 47. Retrieved from http://www.biomedcentral.com/1471-2318/11/47

Hutnik, N., Smith, P., & Koch, T. (2012). What does it feel like to be 100? Socio-emotional aspects of well-being in the stories of 16 centenarians living in the United Kingdom. *Aging and Mental Health, 16*(7), 811–816.

Islam, F. (2013). Examining the "healthy immigrant effect" for mental health in Canada. *The University of Toronto Medical Journal, 90*(4), 169–175.

Johnson, K. J., & Mutchler, J. E. (2013). The emergence of a positive gerontology: From disengagement to social involvement. *Gerontologist, 54*(1), 93–100. doi:10.1093/geront/gnt099

Jonson, H. (2013). We will be different? Ageism and the temporal construction of old age. *Gerontologist, 53*(2), 198–204.

Jung, C. G. (1954). Marriage as a psychological relationship. In W. McGuire, H. Reed, M. Fordham et al. (Eds.), & R. F. C. Hull (Trans.), *Collected works: The development of personality* (Vol. 17). New York, NY: Pantheon Books.

Jung, C. G. (1960). The stages of life. In W. McGuire, H. Reed, M. Fordham et al. (Eds.), & R. F. C. Hull (Trans.), *Collected works: The structure and dynamics of the psyche* (Vol. 8, pp. 387–403). New York, NY: Pantheon Books.

Kahana, E., Bhatta, T., Lovegreen, L. D., et al. (2013). Altruism, helping, and volunteering: Pathways to well-being in late life. *Journal of Aging and Mental Health, 25*(1), 159–187.

Keith, V. M. (2014). Stress, discrimination, and coping in late life. In K. E. Whitfield & T. A. Baker (Eds.), *Handbook of minority aging* (pp. 65–84). New York, NY: Springer.

Kivnick, H. Q., & Wells, C. K. (2013). Untapped richness in Erik H. Erikson's rootstock. *Gerontologist, 54*(1), 40–50. doi:10.1093/geront/gnt123

Knight, B. G., & Losada, A. (2011). Family caregiving for cognitively or physically frail older adults: Theory, research, and practice.

In K. W. Schaie & S. L. Willis (Eds.), *Handbook of the psychology of aging,* (7th ed., pp. 353–365). New York, NY: Elsevier.

Kohn, R. R. (1982). Cause of death in very old people. *Journal of the American Medical Association, 247,* 2793–2797.

Kryla-Lighthall, N., & Mather, M. (2009). The role of cognitive control in older adults' emotional well-being. In V. L. Bengston, M. Silverstein, N. M. Putney et al. (Eds.), *Handbook of theories of aging* (2nd ed., pp. 323–344). New York, NY: Springer.

Lawton, M. P. (1982). Competence, environmental press, and the adaptation of older people. In M. P. Lawton, P. G. Windley, & T. O. Byerts (Eds.), *Aging and the environment: Theoretical approaches* (pp. 33–59). New York, NY: Springer.

Li, P. (2000). *Cultural diversity in Canada: The social construction of racial differences.* Retrieved from http://www.justice.gc.ca/eng/rp-pr/csj-sjc/jsp-sjp/rp02_8-dr02_8/rp02_8.pdf

Lowry, K. A., Vallejo, A. N., & Studenski, S. A. (2012). Successful aging as a continuum of functional independence: Lessons from physical disability models of aging. *Aging and Disease, 3*(1), 5–15.

Madden, C. L., & Cloyes, K. G. (2012). The discourse of aging. *Advances in Nursing Science, 35*(3), 264–272.

Manton, K. G., Gu, X., & Lowrimore, G. R. (2008). Cohort changes in active life expectancy in the U.S., elderly population: Experience from the 1982–2004 National Long-Term Care Survey. *Journal of Gerontology: Social Sciences, 63*(5), S269–S281.

Maslow, A. H. (1954). *Motivation and personality.* New York, NY: Harper & Row.

Melzer, D., Pilling, L. C., Fellows, A. D., et al. (2013). Gene expression biomarkers and longevity. *Annual Review of Gerontology and Geriatrics, 3,* 233–258.

Meyer, M. H., & Parker, W. M. (2011). Gender, aging, and social policy. In R. H. Binstock & L. K. George (Eds.), *Handbook of aging and the social sciences* (7th ed., pp. 323–335). New York, NY: Elsevier.

Morley, J. E. (2009). Successful aging or aging successfully. *Journal of the American Medical Directors Association, 10*(2), 85–86.

Murabito, J. M., Yuan, R., & Lunetta, K. L. (2012). The search for longevity and healthy aging genes: Insights from epidemiological studies and samples of long-lived individuals. *Journals of Gerontology: Biological Sciences and Medical Sciences, 67*(5), 470–479.

New England Centenarian Study. (2014). *Why study centenarians? An overview.* Retrieved from http://www.bumc.bu.edu/centenarian/overview

Peck, R. C. (1968). Psychological developments in the second half of life. In B. L. Neugarten (Ed.), *Middle age and aging* (pp. 88–92). Chicago, IL: University of Chicago Press.

Penningroth, S. L., & Scott, W. D. (2012). Age-related differences in goals: Testing predictions from selection, optimization, and compensation theory and socioemotional selectivity theory. *International Journal of Aging and Human Development, 74*(2), 87–111.

Public Health Agency of Canada. (2010). *The Chief Public Health Officer's Report on the State of Public Health in Canada 2010—The health and well-being of Canadian seniors.* Retrieved from http://www.phac-aspc.gc.ca/cphosphc-respcacsp/2010/fr-rc/cphorsphc-respcacsp-06-eng.php

Rattan, S. (2013). Healthy aging, but what is health? *Biogerontology, 14*(6), 673–677. doi:10.1007/s10522-013-9442-7

Read, S., Braam, A. W., Lyyra, T. M., et al. (2014). Do negative life events promote gerotranscendence in the second half of life? *Aging and Mental Health, 18*(1), 117–124. doi:10.1080/13607863.2013.814101

Riley, M. W., Johnson, M., & Foner, A. (1972). *Aging and society. Vol. 3: A sociology of age stratification.* New York, NY: Russell Sage Foundation.

Rohr, M. K., & Lang, F. R. (2009). Aging well together—A mini review. *Gerontology, 55,* 333–343.

Rose, A. M. (1965). The subculture of the aging: A framework for research in social gerontology. In A. M. Rose & W. Peterson (Eds.), *Older people and their social worlds.* Philadelphia, PA: F. A. Davis.

Sebastiani, P., Bae, H., Sun, F. X., et al. (2013). Meta-analysis of genetic variants associated with human exceptional longevity. *Aging, 5*(9), 653–661.

Sebastiani, P., & Perls, T. (2012). The genetics of extreme longevity: Lessons from the New England Centenarian Study. *Frontiers in Genetics, 30,* 277. doi:10.3389/fgene.2012.00277

Sebastiani, P., Riva, A., Montano, M., et al. (2012). Whole genome sequences of a male and female super-centenarian, ages greater than 114 years. *Frontiers in Genetics, 2,* 90. doi:10.3389/fgene.2011.00090

Statistics Canada. (2013). *Immigration and ethnocultural diversity in Canada.* Retrieved from http://www12.statcan.gc.ca/nhs-enm/2011/as-sa/99-010-x/99-010-x2011001-eng.pdf

Statistics Canada. (2012a). *Life expectancy at birth, by sex, by province.* Retrieved from http://www.statcan.gc.ca/tables-tableaux/sum-som/l01/cst01/health26-eng.htm

Statistics Canada. (2012b). *Deaths—2009 (Catalogue No. 84FO211X).* Ottawa, ON: Government of Canada.

Statistics Canada. (2012c). *Centenarians in Canada, age and sex, 2011 census (Catalogue No. 98-311-X2011003).* Ottawa, ON: Government of Canada.

Taylor, M. G., & Lynch, S. M. (2011). Cohort differences and chronic disease profiles of differential disability trajectories. *Journals of Gerontology: Psychological Sciences and Social Sciences, 66*(6), 729–738.

Tornstam, L. (1994). Gerotranscendence: A theoretical and empirical exploration. In L. E. Thomas & S. A. Eisenhandler (Eds.), *Aging and the religious dimension* (pp. 203–225). Westport, CT: Greenwood.

Tornstam, L. (1996). Gerotranscendence: A theory about maturing into old age. *Journal of Aging & Identity, 1,* 37–50.

Unson, C., & Richardson, M. (2013). Insights into the experiences of older workers and change: Through the lens of selection, optimization, and compensation. *Gerontologist, 5*(3), 484–494.

Vacante, M., D'Agata, V., Motta, M., et al. (2012). Centenarians and supercentenarians: A block swan. Emerging social, medical and surgical problems. *BioMed Central Surgery, 2012, 12*(Suppl. 1), S36. Retrieved from http://www.biomedcentral.com/1471-2482/12/S1/S36

Willcox, D. C., Willcox, B. J., & Poon, L. W. (2010). Centenarian studies: Important contributors to our understanding of the aging process and longevity. *Current Gerontology and Geriatrics Research, 2010* [Article ID 484529]. doi:10.1155/2010/484529

Wolinsky, F. D., Bentler, S. E., Hockenberry, M. P., et al. (2011). Long-term declines in ADLs, IADLs, and mobility among older Medicare beneficiaries. *BioMed Central Geriatrics, 11,* 43. Retrieved from http://www.biomedcentral.com/1471-2318/11/43

Zarit, S. H. (2009). A good old age: Theories of mental health and aging. In V. L. Bengston, M. Silverstein, N. M. Putney et al. (Eds.), *Handbook of theories of aging* (2nd ed., pp. 675–691). New York, NY: Springer.

part 2

Nursing Considerations for Older Adults

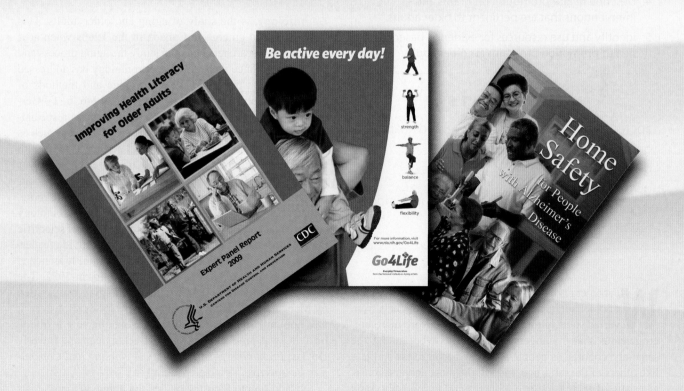

chapter 5

Gerontological Nursing and Health Promotion

LEARNING OBJECTIVES

After reading this chapter, you will be able to:

1. Describe the scope of gerontology and geriatrics.

2. Discuss the practice of gerontological nursing as a specialty for some nurses and a responsibility for all nurses in adult care settings.

3. Identify and use resources for improving competence in care of older adults.

4. Describe health promotion programs and interventions that are pertinent to older adults.

5. Identify and use resources for evidence-based health promotion programs for older adults.

KEY POINTS

appreciative inquiry

geriatrics

gerontology

gerontological nursing

health

health promotion

health-related quality of life

motivational interviewing

Stages of Change model

wellness

What emerges from the information in Part 1 is an image of older adults as a diverse group of individuals from varied sociocultural backgrounds who are more heterogeneous than homogeneous. Clearly, even among the same-age cohorts, as people age, they become less and less like others of the same age. Indeed, the most universal characteristic of increasing age is increasing individuality and diversity. Because the provision of health care and other services to this population is so complicated, several branches

of science have evolved to address the unique issues related to aging and older adults. In recent years, there has been increasing attention to the importance of all nurses becoming competent in addressing the unique health care needs of older adults and applying evidence-based guidelines to nursing practice. There has also been increasing attention to the importance of health promotion interventions and the roles of nurses in promoting wellness.

GERONTOLOGY AND GERIATRICS

Gerontology, is the study of aging and older adults. This field started to emerge in Canada in the 1960s when academics and researchers began to study the aging process and older adults. Since its beginning, gerontology has addressed problems that "transcend the knowledge and methods of any one discipline or profession" (Frank, 1946, p. 1). Gerontology continues to be interprofessional and is a specialized area both within and across various disciplines, such as nursing, psychology, social work and certain allied health professions. Although the initial focus of gerontology was primarily on *problems of aging and older adults*, the focus has shifted to an emphasis on *healthy and successful aging*. Founded in 1971, The Canadian Association on Gerontology (www.cagacg.ca) is a national, interprofessional, scientific and educational organization established to provide leadership in matters related to the aging population. It launched its journal, the *Canadian Journal on Aging*, in 1982. The first Canadian textbook with a focus on aging was written by Marshall and McPhersen in the early 1980s. However, it was not until 1993 that the first Canadian nursing textbook on aging was produced by Ann C. Beckingham and Beverly DuGas, *Promoting Healthy Aging: A Nursing and Community Perspective*.

In addition to focusing on healthy aging, gerontologists are addressing the increasing diversity among older people and the increasing complexity of providing health care for older adults. Consequently, the health care specialties of geriatric medicine and gerontological nursing have emerged. Geriatrics (also called geriatric medicine) is a subspecialty of internal medicine or family practice that focuses on the medical problems of older people. The Canadian Geriatrics Society, which was initially called the Canadian Society of Geriatric Medicine, was established in 1981. While in the past, physicians in North America were called to "alleviate the inevitable deficiencies and limitations inherent in growing old" (Touhy, 1946, p. 17), in recent decades, geriatric practitioners have shifted their focus from curing to caring. This does not mean, however, that decisions about interventions are based primarily on chronologic age. Rather, decisions about interventions are based on a holistic assessment of the individual, with emphasis on quality-of-life issues, interventions to maintain optimal functioning and health promotion as a means of delaying the onset of disability.

In addition to professional associations enhancing the status of gerontology in Canada, there have been a number of other initiatives undertaken to enhance knowledge of aging and older adults in this country. The Canadian Health and Aging Study focused on the epidemiology of dementia, wherein 10,000 older adults were followed from 1991 to 2001. Initiated in 2002, the Canadian Longitudinal Study on Aging (CLSA) is a large, national, long-term study that follows approximately 50,000 men and women between the ages of 45 and 85 for at least two decades. As of February 2014, 35,000 participants had been recruited. More recently, the National Initiative for the Care of the Elderly (NICE) was funded in 2005 under a grant from the Networks of Centres of Excellence. Launched in Canada, NICE is an international network of researchers, practitioners, students and older adults working to improving the care of older adults, both in Canada and abroad.

GERONTOLOGICAL NURSING AS A SPECIALTY AND A RESPONSIBILITY

Although nurses in Canada first recognized the importance of addressing the unique needs of older adults in the early 1900s, gerontological nursing was not considered a specialty until more recently. The Gerontological Nursing Association (GNA) was the first provincial (Ontario) group of nurses who, in 1974, joined together to recognize this nursing specialty. Other provinces and territories followed the example of Ontario and established their own gerontological nursing groups. The term gerontological nursing is commonly used instead of *geriatric nursing*, to more accurately reflect the broader scope of nursing care rather than a focus on disease conditions. Provincial gerontological nursing groups are linked in membership with the national group. For more than thirty years, the Canadian Gerontological Nursing Association (CGNA) has demonstrated strong support of gerontological nursing as a specialty, which includes its 2010 document *Gerontological Nursing Competencies and*

Standards of Practice. This document describes the responsibilities of gerontological nurses, who are the health care professionals consistently responsible for the 24-hour care of older adults in all clinical settings and includes the following expectations:

STANDARD I: Gerontological nurses assist clients to maintain homeostatic regulation through assessment and management of physiological care to minimize adverse events associated with medications, diagnostic or therapeutic procedures, nosocomial infections or environmental stressors.

STANDARD II: Gerontological nurses promote older adults to optimize functional health that includes an integration of abilities that involve physical, cognitive, psychological, social and spiritual status.

STANDARD III: Gerontological nurses provide responsive care that facilitates and empowers client independence through life-course changes. A responsive care approach recognizes that certain behaviours are not necessarily solely related to pathology, but instead may be related to circumstances within the physical or social environment surrounding well older persons and those with dementia, and maybe an expression of unmet need.

STANDARD IV: Gerontological nurses develop and preserve therapeutic relationship care. Relationship-centred care is an approach that recognizes the importance and uniqueness of each health care participant's relationship with every other and considers these relationships to be central in supporting high-quality care, a high-quality work environment and superior organizational performance.

STANDARD V: Gerontological nurses are aware of economic and political influences by providing or facilitating care that supports access to and benefit from the health care delivery system. Systems to support and sustain practice changes should be in place, including ongoing education, policies and procedures, and job descriptions.

STANDARD VI: Gerontological nurses are responsible for assessing the client and the environment for hazards that threaten safety, as well as planning and intervening to appropriately maintain a safe environment.

In addition, CGNA has worked collaboratively with other organizations for several decades to promote gerontological nursing. In 2003, a partnership was initiated with the National Gerontological Nursing Association (NGNA) in the United States to share information and promote mutual goals. Out of this alliance, a position paper on gerontological education was developed. The Canadian Nurses Association (CNA) is another nursing organization that recognizes gerontological nursing as a specialization by offering certification as a gerontological nurse. The first group of registered nurses was certified in gerontology by the CNA in 1999. Currently, this group represent the largest group of certified nurses in Canada.

Opportunities for advance practice nurses in geriatric care settings have been emerging in the recent years.

An advanced practice nurse (APN) who focuses on gerontology holds a degree higher than a baccalaureate and demonstrates clinical expertise in caring for older adults at all levels of wellness and illness. Roles of advanced practice nurses include teacher, researcher, consultant, administrator, expert clinician, independent practitioner, care/case manager, individual/group counsellor and interprofessional team member/leader. In 2004, an 18-month initiative was launched by the CNA to facilitate the sustained integration of the nurse practitioner (NP) role in Canada. There are currently four NP specialty areas in Canada: NP-Primary Health Care, NP-Pediatrics, NP-Adult and NP-Anesthesia. An advanced practice nurse with an interest in gerontology will take either a primary health care or adult route; however, neither option focuses specifically on older adults.

Competencies for Older Adult Care

Baccalaureate nursing programs provide a general nursing education to meet the competencies (jurisdictional) required to practice at an entry level and the five core competencies identified by the Committee of the Health Professions Education Summit (provide patient-centred care, work in interprofessional teams, employ evidence-based practice, apply quality improvement, utilize informatics) (Canadian Associations of Schools of Nursing [CASN], 2011). They may also respond to specific regional health needs. These jurisdictional competencies are linked to the competencies of the CNA, which are grouped under the domains of professional practice, nurse–client partnership, health and wellness, and changes in health. While none are specific to older adults, it is expected that the registered nurse is able to use the standards and the CNA's (2008) Code of Ethics when working with older adults and those important to them. In conjunction with the growth of gerontological nursing as a specialty, there has been increasing recognition that *all nurses who work with adults* need to be competent in addressing the unique health issues of *older adults*. This recognition has evolved from a combination of demographic changes discussed in Chapter 1 and the increasing concerns about quality of care for older adults.

A link to the full document discussing the gerontological nursing competencies is provided in the learning activities.

Initiatives and Resources for Improving Gerontological Nursing Competencies

While there are an increasing number of Canadian resources focused upon gerontological nursing, many of the resources used by nurses in Canada are drawn from the United States. Since the early 1990s, the Hartford Foundation for Geriatric Nursing has demonstrated a major and ongoing commitment to improving nursing care of older adults by funding many initiatives directed toward increased nursing knowledge and evidence-based clinical practice. In 1999, the Hartford Foundation for Geriatric Nursing initiated partnerships with 54 specialty nursing organizations to improve competency

in care of older adults. This initiative has expanded with support from the American Nurses Association and philanthropic organizations and continues to develop and update evidence-based resources related to care for older adults, which Canadian nurses have easy access to. Of particular importance to all nurses and nursing students, the Hartford Foundation for Geriatric Nursing supports the development of evidence-based assessment tools and information related to nursing interventions for older adults. Resources include tools and related material for general assessment, for older adults with dementia and for specialized care, such as pain, caregiving and risks for cardiovascular disease. Periodically, assessment tools are updated and new ones are added, including resources developed in conjunction with specialty nursing organizations. All resources are readily accessible through the ConsultGeriRN section of Hartford Foundation for Geriatric Nursing, which can be accessed through the link in Online Learning Activity 5-1. There is as yet no similar substantive resource development in Canada. However, there are initiatives undertaken by the CNA (NurseONE), RNAO, NICE and the Canadian Coalition for Seniors Mental Health to enhance the use of evidence-based tools, which can be used by nurses.

Figure 5-1 provides a timeline of significant events related to nursing care of older adults as a specialization for some and a responsibility for all nurses in adult care settings.

See **ONLINE LEARNING ACTIVITY 5-1:**
RESOURCES FOR IMPROVING COMPETENCY IN PROVIDING NURSING CARE FOR OLDER ADULTS
at http://thepoint.lww.com/Miller7e

HEALTH, WELLNESS AND HEALTH PROMOTION

Nurses often use the terms *health* and *wellness* interchangeably because of the shifting paradigm from the traditional health–illness continuum to a whole-person model and person-centred care. This paradigm shift is evident in holistic nursing definitions of health and wellness. For example, a holistic nursing definition of **health** is "an individually defined state or process in which the individual (nurse, client, family, group or community) experiences a sense of well-being, harmony, and unity such that subjective experiences about health, health beliefs, and values are honoured; a process of becoming an expanded consciousness" (Mariano, 2013, p. 60). Similarly, a holistic nursing definition of **wellness** is "integrated, congruent functioning aimed toward reaching one's highest potential" (Mariano, 2013, p. 61). In this text, *health* is defined as the ability of older adults to function at their highest capacity despite the presence of age-related changes and risk factors, whereas *wellness* is an outcome (also called a positive functional consequence) for older adults whose well-being and quality of life is improved

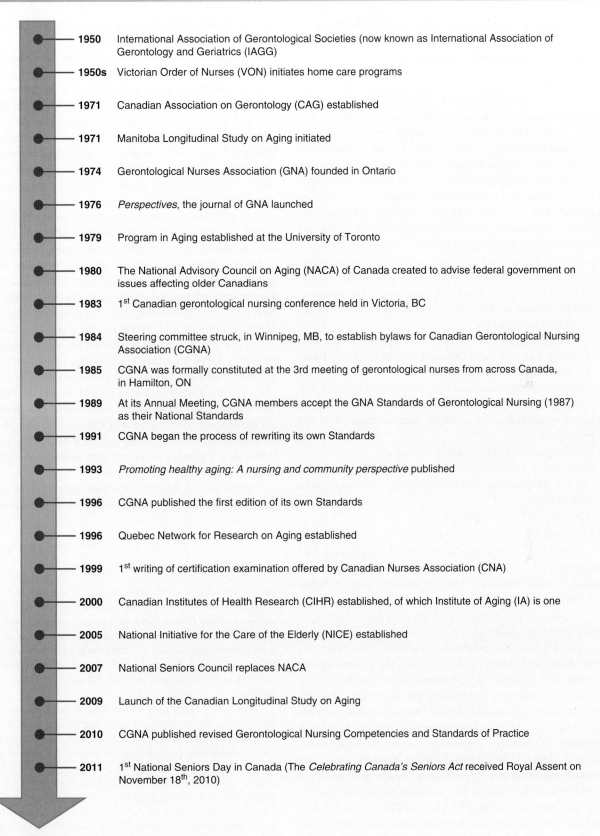

1950 International Association of Gerontological Societies (now known as International Association of Gerontology and Geriatrics (IAGG)

1950s Victorian Order of Nurses (VON) initiates home care programs

1971 Canadian Association on Gerontology (CAG) established

1971 Manitoba Longitudinal Study on Aging initiated

1974 Gerontological Nurses Association (GNA) founded in Ontario

1976 *Perspectives*, the journal of GNA launched

1979 Program in Aging established at the University of Toronto

1980 The National Advisory Council on Aging (NACA) of Canada created to advise federal government on issues affecting older Canadians

1983 1st Canadian gerontological nursing conference held in Victoria, BC

1984 Steering committee struck, in Winnipeg, MB, to establish bylaws for Canadian Gerontological Nursing Association (CGNA)

1985 CGNA was formally constituted at the 3rd meeting of gerontological nurses from across Canada, in Hamilton, ON

1989 At its Annual Meeting, CGNA members accept the GNA Standards of Gerontological Nursing (1987) as their National Standards

1991 CGNA began the process of rewriting its own Standards

1993 *Promoting healthy aging: A nursing and community perspective* published

1996 CGNA published the first edition of its own Standards

1996 Quebec Network for Research on Aging established

1999 1st writing of certification examination offered by Canadian Nurses Association (CNA)

2000 Canadian Institutes of Health Research (CIHR) established, of which Institute of Aging (IA) is one

2005 National Initiative for the Care of the Elderly (NICE) established

2007 National Seniors Council replaces NACA

2009 Launch of the Canadian Longitudinal Study on Aging

2010 CGNA published revised Gerontological Nursing Competencies and Standards of Practice

2011 1st National Seniors Day in Canada (The *Celebrating Canada's Seniors Act* received Royal Assent on November 18th, 2010)

FIGURE 5-1 Significant events in the growth of gerontological nursing.

through nursing interventions. The growing emphasis on wellness recognizes the importance of health promotion and broadens the focus on self-responsibility.

Health Promotion for Older Adults

Health promotion refers to programs or interventions that focus on behaviour changes directed toward improved health and well-being of individuals, groups, communities and nations in relation to their environments. Traditionally, health promotion programs emphasized disease prevention (i.e., risk reduction) and health maintenance (i.e., sustaining a neutral state of health), but more recently health promotion also emphasizes personal responsibility for health and self-care actions to achieve high-level wellness. Based on this broader approach, promoting wellness for older adults inherently involves helping older adults incorporate health-enhancing behaviours into their daily lives. The scope of health promotion interventions for older adults includes all of the following aspects:

- Regularly engaging in several types of physical exercise
- Assuring optimal nutritional intake and avoiding foods associated with risk for disease
- Engaging in recommended screening and preventive services, such as blood pressure checks and vaccinations
- Using stress-reduction methods, such as meditation and relaxation
- Fostering healthy relationships with others
- Engaging in self-wellness actions (e.g., getting adequate rest and sleep, taking time for enjoyable activities alone or with others)
- Attending to spiritual growth
- Engaging in holistic wellness practices (e.g., yoga, tai chi)

In addition, promoting discussions about advance care planning is a topic that is currently receiving attention as an aspect of health behaviour change (Canadian Hospice Palliative Care Association, 2012; Fried et al., 2012).

Because of the importance of reducing health care costs and improving quality of care, health promotion programs increasingly focus on evidence-based interventions to prevent, detect and manage conditions that are leading causes of death and disability (e.g., cardiovascular disease, cancer, stroke). For example, recognizing the urgent need for collective action on vascular health, organizational partners including the Canadian Cardiovascular Society, Canadian Diabetes Association, Canadian Society of Endocrinology and Metabolism, Canadian Stroke Network, Heart and Stroke Foundation and Hypertension Canada have endorsed *Making the connection: A call to action on vascular health.* This document was created by Vascular 2013, Canada's first national congress for knowledge exchange and community building in vascular health. Its recommendations for health care practitioners include maximizing interprofessional collaboration to comprehensively manage vascular risk and prevention, keeping up-to-date on and following best care practices, and collaborating with other sectors to advocate

for and address legislative and social and built environment factors that affect population health.

Another focus of health promotion for older adults is on effective management, including self-management, of chronic conditions such as diabetes that occur more commonly among older adults and affect independent functioning and quality of life. The Conference Board of Canada (2013) has examined the economic costs of health in this country. They report that declines in health and functioning among older adults are due to the following chronic conditions: chronic kidney disease, diabetes, osteoporosis and osteoarthritis/rheumatoid arthritis.

In addition to having an impact on the cost of care, health promotion can have a positive effect on quality of life. A commonly cited goal of gerontological health care is to *add life to years, not just more years to life*, which is synonymous with improved quality of life. The concept of **health-related quality of life** was proposed in the United States by the National Center for Chronic Disease and Health Promotion (at the CDC) in 1993. Health-related quality of life is measured by a standard set of questions, called "Healthy Days Measures," addressing one's perception of physical and mental health and functioning. A Canadian initiative is the Canadian Index of Well-Being developed by the International Initiative for Sustainable Development in all dimensions of life. Statistics Canada also uses the Community Health Survey as an indicator of quality of life, in addition to a number of other health assessment tools available off its website.

Even though health promotion interventions are cost-effective ways of preventing disease and disability and

A Student's Perspective

On our first day at the facility, we interviewed Teri, the registered nurse who oversees all the clinical care. She has been a nurse for about 15 years and she was very animated and passionate about her job. Throughout her years as a nurse, she has worked in settings such as hospitals, the ICU, a dermatologist's office and now in long-term care. She did not think she'd be working in gerontological nursing, but she is very happy and fulfilled.

Terri talked about some of the different ways the staff promotes wellness for residents including things such as life-enriching activities that include health and fitness programs, special outings and cultural events to enhance a resident's mind, body and spirit. Another way they promote wellness that really caught my attention is the fact that the staff of nurses and other employees work hard to keep residents in their current living situation. For example, they will do whatever is necessary to keep clients in the independent living apartment before moving them to assisted living. They strive to help the residents keep their independence as long as possible, and I really enjoyed that aspect of their care.

Molly D.

improving functioning and quality of life for older adults, older adults as a group receive fewer prevention and screening services than other populations. This is due to misperceptions, such as (1) older adults are less responsive to health promotion interventions and (2) preventive services are less effective after the onset of chronic illness. In reality, health promotion is essential for older adults precisely because they have more chronic conditions, have complex health care needs and use considerably more health care services than younger adults. In addition, longitudinal studies show that even after the age of 75 or 80, health-promoting interventions for older adults are effective for improving functioning and quality of life and increasing life expectancy (Gustafsson et al., 2012; Pascucci et al., 2012; Rizzuto et al., 2012). Another current concern is that significant health disparities exist among older adults related to use of clinical preventive services (Box 5-1).

Types of Health Promotion Interventions

Interventions to promote physical and psychosocial well-being include screening programs, risk-reduction interventions, environmental modifications and health education. This section reviews these types of programs in relation to promoting wellness for older adults. All clinically oriented chapters of this text emphasize health promotion because this is a central focus of the functional consequences model for promoting wellness. Thus, nursing interventions are directed toward improved health, functioning and quality of life for older adults, with emphasis on teaching older adults and their caregivers about health-promoting activities.

Screening Programs

Screening programs are an essential component of disease prevention because they may detect serious and progressive conditions as early as possible. The Canadian Task

Force on Preventative Health Care established by the Public Health Agency of Canada, as well as many professional organizations, publish evidence-based recommendations for screening related to conditions such as glaucoma, diabetes, hypertension, hyperlipidemia, osteoporosis, cognitive impairment and many types of cancer. Screening programs focus on conditions that can be accurately detected and effectively treated before they progress to a serious or fatal stage. Cost-effectiveness of a screening test is determined according to criteria such as its ability to detect a condition or risk factor at an early stage and without excessive false-positive or false-negative results. Another requirement for recommending a screening test is that early intervention must be superior to waiting until signs or symptoms of disease are present.

In recent years, attention has been paid to age-based recommendations for certain screening procedures. For example, guidelines for breast, colon, prostate and cervical cancer include a chronologic age for discontinuing the screenings. It is imperative to consider chronological age as only one criterion for decisions about screening for, or treatment of, diseases. Most importantly, decisions need to be based on the individual's current and anticipated status with regard to health, functioning and quality of life.

Risk-Reduction Interventions

Risk-reduction interventions, which are based on an assessment of the risk for developing a particular condition, are directed toward reducing the chance of developing that condition. Some risk-reduction interventions (e.g., vaccinations) apply to all older adults, and other interventions vary according to specific risk factors and the health level of an older person. Risk-assessment tools have been developed for various conditions pertinent to older adults, such as falls, anxiety, depression, heart disease, pressure ulcers and elder abuse and neglect, as discussed in this book. These tools often include a rating scale to identify people who are most likely to develop a particular condition so that health care professionals can plan and implement preventive interventions for them. These tools also serve to identify risk factors that can be addressed through preventive interventions.

Even without formal assessment tools, however, health care professionals can usually identify risk factors that can be addressed to prevent disease or disability. Typically, priority is given to reducing the risk factors that are most dominant or likely to have the most serious negative consequences. For example, health promotion interventions for a relatively healthy older adult with a history of hypertension, hypercholesterolemia and family history of heart attacks would address risk factors for heart disease. Health promotion interventions for a frail older adult who is in a skilled care unit and who is recovering from a fractured hip would focus on risk for falls.

Many organizations disseminate guidelines for health promotion interventions, and they are not always in agreement, especially with regard to recommendations for older

---

Box 5-1 Evidence-Informed Nursing Practice

Background: One consequence of an aging Canadian population is the need for nurses who are educated and prepared to work with older adults.

Question: What are the attitudes of undergraduate nursing students toward older adults?

Method: Three focus groups were conducted with third-year undergraduate students in a generalist nursing program in a small Canadian city. A qualitative descriptive approach was used to analyse the verbatim transcripts.

Findings: Students had positive reactions to caring for older adults, at least when dementia was not present. However, they also identified that they received strong messages from their clinical instructors and other nursing staff that gerontological nursing is not valued or prestigious.

Implications for Nursing Practice: Practising nurses need to understand their influence upon the professional socialization of students and how this can influence the care of older patients.

Source: Gould, O. N., Dupuis-Blanchard, S., & MacLennan, A. (2013). Canadian nursing students and the care of older patients: How is geriatric nursing perceived? *Journal of Applied Gerontology.* Advance online publication. doi:10.1177/0733464813500585

adults. For example, there is much controversy about the use of vitamin D supplements for overall good health or the prevention of fractures. The Government of Canada does not recommend vitamin D supplements; however, it partly funded the Institute of Medicine's (2010) report *Dietary Reference Intakes (DRIs) for vitamin D and calcium*, which recommends that all adults age 50 years and above consume 800 to 1,000 IU of vitamin D daily. Because there are few food sources of vitamin D and exposure to sunlight is necessary for synthesis of vitamin D, daily supplementation is recommended for older adults (Dore, 2013).

For all older adults, risk-reduction interventions include lifestyle factors, such as weight management, optimal nutrition, adequate physical activity, sufficient sleep, avoidance of secondhand smoke and appropriate stress-relieving techniques. Smoking cessation is a risk-reduction activity for all people who smoke. Health promotion activities to reduce risk may also include the use of over-the-counter medications (e.g., low-dose aspirin), nutritional supplements (e.g., vitamins) and complementary and alternative therapies (e.g., yoga).

Vaccinations (also called immunizations) are an important and often overlooked risk-reduction intervention for older adults. In addition to the vaccinations for influenza, pneumonia and tetanus that have been routinely recommended for decades, a herpes zoster vaccination has been recommended for people aged 60 years and older. Figure 5-2 illustrates an easy-to-read educational handout that nurses can use to teach older adults about vaccinations.

Environmental Modifications

Environmental modifications are health promotion activities when they reduce risks or improve a person's level of functioning. The functional consequences model for promoting wellness addresses environmental modifications as health promotion interventions in relation to many aspects of functioning in the clinically oriented chapters of this text. For example, environmental modifications can be effective health promotion interventions when their implementation reduces fall risks (Chapter 22), improves hearing and vision (Chapters 16 and 17) and prevents urinary incontinence (Chapter 19).

Health Education

Health education is an essential component of health promotion because it focuses on teaching people to engage in self-care activities that are preventive and wellness enhancing. Health education interventions address specific conditions, as well as overall health and functioning. For example, engaging in regular exercise is a major focus of health education because lack of physical activity is well recognized as a risk factor that contributes to numerous unhealthy conditions. Additional topics of health education that are important for all adults are nutrition, dental care and avoidance of smoking and secondhand smoke (see Chapters 18 and 21). Clinically oriented chapters of this text contain intervention

boxes with guidelines for teaching older adults and their caregivers about specific aspects of health and functioning (refer to list at the end of the table of contents of this book). It is imperative to incorporate cultural considerations in health education and to address health literacy as discussed in Chapter 2. Nurses can use Box 5-2 as a guide to teaching older adults about the most widely agreed-on guidelines for health promotion interventions.

Resources for Health Promotion

Many national nonprofit and governmental organizations provide publications and web-based information related to prevention of specific conditions, such as cancer and cardiovascular disease. National organizations also provide valuable information related to self-management of chronic conditions (e.g., arthritis and diabetes) that can be used for health promotion. In addition, links to pertinent resources are provided in the Online Learning Activities in this book. Nurses can access resources related to the national programs for health promotion for older adults listed in Box 5-3 through the links in Online Learning Activity 5-2.

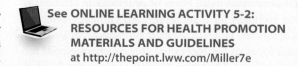

See **ONLINE LEARNING ACTIVITY 5-2:**
RESOURCES FOR HEALTH PROMOTION
MATERIALS AND GUIDELINES
at http://thepoint.lww.com/Miller7e

Promotion of Physical Activity as a Nursing Intervention for Wellness

Articles about the need for increased physical activity are ubiquitous in lay and professional literature, and physical activity has emerged as the most widely heralded health promotion intervention today. In recent years, there is increasing emphasis on the premise that moderate-intensity physical activity can improve overall health and quality of life and lower the risk for disease. Numerous studies identify all the following health benefits of physical activity:

- Weight control
- Decreased risk of cardiovascular disease, diabetes, metabolic syndrome and some cancers
- Strengthening of bones and muscles
- Reduced risk for falls
- Improved mental health and mood, including alleviation of mild depression
- Improved functioning in daily activities
- Increased longevity (e.g., Fortes et al., 2013; Ip et al., 2013; Lee et al., 2013; Public Health Agency of Canada, 2011).

Despite the wealth of well-established evidence about the beneficial effects of physical activity for older adults, less than one third of older people in Canada engage in it regularly. Nurses take many roles in promoting physical activity for older adults, in particular, teaching older adults about the health benefits of physical activity. Nurses also assess for

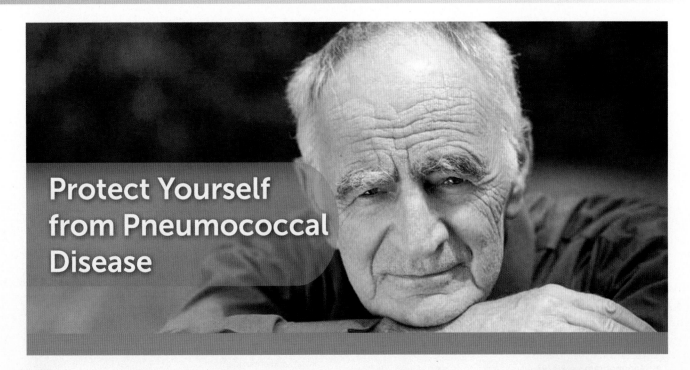

Protect Yourself from Pneumococcal Disease

WHAT IS IT?

Pneumococcal disease (a common complication of influenza) is a bacterial disease that can cause three serious infections:
- meningitis (brain infection)
- bacteremia (bloodstream infection)
- pneumonia (lung infection)

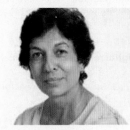

WHO IS AT RISK?

Adults:
- with a chronic illness such as:
  - heart disease   • diabetes   • HIV   • asthma
- who have smoking-related diseases such as COPD
- without a working spleen
- with weakened immune systems
- who are on immunosuppressive therapies
- 65 years of age and older

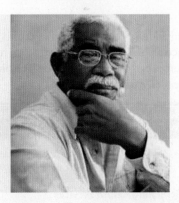

PNEUMOCOCCAL VACCINES ARE SAFE AND EFFECTIVE.

Talk to your family physician, nurse, pharmacist or public health office about being immunized.

For more information, visit immunize.ca

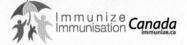
Immunize Immunisation Canada
immunize.ca

FIGURE 5-2 Example of an educational handout to teach older adults about vaccinations.

Box 5-2 Guidelines for Prevention and Health Promotion Interventions for Older Adults

Screening

For Healthy Older Adults

- **Blood pressure:** checks at least annually, more frequently if risk factors are present (e.g., diabetes, race)
- **Serum cholesterol:** every 5 years, more frequently in people with risk, such as personal or family history of cardiovascular disease
- **Fecal occult blood and rectal examination:** screening for colorectal cancer with stool tests, either the fecal occult blood test (FOBT) or fecal immunochemical test (FIT) every 2 years at age 50 and above
- Read more: http://www.cancer.ca/en/cancer-information/cancer-type/colorectal/screening/?region=on#ixzz30zC7COK9
- **Sigmoidoscopy:** every 5 years at age 50–75 years
- **Visual acuity and glaucoma screening:** annually
- **Breast examination:** self-examination monthly, annually by primary care practitioner

For Women

- **Pap smear and pelvic examination:** annually until three consecutive negative examinations, then every 3 years until age 69 years; after age 70, may stop being tested, after three negative Pap tests in a row over 10 years
- **Mammogram:** every 2–3 years at age 50–69 years; at ages 70–74, routinely screening every 2–3 years

For Men

- **Digital rectal examination:** annually

For Older Adults With Risk Factors

- Blood glucose level
- Thyroid function

- Heart function (electrocardiography)
- Bone density
- Mental status assessment
- Screening for dementia, depression, substance abuse
- Urinary incontinence assessment
- Functional assessment
- Screening for adverse medication effects and drug interactions
- Skin cancer assessment
- Fall risk assessment
- Pressure ulcer assessment
- Elder abuse or neglect assessment
- HIV screening
- Abdominal aortic aneurysm

For Men

- Prostate-specific antigen (PSA) blood test

Health Promotion Counselling

For All Older Adults (Unless Contraindicated)

- **Exercise:** at least 30 minutes of moderate-intensity physical activity daily
- **Nutrition:** adequate intake of all vitamins and minerals, especially calcium and antioxidants
- **Dental care and prophylaxis:** every 6 months
- **Protective measures:** seat belts, sunscreens, smoke detectors, fall risk prevention

For Older Adults if Applicable

- **Smoking cessation**
- **Substance abuse cessation**
- **Weight loss**
- **Vitamin supplements or low-dose aspirin**

---

and address other factors that positively or negatively influence an older adult to participate in regular physical activity. Nurses can use Figure 5-3 to teach older adults about recommended exercises.

Box 5-3 National Programs for Health Promotion for Older Adults

Public Health Agency of Canada, Centre for Health Promotion, http://www.phac-aspc.gc.ca/chhd-sdsh/index-eng.php

Screening Health Services

- Breast Cancer Society of Canada, http://www.bcsc.ca/p/48/l/102/t/Breast-Cancer-Society-of-Canada---Regional-Breast-Cancer-Screening
- Canadian Breast Cancer Foundation, http://www.cbcf.org/central/AboutBreastHealth/EarlyDetection/Mammography/Pages/Where-to-Get-a-Mammogram.aspx
- Canadian Diabetic Association, http://guidelines.diabetes.ca/ScreeningAndDiagnosis.aspx
- Canadian Task Force on Preventative Health Care, canadiantaskforce.ca
- Colon-rectal Cancer Screening, http://www.cancerview.ca/idc/groups/public/documents/webcontent/rl_cancer_1crcscreen.pdf
- Public Health Agency of Canada, http://cbpp-pcpe.phac-aspc.gc.ca/interventions/community-based-screening-depression-suicide-prevention/

MODELS OF BEHAVIOUR CHANGE FOR HEALTH PROMOTION

Health promotion interventions for preventing disease often require a change from detrimental health-related behaviours to those that enhance wellness. Even after people adopt new behaviours, they need to maintain these healthier behaviours and not revert to unhealthy ones. The more ingrained and rewarding or pleasurable the behaviours that must be changed, the more difficult it is to refrain from these activities. Some unhealthy behaviours, such as cigarette smoking, have a strong addictive component that increases the difficulty of behaviour change. Similarly, the more comfortable a person is with the absence of healthy behaviours, such as physical activity, the more difficult it will be to develop healthier behaviours.

Initiation and maintenance of healthy behaviours involve both motivation and action steps. The role of gerontological health care professionals in health promotion interventions is to lead and support the older person in replacing unhealthy behaviours with health-promoting behaviours. The **Stages of Change model** (also called the Transtheoretical model) has been widely used by health care professionals to explain stages of behaviour change. During the last three decades,

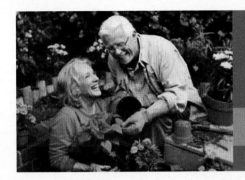

Tips to Get Active

> Physical Activity Tips for Older Adults (65 years and older)

Physical activity plays an important role in your health, well-being and quality of life.
These tips will help you improve and maintain your health by being physically active every day.

1
Take part in at least
**2.5 hours of moderate- to
vigorous-intensity aerobic
activity each week.**

2
Spread out the activities
into sessions of
10 minutes or more.

3
It is beneficial to **add muscle
and bone strengthening activities**
using major muscle groups **at least
twice a week.** This will help your
posture and balance.

Tips to help you get active

☑ Find an activity you like such as
swimming or cycling.

☑ **Minutes count** — increase your activity
level 10 minutes at a time. Every little
bit helps.

☑ **Active time can be social time** — look
for group activities or classes in your
community, or get your family or friends
to be active with you.

☑ Walk wherever and whenever you can.

☑ Take the stairs instead of the elevator,
when possible.

☑ Carry your groceries home.

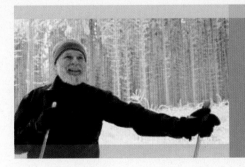
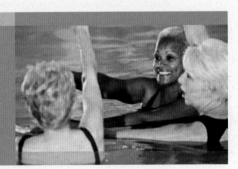

- **Start slowly**
- **Listen to your body**
- **Every step counts**

Public Health   Agence de la santé
Agency of Canada   publique du Canada

Canada

FIGURE 5-3 Example of an educational handout about recommended types of exercise for older adults.

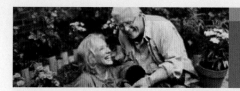

Tips to Get Active

> Physical Activity Tips for Older Adults (65 years and older)

The Health Benefits of Being Active

> IMPROVE YOUR BALANCE
> REDUCE FALLS AND INJURIES
> HELP YOU STAY INDEPENDENT LONGER

> HELP PREVENT HEART DISEASE, STROKE, OSTEOPOROSIS, TYPE 2 DIABETES, SOME CANCERS AND PREMATURE DEATH

Aerobic activity, like PUSHING A LAWN MOWER, TAKING A DANCE CLASS, OR BIKING TO THE STORE, is continuous movement that makes you feel warm and breathe deeply.

Strengthening activity, like LIFTING WEIGHTS OR YOGA, keeps muscles and bones strong and prevents bone loss. It will also improve your balance and posture.

What is moderate aerobic activity?	What is vigorous aerobic activity?	What are strengthening activities?
Moderate-intensity aerobic activity makes you breathe harder and your heart beat faster. You should be able to talk, but not sing.	Vigorous-intensity aerobic activity makes your heart rate increase quite a bit and you won't be able to say more than a few words without needing to catch your breath.	Muscle-strengthening activities build up your muscles. With bone-strengthening activities, your muscles push and pull against your bones. This helps make your bones stronger.
› Examples of moderate activity include walking quickly or bike riding.	› Examples of vigorous activity include jogging or cross-country skiing.	› Examples of muscle-strengthening activities include climbing stairs, digging in the garden, lifting weights, push-ups and curl-ups. › Examples of bone-strengthening activities include yoga, walking and running.

www.publichealth.gc.ca/paguide

Every step counts!
If you're not active now, adding any amount of physical activity can bring some health benefits. Take a step in the right direction. Start now and slowly increase your physical activity to meet the recommendations.

More physical activity provides greater health benefits!
That means the more you do, the better you'll feel. Get active and see what you can accomplish! Move more!

Is physical activity safe for everyone?
The recommended level of physical activity applies to all adults aged 65 years and older who do not have a suspected or diagnosed medical condition. Consult a health professional if you are unsure about the types and amounts of physical activity most appropriate for you.

Canadian Physical Activity Guidelines were developed by the Canadian Society for Exercise Physiology and are available at: www.csep.ca/guidelines

Cat.: HP10-16/4-2011E-PDF   ISBN: 978-1-100-18925-3

FIGURE 5-3 *(continued)*

the Stages of Change has been used successfully in programs for stress management, sun exposure, smoking cessation, medication compliance, alcohol and drug cessation, diet and weight control and screening for cancers. As the name implies, the Stages of Change model describes five specific stages through which a person progresses in accomplishing behaviour changes (Table 5-1).

In the first stage, *precontemplation*, the person is unaware of the problem, is in denial of the need for change,

or is resistant to change. At this stage, the person has no intention of changing his or her behaviours within the next 6 months. Appropriate health promotion interventions for a person in this stage include providing information about the problem behaviour and providing unconditional encouragement for thinking about behaviour change. When working with an older adult in this stage, gerontological nurses can offer information, discuss their own beliefs and help the person identify the personal benefits of the health-promoting

TABLE 5-1 Applying the Stages of Change Model to Mrs. H.

Stage	Nurse	Mrs. H.
I: Precontemplation		
Assessment	"I know you're concerned about preventing heart disease because you've talked with me about your high blood pressure and you pay attention to avoiding high-fat foods. How do you think you rate on a scale of 1–10, with 1 being the lowest level and 10 being the best, in level of physical activity for preventing heart disease?"	"I would rate myself about 10. I take the dog out for a 5-minute walk every morning. My friend says we don't need more than 10 minutes of walking a day after we're 70 years old."
Intervention	"Did you know that there is extremely good evidence that 30 minutes of physical activity every day—even if it's not done all at once—is a good measure for protecting against heart disease? Would you be willing to read this information from the Heart and Stroke Foundation and let me know what you think when I see you again next week?"	"I've seen that before, but I'll try to read it this week if I have a chance."
II: Contemplation		
Assessment	"Now that you've had a chance to read that information, what's your understanding of the role of physical activity in preventing heart problems?"	"I think the Heart and Stroke Foundation is on an exercise kick—they must think we all want to participate in marathons! Maybe they have a point about walking more than 15 min a day, but don't they realize that those of us who are in our 70s have a lot of problems walking? Most of us have arthritis. I think that brochure was written for people in their 20s, but on the other hand, maybe they do know what they're talking about."
Intervention	"From what I know, the Heart and Stroke Foundation focuses on helping people prevent heart disease through healthy habits. They strongly urge everyone to do physical exercise for 30 minutes every day to keep the heart healthy. Many studies of people of all ages support this recommendation. You already walk 5 minutes with your dog every day, so you've gotten a good start on daily exercise. I bet your dog would love to go just a little farther each day and you would be quite capable of increasing your walk by just a little bit."	"Well, the dog is getting pretty fat, and it would probably do her good to get out for another walk in the evening. But it's hard enough for me to get out once a day with the weather as cold as it is right now. With my arthritis, I think I should wait a couple of months until the weather is warmer."
III: Preparation		
Assessment	"Since we met a couple of months ago, what are your current thoughts about increasing your walking?"	"I've been doing a lot of thinking about what we discussed, and now that spring is finally here, I think it's time to increase my walking time by a little bit each day. I just hope my arthritis doesn't get worse if I walk more."
Intervention	"So, have you thought of a plan that might work for you? Can you identify people who might be helpful in supporting your efforts?"	"Well, to begin with, I thought I could walk for 10 minutes every morning instead of 5—my dog sure would like that. I could increase that by 5 minutes every few weeks until I get up to 30 minutes a day. I've told my daughter that I'm trying to do more walking, and she said she might come over and walk with me and the dog on Saturdays. I do worry about my arthritis, though."
IV: Action		
Assessment	"It's so good to hear that you've been increasing your walking time for 3 months now. Congratulations on getting up to 30 minutes a day. How are you feeling about that?"	"My dog sure likes it, but I'm not sure that it's doing any good for me. I guess it feels good to pay attention to my health, but I haven't noticed that I'm feeling any better physically—at least not yet. My daughter came with me for the first few weeks and that was a good chance to see her, but she hasn't been coming for the last 3 weeks."

(continued)

TABLE 5-1 Applying the Stages of Change Model to Mrs. H. *(continued)*

Stage	Nurse	Mrs. H.
Intervention	"You deserve a lot of credit for accomplishing your goal—do you give yourself any rewards? It sounds as though you're disappointed that your daughter stopped walking with you—is there anyone else who might walk with you?"	"I guess I do deserve some credit—I did buy myself a new pair of walking shoes last week. A neighbour lady has talked to me about my walking and she said she'd like to get out there and join me, but I didn't encourage that because I thought my daughter would be coming with me. Maybe I'll invite her along—she could use the exercise, too."
V: Maintenance		
Assessment	"Congratulations on walking for 30 minutes every day for 7 months—that's quite an accomplishment and a nice gift for yourself and your health. You also deserve credit for getting your neighbour to join you at least a couple of days a week. Are you concerned about any temptations to cut down on your walking routine?"	"Thanks for the encouragement—my neighbour says she appreciates me inviting her along, and I enjoy the chance to keep up on neighbourhood happenings by chatting with her when we walk. I am a little concerned about keeping up with the walking during the winter. I don't even take the dog out when it snows."
Intervention	"Have you thought about walking in the mall when the weather is bad? I'm not sure if you can take the dog along, but the mall opens every day an hour before the stores open so that walkers can come. I understand there's quite a group that walks there in the mornings."	"That sounds like a good idea—my neighbour mentioned that we might go there in bad weather. I think I'll try that out—maybe if I went to the mall, I could get my daughter to meet me there on Saturdays."

behaviours. The nurse also can acknowledge the person's perspective and point out the negative consequences of current behaviours.

The second stage, *contemplation*, is characterized by an intention to change in the foreseeable future, on the basis of some acknowledgment of the negative consequences of current behaviours and positive consequences of different behaviours. The person is likely to ask questions and to seek information about the short- and long-term risks and benefits of various behaviours. He or she is likely to be ambivalent about giving up a rewarding activity or taking on an activity that is viewed as difficult or less enjoyable. During this stage, the gerontological nurse can help the person see that the benefits outweigh the disadvantages, even though the person may not experience the benefits immediately. Appropriate health promotion interventions for this stage include providing additional information about the risks and benefits and exploring with the person how he or she can begin establishing personal goals for a healthier lifestyle. Interventions also include increasing the person's sense of self-efficacy by helping the person to see himself or herself practising these new behaviours. When working with an older adult in this stage, it is helpful to express confidence in the person's ability to develop health-promoting behaviours.

Stage three, the *preparation* stage, is characterized by some ambivalence about the unhealthy behaviour but a stronger inclination to change to healthier behaviours. The person acknowledges the need for change, expresses serious intent to adopt the healthier behaviours within the next month and begins to identify strategies for implementing them. During this stage, people usually benefit from support from family and friends, and they are likely to state their intentions and seek help from others in accomplishing their goals. Gerontological nurses can support and provide positive reinforcement for the person's intent to change; they also can point out the progress that the person already has made in developing an action plan. An important role for nurses is to assist with developing a plan and identifying the person's goals and small-step strategies to achieve them. Although discussing the barriers to changing behaviours might be necessary, it is important to focus on the benefits of the new behaviour. Planning strategies for dealing with anticipated difficulties in implementing the plan is also helpful.

Action, the fourth stage, occurs when the person has already made the behaviour change, but the changes have been practised for less than 6 months. At this stage, people usually do not fully experience the benefits of the new behaviour and are vulnerable to resuming prior unhealthy behaviours or giving up the new healthy behaviours. At the same time, they are likely to have high levels of self-efficacy and to feel good about the progress they have made. Health promotion interventions during this stage are directed toward reinforcing the progress that has been made, as well as toward identifying any barriers to continuing the healthy behaviours. Gerontological nurses can help the older adult identify motivators, establish a reward system and plan strategies for overcoming the identified obstacles. They can also ask about support from friends and family and help the person identify ways of extending their support system if necessary.

Stage five, *maintenance*, occurs when the person has continued the healthy behaviours for 6 months or longer. By this time, the person is experiencing positive effects of the healthier behaviour and the risk of relapse is less. During this stage, levels of self-efficacy are usually high and the person is motivated to maintain the healthier lifestyle. Because the person has less need for external support, the role of the gerontological nurse diminishes. Health promotion interventions during this stage include reinforcement of progress and positive feedback about the healthier behaviours. In addition, the nurse can ask about any difficulties in maintaining the progress and help the person identify strategies to overcome any difficulties.

Models of behaviour change that have been developed more recently are based on a positive approach and build on the person's strengths. Motivational interviewing is an example of a positive model in which the health care professional assumes the role of a "change coach" and works in partnership with the person. This model emphasizes all the following:

- Personal autonomy and self-responsibility
- Capacity rather than incapacity
- Actions to facilitate change, rather than reasons for avoiding change
- Communication techniques of affirmation, summarizing, reflective listening, open-ended questions and avoid argumentation or direct persuasion
- Discussion about the person's awareness of the problem, main concerns, intention to change and confidence about changing
- Exploration of goals and the costs and benefits of changing versus not changing
- Communicating empathy, caring and a genuine interest in the person's perspective

Although the full use of motivational interviewing requires extensive training, nurses can apply a brief form to health promotion interventions (Noordam et al., 2013; Stawnychy et al., 2014). Online Learning Activity 5-3 provides a link to an article describing the application of brief motivational interviewing to effectively improve the health behaviours of a challenging patient with heart failure.

See **ONLINE LEARNING ACTIVITY 5-3:**
ARTICLE DESCRIBING APPLICATION OF MOTIVATIONAL INTERVIEWING TO NURSING CARE OF A PATIENT WITH HEART FAILURE
at http://thepoint.lww.com/Miller7e

Appreciative inquiry is another positive model that has recently been applied to promoting behaviour change in health care settings. This model replaces deficit thinking with possibility thinking and uses a set of questions to appreciate and value the best of what is, to envision a future of what might be and to dialogue about and create what will be. The process is divided into four steps designated as discover, dream, design and delivery. Moore and Charvat (2007) proposed that nurses use the appreciative inquiry approach to explore the person's experiences of what works or has worked to promote health, as in the following questions for each of the four steps:

- Discover: Describe a time when you had an exceptionally healthy lifestyle and consider the following questions: What did you appreciate about the experience? How did you make this happen? What people or situational factors supported this positive experience?
- Dream: Imagine that you are so physically active that you feel very fit and healthy and consider the following questions: What would you feel like on a daily basis? What would you be doing? How would you look? What would you be doing for exercise? How do you think it would help your heart?
- Design: What could you do now to be more in charge of your own health and care? Who would you go to for help?
- Delivery: What are we going to do to start this process?

Through this interaction, the nurse and client engage in a cooperative search for strengths, passions and life-giving forces, so the patient is open to new possibilities.

Nurses can apply principles from these models as they work with older adults to promote healthy behaviours related to nutrition, physical activity, weight management and other lifestyle factors that increase the risk for disease and affect the person's health and functioning. Nurses also have applied principles of appreciative inquiry to develop a transitional care coaching intervention to improve care for chronically ill medical patients when they are discharged from hospital to home (Scala & Costa, 2014). Although most nurses are not professional health coaches, all nurses can incorporate communication techniques for encouraging behaviour change such as the following: self-efficacy, values clarification, consciousness raising, restructuring, focusing on benefits and strengthening social support. Box 5-4 briefly describes these interventions and provides examples of communication techniques that can be used to help older adults increase healthy behaviours or decrease those that endanger their health.

Case Study

Mrs. H. is 72 years old and visits the local senior centre three times weekly for meals and social activities. Once a month she comes to see you to have her blood pressure checked. You have recently studied the Stages of Change and are interested in applying it to your clinical work in the senior wellness program. Mrs. H. takes medication for high blood pressure and has expressed concern about heart disease. When you discuss risk factors for heart disease with Mrs. H., she says that she would like to incorporate more physical activity into her daily life, as long as it doesn't worsen her arthritis. She agrees to begin meeting with you regularly to develop a plan. Table 5-1 shows how you might apply the Stages of Change to your work with Mrs. H.

Case Study (continued)

THINKING POINTS

Precontemplation Stage

- From a health promotion perspective, how would you assess Mrs. H.'s understanding of the role of exercise in preventing heart disease? What misconceptions would you want to address?
- What are the goals of your teaching interventions at this stage?

Contemplation Stage

- How would you assess Mrs. H.'s perception of the advantages and disadvantages of increased levels of exercise?
- What are the goals of your teaching interventions at this stage?
- What additional teaching points would you incorporate in your health promotion interventions at this time?

Preparation Stage

- What additional assessment questions would you ask Mrs. H.?
- What are the goals of your teaching interventions at this stage?
- What additional teaching points would you incorporate, particularly with regard to Mrs. H.'s concerns about her arthritis?

Action Stage

- What concerns would you have about Mrs. H. during this stage, and what additional questions would you ask?
- What additional teaching points would you make?

Maintenance Stage

- What additional assessment questions would you ask Mrs. H.?
- What additional teaching points would you make?

Box 5-4 Communication Techniques for Encouraging Behaviour Change

Self-efficacy: increasing the older adult's confidence in accomplishing the desired behaviour
- "You deserve a lot of credit for losing those first 5 pounds. Sometimes those are the hardest ones to lose, so you can be confident that you can keep making progress pound by pound."
- "Think about a time when you were successful in the face of a challenge, even though you weren't confident."
- "Describe a personal characteristic that helps you accomplish your goals."

Values clarification: helping older adults identify values in order to reconcile differences between expectations and behaviours
- "People often have mixed feelings about changing behaviours. For example, you know that being overweight increases the risks to your health, but at the same time, you enjoy eating. Let's talk about the ways in which your health is important to you."
- "It sounds like you have a conflict between believing that getting more exercise is good for your health and believing that you have time for this. Let's talk about how you can use your time to support your health."

Consciousness raising: increasing the older adult's awareness about risks that are identified objectively (e.g., elevated blood pressure or abnormal laboratory values for lipids) but are not associated with immediate symptoms
- "Your blood pressure has been around 156/90 for several weeks lately. Are you aware that the ideal range is below 120/80?"
- "Your weight has been increasing during the last 3 years and it is at the point that you are at an increased risk for diabetes, especially because you also have high blood pressure."

Restructuring: using positive thinking to focus on ways of overcoming barriers

- "I know it's hard to get outside in the winter, so let's try to identify some ways of getting more exercise indoors during your usual activities. For instance, are there times that you could walk in shopping malls or even around your house?"
- "You've identified several barriers to achieving your goal. Can you pick the one that is the easiest to tackle and we'll see if we can find some ways to overcome that. I know that one of your strengths is facing your challenges, so let's look at one of those challenges and come up with a strategy that might work for you."

Focusing on benefits (also called reinforcing rewards): immediately and frequently reinforcing benefits, which are classified as tangible, social or self-generated
- "Describe how you felt the last time you were at your ideal body weight."
- "Can you identify a healthy reward for engaging in physical activity, for example, by treating yourself to fresh fruit after you come back from the park?"
- "Let's talk about the benefits of quitting smoking. For example, within a day of quitting you've already decreased your risk for heart attack. Can you think of another benefit?"

Strengthening social support: involving family and friends in healthy behaviours
- "That's an excellent idea to walk with your friend for a half-hour right after you both come back from the lunch program at the senior centre."
- "When your grandchildren visit, would it be feasible to take them to the park or a playground?"

Adapted from Miller C. A. (2013). *Fast facts for health promotion in nursing: Promoting wellness in a nutshell* (used with permission from Springer).

Chapter Highlights

Gerontology and Geriatrics

- Gerontology and geriatrics are areas of professional specialization that have evolved since the mid-20th century to address the unique needs of older adults.
- The original focus of these specialties was on problems associated with aging, but the current focus is on quality-of-life issues and promoting optimal health and functioning.

Gerontological Nursing as a Specialty and a Responsibility

- Gerontological nursing was first recognized as a specialty in Canada by the Gerontological Nurses Association; major strides have been made in advancing this specialization through professional nursing organizations (Fig. 5-1).
- There is increasing recognition that all nurses in adult health care settings need to be competent in addressing the complex and unique health care needs of older adults.
- The current perspective of health care providers and policy makers recognizes the dual need for specialized gerontological nurses and for all nurses in adult clinical settings to develop skills in caring for older adults.
- Many evidence-based resources are available for nurses and nursing students to develop competency in care of older adults.

Health, Wellness and Health Promotion

- Health promotion programs currently include both the traditional focus on disease prevention and health maintenance and the more recent focus on personal responsibility for health self-care actions to achieve high-level wellness.
- Health promotion programs are effective for reducing health care costs and for improving health-related quality of life.
- Older adults in ethnic and racial minority groups access and receive fewer preventive care services compared with white older adults.

Health Promotion for Older Adults

- Nurses have important roles in health promotion interventions, which are essential for preventing chronic conditions, reducing mortality and improving quality of life for older adults.
- Types of health promotion interventions for older adults include screening programs, risk-reduction interventions, environmental modifications and health education (Box 5-2 and Fig. 5-2).
- Many national nonprofit and governmental organizations provide publications and web-based information for health promotion related to specific conditions (Box 5-2).
- Nurses have important roles in teaching older adults about the benefits of physical activity and promoting exercise (Fig. 5-3).

Models of Behaviour Change for Health Promotion

- The Stages of Change model has been used to address disease prevention and health promotion interventions that require a change in health-related behaviours (Table 5-1).
- Positive models of behaviour change include motivational interviewing and appreciative inquiry.
- Nurses can incorporate communication techniques to address all the following: self-efficacy, values clarification, consciousness raising, restructuring, focusing on benefits and strengthening social support (Box 5-4).

Critical Thinking Exercises

1. Describe the development of gerontological nursing from the 1960s to the present.
2. You are asked to give a presentation to beginning nursing students to recruit them for an elective class called "Nursing for Wellness in Older Adults." What topics would you expect to be covered in this course, and what points would you make to encourage them to enlist in this course?
3. You are discussing with your fellow students the choices you will be making about a practice area after graduation. You tell them that you are planning to specialize in gerontological nursing, and they challenge your decision with statements such as "You'll be bored to death taking care of old folks. Why don't you specialize in something exciting like trauma care? Besides, there's not much to do about the conditions of older folks, and what's the challenge in taking care of people who aren't going to get better?" How do you respond to these statements?
4. Identify one health-related behaviour that you would like to change in your life (e.g., smoking cessation, increased level of exercise, decreased dietary fat intake) and develop a care plan for your behaviour change using the Stages of Change of Health Promotion (as in the case study).

REFERENCES

Canadian Associations of Schools of Nursing. (2011). *Position statement: Baccalaureate education and Baccalaureate programs*. Retrieved from http://www.casn.ca/vm/newvisual/attachments/856/Media/BaccalaureatePositionStatementEnglishFinal.pdf

Canadian Gerontological Nursing Association. (2010). *Gerontological nursing competencies and standards of practice*. Retrieved from http://www.cgna.net/Standards_of_Practice.html

Canadian Hospice Palliative Care Association. (2012). *Advance care planning in Canada: National framework*. Retrieved from http://www.advancecareplanning.ca/media/40158/acp%20framework%20 2012%20eng.pdf

Canadian Nurses Association. (2008). *Code of ethics*. Ottawa, ON: Author.

Dore, R. K. (2013). Should healthy people take calcium and vitamin D to prevent fractures? What the U.S. Preventive Services Task Force and others say. *Cleveland Clinic Journal of Medicine, 80*(6), 341–344.

Fortes, C., Mastroeni, S., Sperati, A., et al. (2013). Walking four times weekly for at least 15 minutes is associated with longevity in a cohort of very elderly people. *Maturitas, 74*, 246–251.

Frank, L. K. (1946). Gerontology. *Journal of Gerontology, 1*(1), 1–11.

Fried, T. R., Redding, C. A., O'Leary, J., et al. (2012). Promoting advance care planning as health behaviour change. *Patient Education and Counselling, 86*(1), 25–32.

Gould, O. N., Dupuis-Blanchard, S., & MacLennan, A. (2013). Canadian nursing students and the care of older patients: How is geriatric nursing perceived? *Journal of Applied Gerontology.* Advance online publication. doi:10.1177/0733464813500585

Gustafsson, S., Wilhelmson, K., Eklund, K., et al. (2012). Health-promoting interventions for persons aged 80 and older are successful in the short term: Results from the randomized and three-armed elderly persons in the Risk Zone study. *Journal of the American Geriatrics Society, 60*(3), 447–454.

Institute of Medicine. (2010). *Dietary reference intakes for calcium and vitamin D.* Washington, DC: National Academies Press.

Ip, E. H., Church, T., Marshall, S. A., et al. (2013). Physical activity increases gains in and prevents loss of physical function: Results from the lifestyle interventions and independence for elders pilot study. *Journals of Gerontology: Biological sciences and Medical Sciences, 68*(4), 426–432.

Lee, H., Lee, J.-A., Brar, J. S., et al. (2013). Physical activity and depressive symptoms in older adults. *Geriatric Nursing, 35*, 37–41.

Mariano, C. (2013). Holistic nursing: Scope and standards of practice. In B. M. Dossey & L. Keegan (Eds.), *Holistic nursing: A handbook for practice* (6th ed., pp. 59–83). Boston, MA: Jones and Bartlett.

Moore, S. M., & Charvat, J. (2007). Promoting health behaviour change using appreciative inquiry: Moving from deficit models to affirmation models of care. *Family & Community Health Nursing, 30*(15 Suppl. 1), S64–S74.

Noordam, J., de Vet, E., van der Weijden, T., et al. (2013). Motivational interviewing within the different stages of change: An analysis of practice nurse-patient consultations aimed at promoting a healthier lifestyle. *Social Sciences & Medicine, 87*, 60–67.

Pascucci, M. A., Chu, N., & Leasure, A. R. (2012). Health promotion for the oldest of old people. *Nursing Older People, 24*(3), 22–28.

Public Health Agency of Canada. (2011). *Physical activity.* Retrieved from http://www.phac-aspc.gc.ca/hp-ps/hl-mvs/pa-ap/index-eng.php

Rizzuto, D., Orsini, N., Qui, C., et al. (2012). Lifestyle, social factors, and survival after age 75: Population based study. *British Medical Journal, 345*, e5568. doi:10.1136/bmj.35568

Scala, E., & Costa, L. (2014). Using appreciative inquiry during care transitions. *Journal of Nursing Care Quality, 29*(1), 44–50.

Stawnychy, M., Creber, R. M., & Riegel, B. (2014). Using brief motivational interviewing to address the complex needs of a challenging patient with heart failure. *Journal of Cardiovascular Nursing, 29*(5), E1–E6.

The Conference Board of Canada. (2013). *Health matters: An economic perspective.* Retrieved from http://www.conferenceboard.ca/e-library/abstract.aspx?did=5309

Touhy, E. L. (1946). Geriatrics: The general setting. *Geriatrics: Official Journal of the American Geriatrics Society, 1*(1), 17–20.

Vascular Health. (2013). *Making the connection: A call to action on vascular health.* Retrieved from http://www.canadianstrokenetwork.ca/wp-content/uploads/2013/10/VascularDeclaration_ENG-1.pdf

chapter 6

Health Care Settings for Older Adults

LEARNING OBJECTIVES

After reading this chapter, you will be able to:

1. Describe commonly available types of community-based services for older adults.

2. Describe the types of home care services and explain how people obtain these services.

3. Explain the difference between skilled nursing home care and long-term nursing home care.

4. Discuss issues related to quality of care in nursing homes and efforts of the nursing home culture change movement to address these issues.

5. Discuss ways in which concerns about quality of care for hospitalized older adults are being addressed.

6. Apply Quality and Safety in Nursing (QSEN) competencies to care of older adults.

7. Discuss ways in which nurses address needs of caregivers.

8. Describe sources of payment for health care services for older adults.

KEY POINTS

acute care for elders (ACE)	medicare
adult day centres	nonmedical home care
continuum of care	quality and safety education for nurses (QSEN)
faith community nursing	
geriatric care manager	resident-centred care
geriatric resource nurse (GRN)	respite care
insurance gap	skilled home care
long-term care insurance	telehealth
	transitional care

Although nurses have always cared for older adults, only relatively recently have programs been developed to address the unique health care needs of older adults. This chapter presents information about the wide array of services that address the needs of older adults, starting with those that are community based and proceeding to those that are institutionally based. However, even this distinction is not always clear because older adults typically receive care in several places, and some services, such as skilled care and hospice, are provided in both community and institutional settings. Because health care providers and policy makers are currently focusing on major concerns related to both quality and coordination of care, this chapter discusses the roles of nurses in addressing these issues.

The federal government works collaboratively with all jurisdictions; however, the management and delivery of health care to Canadians is the responsibility of the provinces/territories. The federal government implemented a universal medicare system in 1972 based upon the Medical Care Act of 1968. The informal name given to this system of **Medicare** (discussed later in this chapter) stimulated major changes in the delivery of health care services to older adults, primarily in terms of increased access to care for older adults. During the 1990s, policy makers and health care providers began raising serious concerns about Medicare because while it provided payment for hospital services, it did not address duplication of services and increasing financial costs related to duplication of services. Consequently, the 1990s was an era of health care reform. More recent provincial and federal health commissions have recommended reforms to the Canada Health Act (CHA) to cover more than "medical" treatment. These concerns have led to the current emphasis on the "triple aim" of improving care, improving health and reducing costs (Ouslander & Maslow, 2012). All jurisdictions and many national organizations are addressing these concerns, resulting in a wave of major changes in delivery of health care services to older adults. See Figure 6-1 for significant actions by governments and national associations that have influenced the care and services provided to older adults.

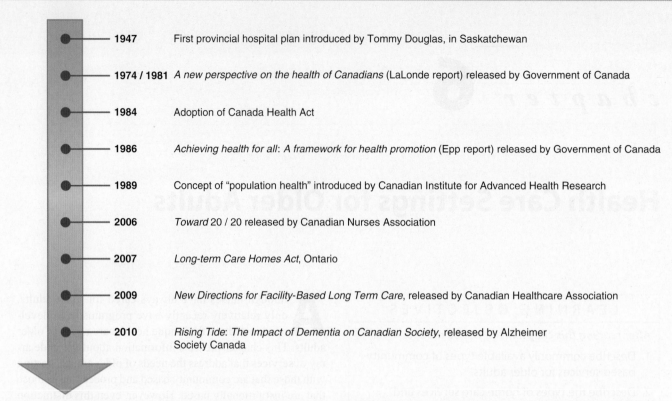

1947	First provincial hospital plan introduced by Tommy Douglas, in Saskatchewan
1974 / 1981	*A new perspective on the health of Canadians* (LaLonde report) released by Government of Canada
1984	Adoption of Canada Health Act
1986	*Achieving health for all: A framework for health promotion* (Epp report) released by Government of Canada
1989	Concept of "population health" introduced by Canadian Institute for Advanced Health Research
2006	*Toward 20 / 20* released by Canadian Nurses Association
2007	*Long-term Care Homes Act*, Ontario
2009	*New Directions for Facility-Based Long Term Care*, released by Canadian Healthcare Association
2010	*Rising Tide: The Impact of Dementia on Canadian Society*, released by Alzheimer Society Canada

FIGURE 6-1 Significant events that have spurred the development of various models of care for older adults. This list is an overview; review the legislation specific to the jurisdiction in which one practices. (http://www.e-laws.gov.on.ca/html/statutes/english/e-laws_statutes_07l08_e.htm)

It is important to recognize that all programs and institutions that receive Medicare funds—which includes virtually all health care facilities and programs—are directly affected by policies of the federal government. Even when services are not covered by insurance, if the providing agency receives public funds, the services must comply with the CHA and its regulations.

COMMUNITY-BASED SERVICES FOR OLDER ADULT

Public and private agencies have provided many types of community support resources for older adults for decades and the range of these services has been broadening in recent decades (see Fig. 6-2). For example, home-delivered meals programs have been available in most metropolitan areas for decades, and in recent years, groceries and prepared meals have become available for delivery within 24 hours through Internet sites or toll-free phone numbers. Although community-based services are widely available, older adults and their caregivers often are not aware of the great variety of services available to meet the health needs of older adults in their own homes. Even when they are aware of such services, they may not know the eligibility criteria for publicly funded services to which they are entitled. Also, if community-based services are not culturally relevant, older adults or their families may not use them, even when they are aware of their existence. For example, South Asian Canadians have higher levels of unmet needs for dementia services because of lack

of awareness of services, reluctance to use public services and lack of problem recognition (McCleary et al., 2012).

Because the use of these resources may improve the health, functioning and quality of life of older adults, nurses need to address any lack of information about these services. In addition, it is important to address other barriers, such as negative attitudes of family caregivers, by teaching about the positive effects of services for both the older adult and family caregivers (Phillipson & Jones, 2012). Box 6-1 summarizes community-based services and resources that are widely available to address needs of older adults. These services are particularly important for older adults living in their own homes or other independent settings, which includes 92% of all adults aged 65 and above (Statistics Canada, 2012). Online Learning Activity 6-1 provides links to additional information about these types of programs.

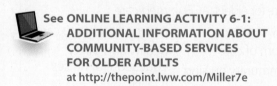

See **ONLINE LEARNING ACTIVITY 6-1: ADDITIONAL INFORMATION ABOUT COMMUNITY-BASED SERVICES FOR OLDER ADULTS** at http://thepoint.lww.com/Miller7e

Health Promotion Programs

Because of the growing emphasis on health and wellness, many community-based programs for older adults incorporate health promotion activities. Senior centres and other places where older adults gather often offer periodic health screenings and health education activities. Among the health

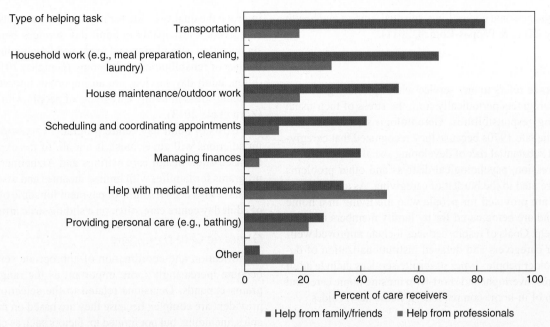

Notes: Includes all activities for which care receiver received help and not only the types of care received from the primary caregiver. Responses of "don't know" and "not stated" are included in the calculation of percentages, but are not shown separately.

FIGURE 6-2 Most common type of care received from family and friends. Includes all activities for which care receiver received help and not only the types of care received from the primary caregiver. Responses of "don't know" and "not stated" are included in the calculation of percentages, but are not shown separately. (Statistics Canada, General Social Survey, 2012)

promotion activities offered by these programs are blood pressure checks; safe driving courses; smoking-cessation classes; health screening (e.g., cancer, vision, hearing); flu shots and other immunizations; medication assessment, management and education; and various types of exercises, such as walking, aerobics, aquatics or tai chi. Health education topics include nutrition, stress management, general health care and seasonal health challenges such as hypothermia, heat-related illness, and colds and flu.

Box 6-1 Community Resources for Older Adults

Senior Information and Referral Service: Local programs, sometimes called an "Infoline," that provide information about agencies to address specific needs

Senior Centres: Community-based centres providing services for older adults, such as meals, limited transportation and social and educational programs

Home-Delivered Meals: Programs that provide home delivery of hot meals to homebound people, sponsored by local senior centres, churches or hospitals

Companions and Friendly Visitors: Programs that offer services such as socially oriented home visits, assistance with errands or accompaniment to appointments

Telephone Reassurance: Service providers make scheduled telephone calls to older people to provide support and reminders

Personal Emergency Response Systems: An emergency response system that involves the use of a "call button" (e.g., necklace or bracelet) to initiate a phone call to designated people when assistance is needed (e.g., if the person falls)

Energy Assistance Programs: Provincial and territorial programs that offer financial assistance for utility bills for people with low incomes

Organized group activities, such as senior wellness programs, frequently take place in, or are sponsored by, community-based senior centres that are available in almost every community. Hospitals and other health care institutions are becoming more involved in providing a broad range of health promotion programs and are employing nurses to address the needs of older adults in the community. Senior centres and health care agencies often co-sponsor programs to address specific health concerns, such as diabetes, glaucoma, cholesterol levels or blood pressure. For example, senior health fairs provide the opportunity for follow-up and referral of identified medical issues. Thus, these programs can provide a valuable health promotion service for older adults and, at the same time, increase the potential patient base for health care providers.

Faith Community Nursing

Faith community nursing (also called parish nursing) formally began in Canada in 1998, with a conference call organized by the Salvation Army and the Catholic Health Organization of Canada. The Canadian Association for Parish Nursing Ministry has been recognized as a specialty interest group by the Canadian Nurses Association. The Canadian Association of Parish Nurses (2013) describes a parish nurse as a nurse with specialized knowledge who is called to the ministry and affirmed by a faith community to promote health, healing and wholeness). Faith community nurses spend 50% to 100% of their time providing services to older adults, such as health education, referrals, health screenings, personal counselling, spiritual support and health advocacy (King & Pappas-Rogich, 2011).

Respite Services

Respite care refers to any service whose primary goal is to relieve caregivers periodically from the stress of their usual caregiving responsibilities. Gerontologists first used this term in the late 1970s because they recognized that caregivers are at substantial risk of developing social isolation, clinical depression, psychological distress and other problems directly related to the burden of caregiving. As such, respite services are provided for people who are living in a home setting and are being cared for by family members or other unpaid help. Goals of respite services include improved well-being for caregivers and delayed institutionalization of dependent older people. Types of respite services include adult day centres, overnight and short-term nursing home care, and provision of in-home companions or home health aides.

Adult Day Centres

Adult day centres have become a major community-based resource for the care of dependent older adults. Baycrest in Toronto opened its adult community day centre in 1959, the first of its kind in Canada (see more at http://www.baycrest. org/care/care-programs/community-programs/adult-day-programs/#sthash.Ea8Wi3fR.dpuf). There are two types of adult day care centres: social and medical. Facilities staffed with medical personnel are sometimes known as adult day health centres. A senior attending an adult day health centre generally requires that a physician complete a health assessment before he or she enters the program. This type of health centre will usually include therapy according to the needs of those in the program, such as physical, speech and occupational therapies. The staff will include registered nurses and other health care professionals.

Social centres provide structured social and recreational activities for functionally impaired older people in a group setting. Both types of adult day centres provide meals and any of the following services: transportation, medication management, assistance with personal care, and other health-related services and therapies. In addition, both types of day centres generally provide supervised care on weekdays for 8 hours a day, with approximately 5 hours of formal programming during that time and 3 hours of social interaction and other unstructured activities. Less commonly, services are available for longer hours and on weekends and holidays.

Participants in adult day centres usually are impaired to the point that they need supervision or assistance in several functional areas. Most participants are cognitively impaired, but depression and physical disabilities are common conditions among adult day centre participants. Participants typically live with a family member, but some live independently or in group settings. The goals of these programs are to maintain or improve the functional abilities of impaired older people, to delay or prevent the need for institutional care, to provide relief for caregivers of dependent older adults and to improve the quality of life for impaired older adults and their caregivers. Participants in adult day services benefit from socialization, stimulation and improved functioning through the use of rehabilitation and therapy (Gaugler, 2014). In addition, adult day services are an important intervention for reducing stress in family caregivers of people with dementia (Zarit et al., 2013).

Costs of adult day centre programs vary widely. Most jurisdictions will cover most, if not all, of the expenses for licensed adult health care settings and Alzheimer's-related programs for families with limited incomes and assets. Families have also been a source of payment for some of the costs of adult day centre care, often on a sliding scale arrangement.

Geriatric Care Managers

Identification and coordination of appropriate services has become increasingly more important as the range of programs expands. Decisions related to the selection of care providers are complex because they are based on many variables, including, but not limited to, factors such as cost, availability and acceptability. Older adults and their families may not be prepared to take on the tasks associated with identifying, arranging and coordinating appropriate services. Two societal trends that have affected the ability and availability of families to manage care for older adults are the entry of more women into the paid workforce and the cross-country, or even international, mobility of adult children families away from their hometowns. These factors, along with the significant increase in the number of people aged 85 years and older, have led to the need for independent, community-based, professional geriatric care management services.

A **geriatric care manager** serves as the primary care coordinator who is responsible for implementing immediate and long-term plans as the needs of the older adult change. Care management services involve comprehensive assessment, care planning, implementation, monitoring and reassessment. Care managers typically work not only with older adults, but also with other professionals, family members, caregivers and support resources. When family members provide care or coordinate services, care managers often provide counselling and education to address the needs of caregivers, who may or may not be older adults themselves. Nurses are in an ideal position to assume the role of a geriatric care manager because they can comprehensively assess the needs for immediate and long-term care services and then plan, coordinate and oversee the services.

Geriatric care managers work either as independent contractors or through nonprofit and for-profit groups and organizations. Although the terms care manager and case manager are sometimes used interchangeably, these roles may be interpreted differently depending upon the setting and jurisdiction in which the older adult resides. Hospitals and community-based agencies (e.g., home care) sometimes use case managers to make sure that patients receive the most appropriate and cost-effective services. Resources for additional information about geriatric care managers are included in Online Learning Activity 6-1.

HOME-BASED SERVICES

Older people and other dependent populations have always received much of their health care at home and visiting nurse services have existed in Canada since the late 19th century. In 1896, Lady Ishbel Aberdeen, wife of Canada's then governor-general, visited Vancouver. During this visit, she heard vivid accounts of the hardship and illnesses affecting women and children in isolated areas of the country. Later that same year, she participated in the annual meeting of the National Council of Women, where she heard similar stories. Lady Aberdeen responded to a resolution passed at this meeting, which asked her to establish an order of visiting nurses in Canada. The order was to be a memorial to the 60th anniversary of Queen Victoria's ascent to the British throne.

The delivery of home care services dramatically changed when Medicare began funding these services through transfer pays to the provinces/territories from the federal government. Although funding was not directly provided for home care services, funds were provided for provinces to use for it at their discretion. (The Canada Health Transfer is the federal government's transfer payment program in support of the health systems of the provinces and territories.) Although home health care services were established as a short-term supplement to acute care services for people who needed skilled care, consumers came to view these services as an extension of long-term care for people with chronic illnesses. In 2009, 25% of older adults reported receiving some level of home-based services in Canada, from either private or public agencies (Statistics Canada, 2012). It is likely that the use of home care is actually greater. Some informal care, for example from a spouse, may not have been reported, since it may be perceived as part of usual support provided to family members.

At the time that the federal government was cutting funds for home care, provincial/territorial governments were addressing the high cost of care in nursing homes—which placed a heavy financial burden on programs—by providing more funds for home- and community-based services. Thus, motivated both by cost containment and by consumer preference, provincial/territorial long-term care policy began shifting to community-based services. Many affordable services have become widely available through public, private and nonprofit agencies.

Over time, two types of home care services—skilled home care and nonmedical home care—have evolved to address different needs. Skilled home care services address the needs of people who are recovering from an illness or injury and have potential for returning to their previous level of functioning. In contrast, nonmedical home care services address needs of people with chronic or declining conditions who do not qualify for skilled care.

Ensuring the availability of home care services in rural areas is particularly important. It is projected that by 2021, one in four older adults will live in a rural setting (Statistics Canada, 2008). Rural home care providers provide care to other groups, such as individuals of all ages recovering from surgeries, with chronic conditions and/or undergoing treatments for cancer and other conditions. In many small rural communities, the visit from the home care provider may be the only access to care that older clients have. Distance, weather, lack of access to or ability to drive or finance transportation, and being ill or in recovery can severely compromise rural older adults' access to care outside their immediate community. Thus rural home care providers are essential to the health of many older adults (Box 6-2).

Box 6-2 Evidence-Informed Nursing Practice

Background: Home care services support older adults remaining within their own homes and in the community instead of entering long-term care facilities prematurely.

Question: What are the gender differences in admission to long-term care facilities from home care services?

Method: A population-based retrospective cohort study was conducted.

Findings: Women were older and outnumbered men; however, men presented with higher levels of needs. While women relied on a child or child-in-law for support, men relied on a spouse. The caregivers of men reported twice as much stress as did those of women.

Implications for Nursing Practice: Nurses need to understand who uses home care services so that programs are developed based upon identified need.

Source: Gruneir, A., Forrester, J., Camacho, X., et al. (2013). Gender differences in home care clients and admission to long-term care in Ontario, Canada: A population-based retrospective cohort study. *BMC Geriatrics, 13,* 48.

Skilled Home Care

Home care services are not mandated by the CHA, although provincial/territorial and sometimes municipal governments provide funding for it. Home care services provided under provincial/territorial health care authorities have always been limited to skilled home care and restricted to people who meet all of the following criteria:

- The person must be homebound (i.e., leaving the home requires considerable and taxing effort).
- The services must be ordered by a primary care provider.
- There must be a need for skilled nursing or rehabilitative services.
- The person must require intermittent, but not full-time, care.

For people who meet these criteria, the following types of home care services may be provided: skilled nursing, physical therapy, occupational therapy, nutrition counselling, speech–language therapy, medical social work, home health aide, and medical supplies and equipment. In addition to nursing assessment and interventions, skilled nursing services can include case management, medication management, infusion therapy, intravenous antibiotics and psychiatric nursing care. Examples of home health aide services that can be provided under the directions of a licensed nurse or therapist include assistance with bathing, linen changes, range-of-motion exercises and assistance with transfers and ambulation. People often qualify for skilled home care after a hospitalization or a stay in a skilled nursing or rehabilitation setting for an acute episode, or they may qualify when they experience a change in their condition, but have not needed

TABLE 6-1 Goals of Home Care in Canada
Goals of Home Care
• Help people maintain or improve their health status and quality of life,
• Assist people in remaining as independent as possible,
• Support families in coping with a family member's need for care,
• Help people stay at or return home and receive needed treatment, rehabilitation or palliative care and
• Provide informal/family caregivers with the support they need.

Source: Health Canada. (2004). *Home and community care.* Retrieved from http://www .hc-sc.gc.ca/hcs-sss/home-domicile/commun/index-eng.php

care in a hospital or nursing home. Table 6-1 identifies the goals of home care.

Because skilled home care services are meant to be short-term, a major focus is on teaching the older person and caregivers about self-care activities. Typical skilled care recipients are (1) people who are homebound but able to manage most of their daily care at some level of independence and (2) people who, although homebound and dependent in many functional areas, receive help from families, friends or paid caregivers to supplement the skilled care services. If people reach a level of independence such that they are no longer homebound, they cannot continue receiving publically funded skilled home care services. Likewise, people no longer qualify for skilled care after they achieve self-care goals. Many people receiving skilled care, however, still need some level of home care services after they no longer qualify for publically funded skilled care and services are discontinued. Private services are available but may not be a financially viable option for some older adults.

With the current emphasis on improving quality and outcomes and reducing costs, health care providers are developing innovative models of care that include skilled home care as an integral component. Examples of such programs are as follows:

● Telepsychiatry service for older adults connecting a university-affiliated geriatric centre to a rural geriatric mental health outreach service in Northwest Ontario (Conn et al., 2013).
● Seniors Centre without Walls Social and Education Program in Manitoba provides free social and educational programming via telephone to older adults (Newall & Menec, 2013).
● The IMPACT clinic (Interprofessional Model of Practice for Aging and Complex Treatments) is a model of interprofessional care for community-dwelling older adults in Ontario (Tracy et al., 2013).

Programs such as these are likely to continue developing as essential components of innovative and comprehensive models of care. Organizations such as the Canadian Nurses Association, the Canadian Home Care Association and the Canadian Medical Association have requested to the federal government that Medicare is expanded to include home care.

Nonmedical Home Care

A wide spectrum of nonmedical home care services are available for the large majority of older adults who need home-based services but do not meet the criteria for skilled home care. At one end of the spectrum is nonskilled care provided by companions, homemakers and home health aides. The most common services are meal preparation, light housekeeping, assistance with personal care, accompaniment to medical appointments, and grocery shopping and other errands. These services are often supplemented by community-based services, such as transportation and home-delivered meals, as described in Box 6-1. Frequency of service ranges from a couple hours monthly to 24 hours daily. A licensed nurse may assess the client and supervise the services, and a registered nurse or licensed practice nurse (registered nursing assistant) usually assists with medication management, if needed.

Sources of Home Care Services

Home care services are available through formal sources (e.g., agencies) or informal sources (e.g., independent caregivers). People who self-pay for home care can obtain services from agencies or from informal sources, but when home care services are covered by insurance or public funds, they traditionally have been provided by agencies under contractual arrangements. Agencies usually provide initial assessments, arrange for services, assign workers, provide ongoing supervision and collect payment for services. They are responsible for hiring, training, directing, scheduling and firing workers. Some agencies provide a wide range of services, including licensed nurses and care managers. Other agencies provide only a limited type of nonmedical service, such as companions or light housekeeping. Some so-called agencies, however, are little more than a registry or referral service. When services are obtained from informal sources rather than from agencies, the care recipient or a surrogate decision maker is responsible for performing the organizational tasks that agencies normally perform (e.g., hiring, firing and supervising the caregiver). In this case, a geriatric care management service (discussed later in this chapter) can be helpful for arranging services and overseeing the care. A common way of finding independent caregivers and other home care resources is through a word-of-mouth network, in which names are obtained from friends, families, churches or local health care agencies.

Roles for Nurses in Home Care

Nurses who provide skilled home care services typically assume a primary coordinating role working with an interprofessional team that can include all or any of the following: primary care providers, psychiatrists, social workers, rehabilitation therapists and home health aides. Nursing responsibilities are usually long-term and involve all of the following skills: assessments, care planning, hands-on care, health education, coordination of care and referrals for additional services. In most home settings, nurses direct their interventions as much toward the caregivers of dependent older people as toward the older people themselves. In this role, they also provide teaching and role modelling about interventions to provide adequate care for the older adult. In addition, they address needs of the caregiver related to information about resources and ways to reduce caregiver stress.

A challenge for nurses working in home care agencies is to keep up-to-date with technological advances that increasingly are an integral part of health care services. In addition to increasing use of electronic health records, technologic advances have significantly influenced the availability of new communication systems that are commonly used in home care. **Telehealth** (also called telemedicine or telecare) is the use of electronic information and communication technologies to provide and support health care when the patient and provider are not in the same proximity. In home care settings, telehealth has been used primarily to collect and transmit assessment information, which is called telemonitoring (or telehealth monitoring). Nurses providing skilled home care services are increasingly incorporating telemonitoring as a tool for improving health outcomes in people with diabetes, hypertension, heart failure and chronic obstructive pulmonary disease (Chang et al., 2013; Fairbrother et al., 2014; Hoban et al., 2013; Nesbitt, 2012). Canada Health Infoway's (n.d.) Telehealth program supports jurisdictional projects that give patients in remote communities better access to timely, relevant health care services. These improvements result from electronic solutions that facilitate the delivery of health information and services between patients and their authorized health care providers, regardless of location. Recent studies have found that use of telemonitoring in home care can improve older adults' ability to manage their care and reduce hospitalization and emergency department visits (Heeke et al., 2014; Woods & Snow, 2013; Zavertnik, 2014).

NURSING HOME SETTINGS

The term **nursing home**, or *long-term care facility,* or *continuing care facility*, refers to a residential institutional setting for people who need assistance with several ADL. Nursing homes are licensed by the province/territory. These facilities are not funded under the CHA, and there are different services, funding levels and definition in each jurisdiction. What is common is that nursing homes are required to have continuous on-site supervision by a registered nurse or a licensed practical nurse. In addition to medical care and nursing services, nursing homes must provide dental, podiatry, medical specialty consultation services and rehabilitation therapies (e.g., physical and occupational therapies). There is some overlap between health care services provided in acute care and nursing home settings, but the care recipients are called *residents* rather than *patients* because these are residential facilities. Nursing home care can be categorized as skilled care.

To qualify *for skilled care in a nursing home*, people must meet the following criteria:
- Have a medical condition that is associated with the need for skilled care
- Have a physician referral for services that must be provided by licensed professionals, such as nurses or therapists
- Require daily skilled care that can be provided appropriately in a skilled nursing facility

Medical costs are covered for people who meet the criteria for skilled care in a nursing facility, *but only as long as the person continues to require the skilled level of services.* Typical diagnoses associated with skilled care in a nursing home are stroke, fractured hip and congestive heart failure. If his or her condition declines, for example with dementia, the person may continue to require a significant level of care without meeting the relatively narrow criteria for skilled care. In these situations, the person usually begins paying for needed care unless family members can provide it.

Long-term care in a nursing home refers to services provided for chronically ill people who need assistance with daily activities. In contrast to admissions for skilled nursing care that usually occur following a hospitalization, admissions for long-term care in a nursing home typically occur after a period of gradual decline in functioning because of a chronic condition, such as dementia. Also, in contrast to skilled nursing home care, insurance programs rarely cover long-term care in a nursing home.

In recent decades, changes in health care services for older adults have significantly influenced both long-term and short-term nursing home care. On any given day, about 5% of older adults are residing in a nursing facility; however, almost half of people older than 65 years are likely to spend some time in a nursing home. These statistics reflect the following major trends in health care for older adults in Canada:
- Account for more than 50% of acute care patient days
- Shorter lengths of hospital stays
- Increased availability of community-based programs that address needs for long-term care
- Increased use of skilled home care services

One result of these trends is that the percentage of long-term residents who are more dependent on assistance with ADL has gradually increased in recent years because people who are less dependent now receive care in other settings, such as assisted-living facilities.

During the 1990s, nursing homes began developing dementia special care units; however, the care in these units was similar to that in other nursing home units. During the early 2000s, Alzheimer Canada and regulatory agencies demanded more accountability for programs that were advertised as dementia special care units. The increasing popularity of assisted-living and other residential care facilities during this same time stimulated the development of dementia special care units within residential care communities.

Quality of Care in Nursing Homes

During the past two decades, health care consumers, providers and organizations have increasingly focused on concerns about quality of care and quality of life for people who need long-term care. This focus stems in part from consumer pressure that began during the 1970s, which addressed the rights of older adults in such facilities. Nursing home residents' rights in Canada have been primarily legislated at the provincial level. In Ontario, for example, the *Long Term Care Homes Act 2007* contains a "Residents' Bill of Rights," including, *inter alia*, the rights to be treated with courtesy and respect, to privacy in treatment, to be informed of one's medical condition and treatment, to consent to or refuse treatment, to confidentiality of medical records and treatment, to receive visitors, and, when near death, to have family members present 24 hours a day. At the same time, many types of community-based residential care facilities, such as assisted-living facilities and residential dementia special care units, were developing. Because of influences such as these, a new era in nursing home care has evolved.

The term **culture change** has been used since 1997 in the United States to describe a major movement toward implementing fundamental reforms in the way that nursing homes provide care. This movement in Canada has been speared in more recent years by the work of the Alzheimer Society of Canada (2012). A major goal of culture change is to transform the philosophy and practice in nursing homes from an overemphasis on safety, uniformity and medical care to a consumer-directed focus on health promotion, quality of life and individualized care. **Resident-centred care**, defined as care that emphasizes personal choices and quality of life, is a core component of the culture change movement.

The culture change movement has been gaining momentum, not only in the private sector but also in the public sector. Box 6-3 provides information about models of long-term care that are based on the culture change movement.

A Student's Perspective

This week in the nursing home, I found it was important to listen to Mrs. R. while allowing her to make her limitations known to me. I asked if she needed help, and didn't just provide it. I paid close attention to her body language and nonverbal communication. After finding her fast asleep sitting up during breakfast, I woke her and allowed her to tell me what was next. She determined that going to the bathroom and then getting washed would be best. After she was ready, I helped her down to the beauty salon to get her hair done, which is something she does every Friday afternoon. It can be easy to fall into the patient care aspect of a nursing home where you expect them to be on a schedule; however, you have to treat it as their home and allow them to pick and choose their activities and rest periods.

Jillian B.

Box 6-3   Long-Term Care Settings Based on the Culture Change Movement

Eden Alternative

- Was developed in the mid-1990s by William Thomas, MD, with the intent of creating small-group neighbourhoods of residents
- Is a comprehensive program to transform the organizational culture as well as the physical, spiritual, psychosocial and interpersonal environments of a facility
- Incorporates pets, plants and children into the environment to create a homelike setting and improve the residents' quality of life
- Also incorporates strategies to engage and empower staff in bringing about environmental change

Green House Project

- Developed in 2003 as a small-house nursing home by William Thomas, MD, the founder of the Eden Alternative
- Typically houses 7 to 12 residents in a home that blends in with neighbouring houses
- In small-house nursing homes, provides a full range of licensed and certified nursing home services in a normal household setting to older people with high levels of disability, including those associated with dementia
- Emphasizes relationships and meaning-making in interventions for dementia-related behavioural disturbances

---

In 2013, the Canadian Institute for Health Information (CIHI) published a report, the purpose of which was to establish a baseline for tracking the quality of care provided to older adults living in nursing homes. It profiled the eight quality indicators derived from the Resident Assessment Instrument–Minimum Data Set collected through the Continuing Care Reporting System at the CIHI. The findings are a starting point for a conversation in this country about the quality of care provided to those who reside in nursing homes. Findings identified that while some homes do better than others, no single facility or jurisdiction performs well on all of the indicators. There is also wide variation in performance of the homes between and within jurisdictions. Higher total nursing and RN hours per resident-day are associated with better care. Thus, nursing hours per resident-day is considered to be one reasonable measure of nursing home quality (Statistics Canada, 2010).

Roles for Nurses in Nursing Home Settings

Nurses have always assumed strong leadership roles in nursing homes and other long-term care settings, and opportunities for role expansion are associated with the increasing complexity of care. Also, because of the focus on improved quality of care in nursing home settings, nurses have many opportunities to implement innovative changes in delivery of care. Roles for registered nurses in long-term care settings include team leader, nursing supervisor, wellness nurse, director of nursing and assistant director of nursing. Nurses also have very strong roles in teaching nursing assistants (sometimes called health care aides) about the best care for nursing home residents. Some provincial health care systems have provided funding that nursing homes may use to employ a nurse practitioner or other advanced practice nursing services. The use of advanced practice nurses promotes improved quality of care. In addition to direct care of residents, advanced practice nurses may provide staff education, assist with program development, act as consultants in planning and implementing care, establish support groups for clients and families and act as advocates for clients and their families.

Models of care based on the culture change movement present many challenges, as well as opportunities, for nurses because culture change involves philosophical and organizational changes that affect all staff. For example, the Green House model conceptualizes nurses and other professionals as members of a visiting clinical support team that order and supervise care within their area of professional practice. Nurses do not supervise the direct care staff, but they often assume administrative and consultant roles. Mueller and colleagues (2013) published 10 competencies for nurses in culture change nursing homes, as in the following examples:

- Models, teaches and uses effective communication skills, including active listening, giving meaningful feedback and addressing emotional behaviours
- Implements and role-models person-directed care practices
- Identifies and addresses barriers to person-directed care
- Maintains consistency of caregivers for residents
- Solves complex problems related to resident choice and risk
- Involves residents, families and all team members in problem-solving, decision-making and planning

Online Learning Activity 6-2 provides links to additional information related to improving the quality of care and quality of life for nursing homes resident.

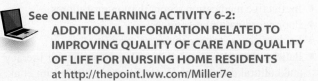

See **ONLINE LEARNING ACTIVITY 6-2:**
ADDITIONAL INFORMATION RELATED TO
IMPROVING QUALITY OF CARE AND QUALITY
OF LIFE FOR NURSING HOME RESIDENTS
at http://thepoint.lww.com/Miller7e

A relatively new care option in Canada, the assisted-living facility (sometimes called designated living) was initially developed by for-profit developers and targeted to upper-middle- and high-income older adults. These facilities accommodate physically and mentally frail older adults who require a protective environment, regular and unscheduled assistance with daily living activities, and some nursing care. Unlike, however, the more medically oriented environment of a nursing home, assisted living offers a "social" or "residential" care model that resembles a hotel in both its appearance and operation. Residents have individual apartments, can lock their doors and have more say in their own care. Moreover, even as they need assistance to cope with their vulnerabilities, they are still able to maintain their dignity and independence.

HOSPITAL SETTINGS

Hospital settings (also called acute care settings) are an important part of the continuum of care because of the complexity of care associated with illnesses in older adults (as discussed in detail in Chapter 27). Older adults constitute the "core business" of hospitals because they account for 40% of inpatient hospital admissions in Canada. Furthermore, the length of stay for older adults is longer than for nonseniors; for instance, in 2009 to 2010, older adults stayed in hospital 1.5 times longer than nonseniors (CIHI, 2011). The increasing awareness of unique needs of hospitalized older adults is leading to the development of programs to address these needs. This section presents information about specialized programs and resources that are currently available. Because issues related to quality of care are multifaceted, they need to be addressed in policies and practices by the institution and by each professional group within the institution. This section discusses current efforts to address concerns about quality of care in hospitals, with attention on roles of nurses.

Acute Care Units for Elders

Since the early 1980s, hospitals in Canada have been establishing comprehensive geriatric assessment units, called **acute care for elders (ACE)** units, based on the underlying premise that older adults have complex and unique needs that can be addressed by a specially trained interprofessional team to prevent functional decline during hospitalization. Reviews of studies show that positive outcomes of ACE units include reduced functional decline, decreased risk of complications and shorter lengths of stay (Fox et al., 2013). Key elements of ACE units are patient-centred care, interprofessional team management, frequent medical review, early discharge planning, a specially adapted physical environment, and assessment and interventions for common geriatric syndromes (e.g., mobility, fall risk, self-care, skin integrity, continence, confusion, depression, anxiety). In addition to gerontological nurses, the health care teams in ACE units typically include a geriatrician, pharmacist, social worker, various rehabilitation therapists (e.g., speech, physical or occupational therapists), mental health professionals (e.g., psychologists or psychiatrists) and supportive therapies such as music or activity. If a dedicated ACE unit is not feasible, nurses in all acute care settings should focus on (1) patient-centred care, including individualized preventive care interventions based on functional assessment; (2) daily review of medications, treatments and planned procedures and (3) referrals for rehabilitation therapists (Fox, 2013).

Resources for Improving Care of Hospitalized Older Adults

In 1992, the Hartford Foundation in the United States funded a major initiative called the Nurses Improving Care to the Hospitalized Elderly (NICHE). The NICHE program is ongoing and is active not only in the United States, but also in

Canadian hospitals. In 2014, The Halton Health Care Services (Ontario) was the first Canadian hospital to be awarded "Exemplar" status for its NICHE program. A unique characteristic of NICHE is its focus on developing a positive nurse practice environment by involving nurses at all levels in decisions regarding care of older adults (Capezuti et al., 2012a). An integral component of NICHE is the **geriatric resource nurse (GRN)**, who serves as a consultant and role model for other nurses. These nurses are skilled at identifying and addressing specific geriatric syndromes, such as falls and confusion, and implementing interventions that discourage using restrictive devices and promote patient mobility. Evaluation of the GRN model has identified reductions in costs and improvements in all of the following areas: nursing knowledge, quality of care, implementation of geriatric protocols and clinical outcomes related to conditions such as delirium (Capezuti et al., 2012b).

In 2011, NICHE published standards of care and information about resources to address needs of hospitalized older adults. Box 6-4 delineates some of these standards that nurses

---

Box 6-4 Examples of Standards of Care for Hospitalized Older Adults Established by the Joint Commission and Nurses Improving Care for Healthsystem Elders (NICHE)

Nursing and Human Resources

- The Geriatric Resource Nurse model is implemented and evaluated.
- Specialized needs of hospitalized older adults are discussed in staff orientation, interprofessional continuing education and competency-based training for nursing staff.
- NICHE coordinator and managers evaluate the learning needs of the staff related to care of hospitalized older adults.

Provision of Care

- The care, treatment and services provided to hospitalized older adults is interprofessional.
- The interprofessional team utilizes evidence-based assessment practices and individualized interventions to prevent and manage pain, falls/related injuries and other geriatric syndromes.
- The unique needs of older adult patients are integrated within palliative care and end-of-life services.
- The learning needs of hospitalized older adults and their families are addressed.
- Policies and practices support alternatives to physical restraints.
- Transitional care needs of older adults and their families are addressed through comprehensive assessment, planning and interventions.

Medication Management

- Administration and prescription of medications for older adults is consistent with evidence-based practice (e.g., using AGS Beers' Criteria).

Environments of Care

- Physical environment reflects aging-sensitive principles to provide for basic safety: nonglare flooring, adequate lights, grab bars, adjustable height beds and appropriate use of alarms.
- All practitioners are familiar with their roles and responsibilities relative to the environment of care.

Source: Adapted from NICHE. (2011). A crosswalk: Joint Commission Standards & NICHE Resources.

---

can implement, even if NICHE or other specialized geriatric resources are not readily available. In addition, nurses can access evidence-based information related to care of older adults through the Internet sites listed in Online Learning Activity 6-3.

 See **ONLINE LEARNING ACTIVITY 6-3: EVIDENCE-BASED INFORMATION AND TOOLS FOR ADDRESSING NEEDS OF HOSPITALIZED OLDER ADULTS** at http://thepoint.lww.com/Miller7e

Concerns About Transition in Care

Because concerns about quality of care in hospitals have escalated in recent years, provincial/territorial health care jurisdictions have supported initiatives to improve care and decrease the cost of care, particularly for older adults.

Of particular concern in hospital settings is the lack of coordination during transitions in care, which refers to the numerous transfers of older adults between health care settings during the course of an illness. Older adults with complex medical problems or combinations of chronic and acute problems (e.g., dementia and heart failure) are particularly vulnerable to experiencing problems as they transfer between care settings. This issue is currently viewed as high priority by organizations such as the Canadian Patient Safety Institute because it is associated with many serious outcomes, such as high rates of readmission to hospitals within 30 days of discharge. Factors that affect transitions in care and compromise patient safety include the following:

- Communication gaps
- Incomplete transfer information
- Inadequate patient education, particularly for older adults and their caregivers
- Ineffective medication reconciliation procedures
- Poor coordination of services
- Lack of access to essential care services
- Patient characteristics, such as language, health literacy and cultural differences (Enderlin et al., 2013; Lim et al., 2012).

Problems with transitions in care occur during transfers within institutions and during transfers from one setting to another, whether those are institutions, homes or community settings.

Many organizations and governmental agencies are addressing issues in transitions in care, but most of these initiatives are in early stages of implementation. One example is drawn from one of the six health authorities in British Columbia. The realization that lack of standardization was resulting in unequal distribution of quality health care services initiated a redesign of the home care liaison role. Employing a program management perspective, the focus of the liaison role became the development a transition plan for clients (Meadows et al., 2014).

Although problems with transitions of care are primarily related to the overall practices of institutions, all professionals within the setting share responsibility for aspects of transitions. Numerous models have been developed to address the contributing factors, and nurses have assumed primary roles in developing and implementing interventions. Programs that successfully reduce readmission rates involve implementation of an enhanced patient-centred discharge process, which addresses all of the following: medication reconciliation, coordination with community-based providers and effective patient self-management of disease (Cloonan et al., 2013).

There is much support for the implementation of **transitional care**. However, there is no one commonly accepted definition of *transitional care* in Canada. It is perhaps best defined by the American Geriatrics Society (2003): "[T]ransitional care encompasses both the sending and the receiving aspects of the transfer is based on a comprehensive plan of care and includes logistical arrangements, education of the patient and family, and coordination among the health professionals involved in the transition" (p. 556).

Nurses have developed an easy-to-use and evidence-based screening tool called the Transitional Care Model (TCM): Hospital Discharge Screening Criteria for High Risk Older Adults to identify older adults who are at risk for poorly managed transitions. Nurses are encouraged to use this tool to identify older adults who need special attention for transitional care interventions (Lim et al., 2012). The Re-engineered Hospital Discharge (RED) model is another evidence-based approach that is implemented to improve care transitions and reduce readmission rates (Poston et al., 2014). This program is multifaceted and includes a strong role for nurses. The three major components of this model are as follows: (1) a nurse discharge advocate whose primary responsibility is to coordinate discharge plans and communicate with patient/family and all care providers; (2) an after-hospital care plan document that is patient-centred, low-literacy level and highly pictorial that includes all pertinent information and (3) telephone follow-up by a clinical pharmacist 3 days post-discharge for teaching and follow-up. Online Learning Activity 6-4 includes an article describing the use of the RED model to reduce the 30-day readmission rate for patients with strokes.

See ONLINE LEARNING ACTIVITY 6-4: ADDITIONAL INFORMATION ABOUT TRANSITIONAL CARE MODELS AND ARTICLE DESCRIBING THE IMPLEMENTATION OF A MODEL TO REDUCE READMISSIONS at http://thepoint.lww.com/Miller7e

BROADER ISSUES RELATED TO CARE FOR OLDER ADULTS

All sectors of health care and the larger society have identified quality and safety issues as a high priority that is being addressed by professional disciplines, including nursing. Another high priority that policy makers and care providers are focusing on is addressing the needs of caregivers. Although these concerns are not specific to older adults, they disproportionately affect nursing care of older adults. Because these are important aspects of gerontological nursing care, this book includes material related to these topics.

Quality and Safety in Nursing

As already mentioned, concerns about quality of health care for older adults need to be addressed at an institutional level, with essential input from all involved professionals. One way in which nurses are addressing this issues is through the rapidly growing network of nurses working toward widespread implementation of a framework called **Quality and Safety Education for Nurses (QSEN)**. The QSEN project evolved from a series of grants from the Robert Wood Johnson Foundation in response to the Institute of Medicine's report, called *To Err Is Human* (Institute of Medicine, 2000). This was the first of a series of reports that addressed aspects of the "quality chasm" that existed in the Canadian health care system. Initiatives such as QSEN are congruent with current national priorities related to health care, which are as follows (Schumann, 2012):

- Making care safer
- Ensuring person- and family-centred care
- Promoting effective communication and coordination of care
- Promoting the most effective strategies for preventing and treating leading causes of mortality, starting with cardiovascular disease
- Promoting wide use of best practices that support healthy living
- Making quality care more affordable

Nurses have developed QSEN competencies with the goal of improving the delivery of health care services in all of the following areas: patient-centred care, teamwork and collaboration, evidence-based practice, quality improvement, safety and informatics. Competencies for each of the six areas are identified for knowledge (K), skills (S) and attitudes (A), or KSA. Some of the competencies apply more directly to the work environment, but all competencies affect direct care of patients in some way. In this book, QSEN competencies that are most directly related to care of older adults are applied to case examples in the clinically oriented chapters. Table 6-2 summarizes QSEN competencies and the associated KSA for patient-centred care, teamwork and collaboration, and evidence-based practice. Although other QSEN competencies are equally important in clinical practice, the application of QSEN to case examples in this textbook focuses on the ones that nurses can most directly incorporate in their care of older adult patients.

Addressing Needs of Caregivers

The term **caregiver burden** is commonly used to describe the financial, physical and psychosocial problems that family members experience when caring for older adults who are impaired or suffering from illness. Specific functional consequences associated with caregiver burden include depression, disturbed sleep, social isolation, family discord, career

TABLE 6-2 Quality and Safety in Nursing (QSEN) Competencies and Related Knowledge, Skills and Attitudes

QSEN Competency	Knowledge/Skill/Attitude
Patient-centred care	(K) Integrate understanding of multiple dimensions of patient-centred care. (K) Describe how diverse backgrounds function as a source of values. (K) Describe strategies to empower patients in all aspects of the health care process. (K) Examine common barriers to active involvement in patients. (K) Discuss principles of effective communication. (K) Examine nursing roles in ensuring coordination, integration and continuity of care. (S) Elicit patient values, preferences and expressed needs. (S) Provide patient-centred care with sensitivity and respect for diversity of the human experience. (S) Assess own level of communication skill in encounters with patients and families. (S) Communicate care provided and needed at each transition in care. (A) Value seeing health care situations "through patients' eyes."
Teamwork and collaboration	(K) Describe scopes of practice and role of health care team members. (K) Recognize contributions of other individuals and groups in helping patient achieve health goals. (K) Describe impact of own communication style on others. (S) Integrate the contributions of others who play a role in helping patient achieve health goals.
Evidence-based practice	(K) Describe how the strength and relevance of available evidence influence the choice of intervention. (S) Base individualized care plan on patient values, clinical expertise and evidence. (S) Read original research and evidence reports related to clinical practice. (A) Value evidence-based practice as integral to determining the best clinical practice.

interruptions, financial difficulties, lack of time for self, poor physical health, psychological/emotional/mental strain, and feelings of anger, guilt, grief, anxiety, hopelessness and helplessness. Lack of choice in assuming the caregiving role, because of kinship or a sense of obligation, is identified as a risk factor for developing symptoms of caregiver burden (Schulz et al., 2012). Although most studies have focused on the burdens of caregiving, caregivers typically experience a combination of negative and positive feelings associated with both the burdens and inconveniences of caregiving and the satisfaction of helping others. Positive outcomes related to the experience of caregiving include feelings of satisfaction and, personal gratification, experiences of social approval and finding meaning in the caregiver role (Lin et al., 2012; Shim et al., 2013). These positive effects, particularly finding meaning in the caregiver

role, can mediate the effects of caregiver burden and improve life satisfaction (Kruithof et al., 2012; Quinn et al., 2012).

For older adults who have dementia or other conditions that cause progressive declines in functioning, the role of caregiver usually evolves gradually and can last for years. Even in situations in which older adults do not have progressively declining conditions, families of older adults frequently deal with intermittent and cumulative conditions that require intense medical care or rehabilitative services. It is not uncommon for families of older adults to take on roles of care managers and find themselves negotiating health care services for at least one and sometimes several parents, grandparents, aunts, uncles and other relatives or friends.

Nurses have important roles in promoting **caregiver wellness**. For example, studies indicate that increased feelings of self-efficacy improve caregiver well-being for family caregivers who provide assistance for older adults with dementia and other chronic illnesses (Giovannetti et al., 2012; Henriksson & Arestedt, 2013; Semiatin & O'Connor, 2012). Thus, relatively simple communication techniques, such as providing positive feedback when teaching caregivers, can improve a caregiver's sense of self-efficacy. Nurses address teaching needs of older adults' families, partners and significant others as an essential nursing responsibility related to continuity of care for patients in all health care settings. Consistent with this responsibility, nurses follow standards of care and document the teaching they provide regarding caregiving instructions, but they do not necessarily address the broader needs of caregivers because of barriers, such as time constraints and perception of this as a nonessential aspect of care. However, when nurses care for dependent older adults, it is important to recognize that even the basic needs of the older adult cannot be met without a strong support system. Thus, nurses need to identify outcomes and interventions to prevent caregiver burnout and enhance the ability of families and other caregivers to provide the necessary care, as discussed in Chapter 27. As with all aspects of caring for older adults, there is great individual variation among families, caregivers and care recipients, so there are many varied interventions to address caregiver issues.

Comprehensive Models

Provincial/territorial governments have funded innovative models of long-term care for people with chronic conditions that are both comprehensive and cost-effective. These types of programs developed slowly, but have gradually expanded. One initiative is the Evercare model, which two nurse practitioners began as a pilot program in 1987 in the United States. There are now Evergreen houses across Canada. The Evercare model is made up of nurse practitioners and care managers who guide patients through the health care system. Core care principles of the Evercare model include the following:

- Nurse practitioners plan and provide care, with attention to the patient's physical, social and psychological needs.
- Transfers between different health care settings are minimized.

- Health care providers focus on prevention and ensure regular assessments and early detection of illness.
- Care teams advocate for patients and help them get the most from their health insurance benefits.
- Families are encouraged to be actively involved with the care.

The Evercare nurse model addresses important deficits in physician care for complex geriatric conditions, such as chronic disease and end-of-life care (Wenger et al., 2011).

The Guided Care model has been implemented as a nurse–physician partnership for promoting evidence-based care and self-management for patients with chronic conditions. Initial studies indicate that this model improves quality and efficiency of care and is feasible and acceptable to physicians, patients and family caregivers (Boult et al., 2013). A specially educated registered nurse works with several primary care to implement the following clinical processes: assessments, monitoring and coaching; provision of evidence-based comprehensive interventions; promotion of self-management; coordination of all care, including transitions; education and support of caregivers; and facilitation of access to community resources. This model has been used to effectively improve quality of care for patients with chronic conditions (Marsteller et al., 2013).

Another model of care is based upon the concept of Creative Aging, Garrison Greens Seniors Community in Calgary, Alberta in one such long-term facility that bases its programming on this concept. Creative Aging is based upon the work of Dr. Gene Cohen, author of *The Creative Age: Awakening Human Potential in the Second Half of Life*. He advocated for a shift in societal thinking about older adults from a deficit approach that stresses losses to an asset approach that emphasizes strengths, potential and achievements. Thus built into the programs for seniors are numerous opportunities for a variety of art and dance/movement experiences.

Continuum of Care

Since the early 1970s, many provinces have created continuum (or integrated) care systems to varying extents (Chappell & Hollander, 2011). This system has a single point of entry, which is initiated by an interprofessional team. A continuum of care perspective is designed to meet the changing needs of the older adult through connecting home, community and long-term care services so that an older adult can move seamlessly through levels of care. It is a direct response to fragmented and disjointed health care services often experienced by older adults and their care providers, and to health care system costs inefficiencies.

PAYING FOR HEALTH CARE SERVICES FOR OLDER ADULTS

Sources of payment for health care services are self-pay, private insurance and government-supported programs such as Medicare, as well as Veterans Affairs Canada. Although health care is free in Canada, there are numerous health care services (such as eye exams or physiotherapy), which are not necessarily free. Because specifics about what is covered by health care and what is not evolves over time, and also because many of the newer programs are available only in certain geographic locations, it is difficult to keep up-to-date on all the options available to older adults today. Despite the complexity and limitations of programs, however, nurses need to know enough about common types of programs so they can understand and address some of the barriers to, and challenges of, implementing nursing care plans and discharge plans. For example, knowing the provincial/territorial criteria for skilled home care services enables the nurse to make referrals for this type of nursing care when appropriate. This section presents information about the programs that most directly influence health care services for older adults, including those that play a major role in the ability of older adults to live in home settings.

Out-of-Pocket Expenses

Despite the major contribution of all levels of government in paying for health care services, out-of-pocket health care expenses have been increasing steadily in recent decades and that burden falls disproportionately on poor people.

Medicare

Canada does not have a national health insurance plan. It does have 13 separate insurance programs run by the provinces and territories, loosely bound together by federal agreements and the CHA. In 1984, the CHA established that the federal and provincial/territorial governments would share the costs 50/50. However, to be eligible for federal funding, provincial/territorial health insurance plans must adhere to the principles of the CHA (publically administered, comprehensive, universal, accessible and portable). Medicare covers primarily hospital and physician services, with limited Medicare coverage for health protection and promotion, disease prevention, and services related to specific groups (e.g., Aboriginal people living on reserves, inmates of federal prisons, military personnel and veterans). Although the federal government works in collaboration with all jurisdictions, the management and delivery of health care to all Canadians is the responsibility of the provinces/territories.

In recent years, numerous problems have been identified with the Canadian health care system, which have direct impact on the health of older adults, such as, excessive wait times for various types of surgeries including hip and knee replacements and cataracts, emphasis upon primary health care with too little on disease prevention and health promotion, the inflation costs of drug research, and the shortage of health care personnel including professional nurses (Canadian Federation of Nurses Unions, 2012; Health Council of Canada, 2005). This has supported the larger discussion of health care reforms in Canada.

Insurance Gap

The many limitations of the original Medicare program has led to the development of insurance gap policies, which are supplemental policies that attempt to fill the gap between the services covered by original Medicare and those that are paid for out-of-pocket health care expenses. All supplemental policies, which are regulated by federal and provincial/territorial legislation, cover the premiums and copayments for services covered by Medicare, but additional benefits vary according to each policy. They have developed 10 standard plans that insurance companies must follow in the provision of Medigap policies. Plan A contains basic benefits, such as coverage for coinsurance payments and additional payments for hospital days. Other plans (B through J) cover Part A deductible and additional services, such as prescription medications, preventive medical care, skilled nursing coinsurance and medical care in foreign countries. Because health insurance choices have become increasingly complex, nurses can encourage older adults and their caregivers to seek information from organizations that are not directly involved with selling insurance policies, such as local senior centres.

Long-Term Care Insurance

Long-term care insurance policies are designed to cover some long-term care expenses that are not covered by health insurance programs. When long-term care insurance policies were first promoted in the late 1980s, they were unregulated and many of the policies contained large loopholes and significant barriers to receiving benefits. Suggested requirements for long-term care insurance policies include inflation protection and caps on rates. A good long-term care policy will provide payment for a range of options, including home care services, assisted-living facilities and nursing home care. In addition, policies should be open enough that they include services that may be developed in the future but are not available at the time the policy is initiated. For example, the first long-term care policies that were developed were limited to nursing home care because few other options were available at that time. A major drawback of this type of insurance for older people is that the premiums are often based on the age of the person when he or she initially signs up for the policy. For most older adults, therefore, the cost of the policy will outweigh the benefits.

Chapter Highlights

Community-based Services for Older Adults

- Public and private agencies have provided many types of services for older adults, with the range of services continually broadening (Table 6-1 and Box 6-1).
- Health promotion programs provide organized screening and health education services in community settings, such as senior centres.
- Faith community nursing is a holistic approach to addressing the physical, emotional and spiritual needs of members of religious congregations.
- Respite care refers to any service whose primary goal is to relieve caregivers periodically from the stress of their usual caregiver responsibilities.

- Adult day centres provide structured activities for functionally impaired older people in a group setting.
- Geriatric care management services involve comprehensive assessment, care planning, implementation, monitoring and reassessment to address immediate and long-term needs of older adults.

Home-Based Services

- Skilled home care services, including nursing, therapies and home health aides, provide skilled care for homebound older adults who meet criteria established by the jurisdictional health authority.
- A wide spectrum of services ranging from housekeeping and companionship to full-time hands-on nursing care are available under the auspices of nonmedical home care.
- Home care services are formal sources, such as agencies, or informal sources, including independent caregivers and family and friends.
- Nurses working in home care agencies have many responsibilities, including using telehealth technology as an integral part of assessment and nursing care.

Nursing Home Settings

- Nursing homes are residential institutional settings for people who need assistance with several daily activities.
- Skilled care in a rehabilitation unit addresses short-term needs of people who need nursing care and/or rehabilitation therapies for people who have had an acute illness and are expected to progress to a higher level of functioning.
- Long-term care in a nursing home refers to services provided for chronically ill people who need significant assistance with daily activities.
- The nursing home culture change movement was initiated in 1997 with the goal of transforming the philosophy and practice in nursing homes to emphasize resident-centred care (Box 6-2).
- Nurses have many roles in addressing issues related to quality of care in nursing homes.

Hospital Settings

- Specialized Acute Care for Elders (ACE) units address the complex needs of hospitalized older adults though interprofessional assessments and interventions.
- The NICHE program offers many resources for implementing standards of care for hospitalized older adults (Box 6-3).
- Transitional care addresses lack of coordinated care when patients are discharged from hospitals.

Broader Issues Related to Care for Older Adults

- Quality and Safety in Nursing (QSEN) competencies have been developed to help nurses address national priorities related to improving quality of health care services (Table 6-3).
- An essential component of nursing care for older adults is addressing needs of caregivers.

Paying for Health Care Services for Older Adults

- Sources of payment for health care services are self-pay (also called out-of-pocket), public funds and insurance policies for people who have them.
- Medicare is the informal name for the provincial/territorial health insurance programs funded by transfer payments that cover hospital and medical care (Box 6-4).
- Provincial/territorial governments have funded innovative models of care that are comprehensive and cost-effective for people with chronic conditions.
- Insurance policies are available from many sources to supplement original Medicare policies.
- Long-term care insurance policies are available to cover the cost of some long-term care services, but the costs outweigh the potential benefits for most older adults.

Critical Thinking Exercises

1. Mrs. S. is 84 years old. She was recently diagnosed with dementia. She is able to care for herself as long as someone reminds her to eat her meals and take her medications. Two months ago, she began living with her daughter who works full-time and is involved with several church-related activities. Three days a week, Mrs. S.'s daughter takes her to an adult day centre at 8:30 AM and picks her up at 4:30 PM Twice weekly, Mrs. S. receives home-delivered meals. Find local resources for the types of services delineated in Box 6-1 and obtain information about four or five additional services that Mrs. S.'s daughter may need to use.

2. Mrs. F. is a resident in the skilled care section of the nursing home where you work. She had been living alone in her own home before being admitted to the hospital with a fractured hip 4 weeks ago. She has regained much of her independence and walks with a walker and one-person assist. She expects to ambulate independently using a walker within 2 weeks, at which time she expects to return to her own home. She asks you what kind of services would be available in her home. What additional information would you want to know before you answered her questions? What information would you give to her? What suggestions would you make?

3. Your great aunt, who is 84 years old, is being admitted to a nursing home for long-term care. Her diagnoses include dementia, arthritis and heart failure. Her daughter (who is your aunt) asks your advice about what to look for when she is selecting a nursing home. Use the resources in Online Learning Activity 6-2 to explore information about culture change and quality of care in nursing homes.

 For more information about topics discussed in this chapter, be sure to check out the interactive Online Learning Activities and other helpful resources at http://thepoint.lww.com/Miller7e

REFERENCES

Alzheimer Society of Canada. (2012). *Creating a culture change in long-term care homes for people with dementia and their families from a person-centred perspective*. Retrieved from www.alzheimer.ca/~/.../Culture-change/culture_steer_committee_e.pdf

American Geriatrics Society. (2003). Improving quality of transitional care for persons with complex care needs. American Geriatrics Society position statement. *Journal of the American Geriatrics Society, 51*(4), 556–557.

Boult, C., Leff, B., Boyd, C. M., et al. (2013). A matched-pair cluster-randomized trial of guided care for high-risk older patients. *Journal of General Internal Medicine, 28*(5), 612–621.

Canadian Association of Parish Nurses. (2013). *Nursing parish fact sheet*. Retrieved from http://www.capnm.ca/fact_sheet.htm

Canadian Federation of Nurses Unions. (2012). *The nursing workforce*. Retrieved from nursesunions.ca/sites/.../2012.backgrounder.nursing_workforce.e_0.pdf

Canada Health Infoway. (n.d.). *Telehealth*. Retrieved from https://www.infoway-inforoute.ca/index.php/programs-services/investmentprograms/telehealth

Canadian Institute for Health Information. (2005). *Exploring the 70/30 split: How Canada's health care system is financed*. Retrieved from https://secure.cihi.ca/estore/productSeries.htm?pc=PCC292

Canadian Institute for Health Information. (2011). *Health care in Canada, 2011: A focus on seniors and aging*. Ottawa, ON: Author. Retrieved from https://secure.cihi.ca/free_products/HCIC_2011_seniors_report_en.pdf

Canadian Institute for Health Information. (2013). *When a nursing home is home: How do Canadian nursing homes measure up on quality?* Retrieved from https://secure.cihi.ca/free_products/CCRS_QualityinLongTermCare_EN.pdf

Capezuti, E., Boltz, M., Cline, D., et al. (2012a). Nurses improving care of Healthsystem Elders: A model for optimizing the geriatric nursing practice environment. *Journal of Clinical Nursing, 21*, 3117–3125.

Capezuti, E., Boltz, M., & Nigolian, C. (2012b). Acute care models. In M. Boltz, E. Capezuti, T. Fulmer, et al. (Eds.), *Evidence-based practice protocols for best practice* (4th ed., pp. 670–681). New York, NY: Springer.

Chang, C.-P., Lee, T.-T., Chou, C.-C., et al. (2013). Telecare for diabetes mellitus. *Computers, Informatics, Nursing, 31*(10), 505–511.

Chappell, N., & Hollander, M. (2011). An evidence-based policy prescription for an aging population. *Health care Papers, 11*(1), 8–18. doi:10.12927/hcpap.2011.22246

Cloonan, P., Wood, J., & Riley, J. B. (2013). Reducing 30-day readmissions. *Journal of Nursing Administration, 43*(7–8), 382–387.

Conn, D., Madan, R., Lam, J., et al. (2013). Program evaluation of a telepsychiatry service for older adults connecting a university-affiliated geriatric centre to a rural psychogeriatric outreach service in Northwest Ontario, Canada. *International Psychogeriatrics, 25*, 1795–1800.

Enderlin, C. A., McLeskey, N., Rooker, J. L., et al. (2013). Review of current conceptual models and frameworks to guide transitions of care in older adults. *Geriatric Nursing, 34*(47–52).

Fairbrother, P., Ure, J., Hanley, J., et al. (2014). Telemonitoring for chronic heart failure: The views of patients and health care professionals—A qualitative study. *Journal of Clinical Nursing, 23*, 132–144.

Fox, M. (2013). Adapting the Acute Care for Elders (ACE) model to your hospital. *Geriatric Nursing, 34*, 332–334.

Fox, M. T., Sidani, S., Persaud, M., et al. (2013). Acute Care for Elders components of acute geriatric unit care: Systematic descriptive review. *Journal of the American Geriatrics Society, 61*, 939–946.

Gaugler, J. E. (2014). The process of adult day service use. *Geriatric Nursing, 35*, 47–54.

Giovannetti, E. R., Wolff, J. L., Xue, Q. L., et al. (2012). Difficulty assisting with health care tasks among caregivers of multimorbid older adults. *Journal of General Internal Medicine, 27*(1), 37–44.

Gruneir, A., Forrester, J., Camacho, X., et al. (2013). Gender differences in home care clients and admission to long-term care in Ontario, Canada: A population-based retrospective cohort study. *BMC Geriatrics, 13*, 48. Retrieved from http://www.biomedcentral.com/1471-2318/13/48

Health Council of Canada. (2005). Health Care Renewal in Canada: Accelerating Change. Retrieved from http://healthcouncilcanada.ca/tree/2.48-Accelerating_Change_HCC_2005.pdf

Heeke, S., Wood, F., & Schuck, J. (2014). Improving care transitions from hospital to home health nursing with remote telemonitoring. *Journal of Nursing Care Quality, 29*(2), E21–E28.

Henriksson, A., & Arestedt, K. (2013). Exploring factors and caregiver outcomes associated with feelings of preparedness for caregiving in family caregivers in palliative care: A correlational, cross-sectional study. *Palliative Medicine, 27*(7), 639–646.

Hoban, M. B., Fedor, M., Reeder, S., et al. (2013). The effect of telemonitoring at home. *Home Health care Nurse, 31*(7), 368–378.

Institute of Medicine. (2000). *To err is human: Building a safer health system*. Retrieved from www.nap.edu

King, M. A., & Pappas-Rogich, M. (2011). Faith community nurses: Implementing Healthy People standards to promote the health of elderly clients. *Geriatric Nursing, 32*, 459–464.

Kruithof, W. J., Visser-Meily, J. M., & Post, M. W. (2012). Positive caregiving experiences are associated with life satisfaction in spouses of stroke survivors. *Journal of Stroke and Cerebrovascular Disease, 21*(8), 801–807.

Lim, F., Foust, J., & Van Cleave, J. (2012). Transitional care. In M. Boltz, E. Capezuti, T. Fulmer, et al. (Eds.), *Evidence-based practice protocols for best practice* (4th ed., pp. 682–702). New York, NY: Springer.

Lin, I. F., Fee, H. R., & Wu, H. S. (2012). Negative and positive caregiving experiences: A closer look at the intersection of gender and relationships. *Family Relationships, 61*(2), 343–458.

Marsteller, J. A., Hsu, Y. J., Wen, M., et al. (2013). Effects of guided care on providers' satisfaction with care: A three-year matched-pair cluster-randomized trial. *Population Health Management, 16*(5), 317–325.

McCleary, L., Persaud, M., Hum, S., et al. (2012). Pathways to dementia diagnosis among South Asian Canadians. *Dementia, 12*, 769–789. doi:10.1177/1471301212444806

Meadows, C. A., Fraser, J., Comus, S., & Henderson, K. (2014). A system-wide innovation in transition services. *Home Health Care Nurse, 32*(2), 78–86. doi:10.1097/NHH.0000000000000016

Mueller, C., Burger, S., Rader, S., et al. (2013). Nurse competencies for person-directed care in nursing homes. *Geriatric Nursing, 34*, 101–104.

Nesbitt, T. S. (2012). *The evolution of telehealth: Where have we been and where are we going?* Washington, DC: National Academy of Sciences.

Newall, N. E. G., & Menec, V. H. (2013). Targeting socially isolated older adults: A process evaluation of the Seniors without Walls Social and Educational Program. *Journal of Applied Gerontology*. Advance online publication doi:10.1177/0733464813510063

Nurses Improving Care for Healthsystem Elders. (2011). *A crosswalk: Joint commission standards & NICHE resources*. Retrieved from www.nicheprogram.org

Ouslander, J. G., & Maslow, K. (2012). Geriatrics and the triple aim: Defining preventable hospitalizations in the long-term care population. *Journal of the American Geriatrics Society, 60*(12), 2313–2318.

Phillipson, L., & Jones, S. C. (2012). Use of day centres for respite by help-seeking caregivers of individuals with dementia. *Journal of Gerontological Nursing, 38*(4), 24–34.

Poston, K. M., Dumas, B. P., & Edlund, B. J. (2014). Outcomes of a quality improvement project implementing stroke discharge advocacy to reduce 30-day readmission rates. *Journal of Nursing Care Quality, 29*(3), 237–244.

Quinn, C., Clare, L., & Woods, R. T. (2012). What predicts whether caregivers of people with dementia find meaning in their role? *International Journal of Geriatric Psychiatry, 27*(11), 1195–1202.

Schulz, R., Beach, S. R., Cook, T., et al. (2012). Predictors and consequences of perceived lack of choice in becoming an informal caregiver. *Aging and Mental Health, 16*(6), 712–721.

Schumann, M. J. (2012). Policy implications driving national quality and safety initiatives. In G. Sherwood & J. Barnseiner (Eds.), *Quality and safety in nursing: A competency approach to improving outcomes*. Hoboken, NJ: Wiley-Blackwell.

Semiatin, A. M., & O'Connor, M. K. (2012). The relationship between self-sufficiency and positive aspects of caregiving in Alzheimer's disease caregivers. *Aging and Mental Health, 16*(6), 683–688.

Shim, B., Barroso, J., Gilliss, C. L., et al. (2013). Finding meaning in caring for a spouse with dementia. *Applied Nursing Research, 26*(3), 121–126.

Statistics Canada. (2008). *Rural and small town Canada* (21-006-X). Retrieved from http://www.statcan.gc.ca/pub/21-006-x/21-006-x2007008-eng.pdf

Statistics Canada. (2010). *Trends in long-term care staffing by facility ownership in British Columbia, 1996 to 2006* (82-003-X). Retrieved from http://www.statcan.gc.ca/pub/82-003-x/2010004/article/11390/findings-resultats-eng.htm

Statistics Canada. (2012). *Living arrangement of seniors* (Catalogue no. 98-312-X2011003). Ottawa, ON: Author.

Tracy, C. S., Bell, S. H., Nickell, L. A., et al. (2013). The IMPACT clinic. *Canadian Family Physician, 59*, e148–e155.

Wenger, N. S., Roth, C. P., Martin, D., et al. (2011). Quality of care provided in a special needs plan using a nurse care manager model. *Journal of the American Geriatrics Society, 59*(10), 1810–1822.

Woods, L. W., & Snow, S. W. (2013). The impact of telehealth monitoring on acute care hospitalization rates and emergency department visit rates for patients using home health skilled nursing care. *Home Health care Nurse, 31*(1), 39–45.

Zarit, S. H., Kim, K., Femia, E. E., et al. (2013). The effects of adult day services on family caregivers' daily stress, affect, and health: Outcomes for the Daily Stress and Health (DaSH) Study. *Gerontologist, 54*(4), 570–579.

Zavertnik, J. E. (2014). Self-care in older adults with heart failure. *Clinical Nurse Specialist, 28*(1), 19–32.

chapter 7

Assessment of Health and Functioning

LEARNING OBJECTIVES

After reading this chapter, you will be able to:

1. Discuss factors that contribute to the complexity of assessing older adults.

2. Use basic nursing assessment and functional assessment tools.

3. Describe how the older adult's environment, use of adaptive and assistive devices, and cognitive abilities can affect functioning.

4. Discuss nursing roles related to function-focused care and comprehensive geriatric assessments.

5. Assess safety of older adults in their home settings.

6. Explain how nurses can assess and address concerns about safe driving by older adults.

KEY POINTS

activities of daily living (ADL)

complexity of assessing health in older adults

comprehensive geriatric assessment

everyday competence

functional assessment

function-focused care

instrumental activities of daily living (IADL)

minimum data set (MDS) for resident assessment and care screening

nursing assessment tools

safe driving

Assessment of health and functioning of older adults is an essential and complex component of nursing care. This chapter discusses approaches to and tools for assessing the older adult's health and functioning. It also discusses currently evolving information about function-focused care. In addition, because health and functioning significantly affect the ability to drive a motor vehicle—which is a major safety concern with implications for society and individual older adults—this chapter discusses how nurses can assess and address risk factors that interfere with safe driving by older adults.

HEALTH ASSESSMENT OF OLDER ADULTS

A major challenge of caring for older adults is the complexity of assessing their health, especially from a comprehensive and holistic nursing perspective. Many factors contribute to the **complexity of assessing health in older adults**:

- Older adults commonly have one or more chronic conditions in addition to any acute health conditions for which they are being assessed. These conditions often interact, causing older adults' health to fluctuate unpredictably.
- Manifestations of illness, even acute illness, tend to be obscure and less predictable in older adults than in younger adults. For example, in older adults, one of the most common manifestations of illness or an adverse medication effect is a change in behaviour or mental status.
- For any one manifestation of illness in an older adult, there are usually several possible explanations. For example, changes in function can be caused by a combination of several conditions, such as acute illness, psychosocial factors, environmental conditions, age-related changes, a new chronic illness, an existing chronic illness, or an adverse effect of medication(s) or other treatments.
- Treatments are often directed toward the symptoms while the source of a problem is obscure and unresolved. This treatment approach can mask the underlying problem even further and cause additional complications (e.g., when adverse medication effects are not recognized as such and are treated with additional medications).
- Cognitive impairments can make it difficult for older adults to accurately report or describe a physiologic problem and reliable sources of information may be scarce or inaccessible.

- In many cases, by the time illness in an older adult is detected and addressed, the underlying physiologic disturbance is in an advanced stage and additional complications have developed.
- Myths and misunderstandings can lead health care providers, family members or older adults to falsely attribute treatable conditions to aging.

Because of these factors, a detective-like approach is needed for assessing older adults. This approach requires nurses to assess all aspects of the person's body, mind and spirit to look for clues—which are usually many and complicated and range from subtle to obvious—to underlying causes of changes in health or functioning.

The Functional Consequences Model for Promoting Wellness in Older Adults (described in Chapter 3) is applied to specific aspects of functioning throughout this book. Nurses can use these detailed guides to assess older adults holistically and to plan and implement nursing interventions directed toward improved functioning and quality of life (refer to the list of assessment and intervention boxes in the front matter of this book). Chapter 27 provides information about unique and atypical manifestations of illness in older adults. Clinically oriented chapters of this text also include information about normal age-related variations that nurses need to consider when assessing specific aspects of health and functioning. In addition, Table 7-1 can be used as a guide to age-related variations in laboratory values that are pertinent to the overall nursing assessment of older adults.

NURSING ASSESSMENT TOOLS

Since the late 1980s, the Hartford Institute for Geriatric Nursing (in the United States) has been in the forefront of developing, promulgating and updating evidence-based and easy-to-use **nursing assessment tools** for use in various settings. These assessment guides, called *Try This: Best Practices in Nursing Care to Older Adults*, and cost-free web-based articles and videos demonstrating the application of these tools can be accessed through the online learning activities in clinically oriented chapters of this book. Within Canada, the RNAO (Registered Nurses' Association of Ontario; http://www.rnao.ca/bpg) has developed and continues to generate and update *Best Practice Guidelines* for nurses working with children, adults and older adults experiencing a myriad of health challenges. For older adults, Best Practice Guidelines have been developed for "Screening for Delirium, Dementia and Depression in the Older Adult," as well as "Caregiving Strategies for Older Adults with Delirium, Dementia and Depression," "Prevention of Constipation in the Older Adult Population" and "Prevention of Falls and Fall Injuries in the Older Adult." In the summer of 2014, the RNAO released Best Practice Guidelines for Abuse and Neglect of Older Adults. Additionally, NICE (The National Initiative for the Care of the Elderly) provides tools for nurses

TABLE 7-1 Age-Related Variations in Laboratory Values

Laboratory Values That Are NOT Affected by Normal Aging

- Hematocrit and hemoglobin
- Electrolytes (sodium, potassium, chloride, bicarbonate)
- Calcium
- Phosphorus
- Liver function tests
- Blood urea nitrogen
- Thyroid tests
- White blood cell count
- Platelet count

Laboratory Values that are Often Abnormal in Older Adults	Clinical Considerations
Sedimentation rate	Elevations between 10 and 20 mm may be within normal for older adults
Glucose	Glucose may be elevated during acute illness and return to normal when the physiologic stress resolves
Albumin	Average values decline slightly with increased age, especially during acute illness, but significant decreases indicate undernutrition
Alkaline phosphatase	May be mildly elevated with normal aging, but significant elevations may occur with serious illness (e.g., liver or Paget disease)
Serum iron, iron-binding capacity, ferritin	Decreased values may usually indicate undernutrition and/or gastrointestinal blood loss
Urinalysis	Hematuria requires further evaluation; slight pyuria or bacteriuria are common and do not necessarily require treatment

Source: Adapted from R. L. Kane, J. G., Ouslander, I. B. Abrass, et al. (2013). *Essentials of clinical geriatrics* (7th ed.). New York, NY: McGraw.

for assessment of older clients pertaining to walking, elder abuse, driving cessation, mental health and the like (http://www.nicenet.ca/tools-mental-health). While these guidelines and tools do not replace a comprehensive assessment, they are nonetheless useful for identifying specific areas to address in the care plan. Also, it is important to consider that the purpose of some assessment guidelines and tools is to screen for indicators of certain conditions, such as depression or dementia, and in these situations, they are a stepping stone to further assessment.

An easy-to-use tool that has been widely used since 1991 to identify common syndromes in older adults that require nursing interventions is the Fulmer SPICES, an acronym for **S**leep disorders, **P**roblems with eating or feeding, **I**ncontinence, **C**onfusion, **E**vidence of falls and **S**kin breakdown

(Fulmer & Wallace, 2012). Online Learning Activity 7-1 provides additional information about the SPICES and other assessment tools. Another easy-to-use assessment tool that can be used to measure changes in level of functioning is called "SHOW ME." Nurses in home care settings can use this tool to assess functioning in the following areas: **S**hirt & shoes, **H**ike to bathroom, **O**rganization and use of grooming utensils, **W**alk through home in all areas needed for ADL/IADL, **M**edications and **E**ating and making meals (Narayan et al., 2009).

> ### Wellness Opportunity
>
> When assessing older adults, nurses try to identify the conditions that affect not only health status and level of functioning, but also quality of life.

FUNCTIONAL ASSESSMENT

A functional assessment is an integral component of a holistic assessment because an essential part of promoting wellness for older adults is identifying areas where function can be improved. **Functional assessment** refers to the measurement of a person's ability to fulfil responsibilities and perform self-care tasks. Functional assessment has its roots in the 1920s when workers' compensation programs needed to determine a cash value to impairments that affected loss of function in jobs. Initially, there were no standards for this and the determination was based solely on a physician's opinion. When rehabilitation services were developed after World War II, tools were needed to measure changes in functional abilities. Functional assessment tools measure **activities of daily living (ADL)**, which are the tasks associated with meeting one's basic needs and **instrumental activities of daily living (IADL)**, which are the more complex tasks that are essential in community-living situations.

In recent years, health care practitioners have increasingly recognized the value of functional assessment, particularly with regard to chronic conditions and geriatric care. In contrast to a medical diagnosis approach, a functional assessment approach focuses on improved functioning in daily life, regardless of diagnosis. In geriatric clinical settings, there is increasing emphasis on using functional assessments as a core component of **function-focused care**, which is a rehabilitative approach to preventing functional decline and improving an older adult's level of functioning. Figure 7-1 lists major trends related to the use of functional assessment approaches in gerontological health care settings today. Details about functional assessment and function-focused care are discussed in the following sections.

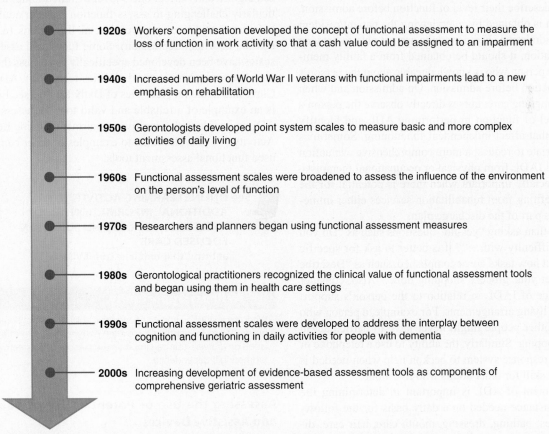

1920s Workers' compensation developed the concept of functional assessment to measure the loss of function in work activity so that a cash value could be assigned to an impairment

1940s Increased numbers of World War II veterans with functional impairments lead to a new emphasis on rehabilitation

1950s Gerontologists developed point system scales to measure basic and more complex activities of daily living

1960s Functional assessment scales were broadened to assess the influence of the environment on the person's level of function

1970s Researchers and planners began using functional assessment measures

1980s Gerontological practitioners recognized the clinical value of functional assessment tools and began using them in health care settings

1990s Functional assessment scales were developed to address the interplay between cognition and functioning in daily activities for people with dementia

2000s Increasing development of evidence-based assessment tools as components of comprehensive geriatric assessment

FIGURE 7-1 Significant trends related to the use of functional assessment approaches in gerontological health care settings today.

A Student's Perspective

During my first week with Mr. M., I was able to sit with him while he was having breakfast, and I used this time to consider his strengths and weaknesses. While studying his interactions with others, I observed that he had difficulty being understood. He struggled to articulate his various wants and needs. This seemed to lead to Mr. M. being more isolated than would otherwise be the case. One of his strengths was his ability to feed himself. Initially, I had hoped to read his chart more before meeting him. However, this interaction allowed me a more accurate assessment of his abilities than what would have been recorded in his chart.

After breakfast, we returned to his room to do oral care and to shave. After this, I helped transfer Mr. M. to his bed and he asked for a drink, which I gave him and he started choking. I was terrified, but fortunately my senior student was with me and together we managed the situation and he was okay. I learned from this experience to assess the person's entire environment before addressing patient needs and desires. Mr. M. choked because I gave him a cup of water that was not thickened.

Kimberly S.

Nurses obtain information for the functional assessment from several sources. When older adults are able to accurately describe their level of function before admission, information is obtained by interviewing the patient/resident soon after admission. If older adults are not able to provide this information, it should be obtained from a family member or other person who is knowledgeable about the person's level of function before admission. On admission and when providing ongoing care, nurses directly observe the person's current level of function in performing ADL and identify conditions that affect independent functioning. Sometimes it is appropriate to request a more comprehensive evaluation of ADL and IADL from physical or occupational therapists. This is especially important when there is potential for the person benefiting from rehabilitation services either immediately or as part of the discharge plan.

Rather than asking "yes-no" questions such as "Do you have any difficulty with…?" it is better to ask for specific details about how tasks are accomplished, such as "Describe how you get your grocery shopping done." Also, consider the relevance of IADL in relation to the person's support system and living arrangements. For example, a person who lives with other people might never have to participate in grocery shopping. Similarly, the ability to use a telephone or emergency response system to beckon help when needed is an essential skill for older adults who live alone.

Assessment of ADL is important in determining the level of assistance needed on a daily basis for the following activities: bathing, dressing, mouth care, hair care, dietary intake, transfer mobility, ambulation, bed mobility and bladder and bowel elimination. When assessing ADL, it is

important to determine whether limitations are attributable, at least in part, to cognitive impairments, rather than primarily to physical limitations. For example, the ability to dress independently can be limited by difficulties with processing information, as is common in people with dementia. Also, it is important to assess any relationship between cognitive impairment and difficulty with maintaining bowel and bladder control because this information is pertinent to planning effective interventions.

IADL include shopping, laundry, transportation, housekeeping, meal preparation, money management, medication management and the use of telephone. Although these IADL are less important for residents or patients in institutional settings, an assessment is essential for discharge planning. When older adults cannot perform IADL and have no caregiver to help with the tasks, community resources, such as home-delivered meals, are available to meet these needs.

Wellness Opportunity

Nurses identify factors that affect the older adult's quality of life by asking a question, such as "Are there enjoyable activities that you used to do but are no longer able to do because of health problems?"

Because cognitive status and psychosocial functioning can significantly affect one's level of functioning, it is particularly challenging to assess function in older adults who have any cognitive or psychosocial limitations (e.g., dementia, delirium, depression). Some functional assessment scales have been developed specifically to address the interplay between cognition and abilities to perform ADL. The Cleveland Scale for Activities of Daily Living (see Fig. 7-2) is an example of a reliable and valid tool for assessing the ADL in people with cognitive impairment. Online Learning Activity 7-1 provides links to examples of other commonly used functional assessment tools.

 See **ONLINE LEARNING ACTIVITY 7-1: ADDITIONAL INFORMATION ABOUT ASSESSMENT TOOLS AND FUNCTION-FOCUSED CARE** at http://thepoint.lww.com/Miller7e

Wellness Opportunity

When assessing the impact of cognitive abilities on functioning, nurses can try to identify simple interventions, such as putting labels on drawers, that can improve the person's self-esteem by promoting independence.

Assessing the Use or Potential Use of Adaptive and Assistive Devices

The actual or potential use of items, such as mobility aids (e.g., canes, walkers, wheelchairs) and adaptive equipment

CLEVELAND SCALE FOR ACTIVITIES OF DAILY LIVING (CSADL)

Name or ID of Subject _____

Date _ _/_ _/_ _ Rater_____
　　　　　　　　　　　　　　　m m d d y y

Name of Informant _____

Relation of Informant to Subject *(Circle one.)*

1 Spouse　　4 Friend or other family

2 Child　　　5 Professional: _____

3 Sibling　　6 Other: _____

Contact with Subject

1　2 days/week

2　3–4 days/week

3　5 or more days/week

Interview Type

1　Visit

2　Telephone

To administer this scale, the rater must be thoroughly familiar with the Manual, which includes the full instructions. Place rating in blank after each item number. Several items have specific rating instructions. In particular, some require special questioning if the subject is rated as dependent (rating of 1, 2, or 3).

Rating	*Meaning of Rating*
0	**Never Dependent.** [S] does this effectively, quite independently, without any direction or help.
1	**Sometimes Dependent.** [S] usually does this independently, but sometimes or in some situations [S] needs direction or help.
2	**Usually Dependent.** [S] usually requires some direction or help, but sometimes or in some situations [S] does it independently.
3	**Always Dependent.** [S] always requires direction or help. [S] never does it independently.
9	Cannot rate because of insufficient information

Bathing

1. ____ Initiates bath or shower with appropriate frequency and at appropriate times

2. ____ Prepares bath/shower (draws water of proper temperature, ensures soap and towel are present, etc.)

3. ____ Gets in and out of tub or shower

4. ____ Cleans self

Toileting

5. ____ Able to physically control timing of urination

6. ____ Able to physically control timing of bowel movements

7. ____ Recognizes need to eliminate

8. ____ After toileting, cleans and re-clothes self appropriately

Personal Hygiene and Appearance

9. ____ Initiates personal grooming with appropriate frequency and at appropriate times

10. ____ Washes hands and face

11. ____ Brushes teeth

12. ____ Combs hair, shaves (as appropriate)

FIGURE 7-2 The Cleveland Scale for Activities of Daily Living (CSADL). This functional assessment form was specifically designed for use with people with Alzheimer's disease. (Used with permission from the University Memory and Aging Centre, Case Western Reserve University, Cleveland, OH. © 1994.)

Dressing

13. _____ Initiates dressing at appropriate time

14. _____ Selects clothes

15. _____ Puts on garments, footwear, etc.

16. _____ Fastens clothing (buttons, shoelaces, zippers, etc.)

Eating

17. _____ Initiates eating at appropriate times of day and with appropriate frequency

18. _____ Carries out physical acts of eating (including using utensils)

19. _____ Eats with acceptable manners, e.g., with appropriate speed, does not speak with food in mouth, etc.

20. _____ Prepares own meals (includes cooking on stove). *This item requires special questioning.*

Mobility

21. _____ Initiates actively moving about the environment, as opposed to sitting, not attempting to get about, etc.

22. _____ Actively moves about environment (with or without assisting device)

22a. Does subject have physical limitations of mobility? *(Circle one of following codes.)*

　　0　No physical limitations of mobility

　　1　Yes, there are physical limitations of mobility. *(Circle all that apply.)*

Needs assistance of other persons to walk	Trouble getting in or out of bed	Other Mobility Problems
Needs cane	Trouble getting in or out of chair	*(describe):*
Needs walker	Trouble getting on or off toilet	
Needs wheelchair	Trouble climbing or descending stairs	

Medications

23. _____ Takes medications as scheduled and in correct dosages. *If subject has taken no medications during prior year, rate item as 9. This item requires questioning.*

Shopping

24. _____ Does necessary grocery shopping, buying appropriate items and quantities. *This item requires special questioning.*

25. _____ Does necessary clothes shopping, buying appropriate items and quantities. *This item requires special questioning.*

Travel

26. _____ Finds way about in familiar surroundings

27. _____ Orients to unfamiliar surroundings without undue difficulty

28. _____ Travels beyond walking distance (i.e., driving own vehicle or using public transportation)

29. _____ Drives motor vehicle. *This item requires special questioning.*

FIGURE 7-2 *(continued)*

Hobbies, personal interests, employment

30. _____ Initiates activities of personal interest (e.g., card playing, woodworking, others). *This item requires special questioning.*

31. _____ Carries out such activities. *This item requires special questioning.*

32. _____ Does subject work for pay? *If subject does not work because of having reached an age appropriate to retirement from his or her occupation, rate 9. This item requires special questioning.*

Housework/home maintenance (as appropriate to individual situation)

33. _____ Initiates work around house as needed. *This item requires special questioning.*

34. _____ Carries out work effectively, e.g., cleanly, neatly, accurately, efficiently. *This item requires special questioning.*

Types of work done *(Don't score, just circle)*

Dish washing	Vacuuming	Mowing lawn
Sweeping	Scrubbing floors	Gardening
Personal laundry	Small home repairs	Minor car care
Other types of work *(Describe):*		

Telephone

35. _____ Looks up numbers

36. _____ Dials numbers

37. _____ Answers phone

38. _____ Takes messages

Money Management

39. _____ Pays for purchases (selecting appropriate amount and determining correct change). *This item requires special questioning.*

40. _____ Manages financial responsibilities beyond paying for immediate purchases (e.g., paying monthly bills, managing checking or savings account, etc.). *This item requires special questioning.*

Communication Skills

41. _____ Spontaneously expresses thoughts and needs to others

42. _____ Responds accurately to spoken instructions and conversation

43. _____ Reads and understands single words and short phrases (signs, lists, etc.)

44. _____ Reads and understands complex material (books, newspapers, etc.)

45. _____ Writes short phrases (lists, brief messages)

46. _____ Writes complex material (letters, diary, etc.)

FIGURE 7-2 *(continued)*

Social Behavior

47. ____   Behaves in a socially appropriate manner. Socially inappropriate behaviors encompass a **wide** range of behavior, including but not limited to such things as making rude remarks, belching, touching private parts, showing little regard for personal privacy, etc. For this item, dependency refers to the extent to which other people must direct or manage the subject to ensure that he or she behaves in a socially appropriate fashion.

Other Problems — Are there any situations in which patient does not behave in an independent and responsible fashion that have not been covered by these questions? *(Circle one of following codes.)*

48.   0   No other dependent behaviors

      1   Yes, there are other dependent behaviors.   *(Please provide details below.)*

QUALITY OF INTERVIEW (Rater's Judgment)

Interview appeared valid   0

Some questions about interview, but it is probably acceptable   1

Information from interview is of doubtful validity   2

Rater should record the basis for judging the interview of questionable or doubtful validity.

Comments:

FIGURE 7-2 *(continued)*

(e.g., grab bars), should be assessed as factors that can significantly affect safety, functioning and quality of life for older adults. Physical, occupational and rehabilitation therapists are skilled in assessing for the use of these aids, but nurses need to be familiar with the array of adaptive and assistive devices so that they can make recommendations or facilitate referrals for further evaluation. Online Learning Activity 7-2 provides information about many helpful and innovative devices that can be used to improve functioning and independence in daily activities. Additional assistive devices are illustrated and discussed in many chapters of this book (e.g., see Chapters 16, 17, 22).

Nurses can also identify problems related to the use of assistive devices and request further evaluation by a qualified therapist. For example, nurses can assess the comfort and function of wheelchairs because improper fit leads to specific problems, such as the ones delineated in Table 7-2. Another nursing responsibility is making sure that wheelchairs are used appropriately for responsible patient care rather than for staff convenience, as is sometimes the case in long-term care facilities.

 See **ONLINE LEARNING ACTIVITY 7-2: RESOURCES FOR INFORMATION ABOUT HELPFUL AND INNOVATIVE DEVICES TO IMPROVE FUNCTIONING AND INDEPENDENCE** at http://thepoint.lww.com/Miller7e

TABLE 7-2 Negative Effects of Improper Wheelchair Fit

Seating Problem	Result on Body	Potential Effect
Wheelchair too high	Feet do not touch the floor	Edema and decreased circulation in legs
	Unable to self-propel	Decreased activity
	Pelvis moves forward	Poor sitting posture
Poor back support	Compression of trunk, chest, abdomen	Skin breakdown on back and sacrum
	Sliding out of chair	Impaired gastrointestinal and respiratory function
	Increased pelvic tilt	
Wheelchair too heavy	Difficulty moving chair	Decreased activity
Wheelchair too wide	Pelvic shifting laterally	Shear stress on skin
	Forward leaning	Poor posture, circulation
	Difficulty using hand rims	Decreased mobility
Seat not firm enough ("sling" effect)	Scoliosis	Poor posture, circulation
	Sliding out of chair	Shear stress on skin
Footrest too high	Poor femoral support	Poor posture
	Unequal pressure distribution	Skin breakdown
	Increased ischial tuberosity	

Source: Rader, J., Jones, D., & Miller, L. (2000). The importance of individualized wheelchair seating for frail older adults. *Journal of Gerontological Nursing, 26*(11), 24–31.

FUNCTION-FOCUSED CARE

Function-focused care, which was previously referred to as restorative care, is an approach to care that focuses both on evaluating a person's underlying capability with regard to functional and physical activity and on implementing interventions to optimize and maintain functional abilities and increase physical activities (Resnick et al., 2013). The philosophy of function-focused care addresses direct care issues, as well as broader considerations, such as environmental factors and staff training. Studies find that this approach is effective in improving outcomes for older adults with acute and chronic conditions, including trauma and dementia (Burket et al., 2013; Galik et al., 2013). In addition, evidence-based practice guidelines for geriatric nursing have incorporated this approach in relation to assessment of physical function and preventing functional decline in acute care settings, as summarized in Box 7-1 (Boltz et al., 2012; Kresevic, 2012).

 Box 7-1 Evidence-Based Practice: Function-Focused Care and Assessment of Physical Function

Statement of the Problem

- Older adults often experience functional decline during hospitalization, and this leads to poor long-term outcomes, which include increased mortality, decreased functional recovery and increased likelihood of being discharged to a nursing facility.
- Some functional decline that occurs during hospitalization is progressive and irreversible, but some can be prevented or ameliorated by prompt and aggressive nursing interventions (e.g., ambulation, toileting schedules, effective communication, use of adaptive equipment, appropriate medication regimens).
- Risk factors for functional decline during hospitalization include pain, depression, malnutrition, decreased mobility, cognitive impairment and adverse medication effects.
- Bed rest and lack of physical activity result in loss of muscle strength and muscle mass, altered sensory awareness, reduced appetite and thirst sensation, and decreased aerobic capacity and pulmonary ventilations.
- Interprofessional care plans are essential for performing functional assessments, evaluating conditions that restrict physical activity (e.g., restraints) and implementing interventions for progressive mobility.

Recommendations for Assessment of Physical Function

- Functional assessment is a critical component of nursing care and involves assessment and documentation of (1) a person's ability to perform activities of daily living (ADL) and instrumental activities of daily living (IADL), with particular attention to mobility, and social activities, (2) level of assistance needed, (3) sensory function and (4) cognitive function.
- Document baseline functional status and information about recent or progressive changes.
- Assess function at appropriate intervals to validate capacity, decline or improvement.
- Assess strengths and abilities of older adults, as well as limitations.

Recommendations for Care Strategies to Improve Functional Status

- Maintain the person's daily routine as much as possible through physical activity and social interaction.
- Minimize bedrest and encourage physical activity (exercise, ambulation, range of motion).
- Avoid restraints.
- Use medication judiciously and in appropriate doses.
- Assess for and manage pain.
- Facilitate referrals for rehabilitation therapy, nutrition counselling and coaching.
- Allow flexible visitation, including pets.
- Teach older adults, families and care givers about the value of independent functioning and strategies to prevent functional decline.

Sources: Boltz, M., Resnick, B., & Galik, E. (2012). Interventions to prevent functional decline in acute care settings; Kresevic, D. (2012). Assessment of physical function. In M. Boltz, E. Capezuti, T. Fulmer, & D. Zwicker (Eds.), *Evidence-based practice protocols for best practice* (4th ed., pp. 89–121). New York, NY: Springer.

COMPREHENSIVE GERIATRIC ASSESSMENTS

As gerontologists and health care providers began addressing the complexity of care for older adults, they recognized the need for assessment models that were more comprehensive than those that focused on particular aspects of health or functioning. A **comprehensive geriatric assessment** includes medical, psychosocial, cognitive and functional components, as described in an article by Wells and Wade (2013), which is available through Online Learning Activity 7-3.

In the United States, the Omnibus Budget Reconciliation Act of 1987 mandated that all Medicaid- and Medicare-funded nursing homes begin using a standardized assessment form, called the **Minimum Data Set (MDS) for Resident Assessment and Care Screening**. In Canada, the RAI-MDS (2.0) began to be used around 2007 and currently is being used by all provinces to assess older adults residing in long-term care facilities, except for New Brunswick and Quebec (Sutherland et al., 2013). The value of the MDS has been internationally recognized and both the nursing home and home care versions have been translated, validated, and implemented in many countries, including Canada, Australia, and Asian and European countries. While the RAI-MDS (2.0) has many strengths, it is weak in its ability to measure mood or behavioural problems (Sutherland et al., 2013). Please note that while the RAI-MDS (3.0) is being used in the United States, as of 2013, Canada still used the RAI-MDS (2.0) (Estabrooks et al., 2013). Box 7-2 summarizes components of the MDS form (3.0), with examples of items related to each topic, and Figure 7-3 shows the section on functional status, with details related to assessment of ADL.

 Box 7-2   Minimum Data Set (MDS) Categories and Examples of Assessment Items

Hearing, Speech, Vision

- Ability to hear, use of hearing aid
- Speech clarity, abilities to make self understood and to understand others
- Ability to see in adequate light, use of corrective lenses

Cognitive Patterns

- Repetition and recall of three words
- Orientation to year, month, day
- Short- and long-term memory
- Ability to make decisions about tasks of daily life
- Signs and symptoms of delirium

Mood (Interview or Self-Assessment)

- Symptoms of depression during the past 2 weeks
- Evidence of depression

Behaviour

- Hallucinations or delusions
- Physical or verbal behavioural symptoms directed toward others
- Rejection of care
- Wandering
- Changes in behaviour

Preferences for Customary Routine, Activities, Community Setting

- Preferred routine for daily activities (e.g., personal care, communication, social and religious activities)
- Potential for returning to the community

Functional Status (see Fig. 7-3)

Bladder and Bowel

- Ability to maintain urinary and bowel continence
- Toileting program for urinary elimination (e.g., scheduled toileting, prompted voiding, bladder training) or bowel continence
- Bowel patterns

Active Disease Diagnosis (i.e., currently listed diagnoses)

- Cancer
- Conditions related to any of the following systems: thermoregulation, circulatory, gastrointestinal, genitourinary, musculoskeletal, pulmonary, neurological or metabolic
- Nutritional conditions
- Infection
- Psychiatric or mood disorder ·

Health Conditions

- Pain management and assessment
- Cough or shortness of breath (dyspnea)

- Chest pain or angina
- Current tobacco use
- Prognosis related to chronic disease that may result in shortened life expectancy
- Falls assessment and history

Swallowing/Nutrition Status

- Swallowing disorder
- Height and weight
- History of weight loss of 5% or more during last month or 10% or more in the past 6 months
- Nutritional approaches (e.g., feeding tube, mechanically altered diet, therapeutic diet)

Oral/Dental Status

- Condition of teeth and gums
- Absence of teeth
- Mouth or facial pain

Skin Conditions

- Presence of pressure ulcers in the past 5 days
- Pressure ulcer stages
- Healed pressure ulcers
- Other skin problems (e.g., venous or arterial ulcers, surgical wounds, burns, open lesions)
- Skin treatments (e.g., pressure-reducing devices, repositioning program, dressings, nutrition or hydration interventions to manage skin problems)

Medications

- Injections
- Use of any of the following medications during the past 5 days: antipsychotic, antianxiety, antidepressant, hypnotic, anticoagulant

Special Treatments and Procedures

- Cancer treatments
- Respiratory treatments
- Dialysis
- Hospice care
- Vaccination status (influenza, pneumococcal)
- Therapies (e.g., speech-language, occupations, physical, respiratory, psychological, recreational)
- Nursing rehabilitation and restorative care
- Physician examination and orders during the past 5 days

Restraints

- Any method that the person cannot remove easily, which restricts freedom of movement or normal access to one's body

Source: Recommended MDS 3.0, available at www.cms.gov

Section G

Functional Status

G1. Activities of Daily Living (ADL) Assistance

Code for most dependent episode in last 5 days:

Coding:

0. Independent—resident completes activity with no help or oversight

1. Set up assistance

2. Supervision—oversight, encouragement, or cueing provided throughout the activity

3. Limited assistance—guided maneuvering of limbs or other non-weight bearing assistance provided at least once

4. Extensive assistance, 1 person assist—resident performed part of the activity while one staff member provided weight-bearing support or completed part of the activity at least once

5. Extensive assistance, 2 + person assist—resident performed part of the activity while two or more staff members provided weight-bearing support or completed part of the activity at least once

6. Total dependence, 1 person assist—full staff performance of activity (requiring only 1 person assistance) at least once. The resident must be unable or unwilling to perform any part of the activity.

7. Total dependence, 2 + person assist—full staff performance of activity (requiring 2 or more person assistance) at least once. The resident must be unable or unwilling to perform any part of the activity.

8. Activity did not occur during the entire period

Enter Codes in Boxes →
→

Enter / Code		
Enter Code	**a.**	**Bed mobility** moving to and from lying position, turning side to side, and positioning body while in bed.
Enter Code	**b.**	**Transfer** moving between surfaces—to or from: bed, chair, wheelchair, standing position (**excludes** to/from bath/toilet).
Enter Code	**c.**	**Toilet transfer** how resident gets to and moves on and off toilet or commode.
Enter Code	**d.**	**Toileting** using the toilet room (or commode, bedpan, urinal); cleaning self after toileting or incontinent episode(s), changing pad, managing ostomy or catheter, adjusting clothes (**excludes** toilet transfer).
Enter Code	**e.**	**Walk in room** walking between locations in his/her room.
Enter Code	**f.**	**Walk in facility** walking in corridor or other places in facility.
Enter Code	**g.**	**Locomotion** moving about facility, with wheelchair if used.
Enter Code	**h.**	**Dressing upper body** dressing and undressing above the waist, includes prostheses, orthotics, fasteners, pullovers.
Enter Code	**i.**	**Dressing lower body** dressing and undressing from the waist down, includes prostheses, orthotics, fasteners, pullovers.
Enter Code	**j.**	**Eating** includes eating, drinking (regardless of skill) or intake of nourishment by other means (e.g., tube feeding, total parenteral nutrition, IV fluids for hydration).
Enter Code	**k.**	**Grooming/personal hygiene** includes combing hair, brushing teeth, shaving, applying makeup, washing/drying face and hands (**excludes** bath and shower).
Enter Code	**l.**	**Bathing** how resident takes full-body bath/shower, sponge bath and transfers in/out of tub/shower (**excludes** washing of back and hair).

G2. Mobility Prior to Admission

↓ **Complete only on admission assessment** ↓

Enter Code	**a.**	Did resident have a **hip fracture, hip replacement, or knee replacement** in the 30 days prior to this admission?
		0. **No** → Skip to G3, Balance During Transitions and Walking
		1. **Yes** → Complete G2b
		9. **Unable to determine** → Skip to G3, Balance During Transitions and Walking
	b.	If yes, check all that apply for tasks in which the resident was independent prior to fracture/replacement.

Check all that apply.

☐ 1. **Transfer**
☐ 2. **Walk across room**
☐ 3. **Walk 1 block on a level surface**
☐ 4. **Resident was not independent in any of these activities**
☐ 9. **Unable to determine**

FIGURE 7-3 Functional Status section of MDS 3.0, available at www.cms.gov. Within Canada, conversations have started to upgrade the assessment tool being used.

Section G — Functional Status

G3. Balance During Transitions and Walking

After observing the resident, code the following **walking and transition items for most dependent** over the last 5 days:

Coding:

0. **Steady at all times**
1. **Not steady, but able to stabilize without human assistance**
2. **Not steady, only able to stabilize with human assistance**
3. **Activity did not occur**

Enter Codes in Boxes

Enter / Code	Item
	a. **Moving from seated to standing** position
	b. **Walking** (with assistive device if used)
	c. **Turning around** and facing the opposite direction while walking
	d. **Moving on and off toilet**
	e. **Surface-to-surface transfer** (transfer from wheelchair to bed or bed to wheelchair)

G4. Functional limitation in range of motion

Code for limitation during last 5 days that interfered with daily functions or placed resident at risk of injury.

Coding:

0. **No impairment**
1. **Impairment on one side**
2. **Impairment on both sides**

Enter Codes in Boxes

Enter / Code	Item
	a. **Lower extremity** (hip, knee, ankle, foot)
	b. **Upper extremity** (shoulder, elbow, wrist, hand)

G5. Gait and Locomotion

Check all that were normally used in the past 5 days:

Check all that apply.

☐	a.	**Cane/Crutch**
☐	b.	**Walker**
☐	c.	**Wheelchair (manual or electric)**
☐	d.	**Limb prosthesis**
☐	e.	**None of the above** were used

G6. Bedfast

Enter / Code

In bed or in recliner in room for more than 22 hours on at least three of the past 5 days.

0. **No**
1. **Yes**

G7. Functional Rehabilitation Potential

↓   **Complete only on admission assessment**   ↓

Enter / Code

a. **Resident believes s/he is capable of increased independence** in at least some ADL's.

0. **No**
1. **Yes**
9. **Unable to determine**

Enter / Code

b. **Direct care staff believe resident is capable of increased independence** in at least some ADL's.

0. **No**
1. **Yes**

FIGURE 7-3 (continued)

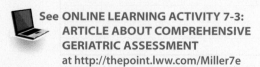

See **ONLINE LEARNING ACTIVITY 7-3:
ARTICLE ABOUT COMPREHENSIVE
GERIATRIC ASSESSMENT**
at http://thepoint.lww.com/Miller7e

Wellness Opportunity

Keep in mind that formal assessment tools fulfil requirements for documentation, but their primary purpose is to improve care and quality of life for older adults.

ASSESSMENT OF SAFETY IN HOME SETTINGS

In addition to assessing the older adult's health and functioning, nurses need to be aware of environmental factors that influence the person's safety, functioning and quality of life. Researchers and practitioners increasingly are addressing the interrelationship between people and their environments, and this is particularly pertinent to care of older adults. In the late 1990s, the term **everyday competence** was used to describe the effects of cultural, physical, cognitive, emotional, social and contextual factors on a person's daily functioning. This is particularly important to consider when assessing older adults because these factors can appreciably hinder or improve functional abilities. For example, environmental factors that significantly affect hearing, vision and mobility are discussed in Chapters 16, 17 and 22, respectively.

Home assessments provide an excellent base for assessing the relationship between older adults and their environments. These assessments are essential not only for identifying fall risks (as discussed in Chapter 22), but also for identifying environmental conditions that positively or negatively affect safety, functioning and quality of life. For example, proper lighting is essential for performing enjoyable activities, such as reading, playing cards and engaging in hobbies. Similarly, the ability to regulate the temperature is important not only as a safety consideration for preventing hypothermia and hyperthermia, but also for comfort. During home visits, it is especially important for nurses to respect autonomy and privacy and be nonjudgmental, and at the same time be able to identify all factors that affect the person's functioning and quality of life. This is particularly important for older adults with significant limitations or who are experiencing dementia (see Box 7-3). It can also be useful for nurses to ask family members about their concerns about the safety of their older members, especially if these older individuals live alone and are cognitively impaired. Nurses can use Box 7-4 as a guide to assessing home environments for safety and optimal functioning.

Wellness Opportunity

In addition to assessing conditions that affect functioning, nurses pay attention to environmental factors that affect quality of life.

DRIVING SAFETY

Nurses are among the health care professionals responsible for addressing complex decisions about driving, not only as a personal safety issue for older adults, but also as an ethical issue to protect society. **Safe driving** is an IADL that is the focus of much attention from health care professionals, as well as all members of society as illustrated in the following examples:

- Geriatricians and occupational therapists discuss criteria for assessing driving abilities of older adults.

Box 7-3 Evidence-Informed Nursing Practice

Background: While there are a number of studies examining family members' concerns about their older members with dementia living alone, there are fewer reports about the concerns of these older adults living alone. As a number of older adults with dementia live alone, it is important to understand the meaning they attribute to living alone.

Methods: Using a phenomenological approach, the researchers interviewed eight women (aged 57–87 years) from Ontario who were living alone and had been diagnosed with mild to moderate dementia. Within these interviews, participants were asked to describe what it was like to live alone with dementia, their thoughts on continuing to live alone, concerns about safety and living alone with dementia, what it was like to ask for help and their concerns for the future.

Findings: Themes related to time emerged in the data. The women spoke of "holding back the time," whereby they were trying to stay independent within their homes as long as they could. They tried to "store time" through taking medications to slow the progression of the dementia. They discussed the "dreaded time" when their disease would be worse and they could no longer function on their own. They identified "now" as the time to stop driving or to register for the Alzheimer Society Safely Home Registry. "Limited time" was discussed in terms of shortened time to remain at home, as well as impending death. However, these women indicated that they feared burdening their families much more than death.

Implications for Nursing Practice: The importance of time is heightened for older adults living alone with dementia. Nurses can be sensitive to the meaning older adults attribute to their dementia including the importance of early diagnosis (so that older adults can commence medication to possibly delay the worsening of symptoms), as well as significance of addressing future concerns.

Source: de Witt, L., Ploeg, J., & Black, M. (2010). Living alone with dementia: An interpretive phenomenological study with older women. *Journal of Advanced Nursing, 66,* 1698–1707.

- Families and health care professionals debate about ethical issues related to forcing older drivers, especially those who have dementia, to stop driving.
- Lawmakers and seniors' advocacy groups (e.g., CARP) question the need for mandatory testing for drivers at the age of 80 or above.
- Geriatric references increasingly point out the need for evidence-based assessment tools and guidelines for families, lawmakers and professionals to address the many issues related to older adult drivers.

Nurses have important roles in collaborating closely with other care providers to address this complex issue from a broad perspective. Psychosocial implications related to driving cessation are discussed in Chapter 12, and in this chapter safe driving is discussed as an IADL.

Wellness Opportunity

Nurses can sensitively address issues about driving by expressing compassionate concern not only for the individual older adult, but also for the safety of others.

Box 7-4 Guidelines for Assessing the Safety of the Environment

Illumination and Colour Contrast

- Is the lighting adequate but not glare producing?
- Are the light switches easy to reach and manipulate?
- Can lights be turned on before entering rooms?
- Are night lights used in appropriate places?
- Is colour contrast adequate between objects, such as a chair and the floor?

Hazards

- Are there highly polished floors, throw rugs or other hazardous floor coverings?
- If area rugs are used, do they have a nonslip backing, and are the edges tacked to the floor?
- Are there cords, clutter or other obstacles in pathways?
- Is there a pet that is likely to be running underfoot?

Furniture

- Are chairs the right height and depth for the person?
- Do the chairs have armrests? Are tables stable and of the appropriate height?
- Is small furniture placed well away from pathways?

Stairways

- Is lighting adequate?
- Are there light switches at the top and bottom of the stairs?
- Are there securely fastened handrails on both sides of the stairway?
- Are all the steps even?
- Are the treads nonskid?
- Should coloured tape be used to mark the edges of the steps, particularly the top and bottom steps?

Bathroom

- Are grab bars placed appropriately for the tub and toilet?
- Does the tub have skid-proof strips or a rubber mat in the bottom?
- Has the person considered using a tub or shower seat?
- Is the height of the toilet seat appropriate?
- Has the person considered using an elevated toilet seat?
- Does the colour of the toilet seat contrast with surrounding colours?
- Is toilet paper within easy reach?

Bedroom

- Is the height of the bed appropriate?
- Is the mattress firm at the edges to provide enough support for sitting?
- If the bed has wheels, are they locked securely?
- Would full or partial side rails be a help or a hazard?
- When side rails are in the down position, are they completely out of the way?

- Is the pathway between the bedroom and bathroom clear of objects and adequately illuminated, particularly at night?
- Would a bedside commode be useful, especially at night?
- Is there a light near the bed, and does the person have sufficient physical and cognitive ability to turn it on before getting out of bed?
- Is furniture positioned to allow safe use of assistive devices for ambulation?
- Is a telephone situated near the bed?

Kitchen

- Are storage areas used to the best advantage (e.g., are objects that are frequently used in the most accessible places)?
- Are appliance cords kept out of the way?
- Are nonslip mats used in front of the sink?
- Does the person know how to use the oven, stove or microwave safely?

Assistive Devices

- Is a call light available, and does the person know how to use it?
- What assistive devices are used?
- Would the person benefit from any assistive devices that are not being used?
- Are assistive devices being used safely and properly, or do they present additional hazards?

Temperature

- Is the temperature of the room(s) comfortable?
- Can the person read the markings on the thermostat and adjust it appropriately?
- During cold months, is the room temperature high enough to prevent hypothermia?
- During hot weather, is the room temperature cool enough to prevent hyperthermia?

Overall Safety

- How does the person obtain objects from hard-to-reach places?
- How does the person change overhead light bulbs?
- Are doorways wide enough to accommodate assistive devices?
- Do door thresholds create hazardous conditions?
- Are telephones accessible, especially for emergency calls? Would it be helpful to use a cordless portable phone?
- Would it be helpful to have some emergency call system available?
- Does the person wear sturdy shoes with nonskid soles?
- Does the person keep a list of emergency numbers by the phone?
- Does the person have an emergency exit plan in the event of fire?
- Are smoke alarms present and operational?
- Is there a carbon monoxide detector in an appropriate place (if the house has gas appliances, wood burning stoves or another object that produces carbon monoxide)?

Risks for Unsafe Driving

When motor vehicle accident rates are adjusted for miles driven, the at-fault crash rate for drivers older than 70 years is comparable to that of drivers below age 25 years, with the casualty rate increasing exponentially after age 75 or 80 (Young & Bunce, 2011). Age-related changes in vision, musculoskeletal function and central and autonomic nervous systems can affect driving abilities even in healthy older adults. In addition, older adults often have other conditions that increase the risk for unsafe driving, such as medical

conditions, cognitive impairment, functional limitations, medication use and alcohol consumption. Two commonly identified concerns related to driving are difficulty with night driving and safely changing lanes (Fortin-McCue et al., 2013).

Risks for unsafe driving are identified by a comprehensive assessment that includes all of the following components (Classen et al., 2013; Flanagan, 2011):

- Full visual examination, including acuity and contrast sensitivity

- Cognitive tests, including skills related to attention, executive function and visuoperceptual processing
- Motor performance, including gait, balance, postural control and speed of walking
- Medication review
- Self-report questions
- Questions for family members and caregivers

Although these specific components have been identified, evidence-based recommendations about criteria for driving cessation are lacking, even among driver rehabilitation specialists (Bowers et al., 2013; Dickerson, 2013; Martin et al., 2013).

Nursing Assessment of Driving

Questions about the older person's perception of or concerns about his or her driving can be used to open the discussion of this important, but sometimes sensitive, topic. Studies indicate that most older adults, including those with mild cognitive impairment and mild dementia, have insight into their driving abilities and appropriately self-regulate by avoiding complex and risky driving situations (O'Connor et al., 2011, 2013). Some older adults, however, have little or no insight and adamantly insist on driving despite evidence that their driving poses serious risks to themselves and others (Wood et al., 2013). Nurses can open the discussion by indicating that questions about driving are routinely incorporated into an assessment so any identified safety concerns can be addressed proactively. The following questions can be used for this part of the assessment:

- Do you have any concerns about your ability to drive safely?
- Have you adjusted your driving patterns to avoid certain situations, such as driving at night, on highways or at intersections involving left-hand turns?
- Has anyone in your family expressed concerns about your driving?
- Have you gotten lost while driving in places that are usually familiar?
- Have you been in any accidents during the past couple of years? (If yes, ask about circumstances.)
- Have you had any citations related to unsafe driving or driving under the influence?

When appropriate, nurses can use these same kind of questions to elicit assessment information from family members who are likely to have observations and concerns.

If answers to any of these questions raise concerns about driving safety, a more comprehensive assessment is warranted, as discussed in the next section. Also, if the older person has any condition that is associated with risks for driving (e.g., dementia, functional impairment, significant vision impairment), arrangements should be made for appropriate assessments, which are usually performed by specialized rehabilitation specialists.

Wellness Opportunity

Nurses can promote personal responsibility by assessing the older adult's awareness of driving issues and their willingness to address these concerns.

Nursing Interventions Related to Safe Driving

Addressing risk factors that affect driving abilities is an important health promotion activity that should be integrated into usual care for older adults, preferably before significant safety concerns arise. Geriatricians have recommended that "advance driving directives" be initiated to facilitate discussions between health care professionals and older drivers as a routine part of care (Betz et al., 2013a, 2013b). Geriatricians also recommend a comprehensive approach to "stages of driving cessation" for people with dementia, which would include individualized interventions that are optimally timed, address grief, provide caregiver support, maintain key relationships and explore alternative means of transportation (Liddle et al., 2013).

Some risks for unsafe driving can be minimized through interventions that address contributing factors, such as vision and hearing impairments and medication-related issues (discussed in Chapters 16, 17 and 8, respectively). When pathologic conditions affect neuromuscular functioning, nurses may suggest a referral for physical or occupational therapy to improve particular aspects of functioning that affect driving. For example, an older person with arthritis or Parkinson's disease may benefit from working with a therapist who has additional training for driving rehabilitation. Even if the therapist does not have special training, the older adult can focus on the goal of improved safety and functioning for driving skills as part of the therapy program. Older adults may be more motivated to participate in exercises prescribed by physical or occupational therapists if they see a connection between the therapies and maintaining safe and independent functioning.

Wellness Opportunity

Nurses can promote quality of life for older adults by creatively identifying appropriate and acceptable ways of improving an older adult's ability to continue driving safely.

Referrals for Driving Evaluation and Recommendations

Families are likely to seek guidance from nurses and other health care professionals to address their safety concerns about driving abilities of an older adult. In Canada, the first means of evaluation for safety in driving is conducted by the physician (or depending upon the province, may also be a nurse practitioner or an occupational therapist). The physician is responsible for conducting a physical exam, visual testing and to utilize a screening tool to assess cognitive intactness or impairment. Where there are concerns, physicians are instructed (by the Canadian Medical Association publication, *Determining Medical Fitness to Operate Medical Vehicles: CMA Driver's Guide*) to refer patients for a road assessment mandated by the provincial motor vehicle board (Laycock, 2011). The provincial motor vehicle board will then review physicians' reports and make a decision regarding what kind of further testing is needed. For instance, when cognitive impairment is suspected, the provincial board may refer older adults for a DriveABLE assessment (Dobbs, 2013; Saskatchewan Society of Occupational Therapists, 2014). When suggesting that an older adult needs to be assessed by his or her family physician, it is important to emphasize that the purpose is not to take away the person's driving privileges but rather to identify interventions to improve safety for the person and others.

Recommendations from the provincial motor vehicle board of driving evaluation results can widely vary and may include modifying vehicles to compensate for physical limitations, participating in driving rehabilitation therapy or refraining from or restricting driving. Examples of adaptive equipment include pedal extenders, distance sensors, left foot accelerators, steering wheel adaptations, touch pads to operate auxiliary controls and spot mirrors to compensate for visual and range-of-motion deficit. Examples of recommendations related to driving restrictions are no highways, short distances or familiar areas only, daytime or fair weather driving only and requiring the presence of a navigator.

Mature drivers' workshops are another type of resource that helps older adults recognize driving issues and improve safety. These programs are available in some communities in Canada and are often advertised through seniors' centres (Jensen, 2010) or through the Canada Safety Council (55 Alive Driver Refresher Course). Use Online Learning Activity 7-4 to find information about resources related to education, evaluation and rehabilitation related to driving.

In addition to suggesting programs that directly address safe driving, nurses can suggest referrals to programs that provide transportation for older adults. For example, senior centres are available in many urban areas of the country and they generally provide transportation services and/or information about local resources.

 See **ONLINE LEARNING ACTIVITY 7-4: RESOURCES RELATED TO EDUCATION, EVALUATION, AND REHABILITATION RELATED TO DRIVING** at http://thepoint.lww.com/Miller7e

Chapter Highlights

Health Assessment of Older Adults

- Assessment of health and functioning in older adults is challenging because of many factors that contribute to the complexity of assessing older adults (e.g., presence of multiple interacting conditions, unique manifestations

of illness, treatments that mask the underlying problem, myths and misunderstandings about aging).
- Consider age-related variations in some laboratory values when assessing older adults (Table 7-1).

Nursing Assessment Tools

- Easy-to-use and evidence-based nursing assessment tools and related resources are available through online learning activities in clinically oriented chapters of this text.

Functional Assessment

- Approaches to functional assessment have evolved since the 1920s, with current emphasis on function-focused care and comprehensive geriatric assessments (Fig. 7-1).
- Functional assessment tools provide a structure for assessing the person's ability to perform ADL and IADL.
- The Cleveland Scale for Activities of Daily Living can be used for older adults who are cognitively impaired (Fig. 7-2).
- Assessing the use of adaptive equipment and assistive devices is important for identifying factors that affect safety, comfort and functioning.

Function-Focused Care

- Function-focused care focuses both on evaluating a person's underlying capability with regard to functional status and physical activity and on implementing interventions to optimize and maintain functional abilities and increase physical activities (Box 7-1).

Comprehensive Geriatric Assessments

- Comprehensive geriatric assessments, such as the Minimum Data Set for Resident Assessment and Care Planning, are used to provide information about all aspects of functioning (Box 7-2 and Fig. 7-3).

Assessment of Safety in Home Settings

- Assessment of the home environment is important for identifying factors that affect safety, comfort, functioning and quality of life (Box 7-4).

Driving Safety

- Nurses have an important role in identifying risk factors that compromise safe driving in older adults.
- Common risk factors include conditions that affect vision, cognition, motor responses and reaction time.
- Nurses incorporate questions about driving to identify the need for a more comprehensive assessment.
- Risks for unsafe driving can be minimized through interventions that address contributing factors (e.g., vision and hearing impairments, medication-related issues).
- Nurses have important roles in facilitating referrals for further evaluation or for programs related to driving safety, education and rehabilitation.

Critical Thinking Exercises

1. Review the factors that contribute to the complexity of assessing health of older adults and apply these to an older adult in a clinical setting or someone you know personally.

2. Using Online Learning Activity 7-1, select a nursing assessment tool that would be easy to use in clinical settings and apply the information to an older adult for whom you have cared.

3. Read the evidence-based information in Box 7-1 and identify ways in which this information is applicable to older adults in hospitals or nursing homes.

4. Identify an older adult (in a clinical setting or someone you know personally) who has some functional impairment, as well as some cognitive impairment, and perform a functional assessment on him or her, using Figure 7-2.

5. Identify an older adult (in a clinical setting or someone you know personally) who has risk factors that affect his or her driving safety; explore one or more of the resources listed in Online Learning Activity 7-4 to find information applicable to addressing concerns about safe driving for this person.

For more information about topics discussed in this chapter, be sure to check out the interactive Online Learning Activities and other helpful resources at http://thepoint.lww.com/Miller7e

REFERENCES

Betz, M. E., Jones, J., Petroff, E., et al. (2013a). "I wish we could normalize driving health": A qualitative study of clinician discussions with older drivers. *Journal of General Internal Medicine, 28*(12), l573–1580. doi:1007/s11606-013-2498-x

Betz, M. E., Lowenstein, S. R., & Schwartz, R. (2013b). Older adult opinions of "advance driving directives." *Journal of Primary Care and Community Health, 4*(1), 14–27.

Boltz, M., Resnick, B., & Galik, E. (2012). Interventions to prevent functional decline in acute care settings. In M. Boltz, E. Capezuti, T. Fulmer, et al. (Eds.), *Evidence-based practice protocols for best practice* (4th ed., pp. 104–121). New York, NY: Springer.

Bowers, A. R., Anastasio, R. J., Sheldon, S. S., et al. (2013). Can we improve clinical prediction of at-risk older drivers? *Accident Analysis and Prevention, 59*, 537–547. doi:10.1016/j.aap.2013.06.37

Burket, T. L., Hippensteel, D., Penrod, J., et al. (2013). Pilot testing of the function focused care intervention on an acute care trauma unit. *Geriatric Nursing, 34*, 241–246.

Classen, S., Wang, Y., Winter, S. M., et al. (2013). Concurrent criterion validity of the safe driving behaviour measure: A predictor of on-road driving outcomes. *American Journal of Occupational Therapy, 67*(1), 108–116.

Dickerson, A. E. (2013). Driving assessment tools used by driver rehabilitation specialists: Survey of use and implications for practice. *American Journal of Occupational Therapy, 67*(5), 564–573.

Dobbs, A. R. (2013). Accuracy of DriveABLE cognitive assessment to determine cognitive fitness to drive. *Canadian Family Physician, 59*, e156–e161.

Estabrooks, C. A., Knopp-Sihota, J. A., & Norton, P. G. (2013). Practice sensitive quality indicators in RAI-MDS 2.0 nursing home data. *BioMedCentral, 6*, 460. doi:10.1186/1756-0500-6-460

Flanagan, N. M. (2011). Driving and dementia: What nurses need to know. *Journal of Gerontological Nursing, 37*(8), 10–13.

Fortin-McCue, L. A., Saleheen, H., McQuay, J., et al. (2013). Implementation of a community-based mature driver screening and referral program. *Accident Analysis and Prevention, 50*, 751–757.

Fulmer, T., & Wallace, M. (2012). Fulmer SPICES: An overall assessment tool for older adults. *Try this: Best Practices in Nursing Care to Older Adults.* Hartford Institute for Geriatric Nursing. Retrieved from www.consultgerirn.org

Galik, E., Resnick, B., Hammersla, M., et al. (2013). Optimizing function and physical activity among nursing home residents with dementia: Testing the impact of function-focused care. *The Gerontologist.* Advance online publication. doi:10.1093/geront/gnt108

Jensen, L. (2010). Senior drivers. *BC Medical Journal, 52*(2), 97.

Kresevic, D. (2012). Assessment of physical function. In M. Boltz, E. Capezuti, T. Fulmer, et al. (Eds.), *Evidence-based practice protocols for best practice* (4th ed., pp. 89–103). New York, NY: Springer.

Laycock, K. M. (2011). Driver assessment: Uncertainties inherent in current methods. *BC Medical Journal, 53*(2), 74–78.

Liddle, J., Bennett, S., Allen, S., et al. (2013). The stages of driving cessation for people with dementia: Needs and challenges. *International Psychogeriatrics, 25*(12), 2033–2046. doi:10.1017/S1041610213001464

Martin, A. J., Marottoli, R., & O'Neill, D. (2013). Driving assessment for maintaining mobility and safety in drivers with dementia. *Cochrane Database, Systematic Reviews, 8*, CDC006222. doi:10.1002/14651858.CD006222.pub4

Narayan, M. C., Salgado, J., & VanVoorhis, A. (2009). SHOW ME: Enhancing OASIS functional assessment. *Home Health care Nurse, 27*(1), 19–23.

O'Connor, M. L., Edwards, J. D., & Bannon, Y. (2013). Self-rated driving habits among older adults with clinically-defined mild cognitive impairment, clinically-defined dementia, and normal cognition. *Accident Analysis and Prevention, 61*, 197–202. doi:10.1016/j.app.2013.05.010

O'Connor, M. L., Edwards, J. D., Small, B. J., et al. (2011). Patterns of level and change in self-reported driving behaviours among older adults: Who self-regulates? *Journals of Gerontology: Psychological Sciences and Social Sciences, 67*(4), 437–446.

Resnick, B., Galik, E., & Boltz, M. (2013). Function focused care approaches: Literature review of progress and future possibilities. *Journal of the American Medical Directors Association, 14*, 313–318.

Saskatchewan Society of Occupational Therapists. (2014). *Mandatory reporting to SGI.* Retrieved from http://www.ssot.sk.ca/mandatory-reporting-to-sgi

Sutherland, J. M., Repin, N., & Crump, R. T. (2013). *The Alberta Health Services patient/care-based funding model for long-term care: A review and analysis.* Retrieved from http://www.albertahealthservices.ca/Publications/ahs-pub-ltc-pcbf.pdf

Wells, M., & Wade, M. (2013). Physical performance measures: An important component of the comprehensive geriatric assessment. *Nurse Practitioner, 38*(6), 49–53.

Wood, J. M., Lacherez, P. F., & Anstey, K. J. (2013). Not all older adults have insight into their driving abilities: Evidence from an on-road assessment and implications for policy. *Journals of Gerontology: Medical Sciences, 68*(5), 559–566.

Young, M. S., & Bunce, D. (2011). Driving into the sunset: Supporting cognitive functioning in older drivers. *Journal of Aging Research*, 2011 [Article ID 918782]. doi:10.4061/2011/918782

chapter 8

Medications and Other Bioactive Substances

Although the topic of medications and older adults is not a distinct category of function in the same sense as physiologic and psychosocial aspects of function (e.g., vision and cognition), it can be addressed from a similar perspective. This chapter presents information within the context of the functional consequences theory for promoting wellness to address issues related to medications and older adults, with particular attention to the role of nurses.

INTRODUCTION TO BIOACTIVE SUBSTANCES

In addition to discussing prescription and over-the-counter (OTC) medications in relation to older adults, this chapter addresses other bioactive substances that are used for therapeutic purposes (e.g., herbs and homeopathic remedies). Bioactive substances that can affect medication action are also addressed in the section on medication interactions. Nurses need to be aware of the special considerations related to commonly used types of bioactive substances so that they can promote safe and effective use for older adults.

Considerations Regarding Medications

Effects of medications in the body are usually considered in relation to **pharmacokinetics** (i.e., how the drug is absorbed, distributed, metabolized and excreted) and **pharmacodynamics** (i.e., how the body is affected by the drug at the cellular level and in relation to the target organ). Absorption refers to the passage of a medication from its site of introduction, usually the gastrointestinal tract, into the general circulation. Absorption of oral medications can be affected by diminished gastric acid, increased gastric pH, delayed gastric emptying and the presence of other substances (e.g., food, nutrients, medication additives). Because most oral medications are absorbed by passive diffusion across the small intestine—a process that is not pH dependent—they are not usually affected by any alterations in gastric acidity. The unique chemical properties of each medication determine

Promoting Safe and Effective Medication Use in Older Adults

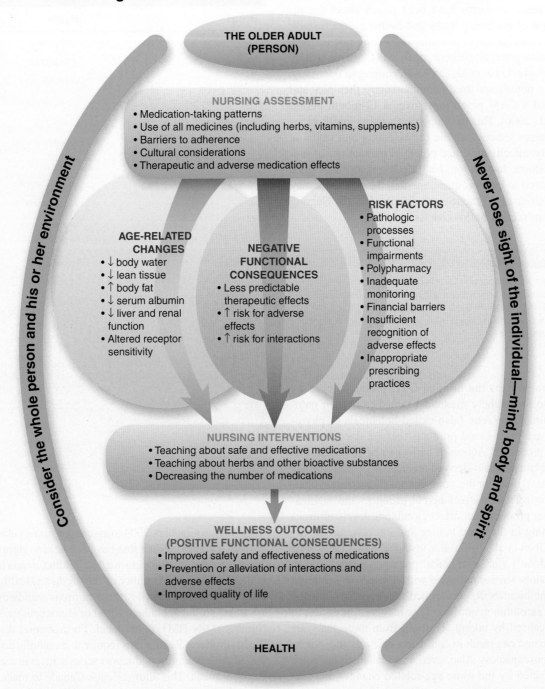

THE OLDER ADULT (PERSON)

NURSING ASSESSMENT
- Medication-taking patterns
- Use of all medicines (including herbs, vitamins, supplements)
- Barriers to adherence
- Cultural considerations
- Therapeutic and adverse medication effects

AGE-RELATED CHANGES
- ↓ body water
- ↓ lean tissue
- ↑ body fat
- ↓ serum albumin
- ↓ liver and renal function
- Altered receptor sensitivity

NEGATIVE FUNCTIONAL CONSEQUENCES
- Less predictable therapeutic effects
- ↑ risk for adverse effects
- ↑ risk for interactions

RISK FACTORS
- Pathologic processes
- Functional impairments
- Polypharmacy
- Inadequate monitoring
- Financial barriers
- Insufficient recognition of adverse effects
- Inappropriate prescribing practices

NURSING INTERVENTIONS
- Teaching about safe and effective medications
- Teaching about herbs and other bioactive substances
- Decreasing the number of medications

WELLNESS OUTCOMES (POSITIVE FUNCTIONAL CONSEQUENCES)
- Improved safety and effectiveness of medications
- Prevention or alleviation of interactions and adverse effects
- Improved quality of life

HEALTH

Consider the whole person and his or her environment

Never lose sight of the individual—mind, body and spirit

the degree to which it is susceptible to any gastrointestinal changes, regardless of age. For example, pH-sensitive medications, such as penicillin and ferrous sulfate, are more likely to be affected by altered gastric acid levels or by prolonged exposure to these acids because of delayed emptying.

Two measures of the efficiency of metabolism and elimination of a drug are elimination half-time and clearance rate. **Elimination half-time** (also called serum half-life) is the time required to decrease the drug concentration by one half of its original value. It takes five half times to reach steady-state concentrations after a drug is initiated or to completely eliminate a drug from the body after a drug is discontinued. The **clearance rate** measures the volume of blood from which the drug is eliminated per unit of time. An increase in serum half-time or a decrease in clearance rate may result in accumulation of the drug. The result is that the therapeutic effect is likely to be altered and the risk of adverse effects is likely to be increased.

Considerations Regarding Herbs and Homeopathy

In recent years, concerns have been raised about the increasing use of medicinal herbs and herbal products, with particular concerns about potential herb–drug interactions. Complementary and alternative medicine (CAM) is widely used in Canada (Quan et al., 2008). According to one study, 50% of the population used complementary therapies and 22% visited a CAM practitioner over a 12-month period (Boon et al., 2006). This has important nursing implications because nurses are responsible for assessing and teaching about safety, effectiveness and potential interactions of medicinal products. In addition, health care practitioners need to be prepared to address questions that their patients may ask about alternative practices, as discussed in the Nursing Interventions section of this chapter.

 DIVERSITY NOTE

As the largest visible minority in Canada, the Chinese report greater use of complementary and alternative medicine use than other minority groups and white Canadians (Lai & Chappell, 2007; Quan et al., 2008).

First Nations people in Canada may use sweat lodges for healing and promoting wellness.

Herbs

Herbs were perhaps the original OTC products, used by people who found these medicinal remedies in their natural environments. **Herbs** (also called botanicals or phytotherapies) are plant-based products that are used for their medicinal properties. Action of herbs can be similar to that of commonly used plant-derived medications (see Table 8-1 for examples). Because the same pharmacokinetic and pharmacodynamic factors affect herbal products and medications, herbal products can affect circulating levels of drugs by interacting in the liver, kidney and intestine and at target sites (Chen et al., 2012). For instance, older adults who ingest St. John's wort—an herbal preparation that is taken for depression—in combination with a selective serotonin reuptake inhibitor (SSRI) prescribed for depression may be at risk for serotonin syndrome. This involves an excess of serotonin caused by taking serotonin from more than one preparation and can result in confusion, seizures and, potentially, unconsciousness. Also, even when taken alone, herbs can be affected by the same age-related changes and risk factors that affect medications in older adults.

Although manufacturers are required to ensure the accuracy of the ingredient list, labels do not necessarily include accurate information about additional ingredients, potential harmful effects, quantity of active ingredients or suitability of form for human use. Despite the lack of strict requirements, however, some safeguards are in place to protect consumers from false claims. Health Canada–Food and Drug Regulations (FDR) is responsible for addressing false claims on product labels, as well as monitoring advertising claims in the media.

There are also additional safeguards in place to address concerns about safety of herbal products and dietary supplements. Health Canada established Natural Health Products

TABLE 8-1 Drugs and Herbs With Similar Bioactivity	
Drugs	**Herbs**
Aspirin	Birch bark
	Willow bark
	Wintergreen
	Meadowsweet
Anticoagulants	Dong quai
	Feverfew
	Garlic
	Ginkgo biloba
	Wintergreen
Caffeine	Guarana
	Kola nut
Ephedrine	Ephedra
Estrogen	Black cohosh
	Fennel
	Red clover
	Stinging nettle
Lithium	Thyme
	Purslane
Monoamine oxidase inhibitors	Ginseng
	St. John's wort
	Yohimbe
Nicotine	Lobelia
Calcium-channel blockers	Angelica

Regulations in January 2004 to assure consumers that they are buying a quality product that has been held to rigorous standards. These regulations ensure that Health Canada has determined the safety and quality of the product (Health Canada, 2012a). Products that meet these rigorous standards display a Natural Product Number (NPN) or Homeopathic Medicine Number (DIN-HM) on the label. Furthermore, the Natural Health Products Regulations require that manufacturers monitor adverse reactions and report serious adverse reactions to Health Canada. This allows Health Canada to make changes in product safety information, warn the public of potential adverse reactions and, in some cases, remove unsafe products from the Canadian market (Health Canada, 2012a).

Although many dietary supplements are safe, if they have been obtained from reliable sources, the risk for adverse effects increases for people with certain conditions, such as a history of stroke, glaucoma, diabetes, hypertension, heart disease and any disorder requiring anticoagulation therapy. Also, surgical care can be complicated by effects of certain herbs, such as those that affect coagulation or electrolyte balance or prolong the effects of anesthetics. Thus, surgeons generally recommend that all herbs and supplements be discontinued at least 2 weeks before surgery.

TABLE 8-2 Potential Adverse Effects of Some Herbs

Herbs	Potential Effect
Black cohosh	Bradycardia, hypotension, joint pains
Bloodroot	Bradycardia, arrhythmia, dizziness, impaired vision, intense thirst
Boneset	Liver toxicity, mental changes, respiratory problems
Coltsfoot	Fever, liver toxicity
Dandelion	Interactions with diuretics, increased concentration of lithium or potassium
Ephedra	Anxiety, dizziness, insomnia, tachycardia, hypertension
Feverfew	Interference with blood-clotting mechanisms
Garlic	Hypotension, inhibition of blood clotting, potentiation of antidiabetic drugs
Ginseng	Anxiety, insomnia, hypertension, tachycardia, asthma attacks, postmenopausal bleeding
Ginkgo biloba	Increased anticoagulation
Goldenseal	Vasoconstriction
Guar gum	Hypoglycemia
Hawthorn	Hypotension
Hops, skullcap, valerian	Drowsiness, potentiation of antianxiety or sedative medications
Kava	Damage to the eyes, skin, liver and spinal cord from long-term use
Licorice	Hypokalemia, hypernatremia
Lobelia	Hearing and vision problems
Motherwort	Increased anticoagulation
Nettle	Hypokalemia
Senna	Potentiation of digoxin
Yohimbe	Anxiety, tachycardia, hypertension, mental changes

Another concern is that herbs and other dietary supplements have the potential for interactions with other drugs, particularly those drugs with a narrow therapeutic range (e.g., digoxin and theophylline). Some of the more serious effects of herbs (listed in Table 8-2) include altered liver function, electrolyte imbalance, elevated blood pressure, diminished blood-clotting mechanisms and alterations of the heart rate and rhythm. Less serious adverse effects include nausea, vomiting and other gastrointestinal symptoms from oral preparations, especially if they are taken with medications that have similar adverse effects.

Homeopathic Remedies

Three concepts are crucial to understanding homeopathy, as it was proposed two centuries ago by the German physician, Samuel Hahnemann. First, according to the law of similars, or "like cures like," homeopathy stimulates the body's self-healing abilities through the use of a small amount of a substance similar to that which caused the illness. For example, quinine can produce symptoms of malaria in a healthy person, and it can cure malaria when administered in minute doses. Second, on the basis of the concept that potency of a substance increases the more it is diluted, homeopathic remedies are diluted repeatedly and shaken vigorously each time. Third, on the basis of the concept that treatment must be individualized to match each episode of illness, homeopathic practitioners focus on treating the person, not the disease. Homeopathy is widely used in India, Russia, Mexico and European countries, and it is gaining acceptance in Canada as a safe alternative to conventional medicine.

Although most homeopathic remedies are now available for self-treatment, a few are available only through health care practitioners. Homeopathic remedies are regulated by the Natural Health Products Directorate in Canada. Remedies come in a variety of single-substance or combination forms, including powders, wafers, small tablets and alcohol-based liquids. Because OTC homeopathic products are too weak to cause adverse effects, there is less concern about these products.

AGE-RELATED CHANGES THAT AFFECT MEDICATIONS IN OLDER ADULTS

Age-related changes that affect medications in older adults are discussed in relation to those that affect therapeutic effects and those that affect the skills involved with taking them. The factors that have the most significant impact on the effectiveness of medications in older adults are not age-related changes, but risk factors, and are considered in the section on risk factors.

Changes That Affect the Action of Medications in the Body

An age-related decline in glomerular filtration rate, which begins in early adulthood and progresses at an annual rate of 1% to 2%, can decrease renal clearance and increase serum levels of medications. This is especially problematic for medications that are highly water soluble and those that have a narrow therapeutic range (see Box 8-1 for examples).

Box 8-1 Effects of Age-Related Changes on Medication Effectiveness

Medications With Decreased Clearance Caused by Renal Changes

Amantadine
Atenolol
Ceftriaxone
Cephalexin
Chlorpropamide
Cimetidine
Ciprofloxacin
Colchicine
Digoxin
Enalapril
Furosemide
Gentamicin
Glyburide
Hydrochlorothiazide
Levofloxacin
Lisinopril
Metformin
Penicillins
Ranitidine

Medications With Decreased Clearance Caused by Hepatic Changes

Acetaminophen
Amitriptyline
Barbiturates
Benzodiazepines
Codeine
Labetalol
Lidocaine
Meperidine
Morphine
Phenytoin
Propranolol
Quinidine
Salicylates
Theophylline
Warfarin

Medications With Increased Concentrations Caused by Changes in Body Composition

Cimetidine
Digoxin

Ethanol (alcohol)
Gentamicin
Morphine
Propranolol
Quinine
Warfarin

Medications With Decreased Concentrations Caused by Changes in Body Composition

Phenobarbital
Prazosin
Thiopental
Tolbutamide

Medications With Increased Potency Caused by Increased Receptor Sensitivity

Angiotensin-converting
  enzyme (ACE)
  inhibitors
Diazepam
Digoxin
Diltiazem
Enalapril
Felodipine
Levodopa
Lithium
Midazolam
Morphine
Temazepam
Verapamil
Warfarin

Medications Whose Signs of Toxicity May Be Delayed Because of Decreased Receptor Sensitivity

β-blockers
Bumetanide
Dopamine
Furosemide
Isoproterenol
Propranolol
Tolbutamide

Hepatic blood flow declines progressively, beginning around the age of 40 years, and this age-related change can increase serum levels of substances that are metabolized more extensively by the liver. In addition, factors such as diet, caffeine, smoking, alcohol, genetic variations and pathologic conditions can affect liver metabolism of substances. In recent years, there has been increasing attention to the role of enzyme systems in the liver that are responsible for the metabolism of bioactive substances, including medications, herbs, nutrients and nicotine. The cytochrome P-450 system is particularly important with regard to interactions because competition at the enzyme sites can cause adverse effects and interactions, as discussed in the section on medication interactions. Box 8-1 lists examples of medications that are affected by age-related hepatic changes.

Age-related changes in body composition (i.e., decreased body water and lean tissue and increased body fat) can affect substances according to their degree of fat or water solubility. Consequently, medications that are distributed primarily in body water or lean body mass may reach higher serum concentrations in older adults and their effects may be more intense. Similarly, the serum concentration of highly fat-soluble substances can increase, so the immediate therapeutic effects are diminished, but the overall effects are prolonged or erratic.

Protein-binding capacity of a medication (i.e., the extent to which their molecules are bound to serum albumin and other proteins) is an important determinant of both therapeutic and adverse effects. Low serum albumin levels, which are common in older adults, lead to an increased amount of the active portion of protein-bound substances. In addition, when two or more protein-bound substances compete for the same binding sites, adverse effects are more likely to occur. Medications that are most likely to have adverse effects when they are taken together or when serum albumin levels are low include aspirin, digoxin, furosemide, nonsteroidal anti-inflammatory drugs (NSAIDs), hypoglycemics, phenytoin, sertraline and sulfonamides.

In addition to changes that affect pharmacokinetics, age-related changes in receptor sensitivity can influence pharmacodynamics and cause older adults to be more or less sensitive to particular substances (see Box 8-1 for examples). For instance, an increased sensitivity of the older brain to centrally acting psychotropic medications may potentiate both the therapeutic and adverse effects of these drugs. This is particularly true for anticholinergic medications, as discussed in the section on inappropriate prescribing practices. Age-related change in homeostatic mechanisms, such as thermoregulation, fluid regulation and baroreceptor control over blood pressure, also can affect pharmacodynamics. For example, inefficient fluid regulation may alter the action of medications, such as lithium, that are particularly sensitive to fluid and electrolyte balance.

Changes That Affect Medication-Taking Behaviours

For any adult, all the following factors affect the appropriate use of medications:

- Motivation
- Knowledge about the purpose of the substance
- Cultural and psychosocial influences
- Ability to obtain correct amounts (influenced by factors such as cost, accessibility)
- Ability to distinguish the correct container
- Ability to read and comprehend directions
- Ability to hear and remember verbal instructions
- Knowledge about correct timing for consumption
- Ability to follow the correct dosage regimen
- Physical ability to remove the substance from the container and administer it
- Ability to swallow oral preparations
- Additional skills related to coordination, manual dexterity and visual acuity for substances that are administered nasally, transdermally, subcutaneously or by other routes

Even for healthy older adults, age-related changes and functional impairments often interfere with these skills. For example, hearing or vision changes can interfere with the ability to understand instructions and read directions and labels on bottles. Any limitations in fine motor movement of the hands may interfere with the ability to remove lids from containers, especially when the lids are tamper resistant. Although age-related change can influence skills related to taking medications, risk factors that commonly occur in older adults exert a stronger influence.

 ### RISK FACTORS THAT AFFECT MEDICATION-TAKING BEHAVIOURS

Risk factors that influence medication-taking behaviours for older adults can arise from the person's own attitudes or level of knowledge and socioeconomic circumstances, or they can be attributed to outside sources (e.g., health care providers). The consumption of more than one bioactive substance greatly increases the potential for adverse and altered therapeutic effects. Because older adults often take several or many medications, they are more likely to experience interactions and adverse effects. Additional risks arise from myths and misunderstandings that affect the medication consumption patterns of older adults. Finally, certain factors unrelated to age, such as weight, sex and smoking habits, combine with age-related changes and risk factors to increase further the risk of adverse and altered effects.

> ### Wellness Opportunity
>
> Nurses provide holistic care when they explore the wide range of factors that affect medications and medication-taking behaviours, with emphasis on identifying those that are most amenable to health promotion interventions.

Pathologic Processes and Functional Impairments

Because the purpose of any medication is to relieve or control symptoms, one can assume that people who take medications have at least one underlying pathologic process. The increased prevalence of chronic conditions in older adults adds complexity to prescribing the safest and most appropriate medication regimen. For example, pain management for many older adults who have both arthritis and hypertension is complicated by the common occurrence of increased blood pressure as an adverse effect of NSAIDs.

Medication–disease interactions manifest themselves in any of the following ways:

- Pathologic processes can exacerbate age-related changes that would otherwise have little or no impact on the medication. For example, malnutrition further decreases serum albumin, thereby increasing both the therapeutic and adverse effects of highly protein-bound medications.
- Pathologic processes can alter therapeutic and adverse effects of substances. For instance, heart failure decreases both the metabolism and the excretion of most medications.
- Medications can cause serious adverse effects for people with pathologic conditions. For example, anticholinergics may cause urinary retention in men with prostatic hyperplasia.

Pathologic conditions not only influence the action of substances in the body but also contribute to nonadherence, especially in combination with functional limitations. For example, dementia can significantly affect the older adult's ability to understand directions, remember instructions and self-manage medication regimens. Dysphagia is an example of a physical limitation that can interfere with the ability to take substances orally.

Behaviours Based on Myths and Misunderstandings

Myths and misunderstandings influence attitudes held by older adults, as well as their caregivers, about the use of medications. An attitude that can be potentially harmful for older adults is that medications provide a "quick fix" for problems that commonly occur during later adulthood. For example, messages promoting medications for overactive bladder can reinforce false beliefs about urinary incontinence and lead to inappropriate use of medications without proper evaluation (as discussed in Chapter 19). Although adults of any age can be influenced by these attitudes, older adults are more likely than their younger counterparts to experience adverse effects and drug interactions.

Another potentially harmful belief is that OTC remedies are always safe, even in extra-strength doses. Although OTC preparations may be relatively safe for healthy younger adults, they can cause problems for older adults, particularly when combined with other substances. For example, OTC preparations for colds and insomnia typically contain anticholinergic ingredients that are strongly associated with delirium and other serious adverse effects in older adults. In these situations, the addition of a seemingly harmless OTC product to an already complex regimen of prescription medications can be the factor that tips the scale of safety and causes a serious effect, such as delirium. NSAIDs are another category of OTC drugs that commonly have serious adverse effects in older adults, either alone or with other substances (e.g., anticoagulants, prednisone). Acetaminophen, also a commonly used OTC product, can have serious adverse effects, including liver failure and death, when used in high doses.

Attitudes and expectations about medications as quick-fix remedies can influence the prescribing patterns of primary care practitioners. For example, a nonpharmacologic remedy may be safer than, and just as effective as, a prescription medication, but these remedies usually demand more of the practitioner's time and some degree of patient motivation. Sleep and anxiety complaints are examples of conditions that respond to evidence-based nonpharmacologic treatments, but these conditions are often addressed by prescription medications because of the attitudes of the patient or primary care practitioner.

> ### Wellness Opportunity
>
> By taking time to identify an older adult's beliefs about illness and treatments (including pharmacologic and nonpharmacologic approaches), nurses pave the way for teaching about the safest and most effective interventions.

Communication Barriers

Another factor that may contribute to an increased use of prescriptions by older adults is their reluctance to challenge or question the primary care practitioner, whom they perceive as "all-knowing." Although the image of the infallible physician is subsiding, older adults are still inclined to accept advice from prescribing practitioners without question. Additional communication barriers include lack of confidence in one's communication skills and fear of appearing ignorant. Hearing and vision impairments also may interfere with patient-directed discussions of a treatment plan. An attitude of impatience on the part of the health care practitioner may also thwart discussion. In addition, language barriers and differences on the part of either the older adult or the health care practitioner can interfere with a discussion of health issues and lead to misunderstandings.

Lack of Information

Despite the fact that older adults are the primary consumers of prescription and OTC medications, our knowledge about medication effects in older adults is insufficient and still in an early phase. Before the 1980s, research on the influence of age-related effects on medications was virtually nonexistent and the few cross-sectional studies that were done identified age differences rather than age-related changes. Efforts are being made, however, to identify medications that may be more likely to cause adverse reactions in some older adults. For instance, the Institute for Safe Medication Practices Canada contains information about the potential dangers of particular medications on older adults (see http://www.ismp-canada.org/beers_list/). Although some progress has been made in this area, a current concern is that evidence-based information is lacking about prescribing for older adults with multiple conditions, which is the group for whom most medications are prescribed (American Geriatrics Society, 2012a; Le Couteur et al., 2012).

Another concern is that some adverse effects and medication–medication interactions are identified only after a medication has been on the market for several years. This is particularly important for older adults because they are most likely to have the highest risk for adverse effects and interactions. Thus, recently approved medication should be used cautiously in older adults because of the increased risk of adverse effects and unpredictable interactions.

Inappropriate Prescribing Practices

During the late 1980s, geriatricians began to address medication-related problems in older adults because of widespread concerns about the quantity and types of drugs prescribed for this population. The phrase **potentially inappropriate medications** refers to medications that pose more risks than benefits for older adults, particularly when safer alternatives exist. In 1991, an international panel of experts used consensus criteria to identify drugs that should not be used by frail older adults (Beers et al., 1991). According to these explicit criteria, known as the **Beers Criteria** (complete title 2012 AGS Beers Criteria for Potentially Inappropriate Medication Use in Older Adults), medications are deemed inappropriate if they are ineffective or have poor safety profiles, or if better drugs are available (Beers et al., 1991). Since the 1990s, the Beers Criteria have been updated several times. They are widely used in Canada, the United States and worldwide to guide research and clinical practice.

In 2012, the American Geriatrics Society published an updated Beers Criteria list that was developed by a team of experts who used an enhanced evidence-based methodology. The updated Beers Criteria summarize evidence-based rationales and ratings for recommendations in the following three categories (American Geriatrics Society, 2012b):

1. Potentially inappropriate medications for use in older adults by organ system/therapeutic category (e.g., anticholinergics, antithrombics, anti-infective, cardiovascular, central nervous system, endocrine, gastrointestinal and pain medications)
2. Potentially inappropriate medications for use in older adults resulting from drug effects that may exacerbate the disease or syndrome (e.g., heart failure, syncope, chronic seizures, delirium, dementia, falls/fractures, insomnia, Parkinson disease, chronic constipation, gastric or duodenal ulcers, chronic kidney disease, urinary incontinence, benign prostatic hyperplasia)
3. Potentially inappropriate medications that should be used cautiously in older adults (e.g., aspirin for primary prevention of cardiac events, certain antipsychotics and vasodilators)

An important theme of the Beers Criteria and other guidelines is that medications are determined to be appropriate or inappropriate in relation to the patient's condition. For example, a study of older adults discharged from intensive care units found that many of the medications were appropriate during the admission but were inappropriate following discharge (Morandi et al., 2013).

In 1997, a Canadian panel extended the work of Dr. Beers by identifying inappropriate prescriptions for older Canadians, as well as examining the rationale for prescribing particular medications, comorbidities and the length of treatment (Institute for Safe Medication Practices Canada, 2014). Based on this review, Naugler and colleagues (2000) developed and tested the Improving Prescribing in the Elderly Tool (IPET).

Developed more recently, the **STOPP/START criteria** is another evidence-based screening tool that is widely used in European countries. The STOPP (Screening Tool of Older Persons' Prescriptions) is useful for identifying potentially inappropriate medications and recent studies indicate that it may be better than earlier versions of the Beers Criteria for predicting adverse events (Hill-Taylor et al., 2013; Petrarca et al., 2012; Yayla et al., 2013). To date, no studies have been published comparing the STOPP tool with the 2012 Revised Beers Criteria. The START (Screening Tool to Alert doctors to Right Treatment) is an evidence-based screening tool used in conjunction with STOPP. A major feature of the START tool is that it lists medications that should be considered for people age 65 or older with certain conditions, as long as there are no contraindications. Studies find that when used together, the STOPP/START criteria are valid, reliable and comprehensive for improving prescribing practices and facilitating decisions about medications that should be discontinued or initiated (Corsonello et al., 2012; Gallagher et al., 2011). Online Learning Activity 8-1 provides links to the Beers Criteria and an article describing the STOPP/START, as well as additional information about this these tools.

 See ONLINE LEARNING ACTIVITY 8-1:
ADDITIONAL INFORMATION ABOUT BEERS CRITERIA AND LINK TO AN ARTICLE ABOUT STOPP/START
at http://thepoint.lww.com/Miller7e

Wellness Opportunity

Nurses have many opportunities to prevent adverse medication effects by raising questions about the use of medications that are potentially inappropriate.

Polypharmacy and Inadequate Monitoring of Medications

There is no one definition of **polypharmacy** but it typically refers to the use of more medications than are clinically indicated. It is important to recognize that it applies more to the appropriateness of medications than to the number of medications, and this is assessed by ensuring that the medication is not causing adverse effects and that the benefits outweigh the risks (Riker & Setter, 2012). Polypharmacy is common in older adults, particularly those in long-term care facilities, with nearly half of older adults taking one or more medications that are not medically necessary (Maher et al., 2014). Although multiple medications may be necessary for older adults with several pathologic conditions, polypharmacy can lead to drug interactions and adverse medication effects.

As the number and sources of medications increase, the need for monitoring becomes more important, from the time of the initial prescription until the termination of treatment. The following risk factors could potentially interfere with medication monitoring in older adults:

- Patient consultations with multiple health care providers, who usually do not communicate with each other about the patient's care
- Health care practitioners' lack of information about medications obtained from a variety of sources (i.e., prescription medications offered by friends and relatives or nonprescription products, such as herbs, nutritional supplements and OTC products)
- Health care practitioners' lack of information about a patient's nonadherence to a treatment regimen
- A patient's fear of disclosing information about folk remedies or medications obtained from sources other than the prescribing health care practitioner
- A patient's reluctance to disclose information about self-directed changes in the medication regimen
- An assumption by the patient or health care practitioner that once most medications are started, they should be continued indefinitely
- An assumption by the patient or health care practitioner that once an appropriate medication dosage is established, it will not need to be changed
- An assumption by the patient or health care practitioner that a lack of adverse effects early in the course of treatment indicates that adverse effects will never occur
- Changes in the patient's weight, especially weight loss, which may affect pharmacokinetic processes
- Changes in the patient's daily habits (e.g., smoking, activity level or nutrient and fluid intake), which may affect pharmacokinetic processes
- Changes in the patient's mental–emotional status, which may affect medication consumption patterns
- Changes in the patient's health status, which may affect medication actions, increasing the potential for adverse effects

Medication Nonadherence

Medication nonadherence refers to medication-taking patterns that differ from the prescribed pattern, including missed doses, failure to fill prescriptions, or medications taken too frequently or at inappropriate times. Reviews of studies indicate that medication nonadherence occurs in about half of older adults and that half of all new medication users will fail to consume at least 80% of prescribed dose during the first year of therapy (Blackburn et al., 2013; Marcum & Gellad, 2012). Medication nonadherence is associated with multiple interacting factors including all the following that are consistently identified in studies: cognitive impairment, social isolation, depression, asymptomatic disease, low health literacy, adverse medication effects, long treatment duration, high number of medications or daily doses, poor communication between the patient and provider, and misunderstandings about the medication or disease (Hugtenburg et al., 2013; Lee, 2013).

Financial Concerns Related to Prescription Drugs

Although each province and territory in Canada has prescription drug coverage for low-income seniors, each jurisdiction has its own care plan, and hence plans vary significantly between the provinces (Lung Association of Saskatchewan, 2012). For older adults who do not qualify for prescription drug coverage, out-of-pocket costs may be significant. More and more, Canadians are using generic prescriptions, rather than brand name. Almost 45% of all prescriptions filled are generic (Health Canada, 2012b), thus reducing the costs for health care consumers.

Insufficient Recognition of Adverse Medication Effects

Another problem specific to older adults is that adverse effects are likely to be misinterpreted or not recognized as such because of their similarity to age-related changes or commonly occurring pathologic conditions. When an older adult experiences an adverse medication reaction, two or three potential causes other than the medication can usually be identified, with medications being a common cause. For example, a study of older patients seeking care for urinary incontinence found that 60.5% were taking medications that potentially contributed to their symptoms, with polypharmacy being a major risk factor (Kashyap et al., 2013). Although adverse effects are not unique to older adults, they occur more commonly with increasing age and are more likely to be attributed erroneously to pathologic conditions or age-related changes and circumstances.

The term **prescribing cascade** has been applied to the following commonly occurring scenario: an adverse drug reaction is misinterpreted as a new medical condition, a drug is prescribed for this condition, another adverse drug effect occurs, the patient is again treated for the perceived additional medical condition, and the sequence perpetuates new adverse events. Table 8-3 summarizes adverse medication effects that are likely to remain unrecognized in older adults because of their similarity to age-related changes.

Wellness Opportunity

Nurses promote wellness when they challenge ageist attitudes and identify adverse effects falsely attributed to aging or pathologic conditions.

TABLE 8-3 Some Adverse Medication Effects That May Remain Unrecognized in Older Adults

Manifestation of Effect	Medication Type	Specific Examples
Cognitive impairment	Antidepressants; antipsychotics; antianxiety agents; anticholinergics; hypoglycemics; OTC cold, cough and sleeping preparations	Perphenazine, amitriptyline, chlorpromazine, diazepam, chlordiazepoxide, benztropine, trihexyphenidyl, cimetidine, digoxin, barbiturates, tolazamide, tolbutamide, chlorpheniramine, diphenhydramine
Depression	Antihypertensives, antiarthritics, antianxiety agents, antipsychotics	Reserpine, clonidine, propranolol, indomethacin, haloperidol, barbiturates
Urinary incontinence	Diuretics, anticholinergics	Furosemide, doxepin, thioridazine, lorazepam
Constipation	Narcotics, antacids, antipsychotics, antidepressants	Codeine, chlorpromazine, calcium carbonate, aluminum hydroxide, amoxapine
Vision impairment	Digitalis, antiarthritics, phenothiazines	Digoxin, indomethacin, ibuprofen, chlorpromazine
Hearing impairment	Mycin antibiotics, salicylates, loop diuretics	Gentamicin, aspirin, furosemide, bumetanide
Postural hypotension	Antihypertensives, diuretics, antipsychotics, antidepressants	Guanethidine, furosemide, propranolol, chlorpromazine, imipramine, clonidine
Hypothermia	Antipsychotics, alcohol, salicylates	Haloperidol, aspirin, alcohol, fluphenazine
Sexual dysfunction	Antihypertensives, antipsychotics, antidepressants, alcohol, antihypertensives	Timolol, clonidine, thiazides, haloperidol, amitriptyline, alcohol, cimetidine, propranolol, methyldopa
Mobility problems	Sedatives, antianxiety agents, antipsychotics, ototoxic medications	Chloral hydrate, diazepam, furosemide, gentamicin
Dry mouth	Anticholinergics, corticosteroids, bronchodilators, antihypertensives	Chlorpromazine, haloperidol, prednisone, furosemide, sertraline, theophylline
Anorexia	Digitalis, bronchodilators, antihistamines	Digoxin, theophylline, diphenhydramine
Drowsiness	Antidepressants, antipsychotics, OTC cold preparations, alcohol, barbiturates	Amitriptyline, haloperidol, chlorpheniramine, secobarbital
Edema	Antiarthritics, corticosteroids, antihypertensives	Ibuprofen, indomethacin, prednisone, reserpine, methyldopa
Tremors	Antipsychotics	Haloperidol, chlorpromazine, thioridazine

MEDICATION INTERACTIONS

Medications can interact with any other biologically active substance, including other medications, herbs, nutrients, alcohol, caffeine and nicotine. These interactions occur not only with prescription medications but also with commonly used OTC products, including antacids, analgesics and remedies for coughs, colds and sleep problems. Interactions result in altered therapeutic effects and an increased potential for adverse effects.

Medication–Medication Interactions

The risk of adverse effects from interactions between two or more medications increases exponentially according to the number of medications being consumed. Because older adults often take two or more medications concurrently, they are at increased risk for medication–medication interactions. Medication–medication interactions are typically caused by competitive action at binding sites, but they can be caused by any mechanism that influences the absorption, distribution, metabolism or elimination of any of the medications. Effects of medication–medication interactions include increased or decreased serum levels of either one or both of the medications, with subsequent altered therapeutic effects and increased risk of adverse or toxic effects. Medication–medication interactions can cause serious functional consequences and are a major cause of unnecessary hospital admissions (Obreli-Neto et al., 2012).

Although it is impossible to know details about all potential medication–medication interactions, nurses can be aware of specific mechanisms that are most commonly associated with these interactions in older adults, as listed in Table 8-4, which also lists examples of each type. It is important to be aware of serious interactions that occur more frequently with certain medications. For example, warfarin (Coumadin) requires close monitoring because serum levels are easily altered by interactions with other medications, foods and herbs.

Medications and Herbs

Many medication–herb interactions have been identified in recent years because of the increased use of herbs and increased attention to interactions. Although the more widely recognized medication–herb interactions are sometimes listed in pharmacology references, the extent of medication–herb interactions is probably not fully recognized, as older adults may be reluctant to tell their health care practitioner that they are using herbal preparations. Medications that are likely to be affected by herbs are warfarin, insulin, aspirin, digoxin, cyclosporin and ticlopidine (de Lima Toccafondo & Huang, 2012; Tsai et al., 2012). Some herb–medication interactions are mild, but a few herbs, such as St. John's wort, can be sufficiently serious to endanger the person's health (Izzo, 2012).

Medications and Nutrients

In the context of medication–nutrient interactions, the term nutrient includes foods, beverages, enteral formulas and dietary supplements. Older adults are likely to experience medication–nutrient interactions because of a combination of age-related changes and other risk factors. For example, changes in the gastrointestinal tract can delay or diminish the absorption of medications. Another widely recognized example is the effect of grapefruit juice on increasing the bioavailability of certain

TABLE 8-4 Types and Examples of Medication–Medication Interactions

Type of Interaction	Interaction Example	Effect
Binding effect (e.g., an oral drug diminishes the absorption of another drug in the stomach)	Magnesium- or aluminum-containing antacids may bind with tetracycline in the stomach	Decreased effects of tetracycline
Metabolism interference effect (e.g., one drug interferes with hepatic metabolism of another drug)	Ciprofloxacin and anticonvulsants inhibit metabolism of warfarin	Increased effects of warfarin
Metabolism-enhancing effect (e.g., one drug activates the drug-metabolizing enzymes in the liver)	Phenobarbital increases metabolism of warfarin	Decreased effects of warfarin
Elimination interference effect (e.g., one drug interferes with the renal elimination of another drug)	Furosemide can interfere with elimination of salicylates	Increased effects of salicylates
Elimination enhancement effect (e.g., renal reabsorption is blocked because of altered urinary pH)	Sodium bicarbonate can enhance excretion of lithium, tetracyclines and salicylates	Decreased effects of lithium, tetracycline or salicylate
Competitive or displacement effect (e.g., two drugs compete at receptor sites)	Diphenhydramine may interfere with effect of cholinergic agents (e.g., donepezil)	Decreased effects of donepezil
Potentiating effect (e.g., two drugs produce greater effects when taken together even though they have different actions)	Acetaminophen taken with codeine has a greater analgesic effect than either medication taken alone	Increased analgesic effect
Additive effect (e.g., two drugs produce greater effect because they have similar action)	Verapamil or diltiazem may have additive effect when taken with a β-blocker	Increased effect on blood pressure

drugs, such as statins, benzodiazepines and calcium-channel blockers (Hanley et al., 2011). Clinically significant nutrient–medication interactions are likely to occur if the following medications are taken with food: biphosphonates, carbidopa/levodopa (Sinemet), ciprofloxacin (Cipro), digoxin (Lanoxin), furosemide (Lasix), glipizide (Glocotrol), levothyroxixin (Synthroid), metformin (Glucophage), metoprolol (Lopressor) and warfarin (Coumadin; Anderson & Fox, 2012). Table 8-5 lists examples of nutrient–medication interactions.

Medications and Alcohol

Alcohol interacts with medications in the same way as other central nervous system depressants, but health care practitioners do not always inquire about a patient's use of alcohol, and even when people are asked, they might not accurately acknowledge the amount of alcohol used. Alcohol is consumed not only in beverages but also in OTC preparations, such as mouthwashes, vitamin and mineral tonics, and liquid cough and cold preparations. When taken with medications, alcohol can alter the therapeutic action of medications and increase the potential for adverse effects. Older adults may be more susceptible to medication–alcohol interactions because age-related changes in receptor sensitivity and body composition lead to higher blood-alcohol levels. Table 8-6

lists some of the medication–alcohol interactions that can occur in older adults.

Medications and Nicotine

Medication–nicotine interactions can be associated with tobacco smoking, smokeless tobacco and the many nicotine-based products that are increasingly being used as substitutes for smoking. Because nicotine can interfere with the therapeutic action of medications, smokers may require higher doses of a medication and it may be necessary to adjust doses when smoking patterns change either voluntarily or involuntarily (e.g., during a hospitalization). Also when nicotine products, such as patches, are initiated or discontinued, doses may need to be adjusted. Table 8-7 lists some common medication–nicotine interactions.

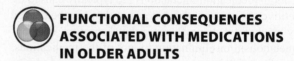

FUNCTIONAL CONSEQUENCES ASSOCIATED WITH MEDICATIONS IN OLDER ADULTS

Age-related changes can alter therapeutic effects of medications and increase the potential for adverse effects even in healthy older adults, as discussed in this section. As already

TABLE 8-5 Medication–Nutrient Interactions

Effect on Medication	Example of Interaction Effect
Delayed absorption rate, no effect on amount absorbed	Ingestion of food may delay absorption of cimetidine, digoxin and ibuprofen
Reduced rate and amount of absorption	Calcium decreases absorption of tetracycline. A high-protein or high-fibre meal decreases absorption of levodopa. Grapefruit juice can decrease absorption of antifungals and antihistamines
Reduced absorption because of nonnutrient components	Caffeinated tea and fibre intake interfere with iron absorption
Increased absorption	High-fat foods increase serum levels of griseofulvin
Decreased therapeutic effect	Vitamin K decreases the effectiveness of warfarin. Charcoal broiling of foods diminishes the effectiveness of aminophylline or theophylline
Increased rate of metabolism	A high-protein diet increases the metabolism of theophylline
Increased concentrations and bioavailability	Potential effect of grapefruit juice and amiodarone, atorvastatin, buspirone, calcium-channel blockers, carbamazepine, diazepam, lovastatin, simvastatin and triazolam

TABLE 8-6 Medication–Alcohol Interactions

Type of Interaction	Example of Interaction Effect
Altered metabolism of benzodiazepines when combined with alcohol	Increased psychomotor impairment and adverse effects
Altered metabolism of barbiturates and meprobamate when combined with alcohol	Central nervous system depression
Altered metabolism of alcohol when combined with chlorpromazine	Increased serum levels of alcohol and acetaldehyde; increased psychomotor impairment
Enhanced vasodilation as a result of a combination of alcohol and nitrates	Severe hypotension and headache, enhanced absorption of nitroglycerin
Altered metabolism of oral hypoglycemics in the liver	Potentiation of oral hypoglycemics by alcohol

TABLE 8-7 Medication–Nicotine Interactions

Effect of Nicotine	Example of Interaction Effect
Altered metabolism	Decreased efficacy of analgesics, lorazepam, theophylline, aminophylline, β-blockers and calcium-channel blockers
Vasoconstriction	Increased peripheral ischemic effect of β-blockers
Central nervous system stimulation	Decreased drowsiness from benzodiazepines and phenothiazines
Stimulation of antidiuretic hormone secretion	Fluid retention, decreased effectiveness of diuretics
Activation of neuroendocrine pathways	Interacts with insulin, aggravates insulin resistance, interferes with α-blockers
Increase in platelet activity	Decreased anticoagulant effectiveness (heparin, warfarin); increased risk of thrombosis with estrogen use
Increased gastric acid secretion	Decreased or negated effects of H2 antagonists (cimetidine, famotidine, nizatidine, ranitidine)

discussed in the section on risk factors, when adverse effects are not recognized in older adults, serious consequences may result. This section discusses additional functional consequences that are more uniquely associated with medications in older adults and have implications for nurses.

Altered Therapeutic Effects

Age-related changes alone can alter the therapeutic action of some substances; however, most of the altered therapeutic effects that occur in older adults are caused by risk factors, such as polypharmacy. Consequently, the therapeutic effectiveness of substances is less predictable, even in healthy older adults. The main implication is that medications need to be monitored more closely in older adults, especially initially and when there is any change in the person's medical status or treatment regimen. Thus, the commonly accepted principle for geriatric drug prescribing is "start low and go slow."

Increased Potential for Adverse Effects

Adverse drug events (also called adverse drug reactions or adverse medication effects) are the unintended and undesired outcomes of a medication that occur in doses normally used in humans. Consequences of adverse drug events include a decline in function, an increased risk for falls and fractures, an increased number of visits for health care services, admission to a hospital or prolongation of a hospital stay, and death. Up to 13% of patients taking two medications and 82% of those taking six medications experience an adverse drug event (Little & Morley, 2013). There is much agreement that adverse medication events occur commonly, have serious consequences and frequently are avoidable. Box 8-2 lists some of the factors that can increase the risk for adverse drug events.

In recent years, there has been increasing attention on adverse drug events as a preventable cause of hospitalizations for older adults. Medications most frequently cited as causes of emergency hospitalizations are warfarin, antiplatelet drugs and antidiabetic drugs, including insulin and oral hypoglycemics (Budnitz et al., 2011). Attention is also focusing on adverse drug events that occur during hospitalization. Some conditions associated with increased risk for adverse drug events

Box 8-2 Factors That Increase the Risk for Adverse Medication Effects

- Increased numbers of medications
- Frailty
- Malnourishment or dehydration
- Multiple illnesses
- An illness that interferes with cardiac, renal or hepatic function
- Cognitive impairment
- History of medication allergies or adverse effects
- Fever that can alter the action of certain medications
- Recent change in health or functional status
- Medications in any of the following categories: anticoagulant/antiplatelet, antidiabetics, NSAIDs, central nervous system drugs

during hospitalization include renal failure, increasing number of medications, inappropriate medications, age 75 years and older and use of central nervous system drugs and antiinfectives (Dupouy et al., 2013; O'Connor et al., 2012).

Several aspects of adverse medication effects are particularly important for the care of older adults. As discussed in the section on risk factors, adverse effects may not be recognized as such because they are similar to the manifestations of pathologic conditions or they are mistakenly attributed to aging. Three concerns of particular importance are anticholinergic adverse effects, changes in mental status and tardive dyskinesia.

Anticholinergic Adverse Effects

In recent years, geriatricians have increasingly recognized that older adults are particularly susceptible to the **anticholinergic adverse effects** from medications, including some medications that are not widely recognized as having anticholinergic effects in the body. Many OTC agents commonly used for coughs, colds and sleep problems contain anticholinergic ingredients. Anticholinergic adverse effects can also occur from systemic absorption of commonly used topical medications or ophthalmic agents (e.g., mydriatics and cycloplegics). Common types of medications with anticholinergic properties include antidepressants, antihistamines, antiparkinson agents, antipsychotics, cardiovascular

Box 8-3 Examples of Medications with Anticholinergic Effects

Antidepressants

Amitriptyline
Desipramine
Imipramine
Mirtazapine
Nortriptyline
Paroxetine
Trazodone

Antihistamines

Chlorpheniramine
Diphenhydramine
Hydroxyzine
Loratadine
Meclizine
Promethazine

Antiparkinson Agents

Benztropine
Trihexyphenidyl

Antipsychotics

Chlorpromazine
Clozapine
Fluphenazine
Haloperidol
Prochlorperazine
Promethazine

Quetiapine
Risperidone

Cardiovascular Agents

Captopril
Digoxin
Dipyridamole
Isosorbide dinitrate
Nifedipine

Gastrointestinal Agents

Belladonna
Cimetidine
Dicyclomine
Hyoscyamine
Loperamide
Ranitidine

Urinary Antispasmodics

Oxybutynin
Tolterodine

Miscellaneous Agents

Amantadine
Atropine
Meclizine
Theophylline
Warfarin

agents, gastrointestinal agents and urinary antispasmodics (see Box 8-3 for examples).

Longitudinal studies conducted in a number of countries have consistently identified anticholinergic agents as a causative factor for significant and long-term cognitive impairment in older adults, including delirium and mild cognitive impairment (e.g., Cai et al., 2013; Pasina et al, 2013; Puustinen et al., 2012; Uusvaara et al., 2013). Another concern related to anticholinergic agents is that their pharmacologic action can counteract the effects of cholinesterase inhibitors, which are prescribed as a primary treatment for dementia. The Beers Criteria and guidelines emphasize the importance of avoiding medications with anticholinergic effects because they are inappropriate for use in older adults and safer alternatives are usually available.

Altered Mental Status

Although medications can cause mental changes in anyone, older adults are at increased risk for medication-related altered mental status. In addition, when older adults experience changes in their mental status, these changes are likely to be attributed to dementia or another pathologic condition, rather than being recognized as adverse medication effects. Nurses need to be alert to the possibility that even a simple OTC product, such as diphenhydramine, is a common cause of mental changes in older adults.

Delirium is an acute confusional state that can be precipitated by any medication or by medication interactions (refer to Chapter 14 for further discussion of delirium). Older adults are particularly susceptible to medication-induced delirium because of altered neurochemical activity in the brain. Moreover, some pathologic conditions (e.g., dementia, dehydration, malnutrition, head injury or central nervous system infection) can increase the risk for medication-induced delirium. Even at nontoxic serum levels, or at doses considered normal, medications can cause mental changes in older adults. It is important to keep in mind that medication-induced mental changes do not always subside immediately after the offending medication is discontinued. In some cases, it may take several weeks or even months after the medication is decreased or discontinued for mental function to return to the premedication level. Some medications that are likely to cause mental changes in older adults, as well as the mechanisms underlying these adverse actions, are listed in Table 8-8.

Antipsychotics in People With Dementia

The use of psychotropic drugs in long-term care facilities has been a particular focus of concern for some time. While in the United States there are limitations placed on the administration of medications, this is not the case in Canada (Fischer et al., 2011). (Due to the OBRA reforms in 1987, nursing homes in the United States were restricted in prescribing antipsychotic medications for psychotic symptoms only, not for wandering, insomnia or anxiety.) Although there is greater awareness about the dangerous side effects of antipsychotic medications for older adults with dementia, these medications continue to be prescribed unnecessarily, and studies continue to identify serious consequences related to antipsychotics

TABLE 8-8 Mechanisms of Action for Mental Changes Caused by Adverse Medication Effects

Mechanism of Action	Examples
Anticholinergic effects	Atropine, scopolamine, antihistamines, antipsychotics, antidepressants, antispasmodics, antiparkinsonian agents
Decreased cerebral blood flow	Antihypertensives, antipsychotics
Depression of respiratory centre	Central nervous system depressants
Fluid and electrolyte alterations	Diuretics, alcohol, laxatives
Altered thermoregulation	Alcohol, psychotropics, narcotics
Acidosis	Diuretics, alcohol, nicotinic acid
Hypoglycemia	Hypoglycemics, alcohol, propranolol
Hormonal disturbances	Thyroid extract, corticosteroids
Depression-inducing action	Methyldopa, indomethacin, barbiturates, fluphenazine, haloperidol, corticosteroids

in people with dementia (Allen, 2012; Colloca et al., 2012; Senft, 2012). Unfortunately, medications used to treat the side effects, such as using benztropine (Cogentin) to treat extrapyramidal side effects, also have anticholinergic side effects, which can increase the risks of orthostatic hypotension and falls. Also, adding medications to treat side effects increases the risk for polypharmacy and possible delirium in older adults. The strong association between serious adverse effects and the first-generation antipsychotics (e.g., haloperidol and thioridazine) led to the development of second-generation (also called atypical) antipsychotics, which include risperidone, olanzapine, quetiapine, aripiprazole and ziprasidone.

During the past two decades, studies have focused on both the therapeutic effectiveness and the risk of adverse effects related to the use of atypical antipsychotics. Recent reviews have concluded that atypical antipsychotics are associated with serious adverse effects, including death, stroke, falls, delirium, hip fractures, cognitive decline and movement disorders, and these adverse effects occur in community-dwelling older adults as well as those in nursing homes (Brandt & Pyhtila, 2013; Seitz et al., 2013; Steinberg & Lyketsos, 2012). The concern about adverse effects is serious enough that in 2005, Health Canada issued a warning about the use of atypical antipsychotics with older adults with dementia (Alessi-Severini et al., 2013). Because of major concerns about adverse effects, there is increasing emphasis on nonpharmacologic management of neuropsychiatric symptoms in people with dementia, as discussed in Chapter 14. Research suggests, however, that atypical antipsychotics are still being used frequently within long-term care (see Box 8-4).

Studies also confirm the need for education of nursing staff to improve knowledge, attitudes and beliefs about antipsychotic use for nursing home residents (Lemay et al., 2013). While it is understandable that staff in long-term care need ways to manage agitated behaviours in those with dementia, antipsychotic medication should not be the first line of treatment (BC Ministry of Health and BC Medical Association, 2007). Rather, staff in long-term care need education on how to provide individualized care to older adults that allows for some self-determination around personal care decisions (such as showering or bathing), as well as engaging residents in meaningful activities (Alzheimer Society of Canada, 2011). Learning Activity 8-2 provides the link for the Alzheimer Society of Canada, 2011 Guidelines for Care.

See **ONLINE LEARNING ACTIVITY 8-2: ADDITIONAL INFORMATION IN THE GUIDELINES FOR CARE: PERSON-CENTRED CARE OF PEOPLE WITH DEMENTIA IN CARE HOMES (ALZHEIMER SOCIETY OF CANADA, 2011)** at http://thepoint.lww.com/Miller7e

Tardive Dyskinesia and Drug-Induced Parkinsonism

Tardive dyskinesia refers to a constellation of rhythmic and involuntary movements of the trunk, extremities, jaw, lips,

---

Box 8-4 Evidence-Informed Nursing Practice

Background: Despite the fact that health agencies in Canada including the Canadian Mental Health Association have issued warnings about the use of atypical antipsychotic medications for individuals with dementia, and guidelines have suggested the importance of only using these medications when the benefits are deemed to be greater than the risks, they are still being used.

Questions: What is the utilization of antipsychotic medications and benzodiazepines within older adults living in Manitoba between the years of 1997/98 and 2008/09? How does the usage of these medications differ between older adults living within the community and those residing in long-term care facilities?

Method: Researchers compared the utilization of atypical antipsychotic medications and benzodiazepines of community-dwelling older Manitobans (greater than 65 years of age) with those in long-term care facilities between 1997/98 and 2008/09.

Findings: Older adults living in long-term care were almost 20 times more likely to receive atypical antipsychotics than those in the community. Those most likely to receive antipsychotic medications were male and had dementia. Individuals who were very old and received many medications were less likely to be treated with high doses of atypical antipsychotics. The researchers concluded that while older adults in long-term care are receiving lower doses of atypical antipsychotic medications (compared with those administered before the Health Canada warning), the usage of these medications in facilities is still high.

Implications for Nursing Practice: Nurses should observe older adults with dementia who are receiving atypical antipsychotics for adverse effects. As much as possible, behavioural strategies should be attempted to help older adults with agitation, rather than the use of these medications.

Source: Alessi-Severini, S., Dahl, M., Schultz, J., et al. (2013). Prescribing psychotropic medications to the elderly population of a Canadian province: A retrospective study using administrative databases. *PeerJ*, 1, e168. doi:10.7717.peerj.168

---

mouth or tongue. The earliest signs are usually fine, wormlike movements of the tongue. Other early signs include chewing, grimacing, lip smacking, jaw clenching, eye blinking and side-to-side jaw movements. Manifestations can begin as early as 3 to 6 months after initiation of antipsychotic medications, and they usually persist even after the causative agent is discontinued. It is considered an adverse effect of dopamine receptor-blocking agents and serotonin–norepinephrine reuptake inhibitors (i.e., certain antipsychotics and antidepressants; Lee et al., 2013; Waln & Jankovic, 2013). Tardive dyskinesia deserves special attention with regard to older adults because advanced age correlates with both an earlier onset and increased severity of tardive dyskinesia. Moreover, when combined with age-related changes and risk factors, tardive dyskinesia can seriously impair the older adult's ability to perform activities of daily living (ADLs).

Drug-induced parkinsonism is the occurrence of Parkinson-like manifestations as an adverse medication effect. Manifestations can be reversed if the offending drug is stopped, but many times the condition is misdiagnosed as Parkinson disease and treated inappropriately with an antiparkinson medication. Main causative drugs identified in studies include antipsychotics, calcium-channel antagonists, valproic acid and antiepileptic agents (Bohlega &

Al-Foghom, 2013; Silver & Factor, 2013). Despite its common occurrence, this condition is often not diagnosed correctly and is treated inappropriately with medications rather than with the more effective approach of discontinuing the causative drug (Lopez-Sendon et al., 2013).

NURSING ASSESSMENT OF MEDICATION USE AND EFFECTS

Nurses assess medication regimens and medication-taking behaviours of older adults to accomplish the following:
- Determine the effectiveness of the medication regimen.
- Identify any factors that interfere with the correct regimen.
- Ascertain risks for adverse effects or altered therapeutic actions (with particular attention to older adults at increased risk).
- Detect adverse medication effects.
- Identify teaching needs with regard to medications.

During a medication assessment, nurses should clarify the prescribed medication regimen and identify actual medication-taking behaviours so that they can assess for adherence to the treatment regimen.

Communication Techniques for Obtaining Accurate Information

Some of the many barriers to obtaining accurate information about medications and medication-taking behaviours include time limitations, complex medication regimens and lack of a trusting relationship. Because medication assessments can be time-consuming, and because the older adult may not think of all the information during the first interview or may initially be reluctant to reveal accurate information, it may be necessary to conduct the medication assessment over the course of two or more visits. Many older adults have learned not to ask questions about their health care because they are unsure of what to ask or they falsely believe that they are not entitled to medical information. Reluctance to openly discuss medications may be caused by fear of being judged, especially if the prescribed regimen is not being followed exactly or if the person uses folk remedies, alternative therapies or OTC medications. When people do not follow the medication regimen exactly as prescribed, they are likely to recite the orders rather than describe their actual medication-taking behaviours. Another factor that contributes to this reluctance is anxiety about discussing the underlying reason for not following the regimen. For example, older adults who cannot afford medications may be embarrassed to discuss their limited finances.

Nurses can address the barriers by asking open-ended questions in a matter-of-fact way and conveying a nonjudgmental attitude during the medication interview. Keep in mind the importance of eliciting information about the use of herbs, folk remedies, OTC preparations and complementary and alternative care practices. For example, "What do you do to help you sleep?" is more open-ended than "Do you take any medications for sleep?" because the latter may be interpreted only in relation to prescription medications.

Another interview technique is to use leading questions related to potential risk factors that interfere with the older person's ability to adhere to the prescribed regimen. For example, if the cost of medications is a problem, ask a question such as "I know that some of these prescribed medications can be quite expensive; do you have any problems with getting them?" Similarly, asking a question such as "I know you don't drive, do you have someone who helps you get them from the pharmacy?" may elicit information about transportation barriers.

Nurses should ask additional questions about the person's ability to take his or her medications as prescribed based on specific observations. For example, if the older adult has limited hand strength, an appropriate assessment question would be "Do you have any difficulty getting the caps off your medication bottles?" Another technique for eliciting information is to ask about the person's method of organizing medications. For example, people taking medications often have a method of organizing their regimen by using divided medication boxes or written charts or schedules. They are usually willing to show this organizational system to the nurse and, in fact, may be proud to discuss their method with the nurse during the medication assessment.

> **Wellness Opportunity**
>
> Nurses can build on their trusting relationship with older adults to encourage open discussion of factors that interfere with adherence to medication regimens.

Scope of a Medication Assessment

Medication assessments include information about all of the following:
- Prescription and OTC medications, used orally and by all other routes (e.g., nasal, aural, topical, optical, injectable, dermal methods)
- Medications that are used only sporadically or as needed
- Vitamins, minerals and dietary supplements (including dosages and frequency)
- Alcohol, caffeine
- Tobacco smoking, use of nicotine products (including information about recent changes)
- Folk remedies and complementary and alternative modalities, including all herbal products and homeopathic remedies

Information about doses of vitamins and minerals is important because megavitamins can be harmful, and even low doses can cause interactions or produce adverse effects (e.g., iron or calcium carbonate can be constipating). Information about the brand names of OTC medications can help identify additives that may be causing problems or increasing the risk of altered medication action (e.g., analgesics with caffeine, antacids with lactose or bronchodilators with sulfites). Information about folk remedies and complementary and alternative health care practices can help identify health beliefs that affect adherence and other aspects of medication-taking behaviours.

Nurses also need to assess the person's understanding of the purpose of medications; doing so provides information about his or her understanding of health status and medical conditions. As with other parts of the medication assessment, it is essential to phrase questions in as open-ended and non-judgmental a manner as possible. Asking "What do you take this pill for?" with a tone of curiosity will likely elicit more information than asking questions such as, "What do you take for your heart?" or "Why do you take furosemide?"

Obtaining information about allergies and adverse reactions is essential because anyone with a history of medication-related problems will need to be closely monitored, especially if the medications being administered are similar to those that caused the reaction. Sometimes people state that they are allergic to a medication, but when they are asked about the symptoms, they describe an adverse effect rather than an allergic reaction. Therefore, rather than simply documenting that the person is allergic to a certain medication, nurses should document the specific reaction that occurred. Nurses can use Box 8-5 as a guide to assessing medications regimens and medication-taking behaviours.

Nurses should also obtain and document information about the person's perception of and preferences for various forms of medications because this information can influence prescribing decisions, especially when there are several options that may be equally effective. Similarly, nurses should identify any cultural factors that might influence medication-taking behaviours. For example, according to some Asian traditions, illness is perceived as an imbalance of hot and cold forces. If the illness makes the body hot, then the remedy should make it cooler. Box 8-6 lists some cultural factors that are pertinent to a medication assessment.

Another aspect of a comprehensive medication assessment is the identification of biocultural variations that can affect the metabolism of medications. These variations can have important implications related to doses of medications and assessment of both therapeutic and adverse effects. Nurses can use the information in Box 8-6 to be aware of ways in which some groups may respond differently to certain medications. Keep in mind that these are only examples of biocultural variations that have been identified in some studies. As with all aspects of cultural variations, it is imperative to be aware of possible influence of biologically based differences while at the same time avoiding generalizations.

Another component of a comprehensive medication assessment is obtaining information about various sources of health care. This information is particularly important when someone receives care from more than one health care practitioner, as is often the case. Nurses can ask nonjudgmentally about whether the person receives care from non-Western health care practitioners, such as herbalists, spiritual healers, naturopathic practitioners or Ayurvedic doctors. Box 8-7 summarizes some culturally specific sources of health care and treatment modalities that older adults might use.

 Box 8-5 Guidelines for Medication Assessment

Information About the Therapeutic Agents

- Prescription pills, liquids, injections, eye drops, ear drops, nasal sprays, transdermal methods and topical preparations
- Over-the-counter preparations that are used regularly or occasionally
- Vitamins, minerals and nutritional supplements
- Pattern of alcohol, caffeine or tobacco use
- Herbs and herbal preparations
- Homeopathic remedies
- Home folk remedies
- Sources of health care, including complementary and alternative practitioners

Interview Questions to Assess Medication-Taking Behaviours

- How would you describe your usual daily routine for taking medications and remedies, beginning when you get up in the morning?
- Is there anything else you do or use to treat illness or to maintain your health, such as using herbs, ointments, home remedies or nutritional supplements?
- Are you taking anyone else's medications?
- What do you do when you miss a dose of medication?
- What do you take for constipation? What do you do to help you sleep (or to alleviate any other identified problem)?
- How do you get your prescriptions filled? (Where do you get your remedies?)
- Do you have any difficulty taking your pills?
- What method do you use to keep track of your medications and remedies?
- Is there anything you do to help you remember to take your medicines or remedies at the appropriate time?

Interview Questions to Assess the Person's Understanding of the Purpose of Medications and Other Remedies

- What is this medication (or herb, etc.) for?
- For medications (or remedies) that are used as needed (PRN): How do you decide when to take this pill (or remedy)?
- What did your health care practitioner tell you about this medication (or herb, etc.)?
- What problems were you having when the health care practitioner prescribed this medication (or suggested that you use this remedy)?

Interview Questions to Elicit Additional Information

- Are there any medications or remedies you were taking at one time but are no longer taking?
- Have you ever had an allergic reaction, or any other bad reaction, to a medication or remedy? (If yes, describe what happened.)
- Where do you store your medications and remedies?

Questions and Observations Based on Reading of Prescription Labels

- Who is the prescribing health care practitioner?
- If there is more than one health care practitioner, does each practitioner know all the medications that are being used?
- Are any medications the same or similar and prescribed by different health care practitioners?
- If the dates on various prescriptions are different, were the later medications supposed to be added to the medication regimen or were they intended to replace previously prescribed medications?
- Are the date of the last refill and the number of pills in the bottle consistent with the prescribed regimen?

Wellness Opportunity

Nurses promote personal responsibility for health by encouraging discussion of various sources of care.

Box 8-6 Cultural Considerations: Culturally Competent Medication Assessment and Interventions

Overview

- Teaching about medications should be done in the context of culturally based beliefs about health, illness and remedies.
- Medications that are not readily available or that are available by prescription only in Canada may be available over the counter in other countries, such as the United States, Mexico and Latin America.
- People of Vietnamese and other cultural groups may view injections as being more effective than pills and pills as being more effective than drops.
- People of Asian, Latino and Middle Eastern heritage believe it is important to take medicine with certain foods or beverages (e.g., tea or warm water rather than cold water) to provide the necessary balance.
- Some Chinese and other Asian people may have the following preferences:
  Balms and ointments rather than pills for local pain
  Teas and soups rather than antacids for indigestion
  Herbs rather than prescription drugs

Biocultural Variations in the Metabolism of Medications

Biocultural variations may affect the metabolism of medications in the following groups:

African Canadians

- Increased risk for adverse effects from psychotropics (e.g., lithium toxicity, delirium from tricyclic antidepressants, agranulocytosis from clozapine)
- Increased risk for angioedema due to angiotensin-converting enzyme (ACE) inhibitors
- Diminished therapeutic response to propranolol and ACE inhibitors
- Respond best to diuretics, calcium antagonists and α-blockers for hypertension
- Increased incidence of adverse effects, such as depression, with thiazides
- Decreased therapeutic response to analgesics and increased risk of adverse gastrointestinal effects, especially with acetaminophen
- Diminished eye dilatation in response to mydriatic drug

Arab Canadians

- Require lower dose of antiarrhythmics, antihypertensives, neuroleptics and psychotropics
- May need a higher dose of opioids for adequate analgesic effects

Asian/Pacific Islanders

- Sensitivity to propranolol and other β-blockers, manifest by decreased blood levels accompanied by seemingly more profound response
- Respond best to calcium antagonists for hypertension
- Require lower doses of antidepressants and neuroleptics (e.g., benzodiazepines, haloperidol)
- Increased gastrointestinal adverse effects associated with analgesics
- Decreased therapeutic effects of opiates
- May require dose adjustment for fat-soluble vitamins and other drugs
- Increased sensitivity to alcohol

Filipino

- Increased sensitivity to central nervous system depressants (e.g., haloperidol)

Sources: Andrews, M. M. (2012). Cultural competence in the health history and physical examination. In M. M. Andrews & J. S. Boyle. *Transcultural concepts in nursing care* (6th ed.). Philadelphia, PA: Lippincott Williams & Wilkins; Purnell, L. D. (2013). *Transcultural health care: A culturally competent approach* (4th ed.). Philadelphia, PA: F. A. Davis.

Box 8-7 Cultural Considerations: Culturally Specific Health Care Sources and Practices

Cultural Group	Sources of Care[a]	Health Practices[a]
Aboriginals (First Nations)	Natural medicines, traditional foods, including berries	Ceremonies, such as sweat lodges
African Canadians	Home remedies, faith and root healers (herbalists)	Folk remedies (e.g., teas, herbs); magic or voodoo (especially in rural areas)
Chinese	Herbalists, acupuncturists	Herbs, food, beverages and other remedies to balance yin and yang
Filipino	Folk healers (hilot)	Prayer, exorcism, hot/cold balance
Hindu	Traditional healers (nattuvaidhyars)	Ayurvedic medicine (herbs and roots)
Japanese	Herbalists	Herbs, prayer at temple, church or small shrines at home
Russians	Folk remedies	Herbal teas, sweet liquor, physical modalities (oils, ointments, enemas, mud baths)
Vietnamese	Asian physicians, folk healers, spiritual healers, magicians (sorcerers)	Herbs, acupuncture, cup suctioning, skin pinching

[a]In North America, Western practitioners and medicine often are used with these sources of care and health practices.
Sources: National Advisory Committee on Prescription Drug Misuse. (2013). *First do no harm: Responding to Canada's prescription drug crisis.* Ottawa, ON: Canadian Centre on Substance Abuse.
Purnell, L. D. (2013). *Transcultural health care: A culturally competent approach* (4th ed.). Philadelphia, PA: F. A. Davis.

Observing Patterns of Medication Use

In addition to using good communication techniques, nurses obtain essential assessment information by reviewing the person's array of medications. When nurses conduct the medication assessment in the home setting, they can ask to see all the medications that the older person uses. In settings other than the home, the nurse can ask the older adult ahead of time to bring in all of his or her medications. In community settings, nurses might sponsor a "brown bag" medication review session. Program participants are asked to bring all their medications to an educational session, during which the nurse provides group education and individual assessment and counselling regarding the medications. Because older people often are very comfortable discussing medications with their peers, this method is both nonthreatening and quite effective.

Direct observation of medication containers provides useful information about adherence, dates of original prescription and refills, duplication of similar medications and pharmaceutical treatments for pathologic conditions. For example, if three types of antihypertensive medications have been prescribed at different times, inquire whether the second or third medication was supposed to replace or supplement the original medication. Also assess whether the bottles contain the original medications, and ask additional questions when the contents are not consistent with expectations. For example, if the label indicates that the original prescription was for 30 pills, but it has not been refilled for 1 year, the nurse might inquire about the reason. Patients may explain that they cannot afford the prescription or they cannot manipulate the childproof lid. Another purpose for examining medication containers is to discover information about sources of care and duplication of medications. It is not unusual to find that patients are getting prescriptions from more than one health care practitioner, with the same or similar medications from different sources or under more than one name (e.g., generic and brand names).

Linking the Medication Assessment to the Overall Assessment

The nurse uses information from the medication interview with the overall health assessment in several ways. First, information about past and present medication patterns can provide clues to identified problems or complaints. For example, if the person complains of morning lethargy or experiences mental changes, the nurse can inquire about the use of medications with anticholinergic properties, including OTC products (e.g., diphenhydramine). Information about changes in health-related behaviours can also shed light on current problems, such as the recurrence of symptoms that were once controlled by medications. For example, if an insulin-dependent diabetic stopped smoking, it is important to consider whether the dose of insulin needs to be decreased. Recent medication-taking behaviours also may account for health problems that are residual or latent adverse medication effects. A common example of a residual adverse effect is the onset of diarrhea after a course of antibiotics.

Second, nurses use the overall health assessment as a base of information to determine the expected and actual outcomes of medications. These outcomes are evaluated through subjective and objective assessment information. For example, analgesic effectiveness is measured according to reported level of pain relief, and the effectiveness of antihypertensive medications is judged according to lowered blood pressure readings.

Third, the overall assessment, including functional aspects, helps answer the question "Can the person or caregivers safely and effectively administer medications?" This complex question involves an assessment of all aspects of medication-taking behaviours, as described in the sections on age-related changes and risk factors. The environment also should be assessed in relation to certain conditions, such as the accessibility of water and the availability of a refrigerator (if necessary for medication storage) that can affect medication-taking behaviours. The overall assessment also might provide information about financial limitations,

mobility or transportation problems that interfere with obtaining medications.

Fourth, if the home environment can be observed as part of the overall assessment, important clues to health problems and medication-taking behaviours may be disclosed. For example, observing that nitroglycerin is stored on a sunny window sill may explain why the medication is not effective in relieving angina. An assessment of the home environment may lead to additional pertinent information. For example, when the nurse observes OTC preparations and folk remedies in the home, she or he has the opportunity to ask about the use of these items.

Finally, the overall health assessment serves as the basis for identifying many factors that can increase the risk for nonadherence, altered therapeutic effects and adverse medication effects. For example, the nursing assessment of the older adult's cognitive abilities and abilities to perform daily activities provides valuable information about factors that can significantly influence medication-taking behaviours. Similarly, the nursing assessment of depression and other psychosocial aspects of functioning can provide important information about motivational and behavioural factors that can influence medication-taking behaviours.

Identifying Adverse Medication Effects

The first, and sometimes most difficult, step in alleviating adverse medication effects is to recognize their existence. Because many adverse effects are subtle and superimposed on one or more symptoms of illness, they may be attributed to pathologic conditions rather than to the treatment of the condition. Nurses are often the first to recognize adverse medication effects because they generally spend more time with patients than do primary care practitioners. Nurses are also more attentive to long-term monitoring of changes in day-to-day function, in contrast to the medical practitioner's focus on acute illness. Particularly in long-term care and home settings, the nurse is the health professional most likely to notice subtle changes in function that may be attributable to adverse medication effects.

Health care practitioners may hesitate to discuss adverse medication effects with patients for several reasons: (1) They may be uncertain about the potential adverse effects of a prescribed drug, especially when newer medications are prescribed; (2) they may assume that the power of suggesting possible adverse effects will become a self-fulfilling prophecy or (3) they may fear that the patient will choose not to take the medication. The nurse can serve as an "interpreter" between the prescribing practitioner and the patient by emphasizing the medication's benefits, as well as pointing out the problems that are most likely to arise. The nurse can also provide health education about ways to avoid adverse effects. For example, if a medication is likely to cause stomach irritation, taking the medication after meals or with milk may prevent this effect. Nurses do not automatically initiate a discussion of all the potential adverse effects of a medication, but when a change in health status is potentially related to adverse medication effects, nurses can raise that possibility.

Changes in mental status are a potentially devastating adverse medication effect that is often overlooked as such, especially when superimposed on existing dementia. Medication-induced mental status changes (e.g., confusion, lethargy, depression, agitation) can be sudden and obvious, or subtle and gradual. For example, delirium or hallucinations are usually obvious, but they may be attributed mistakenly to pathologic processes rather than to medication effects. Thus, whenever an older person experiences an alteration in mental status, medication intake must be assessed carefully. Besides considering all prescription drugs, alcohol and OTC medications (especially those with anticholinergic properties) must be considered as potential contributing factors. When medications are a potential cause of altered mental status, consideration must be given to discontinuing or lowering the dose of the medication. Assessment also addresses the possibility that the altered mental state interferes with proper dosing (e.g., when memory impairment contributes to overdosing or underdosing). Another aspect of assessing the relationship between mental changes and medications is to recognize that it may take days or even months after discontinuation of the medication before mental status returns to baseline. The resolution time depends on the particular medication involved, the length of time it was consumed and the person's general health status.

NURSING DIAGNOSIS

When the nursing assessment identifies factors that interfere with safe and accurate medication self-administration (e.g., cognitive or functional impairments affecting medication-taking ability), an applicable nursing diagnosis is Ineffective Self-Health Management. This diagnosis is defined as a "pattern of regulating and integrating into daily living a therapeutic regimen for the treatment of illness and its sequelae that is unsatisfactory for meeting specific health goals" (Herdman, 2012, p. 161). Related factors that might be identified include complex medication regimens, inadequate social supports, adverse effects of medication(s), lack of money or transportation, and lack of understanding of instructions.

If the nursing assessment identifies adverse effects of medications, particularly those that affect one's safety or quality of life, the nurse might address these through a nursing diagnosis that is specific to the adverse effect. Examples of these diagnoses include Confusion, Constipation, Urinary Incontinence, Imbalanced Nutrition, Impaired Memory and Risk for Falls.

Wellness Opportunity

Nurses can use the wellness nursing diagnosis of Readiness for Enhanced Self-Health Management when caring for older adults who are interested in addressing potential adverse effects.

PLANNING FOR WELLNESS OUTCOMES

The following Nursing Outcomes Classification (NOC) terminology can be used in care plans to identify wellness outcomes that are pertinent to medications and older adults: Adherence Behaviour, Health-Promoting Behaviour, Knowledge: Medication, Medication Response, Risk Detection, and Self-Care: Non-Parenteral Medication, and Self-Management: Chronic Disease.

Wellness Opportunity

Participation in health care decisions is an outcome that is applicable when nurses empower older adults to make responsible decisions about the use of OTC products, such as herbs and medications.

NURSING INTERVENTIONS TO PROMOTE SAFE AND EFFECTIVE MEDICATION MANAGEMENT

Promoting safe and effective medication-taking patterns in older adults is multidimensional and depends on coordinated efforts from several health care providers, including nurses, pharmacists and prescribing practitioners. In community settings, nurses have major roles in teaching older adults about medications and identifying interventions to support adherence to the therapeutic regimen. In all settings, nurses have major roles in preventing and identifying adverse effects. Box 8-8 summarizes a protocol for reducing adverse drug events developed by Zwicker and Fulmer (2012), and Learning Activity 8-3 provides additional information related to this protocol. The following sections describe practical interventions that nurses can use to promote adherence, prevent adverse effects and encourage safe and effective medication-taking behaviours in older adults.

See **ONLINE LEARNING ACTIVITY 8-3: PROTOCOL FOR REDUCING ADVERSE DRUG EVENTS** at http://thepoint.lww.com/Miller7e

Medication Reconciliation

Medication reconciliation is an evidence-based intervention that has been implemented in health care settings and, since 2011, is considered one of the top patient safety priorities in Canada by the Canadian Patient Safety Institute (Accreditation Canada, The Canadian Institute for Health Information, The Canadian Patient Safety Institute, and the Institute for Safe Medication Practices in Canada, 2012). Medication reconciliation is the process of identifying a patient's medication errors, such as omissions, duplications, dosing errors or drug interactions during transitions in care. The three steps involved in the process follow: (1) verification by collecting an accurate list; (2) clarification of questions about drugs, dosages, frequency and other pertinent information and (3) reconciliation of any discrepancies or concerns

Box 8-8 Evidence-Based Practice: Reducing Adverse Drug Events

Statement of the Problem

- About 35% of older adults experience adverse drug events with almost half of these being preventable.
- Reasons for medication-related problems: age-related physiologic changes that alter pharmacokinetics and pharmacodynamics, polypharmacy, incorrect doses of medications, inappropriate prescribing practices (e.g., use of medications to treat symptoms that are not disease specific), adverse drug reactions and interactions, nonadherence and medication errors

Recommendations for Nursing Assessment

- A comprehensive medication assessment includes all of the following: thorough drug history, focused questions about nicotine, alcohol, vitamins, herbs, folk remedies and all nonprescription products.
- Use assessment tools to (1) evaluate ability to self-administer medications, (2) identify potential inappropriate medications and drug–drug or drug–disease interactions and (3) assess renal function.
- Consider age-related changes in pharmacokinetics and pharmacodynamics: absorption, distribution, metabolism, clearance.
- Assessment strategies: brown bag method, medication reconciliation process.
- Identify medications associated with high risk for adverse drug reactions using Beers Criteria.
- Identify patient characteristics associated with potential adverse medication effects, such as dementia, polypharmacy, renal insufficiency and multiple chronic conditions.

- Identify potential interactions with other prescriptions and with all nonprescription products.

Nursing Interventions for Reducing Adverse Drug Events During and After Hospitalization

- Empower patients by providing information and involving them in decisions.
- Collaborate with interprofessional team for the following interventions: discontinuing unnecessary drugs, using safer drugs, optimizing the regimen, avoiding the prescribing cascade, avoiding inappropriate medications and using nonpharmacologic approaches for symptoms.
- Consider any new symptoms as a possible adverse medication effect.
- Follow the prescribing principle of "start low and go slow."

Nursing Interventions for Reducing Adverse Drug Events at Discharge

- Use medication reconciliation during transitions in care.
- Assess patient's abilities and limitations with regard to self-administration of medications.
- Address adherence issues that are likely to occur.
- Provide patient and caregiver education about safe and effective medication management.

Source: Zwicker, D. E., & Fulmer T. (2012). Reducing adverse drug events. In E. Capezuti, D. Zwicker, M. Mezey, & T. Fulmer (Eds.), *Evidence-based geriatric nursing protocols for best practice* (4th ed., pp. 324–362). New York, NY: Springer.

---

by communicating with prescribing practitioners. This process is warranted because studies confirm that medication discrepancies occur frequently during transitions in care, including admission to and discharge from acute care and long-term care settings (Harris et al., 2013; Sinvani et al., 2013). Although the initial focus of medication reconciliation was on hospital admissions and discharges, it is imperative that this process be performed during any transition, even within the same facility. Important nursing interventions for a successful medication reconciliation have been described by Pincus (2013) as follows:

- Determine who administers medications.
- View all the medications.
- Be aware of medications that are commonly implicated in discrepancies (e.g., as-needed medications, medications used prophylactically during hospitalization).
- Address ability to get prescriptions filled.
- Address issues that affect adherence (e.g., administration difficulties).
- Allow the patient to ask questions.

Online Learning Activity 8-4 provides links to resources related to medication reconciliation.

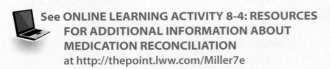

See **ONLINE LEARNING ACTIVITY 8-4: RESOURCES FOR ADDITIONAL INFORMATION ABOUT MEDICATION RECONCILIATION** at http://thepoint.lww.com/Miller7e

Teaching About Medications and Herbs

Medications are safest and most therapeutic when they are taken as prescribed and when the regimen is periodically reevaluated for maximum effectiveness and minimal risk of adverse reactions. An effective way to initiate health education about medications is to have the person write a list of all medications and OTC agents taken and to include a history of medication allergies and adverse effects. Emphasize that this information should be available to health care practitioners during all interactions because it is essential that all practitioners keep track of the person's medications. This list is especially important when more than one health care practitioner is involved. Nurses should explain that a medication list facilitates communication and reminds the health care practitioner periodically to reevaluate the medication regimen.

It is imperative to discuss each medication on the list and provide appropriate information on the basis of assessment of the person's knowledge and understanding. Morrow and Conner-Garcia (2013) have summarized the following recommendations for communicating with older adults about medications:

- Use concrete, active and direct language with emphasis on how the medication helps the person.
- Use patient education materials that are concrete, matched to patient needs and reinforced with graphics.
- Explore patient concerns by empathic listening.

● Verify patient understanding by "teachback" techniques, such as asking older adults to state information in their own words or having them demonstrate how they take/organize their medications.

Because older adults may be reluctant to question their health care practitioners, nurses can suggest pertinent questions for discussion with prescribing practitioners. In addition, nurses can teach older adults and their caregivers about obtaining medication-related information from knowledgeable sources, such as pharmacists. People need to understand that prescribing practitioners are skilled in diagnosing illnesses and deciding the most appropriate interventions and that pharmacists are the health care practitioners who are often the most knowledgeable about the specific actions and interactions of medications. Nurses can use Box 8-9 to teach older adults about which medication questions are best answered by prescribing practitioners and which are best addressed by pharmacists.

Because good communication skills are essential to obtaining answers to the questions listed in Box 8-9, nurses can suggest ways of communicating effectively with pharmacists and other health care practitioners. For example, nurses can help older adults develop a list of questions about specific medications that they can discuss with pharmacists or health care practitioners. In home settings, nurses can serve as role models of appropriate communication by calling the pharmacist or prescribing practitioner to discuss medications in the presence of the older adult or caregiver.

Wellness Opportunity

Nurses find opportunities to empower older adults by teaching them effective ways of communicating with health care providers so that they can knowledgeably observe for therapeutic and adverse medication effects.

As discussed in the Nursing Assessment section, nurses need to ask about the use of herbs and other bioactive substances so that they can observe for and teach about interactions and adverse effects, when appropriate. Although information about the use of complementary and alternative therapies needs to be an integral part of the assessment, nurses cannot know all the details about these products. At a minimum, however, they need to know how to teach about these remedies, just as they teach about pharmacologic and medical interventions. Nurses can use Box 8-10 as a tool to teach their patients about general precautions for the use of herbs and homeopathic remedies, such as being aware of potential interactions and adverse effects and making sure that all health care practitioners are aware of all OTC products that are used.

Another important nursing role—and a way of promoting personal responsibility—is teaching patients and caregivers about reliable sources of information on which they can base decisions. Within the United States, the National Institutes of Health (NIH) established the National Centre for Complementary and Alternative Medicine to fund research

Box 8-9 Tips for Safe and Effective Medication Use

Nurses are in a key position to teach patients ways to ensure safe and effective ways to take their medications. Some tips for patients follow.

Carry an up-to-date list of all your medications, including herbs and OTC preparations, and show the list to your health care practitioner(s).

When your health care practitioner suggests a medication, ask if there is any way to take care of the problem without medication.

Ask your health care practitioner the following questions about each new, regularly scheduled medication:

● What is the reason for taking the medication?
● How will I know if it's doing what it's meant to do?
● How soon can I expect to feel the beneficial effects?
● What will happen if I don't take it?
● How often am I supposed to take it?
● How long should I continue taking it?
● What should I do if I miss a dose?
● When will you want to see me again, and what will you want me to tell you so that you can determine whether the medication is effective?

Ask your health care practitioner the following questions at follow-up visits:

● Do I still need to take this medication?
● Can the dosage be reduced?

Ask your health care practitioner the following questions about each medication that is prescribed on an "as-needed" (PRN) basis:

● What is the reason for taking the medication, and how should I determine whether I need the medication?
● How often can I take it? Is there a range of frequency?
● What is the maximum dose I can take within 24 hours?
● What should I do if the medication does not relieve the symptoms (e.g., if chest pain continues after taking several nitroglycerin tablets)?

Ask your pharmacist the following questions:

● What are the generic and brand names for this medication?
● Is it likely to interact with the other medications I'm taking?
● Is it likely to interact with herbs, cigarettes, alcohol or any nutrient?
● What is the best time of day to take it?
● Does it matter if I take it before or after meals?
● Are there any side effects I should watch for?
● Is there anything I can do to minimize the risk of side effects (e.g., taking the medication with milk or meals to reduce stomach irritation)?
● Is there anything I should avoid while I'm taking this medication (e.g., milk, certain foods, driving)?
● Are there any special instructions for storing this medication?

and provide evidence-based information about herbs. In Canada, this responsibility falls under the responsibility of Health Canada (see http://www.hc-sc.gc.ca/dhp-mps/prodnatur/index-eng.php), although the site is not as well developed as the NIH one. This and other resources for reliable information are described in Online Learning Activity 8-5.

See **ONLINE LEARNING ACTIVITY 8-5: RESOURCES FOR HEALTH EDUCATION MATERIALS FOR TEACHING OLDER ADULTS ABOUT MEDICATIONS AND HERBS** at http://thepoint.lww.com/Miller7e

Box 8-10 Tips on the Use of Herbs

- Before treating any symptom with a nonprescription product, make sure you are not overlooking a condition that requires medical attention.
- Discuss the use of any nonprescription product with your primary health care provider(s).
- Be cautious about substituting herbs or any OTC product for prescribed medications.
- Seek information from objective sources and check any warnings on the label or package.
- Keep in mind that dietary supplements are not fully regulated by Health Canada.
- Look for a recognized mark of quality verification on the label before purchasing herbs or other dietary supplements.
- Observe for beneficial and harmful effects (it may take several months before these are noticed).
- Report any possible side effects to your primary health care provider for evaluation.
- Herbs can interact with all of the following: other herbs, food, beverages, nutrients, prescription medications and OTC medications.
- Some herbs are contraindicated in people with the following conditions: stroke, glaucoma, diabetes, hypertension, heart disease, thyroid disorder, and any bleeding disorder or condition requiring anticoagulation.
- Common side effects of herbs include stomach problems, skin rashes or allergic reactions.
- Herbs that are used for anxiety or insomnia should not be taken before driving a car.
- Be sceptical about exaggerated claims; if it sounds too good to be true, it probably is!

Source: U.S. Food and Drug Administration.

Addressing Factors That Affect Adherence

When older adults have trouble adhering to their medication regimen, nurses can work with them and their caregivers to identify ways to improve adherence. For example, unit-dose medication systems, which have been widely used in institutional settings, are becoming more available for use in home settings and may be helpful in improving medication adherence, especially when medication regimens are complex. A variety of simple pill organizers (i.e., containers with separate compartments designated for each day of the week and with one or more compartments for each day) are widely available in stores. In addition, more sophisticated devices to enhance independence and improve adherence are available and may be particularly helpful for people with cognitive or functional impairments. For example, human voice recordings, telephone–computer services and beeping watches or key chains can be used to remind the person to take medications at designated times. Nurses can encourage older adults and their caregivers to investigate different types of devices and systems that can be used to improve medication adherence.

Wellness Opportunity

Nurses promote self-responsibility by addressing factors that interfere with adherence and, at the same time, supporting independence.

Even with the increased availability of prescription drug benefits through Medicare, older adults and people with chronic conditions are burdened by the high cost of prescription medications. Thus, nurses often need to address financial barriers that affect adherence to medication regimens because even a person who has an adequate income may decide that a medication is not worth the high cost, especially on an ongoing basis. Nurses can encourage older adults to be candid with their health care practitioners and ask about the availability of less costly but equally safe and effective medications. One way of addressing high costs is to use generic medications, which are regulated by Health Canada and required to be bioequivalent (i.e., identical) to their brand-name counterparts in dosage form, safety, purity, strength, quality, intended use, performance characteristics and route of administration.

Decreasing the Number of Medications

Because the chance of adverse medication effects increases in proportion to the number of medications consumed, a key intervention is to decrease the number of medications to as few as possible. Nurses accomplish this by coordinating the efforts of the prescriber(s) to discontinue duplicate medications or medications that are no longer appropriate and by educating the older person about the judicious use of medications that are not medically necessary. In home and community-based settings, nurses can teach older adults to review their medications with their health care practitioners at every visit.

When older adults are admitted to the hospital, they are often under the care of primary care practitioners who were not the ones who prescribed the medications taken before the admission. Nurses usually obtain the medication history and the prescribing practitioner may automatically order the medications that are listed on the admission assessment. Because the hospital admission is an ideal time to reevaluate the safety, efficacy and necessity of medications, nurses should ask older adults or their caregivers about the purpose and potential adverse effects of each medication. This assessment, which should be done with the medication reconciliation process, may provide important clues to medications or interactions that contributed to or directly caused the problem for which the patient is hospitalized.

When medications are prescribed for behavioural reasons rather than for a medical condition, nurses can teach older adults and their caregivers about these medications and about nonpharmacologic alternatives. For example, caregivers of people with dementia may use medications to address behaviours that might respond equally well to nonpharmacologic interventions that do not have any risk of adverse effects. Once these medications are prescribed, they are likely to be used over long periods without reevaluation. Nurses need to recognize that the efficacy may diminish (e.g., with hypnotics), the underlying reason may resolve or change (e.g., with situational anxiety) and adverse effects may develop gradually and not be recognized (e.g., with anticholinergic agents). Thus, it is imperative to review periodically all medications and to consider whether nonpharmacologic approaches could be used to address the symptoms or behaviours. Behavioural problems are one example of the types of symptoms that can be managed medically but might be managed just as well, and with fewer risks, through nonpharmacologic interventions. Other types of problems that can often be managed without pharmacologic agents are those related to sleep, comfort, anxiety and chronic illnesses.

In community settings, it is important to make sure that older adults and caregivers understand the appropriate use of medications that are prescribed as needed (i.e., they are used as needed). For example, a caregiver of someone with dementia may be instructed to give a behaviour-modifying medication when the person becomes agitated. Although the episodes of agitation may be precipitated by environmental factors (e.g., noise or overstimulation), the caregiver might not realize that nonpharmacologic interventions could be equally effective and carry no risk of adverse effects. In contrast to this situation, a caregiver may withhold medications that could improve the quality of life for the older person and for himself or herself because of misunderstandings or lack of information about the appropriate use of medications. Nurses can teach caregivers about nonpharmacologic interventions, as well as the appropriate use of medications for behaviour management, particularly for people with dementia (discussed in Chapter 14).

> ### Wellness Opportunity
>
> Nurses promote wellness by talking with older adults and their caregivers, when appropriate, about choosing interventions, such as relaxation techniques, that can improve health and quality of life, rather than using medications.

EVALUATING EFFECTIVENESS OF NURSING INTERVENTIONS

Nurses evaluate interventions related to medication management according to the degree to which the older adult follows a safe and effective medication regimen. This process involves an evaluation of medication-taking behaviours, as well as an evaluation of the therapeutic effects of the medication. Another evaluation criterion is the extent to which negative functional consequences, such as interactions and adverse effects, are prevented, alleviated or controlled. In home settings, nurses can evaluate the effectiveness of their interventions by observing the medication-taking patterns of the older adult. In any setting, nurses can evaluate the knowledge of safe and effective use of prescription and OTC medications. Another measure of effectiveness is the degree to which barriers to adherence are eliminated or addressed.

Case Study

Mrs. M., who is 76 years old, is being discharged to her home after a stay in a rehabilitation facility after a stroke. Residual problems from the stroke include left-sided weakness and visual–perceptual difficulties. In addition to the stroke, Mrs. M.'s diagnoses include glaucoma, depression and heart failure. Her medications include the following: multivitamin, one tablet daily; furosemide (Lasix), 20 mg, two tablets daily; aspirin (Ecotrin), 81 mg daily; clopidogrel (Plavix), 75 mg daily; diltiazem (Cardizem), 60 mg, three times daily; metoprolol (Lopressor), 50 mg twice daily; simvastatin (Zocor), 40 mg at bedtime; sertraline (Zoloft), 50 mg at bedtime; and timolol ophthalmic (Timoptic), 0.25% twice daily. The facility's regimen for administering the medications is as follows:

7:30 AM	Cardizem 60 mg Furosemide 20 mg, 2 tablets Ecotrin 81 mg Timoptic, 0.25% in each eye
9:00 AM	Lopressor 50 mg
1:00 PM	Multivitamin, 1 tablet Cardizem 60 mg
3:30 PM	Furosemide 20 mg, 2 tablets
7:30 PM	Timoptic, 0.25% in each eye Cardizem 60 mg Plavix 75 mg
9:00 PM	Lopressor 50 mg Zoloft 50 mg Zocor 40 mg daily

NURSING ASSESSMENT

Your assessment reveals that, before her hospitalization and rehabilitation facility stay, Mrs. M. administered her medications independently, but the only medications she took were the eye drops, furosemide (20 mg once daily) and digoxin, which she is no longer taking. The functional assessment indicates that Mrs. M. has weakness and limited use of her left arm and hand, causing difficulty performing tasks that require fine motor movements. She has full use of her right upper extremity, and she is right-hand dominant. She ambulates independently, but slowly, with a walker. A mental status assessment reveals that Mrs. M. is alert, oriented and has no memory deficits; however, her abstract thinking and time perception have been impaired by the stroke. She has some expressive aphasia, but she seems to understand instructions, especially if ideas are reinforced with concrete examples and demonstrations.

Mrs. M. expresses motivation to take her medications, but she admits to being overwhelmed by the complexity of the regimen, stating that at the rehabilitation facility, they administered her medications at six different times. She is also concerned about self-administering her eye drops because she used to use her left hand to hold her eyelids open. With regard to furosemide, she says she does not like taking it twice a day because it makes her go to the bathroom too much. While at the rehabilitation facility, she has not had any trouble with incontinence, but she worries about what she'll do at home because there is no bathroom on the first floor. She asks whether she can take the entire dose of furosemide at night so that she will only have to get up during the night to go to the bathroom, which is located near the bedroom.

In response to your questions about medication management routines before her stroke, Mrs. M. reports using a compartmentalized medication container and taking her two medications and the eye drops after breakfast, around 9:30 AM. She would administer the second dose of eye drops around 9:30 PM, before getting ready for bed. She had no difficulty remembering the medications because she kept the pill container and one bottle of eye drops near the toaster, and she kept a second bottle of eye drops on her nightstand. Now, however, she expresses concern about the number of times she must take medications if the regimen remains the same as in the rehabilitation facility, and she thinks she will need six pill containers but is not sure where she should put all of them. Mrs. M. also tells you that she is worried about paying for so many medications. Now that she is on so many new pills—and she knows that some are very expensive—she needs to have her medication regimen reviewed and perhaps changed.

Mrs. M. lives with her husband, who is physically healthy but has early-stage Alzheimer disease. Their daughter lives nearby and visits two or three times weekly to assist with grocery shopping, laundry and household chores. She also provides transportation to stores and appointments.

NURSING DIAGNOSIS

You decide on a nursing diagnosis of Noncompliance because Mrs. M. expresses a desire to take her medications, but several factors deter adherence to the current regimen. Related factors include functional impairments, complex medication regimens, negative side effects of furosemide and concern about the cost of medications.

NURSING CARE PLAN FOR MRS. M.

Expected Outcome	Nursing Interventions	Nursing Evaluation
Mrs. M.'s medication routine will be simplified.	• Work with the pharmacist and the prescribing practitioner to simplify the medication regimen. • Discuss with Mrs. M.'s prescribing practitioner the problem of the complexity of the regimen and the cost of medications. Ask Mrs. M.'s prescribing practitioner if she can take Cardizem CD, 180 mg daily, rather than Cardizem, 60 mg three times a day. (This may be less expensive and will eliminate two doses of medication daily.) • Ask the pharmacist about combining medications to allow twice-daily administration. • Assist Mrs. M. in establishing a routine for self-administering medications that will fit in with her usual activities. • At least 3 days before discharge from the rehabilitation facility, arrange for Mrs. M. to assume responsibility for her own medication management, using pill containers that she herself fills.	• Mrs. M. will be able to follow a twice-daily medication dosing schedule.
Mrs. M.'s concerns about furosemide will be addressed.	• Explain the importance of taking furosemide, as ordered, to control heart failure effectively. • Suggest that Mrs. M. obtain a portable commode for use downstairs during the day.	• Mrs. M. will take furosemide as directed and will not experience difficulty with urinary incontinence.

Expected Outcome	Nursing Interventions	Nursing Evaluation
Mrs. M.'s concerns about the cost of medications will be addressed.	• Encourage Mrs. M. to talk with her primary care practitioner about her concerns over the cost of the prescribed medications.	• Mrs. M. will be able to afford her prescribed medications.
A system for self-administering eye drops will be identified.	• Ask an occupational therapist to evaluate Mrs. M.'s ability to self-administer her eye drops and to identify any assistive devices that may increase her independence and reliability in performing this task. • Have Mrs. M. practice self-administering her eye drops before she is discharged from the rehabilitation facility, with staff providing whatever assistance is necessary. • Talk with Mrs. M. about the possibility of her husband assisting with the eye drop procedure if she is unable to do this independently. • Ask Mrs. M.'s ophthalmologist whether the eye drop regimen can be simplified to once-daily dosing by prescribing an extended-action eye drop formula.	• Mrs. M. will self-administer her eye drops or will receive the assistance she needs for eye drop administration from her husband.

THINKING POINTS

- What are the factors that influence Mrs. M.'s ability to manage her medications independently?
- What additional assessment information would be helpful in establishing a plan for Mrs. M. to manage her medications independently?
- What health education would you provide to address Mrs. M.'s concerns about the cost of her medications?
- What steps would you take to ensure that expected outcomes are achieved after Mrs. M. is back in her own home?

Chapter Highlights

Introduction to Bioactive Substances

- Pharmacokinetics, pharmacodynamics and elimination half-time
- Herbs and homeopathic remedies
- Herbs and medications with similar bioactivity (Table 8-1)
- Potential adverse effects of herbs (Table 8-2)

Age-Related Changes That Affect Medications in Older Adults

- Age-related changes that affect medications in the body (Box 8-1)
- Changes that affect medication-taking behaviours

Risks Factors That Affect Medication-Taking Behaviours

- Pathologic processes and functional impairments
- Behaviours based on myths and misunderstandings (e.g., attitudes about and expectations for medications)
- Communication barriers between older adults and prescribing practitioners
- Lack of information
- Inappropriate prescribing practices (Beers Criteria, STOPP/START)
- Polypharmacy and inadequate monitoring
- Medication nonadherence
- Financial concerns related to prescription drugs
- Insufficient recognition of adverse effects (Table 8-3)

Medication Interactions

- Medication–medication interactions (Table 8-4)
- Medication–herb interactions
- Medications and nutrients (Table 8-5)
- Medications and alcohol (Table 8-6)
- Medications and nicotine (Table 8-7)

Functional Consequences Associated With Medications in Older Adults

- Altered therapeutic effects
- Increased potential for adverse drug events (Box 8-2)
- Anticholinergic adverse effects (Box 8-3)
- Increased potential for altered mental status (Table 8-8)
- Antipsychotics in people with dementia
- Tardive dyskinesia and drug-induced parkinsonism

Nursing Assessment of Medication Use and Effects

- Communication techniques for obtaining accurate information
- Scope of a medication assessment (all bioactive substances, older adult's understanding of regimen, preferences) (Box 8-5)
- Cultural considerations (factors that influence medication-taking behaviours, culturally specific health care sources and practices) (Boxes 8-6 and 8-7)
- Patterns of medication use
- Medication assessment as it relates to the overall assessment
- Identifying adverse medication effects

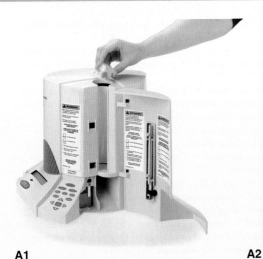

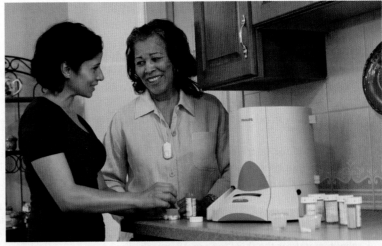

A1   **A2**

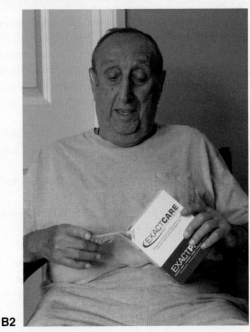

JOE SAMPLE   1/1
Take April 16, 2009   @09:00 AM

Colace   **100MG**   Qty 1
red oval capsule n 512

Glucophage   500MG   Qty 1
white round tablet BMS 6060

Motrin   600MG   Qty 1
white oblong tablet 600

Norvasc   5MG   Qty 1
white octagonal tab NOR

Prilosec   20MG   Qty 1
purple oblong capsule 742

B1   **B2**

FIGURE 8-1 Examples of devices and systems designed to improve medication adherence and independence. (**A**) An automatic pill dispenser with a tamper-proof locking system and an audible alarm, with 28 compartments that can be programmed for taking medications up to four times a day. (**B**) An individualized dosing system for prescription and nonprescription medications, for use in homes and institutions, with each tear-apart compartment printed with patient name, date and time of administration, medication name and dose, and pill description. *(Figure A used with permission from Philips Health care.com. Figure B used with permission from ExactCarepharmacy.com.)*

Nursing Diagnoses
- Ineffective self-health management
- Adverse effects: Confusion, risk for falls, instrumental self-care deficit
- Readiness for enhanced self-health management

Planning for Wellness Outcomes
- Knowledge: Medication
- Self-care: Nonparenteral medication

Nursing Interventions to Promote Safe and Effective Medication Management
- Implementing evidence-based interventions (Box 8-8)
- Medication reconciliation

- Teaching about medications and herbs (Boxes 8-9 and 8-10 patient-teaching tools)
- Addressing factors that affect adherence (Fig. 8-1)
- Decreasing the number of medications

Evaluating Effectiveness of Nursing Interventions
- Medication-taking behaviours that are safe and effective
- Prevention, alleviation or control of negative functional consequences (e.g., interactions, adverse effects).

Critical Thinking Exercises

1. You are asked to give a half-hour presentation titled "Medications and Aging" to a local senior citizens group. Describe the following:

- What points would you cover about age-related changes in terms that would be easily understood by older adults?
- How would you address the risk factors that affect medication action and medication-taking behaviours?
- What tips would you give about taking medications?
- What educational materials would you use?
- How would you promote group participation in the discussion?

2. Carefully read the interview questions in Box 8-5 and decide which questions you would use and how you would phrase the questions in your own words for each of the following situations:
   - You are doing an admission interview for a 78-year-old man who lives alone and has been admitted to the hospital for the third time in 18 months for heart failure.
   - You are working in a senior wellness program in an urban setting with a large number of older adults who were born in Southeast Asia. You are preparing for 15-minute interviews with older adults who have agreed to participate in an educational session to which they must bring all their pills in a bag and ask the nurse about them.

3. Carefully read the information in Boxes 8-9 and 8-10 and describe what information you would be likely to use in each of the following situations.
   - Discharge planning for the 78-year-old man described in Exercise 2, bullet 1.
   - Health education for people described in the senior wellness program in Exercise 2, bullet 2.

For more information about topics discussed in this chapter, be sure to check out the interactive Online Learning Activities and other helpful resources at http://thepoint.lww.com/Miller7e

REFERENCES

Accreditation Canada, the Canadian Institute for Health Information, the Canadian Patient Safety Institute, and the Institute for Safe Medication Practices Canada. (2012). *Medication reconciliation in Canada: Raising the bar.* Ottawa, ON: Author.

Alessi-Severini, S., Dahl, M., Schultz, J., et al. (2013). Prescribing of psychotropic medications to the elderly population of a Canadian province: A retrospective study using administrative databases. *PeerJ, 1,* e168. doi:10.7717/peerj.168

Allen, J. (2012). Avoiding overuse of antipsychotic medications. *Geriatric Nursing, 33*(4), 327–328.

Alzheimer Society of Canada. (2011). *Guidelines for care: Person-centred care of people with dementia living in care homes.* Retrieved from http://www.alzheimer.ca/~/media/Files/national/Culture-change/culture_change_framework_e.ashx

American Geriatrics Society. (2012a). Guiding principles for the care of older adults with multimorbidity. *Journal of the American Geriatrics Society, 60*(10), E1–E25. doi:10.1111/j.1532-5415.2012.04188.x

American Geriatrics Society. (2012b). American Geriatrics Society updated Beers Criteria for potentially inappropriate medication use

in older adults. *Journal of the American Geriatrics Society, 60*(4), 616–631. doi:10.1111/j.1532-5415.2012.03923.x

Anderson, J. K., & Fox, J. R. (2012). Potential food–drug interactions in long-term care. *Journal of Gerontological Nursing, 38*(4), 38–46.

Andrews, M. M. (2012). Cultural competence in the health history and physical examination. In M. M. Andrews & J. S. Boyle (Eds.), *Transcultural concepts in nursing care* (6th ed., pp. 38–72). Philadelphia, PA: Lippincott Williams & Wilkins.

BC Ministry of Health and BC Medical Association. (2007). *BC Clinical Practice Guidelines: Cognitive impairment in the elderly—Recognition, diagnosis and management.* Retrieved from http://www.bcguidelines.ca

Beers, M. H., Ouslander, J. G., Rollingher, J., et al. (1991). Explicit criteria for determining potentially inappropriate medication use by the elderly. *Archives of Internal Medicine, 151,* 1825–1832.

Blackburn, D. F., Swidrovich, J., & Lemstra, M. (2013). Non-adherence in type 2 diabetes: Practical considerations for interpreting the literature. *Patient Preference and Adherence, 7,* 183–189.

Bohlega, S. A., & Al-Foghom, N. B. (2013). Drug-induced Parkinson's disease: A clinical review. *Neuroscience, 18*(3), 215–221.

Boon, H. S., Verhoef, M. J., Vanderheyden, L. C., et al. (2006). Complementary and alternative medicine: A rising health care issue. *Health care Policy, 3,* 19–30.

Brandt, N. J., & Pyhtila, J. (2013). Psychopharmacological medication use among older adults with dementia in nursing homes. *Journal of Gerontological Nursing, 39*(4), 8–14.

Budnitz, D. S., Lovegrove, M. C., Shehab, N., et al. (2011). Emergency hospitalizations for adverse drug events in older Americans. *The New England Journal of Medicine, 365,* 2002–2012.

Cai, X., Campbell, N., Khan, B., et al. (2013). Long-term anticholinergic use and the aging brain. *Alzheimers Dementia, 9*(4), 377–385.

Chen, X. W., Sneed, K. B., Pan, S. Y., et al. (2012). Herb–drug interactions and mechanistic and clinical considerations. *Current Drug Metabolism, 13*(5), 640–651.

Colloca, G., Tosato, M., Vetrano, D. L., et al. (2012). Inappropriate drugs in elderly patients with severe cognitive impairment: Results from the SHELTER Study. *PLOS One, 7*(10), e46669. doi:10.1371/journal.pone.0046669

Corsonello, A., Onder, G., Abbatecola, A. M., et al. (2012). Explicit criteria for potentially inappropriate medications to reduce the risk of adverse drug reactions in elderly people: From Beers to STOPP/START criteria. *Drug Safety, 35*(Suppl. 1), 21–28.

de Lima Toccafondo, V. M., & Huang, S.-M. (2012). Botanical-drug interactions: A scientific perspective. *Planta Medica, 78,* 1400–1415.

Dupouy, J., Moulis, G., Tubery, M., et al. (2013). Which adverse events are related to health care during hospitalization in elderly inpatients? *International Journal of Medical Sciences, 10*(9), 1224–1230.

Fischer, C. E., Cohen, C., Forrest, L., et al. (2011). Psychotropic medication use in Canadian long-term care patients referred for psychogeriatric consultation. *Canadian Geriatrics Journal, 14,* 73–77. doi:10.5770/cgj.v14i13.18

Gallagher, P. F., O'Connor, M. N., & O'Mahony, D. (2011). Prevention of potentially inappropriate prescribing for elderly patients: A randomized controlled trial using STOPP/START criteria. *Clinical Pharmacology and Therapeutics, 89*(6), 845–854.

Hanley, M. J., Cancalon, P., Widmer, W., et al. (2011). The effect of grapefruit juice on drug disposition. *Expert Opinion in Drug Metabolism and Toxicology, 7*(3), 267–286.

Harris, C., Sridharan, A., Landis, R., et al. (2013). What happens to the medication regimens of older adults during and after an acute hospitalization? *Patient Safety, 9*(3), 150–153.

Health Canada. (2012a). *Drugs and health products—About natural health product regulation in Canada.* Retrieved from http://www.hc-sc.gc.ca/dhp-mps/prodnatur/about-apropos/index-eng.php

Health Canada. (2012b). *The safety and effectiveness of generic drugs.* Retrieved from http://www.hc-sc.gc.ca/hl-vs/alt_formats/pdf/iyh-vsv/med/med-gen-eng.pdf

Herdman, T. H. (Ed.). (2012). *NANDA International Nursing Diagnoses: Definitions and classification 2012–2014*. Oxford, England: Wiley-Blackwell.

Hill-Taylor, B., Sketris, I., Hayden, J., et al. (2013). Application of the STOPP/START criteria: A systematic review of the prevalence of potentially inappropriate prescribing in older adults, and evidence of clinical, humanistic, and economic impact. *Journal of Clinical Pharmacology and Therapeutics, 38*(5), 360–372.

Hugtenburg, J. G., Timmers, L., Elders, P. J. M., et al. (2013). Definitions, variants, and causes of nonadherence with medication: A challenge for tailored interventions. *Patient Preference and Adherence, 13*(7), 675–682.

Institute for Safe Medication Practices Canada. (2014). *Safer medication use in older persons information page*. Retrieved from http://www.ismp-canada.org/beers_list/

Izzo, A. A. (2012). Interactions between herbs and conventional drugs: Overview of the clinical data. *Medical Principles and Practice, 21*, 404–428.

Kashyap, M., Tu, M., & Tannenbaum, C. (2013). Prevalence of commonly prescribed medications potentially contributing to urinary symptoms in a cohort of older patients seeking care for incontinence. *BioMed Central Geriatrics, 13*(1), 57.

Lai, D., & Chappell, N. (2007). Use of traditional Chinese medicine by older Chinese immigrants in Canada. *Family Practice, 24*(1), 56–64.

Le Couteur, D. G., McLachlan, A. J., & de Cabo, R. (2012). Aging, drugs, and drug metabolism. *Journals of Gerontology: Biological Sciences, 67*(2), 137–139.

Lee, V. K. T. (2013). Formulating medication adherence strategies using the PASSAction framework. *Canadian Pharmacists Journal, 146*(1), 30–32. doi:10.1177/1715163512472320

Lee, Y., Lin, P. Y., Chang, Y. Y., et al. (2013). Antidepressant-induced tardive syndrome: A retrospective epidemiological study. *Pharmacopsychiatry, 46*(7), 281–285.

Lemay, C. A., Mazor, K. M., Field, T. S., et al. (2013). Knowledge of and perceived need for evidence-based education about antipsychotic medications among nursing home leadership and staff. *Journal of the American Medical Directors Association, 14*(12), 895–900. doi:10.1016/j.jamda.2013.08.009

Little, M. O., & Morley, A. (2013). Reducing polypharmacy: Evidence from a simple quality improvement initiative. *Journal of the American Medical Directors Association, 14*, 152–156.

Lopez-Sendon, J., Mena, M. A., & de Yebenes, J. G. (2013). Drug-induced parkinsonism. *Expert Opinion in Drug Safety, 12*(4), 487–496.

Lung Association of Saskatchewan. (2012). *Access to prescription drugs in Canada*. Retrieved from http://www.sk.lung.ca/drugs/2005.04.04.prescriptions.faq.html

Maher, R. L., Hanlon, J., & Hajjar, E. R. (2014). Clinical consequences of polypharmacy in elderly. *Expert Opinion in Drug Safety, 13*(1), 57–65. doi:10.1517/14740338.2013.82766

Marcum, Z. A., & Gellad, W. F. (2012). Medication adherence to multi-drug regimens. *Clinical Geriatric Medicine, 28*(2), 287–300.

Morandi, A., Vasilevskis, E., Pandharipande, P. P., et al. (2013). Inappropriate medication prescriptions in elderly adults surviving and intensive care unit admission. *Journal of the American Geriatrics Society, 61*(7), 1128–1134.

Morrow, D. G., & Conner-Garcia, T. (2013). Improving comprehension of medication information. *Journal of Gerontological Nursing, 39*(4), 22–29.

Naugler, C. T., Brymer, C., Stolee, P., et al. (2000). Development and validation of an improving prescribing in the elderly tool. *Canadian Journal of Clinical Pharmacology, 7*(2), 103–107.

O'Connor, M. N., Gallagher, P., Byrne, S., et al. (2012). Adverse drug reactions in older patients during hospitalization: Are they predictable? *Age and Ageing, 41*(6), 771–776.

Obreli-Neto, P. R., Nobili, A., de Oliveira, B. A., et al. (2012). Adverse drug reactions caused by drug–drug interactions in elderly outpatients: A prospective study. *European Journal of Pharmacology, 68*(12), 1667–1676.

Pasina, L., Djade, C. D., Lucca, U., et al. (2013). Association of anticholinergic burden with cognitive and functional status in a cohort of hospitalized elderly. *Drugs and Aging, 30*(2), 103–112.

Petrarca, A. M., Lengel, A. J., & Mangan, M. N. (2012). Inappropriate medication use in the elderly. *Consult Pharmacology, 27*(8), 583–586.

Pincus, K. (2013). Transitional care management services. *Journal of Gerontological Nursing, 39*(10), 10–15.

Purnell, L. D. (2013). *Transcultural health care: A culturally competent approach* (4th ed.). Philadelphia, PA: F. A. Davis.

Puustinen, J., Nurminen, J., Vahlberg, T., et al. (2012). CNS medications as predictors of precipitous cognitive decline in the cognitively disabled aged: A longitudinal population-based study. *Dementia & Geriatric Cognitive Disorders, 2*, 57–68.

Quan, H., Lai, D., Johnson, D., et al. (2008). Complementary and alternative medicine use among Chinese and white Canadians. *Canadian Family Physician, 54*(11), 1563–1569.

Riker, G. I., & Setter, S. M. (2012). Polypharmacy in older adults at home: What it is and what to do about it: Implications for home health care and hospice. *Home Health care Nurse, 30*(8), 474–485.

Seitz, D. P., Gill, S. P., Herrmann, N., et al. (2013). Pharmacological treatment for neuropsychiatric symptoms of dementia in long-term care: A systematic review. *International Psychogeriatrics, 25*(2), 185–203.

Senft, D. J. (2012). Antipsychotic drug use: Understanding the recent attention and response to the increased scrutiny. *Geriatric Nursing, 33*(5), 387–390.

Silver, M., & Factor, S. A. (2013). Valproic acid-induced Parkinsonism: Levodopa responsiveness with dyskinesia. *Parkinsonism and Related Disorders, 19*(8), 758–760.

Sinvani, L. D., Beizer, J., Akerman, M., et al. (2013). Medication reconciliation in continuum of care transitions: A moving target. *Journal of the American Medical Directors Association, 14*(9), 668–672. doi:10.1016/j.jamda.2013.02.021

Steinberg, M., & Lyketsos, C. G. (2012). Atypical antipsychotic use in patients with dementia: Managing safety concerns. *American Journal of Psychiatry, 169*(9), 900–906.

Tsai, H.-H., Lin, H.-W., Simon, P. A., et al. (2012). Evaluation of documented drug interactions and contraindications associated with herbs and dietary supplements: A systematic literature review. *International Journal of Clinical Practice, 66*(11), 1056–1078.

Uusvaara, J., Pitkala, K. H., Kautiainen, H., et al. (2013). Detailed cognitive function and use of drugs with anticholinergic properties in older people: A community-based cross-sectional study. *Drugs and Aging, 30*(3), 177–182.

Waln, O., & Jankovic, J. (2013). An update on tardive dyskinesia: From phenomenology to treatment. *Tremor and Other Hyperkinetic Movements*. Retrieved from http://tremorjournal.org/article/view/161

Yayla, M. E., Bilge, U., Binen, E., et al. (2013). The use of START/STOPP criteria for elderly patients in primary care. *The Scientific World Journal, 2013* [Article ID 165873]. doi:10.1155/2013/165873

Zwicker, D., & Fulmer, T. (2012). Reducing adverse drug events. In M. Boltz, E. Capezuti, T. Fulmer, et al. (Eds.), *Evidence-based practice protocols for best practice* (4th ed., pp. 324–362). New York, NY: Springer.

chapter 9

Legal and Ethical Concerns

For the past several decades, various legislative efforts have addressed the rights of older adults with issues pertaining to older adults including end-of-life decisions, the rights of patients and nursing home residents and the quality of care provided to seniors who are vulnerable. Currently, autonomy and decision-making are emphasized, particularly with regard to life-sustaining medical interventions. Many of these legislative and policy initiatives involve ethical issues for gerontological health care practitioners. For example, nurses commonly address questions about the extent to which an older person is able to make decisions about his or her health care. Although legislation provides guidelines, laws do not resolve ethical dilemmas that arise when no advance directive is provided or when conflicts exist about how an advance directive should be interpreted or implemented. The next sections review some of the pertinent legal and ethical issues that are relevant to nursing care of older adults. Additional legal and ethical considerations regarding vulnerable or abused elders are addressed in Chapter 10.

AUTONOMY AND RIGHTS

Autonomy is the personal freedom to direct one's own life as long as it does not infringe on the rights of others. An autonomous person is capable of rational thought and is able to recognize the need for problem solving. In addition, an autonomous person is capable of identifying the problem, searching for alternatives and selecting a solution that allows his or her continued personal freedom. People may be denied the right to autonomy if the outcome of their decisions or their lack of decision-making ability jeopardizes their safety, or the rights, safety or property of others. Loss of autonomy and, therefore, loss of independence, is a very real fear among older adults. Moreover, for older adults with dementia and other conditions that affect decision-making abilities, loss of autonomy is a challenge that is frequently addressed by families and health care professionals throughout the course of the condition, which can last for many years.

Because autonomy is highly valued in many European and North American cultures and there is no easy way to evaluate decision-making abilities—which can fluctuate from day to day—questions often arise about medical interventions and health care decisions. Thus, nurses need to be familiar with legal and ethical guidelines related to competency and decision-making capacity. Nurses are responsible for assisting older adults and their families, often as impartial mediators, when issues concerning personal autonomy arise. However, if the safety of the older person is threatened because of risky behaviours arising from impaired decision-making abilities, nurses must refer older people to the appropriate community agencies (e.g., adult protective services) for further evaluation, as discussed in Chapter 10.

Competency

Competency is a *legal term* that refers to the ability to fulfil one's role and handle one's affairs in a responsible manner. All adults are presumed to be competent, and jurisdictional laws designate the age of competency—usually 18 years—for participating in legally binding decisions. Because competent people are guaranteed all the rights granted by the Canadian constitution and provincial/territorial laws, all adults who have not been declared **incompetent** by a judge have the legal right to make their own decisions about medical treatment and health care. However, in reality, families and health care providers often raise questions about an older person's ability to make reasonable decisions, particularly when the person is cognitively impaired.

When questions are raised about a person's ability to participate in health care decisions, a legally appointed, surrogate decision maker, if one has been designated, assumes decision-making responsibility (see the discussion of health care proxy in the section on advance directives). In the absence of a surrogate decision maker or when conflicts exist among the people involved with making and implementing decisions, a petition can be filed with probate court to determine whether the person is competent. Often, these petitions are filed because a health care provider (usually a physician) is concerned that appropriate decisions be made for a person who is not making safe and reasonable medical decisions independently. Usually a family member files the petition, but if no qualified family member is available, or if family members are in conflict about the petition, an attorney or other person may file. If the court determines that the person is incompetent (i.e., incapable of making decisions on his or her own behalf), the judge assigns either a partial or a full **guardianship.**

With a partial guardianship, the incompetent person continues to make limited decisions; with a full guardianship, the person loses all of his or her rights to make decisions. Although additional court action can revoke or reverse a guardianship after it has been granted, the guardianship typically remains in place until the incompetent person dies. Usually, guardianship is initiated only as a last resort when no other legal intervention is appropriate because it is a drastic measure that takes away rights and entails court proceedings and ongoing court monitoring. Most often the need for guardianship can be avoided if a person makes his or her wishes known in a comprehensive and legally binding manner, including the appointment of a surrogate decision maker, before any questions arise about his or her mental capacities. In the absence of these documents, however, or when conflict arises about the ability of designated people to honour the person's wishes, legal and ethical issues are generally addressed through court proceedings, such as guardianship.

Trusteeship applies when an older adult no longer has the capacity to make a decision on financial matters. An individual who is the subject of a trusteeship order is called a "represented adult"; while, the person authorized to make personal decisions for the represented adult is called the "trustee." A trustee, once appointed by the court, has the legal responsibility to make financial decisions for the represented adult. While trusteeship is an option in Canada, families with older adults are being counselled to consider enduring power of attorney in advance of complete mental incapacitation of the older adult. In these situations, the older adult (who is still mentally competent enough to understand what he or she is doing) signs a legal document appointing someone to manage his or her finances when deemed incompetent by one or two physicians. When the physician(s) signs the form to indicate that the older adult is no longer able to manage finances, enduring power of attorney is activated.

Decision-Making Capacity

Decision-making capacity is a measure of a person's ability to make an informed and logical decision about a particular aspect of his or her health care. It is a *clinical term* that describes the person's ability to understand, make, and be responsible for the consequences of health care decisions. In contrast to competency—which is determined by a court of law—decision-making capacity is determined by health care practitioners and it relates to a single decision rather than a global determination of one's ability to manage one's own affairs. Decision-making capacity requires that the person be able to do all the following:

- Understand and process information that is relevant to the decisions about diagnosis, prognosis and treatment options
- Weigh the relative risks, benefits and outcomes of decisions in relation to one's own situation
- Apply personal values to the situation
- Arrive at a decision that is consistent over time
- Communicate the decision to others

Another term is **mental capacity**, which is a legal construct. The definition varies slightly across provincial and territorial jurisdictions in Canada. An individual is assumed to have capacity unless there is evidence to the contrary. It is generally described as the ability to understand the information needed to make a decision and to appreciate the consequences of that decision (BC Centre for Elder Law, n.d.).

It is important to recognize the influence of differing religious and culturally based beliefs when assessing the rationality of the person's conclusions and decision-making capacity. For example, a belief in miracles may be culturally appropriate for some clients/patients but seem to be delusional to a Western-trained care provider. Within First Nations groups, consensus (i.e., family/community) decision-making is common versus individual autonomy. Older adults are likely to have treatment preferences that are strongly based on religious or cultural beliefs and be unable to provide logical reasons for their decisions (Chettih, 2012).

An additional consideration pertinent to older adults is that determination of decision-making capacity should not be based on chronological age or a particular diagnosis. This is especially important with regard to older adults who have dementia because they may retain the ability to make safe and sufficient decisions during early stages. Moreover, people with dementia express a strong desire to remain involved in decisions about their care for as long as possible and are aware of the gradual loss of this ability as their condition progresses (Fetherstonhaugh et al., 2013). During mild-to-moderate stages of dementia, assessment of decision-making ability is based on the person's ability to describe the importance or implications of the choice on his or her future health (Mitty & Post, 2012). As dementia progresses from early to later stages, everyday decision-making processes usually transition from supportive decision-making, which involves shared decision-making by the person with dementia and family caregivers, to substituted decision-making, which is done by family caregivers (Samsi & Manthorpe, 2013).

Rather than basing conclusions on a person's age or diagnosis, health care professionals focus on a specific situation and evaluate the person's ability to understand the issues involved, to weigh the pros and cons of choices and to communicate about them. For example, a person with dementia may be able to decide about the appointment of a surrogate decision maker but may not be able to participate in a complex decision about medical treatment options for cancer. In this situation, it might be reasonable for the person to designate a family member to make the treatment decision.

It is important to recognize that rather than being an "all or nothing" process, decision-making typically involves considerations related to both the individual and his or her family and others whose opinions the person values. More often than not, decision-making is a complex process in which information is shared between patients and clinicians and among family and others who are affected by the outcomes. Another consideration is that rather than being based primarily on logic and deliberation, decisions are strongly influenced by needs, values, habits, emotions and cultural factors (discussed in the section on Cultural Aspects of Legal and Ethical Issues). Because the ability to value is independent of cognition, people with significant cognitive impairment—as is the case with mild to moderate dementia—are able state their preferences and be involved with decisions (Smebye et al., 2012).

Nurses have dual roles in helping surrogate decision makers involve the older adult as much as possible and while simultaneously supporting shared or surrogate decision makers in assuming responsibility for decisions. This role is especially complex when decisions involve conflicting needs and values of the older adult and the caregivers. For example, spouses and families of people with dementia may experience conflict related to the value of caring for the person at home—a decision that involves sacrifices for the caregiver, as well as benefits for the care recipient—and the decision to have care provided in an assisted living or nursing facility. Additional responsibilities of nurses include documenting the person's specific abilities and limitations in the care plan and ensuring that decision-making abilities are periodically reevaluated.

It is also important to recognize that decision-making capacity can fluctuate from day to day and hour to hour and may be significantly influenced by factors that can be addressed, such as delirium, depression, polypharmacy and sleep deprivation. Thus, an important role of nurses is to promote optimal decision-making capacity by identifying and addressing the factors that influence cognitive functioning and is within the realm of nursing responsibilities. For example, even such a relatively simple measure as ensuring that a hearing-impaired person uses his or her hearing aid may improve communication and thereby have a positive effect on decision-making abilities. Similarly, if a person with dementia has better cognitive abilities in the morning or when rested, then efforts can be made to discuss health care decisions during this time, rather than when the person is more confused.

The phrases *decisional autonomy* and *executional autonomy* are sometimes used in relation to decision-making capacity. Decisional autonomy refers to the ability and freedom to make decisions without external influence, whereas executional autonomy (also called executive autonomy) refers to the ability to implement the decisions. These concepts call attention to the complexity of assessing decision-making capacity and the importance of evaluating a person's ability not only to make reasonable decisions but also to carry out all of the actions necessary for implementing them. This point is particularly important in relation to people with impaired **executive control functions**, which are the cognitive skills involved in successfully planning and carrying out goal-oriented behaviour, such as self-care tasks. Conditions that are likely to cause impaired executive control functions include stroke, dementia, major depression, Parkinson disease, traumatic brain injury and any conditions affecting frontal lobe functioning. These situations are particularly difficult to evaluate because the person may retain the capacity to understand and make decisions (decisional autonomy), but may not have the capacity to carry them out (executive autonomy). Chapter 13 discusses guidelines for nursing assessment of executive control functions, and this topic is addressed in Online Learning Activity 9-1.

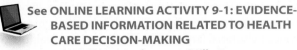

See ONLINE LEARNING ACTIVITY 9-1: EVIDENCE-BASED INFORMATION RELATED TO HEALTH CARE DECISION-MAKING
at http://thepoint.lww.com/Miller7e

ADVANCE DIRECTIVES

Advance directives are legally binding documents that allow competent people to document what medical care they would or would not want to receive if they were not capable of making decisions and communicating their wishes. In the mid-1990s, the Joint Commission on Advance Care Directives by the Canadian Nurses Association, the Canadian Medical Association and the Canadian Health Care Association documented the right of individual patients to self-determination (Canadian Nurses Association, Canadian Medical Association, & Canadian Hospital Association, 1994). Advance directives also enable a person to appoint a **health care proxy** (also called a proxy decision maker or surrogate decision maker), who is responsible for communicating the person's wishes if he or she becomes incompetent or unable to communicate them.

Advance directive documents must be drawn up when the person is capable of understanding their intent, and they become effective only when the person lacks the capacity to make a particular health-related decision. Thus, it is imperative to address advance directives before the onset of any condition, such as dementia, that can affect functioning and cognitive abilities. When the diagnosis of dementia has already been made, it is imperative that decision-making capacity be evaluated and documented as early in the process as possible and specifically in relation to the task of executing advance directive documents. This often requires a comprehensive assessment by an interprofessional team including a mental health professional such as a geriatric psychiatrist. An important nursing responsibility is to facilitate referrals for comprehensive assessments, particularly when conflicts among family members or decision makers exist or are probable in the future. Keep in mind that it may be prudent to periodically reassess decision-making abilities as the older adult's condition changes.

Federal and provincial/territorial laws do not require that people have advance directive documents but their intent is to encourage discussions about health care decisions. Studies indicate that Canadian adults in the general population have completed these documents (Goodridge, 2013) (Box 9-1).

A study of older adults receiving long-term care services found that two factors that were predictive of having advance directives. These factors included having more than 12 years of education and having had a significant health change during the last 6 months (Hirschman et al., 2012).

In Canada, the details of everything from the formal requirements for a valid advance care plan, the authority that such a plan may give to a surrogate decision maker, how and when the advance plan comes into effect, and who takes direction from the advance plan (the surrogate

---

Box 9-1   Evidence-Informed Nursing Practice

Background: The researchers were interested in identifying what proportion of the public completed advance directives in Western Canada. Results would shape public education programs addressing advanced directives.

Question: The question was asked "do you have a living will or a personal directive?"

Method: A telephone survey was conducted with 1,204 Albertans above the age of 18 using the Population Research Laboratory of the University of Alberta.

Results: Of participants above the age of 65, 68.2% had completed advance directives. Results were similar for males and females. The experience of having a family member or friend pass away was strongly related to directive completion.

Nursing Practice Implications: Promoting completion of advance directives promotes autonomy for older adults. Nurses can work with their older clients to educate them on the importance of maintaining their decision-making capacities through the use of advanced directives.

Source: Wilson, D. M., Houttekier, D., Kunju, S. A., et al. (2013). A population-based study on advance directive completion and completion intention among citizens of the western Canadian province of Alberta. *Journal of Palliative Care, 29,* 5–12.

---

decision maker only or the health providers only or both) are all subject to provincial law (Wahl, 2006). There are differences in this type of legislation across Canada. Because of legislation, nurses in all settings should routinely inquire about advance directives and facilitate communication about the older adult's wishes. Provincial/territorial laws vary regarding details (e.g., scope, type of document, conditions for application of advance directives, requirements for updates) of advance directives, and not all jurisdictions honour out-of-province/territorial advance directives. This policy is particularly problematic for older adults who travel between or reside in more than one geographic jurisdiction. Up-to-date information about provincial/territorial laws related to advance directives can be found by using Online Learning Activity 9-2. Common types of advance directives are discussed in the following sections.

See ONLINE LEARNING ACTIVITY 9-2: RESOURCES FOR INFORMATION ABOUT PROVINCIAL/TERRITORIAL LAWS RELATED TO ADVANCE DIRECTIVES
at http://thepoint.lww.com/Miller7e

Power of Attorney for Personal Care (Health Care)

Power of attorney for personal care (health care) is an advance directive that takes effect whenever someone cannot, for any reason, provide informed consent for health care treatment decisions. Because it enables a surrogate health care decision maker, also called a health care proxy (as previously discussed), to represent the person during any time of incapacity, it is often considered the most important advance directive. Like enduring power of attorney (for finances), the power of attorney for health care must be initiated when the person is competent, and it takes effect only when the person is incapacitated. When used with other advance directives, this document provides written guidelines stating the person's wishes on issues, such as termination of life support measures. It is imperative that the health care proxy has a copy of all advance directives and periodically discusses the person's wishes about medical treatments and end-of-life issues. Because language in advance directive documents can sometimes be vague, nurses should encourage older adults to discuss their wishes with their primary care provider, other health care workers and their designated surrogate before a crisis develops.

Do Not Resuscitate (DNR) Orders

A **do not resuscitate (DNR) order** is a very specific type of advance directive that compels health care providers to refrain from cardiopulmonary resuscitation if the person is no longer breathing and has no heartbeat. Sometimes, families, as well as health care professionals, mistakenly associate DNR orders with directives to withhold other medical treatments. For example, questions may arise about not sending someone to a hospital or not requesting certain diagnostic or treatment procedures simply because a DNR order is in place. Other times, DNR orders are overlooked, particularly in emergencies or when the health care power of attorney is not immediately available.

Nurses have important roles in discussing this document with the patient and the health care proxy so that additional and appropriate advance medical directives, or variations of DNR orders, are in place to cover the circumstances that are most likely to arise. It is also imperative to teach older adults, all care providers and health care powers of attorney to have copies of DNR orders readily accessible. The development of guidelines for resuscitation, *Joint Statement on Terminal Illness*, has been supported through a joint statement of the Canadian Nurses Association, Canadian Medical Association, Canadian Hospital Association and the Canadian Bar Association (Canadian Nurses Association, Canadian Medical Association, & Canadian Hospital Association, 1984). These guidelines were replaced in 2009 by a new joint statement.

In 2000 in the United States, the Reverend Chuck Meyers, a nationally recognized expert on ethics and end-of-life issues, proposed the designation of **allow a natural death (AND)** with the intent of replacing negative terms (i.e., "do not") with a positive statement. Patients, families and health care professionals have indicated that they prefer this term to DNR terminology and advocacy groups are working toward legislative changes to include this designation (Whitcomb & Ewing, 2012; Wittmann-Price & Celia, 2010). One such Canadian advocacy group is Dying with Dignity (http://www.dyingwithdignity.ca/2012/08/07/allowing-vsdo-not-language-makes-a-huge-difference-in-end-of-life-decisions.php). Proponents of this change suggest three codes: (1) full support, (2) intermediate support (i.e., continue medical procedures for a short term) and (3) comfort support, allow

natural death (Hospice Patients Alliance, 2013). Although the designation of allow natural death is not recognized in provincial/territorial laws, many jurisdictions and health care institutions allow—and even encourage—variations of the DNR order, such as Comfort Care DNR (also called DNR-Comfort Care, CC/DNR or Comfort Care Only DNR). These legal interventions direct health care professionals (including emergency care workers and first responders) to provide designated comfort care measures but not resuscitative therapies (e.g., cardioversion, chest compression, artificial airway, resuscitative drugs, drugs to correct heart rhythm) if the person is in full respiratory or cardiac arrest or if the person is near this condition. Comfort care measures defined in these documents include oxygen therapy, positioning, airway suctioning, pain medication, control of bleeding and emotional support of patient and family. Jurisdiction-specific procedures for implementing these documents usually require that they be signed by a primary care practitioner and encourage people to make sure these directives are readily available whenever they may be needed. Some provinces/territories have also implemented identification procedures with the use of officially recognized bracelets, wallet cards or other items.

Living Wills

Living wills are a type of advance directive whose purpose is to guide decisions about care that is provided or withheld under certain circumstances, usually at the end of life or when the person is considered terminally ill. In Canada, the generic term is *advanced healthcare directive*. This is a personal care, predeath document and varies in name depending on province/territory. In Ontario it is called *power of attorney for personal care*, in British Columbia a *representation agreement* and in Alberta it is called a *personal directive*. This document's powers are triggered by an incapacity caused by an unforeseen health crisis such as a stroke, heart attack, accident, Alzheimer disease or any other mental or physical disability that deems one unable to make decisions about personal care and healthcare. People must be competent to initiate a living will and they can revoke or change it at any time as long as they remain competent. It is imperative that living wills, and all advance directives, reflect the person's values and goals. A major goal of living wills is to affirm the right of a person to receive or refuse treatment; a limitation is that they do not cover all foreseeable options.

Living wills are not the same as DNR orders because these documents address preferences for a broad range of medical treatments that the person wishes to have or not have in certain circumstances. For example, these advance directives can provide instructions about specific interventions, such as antibiotics, food and nutrition and admission to the hospital. These documents afford reassurance to people who fear that treatments or pain control and comfort measures will not be provided when they are sick and cannot express their own wishes. Although advance directives cannot guarantee that a medical intervention will be provided regardless of the circumstances, they provide legal assurance that the person's preferences will be considered. Because of the inability to predict medical treatments that might become available, and because of the changing health condition of the person executing the document, medical directives should be reviewed and updated periodically.

An important consideration is that living wills typically apply only to situations in which the person is considered terminally ill, whereas other advance directives may apply to a broader range of circumstances, such as irreversible brain damage or temporary incapacity. Another limitation is that definitions of terminal illness are not always clear, and there may be disagreement about whether the person is terminally ill. In general, someone is considered to be terminally ill when a physician determines that his or her predictable life expectancy is 6 months or less. Some laws or policies require that two physicians document that the person is terminally ill.

Most provinces/territories recognize the validity of living wills, but the scope and details of living wills differ across jurisdictions. For example, some provinces/territories require that living wills specifically address certain procedures, such as the withholding or withdrawal of artificial sustenance. Advocacy groups and health care professionals are encouraging all adults to draw up living wills and to take steps to ensure that all their health care providers have copies of these documents.

Medical Orders for Life-Sustaining Treatment

The **Physician Orders for Life-Sustaining Treatment (POLST)** is a recent and evolving development in Canada. Several jurisdictions use the term *Medical Orders for Life-Sustaining Treatment* (MOLST) or *Medical Orders for Scope of Treatment* (MOST) with the same intent as POLST. These medical directives are effective for ensuring that patient preferences are known and honoured in all settings and situations, including emergencies and long-term care (Araw et al., 2013; Hammes et al., 2012; Wenger et al., 2012).

POLST directives are used for people who have advanced chronic progressive illness and/or frailty, those who might die or lose decision-making capacity during the next year, and older adults who have a strong desire to further define their preferences of care (Muller, 2012). POLST addresses the following questions about treatment at the end of life: (1) Will treatment make a difference? (2) Do burdens of treatment outweigh its benefits? (3) Is there hope for recovery and if so, what will life be like afterward? and (4) What does the patient value and what is the patient's goal for care? (Bomba et al., 2012).

In contrast to advance directives, which are initiated and *completed by individuals* to guide decisions about their care in the future, POLST documents are *completed by health care professionals* and serve as a *medical order* for providing or withholding treatment under any circumstances. The document was developed to translate advance directives into physicians' orders that are followed by all clinicians whenever

patients cannot speak for themselves. Thus, they apply to all immediate medical care providers, ranging from emergency medical providers to long-term care facilities, even if these health care professionals have not been involved with the development of the document. POLST documents usually are printed on brightly coloured forms and are transferred across settings.

Citing from work done by the Health Law Institute of Dalhousie University (http://eol.law.dal.ca/?page_id=366), the law in Canada on the unilateral withholding and withdrawal of potentially life-sustaining treatment by a healthcare provider is unclear. Some courts have held that healthcare providers do not have the authority to unilaterally withhold or withdraw potentially life-sustaining treatment, others have said that they do and still others have said that the law is unclear. On October 18, 2013, some clarity was brought to the issue when the Supreme Court of Canada released its decision in *Brian Cuthbertson et al. v Hassan Rasouli* by his litigation guardian and substitute decision maker. The majority of the court found that Ontario's health care consent legislation requires consent from a patient's substitute decision maker before the withdrawal of potentially life-sustaining treatment. However, this decision provides little guidance for provinces and territories other than Ontario as it was based on an interpretation of the Ontario legislation (which others do not share). More clarity in legislation is needed to resolve the ongoing confusion and controversy.

Although there is increasing use of POLST and similar documents, the following ethical issues have been raised about this type of directive (Brugger et al., 2012):

- They may be implemented without the person being terminally ill.
- Not all provinces/territories require the signature of a patient or health care power of attorney for implementation.
- Not all provinces/territories require the signature of the attending physician for implementation.
- Orders accompany the patient across all health care facilities.
- Orders are effective immediately and do not require consultation with the primary care practitioner or health care power of attorney.
- Documents can be drawn up by trained nonphysician "facilitators," including nurses, social workers, admissions coordinators and nursing home administrators.
- Documents use a simplistic check-box format that is not appropriate for complex decisions.

In contrast, ethical arguments in support of POLST emphasize that if these orders are based on a complex decision-making process involving the individual and the health care practitioner they are a tool for communicating *about* life-sustaining interventions rather than simply an order to *forgo* these interventions (Tuohey & Hodges, 2011). The position of the Canadian Medical Association (2013) is that in cases of disagreement between the health care team and the patient or his/her proxy regarding noninitiation or discontinuation of a life-saving or -sustaining intervention, a second medical opinion should be obtained. It is imperative that all nurses are well informed about both the legal and ethical aspects of all types of advance directives. Online Learning Activity 9-3 provides links to useful information about POLST and ethical issues related to medical orders for life-sustaining treatment.

E-planning Web Sites

Most recently, technologic advances are helping people engage in advance care planning as a self-learning and ongoing process through interactive "e-planning" websites. Caring Conversations, offered by the Canadian Palliative Care Association, is an example of a comprehensive website that includes multimedia materials, tailored education and interactive decision-support tools that help individuals to (1) break down complex decisions into more manageable components, (2) identify inconsistencies and/or incompatibilities in stated values and goals, (3) apply personal goals and values to potential clinical situations and (4) translate this information into comprehensible and practical directives to guide surrogates in decision-making (Green & Levi, 2012). Moreover, studies have found that this e-planning tool generates an advance directive that reliably reflects the person's values and goals (Schubart et al., 2012) and makes one's personal wishes known to others. Online Learning Activity 9-3 provides detailed information about this and other e-planning tools that nurses can use to discuss advance care documents with older adults and their caregivers (as discussed in the section on nursing interventions).

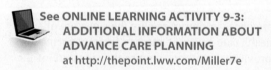

See **ONLINE LEARNING ACTIVITY 9-3:**
ADDITIONAL INFORMATION ABOUT
ADVANCE CARE PLANNING
at http://thepoint.lww.com/Miller7e

LEGAL ISSUES SPECIFIC TO LONG-TERM CARE SETTINGS

Canada's commitment to care for disabled and aging older adults is a long-standing one. The delivery of long-term care is a provincial/territorial responsibility. All jurisdictional health systems in Canada provide some level of residential care support in licensed or regulated facilities. The assessment and placement process to access most long-term care facilities is managed by health authorities.

Within Canada, the **Minimum Data Set (MDS)** for Resident Assessment and Care Planning is used for all long-term care residents. This form includes a Resident Assessment Instrument (RAI), which is a structured, multidimensional resident-assessment and problem-identification system.

In the United States, the RAI was being used in all Medicaid- and Medicare-funded nursing homes by 1991. However, it was not introduced into Canada until 1996. While version 3 of this tool is being utilized within the United States, version 2 is still being used within Canada. During its first year of implementation, MDS 3 has been successful in meeting the guidelines of the World Health Organization and the International Association of Gerontology and Geriatrics consensus group as an effective tool for improving quality of care for nursing home residents if the information is addressed in care plans (Morley, 2013).

In Canada, the Continuing Care Reporting System (CCRS) supports the collection and analysis of nursing home information from the RAI in the Yukon, Newfoundland and Labrador, Ontario, Saskatchewan, Manitoba, Alberta and British Columbia. The information is obtained electronically via the RAI for the Canadian Institute for Health Information (2013), which provides a report. All personal identifiers are removed. It holds information from more than 1,000 nursing homes in Canada, providing a unique tool to measure quality of care. Individual facilities can access aggregate data to compare their performance against benchmarks.

The Nursing Home Residents' Bill of Rights is legislation protecting the rights of nursing home residents within the United States. This bill of rights confers rights on users of nursing homes and similar long-term care facilities and place obligations on providers of those services. This bill of rights provides, through an independent ombudsperson, a process for residents who believe that their rights have been breached to make a complaint. The ombudsperson also has powers of investigation and enforcement. Within Canada, we do not have the same national bill of rights. However, there is still legislation in place to protect older adults living in long-term care; this protection of nursing home residents is sometimes subsumed under other legislation.

Nursing home residents' rights in Canada are primarily legislated at the provincial/territorial level. For example, in Ontario, for instance' the *Long Term Care Homes Act 2007* contains a "Residents' Bill of Rights," including, *inter alia*, the rights to be treated with courtesy and respect; to privacy in treatment; to be informed of one's medical condition and treatment; to consent to or refuse treatment; to confidentiality of medical records and treatment; to receive visitors; and, when near death, to have family members present 24 hours a day. In British Columbia, legislation was passed in 2009 that addressed residents' rights in all types of residential care facilities, including long-term care and supportive-living facilities.

Additionally, a number of provinces/territories have established a "patients' bill of rights" which may be applied to residents of nursing homes. For example, in New Brunswick, the government introduced a bill that would establish a health charter of rights and responsibilities. The introduction of a patients' bill of rights has also been considered in Saskatchewan and Manitoba. There are also a number of nongovernmental agencies that provide information about rights for older adults. In 2010, the Canadian Medical Association endorsed a proposal for a national charter of patients' rights (Vogel, 2010). A draft, Charter for Patient-Centred Care contains rights pertaining not only to the provider–patient relationship, but also to the relationship between the patient and the health care system at large, such as continuity of care between providers, transparency in government decision-making on the delivery of health care, and proactive monitoring and quality improvement. Other examples include the Advocacy Centre for the Elderly in Toronto (http://www.advocacycentreelderly.org/) or Public Legal Education and Information Service of New Brunswick (http://www.legal-info-legale.nb.ca/). Box 9-2 lists some of the rights that might be included in such legislation or other documentation.

ETHICAL ISSUES COMMONLY ADDRESSED IN GERONTOLOGICAL NURSING

Although ethical questions are often associated with major issues as already discussed, many daily care issues related to patients' values, preferences and quality of life involve ethical dilemmas. These issues are omnipresent in health care settings, and they range from seemingly inconsequential concerns like being able to choose the time that meals are served to decisions about how to provide nutrition and hydration to people who are at risk for aspiration. As with all ethical questions, answers are more often in the "grey area" rather than being "black and white." This section first provides an overview of a nursing approach to addressing these issues and then discusses issues commonly encountered when caring for older adults.

Holistic Nursing Ethics

Principles underlying holistic nursing ethics, which emphasize the caring process when curing is not possible, are particularly appropriate in relation to gerontological nursing. Questions such as the following can guide nurses in holistic decision-making about ethical issues (Burkhardt & Keegan, 2013):

- Am I wise and courageous enough to perceive and respect others' differences and honour them as I honour my own beliefs?
- What does the patient want?
- Does the patient understand his or her choices?
- Is the patient being coerced?
- What does quality of life mean for this patient?
- How are others responding to the patient's perceptions of quality of life?
- Does having the technology always mean it should be used?

Although answers to these questions may not be evident, a process of values clarification can be used to guide nurses in ethical decision-making. **Values clarification** is an

---

Box 9-2 Some Rights of Nursing Home Residents

The Right to Be Fully Informed

- The right to daily communication in their language
- The right to assistance if they have a sensory impairment
- The right to be notified in advance of any plans to change their room or roommate
- The right to be fully informed of all services available and the charge for each service

The Right to Participate in Their Own Care

- The right to receive adequate and appropriate care
- The right to participate in planning their treatment, care, and discharge
- The right to refuse medications, treatments, and physical and chemical restraints
- The right to review their own record

The Right to Make Independent Choices

- The right to make personal choices, such as what to wear and how to spend their time
- The right to reasonable accommodation of their needs and preferences
- The right to participate in activities, both inside and outside the nursing home
- The right to organize and participate in a resident council

The Right to Privacy and Confidentiality

- The right to private and unrestricted communication with any person
- The right to privacy in treatment and in personal care activities
- The right to confidentiality regarding their medical, personal or financial affairs

The Right to Dignity, Respect and Freedom

- The right to be treated with the fullest measure of consideration, respect and dignity
- The right to be free from mental and physical abuse
- The right to self-determination

The Right to Security of Possessions

- The right to manage their own financial affairs
- The right to be free from charge for services covered by provincial/territorial health care plans

Rights During Transfers and Discharges

- The right to remain in the facility unless a transfer or discharge is necessary, appropriate or required
- The right to receive a 30-day notice of transfer or discharge

The Right to Complain

- The right to present grievances without fear of reprisal
- The right to prompt efforts by the nursing home to resolve grievances

The Right to Visits

- The right to immediate access by their relatives
- The right to reasonable visits by organizations or individuals providing health, social, legal or other services

Adapted from the Community Legal Education Ontario. Retrieved from http://www.cleo.on.ca/en/publications/everyres; Respecting Your Rights a Guide to the Rights of People Living in British Columbia Long Term Care Facilities. Retrieved from http://www.canadianelderlaw.ca/Residents%20Rights%20%20booklet.pdf

ongoing process in which an individual becomes increasingly aware of what is important and just—and why (Burkhardt & Keegan, 2013). Burkhardt and Keegan (2013) suggest the following ways in which nurses can facilitate this process for patients: (1) listen carefully and reflect back so the patient clarifies what is personally important and (2) list several health behaviours or values, such as health, happiness, independence and good relationships, and ask patients to rank them or identify how they incorporate them into their lives.

Decisions About the Use of Restraints

Since the late 1990s, governmental and health care organizations have addressed the use of physical restraints as a major ethical issue that is relevant to older adults in acute and long-term care settings. A **physical restraint** is any device, method or equipment that immobilizes or reduces the ability of the patient to move his or her arms, legs, body or head freely. Examples of physical restraints are belts, hand mitts, soft wrist or leg restraints, certain types of chairs and full side rails in certain circumstances. In recent years, the use of physical restraints is an indicator of quality of care in institutional settings and health care organizations are initiating major initiatives to limit or eliminate the use of any restrictive devices that infringe upon patient rights.

Although restraints have been used for decades, presumably to protect patients from harm, studies find that these measures are associated with serious harm including increased risks for fractures, delirium, soft tissue injury and even death (Bradas et al., 2012). Increasingly, physical restraints are viewed as an ethical issue related to preservation of autonomy and dignity versus patient safety and protection. A study of nurses' decision-making process related to the use of physical restraints for older patients in acute care found that the complex process requires that nurses obtain a good overall picture of the patient, maintain constant observations and assess and reassess the situation (Goethals et al., 2013). Reducing the use of restraints for older adults requires a multicomponent intervention that includes institutional policy change, staff education, consultation and availability of alternative interventions (Gulpers et al., 2013). Alternatives to physical restraints are addressed in this text in Chapter 8 on delirium and Chapter 22 on fall prevention. Online Learning Activity 9-4 provides a link to evidence-based guidelines and a case study about restraints.

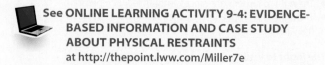 **See ONLINE LEARNING ACTIVITY 9-4: EVIDENCE-BASED INFORMATION AND CASE STUDY ABOUT PHYSICAL RESTRAINTS**
at http://thepoint.lww.com/Miller7e

Issues Related to Artificial Nutrition and Hydration

Nurses frequently address ethical issues about artificial nutrition and hydration when they care for older adults who have poor nutritional intake or limited ability to chew and swallow. **Artificial nutrition and hydration (ANH)** refers to methods of bypassing the upper gastrointestinal to deliver nutritional substances. A percutaneous endoscopic gastrostomy (PEG) tube (sometimes referred to as a "feeding tube") is a surgically inserted tube that is used to deliver nutrients directly to the stomach. In addition to PEG tubes, methods of ANH include jejunostomy tubes, nasogastric (NG) tubes, hypodermoclysis through the subcutaneous tissue and total parenteral nutrition (TPN) delivered through a central or peripheral vein.

In recent years, ANH has become widely used as a life-sustaining treatment that is considered for patients who cannot meet their nutritional needs by mouth or for people with conditions that gradually affect their ability to chew and swallow safely. Because PEG tubes are considered in a variety of circumstances, many studies have addressed safety, efficacy and outcome issues associated with this commonly used intervention. Of particular concern is the fact that about one third of nursing home residents with advanced dementia have PEG tubes, despite the lack of evidence to support this practice (American Geriatrics Society, 2013). Concerns also have been raised about inserting feeding tubes in nursing home residents with advanced cognitive impairment during a hospitalization for an acute illness because this practice does not improve survival (Cai et al., 2013).

Discussions about ANH are often initiated because the person is losing weight or requires considerable and time-consuming assistance with feeding. Another reason these issues arise is because families and caregivers may have unrealistically optimistic expectations about benefits of a feeding tube. Also, families sometimes receive well-intentioned but not evidence-based information about potential benefits of ANH. In all these situations, nurses are responsible for providing up-to-date and evidence-based information about the advantages and disadvantages of ANH. Fortunately, a strong foundation of evidence-based information is now available in position statements of major organizations including the Canadian Nurses Association, the Canadian Hospice and Palliative Care Association and the Canadian Virtual Hospice. Information in Box 9-3 can be used as an evidence-based guide to decisions about ANH and alternative methods of meeting nutritional needs.

Even with the broad base of currently available information, however, decisions related to ANH are complex and emotional for families, caregivers and professionals. A position paper of the Academy of Nutrition and Dietetics emphasizes the complexity of these decisions and affirms that self-determination generally takes precedence over the beliefs of health care providers. The statement further recognizes that "each person approaches end of life with different cultural, religious, philosophical and personal attitudes and values." For some people, "every moment of life, no matter how painful and limited, is of inestimable value" (Academy of Nutrition and Dietetics, 2013, p. 828). One way of addressing the complexity of this issue is to encourage families to use an interactive and educational "decision aid" that is effective for improving decisions about feeding

Box 9-3 Evidence-Based Practice: Key Points About Artificial Nutrition and Hydration (ANH)

Evidence-Based Recommendations Related to the Use of ANH

- The preponderance of evidence *does not support* the effectiveness of ANH in people with advanced dementia or other serious progressive conditions.
- ANH can be beneficial for patients with a potentially reversible condition or with mechanical blockage of the upper gastrointestinal tract.
- Numerous studies have shown that tube feeding in patients with serious progressive conditions does not prolong life and in fact is associated with increased risk of mortality, medical complications (including increased risk for infections), fluid overload and skin excoriation around the tube.
- ANH does *not* protect against aspiration, and in some patient populations may increase the risk of aspiration and its complications.
- Contrary to common beliefs, ANH is associated with an increased risk of developing new pressure ulcers and slower rate of healing for existing pressure ulcers.
- Patient outcomes, such as weight gain, increased caloric intake or improved laboratory values, are *not* adequate reasons for ANH in the absence of improved overall well-being.
- Patients with advanced illness often experience a loss of interest in eating and drinking and some may experience dysphagia; at some point, most patients with advanced illness will refuse food.
- Families and caregivers fear that undernourished patients experience hunger and other troublesome symptoms; however, studies show that most actively dying patients do not experience hunger even if they have poor intake.
- Terminally ill patients may experience thirst or dry mouth, but this symptom is associated with factors other than fluid intake, so ANH is unlikely to alleviate that.

Issues Regarding Decisions Related to ANH

- ANH is a medical therapy that can be declined or accepted by the patient's surrogate decision maker in accordance with advance directives or other indicators of the patient's wishes.

- Decisions to initiate, withhold or withdraw ANH are made by the patient and family with accurate and nonjudgmental input from the health care team.
- ANH is incorporated into the patient's plan only when medically appropriate and consistent with the patient's beliefs.
- Health care providers are responsible for promoting choices, endorsing shared and informed decision-making and honouring patient preferences.
- Perspectives of the patient, family and surrogate decision makers should be assessed with cultural sensitivity by an interprofessional team.

Evidence-Based Recommendations Related to Care

- Nurses and all members of the health care team are responsible for understanding and implementing a care plan that is consistent with the previously expressed wishes of the patient.
- Primary responsibilities of nurses include teaching about evidence-based information related to ANH, supporting surrogate decision makers, promoting the use of advance directives and facilitating early discussions about goals of care and treatment choices.
- Usual care of people with advanced dementia should include efforts to enhance oral feeding by altering the environment and creating patient-centred approaches to feeding.
- Food and water offered to patients by mouth is the usual means of providing nutrition and hydration to patients.
- Good oral care, ice chips and moistening the mouth are interventions that are likely to relieve thirst.

Sources: American Geriatrics Society (2013); American Nurses Association. (2011). *Position statement on forgoing nutrition and hydration*. Retrieved from www.ana.org; Hospice and Palliative Nurses Association. (2011). *HPNA Position Statement: Artificial nutrition and hydration in advanced illness*. Retrieved from www.hpna.org; Teno, Gozalo, Mitchell, et al. (2012). Feeding tubes and the prevention or healing of pressure ulcers. *Archives of Internal Medicine, 172*(9), 697–701.

---

options for people with dementia (Snyder et al., 2013). This type of decision aid is described in Online Learning Activity 9-5. An important nursing responsibility is to involve other team members in decisions and care plans related to meeting nutritional needs of people who have difficulty with oral intake. Speech-language therapists are a major resource for evaluating and advising about the safest and most effective ways of providing nutrients by mouth. They also are an excellent resource for addressing the many issues that arise when safe oral feeding is threatened, as described by Grober and Grober (2012) and available at Online Learning Activity 9-5. Registered dieticians are another resource because they make recommendations on providing, withdrawing or withholding nutrition for individual situations, and they also serve as active members of institutional ethics committees.

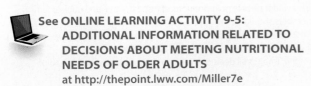 See **ONLINE LEARNING ACTIVITY 9-5:**
ADDITIONAL INFORMATION RELATED TO DECISIONS ABOUT MEETING NUTRITIONAL NEEDS OF OLDER ADULTS
at http://thepoint.lww.com/Miller7e

Issues Specific to Long-Term Care Settings

The increasing attention to quality of care in long-term care settings in recent years has led to more emphasis on autonomy, individual rights and quality of life for residents (as discussed in Chapter 6). Ethical issues are often associated with this approach because it is not always easy to balance needs of individual residents with those of others and the institution itself. Ethical issues also are associated with questions about safety versus freedom. For example, conflicts arise when a resident with a history of falls desires to walk freely around the facility, but staff members want to limit that person's activity. Additional examples of ethical decisions that nurses in long-term care settings commonly address are given below:

- Using restrictive measures to address potential risks to safety (discussed in the following section)
- Restricting cigarette smoking
- Allowing residents to refuse therapies, social activities, and food or fluid
- Providing more care assistance than necessary because it is more time-efficient for the staff (e.g., a nursing home staff member dressing the older individual, rather than

aiding the older adult to dress him- or herself through encouragement and cuing)

- Scheduling resident care practices for the convenience of the staff rather than according to individual preferences
- Accommodating residents who wish to express sexual interests and activities

Long-term care settings address these ethical issues by establishing policies and procedures that are based on best practices. An important nursing responsibility is to involve residents and their surrogate decision makers in developing a plan that is safe, individualized, respectful of the person's preferences and appropriate for addressing everyday ethical issues.

CULTURAL ASPECTS OF ETHICAL ISSUES

Religious teachings and other cultural factors have a strong influence on ethical issues, particularly with regard to advance directives and decisions about ANH and end-of-life care. Because cultural factors influence health care providers as well as their patients/clients, examining one's own biases and assuring culturally competent care (as discussed in Chapter 2) is especially important when addressing ethical issues. A major issue is that legal requirements related to advance directives are strongly biased toward Anglo-centric cultures, with emphasis on individual autonomy. This is in stark contrast to cultural groups that value family-centred decision-making or other approaches to health care decisions. For example, some families may believe that it is a sign of respect to protect an elder from the burdens of receiving information about his or her health status or from making decisions about medical interventions and long-term

care plans. This attitude may be in conflict with that of health care professionals who believe that all competent adults are entitled to information about their own health. Thus, nurses need to identify and accept individual and family decision-making preferences when they discuss advance directives and other aspects of health care decisions.

Another concern is that in general, lower income and education are two conditions that are consistently associated with not having advance directives completed (Carr, 2012; Ko & Lee, 2013). Studies in Canada and westernized countries are identifying significant cultural differences in preferences for life-sustaining treatments (Teixeira et al., 2013). For example, while white North Americans (including Canadians) and those from Europe are less likely to desire intensive end-of-life care (Frost et al., 2011), those of Korean heritage may go to greater extents to lengthen their parents' lives, due to the value of filial piety in combination with the belief that children have a duty to care for their parents and save their parents' lives (Ko et al., 2012).

Another major area of concern in Canada is the need to accommodate people who do not speak English. Language barriers can significantly increase the difficulty of understanding advance directives and participating in complex decisions about treatment and other aspects of care. Even when advance directives are available in the person's primary language, it is difficult to communicate the intent of these documents when there are conflicting cultural views on decisions about health care choices. Interventions to address language barriers are discussed in Chapter 2.

The importance of applying principles of cultural competency to all legal and ethical aspects of nursing care cannot be overemphasized, nor is this a simple process. Box 9-4

 Box 9-4 Cultural Considerations: Legal and Ethical Aspects of Care

Cultural Factors That Influence Ethical Decision-Making

- The intent of advance directives is based on Western values of individual autonomy, but many cultures believe that the fate of human beings is beyond their control.
- Values of filial piety and respect for authority of one's elders—rather than the model of individual autonomy—guide decisions about care in traditional Asian cultures.
- In collectivist cultures (e.g., the Xhosa tribe in South Africa), tribal elders make decisions about care of their members on the basis of distribution of human and material resources.
- Traditional Chinese and many other cultures rely on family members and their physicians to make decisions, rather than expecting to receive information and being involved in decision-making.
- Ethnoreligious groups, including Jews, Muslims and Hindus, are likely to base end-of-life decisions on their beliefs on the sanctity of life.
- Religious beliefs may take precedence over scientific reasoning (e.g., opposition of blood transfusions as a life-saving measure by members of Jehovah's Witnesses).
- Some groups may prefer their own religious and spiritually based healing practices to those of scientific medicine (e.g., Christian scientists).

Cultural Considerations Related to Ethical and Legal Issues in Specific Groups

- *African Canadians/Americans:* It is important to include women and extended family members in decision-making and dissemination of health information.
- *Arab:* Older males assume decision-making roles; most patients expect physicians to select treatments.
- *Chinese:* Each family has a recognized male head who has great authority and assumes all major responsibilities.
- *European Canadian/American:* There is great variation among families, but high value is generally placed on egalitarian relationships and decision-making; advance directives allow patients to specify their wishes and designate a decision maker.
- *Filipino:* Because planning for one's death is taboo, many are adverse to discussing advance directives or living wills.
- *German:* Extended family should be included in decision-making.
- *Greek:* Older people hold positions of respect; extended nuclear family members should be included in decision-making.
- *Hindu:* The patriarchal joint family, based on the principle of superiority of men over women, is the primary authority for decisions.
- *Hmong:* Traditional decision-making requires that the male head of

Box 9-4 *(continued)*

the family or clan make decisions for family members; individuals do not have the right to make their own decisions about health care.

- *Iranian:* The father and/or older male siblings have authority to make decisions for family.
- *Irish:* Families make end-of-life decisions, and these are usually influenced by all the following: their definition of extraordinary means, financial considerations, quality of life and effects on the family.
- *Italian:* Traditional families recognize the father's absolute authority and they accept his decisions as law.
- *Japanese:* Discussion of serious illness and death is taboo, so it is difficult to obtain information.
- *Jewish:* Rabbis may be included in making decisions about health care (e.g., organ donation or transplant).

- *Korean:* Older adults are frequently consulted on important family matters as a sign of respect for their experience.
- *Russian:* It is important to ask clients whom they want to include in medical decisions because extended family is very important.
- *Somali:* Discussing advance directives and end-of-life care is taboo because faithful Muslims believe that Allah will determine how long a person will live; thus, these issues should be addressed indirectly.
- *Turkish:* Traditional families are patriarchal but less traditional ones are more egalitarian, so it is important to identify the family spokesperson and accept decision-making patterns without judgment.
- *Vietnamese:* Women often make family health care decisions.

Source: Purnell, L. D. (2013). *Transcultural health care: A culturally competent approach* (4th ed.). Philadelphia, PA: F. A. Davis.

---

describes characteristics of some cultural groups that potentially influence legal and ethical issues related to care of older adults in Canada and the United States. This information is not intended to promote stereotypes; rather, it is meant as a brief guide to culturally based beliefs that should be considered when developing care plans. In all situations, it is imperative to use excellent communication skills to nonjudgmentally assess and discuss issues related to health care decisions (see Chapter 2 for a guide to culturally sensitive communication).

A Student's Perspective

In working with "G.," an 82-year-old Chinese woman, I have learned a lot about her background. She and her three brothers, two sisters and parents were all born in China. Her parents moved the children to Jakarta, a city in Indonesia, which was a Dutch colony at the time, to get a better education. Chinese culture emphasizes respect for elders, especially the father, who is head of the family. G. giggles and comments, "When father said 'eat that,' we ate it, whether we liked it or not." As an adult, she worked for a time in the front lobby of the Canadian embassy as a translator. Her position led her on many journeys throughout the world, working in Russia, Germany, France and eventually to Canada. G. didn't marry until she was 70, when she married a Canadian. She now lives in a quiet neighbourhood with her husband.

A difficulty in learning more about G. and her culture regarding health care has been her acceptance of her disease process. Her cultural background taught her to view authority figures such as physicians with incredible esteem. Until I learned more about her culture, I wasn't always certain she understood what was being said because she would sit with her head down and only nod, or simply say, "yes." I now realize those behaviours are her way of showing respect to an authority figure. She seldom looks you in the eye, another form of showing respect. She is also hesitant to ask questions so as not to appear disrespectful. G. looks to her husband many times to make decisions for her.

Deborah L.

ROLES OF NURSES REGARDING LEGAL AND ETHICAL ISSUES

Nurses have important roles with regard to implementing advance directives and facilitating decisions about care. Although these issues are often addressed within the context of an interprofessional team and always with the primary care practitioner, nurses have unique and important responsibilities, which are reviewed in the following sections.

Promoting Advance Care Planning

Advance care planning is a complex process that is much broader than simply including certain documents in patient charts when they are admitted to hospitals and facilities. Rather, advance care planning describes a combination of activities that involve thinking and communicating about preferences for future care. Advance care planning is most effective when

- It is an ongoing process that is initiated when the person is healthy as a routine part of care without distractions of other issues
- It includes learning about medical conditions that may occur, treatment options for addressing them and thinking about relevant goals, beliefs and values related to treatment decisions
- It involves formulating and communicating about preferences with all those who will potentially be involved with decisions about the person's care (e.g., family, health care power of attorney, primary care practitioner, specialists)
- All relevant documents are prepared in accordance with legal requirements
- Copies of all appropriate legal documents, such as health care power of attorney, living will, and DNR or modified DNR documents are readily accessible to all who are involved with decisions about the person's care
- All documents are periodically reviewed and updated as necessary (Aw et al., 2012; Green & Levi, 2012)

Additional steps recommended for advance care planning are (1) using past experiences to clarify values, (2) verifying that surrogate decision makers understand their role, (3) deciding about the degree of leeway, if any, to give the surrogate and (4) informing other family and friends of one's wishes (McMahan et al., 2013). Outcomes of effective advance care planning include increased feelings of autonomy, maintenance of control, increased patient satisfaction, improved quality of care, and reduced stress, anxiety and depression in family members (Poppe et al., 2013). Additional outcomes of advanced care planning related to end-of-life care are increased use of hospice, fewer in-hospital deaths, less time in the hospital during the last year, better patient-family satisfaction and improved family–provider communication (Abel et al., 2012; Bischoff et al., 2013; Waldrop & Meeker, 2012).

Although advance care planning is commonly incorporated into usual care when people begin receiving hospice care or have been diagnosed with a serious or terminal illness, the importance of initiating the discussion when people are healthy cannot be overemphasized. For example, nurses can introduce the topic with a hypothetical question such as "Have you designated someone to make decisions for you if you were brought to the emergency room and could not make decisions for yourself at that time?" This approach is unrelated to any diagnosis and can facilitate a transition to additional questions about advance directives.

Implementing Advance Directives

Evidence-based guidelines emphasize the important role of nurses in communicating with and teaching older adults about advance directives and dispelling myths and misperceptions about these documents (Mitty, 2012). Legal and health care professionals are currently emphasizing that implementation of advance directives is an ongoing process that includes teaching and listening and incorporates discussions about personal values and goals of care. Nurses can open the conversation by helping older adults and their health care proxies discuss what quality of life means for the patient, the importance of preserving life and the effects of the patient's illness and death on others (Mitty, 2012).

When care is provided over long periods, documents and preferences need to be reviewed periodically and updated as appropriate, and at all times current documents need to be included in patient charts. In addition, nurses encourage people to provide copies of advance directives to their family members, designated surrogate and anyone likely to be involved with decisions about their medical care. If written advance directives have not been completed, it is important to initiate a discussion of relevant medical care and end-of-life treatment preferences and document any statements made that express a patient's wishes. Boxes 9-5 and 9-6 can be used as

---

Box 9-5 Caregiver Wellness: Information About Health Care Decisions

Advance Care Planning

Advance care planning is an ongoing process that involves learning about types of decisions related to health care, discussing these decisions with family members and health care providers and making your wishes known in legal documents called advance directives.

Actions to Take if You Are a Family Caregiver

- Recognize that it is imperative to engage in advance care planning before any questions arise about the person's ability to express his or her wishes related to health care decisions.
- Explore the resources listed below to obtain information and engage in interactive educational activities related to advance care planning.
- Initiate discussions about advance directives.
- Facilitate the process of preparing appropriate documents and make sure that a health care power of attorney is designated.

What Are Advance Directives?

- *Advance directives* are legal documents that direct decisions about medical care that is provided or withheld.
- Common types of advance directives include living will, do-not-resuscitate orders and power of attorney for personal care (health care).
- The *power of attorney for personal care (health care)* (also called *proxy decision maker*) is extremely important because this gives authority for all health care decisions to a trusted surrogate; it is used only when someone is not able to express his or her own wishes.
- A *living will, do-not-resuscitate order* and other advance directive documents provide guidelines on which the power of attorney for health care can base decisions about treatments.
- Examples of medical care that are addressed in advance directives are cardiopulmonary resuscitation, ventilator use, artificial nutrition and hydration, and comfort care.

How Are Advance Directives Prepared?

- Advance directives must be prepared when the person is competent to make decisions.
- It is best to prepare advance directives before the actual need arises.
- Because requirements for advance directives are determined by each province/territory, legally recognized documents must be obtained from each person's place of residence.
- Appropriate forms and information about preparation of advance directives are readily available from the websites listed in the next section and from any health care institution.
- Although advance directives do not need to be notarized or drawn up by an attorney, if conflicts among family members are likely to arise, it may be advisable to seek legal advice.

What to Do After Preparing Advance Directives

- Make sure that copies of all advance directives are readily available for health care providers and all those who will be involved with decision-making (i.e., health care power of attorney).
- Periodically review the advance directives and update them when there are major changes in health status.
- Initially and periodically discuss the documents with anyone who will be involved with health care decisions.

Resources for Information About Health Care Decisions and Advance Care Planning

- *Advocacy Centre for the Elderly*, http://www.advocacycentreelderly.org/
- *Canadian Centre for Elder Law*, http://www.bcli.org/ccel
- *CARP*, http://www.carp.ca/2013/01/11/a-guide-to-end-of-life-care-for-seniors/
- *Canadian Researchers at the End of Life Network*, http://www.thecarenet.ca/index.php?option=com_content&view=article&id=85

Box 9-6 Examples of Communication Strategies for Discussing Goals of Care

Questions to Assess the Person's Understanding of the Diagnosis and Prognosis

- What is your understanding of what has happened?
- What have the doctors told you about your condition?
- What information would be helpful now?

Exploratory Questions

- Can you explain what you mean?
- Can you talk more about your concerns?
- You indicated that you are concerned about … Can you tell me more about this?
- How can I be of help to you?

Questions to Assess the Person's Supports and Coping Mechanisms

- How have you handled stress in the past?
- Whom can you rely on for support?
- What or who is helping you the most?
- How does your family communicate with each other?
- What are the potential areas of concern for your family?
- Is there anyone you rely on to help make important decisions?

Questions to Identify the Person's Goals

- What do you hope for most in the next few months?
- What is important to you right now?
- Is there anything you are afraid of?

Questions for Families When the Person Cannot Make Independent Decisions

- Tell me about _____ so I know more about him/her.
- What was important to _____.
- What do you know about his/her wishes at end of life from a quality-of-life point of view?

Source: Peereboom, K., & Coyle, N. (2012). Facilitating goals-of-care discussions for patients with life-limiting disease: Communication strategies for nurses. *Journal of Hospice and Palliative Nursing, 14*(4), 251–258.

guides to communication strategies for discussing advance directives and goals of care when decisions are complex.

Facilitating Decisions About Care

Nurses play key roles not only in implementing advance directives but also in working with family members and other caregivers who are involved with making decisions related to care and treatment issues. Advance directives designate surrogate decision makers, but the surrogates do not always have a good understanding of the person's wishes, and this can be a barrier to appropriate implementation. Studies have found that family members feel burdened when they need to make surrogate decisions, and this perception of burden is compounded when they are uncertain about the patient preferences (Majesko et al., 2012). Nurses facilitate these discussions by providing accurate information on rights and statutes, addressing questions about care options, listening to the needs and concerns of all involved, attending to concerns about treatment options and end-of-life care and acting as liaisons with primary care providers when necessary.

As discussed previously, decisions about care are particularly complicated when working with older adults who have cognitive impairments. Evidence-based guidelines for nurses summarize the following nursing care strategies for health care decision-making (Mitty & Post, 2012):

1. Communicate with patient, family and surrogate decision makers to enhance their understanding of treatment options.
2. Be sensitive to racial, ethnic, religious and cultural influences with regard to care decisions, disclosure of information and end-of-life planning.
3. Be aware of available resources for conflict resolution.
4. Observe, document and report the patient's ability to state preferences, follow directions, make simple choices and communicate consistent care wishes.
5. Observe and document fluctuations in patient's mental status and factors that affect it.
6. Assess the patient's understanding specifically in relation to a particular decision (e.g., ask what the patient understands about the risks and benefits of the intervention).
7. Use appropriate decision aids.
8. Help the patient express what he or she understands about the clinical situation and the potential outcomes.
9. Help the patient identify who should participate in discussions and decisions.

Another important role of nurses is to involve other professionals and support resources when complex decisions must be made or when the decision makers seek additional help. In some settings, an interprofessional team—composed of a social worker, a religious leader, therapists, nurses and a primary care provider—may provide information and support to proxy decision makers. Decision-making assistance from professionals may relieve families and proxy decision makers of some of the guilt they could experience when making and implementing decisions, particularly difficult end-of-life decisions. Hospitals and long-term care facilities that are accredited by Accreditation Canada are required to have ethics committees (or access to these committees) that provide a formal mechanism for addressing medical ethical dilemmas within their institutions.

A model for a nurse-led intervention that is used successfully to improve surrogate decision-making involves the following roles for bedside nurses in acute care settings:

1. Prepare the family to be the decision maker by educating them about the responsibilities of the surrogate.
2. Organize regular interprofessional meetings including family and clinicians.
3. Prepare the family for the meeting by helping them formulate questions and understand the issues.

4. Share the information from the family with the other members of the interprofessional team before the meeting.
5. Assure that all pertinent topics are addressed and provide support and encouragement for the family during the meeting.
6. Provide postmeeting support and clarification for family (Erickson, 2013; White, 2011).

When this model is applied to situations involving end-of-life decisions or uncertainty about patient outcomes, nurses also provide anticipatory grief support by encouraging families to think about what it would mean to "hope for the best and prepare for the worst" (White et al., 2012).

Nurses also take a strong role in supporting and facilitating decisions about care during chronic conditions and end-of-life care. In particular, nurses provide information about the best types of services (e.g., hospice programs, palliative care) or place of care (e.g., hospital admission for nursing home residents when medical problems arise). Box 9-7 summarizes a nursing model for facilitating decisions about long-term care for people with dementia.

Promoting Caregiver Wellness

As discussed previously, decisions about medical treatments are usually stressful and complex, not only for the older adult but also for families and caregivers. Stress is magnified when caregivers are responsible for decisions—including decisions that shorten life expectancy—with little or no input from the older adult. For example, when an older person is cognitively impaired and the surrogate decision makers have not previously discussed the care alternatives, the caregiver's stress is compounded by feelings of guilt and uncertainty. Similarly, stress is magnified when family decision makers (e.g., siblings, spouses, in-laws) have differing perspectives or hold conflicting values about treatments. In all situations, nurses are the health care professionals who assume key support roles for caregivers, including teaching and advocacy. In addition to applying information already discussed in this chapter (e.g., learning activities, communication strategies in Box 9-3). Box 9-5 can be used to teach caregivers about health care decision-making; it includes a list of helpful resources that caregivers can be encouraged to explore for additional information.

Box 9-7 Model for Facilitating Decisions About the Care of People With Dementia

Step I: Assess the Decision-Making Situation

- What is the decision-making ability of the person with dementia?
- What are the typical decision-making patterns in the family?
- Who influences the decision-making, either directly or indirectly?
- How do family relationships help or hinder the decision-making process?
- Are there patterns of passive nondecisions, as well as active decisions?
- What is each person's perception of the situation?
- How objective are the perceptions of the various decision makers?
- What does each person in the decision-making process have to gain or lose on the basis of various decisions?

Step II: Obtain Consensus About Problems and Needs

- Have each person involved with the care describe the problems and needs from their perspective.
- Provide additional assessment information about the needs of the person with dementia.
- Address the needs of the caregivers, as well as the needs of the person with dementia.
- Summarize the identified needs of the older adult and the caregivers.

Step III: Discuss Potential Resources

- Ask caregivers to suggest potential solutions and resources.
- Identify resources for the caregivers' needs, as well as for those of the person with dementia.
- Supplement the family's knowledge about resources and potential solutions.
- Discuss the positive and negative consequences of each option for the person with dementia and for the caregivers.
- As the family members discuss solutions, assess their attitudes about using various services and spending family resources to purchase services.

- Provide information about the long-range benefits that the caregivers might not perceive.
- Summarize important points on paper or a blackboard for all participants to review.

Step IV: Agree on a Plan of Action

- Obtain agreement about the most appropriate actions to take.
- Emphasize the fact that any plan of action will be given a trial period and should not be viewed as a permanent decision.
- Suggest a time frame and criteria for evaluating the plan of action.
- Identify one or two people who will evaluate the plan and make appropriate changes.

Step V: Involve the Person With Dementia

- Discuss the ability of the person with dementia to understand the decision.
- Identify the most realistic level of involvement for the person with dementia.
- Identify the best approach to take in involving the person with dementia.
- Identify the roles of caregivers and professionals in assisting the person with dementia to understand the decision.

Step VI: Summarize the Plan and Clarify Roles

- Review and summarize the plan of action.
- Have the caregivers state their roles in very specific terms.
- Clarify the role of the nurse and other professionals.
- Assure caregivers that you will be available for further discussion and problem solving, or provide the name of someone who can assume this role.

Chapter Highlights

Autonomy and Rights

- Autonomy is the personal freedom to direct one's own life as long as it does not infringe on the rights of others.
- Adults are presumed to be competent and have the right to make health-related decisions unless they have been declared incompetent by a judge.
- Decision-making capacity describes one's ability to understand and process information, weigh alternatives, apply personal values, arrive at a decision and communicate that decision to others.
- If an adult's decision-making capacity is questionable or compromised, his or her rights can be protected through legal documents, such as advance directives.

Advance Directives

- Advance directives (e.g., power of attorney for health care, DNR orders, living wills) are legal documents that make a person's wishes about medical treatments known to care providers and surrogate decision makers.
- Legal requirements for advance directives are specified in provincial/territorial laws.
- Advance directives must be drawn up when a person is competent, and they need to be available when questions arise about the person's wishes.
- Nurses have essential roles in teaching older adults and their caregivers about advance directives and respecting each person's values related to health care decisions.

Legal Issues Specific to Long-Term Care Settings

- Provincial/territorial legislation requires nursing homes to meet certain standards of care, to perform and document assessments and to implement interprofessional care plans that comprehensively address residents' needs.
- Improvements in nursing home care that are attributed to the implementation of federal legislation include decreased use of indwelling catheters, reduced use of physical and chemical restraints, fewer cases of dehydration and pressure ulcers and increased use of geriatricians and nurse practitioners.
- A national Nursing Home Bill of Rights in Canada might include principles such as residents being entitled to dignity, self-determination and the opportunity to communicate (Box 9-2).

Ethical Issues Commonly Addressed in Gerontological Nursing

- Values clarification is a process that can be applied when addressing ethical issues in everyday care of older adults.
- Decisions about use of restraints are complex and must be based on evidence-based guidelines.
- ANH is a widely recognized life-sustaining treatment that involves complex ethical issues, as described in Box 9-3.

Cultural Aspects of Legal and Ethical Issues

- Language barriers and cultural influences are important to consider when discussing advance directives.
- Nurses should identify culturally influenced patterns of decision-making when discussing advance directives and end-of-life care with patients and their families (Box 9-4).

Roles of Nurses Regarding Legal and Ethical Issues

- Advance care planning is a complex process that involves ongoing communication about health care decisions that realistically reflect the person's values and preferences for treatments.
- Nurses have essential roles in working with older adults, their families, their health care proxies and all health care professionals to implement advance directives.
- Nurses facilitate decision-making about advance directives by providing information about advance directives and care options to older adults and to proxy decision makers (Box 9-5).
- Nurses facilitate decisions about care of people with dementia by using the model in Box 9-7.

Critical Thinking Exercises

1. You have been assigned to work with Mrs. M., an 85-year-old, white, widowed woman who is in the hospital with congestive heart failure. Her son and daughter tell you that they would like to arrange for her to be discharged to a nursing home because they don't think she takes her medications correctly, and they are tired of her being admitted to the hospital every couple of months "to get her straightened out." The son and daughter live in another province and visit only when their mother is in the hospital. Mrs. M. has told you that she thinks her son and daughter would like to have her "put away in one of those homes" but she is adamantly opposed to leaving her home. She also has told you that they think she is "senile" and that she should stop driving her car, but she thinks she is quite capable of living alone, driving her car and taking care of herself. Your observations are that she needs a lot of direction to take medications and participate in self-care activities, and she seems to be somewhat confused later in the day. What steps would you take to address her competency and decision-making abilities?

2. A 78-year-old Filipino Canadian woman, is being admitted to the hospital with hemiplegia after a stroke. There are no advance directives on her chart. What information would you want to know before you approached her about a living will and power of attorney for health care? How would you explain these documents to her?

3. Mr. S. is 78 years old and has been admitted for hip surgery after a fall-related fracture. He has had dementia for 5 years and his family provides care for him in his home. His son is his power of attorney for health care, but he will not make any decisions unless his three sisters agree to them. Mr. S. does not have any other advance directives, and the family says he never talked much about what medical care services he would want.

He always told his family that they could make whatever decisions are best for him. The physician has asked the family to consider placement of a PEG tube because Mr. S.'s food and fluid intake are inadequate to meet his needs and one pressure area is beginning to develop on his buttocks. Mr. S.'s son and one daughter think that their father would have wanted to have every intervention possible in such a situation, and they think the PEG tube will improve his comfort and prevent the pressure ulcer. The other two daughters adamantly state that their father would never agree to such an invasive procedure and they are not sure it will make him any more comfortable. They also worry about complications from having the tube. You are a member of the interprofessional team that is meeting with the family to help them come to a decision about a PEG tube. What points would you want to make during this family conference?

For more information about the topics discussed in this chapter, be sure to check out the interactive Online Learning Activities and other helpful resources at http://thepoint.lww.com/Miller7e

REFERENCES

Abel, J., Pring, A., Rich, A., et al. (2012). The impact of advance care planning of place of death, a hospice retrospective study. *British Medical Journal Supportive and Palliative Care, 3*, 168–173.

Academy of Nutrition and Dietetics. (2013). Position of the Academy of Nutrition and Dietetics: Ethical and legal issues in feeding and hydration. *Journal of the Academy of Nutrition and Dietetics, 113*(6), 828–833. doi:10.1016/j.jand.2013.03.020

American Geriatrics Society. (2013). *Feeding tubes in advanced dementia position statement.* Retrieved from www.ags.org

American Nurses Association. (2011). *Position statement on forgoing nutrition and hydration.* Retrieved from www.ana.org

Araw, A. C., Araw, A. M., Pekmezaris, R., et al. (2013, May 13). Medical orders for life-sustaining treatment: Is it time yet? *Palliative and Supportive Care,* 1–5.

Aw, D., Hayhoe, B., Smajdor, A., et al. (2012). Advance care planning and the older patient. *Quarterly Journal of Medicine, 105*, 225–230.

BC Centre for Elder Law. (n.d.). *Legal capacity.* Retrieved from http://bc-ceas.ca/information/introduction-to-older-adults-in-bc/capacity/

Bischoff, K. E., Sudore, R., Miao, Y., et al. (2013). Advance care planning and the quality of end-of-life care in older adults. *Journal of the American Geriatrics Society, 61*(2), 209–214.

Bomba, P. A., Kemp, M., & Black, J. S. (2012). POLST: An improvement over traditional advance directives. *Cleveland Clinic Journal of Medicine, 79*(7), 457–464.

Bradas, C. M., Sandhu, S. K., & Mion, L. C. (2012). Physical restraints and side rails in acute and critical care settings. In M. Boltz, E. Capezuti, T. Fulmer, et al. (Eds.), *Evidence-based practice protocols for best practice* (4th ed., pp. 229–245). New York, NY: Springer.

Brugger, E. C., Pavela, S., Toffler, W., et al. (2012). POLST and catholic health care. *Ethics & Medics, 37*(1), 1–4.

Burkhardt, M. A., & Keegan, L. (2013). Holistic ethics. In B. M. Dossey & L. Keegan (Eds.), *Holistic nursing: A handbook for practice* (6th ed., pp. 129–141). Boston, MA: Jones and Bartlett.

Cai, S., Gozalo, P. L., Mitchell, S. L., et al. (2013). Do patients with advanced cognitive impairment admitted to hospitals with higher rates of feeding tube insertion have improved survival? *Journal of Pain & Symptom Management, 45*(3), 524–533.

Canadian Institute for Health Information. (2013). *When a nursing home is a home: How do Canadians nursing homes measure up?* Retrieved from https://secure.cihi.ca/free_products/CCRS_QualityinLongTermCare_EN.pdf

Canadian Medical Association. (2013). *CMA statement on life-saving and life-sustaining interventions.* Retrieved from http://policybase.cma.ca/dbtw-wpd/Policypdf/PD14-01.pdf

Canadian Nurses Association, Canadian Medical Association, & Canadian Hospital Association. (1984). *A protocol for health professionals regarding resuscitative intervention for the terminally ill.* Ottawa, ON: Author.

Canadian Nurses Association, Canadian Medical Association, & Canadian Hospital Association. (1994). *Joint statement on advance care directives.* Ottawa, ON: Author.

Carr, D. (2012). Racial and ethnic differences in advance care planning: Identifying subgroup patterns and obstacles. *Journal of Aging and Health, 24*(6), 923–947.

Chettih, M. (2012). Turning the lens inward: Cultural competence and providers' values in health care decision making. *The Gerontologist, 52*(6), 739–747.

Erickson, J. (2013). Bedside nurse involvement in end-of-life decision making. *Dimensions of Critical Care Nursing, 32*(2), 65–68.

Fetherstonhaugh, D., Tarzia, L., & Nay, R. (2013). Being central to decision making means I am still here!: The essence of decision making for people with dementia. *Journal of Aging Studies, 27*, 143–150.

Frost, D. W., Cook, D. J., Heyland, D. K., et al. (2011). Patient and health-care professional factors influencing end-of-life decision-making during critical illness: A systematic review. *Critical Care Medicine, 39*, 1174–1189.

Goethals, S., de Casterle, B. D., & Gastmans, C. (2013). Nurses' decision-making process in cases of physical restraint in acute elderly care: A qualitative study. *International Journal of Nursing Studies, 50*, 603–612.

Goodridge, D. (2013). Planning for serious illness amongst community-dwelling older adults. *Nursing Research and Practice, 2013*, 1–7. doi:10.1155/2013/427917

Green, M. J., & Levi, B. H. (2012). The era of "e": The use of new technologies in advance care planning. *Nursing Outlook, 60*, 376–381.

Grober, M. E., & Grober, T. P. (2012). When safe oral feeding is threatened: End-of-life options and decisions. *Topics in Lung Disease, 32*(2), 149–167.

Gulpers, M. J., Bleijlevens, M. H., Ambergen, T., et al. (2013). Reduction of belt restraint use: Long-term effects of EXBELT intervention. *Journal of the American Geriatrics Society, 61*(1), 107–112.

Hammes, B. J., Rooney, B. L., Gundrum, J. D., et al. (2012). The POLST program: A retrospective review of the demographics of use and outcomes in one community where advance directives are prevalent. *Journal of Palliative Medicine, 15*(1), 77–85.

Hirschman, K. B., Abbott, K. M., Hanlon, A. L., et al. (2012). What factors are associated with having an advance directive among older adults who are new to long-term care services? *American Journal of Medical Directors Association, 13*(1), 82.e7– 82.e11.

Hospice and Palliative Nurses Association. (2011). *HPNA Position Statement: Artificial nutrition and hydration in advanced illness.* Retrieved from www.hpna.org

Hospice Patients Alliance. (2013). *New designation for Allowing a Natural Death ("A.N.D.") would eliminate confusion and suffering when patients are resuscitated against their wishes.* Retrieved from www.hospicepatients.org/and.html

Ko, E., & Lee, J. (2013, April 25). Completion of advance directives among low-income older adults: Does race/ethnicity matter? *American Journal of Hospice and Palliative Care, 31*(3), 247–253.

Ko, E., Cho, S., & Bonilla, M. (2012). Attitudes towards life-sustaining treatment: The role of race/ethnicity. *Geriatric Nursing, 33*(5), 341–349.

Majesko, A., Hong, S. Y., Weissfeld, L., et al. (2012). Identifying family members who may struggle in the role of surrogate decision maker. *Critical Care Medicine, 40*(8), 2281–2286.

McMahan, R. D., Knight, S. J., Fried, T. R., et al. (2013). Advance care planning beyond advance directives: Perspectives from patients and surrogates. *Journal of Pain Symptom Management, 46*(3), 355–365. doi:10.1016/j.jpainsymman.2012.09.006

Mitty, E. L. (2012). Advance directives. In M. Boltz, E. Capezuti, T. Fulmer, et al. (Eds.), *Evidence-based practice protocols for best practice* (4th ed., pp. 579–599). New York, NY: Springer.

Mitty, E. L., & Post, L. F. (2012). Health care decision making. In M. Boltz, E. Capezuti, T. Fulmer, & D. Zwicker (Eds.), *Evidence-based practice protocols for best practice* (4th ed., pp. 562–578). New York, NY: Springer.

Morley, J. E. (2013). Minimum Data Set 3.0: A giant step forward. *Journal of the American Medical Directors Association, 14*, 1–3. doi:10.1016. jamda.2012.10.014

Muller, L. S. (2012). Legal & regulatory issues: POLST: Something new has been added. *Professional Case Management, 17*(2), 90–93.

Peereboom, K., & Coyle, N. (2012). Facilitating goals-of-care discussions for patients with life-limiting disease: Communication strategies for nurses. *Journal of Hospice and Palliative Nursing, 14*(4), 251–258.

Poppe, J., Burleigh, S., & Banerjee, S. (2013). Qualitative evaluation of advanced care planning in early dementia. *PLoS One, 8*(4), e60412.

Purnell, L. D. (2013). *Transcultural health care: A culturally competent approach.* Philadelphia, PA: F. A. Davis.

Samsi, K., & Manthorpe, J. (2013). Everyday decision-making in dementia: Findings from a longitudinal interview study of people with dementia and family carers. *International Psychogeriatrics, 25*(6), 949–961.

Schubart, J. R., Levi, B. H., Camacho, F., et al. (2012). Reliability of an interactive computer program for advance care planning. *Journal of Palliative Medicine, 15*(6), 637–642.

Smebye, K. L., Kirkevold, M., & Engedal, K. (2012). How do persons with dementia participate in decision making related to health and daily care? A multi-case study. *BMC Health Services Research, 12*, 241.

Snyder, E. A., Caprio, A. J., Wessell, K., et al. (2013). Impact of a decision aid on surrogate decision-makers' perceptions of feeding options for patients with dementia. *Journal of the American Medical Directors Association, 14*, 114–118.

Teixeira, A. A., Hanvey, L., Tayler, C., et al. (2013). What do Canadians think of advanced care planning? Findings from an online opinion poll. *BMJ Supportive & Palliative Care.* doi:10.1136/bmjspcare-2013-000473

Teno, J. M., Gozalo, P., Mitchell, S. L., et al. (2012). Feeding tubes and the prevention or healing of pressure ulcers. *Archives of Internal Medicine, 172*(9), 697–701.

Tuohey, J., & Hodges, M. O. (2011, March–April). POLST reflects patient wishes, clinical reality. *Health Progress,* 60–64.

Vogel, L. (2010). Doctors endorse development of patient charter. *CMAJ, 182.* Advance online publication. doi:10.1503/cmaj.109-3354

Wahl, J. (2006). *Advance care planning: The legal issues.* Retrieved from http://demo.swpalliativecare.ca/infonetwork_docs/AdvanceCarePlanning_Legal.pdf

Waldrop, D. P., & Meeker, M. A. (2012). Communication and advanced care planning in palliative and end-of-life care. *Nursing Outlook, 60,* 365–369.

Wenger, N. S., Citko, J., O'Malley, K., et al. (2012). Implementation of physician orders for life sustaining treatment in nursing homes in California: Evaluation of a novel statewide dissemination mechanism. *Nursing Research and Practice, 28*(1), 51–57. doi:10.1007/s11606-012-2178-2

Whitcomb, J. J., & Ewing, N. (2012). A closing word: Do not resuscitate versus allow natural death and should we change our approach. *Dimensions of Critical Care Nursing, 31*(4), 265–266.

White, D. B. (2011). Rethinking interventions to improve surrogate decision making in intensive care units. *American Journal of Critical Care, 20*(3), 252–257.

White, D. B., Cua, S., Walk, R., et al. (2012). Nurse-led intervention to improve surrogate decision making for patients with advanced critical illness. *American Journal of Critical Care, 21*(6), 396–409.

Wilson, D. M., Houttekier, D., Kunju, S. A., et al. (2013). A population-based study on advance directive completion and completion intention among citizens of the western Canadian province of Alberta. *Journal of Palliative Care, 29*, 5–12.

Wittmann-Price, R., & Celia, L. M. (2010). Exploring perceptions of "Do Not Resuscitate" and "Allowing Natural Death" among physicians and nurses. *Holistic Nursing Practice, 24*(6), 333–337.

chapter 10

Elder Abuse and Neglect

Elder abuse and neglect is one of the most complex and serious functional consequences that affects vulnerable older adults—and one of the most challenging aspects of gerontological nursing. Situations of elder abuse and neglect require an interprofessional approach, with nurses assuming essential roles in detection, assessment and interventions. This chapter presents the topic with emphasis on the key roles of nurses in addressing this complex issue.

OVERVIEW OF ELDER ABUSE AND NEGLECT

Certain members of any population are vulnerable to abuse and neglect by virtue of being physically or psychosocially impaired or subjugated. In industrialized societies today, vulnerable groups are protected and cared for through legislative mandates and social programs. In Canada and many other countries, for example, children and people with developmental/intellectual disabilities have been protected for many decades. In recent decades, additional groups have been recognized as needing protection: victims of domestic violence and abused or neglected older people. Although abuse or neglect of older adults is not new, elder abuse has received increased attention as a social problem, crime and health concern.

Definitions and Characteristics of Elder Abuse

Definitions of elder abuse have changed over time in response to shifts in political climate, public sentiment, available funding and increasing knowledge and professional interest. This section discusses definitions and characteristics of elder abuse, and the following section provides a historical perspective on elder abuse. It is important to recognize that the terms *elder abuse* and *elder mistreatment* are often used interchangeably. This is consistent with the common practice of using both terms in the same context and including types that have a perpetrator (e.g., family, caregiver, acquaintances, strangers), as well as self-neglect, where there is no perpetrator. In Canada, First Nations people have asked that the term "elder abuse" is used with caution because of the cultural implications of the word "elder."

To date, there is not a single reported Canadian court decision containing a definition of elder abuse. In considering elder abuse, Aging and the Law in Canada (n.d.) uses the language of "senior abuse" and states, "Senior abuse is a generic term referring to a wide variety of harms to older adults that are committed by a person or persons they know and would normally have a reason to trust. It is considered different than harm from strangers." This description was developed to address ambiguities over what constitutes elder abuse and to foster empirical investigation of the subject using comparable research design. Although an admirable goal, the definition does not address issues identified by clinicians and evident in jurisdictional legislation. In consideration of these issues, Anetzberger (2012) proposed an elder abuse definition taxonomy. It builds upon the classic work of Margaret Hudson (1991) and reflects prevailing understanding of elder abuse as a construct. As such, it recognizes that current research-to-date suggests significant variation among elder abuse forms, settings and victim–perpetrator relationships. Therefore, each variation set should be studied separately to reveal fully its etiologies and dynamics. The taxonomy begins by identifying the elder abuse perpetrator (i.e., victim himself/herself, trusted other, or stranger or acquaintance) and then the setting for elder abuse occurrence (i.e., domestic or institutional). Therein elder abuse takes the form of either abuse or neglect (either intentionally or unintentionally motivated), with the locus of harm being physical, psychological, social, financial or sexual.

The National Seniors Council established by the Government of Canada (2007) recognizes elder abuse may take the different forms noted above, but also suggests further forms: financial, physical, emotional or psychological, sexual, systemic (e.g., ageism), spiritual and neglect (either self-neglect by older adults or neglect by others). Self-neglect in this classification includes behaviours of older adults that threaten their health or safety.

Efforts are currently underway to provide greater clarity to the meaning and dimensions of elder abuse. In the United States, Conrad and his associates (2011a, 2011b), for example, have applied sophisticated research methods, such as concept mapping, to psychological abuse and financial exploitation. After national and local groups of elder abuse experts identified relevant statements for the construct, the statements were sorted, rated and depicted as conceptual maps. Then focus groups of practitioners and older adult service consumers reviewed these items, and elder abuse victims refined them before the items were subjected to tests of validity and reliability. The resulting older adult psychological abuse and financial exploitation measures are intended to aid the assessment of the problem by both clinicians and researchers. Within Canada, the National Network for the Care of the Elderly (NICE) recently completed a large pilot study, the first step of which was to explore with key informants and stakeholders what constituted elder abuse and what term (e.g., abuse, mistreatment, maltreatment) was most appropriate to use.

Emerging within public and health care awareness is the challenge of **resident-to-resident abuse** (RRA). Pillemer et al. (2012) described this as negative and aggressive physical, sexual or verbal interactions between long-term care residents that in a community setting would be unwelcome and potentially cause physical or psychological distress to the recipient. This study was conducted in the United States, and to date there is no prevalent study of RRA in Canada; however, in 2014, The Institute for Life Course & Aging (University of Toronto) initiated a CIHR-funded meeting of recognized experts in elder abuse to develop a research agenda on RRA.

Historical Recognition of a Social Problem

Awareness of elder abuse as a social problem began in the 1950s and 1960s as the writings of Geneva Mathiasen and Gertrude Hall in the United States and the United Kingdom introduced the concept of granny-battering, which was discussed in a letter printed in the *British Medical Journal* in 1975 (Burston, 1975). The late 20th century witnessed the growing criminalization of elder abuse, a movement that continues today. With it, consumer fraud aimed at older adults, including scams and con games, was subsumed under elder abuse. Concurrently, recognition of domestic violence in later life as an elder abuse form served to shift the practice paradigm to empowering victims and holding perpetrators accountable. There was a medicalization of elder abuse, with physicians increasingly dominating problem intervention, sometimes with a criminal justice twist, as in the establishment of forensic centres and markers related to elder abuse. In this context, elder abuse is viewed as a public health matter, with interventions assuming a prevention lens.

Elder abuse has become a global concern. First recognized in the United States, Great Britain and Canada, elder abuse gained international attention with the establishment of the International Network for the Prevention of Elder Abuse in 1997. Since the early 2000s, the United Nations World Assembly has focused on elder abuse as a major international concern that encompasses virtually anything that causes harm or distress to an older person, ranging from direct forms of aggression to denial of dignity to older people (United Nations Economic and Social Affairs, 2008). As a global concern, elder abuse is typically seen as a violation of human rights or an act of oppression, with interventions often aimed at reforming national public policy to delineate and defend the rights of older people (Dow & Joosten, 2012).

Awareness of elder abuse has been increasing, and it is now recognized as a major social and health problem and a significant aspect of family violence. One indicator of increased global attention to elder abuse is the fact that World Elder Abuse Awareness Day has been commemorated in countries worldwide on June 15 every year since 2006. The Canadian Network for the Prevention of Elder Abuse (CNPEA) was an initial participant in the launching of the Awareness Day. This increasing attention can be attributed to reasons such as the following:

- The older adult population has been increasing rapidly, with the most vulnerable groups of older people (i.e., those who are 85 years of age and older) increasing at the fastest rate.
- Adult children increasingly are called upon to care for their elderly parents; however, some lack the capacity,

skills, resources, availability or physical proximity to undertake this responsibility successfully.

- Researchers and clinicians are directing more attention to the problems that affect the most vulnerable older adults, leading to more information and publications.
- Educational efforts have made professionals and the public more aware of reporting laws and adult protective services.
- Congressional hearings and educational programs have stimulated public and professional interest in the issue.
- Organizations, such as the Canadian Network for the Prevention of Elder Abuse and the National Initiative for the Care of the Elderly have promoted professional networking and advocated for public policy addressing elder abuse.

Gerontological nurses have been in the forefront of research, publications and practice innovations in elder abuse. Nursing journals have featured articles on elder abuse since the 1970s, and clinically oriented nursing texts on elder abuse have been coauthored by nurses since the 1980s. Since the early1990s, nursing has been represented in the field of elder abuse through the research of such Canadian scholars as Elizabeth Podnieks and Lynn McDonald. Nurses and Social Workers also have developed important clinical tools and protocols, particularly in the areas of screening and assessment. There is evidence of similar responses to elder abuse among nurses cross-culturally, suggesting a global humanitarian and nursing perspective to the problem (Erlingsson et al., 2012; Sandmoe et al., 2011).

Prevalence and Causes

Elder abuse is neither a rare nor an isolated phenomenon, with all indicators suggesting that mistreatment of vulnerable older adults is widespread and occurs among all subgroups. Although estimates of elder abuse worldwide range from a low of 4% to a high of 47%, these estimates vary because of significant underreporting and differing definitions (Sooryanarayana et al., 2013). In 1990, Elizabeth Podnieks and associates conducted the "National Survey on Abuse of the Elderly in Canada." This landmark survey was the first to be national in scope and is an important step for understanding the nature and extent of the problem in this country. She documented that 4% of older adults in their telephone survey reported abuse.

Among the various abuse forms, financial exploitation and emotional abuse were the most common and sexual abuse the least. Currently, the National Initiative for the Care of the Elderly is conducting a national prevalence study, funded by Employment and Social Development Canada (formerly Human Resources and Skill Development Canada) (Box 10-1).

Globally, 53 countries representing all six regions of the World Health Organization responded to a questionnaire and acknowledged elder abuse as a major local concern (Podnieks et al., 2010). Although elder abuse research is underway in both developed and developing countries,

Box 10-1 Evidence-Informed Nursing Practice

Background: Little is known about the prevalence of elder abuse in Canada.
Question: Would a life-course perspective be useful for examining elder abuse?
Method: Older adults aged 55 and older completed a cross-sectional telephone survey, comprising five types of elder abuse (neglect, physical, psychological, financial, sexual) and their occurrence over the life course.
Findings: More than half (55%) reported abuse during childhood, and more than one third (34%) reported it during young adulthood. Almost half (43%) reported it during mature adulthood, and a quarter (24%) reported experiencing abuse since age 55.
Implications for Nursing Practice: Considering the occurrence of abuse from a life-course perspective may be useful for nurses to help promote understanding of the older adult's life experiences. Interventions may then be client specific.

Source: McDonald, L., & Thomas, C. (2013). Elder abuse through a life course lens. *International Psychogeriatrics, 25*(8), 1235–1243.

most countries report a need for more studies, particularly on prevalence. Some examples of studies on prevalence and types of elder abuse in countries are as follows:

- Ireland: 2.2%, with financial abuse most frequent (Naughton et al., 2012)
- United Kingdom: 2.6%, where neglect was most common (Biggs et al., 2009)
- Israel: 18.4%, where verbal abuse and financial exploitation dominated (Lowenstein et al., 2009)
- Older women in five European countries, viz., Finland, Austria, Belgium, Lithuania and Portugal: 18.1% (DeDonder et al., 2011)
- Rural community in People's Republic of China: 36.2%, with caregiver neglect and physical mistreatment being the most commonly cited forms (Wu et al., 2012).

The work being done in Canada and in other countries (e.g., India) are laying the foundation for improved elder abuse prevalence research (Podnieks et al., 2012; Shankardass, 2013).

Although the problem can affect any older person, the typical reported elder abuse victim is a socially isolated and physically or cognitively impaired woman of advanced age who lives alone or with the abuser and depends on the abuser for care. Studies have identified profiles of abused elders by type of abuse. For example, victims of self-neglect are likely to have the following characteristics: older age, chronic illness, functional limitations, solo living arrangements, social isolation, inadequate economic resources, and dementia, mental illness, substance abuse or hoarding behaviours (Day et al., 2013; Ernst & Smith, 2011; Mosqueda & Dong, 2011). Finally, there may be some association between type of abuse and the sex of the perpetrator, with men being more likely to exploit or physically abuse elders and women being more likely to physically neglect or psychologically abuse elders.

Studies of specific types of mistreatment indicate that elder abuse results from multiple, interrelated variables.

Box 10-2 Elder Abuse Risk Factors

Perpetrator Risk Factors

- Mental illness
- Alcoholism
- Hostility
- Financial dependency on the victim

Victim Risk Factors

- Dementia
- Problem behaviours
- Disability

Perpetrator/Victim Environment Risk Factors

- Shared living arrangements
- Social isolation or lack of social support

 Box 10-3 Cultural Considerations: Studies Related to Cultural Aspects of Elder Abuse

Those of African origins and working-class Caucasian older women are more likely than Latina and upper-income Caucasian women to identify financial abuse as an aspect of elder mistreatment (Daykin & Pearlmutter, 2009).

Psychological abuse was found to be the most common form of elder mistreatment in a sample of 2,272 Chinese aged 55 years and older in seven Canadian cities, including being scolded, ridiculed, yelled at and threatened (Lai, 2011).

Focus group interviews with older lesbians in Canada identified concern about losing their sexual orientation and experiencing discrimination and extreme isolation if they moved into an institutional setting (Walsh et al., 2011).

Anetzberger (2013) summarized the risk factors associated with perpetrators, victims and perpetrator/victim environments (Box 10-2), emphasizing that perpetrator risk factors were more powerful predictors of abuse occurrence than were victim risk factors. Research on the risk factors of elder abuse points in the following directions:

- Risk factors vary by form of abuse.
- The etiology of any form of abuse is a composite of several interrelated variables.
- The origins of elder abuse are found in both the victim and the perpetrator, as well as in the relationship between the two.
- The etiology of elder abuse differs from that suggested for other abused populations in important ways (e.g., elder abuse is uniquely associated with ageism).

Cultural Considerations

As a worldwide issue, elder abuse is being addressed in the context of the basic human right to be free from violence in the home. Cultural factors strongly influence how elder abuse is defined and perceived, as well as broader aspects of elder abuse. For example, the value of *familism*, which emphasizes needs of the family over those of the individual, can hinder the reporting of elder abuse, as well as the use of support services by Latino immigrants who depend on their families for care (DeLiema et al., 2012). Even the definition of financial abuse can vary according to cultural expectations. For example, elderly Korean immigrants to Canada may hold traditional values about family financial support that could be perceived as exploitation or abuse (Lee et al., 2012). In addition, cultural variations in perceptions of autonomy and decision making (as discussed in Chapter 9) can have an effect on legal and ethical aspects of elder abuse and neglect.

Studies of cultural aspects of elder abuse and neglect are limited, and culturally diverse groups are generally underrepresented in elder abuse research. This includes view of elder abuse in Aboriginal communities (Anisko, 2009). In particular, there is little research on older adults who are vulnerable to self-neglect because of social isolation, such as those who live in rural or remote areas or immigrants who do not speak English. Similarly, older adults who experience stigma, such as lesbian, gay, bisexual and transgender (LGBT) elders, may place a high value on independence and avoid contact

with senior service providers. For example, studies indicate that 65% of LGBT older adults reported victimization due to sexual orientation, 8.3% reported they had been abused by a senior service provider because of homophobia and 8.9% experienced blackmail or financial exploitation (National Center on Elder Abuse, 2013).

Other governmental and nonprofit agencies are addressing cultural aspects of abuse in specific groups, as described in Online Learning Activity 10-1. Box 10-3 lists findings from some of the more recent studies that address cultural aspects of elder abuse. As with all aspects of cultural competency, it is imperative to consider individual variations and avoid generalizations because not all members of a cultural, religious or minority group behave according to reported trends.

 See **ONLINE LEARNING ACTIVITY 10-1: CULTURAL CONSIDERATIONS RELATED TO ELDER ABUSE** at http://thepoint.lww.com/Miller7e

 ## RISK FACTORS FOR ELDER ABUSE AND NEGLECT

Because risk for elder abuse and neglect is associated with a combination of characteristics and circumstances in the victim and perpetrator, identification of all risk factors is very complex. Most often, several risk factors are present and these generally develop over a long period. Risk factors that tend to be common to most elder abuse situations are invisibility of the problem, vulnerability of the older person and psychosocial and caregiver risk factors.

Invisibility and Vulnerability

In contrast to most problems affecting older adults, one of the major risk factors for elder abuse is its invisibility. Despite the increasing attention given to elder abuse, the vast majority of cases are unreported, even in jurisdictions with good reporting and intervention models. Factors that contribute to this invisibility and underreporting include the following:

- Older people generally have less contact with the community than do other segments of the population.

- Older people are reluctant to admit to being abused or neglected because they fear reprisal or believe that alternative situations may be worse than the abusive one.
- Many myths and negative stereotypes associated with old age foster a strong denial of aging and an even stronger denial of the social problems associated with vulnerable older people.

Vulnerability is associated with a combination of social, personal, situational and environmental factors. For example, older adults may have significant psychosocial limitations resulting from conditions such as dementia, depression and mental illness. These conditions can increase their vulnerability to self-neglect or abuse or exploitation by others; they also can affect the ability to seek help from others. Another factor that leads to vulnerability is the absence of close relatives or other support people who are able and willing to provide adequate and appropriate assistance.

Wellness Opportunity

By sensitively communicating care and concern, nurses encourage vulnerable older adults to talk about conditions that can be addressed to prevent abuse or neglect.

Dementia and Psychosocial Factors

Because impaired cognitive function is a common characteristic of abused older adults, considerable attention has been focused on dementia as a risk factor for self-neglect and other types of abuse. Impaired judgment, lack of insight, inability to make safe decisions and loss of contact with reality are specific impairments that can lead to abuse and self-neglect. Within the United States, the National Center on Elder Abuse (2012) reported the following statistics about types of abuse reported by caregivers of people with dementia: 60% verbally abusive, 14% neglectful and between 5% and 10% physically abusive. One study found that mistreatment was detected in 47.3% of a sample of 129 persons with dementia, with the following variables associated with increased occurrence of abuse: aggressive behaviours of the person with dementia and caregiver's anxiety, depression, lower education and higher perceived burden (Wiglesworth et al., 2010). In addition to dementia, depression and delirium are other conditions that can increase the risk for elder abuse and neglect.

Characteristics of depression that contribute to its role in self-neglect include social isolation, a negative outlook and lack of interest in self-care.

When the older adult denies the cognitive impairment or refuses help or evaluation, the risk for elder abuse increases. Older people who live alone may be afraid of acknowledging impairments because they fear that they will be required to receive services or move to a long-term care facility. This fear may lead to social isolation, the overlooking of treatable or reversible causes of impairment or a progressive but unnecessary decline in function.

Long-term mental illness also may predispose an older adult to abuse or neglect, especially in combination with other factors, such as dementia or the loss of a significant social support. Additional risk factors arise from social and environmental sources. The absence of a support system is one of the most common contributing factors to self-neglect and psychological abuse (Melchiorre et al., 2013). For example, older adults in their 80s, 90s or older may have outlived most of the people who once provided support and tangible services. This is particularly problematic for people who have been lifelong recluses or who have no children or extended family.

Caregiver Factors

Caregiving itself does not cause elder abuse; however, it can lead to abuse when those assuming the caregiving role are incapable of doing so because of life stresses, pathologic characteristics, personality characteristics, insufficient resources or lack of understanding of the older adult's condition. Caregivers who perpetrate abuse often exhibit some of the same risk factors associated with abused elders, particularly if the caregivers themselves are older adults. Caregiver factors associated with elder abuse include poor health, cognitive impairment, substance abuse, social isolation, dependence and co-residence, and poor interpersonal relations with the dependent elder. It is not unusual to have a mutually neglectful or abusive situation when an older married couple has several of the psychosocial risk factors just identified and is, in addition, socially isolated. For example, a couple who both have dementia may unintentionally abuse each other and neglect themselves.

Unfolding Case Study

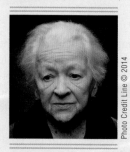

Photo Credit Line © 2014

Part 1: Mrs. B at 82 Years of Age

Mrs. B. is an 82-year-old divorced and widowed mother of four. She lives in a senior citizens' apartment located in the downtown area of a large city. The building is regularly serviced by subsidized transportation to grocery stores and shopping malls and has a nutrition centre on the ground floor. Mrs. B.'s eldest son died in an accident 12 years ago. Her daughter lives 76 km away but visits once a week to do the grocery shopping and other errands. Two sons live within 4 km of their mother's apartment. Mrs. B. lived in the home of one son and his wife until they argued 1 year ago. The other son lives alone in a small apartment and visits his mother two or three times weekly and frequently takes her to lunch or dinner. Mrs. B. has been hospitalized for major depression eight times since her eldest son's death. She also has been diagnosed as having hypertension, rheumatoid arthritis and type 2 diabetes.

Mrs. B. was referred to a home care agency for follow-up after her last hospital stay because her medication regimen, which she had followed for 6 years, had been changed while she was in the hospital. At the time of discharge, Mrs. B. was given a 30-day supply of medications set out in daily-dose medication containers for her. She was to take glyburide, 2.5 mg once a day; propranolol, 40 mg twice a day; paroxetine, 25 mg once a day; folic acid, 1 mg once a day; and methotrexate, four 2.5-mg tablets each Wednesday. Scheduled medication times were 8 AM and 8 PM. The home care nurse was to instruct Mrs. B. in her medication regimen, including what medications she was to take, how she was to take them, what each medication was expected to do and possible side effects. The nurse was also to assess Mrs. B.'s ability to follow instructions and her adherence to the medication regimen.

Because Mrs. B.'s vision was impaired from diabetes, she had difficulty managing her complex medication regimen. The visiting nurse arranged for unit-dose packaging for Mrs. B.'s prescriptions and visited twice a day for 2 days to observe Mrs. B.'s ability to take her medications accurately. On the third morning, the nurse telephoned Mrs. B. at 8:15 AM and asked Mrs. B. if she had any problems taking her pills. Mrs. B. happily reported that she had taken all the pills, including the four methotrexate tablets, without any difficulty. The nurse then scheduled Mrs. B. to be seen three times a week for ongoing assessment for several weeks.

THINKING POINTS

- What are the factors that contribute to the risk of Mrs. B. becoming abused or neglected?
- What are the factors that protect Mrs. B. from becoming abused or neglected?

- As the visiting nurse, what concerns would you have about Mrs. B. when you discharge her from home care, and how would you address these concerns?

ELDER ABUSE AND NEGLECT IN NURSING HOMES

Although most elder abuse occurs in home settings, it also occurs in long-term residential care settings. Elder abuse in nursing homes was first brought to public attention during the early 1970s when several exposés about poor care in nursing homes were published. By the end of the decade, overall nursing home care had improved but neglect and physical abuse of nursing home residents was an ongoing concern.

Recent studies indicate that elder abuse in nursing homes and other institutional settings is a widespread and hidden problem (Hirschel & Anetzberger, 2012; McDonald et al., 2012). Following are examples of studies about prevalence and types of elder abuse in nursing home and other long-term residential care facilities:

- Abuse, gross neglect and exploitation represent more than 7% of all complaints investigated by long-term care ombudsman programs, with physical abuse most common, followed by psychological abuse and resident-to-resident abuse (Miller, 2012).
- A random sample survey of family members with an elderly relative in a nursing home found that 24.3% reported that their elderly relative was abused and about 21% reported neglect on at least one occasion in the past year (Schiamberg et al., 2012; Zhang et al., 2011).

- Families of nursing home residents identified neglect and caretaking mistreatment as the two most frequent types of abuse reported (Griffore et al., 2009).
- Nursing assistants in nursing homes identified psychological abuse as most common, illustrated by argumentative behaviour and intimidation (Castle, 2012a).

Although research is just beginning to unravel elder abuse risk factors in nursing homes, many factors stem from administrative problems within the institution, such as lack of abuse prevention policies, insufficient staff screening, inadequate staff education and training, and staff shortages and turnover. Staff competencies for preventing elder abuse identified by direct care workers include understanding elder abuse risk factors along with acquiring communication, relationship-building and coping skills (DeHart et al., 2009). Another contributing condition that is common in nursing homes is the challenge of dealing with resident-to-staff aggression. For example, a 2-week prevalence study of 1,552 residents in large urban nursing homes found that 15.6% were aggressive toward staff during that period, with verbal abuse (12.4%) and physical aggression (7.6%) being the most common types (Lachs et al., 2013). Hirschel and Anetzberger (2012) reviewed the literature on risk facts for elder abuse in long-term care facilities and found that these can be divided into staffing characteristics (e.g., leading stressful lives and having negative attitudes toward residents), facility characteristics (e.g., inadequate supervision and harsh management practices) and resident characteristics, including social isolation and exhibiting difficult behaviours. Ultimately, effective strategies to address elder abuse in long-term care facilities must focus on all three areas of risk, as well as their interrelationships.

As with elder abuse in community settings, it is rarely reported when it occurs in institutional settings, despite the existence of provincial and federal laws aimed at protecting residents from mistreatment (Ulsperger & Knottnerus, 2011). Studies of nursing home employees found that when elder abuse was not reported, it was typically for one of the following reasons: staff stress and burnout; inadequate staff education or training on elder abuse; difficulty in making a determination about whether or not a situation should be reported; barriers to making a report; or a belief that some elder abuse situations happen because staff are overworked, inexperienced or frustrated in handling difficult residents (McCool et al., 2009; Shinan-Altman & Cohen, 2009).

Resident-to-resident aggression is a type of elder abuse that occurs in nursing homes with a scope and incidence that has serious effects on safety and quality of life of many residents (Castle, 2012b; Teresi et al., 2013). Resident-to-resident aggression is defined as "negative and aggressive physical, sexual or verbal interaction between long-term care residents that in a community setting would likely be construed as unwelcome and have high potential to cause physical or psychological distress in the recipient" (Pillemer et al., 2012, p. 25).

In addition to the federal and provincial laws that apply to elder abuse in all settings, elder abuse in institutional settings is addressed by Medicare regulations, provincial/territorial licensing laws, federal and provincial/territorial health care fraud and abuse laws and long-term care ombudsman laws. Although jurisdictional reporting laws vary, the local adult protective services agency and the nursing home ombudsman program investigate the report. When an abuse report is substantiated, further investigation is carried out by the state agency responsible for licensure and certification and also by the state professional licensing authority when the abuse is committed by a professional.

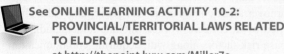

See **ONLINE LEARNING ACTIVITY 10-2:**
PROVINCIAL/TERRITORIAL LAWS RELATED
TO ELDER ABUSE
at http://thepoint.lww.com/Miller7e

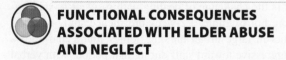

FUNCTIONAL CONSEQUENCES ASSOCIATED WITH ELDER ABUSE AND NEGLECT

Older people who have several risk factors are likely to become victims of elder abuse, as illustrated by the following case examples:

1. A middle-aged alcoholic man hit his aged father during an argument. In turn, both were beaten by their sons/grandsons, who wanted money for drugs.

2. An elderly woman never left home because she feared her memory lapses would prevent her from finding the way back. When she did venture out, she fell on the porch, and the police were called. Outreach workers found she had no food in the house and was malnourished.

3. An unemployed couple kept their impaired grandparents confined to the house, refusing them visitors, abandoning them for days without adequate food and denying them help for fear of losing access to their Old Age Security cheques.

4. A son visited his mother in the nursing home and sexually assaulted her when staff members were not present.

5. A depressed elderly woman refused to take a needed medication with the result that her legs became so swollen that she could not leave her chair.

6. A woman in her 80s—who was weak, incontinent and hypertensive—was abandoned in an emergency department with a note reading "Totally dependent! Handle with care."

These situations illustrate various forms of abuse, which are defined below (National Seniors Council, 2007; The Ontario Network for the Prevention of Elder Abuse, n.d.):

- **Physical abuse:** inflicting, or threatening to inflict, physical pain or injury on a vulnerable elder, or depriving him or her of a basic need
- **Sexual abuse:** nonconsensual sexual contact of any kind, coercing an elder to witness sexual behaviours
- **Emotional (psychological) abuse:** inflicting mental pain, anguish or distress on an elder person through verbal or nonverbal acts
- **Exploitation:** illegal taking, misuse, or concealment of funds, property or assets of a vulnerable elder
- **Neglect:** refusal or failure by those responsible to provide food, shelter, health care or protection for a vulnerable elder
- **Abandonment:** the desertion of a vulnerable elder by anyone who has assumed responsibility for care or custody of that person
- **Self-neglect:** behaviour of an elderly person that threatens his or her own health or safety, such as failure to provide adequate food and nutrition for oneself or failure to take essential medications

Specific actions that are defined in legislation include undue influence, unreasonable confinement, violation of rights and denying privacy or visitors.

Self-neglect and self-abuse are forms of elder abuse that differ from other types in that they have no perpetrator other than the older person himself or herself. In cases of self-abuse, the older person causes injury or pain to herself or himself, including body mutilations. In cases of self-neglect, the older person fails to meet essential needs to the point that his or her health and safety is threatened, usually because of such factors as serious functional impairments or the desire to die (Day et al., 2012). Studies indicate that prevalence of self-neglect is between 10% and 15% (Dong et al., 2012). Self-neglect develops gradually and is often associated with lack of resources, such as food, money and housing; other times adequate resources are available but the older adult does not access appropriate resources. Many self-neglected older adults have underlying problems, such as dementia, depression, psychosis or substance abuse disorders that affect their ability to seek assistance and accept help (Bond & Butler, 2013). Still other times, the person may refuse services because of a desire for privacy or fear of being forced to move or accept unwanted services.

Although elder abuse literature has not focused on situations that are mutually abusive or neglectful, nurses working in home settings have long encountered situations in which two people, often a married couple, abuse each other or are both neglected. These situations may be rooted in a long-term, mutually abusive relationship but usually evolve because of gradual declines in the functional abilities of both people. They may also be associated with the poor coping skills of a spouse or caregiver who is faced with increasing demands and little or no outside help. Many of these situations are now being recognized as aspects of domestic violence (Roberto et al., 2013).

Since the late 1980s, domestic violence in later life has been recognized as another aspect of elder abuse, with much of the focus on older women's experiences of intimate partner violence. Although this is a recognized and unique aspect of elder abuse, attention to and research about this topic remains limited. Some findings from a review of 32 studies by Weeks and LeBlanc (2011) are as follows:

- Abuse of women by their partners is a problem across all ages, races, religions and socioeconomic classes.
- Between 15% and 26.5% of women in midlife and older report intimate partner violence, with one study finding 3.5% of women aged 65 and older experiencing this in the past 5 years.
- Between 48% and 72% of abused older women do not report the abuse.
- Abuse of older women by their partners occurs in several contexts, including longstanding relationships, new relationships or across several relationships, with the most common perpetrators being spouses (62%), current boyfriends (26%) and former spouses (12%).
- When intimate partner violence develops in later life, this may be associated with changes in health status or other aging-related events (e.g., some men become more controlling after retirement).
- When abuse occurs throughout a long-term relationship, it may shift from physical to emotional and financial abuse over time.
- Between 7.9% and 9% of women experiencing intimate partner violence reported that gun ownership and the presence of firearms greatly influenced the relationship dynamics.

Programs that address domestic violence as an aspect of elder abuse are few and rare, especially in rural areas. Barriers to the use of available services include inaccessibility of programs, feelings of self-blame and shame, lack of information, reluctance of older victims to leave long-term relationships and lack of support from family and friends (Weeks & LeBlanc, 2011). Cultural expectations and norms also present barriers to reporting abuse and seeking help, particularly with regard to beliefs about traditional roles of women and the permanency of marriage. It is imperative that domestic violence services are suitable to the needs, beliefs, values and demographic and situational characteristics of individual older victims (Newman et al., 2013).

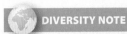
DIVERSITY NOTE

Rural culture can affect help-seeking behaviours in domestic violence situations. For instance, victims may stay in abusive relationships because they live in small, insulated communities with nearby family and strong social networks, especially if violence is an accepted part of life.

Although rape and other sexual violence perpetrated against older people received some attention during the late 1970s, the focus at that time was on sexual assault by strangers. During the 1990s, sexual assault by family members and paid caregivers became a widely recognized aspect of elder abuse. A landmark study of sexual abuse in care facilities found that the typical perpetrator was a man (78.4%), aged 56 (range 19 to 96) and almost as likely to be another resident (41%) as facility staff (43%). The victims were cognitively or physically impaired, with nearly half of the victims requiring assistance in all activities of daily living (ADLs). Sexual abuse most often was represented by molestation, which was four times more frequent than vaginal rapes, the second usual form (Ramsey-Klawsnik et al., 2008). Dementia increases the risk for sexual assault of older adults, both in long-term care and community settings (Connolly et al., 2012). Among the many barriers to the effective prevention of and response to elder sexual abuse—particularly for cognitively impaired victims—is the fact that many cases are not reported and very few are prosecuted (Payne, 2010).

Case Study

When Mr. P.'s wife died, Mr. P., a frail man, sought care in the home of a neighbour who offered both board and care in exchange for his monthly Old Age Security cheque. In reality, the neighbour provided neither, but locked Mr. P. in the basement and gave him little food. If Mr. P. complained about the treatment or refused to sign over the income or property, the caregiver hit or kicked him. After 4 years, the situation was discovered and reported to the city's protective services agency. Mr. P. later sat in the social worker's office and sadly commented, "So this is what it's like to be a protective case."

THINKING POINTS

- What type(s) of abuse does this case represent?
- What are some of the psychosocial consequences that Mr. P. is likely to have experienced in the past 4 years?
- What are some factors that contribute to this situation going on for 4 years?

See **ONLINE LEARNING ACTIVITY 10-3: CASE EXAMPLES OF ELDER ABUSE** at http://thepoint.lww.com/Miller7e

NURSING ASSESSMENT OF ABUSED OR NEGLECTED OLDER ADULTS

Elder abuse is not so much *assessed* as it is *detected,* so nurses often must assume the role of detective putting together clues. Because elder abuse by its very nature is a hidden problem, assessment begins with a suspicion about its existence. Information may be purposefully withheld, and it is rarely volunteered, except in situations in which the older person or caregiver is desperate for help. Clues to elder abuse might first be noted when an older person is seen in an emergency department or admitted to a hospital. Most often, a home visit is an essential component of the assessment process, and gaining admission to the home usually is the first assessment challenge. Many times, the situation deteriorates so gradually that it is hard to determine the onset of abuse. In questionable situations, people who suspect that elder abuse is occurring may ignore the clues in hopes that the situation will resolve by itself.

> **Wellness Opportunity**
>
> Nurses pay particular attention to the older adult's relationships with others so that they can detect clues to elder abuse.

UNIQUE ASPECTS OF ELDER ABUSE ASSESSMENT

Assessment of elder abuse differs from usual nursing assessment in several respects. First, a major goal is to determine whether legal interventions are appropriate or necessary for protection of the older adult, in contrast to situations in which the primary focus is on specific health needs. In situations of suspected abuse, assessment initially focuses on the safety of the older person. This approach is similar to critical care nursing, in which basic life-sustaining needs are addressed immediately and other needs are considered later.

Second, realistic goals for elder abuse situations often are quite limited. For example, in many situations, basic safety is the only goal, especially when the elder and caregiver insist on choices that are not consistent with those recommended by health care workers. An assessment of risks to safety is essential because choice of legal interventions is influenced by the degree of risk. Because the determination of safety often is based on medical and nursing information, the role of the nurse is especially important. In home settings in particular, the nurse may be the only health care professional who directly assesses the situation, and the nursing assessment may be the major determinant of recommendations for legal intervention.

Third, cases of elder abuse generally involve some element of resistance from the older person or caregiver(s).

Only in rare situations do abused elders or their caregivers seek assistance from health care professionals. Although it might be impossible to establish a trusting relationship, the nurse must try, at the very least, to establish an accepting relationship. The initial assessment, therefore, is aimed at identifying ways of gaining access and at least passive acceptance.

Fourth, in contrast to most health care situations, the nurse may be viewed as a threat rather than a help. Thus, it may be difficult to gain access or to obtain adequate assessment information. When this is the case, it is important to minimize the perceived threat even before the initial contact. This can be achieved by identifying someone who acknowledges that a problem exists and is willing to facilitate the assessment process. Any of the following people can be helpful in gaining access and acceptance:

- Neighbours or friends
- Relatives (especially family members who do not live in the problematic home setting)
- Staff from senior centres, offices on aging, or health care or community agencies
- Physicians or any other health professionals
- Faith-based people (e.g., clergy, parish nurses, rabbis)

Fifth, when legal interventions are being considered, the legal rights of the person and the caregivers must be addressed, even when this is beyond the usual scope of nursing. In institutional settings, legal and ethical decisions are guided by medical information and institutional policies, and the role of the physician usually is the most important. In home settings, however, there may be little or no physician input, and nursing input is often the most important.

Finally, the nurse's personal safety is an assessment consideration in many elder abuse situations, especially when visits involve contact with a known or suspected perpetrator. In any situation that places a nurse at risk, it is essential to ensure that appropriate protections and precautions are in place. For example, nurses can arrange their visits in conjunction with protective service workers' visits or, if warranted, law enforcement officers. Some communities have law enforcement officers who are specially trained to deal with elder abuse situations. In addition, it is imperative that nurses are vigilant about potential risks and attentive to an escape route.

> **Wellness Opportunity**
>
> When making home visits, nurses pay particular attention to self-wellness by protecting themselves from risks.

Physical Health

Nursing assessment of physical abuse and neglect focuses on the following: nutrition, hydration, bruises and injuries, degree of frailty and presence of pathologic conditions. The following sections discuss each of these aspects in relation to elder abuse and neglect.

Nutrition and Hydration

Nutrition and hydration are important in determining not only the existence of physical neglect but also the seriousness and urgency of the situation. In community settings, nutrition and hydration status are often a key factor in determining the need for immediate interventions. Nursing assessment of nutrition and hydration status is discussed in Chapter 18 (see the section on using physical assessment and laboratory information, Table 18-1, and Box 18-5).

When indicators of malnutrition or dehydration are identified, the next step is to determine whether the hydration or nutritional status can be improved adequately without removing the person from the setting. The role of the nurse can be especially important in assessing not only the nutrition and hydration status but also the measures required to alleviate these risks immediately. Sometimes, the provision of water and food is the most important intervention in neglect situations. In addition, this intervention is inexpensive and readily available and can be quite effective in establishing a relationship with a hungry or thirsty person.

Injuries, Bruises and Other Physical Harm

Assessment of indicators of physical harm is an important aspect of the detection of neglect or physical abuse. Any of the following conditions can be indicators of abuse or self-neglect: leg ulcers; pressure ulcers; dependent edema; poor wound healing; burns from stoves, cigarettes or hot water; and bruises, swelling or injuries from falls, especially repeated falls. More than one of these indicators at the same time, or over a short period of time, should raise high levels of suspicion about neglect. The possibility of alcohol abuse should also be considered when any of these indicators is identified, especially if the person is also depressed or socially isolated. To detect physical abuse, look for evidence of injury caused by others, such as marks from cuts, bites, burns or punctures; bruises or injuries, especially of the face, head or trunk; bruises on both upper arms, as would result from being grabbed or shaken harshly; or bruises that reflect the shape of objects, like belts or hairbrushes. With evidence of injuries from falls, consider the possibility that the person was shoved or otherwise caused to fall by someone else.

Characteristics of bruises are routinely assessed for information about onset and progression. For example, colour of bruises typically progresses from blue/black to green, then yellow, with red appearing at any time. Although some studies have addressed bruises in child abuse, research on bruises in older adults began only during the mid-2000s, with a landmark study on the life cycle of bruises in older adults (Mosqueda et al., 2005). Trained research assistants performed daily head-to-toe examinations of 101 older adults during the initial 14-day inspection period to identify the onset of new bruises. Researchers examined and documented 108 bruises on 73 participants every day for up to 6 weeks. Subjects were screened to exclude the possibility of abuse and the study considered variables such as medications, fall history and medical conditions. The following findings from this study are pertinent to a nursing assessment of bruises in older adults (Mosqueda et al., 2005):

- Accidental bruises occur in a predictable pattern in older adults, with 89% on extremities, 76% on the dorsal aspect of the arms and none being observed on the neck, ears, genitalia, buttocks or soles of the feet.
- Bruise duration varied from 4 to 41 days, with 81% resolving by day 11.
- Colour of a bruise was not a good indicator of its age.
- The most commonly reported cause was bumping into something.
- Subjects with compromised function and those on medications known to affect coagulation were more likely to have multiple bruises.

A second bruising study (Wiglesworth et al., 2009) investigated the characteristics of bruises sustained by physically abused older adults, as illustrated in Figure 10-1. A review of 839 injuries reported in nine studies, which included the study by Wiglesworth and colleagues, identified the following anatomic distribution of injuries related to elder physical abuse: upper extremity, 44%; head, neck, skull, brain, dental and maxillofacial area, 35%; lower extremity, 11%; and torso, 10% (Murphy et al., 2013).

In recent years, there is increasing attention to the evaluation and documentation of bruises and patterns of injuries as an indicator of physical abuse. In particular, researchers are trying to identify characteristics of injuries caused by a perpetrator, in contrast to those sustained accidentally. This is especially pertinent to identifying forensic markers of elder abuse that are needed to aid in the prosecution of perpetrators. Researchers are also investigating the causes of injuries sustained by abused older adults in relation to location of bruises, as in the following relationships gleaned from data analysis of 67 confirmed case of physical elder abuse (Ziminski et al., 2013):

- Those who reported being choked: lumbar region, head and neck, and left anterior upper arm
- Those who reported being punched or hit: head and neck, right lateral upper arm
- Those who reported being grabbed: lateral or anterior arms, including left anterior upper and lower arm
- Those who reported being beaten: head and neck
- Those who reported being slammed against a wall: lumbar region

Nurses also assess for indicators of abuse caused by excessive amounts of alcohol or drugs, especially psychoactive medications. Sometimes caregivers who abuse drugs or alcohol will give these substances to the people for whom they care, especially if the dependent person is not able or willing to refuse. Another sign of abuse is excessive use of psychoactive medications solely for the caregiver's benefit so that the elder is more easily managed. Nurses are likely to observe any of the following indicators of overmedication in an elder: ataxia, somnolence, clouded mentation, slurred speech, staggering gait or extrapyramidal manifestations.

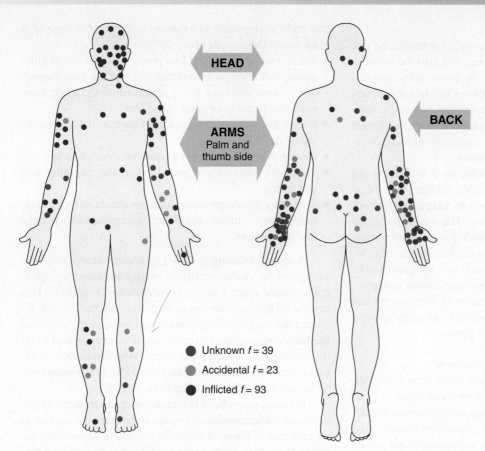

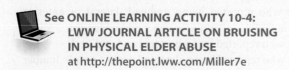

FIGURE 10-1 Bruising in older adults as reported by abused elders. (From Wiglesworth, A., Austin, R., Conona, M., et al. [2009]. *Journal of the American Geriatrics Society, 57*[7], 1191–1196. Used with permission from Wiley-Blackwell.)

Aspects of physical neglect may include withholding therapeutic medications or interfering with medical care. For example, caregivers may decide not to purchase prescriptions or provide nursing care, medical equipment or comfort items because they do not want to spend the money, even though this care is necessary. If the older adult has not freely chosen to forgo treatments, medications or assistance, then this may constitute neglect. If the caregiver is likely to inherit the money that is being saved, this may represent financial exploitation as well.

See ONLINE LEARNING ACTIVITY 10-4:
LWW JOURNAL ARTICLE ON BRUISING IN PHYSICAL ELDER ABUSE
at http://thepoint.lww.com/Miller7e

Degree of Frailty

The degree of frailty of the older adult is another consideration in assessing actual or potential abuse or neglect. For example, an older adult who is physically healthy and fully ambulatory would not have the same degree of risk for fall-related injuries as one who weighs only 36 kg and ambulates unsteadily with a walker. Similarly, if the 75-year-old wife of an alcoholic man can easily escape to safety when he becomes violent, and she chooses to remain in the situation, she would not necessarily be considered a protective case. In contrast, if the woman is cognitively impaired, physically

frail or unable to move quickly and is the target of violence when her husband is inebriated, the situation could be defined as elder abuse.

Pathologic Conditions

In certain medical conditions, it is essential to assess the ability to follow medical regimens and the consequences of noncompliance. For example, consequences can be quite serious when a person with diabetes or congestive heart failure does not take medications correctly. When medication regimens are complex, it is important to determine if it can be simplified to improve adherence and support the person's ability to remain in an independent setting. For example, in an institutional setting, medications might be administered four or more different times during a 24-hour period. However, even though this might be ideal, people in home settings may not be able to follow this regimen, particularly if the older adult lives alone and requires assistance with medications. A thorough nursing assessment can lead to interventions, such as the use of medication organizers (described in Chapter 8), to achieve adequate adherence.

Activities of Daily Living

A major focus of assessment in elder abuse situations is to determine the necessity for legal interventions. Therefore, a nursing assessment of the person's potential for safe performance of activities of daily living (ADLs) is extremely important. This is particularly important when assessing self-neglect because impairments in instrumental ADLs are strongly associated with this type of abuse.

For community-living older adults, it is essential to assess the home environment and the elder's level of functioning in that environment. In addition, nurses often need to obtain information from caregivers. Home care workers provide valuable information, and they provide a different perspective than family members do. In some circumstances, it may be appropriate to involve occupational or physical therapists in the home assessment. When a difference of opinion exists, or when it is difficult to determine the safety of the situation, it may be helpful to have a team conference that includes all of the people who function in assessment or caregiving capacities and who have some degree of objectivity. In cases of suspected elder abuse, the assessment team often includes input from many informal sources of help, such as family and neighbours, as well as formal sources of help, such as nurses, home care workers and social workers.

Personal dress, hygiene and grooming are among the most visible and commonly appraised aspects of daily function. People are often viewed as neglected when they do not comply with socially defined standards of cleanliness, particularly when an unpleasant odour is noted. In self-neglect situations, poor hygiene and grooming are important indicators of underlying problems, but they do not necessarily affect the person's safety. Although health care workers may be inclined to focus initial services on providing assistance with bathing and grooming, the older adult may perceive this as a threat to his or her pride and independence. Thus, nurses assess not only the health effects of poor hygiene but also the consequences of imposing assistance on someone who is unwilling to accept help or acknowledge a hygiene problem. The nurse may determine that efforts to deal with personal hygiene would interfere with the short-term goal of establishing a relationship and the long-term goal of assisting with other aspects of daily function. Thus, it may be appropriate to begin by addressing nutrition, hydration and safety, while deferring attention to personal care issues associated with the most resistance.

Adequate nutrition, hydration and the ability to obtain help in an emergency are the basic human needs that are most often called into question in cases of elder abuse. Other basic needs may also be compromised, usually in relation to specific functional impairments and environmental circumstances. For instance, it is imperative to address bowel and bladder elimination for people who are confined to bed or a chair. For people with mobility limitations or serious vision impairments, safe ambulation and the ability to avoid falls are important considerations. Table 10-1 summarizes some of the specific functional and environmental conditions that present risks to basic needs.

Psychosocial Function

Information in Chapters 13, 14 and 15 are pertinent to assessing psychosocial function in relation to elder abuse. In

TABLE 10-1 Risks to Safety Associated With Functional Limitations

Functional Limitation	Risks to Safety
Any mental or physical impairment, especially combined with social isolation and lack of a support system	Nutrition and hydration
Mobility limitations or seriously impaired vision, especially combined with poor judgment	Falls
Cognitive impairments in ambulatory people	Wandering, getting lost
Compromised mobility	Pressure sores
Cognitive impairment, especially poor judgment	Inability to get help
Poor judgment, especially when living in an unsafe neighbourhood	Basic safety and security

addition, an important aspect of psychosocial function for abuse situations is assessment of the older adult's capacity for reasonable judgments about self-care. This is difficult because the determination of someone's ability to make appropriate judgments is influenced by subjective criteria and opinions. People whose judgment is impaired to the point that they are at serious risk, especially if they do not acknowledge the risk, are usually considered incompetent or incapacitated. Thus, the crucial element of psychosocial assessment for elder abuse cases is a determination of *risk* (i.e., danger to the person) rather than a determination of whether other people would judge the decision as *good* or *appropriate*. When the competence of an older adult to make safe decisions regarding self-care is in doubt, nurses may be legally bound to make reports or consider other legal interventions. There are no federal guidelines for determining the mental capacity of abused or neglected older adults, and the legal criteria differ among provincial/territorial jurisdictions. The ethical and legal considerations related to elder abuse are discussed later in this chapter and more extensively in Chapter 9.

Wellness Opportunity

Nurses promote self-determination for older adults by respecting their rights to make decisions about their care, as long as their actions do not jeopardize safety for themselves or others.

Support Resources

Support resources include those people, such as caregivers and friends, who influence a person's physical and psychosocial function. Some or all of the support people may directly cause the abusive situation or may actively or passively contribute to it. Therefore, nurses assess the support resources in terms of both helpful and detrimental effects. In addition, support resources not currently being used are identified as potential sources of help.

When the caregivers who perpetrate the abuse are also the support resources, nurses assess the potential for working with them to alleviate the negative consequences. Although it is not always easy to work with abusive caregivers, it may be even more difficult to eliminate their influence over an older adult. For example, it is not unusual to address situations in which an alcoholic son or daughter lives with a parent and provides emotional support while at the same time neglecting the parent's needs and financially exploiting the situation. During the assessment, therefore, nurses identify any strengths of the caregiver and any willingness to change the situation voluntarily. If the caregiver is extremely stressed, then respite, along with individual or group support and counselling, may be effective interventions. In mutually abusive situations in which the designated caregiver, often a spouse, is also abused or neglected, the nurse tries to identify any outside sources of support that have not been tapped. For example, in a mutually abusive situation involving a socially isolated married couple, the nurse might identify a relative, friend or paid caregiver who is willing to provide appropriate assistance.

Because a caregiver's lack of knowledge can be an underlying factor in elder abuse, nurses assess the caregiver's understanding of the older adult's needs. For example, caregivers may have good intentions when they use adult briefs for the control of incontinence and do not change them frequently, but they may not understand the potential for skin breakdown. Caregivers may administer excessive amounts of psychoactive medications because they do not understand the correct dosing schedule or the potential adverse effects. This is especially common when medications are ordered on an as-needed basis and the caregiver has not been given clear guidelines for determining when the medication is needed or what the most effective dosage is. In these situations, nursing assessment of the caregiver's knowledge is especially important because educational interventions, role modelling or the provision of additional services may alleviate the abuse.

In situations of neglect, there are usually very few support services to assess, and the major nursing task is to identify potential sources of help and the barriers that interfere with the use of these resources. The assessment of barriers to the use of resources is discussed in Chapter 13 and is summarized in Box 13-8. It is especially important to identify these barriers because simple interventions, such as provision of information or assistance with transportation, may be effective in eliminating them. Cultural influences must also be assessed in relation to the use of support resources, as discussed in Chapter 2.

Environmental Influences

As with other aspects of elder abuse, the primary purposes of assessing the environment are to identify the factors that create risks and to determine which of these factors can be alleviated through interventions. With regard to the immediate living conditions, assess whether minimal standards of safety and cleanliness are being maintained. When home environments are extremely cluttered, it is important to assess both the meaning and the consequences of the clutter. For example, a massive and long-developing collection of clutter from hoarding may be indicative of an underlying disorder and may or may not be a risk to safety that requires immediate attention. Because consequences of hoarding range from socially unacceptable appearances to serious risks to health and safety, it is important to assess the person's ability to safely manoeuvre in the environment during daily activities, as well as during emergency situations, such as a fire. When nurses and other workers are initially exposed to massive amounts of clutter, their first inclination may be to think of a way to eliminate some of it. If this reaction is communicated to the resident of the cluttered home, however, it may become impossible to establish an accepting relationship, and the older adult may reject any further interventions. Thus, it is imperative to communicate a nonjudgmental approach, while at the same time addressing the risks that require immediate action.

Another assessment aspect for community-dwelling older adults is to identify risks to safety in the neighbourhood environment. This is especially important when the older person lives in an area of high crime or extreme isolation and is vulnerable by virtue of impaired judgment, physical frailty, or a combination of physical and psychosocial impairments. For example, people who are only moderately forgetful may be safe in an apartment or a suburban neighbourhood where neighbours watch out for them. In a high-crime neighbourhood, however, forgetting to lock the doors or to take other precautions may place the person at increased risk for physical harm, financial exploitation or other serious abuses. Likewise, in a rural environment, social isolation may increase the risks for vulnerable older adults.

Finally, seasonal conditions can influence the degree of risk for self-neglect in people who are cognitively impaired and live in climates characterized by extreme heat or cold. For example, people who do not pay utility bills may not be in any danger as long as the weather is mild, but when the temperature turns cold, they would be at risk for hypothermia. The same is true for people who occasionally wander outside without dressing appropriately. As long as the neighbourhood is safe and the weather is mild, they may be relatively safe; however, they may be at increased risk during the cold months or very hot months, especially if they do not wear proper clothing. Nursing assessment of risk factors for hypothermia or heat-related illness is discussed in Chapter 25.

Threats to Life

The most immediate consideration in determining whether legal interventions are necessary is the identification of life-threatening situations or serious medical risks. When situations are viewed as critical when they are first discovered, the initial reaction of the person who discovers the situation may be to remove the person from the environment. Many times, however, the person may not want to leave, or there may be no better setting in which the person can receive care immediately. In these situations, nurses may be asked to assess the urgency and seriousness of the situation and to provide an opinion about whether legal interventions are justified. In addition, the nurse often is the person who can either convince the older adult to accept help or convince the caregivers and social workers that the present situation is tolerable. For instance, when nurses determine that the situation is not life-threatening, they can reassure the person that they are trying to improve the situation and support the person remaining as safe and independent as possible. Examples of threats that nurses commonly assess in elder abuse situations include the following:

- History of physical violence on the part of the caregiver, especially when the older adult is unable to escape or otherwise be protected
- Untreated wounds or infections
- Inability to administer insulin correctly
- Progressive gangrene or ulcerated conditions
- Inability to adhere to therapeutic regimens
- Consistent wandering in unsafe neighbourhoods or in very cold weather
- Misuse (usually unintentional) of medically necessary medications, such as those for diabetes or cardiac conditions
- Excessive use of drugs or alcohol, either self- or caregiver induced.

In situations in which the caregiver is the abuser, it is imperative to assess the degree to which the caregiver presents a threat to the life of the dependent older person.

When nurses are notified of a serious situation but they do not have firsthand knowledge of the abused or neglected older person, their first consideration is whether this is an objectively urgent situation or primarily a "crisis" from the perspective of the person who just discovered the situation. Situations that appear the most appalling may actually represent a gradual deterioration over months or years. Therefore, the initial assessment is aimed at determining any immediate threats to the life of the abused adult, such as malnutrition, dehydration, serious injury, untreated medical condition or injury from others. Finally, suicide potential is assessed, especially in self-neglected older adults who are also depressed and expressing feelings of hopelessness. All the principles of suicide assessment that are discussed in Chapter 15 can be applied to elder abuse situations.

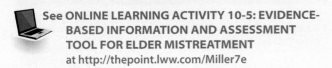

See ONLINE LEARNING ACTIVITY 10-5: EVIDENCE-BASED INFORMATION AND ASSESSMENT TOOL FOR ELDER MISTREATMENT at http://thepoint.lww.com/Miller7e

Cultural Aspects

Definitions and perceptions of elder abuse and neglect are influenced to a great extent by cultural norms. For example, Asian Indians may consider not visiting an older family member to be a form of psychological neglect, but Anglo Canadians may consider it a way of respecting privacy and autonomy. In a qualitative study of their personal experiences of abuse, older Sri Lankan Tamil women in Toronto spoke of the control exerted over them by their adult children and children-in-law, as well as a lack of social and financial support and respect (Guruge et al., 2010). Ploeg et al. (2014) reported that perceptions of elder abuse among marginalized Canadian populations (e.g., Aboriginals, immigrants, refugees, lesbians) had both similarities and differences. For all groups, verbal abuse was the most common experience; however, Aboriginal participants spoke more of financial abuse than did other groups, citing theft as "governmental abuse." Cultural factors also have a strong influence on caregiver roles and responsibilities. Most families have culturally influenced expectations about which family members should provide care to dependent older adults and about whether it is acceptable to enlist the aid of paid caregivers. In some families, there may be conflicts about these expectations, particularly between older and younger generations. Sometimes, these conflicts may need to be identified and addressed before elder abuse or neglect can be resolved.

Nurses identify cultural factors that influence the care that is provided—or not provided—to older adults. When assessing family caregiver relationships, it is important to be sensitive to cultural variations in perspectives on family caregiving and respect differences, while also addressing abusive situations. Box 10-4 lists some assessment questions related to identifying cultural influences. In addition, cultural assessment information on the following topics should be considered: communication and psychosocial assessment (see Chapter 13), nutrition (see Chapter 18), dementia (see Chapter 14) and depression (see Chapter 15).

Box 10-4 Cultural Considerations: Assessing Elder Abuse and Neglect

- What are the family and cultural expectations concerning family caregivers? (e.g., Is it acceptable to employ paid caregivers, or are family members expected to provide all the care?)
- Do family members differ in their perceptions about caregiving responsibilities?
- What are the family and cultural perspectives on autonomy and independence?
- Do family members differ in their perspectives on autonomy and independence?
- How are decisions made about care of the older adult? (e.g., Is it a patriarchal or matriarchal family?)
- Who are the acceptable sources of social support and personal assistance?
- Who are the acceptable sources of health care (e.g., herbalists, spiritual healers, Aboriginal practitioners)?
- What are the acceptable health care practices (e.g., herbs, homeopathy, acupuncture, faith healing, folk remedies)?
- Are there language barriers that influence the care that is provided or that limit the number of care providers?
- How does skin colour affect assessment of bruises, pressure sores and other skin changes?

Case Study

Mrs. K. is 80 years old and had resided in a nursing facility for 1 year until she was recently discharged at her request but "against medical advice" with no prescriptions for her medications or medical referral for home care. She has complex health conditions, including osteoarthritis, coronary artery disease, congestive heart failure, chronic obstructive pulmonary disease (COPD), depression and insulin-dependent diabetes. Although alert and oriented, Mrs. K. has major deficits in her ability to perform daily living tasks. She also depends on a walker for ambulation and has a history of falling, including a fall that resulted in a hip fracture and her admission to a nursing facility.

Mrs. K.'s support system is limited. Her son lives in another province but functions as power of attorney and provides some telephone reassurance. Her daughter is estranged from Mrs. K., and at their last meeting was verbally abusive to her. Mrs. K.'s older brother visits a few times weekly to help with meal preparation, grocery shopping, transportation and medication pickups; however, his own health problems prevent him from providing more help.

Shortly after returning home, Mrs. K.'s precarious health status rapidly deteriorated. She became severely short of breath, requiring continuous oxygen. She began to hallucinate in the evening, believing that she alone had the responsibility of feeding all of the children in the neighbourhood. As her fears increased, so too did the calls to her brother. Eventually, she made several calls every night, overwhelming and exhausting him.

THINKING POINTS

- What form(s) of elder abuse is (are) represented?
- What are signs or indicators of abuse that you as a nurse would be able to identify?
- What factors contribute to Mrs. K.'s current risks?
- How will you proceed in conducting a nursing assessment of Mrs. K.?
- What barriers might you encounter in conducting the assessment? How will you overcome them?

NURSING DIAGNOSIS

Because elder abuse and neglect is so broad and complex, various nursing diagnoses are applicable, depending on the situation. A nursing diagnosis that would apply to many elder abuse situations where family members are caregivers is Compromised Family Coping, defined as

a usually supportive primary person (family member, significant other or close friend) provides insufficient, ineffective or compromised support, comfort, assistance or encouragement that may be needed by the older adult to manage or master adaptive tasks related to his or her health challenge. (Herdman, 2012, p. 352)

In more serious cases of elder abuse, the nursing diagnosis of Disabled Family Coping might be applicable. This is defined

as "behaviour of primary person (family member, significant other or close friend) that disables his or her capacities and the older adult's capacities to effectively address tasks essential to either person's adaptation to the health challenge" (p. 354).

If stress is a contributing factor related to family caregiving, the nursing diagnosis of Caregiver Role Strain, or Risk for Caregiver Role Strain, might be applicable. Related caregiver factors include ineffective coping patterns, functional or cognitive impairments and insufficient resources (e.g., respite, financial assets, assistance with care). Related factors involving the dependent older adult include increased dependence and the presence of difficult or unsafe behaviours (e.g., paranoia, wandering, incontinence).

The nursing diagnosis of Risk for Injury is applicable when older adults are in self-neglecting situations, especially if the person lives alone and is functionally and cognitively impaired. The nursing diagnosis of Decisional Conflict might apply to abused or neglected older adults who live in an environment that places them at risk for harm because they are unable to make decisions about alternative environments. Related factors include fear, lack of information about alternatives and impaired decision-making ability.

Wellness Opportunity

Nurses address body–mind–spirit interrelatedness by identifying nursing diagnoses that address fear and other psychosocial consequences of abuse or neglect.

PLANNING FOR WELLNESS OUTCOMES

Nurses direct care for abused or neglected older adults toward addressing the complex needs of the older adult, as well as those of the family caregivers. Some Nursing Outcomes Classification (NOC) terminology that is likely to pertain to the abused older adult includes Abuse Cessation, Abuse Protection, Abuse Recovery (Emotional, Financial, Physical, Sexual), Neglect Cessation, Neglect Recovery, Self-Care Status and Social Support. Outcomes related to abusive caregivers or family members include Abusive Behaviour Self-Restraint, Caregiver Emotional Health, Caregiver–Patient Relationship, Caregiver Stressors, Caregiver Well-Being, Family Coping, Family Social Climate, Knowledge: Health Resources, Role Performance and Stress Level.

Wellness Opportunity

Quality of Life is a wellness outcome that is applicable to older adults and their caregivers when conditions contributing to abuse or neglect are alleviated.

NURSING INTERVENTIONS TO ADDRESS ELDER ABUSE AND NEGLECT

From a health care perspective, abused older adults can be described as the intensive care patients of the community because they require the highest level of skill from a variety of professionals. Unlike intensive care patients in hospitals, however, not all the team members are specialized health care professionals and many are community-based workers and people who provide informal support. Nurses often assume the role of coordinator or team leader in implementing interventions that address the older adults, the caregivers, and the environment for these inherently complex and challenging situations.

Because of the extensive scope of elder abuse, there are numerous Nursing Interventions Classification (NIC) terms that could be applicable to both the abused or neglected older adult and the caregiver. Some that would be appropriate in most situations are Abuse Protection Support: Elder; Crisis Intervention; Referral; Risk for Injury; Caregiver Support; Coping Enhancement; and Decisional Conflict.

Elder abuse interventions often involve legal actions when decision-making abilities of the older adult are impaired or when reliable and competent caregivers are not available to act in the best interest of the older adult. Thus, many cases of elder abuse involve legal and ethical questions about the competency of the older adult and the caregivers. Nurses often have a key role in advocating for the older adult and may feel unprepared or uncomfortable either making or participating in decisions that affect the rights of others. Similarly, nurses may feel torn between the right of the person to refuse treatment and the obligation to report abuse and neglect situations, as discussed later in this chapter.

Interventions for elder abuse are implemented in community settings over a long period of time by a team of formal and informal care providers. Nurses working in home and community settings have the most direct opportunities for both the prevention of and interventions for elder abuse. Home-delivered meals and nursing and medical strategies are interventions that are usually readily accepted and effective for addressing abused older adults in community settings. In institutional settings, commonly used nursing interventions include education and support of caregivers and facilitation of referrals to appropriate community agencies. Because the opportunities for intervention in institutional settings are quite different from those in community settings, each of these areas is discussed separately in the following sections.

Interventions in Institutional Settings

Nurses in acute and long-term care settings can intervene in cases of elder abuse when they interact with caregivers, who often seek advice from nurses about ways of providing care. For example, nurses can encourage caregivers to use a period of institutionalization to reevaluate the demands of the situation and to consider resources for support and assistance. Family may express ambivalence about managing the older adult's care at home, or they may be unsure or unrealistic about their own ability to provide appropriate care or to cope with the stress of the situation. In some cases, caregivers may be seeking approval for not providing

care at home. In these situations, nurses can facilitate communication among all the decision makers, including the primary care provider, the older adult (as appropriate) and the various family members who are responsible for care. Sometimes, it is appropriate to suggest individual counselling or support groups or make referrals for social services, particularly when caregivers are very stressed about care-related decisions.

When elder abuse is rooted in the caregiver's lack of information, nurses can teach about appropriate caregiving measures and, in some situations, can also serve as a role model. When caregivers need additional health education or support services, a referral to a home care agency for follow-up can be initiated. An important nursing role is to identify needs for skilled nursing care or rehabilitation therapies because health insurance usually covers these services or a portion of these services. If there are serious questions about the adequacy of a discharge plan, a referral for community-based services or a protective service agency for further assessment and ongoing services should be initiated.

Wellness Opportunity

When vulnerable older adults are in an acute or long-term care setting, nurses address psychosocial needs of family caregivers by providing support and education; these are effective tools for preventing elder abuse.

Interventions in Community Settings

In home settings, professional advice about managing difficult behaviours of people with dementia is an important intervention for preventing elder abuse. Nurses in community settings have many opportunities for teaching caregivers about adequate care through role modelling and verbal and written instruction. For example, nurses may suggest innovative ways of meeting the nutritional requirements of an older person who does not eat (use Online Learning Activities 18-3 and 18-6 in Chapter 18 to explore information about this topic).

When elder abuse is rooted in caregiver stress, nurses can suggest services and help find ways of providing care so that the caregiver can use these resources for self-care. The following are examples of services aimed at reducing caregiver stress or dealing with caregiver problems:

- Local Alzheimer Society chapters for support and education groups
- Individual counselling to learn coping skills
- Alcoholics Anonymous for caregivers with alcoholism
- In-home or day care for respite

Home care aides and paid companions are the service providers who are most likely to care for abused older adults in home settings, but they often are ill prepared to detect or address elder abuse. Nurses who provide home-based services, therefore, have a tremendous responsibility to help home care workers recognize and intervene in elder abuse situations. For example, nurses can teach about detecting clues to elder abuse, and they can address concerns about questionable conditions. If nurses cannot openly discuss the situation during home visits, they may have to arrange for a phone conversation with the home care worker. In situations in which the older adult requires a significant degree of physical care or supervision, the services of home care workers may be effective for addressing situations of actual or potential elder abuse. Often, however, the retention of a home care worker in challenging situations depends largely on the degree of support and guidance provided by a professional nurse.

Nurses in other community settings, such as clinics or senior centres, have opportunities to intervene in elder abuse. For example, parish nurses may be the only contact for older adults who neglect themselves or care for a dependent spouse and are not aware of the many resources to address their needs. Nurses can prevent or alleviate elder abuse by facilitating referrals for appropriate community-based resources, such as adult day care or group or home-delivered meals. Even if nurses are not familiar with specific community services, they can discuss the advantages of various types of services and encourage older adults to call their local health agency or seniors' centre. At a minimum, nurses need to be familiar with the phone number for the police or jurisdictional reporting line.

Wellness Opportunity

Nurses help caregivers maintain self-wellness by identifying ways of alleviating stress associated with the demands of caregiving.

Interventions in Interprofessional Teams

Nurses serve as essential members of interprofessional teams (also called interdisciplinary teams) that are responsible for initial and ongoing assessment and implementation of plans to address complex elder abuse situations. Interprofessional teams for elder abuse generally include professionals who offer the perspectives of law, nursing, medicine, psychiatry, social work and rehabilitation therapy, with additional disciplines included when required. When legal interventions are being considered, the interprofessional team conducts a comprehensive assessment, including all aspects of the person's functioning and decision-making capacity, the involvement of the family and significant others in meeting basic needs and the ability of the older person to participate in developing a safe and realistic plan of action.

If nurses do not have access to the resources of an interprofessional team, they need to be creative in finding other professionals with whom they can work. For example, when working with homebound older adults, nurses may need to identify resources for an initial and ongoing medical evaluation and care. In some areas of the country, primary care providers are resuming the practice of making home visits. In addition, with the growing demand for home care services,

an increased number of diagnostic tests are performed in the home (e.g., radiography, blood tests, electrocardiography). In many situations, these diagnostic tests are essential for determining whether involuntary care measures are justified. For instance, if the older adult refuses to go out of the home, blood tests or radiography done in the home may provide the evidence needed to determine whether a hospitalization is warranted.

Interprofessional teams provide a holistic perspective, which is essential for thoroughly assessing the problem and determining appropriate solutions. In addition, team members collaborate in handling complex and difficult cases and they can establish effective approaches to elder abuse prevention and treatment (Anetzberger, 2011; Wilson et al., 2011). In recent years, specialized teams have evolved to address particular elder abuse forms or situations, such as older adult hoarding (Koenig et al., 2013) and financial exploitation (Navarro et al., 2012).

Referrals

An important nursing role is to initiate and facilitate referrals for services that improve functioning for the older adult and decrease the burden of caregiving responsibilities. For instance, speech, physical and occupational therapies may be useful in improving the older person's ability to communicate, ambulate and perform ADLs. Referrals for skilled home care services are usually made at the time of discharge from an institution; however, the older adult or family may have refused the services at that time. Older adults who are not admitted to health care facilities may not know they qualify for skilled home care services, and a nurse making a home visit may be the first health professional to suggest these resources. Although older adults or their families may not know about or may have refused such services, nurses need to assess their willingness to accept help as conditions change.

Nurses also assess whether recent changes in the older adult qualify the person for skilled home care services. For example, a change in medications might qualify a person for skilled nursing care, and a fall might qualify a person for skilled physical therapy. Staffs in home care agencies usually are happy to discuss skilled care services with anyone who calls for information. Nurses also can advise about the possibility of having services covered by health insurance, and they can obtain orders from the primary care provider for those services that are covered under Medicare or health insurance programs (e.g., Blue Cross). Another important role for nurses is suggesting types of medical equipment, disposable supplies and assistive devices to improve function and safety for the older adult and ease caregiver burden. For example, caregivers may respond positively to suggestions from the nurse about obtaining and using grab bars for preventing falls in the bathroom. Some medical equipment is covered by jurisdictional health plans and personal supplemental health insurance, and home care

Prevention and Treatment Interventions

Abused older adults and their caregivers or abusers typically need a wide range of interventions, which can be categorized according to basic function:

- Core, or essential, integrative services
- Emergency services, during crises or just before or after abuse or neglect occurs
- Support services for managing the problem and improving the situation
- Rehabilitative services to address problems of either the victim or the perpetrator
- Preventive services, including programs directed toward changing society in ways that diminish the likelihood of mistreatment or self-neglect

Figure 10-2 identifies some of the specific types of services, arranged by function that may be needed in elder abuse situations. Nurses are the health care professionals who are most accepted and qualified for implementing or arranging for many of the services for both the caregivers and abused or neglected older person(s).

Financial exploitation is an aspect of elder abuse that can be prevented through relatively simple and widely available measures to protect assets. For example, nurses can suggest that a trusted family member establishes a joint account with the older adult and keep track of all transactions. Out-of-town families can oversee financial transactions through online banking.

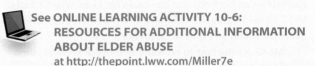
See **ONLINE LEARNING ACTIVITY 10-6:**
RESOURCES FOR ADDITIONAL INFORMATION
ABOUT ELDER ABUSE
at http://thepoint.lww.com/Miller7e

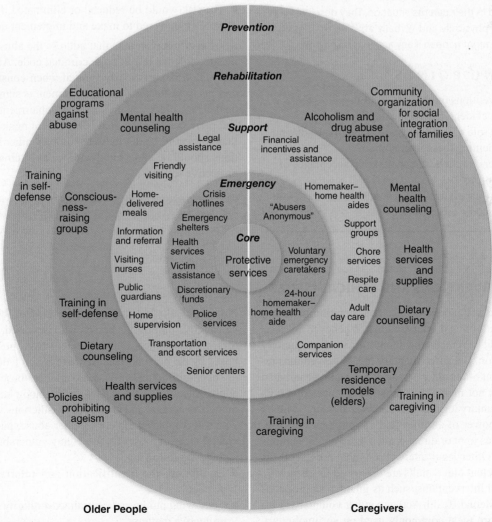

FIGURE 10-2 Types of services needed by abused older adults and their caregivers. (Used with permission from Anetzberger, G. J. [2010]. *Report of the Elder Abuse Project: Recommendations for addressing the problem of elder abuse in Cuyahoga County.* Cleveland, OH: Federation for Community Planning. Originally published in 1982.)

Case Study

Mr. and Mrs. G. have been married for more than 50 years and have six children, four of whom live in their area. Because of Mrs. G.'s memory loss in recent years, Mr. G. has allowed home care workers into the house to assist with activities of daily living and provide care at night because she does not sleep much. The workers report that Mr. G. yells at his wife when she forgets things. On more than one occasion, they witnessed him attempting to force feed her when she failed to eat an entire meal. When the couple is in their bedroom, workers have reported hearing screams, crying and slapping sounds coming from behind the closed door. In the morning, Mrs. G. had bruises on her body and bumps on her head. When asked, Mr. G. denied hitting his wife. Mrs. G. cried when questioned, never providing an explanation for her injuries.

Mr. G. is reluctant to consider additional services, such as adult day care, fearing that the couple's savings will evaporate. He had Mrs. G. change doctors several times in recent years because "they don't do anything to really help her." The children who live nearby have said that they do not want to get involved in their parents' situation. They describe years of their father physically and verbally abusing their mother and fear what might happen if any action is taken now.

THINKING POINTS

- What interventions might be helpful in addressing the elder abuse evident in this situation?
- What is the role of the home care nurse in introducing and implementing these interventions?
- What barriers might be encountered in acceptance of the interventions?
- As the home care nurse in this situation, how will you help to overcome these barriers?

LEGAL INTERVENTIONS AND ETHICAL ISSUES

Most elder abuse situations require consideration of voluntary or involuntary legal interventions. Whenever feasible, problems should be remedied without the use of involuntary legal intervention. Because voluntary legal interventions require the consent of the older person, they cannot be initiated if the person is not mentally competent. Competent adults can revoke voluntary legal interventions at any time. Money management, power of attorney and various types of bank accounts, such as joint or direct deposit, are all interventions of this nature. Other legal interventions that are useful for mentally competent older adults are discussed in Chapter 9.

Some legal interventions, such as guardianship or civil commitment (Mental Health Act), are either voluntary or involuntary but are most commonly used on an involuntary basis when the older person's safety or property is in jeopardy. Because these legal interventions involve a much more extensive loss of personal freedom than do voluntary ones, they should be used with extreme caution. A key consideration in the choice of legal interventions is determining the competency of the person to make decisions, as discussed in Chapters 9 and 13. Some measures, such as guardianship, may be easier to initiate than to discontinue. Others, such as civil commitment (involuntary hospitalization under the Mental Health Act), may be accompanied by long-term stigma, even when the intervention is terminated.

Involuntary legal interventions are used when mental impairments, such as limited insight, judgment, memory or cognition, affect the ability of older people to function safely and meet their basic human needs. In general, involuntary legal intervention is indicated when assessment reveals all of the following conditions:

- Decisions must be made about the older person's health, living arrangements, money or property.
- The older person is not capable of making reasonable decisions.
- There is a risk to the older person's health, safety, money or property.
- The risk would be reduced or eliminated if someone else were empowered to make and implement decisions.

Legal interventions that address the abuser include domestic violence law and the criminal code. Adult protective legislation is particularly limited when considerable property needs protection, the mistreatment is significant and repeated, the older person's mental impairment is substantial and permanent, or the goal is to prevent mistreatment rather than to treat it. Under these conditions, other legal interventions should be considered with, or as alternatives to, adult protective services.

Wellness Opportunity

Nurses support autonomy for older adults by identifying the least invasive legal interventions, while also ensuring the least amount of endangerment.

Adult Protective Services

Philosophically, **adult protective services legislation** provides protection for the person who is abused, for the person offering assistance and for society from possible dangers posed by the person. Because there are no federal guidelines or specific funding, provisions of elder abuse reporting and adult protective services laws differ among jurisdictions. Although provincial and territorial jurisdictions vary in dealing with the complex problem of elder abuse, purposes of provincial/territorial laws for protecting vulnerable older people include the following:

- Facilitating the identification and referral of abuse or neglect
- Conveying public and centralized authority for addressing protective matters
- Establishing a system of protective services to prevent, correct or discontinue abuse or neglect

- Permitting, under certain circumstances, involuntary access to the suspected victim of abuse for the purpose of investigation and service delivery

Usually, local departments of health receive reports of abuse, but in some jurisdictions, police officers receive them.

The scope of reports includes neglect, exploitation, and physical, sexual and psychological abuse. In several provinces/jurisdictions, laws include abandonment and cruel punishment. In most provinces/territories, reporting suspected abuse is mandatory for health, social service and safety professionals and paraprofessionals. Most laws protect the confidentiality of reports and the identity of all people involved in making them. The typical penalty for failure to report is a charge of a misdemeanour, with or without financial penalty. In some provinces/territories, however, failure to report can result in civil liability for damages or notification of the provincial licensing board.

The public authority responsible for implementation must investigate promptly; sometimes, the law mandates a response within 24 to 72 hours. Investigation generally includes a home visit with the alleged victim and consultation with people knowledgeable about the situation. Interventions for at-risk older people can include health care, support services, protective placement, emergency care or financial management. Most laws emphasize due process, self-determination, least restrictive interventions and voluntary acceptance of services by mentally competent adults. Although protective service workers have the primary responsibility for implementing elder abuse laws, nurses have essential roles in reporting and collaborating, assessing, consulting, testifying in court and providing care. Nursing responsibilities associated with each of these roles are discussed in the next sections.

Reporting and Collaborating

Nurses are the health care workers most commonly identified as mandatory reporters in adult abuse and protective services laws. This is appropriate because the usual duties assumed by nurses place them in a key position for witnessing the consequences of abuse and neglect. In addition, a primary role of nurses is to foster collaboration between health care professionals as abuse reporters and adult protective service or law enforcement officials as abuse investigators or service providers.

Mandatory reporting laws do not require reporters to *know* whether abuse or neglect has occurred, but merely to report it if they *suspect* its occurrence. The responsibility for problem verification rests with the public agency charged with law implementation, not with the reporter or referral source. Suspecting elder abuse means detecting signs of violence, such as bruises, welts or fractures. It also means recognizing conditions associated with neglect or deprivation, such as frostbite, malnutrition, dehydration, oversedation, mental changes or uncontrolled medical conditions.

Because most reporting laws provide immunity for mandatory reporters, nurses who act in good faith and without malicious intent can report suspected cases without fear of liability. Some laws offer immunity in the workplace; in these cases, nurses cannot be fired, transferred or demoted for making a report. In all jurisdictions, responsibility for making the report rests with the individual nurse, so nurses cannot delegate reporting to anyone else. The nurse alone has the responsibility for reporting, and for the consequences—both legal and moral—of failing to do so. Even though individual nurses are responsible for reporting, most agencies and hospitals have established protocols to clarify roles and enhance the credibility of the report. Excellent examples of elder abuse detection protocols are available, and they should be considered for use by nurses in all health care settings involving multiple professions and levels of authority. Box 10-5 illustrates a typical protocol for hospital- or agency-based nurses.

Assessing

Protective service workers often call upon nurses to assess their older adults, especially when there is concern about endangerment or questions about the effects of neglect or abuse. Nurses commonly are involved with assessments of older adults who are newly referred or experiencing a change in health status. Nurses are the preferred health care worker for such assessments because of their holistic approach, their availability through nursing agencies, their willingness to make home visits and the relative ease with which older people usually accept nurses.

Because assessment was discussed earlier in this chapter, only one aspect requires further examination here. Formal elder abuse assessment instruments are used to collect and organize all pertinent information, summarize observations and provide a base for planning referrals, services or

---

Box 10-5 Sample Protocol for Nurses With Regard to Elder Abuse

Assessment

- Use usual assessment forms and observe for clues to elder abuse.
- If there is reason for suspicion, use a formal elder abuse assessment tool.
- Observe and interview caregivers and caregiver–older adult interactions.
- Analyze data that raise a suspicion of abuse, neglect or exploitation.
- Consider whether objective findings fit the explanation.

If Abuse and/or Neglect Are Suspected, Consult the Abuse Detection Team

- Report pertinent findings to the team leader and the primary care provider as soon as possible.
- Summarize findings from the assessment guide on progress notes.
- Determine the need to report abuse or neglect to authorities.
- Document additional facts, and whether a report was made, in the progress notes.
- Document discussions with the older adult and caregivers.

Follow-up Actions

- Summarize action steps taken and recommended by team.
- Implement any security measures to protect the older adult.
- Implement appropriate interventions.

legal actions. These tools assess and document all of the following:

- Background data (e.g., older adult's name and address)
- Signs of mistreatment or self-neglect according to type (e.g., bruises or welts in cases of suspected physical abuse)
- Severity of signs (e.g., an immediate life threat)
- Indicators of mistreatment intentionality (e.g., a caregiver who will not allow the nurse to be alone with the older adult)
- Symptoms of acute or chronic illness or impairment (e.g., incontinence)
- Functional incapacity (e.g., an inability to dress or toilet without assistance)
- Aggravating social conditions (e.g., an older adult who lives alone and is socially isolated)
- Source of information (e.g., agency referral)
- Recommended action (e.g., referral of the case to home care service providers)

Online Learning Activity 10-5 provides links to evidence-based assessment tools and guidelines related to elder abuse.

Consulting

In addition to providing direct assessment, nurses often provide consultation when questions arise regarding the health status of older adults. Typical questions relate to medications, continence, nutrition and hydration, and disease signs. Often, consultation services are part of networks among service providers in a given community. Sometimes, they are formally organized through clinical consultation teams that are integral parts of protective services coalitions. Another role for nurses is in staff education for protective services workers on topics such as health assessment, recognition of endangerment and disease prevention and detection.

Testifying in Court

Although very few cases of elder abuse involve court actions, adult protective service workers may need legal assistance to gain access, deliver services or obtain a comprehensive assessment. In these situations, the older person usually is mentally impaired and unable to make decisions that would alleviate or eliminate the neglect or abuse. Legal intervention may also be appropriate when older adults in life-endangering circumstances refuse help. Before legal interventions are permitted, the protective service worker must present evidence to a judge or referee about all of the following:

- Abuse or neglect
- Need for protective services
- Inability to gain voluntary cooperation
- No other way to alleviate the problems

Most of the evidence is provided by physicians, mental health providers and protective service workers; however, nurses are sometimes asked to testify or submit reports about their assessments or services.

Testimony involves two types of evidence: direct observation and expert opinion. Nurses may be called upon to provide in-person testimony about their direct observations because they can provide a professional assessment of the health status or function of the older person. In addition, nursing documentation about assessments and care plans may be used as evidence in court proceedings. Thus, nurses need to carefully, accurately and objectively document all pertinent information with the understanding that their documentation may be used in legal proceedings.

Providing Care

As discussed in the nursing interventions section of this chapter, nurses provide essential care and treatment for abused and neglected older people. They help correct conditions caused by mistreatment and self-neglect, and they prevent their recurrence through such activities as treating injuries, monitoring medication, educating caregivers, obtaining assistive devices and facilitating service referrals. In this role, as in others, nurses work cooperatively with other professionals and with paraprofessionals and use their knowledge and expertise to help the victims of elder abuse.

Ethical Issues

Ethical issues related to abused and neglected older adults are similar to ethical issues in medicine and other fields. Rather than having clear answers and absolute rights and wrongs, there are usually differing perspectives and different implications, depending on what course of action is taken. Law, community pressures and personal concepts of professionalism lead to the erroneous assumption that a problem, such as mistreatment or self-neglect, can be easily or simply resolved. Protective situations involving older people are rarely easily resolved.

Surrounding ethical issues in adult protective services is the fact that all adults in Canadian society have rights—including freedom from intrusion, the right to fair treatment, freedom from unnecessary restraint and the right to self-determination—but these rights can be taken away through the use of legal measures. Professionals often face a dilemma when they need to initiate legal measures that take away the rights of other adults. For example, unless an older adult has been judged to be incompetent by a court of law, he or she has the right to be protected from intrusion, even by well-intentioned professionals. In adult protective service situations, this right is threatened and services can be imposed on an older person who does not willingly agree to assistance.

Another dilemma involves the characteristics of protective situations that sometimes make respecting personal rights so difficult. The following are examples of situations that present ethical dilemmas in relation to respecting personal rights:

- In situations that are urgent or dangerous, it is hard to walk away, even when the older person asks to be left alone.
- Public pressure to do something, no matter what, places pressure on care providers who are trying to resolve the situation while respecting the rights of the older person.

- Contradictory societal values may pit individual rights against other values, such as paternalism and protectionism.
- Because nursing is directed toward helping others, it is difficult to deal with vulnerable older adults who do not accept help, especially when the lack of help has detrimental consequences.
- It may be necessary to make a serious decision based on little information because the older adult may be cognitively impaired, the situation may require immediate actions or pertinent information may be withheld by the older person or the caregivers.
- The questionable mental status of many abused or neglected older adults places decision-making responsibility in the hands of other people. Involuntary legal interventions may unnecessarily deprive the person of certain rights, but inaction can mean that basic human needs are not being met adequately, or at all.
- The intrusive nature of legal interventions, including mandatory reporting, can deprive people of their fundamental rights.

Nurses can apply the hierarchy of principles summarized in Box 10-6 to address ethical dilemmas about particular situations. These principles of adult protective services are arranged from the most to the least important considerations

---

Box 10-6 Hierarchy of Principles of Adult Protective Services

I. *Freedom Over Safety:* The older adults has a right to choose to live at risk of harm, provided she or he is capable of making that choice, harms no one and commits no crime.

II. *Self-Determination:* The older adult has a right to personal choices and decisions until such time that she or he delegates, or the court grants, the responsibility to someone else.

III. *Participation in Decision Making:* The older adult has a right to receive information to make informed choices and to participate in all decisions affecting her or his circumstances to the extent that she or he is able.

IV. *Least Restrictive Alternative:* The older adult has a right to service alternatives that maximize choice and minimize lifestyle disruption.

V. *Primacy of the Adult:* The practitioner's primary responsibility is to serve the older adult, not anyone else (e.g., community people concerned about appearances or a family member concerned about finances).

VI. *Confidentiality:* The older adult has a right to privacy and confidentiality.

VII. *Benefit of Doubt:* If there is evidence that the older adult is making a reasoned choice, the practitioner has a responsibility to assure that the benefit of doubt is in her or his favor.

VIII. *Do No Harm:* The practitioner has a responsibility to take no action that places the older adult at greater risk of harm.

IX. *Avoidance of Blame:* The practitioner has a responsibility to understand the origins of any mistreatment and to commit no action that would antagonize the perpetrator and so reduce the chances of terminating the mistreatment.

X. *Maintenance of the Family:* If the perpetrator is a family member, the practitioner has a responsibility to deal with the mistreatment as a family problem and to try to find appropriate services to resolve the problem.

---

with regard to interventions for abused or neglected older adults.

Adult protective services are fraught with ethical dilemmas. Some of these dilemmas are related to the five basic roles—reporter, investigator, service provider, administrator and planner—assumed by professionals. Each role has a particular sphere of responsibility in addressing elder abuse and neglect. The reporter detects the situation and describes it to someone authorized by law to deal with it. The investigator is the legal agent who assesses the situation and determines the need for protective services. The service provider offers interventions for correcting or discontinuing mistreatment or self-neglect. The administrator manages a protective services program. Finally, the planner develops policies and programs, as well as community education initiatives, aimed at preventing or treating the problem.

Professional workers in each of these roles face different ethical issues. Issues of the reporter role include questions about making a report and the consequences of doing so. The role of the investigator involves confronting questions about privacy, openness and confidentiality. The service provider deals with issues about the rights of the older adult, the rights of the caregivers and the degree of risk for the older person. Program planners and administrators face dilemmas about service priorities and funding, staff and other critical resources. Nurses most often deal with ethical issues in their roles as reporters, investigators and service providers. Table 10-2 identifies some of the ethical problems, as well as related solutions, that nurses may encounter in their roles in adult protective services.

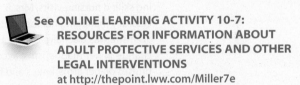

See ONLINE LEARNING ACTIVITY 10-7: RESOURCES FOR INFORMATION ABOUT ADULT PROTECTIVE SERVICES AND OTHER LEGAL INTERVENTIONS at http://thepoint.lww.com/Miller7e

EVALUATING EFFECTIVENESS OF NURSING INTERVENTIONS

Nursing care of abused or neglected older adults is evaluated by the extent to which nursing goals are achieved. If a nursing goal is to alleviate the contributing factor of unnecessary dependence, the care is evaluated by whether the older adult is functioning at a higher level of independence. If a nursing goal is to address caregiver stress, the nursing care might be evaluated by the caregiver accepting help with the care, attending caregiver support groups and expressing less stress about his or her caregiving responsibilities. When the nursing goal is to protect an incompetent older adult from harm, nursing care might be evaluated by the extent to which the least restrictive legal interventions are implemented. In such cases, nursing care is evaluated in terms of protecting the older adult from harm while also protecting his or her rights.

TABLE 10-2 Ethical Questions and Suggested Solutions Regarding Abused Elders

Ethical Question/Implications	Suggested Solution
When do I report elder abuse? (If I report too soon, I may needlessly invade someone's privacy. If I wait, the situation may worsen.)	Report elder abuse when you believe that, without intervention, the situation will deteriorate or endanger the elder.
What if my report places the elder in more danger, or labels someone inaccurately? What if it causes the elder to shy away from me and my agency?	Report elder abuse if you believe that the protective services system can reduce the risk better than the current interventions.
How do I decide if the elder or the caregiver receives priority? (If my priority is the elder, I may alienate his or her family members, who serve as the primary sources of care. If my priority is the family, then the care plan may be contrary to the elder's wishes and may not adequately respect his or her rights.)	With certain exceptions, the elder should receive priority. These exceptions are limited to circumstances in which the elder has been judged to be incompetent by a court of law or is endangering others by his or her behaviour.
Is it more important to maintain standards of confidentiality than to comply with a reporting law?	Provincial/territorial law takes precedence over professional standards.
Does the right of an elder to refuse services extend to total self-neglect and intentional suicide? How can I know that endangered elders clearly understand the consequences of their self-neglect? How can I accept abandoning the situation?	Ethical dilemmas such as these often can be resolved through the use of a hierarchy of values or principles, such as those summarized in Box 10-6.
Can emergency services be thrust upon an elder who would have refused them under ordinary circumstances? If the elder's life is endangered, then is it not my primary responsibility to use my nursing skills in life-saving ways, no matter what the elder chooses? Even if the elder might have refused services in the past, does that mean he or she absolutely would refuse them now?	If the elder is incapable of deciding whether to accept or reject emergency services, then these services should be provided, subject to the constraints of the protective services law. This offers the elder essential protection, but recognizes his or her right to refuse ongoing services when the emergency has subsided and he or she is capable of making decisions on his or her own behalf.

Unfolding Case Study

Part 2: Mrs. B. at 82 Years, 2 Months of Age

Recall that Mrs. B. is 82 years old and lives in a senior citizens apartment. After 2 months of receiving skilled nursing visits, Mrs. B. was discharged from the home care agency because she was successfully managing her medications and other aspects of functioning adequately. Several months after she was discharged, the nurse in the wellness clinic at the senior citizens apartment noted a change in her mannerisms, accompanied by slurred speech and an unbalanced gait. Mrs. B. had bruises on her arms, knees and forehead, but insisted that she had not fallen. After further investigation, the nurse found that her blood pressure was 210/104 mm Hg and that her blood glucose level was 22.5 mg/dL on the glucometer that the nurse kept in the clinic. A pill count revealed that Mrs. B. had not taken her medications for 2½ days. After a consultation with her primary care provider, Mrs. B. was admitted to the hospital. Tests revealed that she had suffered a stroke, resulting in left-sided weakness and short-term memory loss.

Mrs. B. left the hospital against medical advice and returned to her apartment, initially refusing visits from the home care nurse. She insisted that her children come and administer her medications and prepare her meals because she was unable to do this for herself. Mrs. B. reasoned that she had cared for her children when they were young, so they should come when she needed them. The children tried to assist Mrs. B. for 4 days but were unable to meet both her demands and those of their jobs and families. Mrs. B. reluctantly agreed to a visit from the home care nurse who had visited her before. She expected that she would see the nurse once and that the nurse would "make my children do right."

Mrs. B.'s children were present for the initial assessment. Mrs. B. was unable to stand or transfer to the commode without help. She could not use her chart and colour-coded boxes to take her pills. Mrs. B. flatly refused to consider admission to a rehabilitation unit to receive therapy to regain her strength, and she would not consider living with her daughter or either son. The family told the nurse that they were exhausted and on the "verge of a breakdown" and could not continue to provide the care that Mrs. B. needed. The nurse explained to Mrs. B. that it was not safe for her to remain in her apartment without assistance. She suggested that she hire an aide until other arrangements could be made because her children were not obligated to lose their jobs or jeopardize their family relationships to care for her. Mrs. B. accused her children of being greedy and caring only about themselves. She said that children have a duty to care for their parents and that she wasn't going to "have strangers doing the things that decent children should be doing." She directed her concluding remarks at the nurse, stating, "What's more, I don't need you to come back either, because all you want to do is side with my children."

THINKING POINTS

- What strategies would you use to establish a relationship with Mrs. B.?
- What additional assessment information would you want to obtain, and how would you obtain it?
- What would your next steps be in working with Mrs. B.?

- How would you work with the family?
- What other resources would you involve in planning and providing care for Mrs. B.?
- What criteria would you use for making a referral for adult protective services?

Chapter Highlights

Overview of Elder Abuse and Neglect

- Major forms of elder abuse include physical abuse, sexual abuse, emotional or psychological abuse, neglect, abandonment, financial or material exploitation and self-neglect.
- Awareness of elder abuse is widely recognized as a major social and public health problem that has serious consequences for older adults.
- Studies of causes of elder abuse indicate that it differs from other forms of abuse and is complex (Box 10-2).
- Cultural differences in family and caregiver roles affect definitions of elder abuse (Box 10-3).

Risk Factors for Elder Abuse and Neglect

- Elder abuse is usually related to multiple risk factors that develop over a long period.
- Invisibility and vulnerability are two risk factors that occur in most situations of abuse or neglect.
- Common psychosocial risk factors: impaired cognition, long-term mental illness, social isolation, depression
- Caregiver factors: stress, poor health, cognitive impairment, substance abuse, personality characteristics

Elder Abuse and Neglect in Nursing Homes

- Elder abuse is recognized as a problem in nursing homes, and studies indicate that it is widespread and underreported in all types of long-term care residential facilities.

Functional Consequences Associated With Elder Abuse and Neglect

- Definitions and examples of neglect: physical abuse, sexual abuse, emotional or psychological abuse, abandonment, self-neglect
- Domestic violence and sexual abuse are types of elder abuse with unique characteristics.

Nursing Assessment of Abused or Neglected Older Adults

- Unique aspects of elder abuse assessment: safety, limited goals, resistance, nurse viewed as threat, legal and ethical considerations, safety of nurse
- Physical health assessment: nutrition, hydration, indicators of physical harm (Fig. 10-1), degree of frailty, pathologic conditions
- Assessment of functional abilities in relation to safety, basic needs and vulnerability (Table 10-1)
- Psychosocial function: impaired cognition, ability to make safe decisions about personal safety and self-care
- Support resources: caregivers who also are perpetrators, actual and potential resources, barriers to using services
- Environmental influences: home, neighbourhood, seasonal factors
- Threats to life: degree of endangerment and ability to alleviate risks
- Cultural aspects: family and cultural expectations, perspectives on caregiving, barriers to assessment (Box 10-4)

Nursing Diagnosis

- Compromised (or Disabled) Family Coping
- Caregiver Role Strain (or Risk for)
- Risk for Injury
- Decisional Conflict

Planning for Wellness Outcomes

- Quality of Life
- Abuse Cessation, Protection, Recovery
- Neglect Cessation
- Caregiver Stressors, Emotional Health
- Family Coping
- Social Support

Nursing Interventions to Address Elder Abuse and Neglect

- Role of the nurse in institutional settings: teaching caregivers, discharge planning, addressing caregiver stress
- Role of the nurse in community settings: teaching, supervising, providing direct care, working with home care aides, facilitating referrals
- Role of the nurse on interprofessional teams
- Facilitating referrals (services for older adults and caregivers, medical equipment)
- Prevention and treatment interventions (types of core services, programs for preventing financial abuse; Fig. 10-2)

Legal Interventions and Ethical Issues

- Voluntary and involuntary types of legal interventions
- Roles of nurses in adult protective services: reporting and collaborating, assessing, consulting, testifying in court, providing care (Box 10-5)
- Ethical issues: principles of adult protective services (Box 10-6)
- Ethical questions and suggested solutions (Table 10-2)

Evaluating Effectiveness of Nursing Interventions

- Higher level of functioning of older adult
- Alleviation of caregiver stress
- Use of least restrictive legal interventions
- Protection of the older adult

Critical Thinking Exercises

1. Identify factors in each of the following categories that currently contribute to elder abuse and neglect in Canada:
   - Demographic statistics
   - Changes in families
   - Health care systems
   - Health status and other characteristics of older adults
   - Social awareness
2. What is different about the nursing assessment of abused or neglected older adults compared with the nursing assessment of other older adults?
3. What do you believe about family caregiving responsibilities? How would you deal with a family whose values about caregiving differ significantly from yours?
4. What are your beliefs about the degree of risk a frail older adult should be allowed to take?
5. Under what circumstances should an older adult be denied the right to remain in his or her own home?

For more information about the topics discussed in this chapter, be sure to check out the interactive Online Learning Activities and other helpful resources at http://thepoint.lww.com/Miller7e

REFERENCES

Aging and the Law in Canada. (n.d.). Retrieved from http://www.canadi-anelderlaw.ca/Senior%20Abuse.htm

Anetzberger, G. J. (2011). The evolution of an interdisciplinary response to elder abuse. *Marquette Elder's Advisor*, 13(1), 107–128.

Anetzberger, G. J. (2012). An update on the nature and scope of elder abuse. *Generations*, 36(3), 12–30.

Anetzberger, G. J. (2013). Elder abuse: Risk. In A. Jamieson & A. A. Moenseens (Eds.), *Wiley encyclopedia of forensic science*. Chichester, England: John Wiley.

Anisko, B. (2009). Elder abuse in American Indian communities. *American Indian Culture and Research Journal*, 33, 43–51.

Biggs, S., Manthorpe, J., Tinker, A., et al. (2009). Mistreatment of older people in the United Kingdom: Findings from the first national prevalence study. *Journal of Elder Abuse & Neglect*, 21(1), 1–14.

Bond, M. C., & Butler, K. H. (2013). Elder abuse and neglect: Definitions, epidemiology, and approaches to emergency department screening. *Clinical Geriatric Medicine*, 29, 257–273.

Burston, G. R. (1975). Granny-battering, *British Medical Journal*, 3(5983), 592.

Castle, N. (2012a). Nurse aides' reports of resident abuse in nursing homes. *Journal of Applied Gerontology*, 31(3), 402–422.

Castle, N. (2012b). Resident-to-resident abuse in nursing homes as reported by nurses aides. *Journal of Elder Abuse & Neglect*, 24(4), 340–356.

Connolly, M.-T., Breckman, R., Callahan, J., et al. (2012). The sexual revolution's last frontier: How silence about sex undermines health, well-being, and safety in old age. *Generations, Journal of the American Society on Aging*, 36(3), 43–52.

Conrad, K. J., Iris, M., Ridings, J. W., et al. (2011a). Conceptual model and map of psychological abuse of older adults. *Journal of Elder Abuse & Neglect*, 23(2), 147–168.

Conrad, K. J., Ridings, J. W., Iris, M., et al. (2011b). Conceptual model and map of financial exploitation of older adults. *Journal of Elder Abuse & Neglect*, 23(4), 304–325.

Day, M. R., Leahy-Warren, P., & McCarthy, G. (2013). Perceptions and views of self-neglect: A older adult-centered perspective. *Journal of Elder Abuse & Neglect*, 25(1), 76–94.

Day, M. R., McCarthy, G., & Leahy-Warren, P. (2012). Professional social workers' views on self-neglect: An exploratory study. *British Journal of Social Work*, 42(4), 725–743.

Daykin, E., & Pearlmutter, S. (2009). Older women's perceptions of elder mistreatment and ethical dilemmas in adult protective services: A cross-cultural, exploratory study. *Journal of Elder Abuse & Neglect*, 21, 15–57.

DeDonder, L., Lang, G., Luoma, M.-L., et al. (2011). Perpetrators of abuse against older women: A multi-national study in Europe. *Journal of Adult Protection*, 13(6), 302–314.

DeHart, D., Webb, J., & Cornman, C. (2009). Prevention of elder mistreatment in nursing homes: Competencies for direct-care staff. *Journal of Elder Abuse & Neglect*, 21(4), 360–378.

DeLiema, M., Gassoumis, Z., Homeier, D., et al. (2012). Determining prevalence and correlates of elder abuse using promotores: Low income immigrant Latinos report high rates of abuse and neglect. *Journal of the American Geriatrics Society*, 60(7), 1333–1339.

Dong, X., Simon, M., & Evans, D. (2012). Elder self-neglect and hospitalization: Findings from the Chicago Health and Aging Project. *Journal of the American Geriatrics Society*, 60(2), 202–209.

Dow, B., & Joosten, M. (2012). Understanding elder abuse: A social rights perspective. *International Psychogeriatrics*, 24(6), 853–855.

Erlingsson, C., Ono, M., Sasaki, A., et al. (2012). An international collaborative study comparing Swedish and Japanese nurses' reactions to elder abuse. *Journal of Advanced Nursing*, 68(1), 56–68.

Ernst, J. S., & Smith, C. A. (2011). Adult protective services older adults confirmed for self-neglect: Characteristics and service use. *Journal of Elder Abuse & Neglect*, 23(4), 289–303.

Griffore, R. J., Barboza, G. E., Oehmke, L. B., et al. (2009). Family members' reports of abuse in Michigan nursing homes. *Journal of Elder Abuse and Neglect, 21,* 105–114.

Guruge, S., Kanthasamy, P., Jokajasa, J., et al. (2010). Older women speak about abuse and neglect in the post-migration context. *Women's Health & Urban Life, 9,* 15–41.

Herdman, T. H. (Ed.). (2012). *NANDA international nursing diagnoses: Definitions and classification 2012–1014.* Oxford, England: Wiley-Blackwell.

Hirschel, A., & Anetzberger, G. J. (2012). Evaluating and enhancing federal responses to abuse and neglect in long-term care facilities. *Public Policy & Aging Report, 22*(1), 22–27.

Hudson, M. F. (1991). Elder mistreatment: A taxonomy with definitions by Delphi. *Journal of Elder Abuse & Neglect, 3*(2), 1–20.

Koenig, T. L., Leiste, M. R., Spano, R., et al. (2013). Interdisciplinary team perspectives on older adult hoarding and mental illness. *Journal of Elder Abuse and Neglect, 25*(1), 56–75.

Lachs, M. S., Rosen, T., Teresi, J. A., et al. (2013). Verbal and physical aggression directed at nursing home staff by residents. *Journal of General Internal Medicine, 28*(5), 660–667.

Lai, D. W. L. (2011). Abuse and neglect experienced by aging Chinese in Canada. *Journal of Elder Abuse & Neglect, 23*(4), 326–347.

Lee, H. Y., Lee, S. E., & Eaton, C. K. (2012). Exploring definitions of financial abuse in Korean immigrants: The contribution of traditional cultural values. *Journal of Elder Abuse & Neglect, 24*(4), 293–311. doi:10.1080/08946566.2012.661672

Lowenstein, A., Eisikovits, A., Band-Winterstein, T., et al. (2009). Is elder abuse and neglect a social phenomenon? Data from the first national prevalence survey in Israel. *Journal of Elder Abuse & Neglect, 21*(3), 253–277.

McCool, J. J., Jogerst, G. J., Daly, J. M., et al. (2009). Interdisciplinary reports of nursing home mistreatment. *American Medical Directors Association, 10*(3), 174–180.

McDonald, L., & Thomas, C. (2013). Elder abuse through a life course lens. *International Psychogeriatrics, 25*(8), 1235–1243.

McDonald, L., Beaulieu, M., Harbison, J., et al. (2012). Institutional abuse of older adults: What we know, what we need to know. *Journal of Elder Abuse & Neglect, 24*(2), 138–160.

Melchiorre, M. G., Chiatti, C., Lamura, G., et al. (2013). Social support, socio-economic status, health and abuse among older people in seven European countries. *PLoS ONE, 8*(1), e54856. doi:10.1371/journal.pone.0054856

Miller, M. (2012). Ombudsmen on the front line: Improving quality of care and preventing abuse in nursing homes. *Generations, 36*(3), 60–63.

Mosqueda, L., Burnright, K., & Liao, S. (2005). The life cycle of bruises in older adults. *Journal of the American Geriatrics Society, 53,* 1339–1343.

Mosqueda, L., & Dong, X. (2011). Elder abuse and self-neglect: "I don't care anything about going to the doctor, to be honest…" *Journal of the American Medical Association, 306*(5), 532–540.

Murphy, K., Waa, S., Jaffer, H., et al. (2013). A literature review of findings in physical elder abuse. *Canadian Association of Radiology Journal, 64*(1), 10–14.

National Center on Elder Abuse. (2012). *Research brief: How at risk for abuse are people with dementia?* Retrieved from www.ncea.aoa.gov

National Center on Elder Abuse. (2013). *Research brief: Mistreatment of lesbian, gay, bisexual, and transgender (LBGT) elders.* Retrieved from www.ncea.aoa.gov/Library/Review/Brief/Index.aspx

National Seniors Council. (2007). *Report of the National Seniors Council on Elder Abuse.* Retrieved from http://www.seniorscouncil.gc.ca/eng/research_publications/elder_abuse/2007/hs4_38/hs4_38.pdf

Naughton, C., Drennan, J., Lyons, I., et al. (2012). Elder abuse and neglect in Ireland: Results from a national prevalence survey. *Age & Ageing, 41*(1), 98–103.

Navarro, A. E., Gassoumis, A. D., & Wilber, K. H. (2012). Holding abusers accountable: An elder abuse forensic center increases criminal prosecution of financial exploitation. *The Gerontologist, 53*(2), 303–312.

Newman, F. I., Seff, L. R., Beaulaurier, R. L., et al. (2013). Domestic abuse against elder women and perceived barriers to help-seeking. *Journal of Elder Abuse & Neglect, 25*(3), 205–229.

Payne, B. K. (2010). Understanding elder sexual abuse and the criminal justice system's response: Comparisons to elder physical abuse. *Justice Quarterly, 27,* 206–224.

Pillemer, K., Chen, E. K., Van Haitsma, K. S., et al. (2012). Resident-to-resident aggression in nursing homes: Results from a qualitative event reconstruction study. *The Gerontologist, 52*(10), 24–33.

Ploeg, J., Lohfield, L., & Walsh, C. (2014). What is "elder abuse"? Voices from the margin: The views of underrepresented Canadian women. *Journal of Elder Abuse & Neglect, 25*(5), 396–424. doi:10.1080/08946566.2013.780956

Podnieks, E., Anetzberger, G. J., Wilson, S. J., et al. (2010). Worldview environmental scan on elder abuse. *Journal of Elder Abuse & Neglect, 22*(1–2), 164–179.

Podnieks, E., Pillemer, K., Nicholson, J. P., et al. (1990). *National survey on abuse of the elderly in Canada: The Ryerson study.* Toronto, ON, Canada: Ryerson Polytechnic Institute.

Podnieks, E., Rietschlin, J., & Walsh, C. A. (2012). Introduction: Elder abuse in Canada—Reports from a national roundtable discussion. *Journal of Elder Abuse & Neglect, 24*(2), 85–87.

Ramsey-Klawsnik, H., Teaster, P. B., Mendiondo, M. S., et al. (2008). Sexual predators who target elders: Findings from the first national study of sexual abuse in care facilities. *Journal of Elder Abuse & Neglect, 20,* 353–376.

Roberto, K. A., McCann, B. R., & Brossoie, N. (2013). Intimate partner violence in late life: An analysis of national news reports. *Journal of Elder Abuse & Neglect, 25*(3), 230–241.

Sandmoe, A., Kirkevold, M., & Ballantyne, A. (2011). Challenges in handling elder abuse in community care: An exploratory study among nurses and care coordinators. *Journal of Clinical Nursing, 20*(23–24), 3351–3363.

Schiamberg, L. B., Oehmke, J., Zhang, Z., et al. (2012). Physical abuse of older adults in nursing homes: A random sample of adults with an elder family member in a nursing home. *Journal of Elder Abuse & Neglect, 24*(1), 65–83.

Shankardass, M. K. (2013). Addressing elder abuse: Review of societal responses in India and selected Asian countries. *International Psychogeriatrics, 25*(8), 1229–1234.

Shinan-Altman, S., & Cohen, M. (2009). Nursing aides' attitudes to elder abuse in nursing homes: The effect of work stressors and burnout. *The Gerontologist, 49,* 674–684.

Sooryanarayana, R., Choo, W. H., & Hairi, N. N. (2013). A review of prevalence and measurement of elder abuse in the community. *Trauma Violence & Abuse, 14*(4), 316–325.

Teresi, J. A., Ramirez, M., Ellis, J., et al. (2013). A staff intervention targeting resident-to-resident elder mistreatment in long-term care increased staff knowledge, recognition and reporting: Results from a cluster randomized trial. *International Journal of Nursing Studies, 50*(5), 644–656.

The Ontario Network for the Prevention of Elder Abuse. (n.d.). *Forms of elder abuse.* Retrieved from http://www.onpea.org/english/elderabuse/formsofelderabuse.html

Ulsperger, J. S., & Knottnerus, J. D. (2011). *Elder care catastrophe: Rituals of abuse in nursing homes and what you can do about it.* Boulder, CO: Paradigm.

United Nations Economic and Social Affairs. (2008). *Guide to the national implementation of the Madrid International Plan of Action on Aging.* New York, NY: Author.

Walsh, C. A., Olson, J., Ploeg, J., et al. (2011). Elder abuse and oppression: Voices of marginalized elders. *Journal of Elder Abuse and Neglect, 23*(1), 17–42.

Weeks, L. E., & LeBlanc, K. (2011). An ecological synthesis of research on older women's experiences of intimate partner violence. *Journal of Women & Aging, 23,* 283–304.

Wiglesworth, A., Austin, R., Corona, M., et al. (2009). Bruising as a marker of physical elder abuse. *Journal of the American Geriatrics Society, 57*(7), 1191–1196.

Wiglesworth, A., Mosqueda, L., Mulnard, R., et al. (2010). Screening for abuse and neglect of people with dementia. *Journal of the American Geriatrics Society, 58*, 493–500.

Wilson, D. M., Ratajewicz, S. E., Els, C., et al. (2011). Evidence-based approaches to remedy and also to prevent abuse of community-dwelling older persons. *Nursing Research and Practice, 2011* [Article ID 861484, 5 pages]. doi:10.1155/2011/861484

Wu, L., Chen, H., Hu, Y., et al. (2012). Prevalence and associated factors of elder mistreatment in a rural community in People's Republic of China: A cross-sectional study. *PLoS ONE*, e33857. doi:10.1371/journal.pone.0033857

Zhang, Z., Schiamberg, L. B., Oehmke, J., et al. (2011). Neglect of older adults in Michigan nursing homes. *Journal of Elder Abuse & Neglect, 23*(1), 58–74.

Ziminski, C. E., Wiglesworth, A., Austin, R., et al. (2013). Injury patterns and causal mechanisms of bruising in physical elder abuse. *Journal of Forensic Nursing, 9*(2), 84–91.

part 3

Promoting Wellness in Psychosocial Function

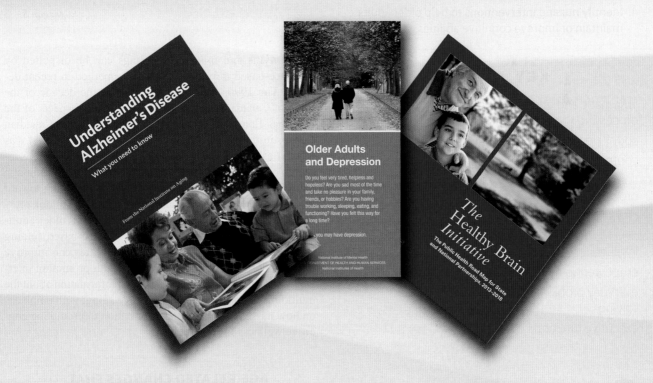

Cognitive Function

LEARNING OBJECTIVES

After reading this chapter, you will be able to:

1. Describe age-related changes that affect cognitive abilities.
2. List risk factors that influence cognitive function in older adults.
3. Discuss the functional consequences associated with cognition in older adults.
4. Identify nursing interventions to help older adults maintain or improve cognitive abilities.

A Student's Perspective

The residents at Heritage continue to amaze me with their stories. There is so much one can learn just by listening, and the residents just want to share their stories and have our company more than anything—at least that is the impression I continually receive from them. They are all friendly, open people who are no different than the rest of us, but they have gained a large amount of knowledge over the years that many of us who are students probably have not acquired yet.

Megan S.

KEY POINTS

automatic and effortful processing theory

cognitive reserve

contextual theories

continuum of processing

crystallized intelligence

developmental intelligence

empowering model

everyday problem solving

executive function

fluid intelligence

memory

metamemory

mild cognitive impairment (MCI)

neuroplasticity

paradox of well-being

scaffolding theory of aging and cognition

socioemotional selectivity

stage theories

wisdom

many myths and misunderstandings can be dispelled by evidence-based information that has emerged in recent decades. The 1990s were considered to be the decade of the brain in Canada. As such, research on many aspects of the brain has flourished. Within the 21st century, the Canadian Consortium on Neurodegeneration in Aging (CCNA) was formed as a research nexus to strengthen collaborative research on Alzheimer disease and other dementias. Although many questions remain unanswered, we are moving toward a better understanding of—and a more positive outlook on—maintaining optimal cognitive function during older adulthood. An exciting and significant evidence-based finding from recent studies is that cognitive abilities can improve throughout older adulthood through health promotion interventions. This chapter presents current information about the multidimensional aspects of cognitive aging, with emphasis on how nurses can apply this information to promoting cognitive wellness for older adults.

Cognition involves many processes, including those involved with thinking, learning and remembering. Myths, such as the one exemplified in the adage "you can't teach an old dog new tricks" are pervasive, long-standing, and detrimental to older adults. Fortunately,

 AGE-RELATED CHANGES THAT AFFECT COGNITION

The first theories about aging and cognition, which were proposed during the 1960s, were based on results of cross-sectional studies using tests designed to predict school

Promoting Cognitive Wellness in Older Adults

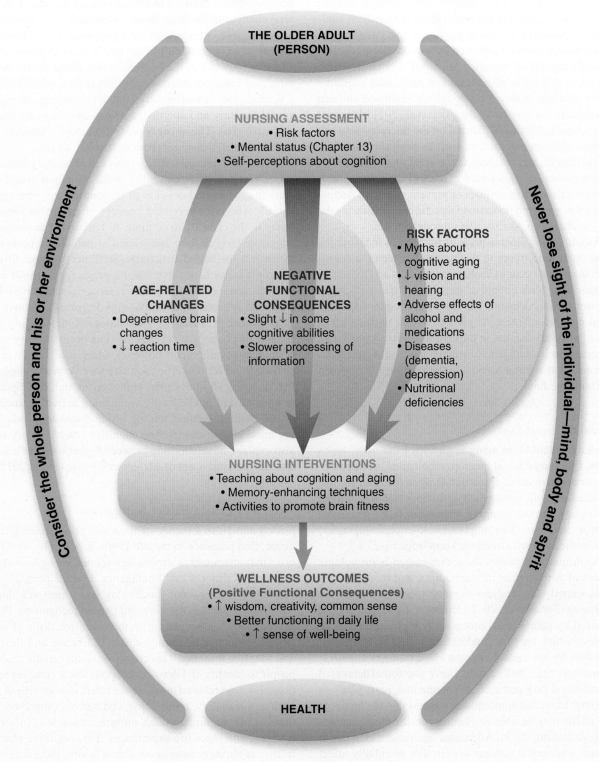

THE OLDER ADULT (PERSON)

NURSING ASSESSMENT
- Risk factors
- Mental status (Chapter 13)
- Self-perceptions about cognition

AGE-RELATED CHANGES
- Degenerative brain changes
- ↓ reaction time

NEGATIVE FUNCTIONAL CONSEQUENCES
- Slight ↓ in some cognitive abilities
- Slower processing of information

RISK FACTORS
- Myths about cognitive aging
- ↓ vision and hearing
- Adverse effects of alcohol and medications
- Diseases (dementia, depression)
- Nutritional deficiencies

NURSING INTERVENTIONS
- Teaching about cognition and aging
- Memory-enhancing techniques
- Activities to promote brain fitness

WELLNESS OUTCOMES
(Positive Functional Consequences)
- ↑ wisdom, creativity, common sense
- Better functioning in daily life
- ↑ sense of well-being

HEALTH

Consider the whole person and his or her environment

Never lose sight of the individual—mind, body and spirit

performance in children. These theories suggested that a global decline in cognitive abilities was a normal and expected part of aging. By the mid-1980s, longitudinal studies pointed toward a decline in peak cognitive development during young adulthood followed by a steady linear decline in specific aspects of cognitive functions. Current research emphasizes that brain maturation and associated cognitive abilities continue to develop throughout adulthood and can be improved even in older adults (Aine et al., 2011). In recent decades, researchers have focused on the interplay between cognitive abilities and factors, such as health, personality, life experiences, and socioeconomic conditions. Gerontologists are particularly interested in identifying interventions that improve cognitive abilities or prevent cognitive decline because it is now well understood that the brain maintains the ability to change in positive ways throughout life.

As with many other aspects of function in older adults, gerontologists are trying to distinguish between the cognitive changes that occur in healthy older adults and those that are associated with cognitive impairment and pathologic processes such as dementia (discussed in Chapter 14). Age-related changes affecting cognition can be understood in terms of physical changes in the central nervous system and in theories about intelligence, memory and psychological development that attempt to explain the relationship between aging and cognition.

Central Nervous System

Knowledge about brain aging is gleaned from many types of data, including clinical, neuropsychological, neuropathologic, neurochemical and neuroimaging investigations. Initial studies of brain aging relied on autopsy findings, but the evolving use of neuroimaging techniques (e.g., functional magnetic resonance imaging, magneto-encephalography) have significantly broadened the knowledge base.

Brain imaging studies show diminished brain volume and loss of white matter in older adults, and these changes are associated with declines in some aspects of cognitive functioning (Farias et al., 2012). However, these changes can be caused by pathological processes (e.g., hypertension or diabetes), which are often undetected in study participants, rather than by age-related changes alone (Aine et al., 2011; Geldmacher et al., 2012). Studies have also found decreased cerebral blood flow and cortical volume loss, particularly in the frontal lobes, but some studies suggest that the brains of older adults may be able to compensate for these changes (Willis & Hakim, 2013). Additional age-related changes in the brain and central nervous system that potentially affect cognitive abilities are reduced brain weight, enlarged ventricles and wider sulci, loss and shrinkage of neurons, reduced neurotransmitters or their binding sites, and accumulation of lipofuscin in nerve cell bodies. Recent studies also focus on age-related changes in brain connectivity that interfere with communication among regions of the brain (Chou et al., 2013; Goh, 2011).

Gerontologists emphasize that because the brain and nervous system continue to develop during adulthood, structural changes in the brain do not necessarily determine cognitive abilities. Researchers have proposed the **scaffolding theory of aging and cognition** as a way of explaining the adaptive response of the brain to the declining neural structures and function. According to this theory, scaffolding is a normal process that involves the development and use of complementary and alternative neural circuits to achieve a cognitive goal. This process protects cognitive abilities despite age-related changes (Park & Bischof, 2011).

The term **neuroplasticity** (also called *neural plasticity*) refers to the physiologic ability of the brain and neural circuits to change and develop in response to environmental stimuli. The closely related concept of **cognitive reserve** refers to the capacity to continue to function at an adequate cognitive level despite age-related or pathologic processes that affect the neural structures (Steffener & Stern, 2012). Neuroplasticity is positive when it promotes neuronal connections and increases cognitive reserve; it is negative when it inhibits neuronal connections and decreases cognitive reserve (Vance et al., 2012). Gerontologists increasingly emphasize that cognitive development can occur at every stage of human development; however, older adults have more challenges to address. The cognitive reserve model suggests that cognitive abilities can be improved through participation in creative and intellectually stimulating activities, such as art, storytelling, reading, writing, group discussions and playing musical instruments. The cognitive reserve theory may also explain the relationship between higher levels of education and delayed onset of Alzheimer disease (Stern, 2012).

Fluid and Crystallized Intelligence

Cattell and Horn's theory of fluid and crystallized intelligence, first proposed in the late 1960s, is one of the first theories that attempted to explain age-related changes in some cognitive abilities. Fluid intelligence depends primarily on central nervous system functioning and a person's inherent abilities, such as memory and pattern recognition. **Fluid intelligence** is associated with the cognitive skills of integration, inductive reasoning, abstract thinking, and flexible and adaptive thinking. This cognitive characteristic enables people to identify and draw conclusions about complex relationships. **Crystallized intelligence** refers to cognitive skills, such as vocabulary, information, and verbal comprehension that people acquire through culture, education, informal learning, and other life experiences. This cognitive characteristic is strongly associated with wisdom, judgment, and life experiences.

According to this theory, fluid and crystallized intelligence develop concurrently during infancy and childhood and are indistinguishable as the central nervous system is maturing. Age-related changes in neural structures cause a decline in fluid intelligence. However, a recent study found that changes in fluid intelligence are more closely associated with pathologic conditions of the circulatory and nervous system than with age-related changes alone (Bergman & Almkvist, 2013). Crystallized intelligence continues to develop during adulthood because of accumulated experiences and learning. Crystallized intelligence, except for those processes that depend on the speed of response, does not decline with age, and it may even increase because of experiences that improve wisdom. Although fluid intelligence is thought to decline with increased age, studies have found that cognitive training activities can improve some components, including memory skills (Gross et al., 2013).

Memory

Memory is often conceptualized as a computer-like information-processing system in which information is first perceived, then stored, and finally retrieved when needed or wanted. *Primary memory* has a short duration and a very small capacity, and it serves as a holding tank for events of the immediate past few seconds rather than as a true memory storage system. Information in the primary memory can be either recalled for a brief time or transmitted to long-term storage. *Secondary memory* has longer duration and, therefore, is more important in terms of retrieval, as well as storage, of information. Retrieval of information from storage is referred to as remote, tertiary, or very-long-term memory processing, and skills involved are classified as *recall memory* and *recognition memory*. Some theories associated with these concepts suggest that older people remember events of long ago better than recent events; however, studies indicate that both types of memory decline equally but older adults have a larger store of information about events of long ago (Botwinick, 1984).

More recently, gerontologists have viewed the information-processing model as too simplistic because it ignores the milieu in which the memory operates. Thus, newer **contextual theories** address variables that can affect memory, including all of the following: health, motivation, expectations, experiences, education, personality, task demands, learning habits, sociocultural background and style of processing information. This theory suggests that memory and other cognitive skills of older adults are better than those of younger adults under some conditions. For example, memory skills in older adults are better when the information is highly interesting, emotionally positive or personally relevant (Stine-Morrow & Basak, 2011).

Another theoretical approach emphasizes encoding and analysing rather than storage and retrieval aspects of memory. According to this perspective, memory is a **continuum of processing**, ranging from shallow to deep levels; the deeper the level at which information is stored, the longer the memory will last. Any of the following variables can affect the depth of storage (Botwinick, 1984):

- Processing techniques, ranging from the shallowest levels used for sensory information to the deepest levels used for highly abstract information

- Elaboration, or quality, of processing conducted at any depth level
- Distinctiveness of the information, which depends partially on how well it is learned
- Depth and elaboration of retrieval processes

This framework suggests that poor memory function in older adults is associated with faulty processing mechanisms.

Another theoretical perspective that views memory as a continuum is the **automatic and effortful processing theory**, which was proposed by Hasher and Zacks (1979). At one end of the continuum is automatic processing, or those tasks that do not require attention or awareness and do not improve with practice. At the other end is effortful processing, or those tasks that demand high levels of attention and cognitive energy. With practice, effortful tasks require less attention and become more automatic. According to this theory, older adults maintain skills related to procedural memory tasks, which require little or no cognitive energy. However, memory tasks that require effortful processes (e.g., selective attention, mental imagery, verbal fluency, language production) decline in older adults (Hayes et al., 2013).

Metamemory refers to self-knowledge and perceptions about memory, cognitive function and development of memory. Metamemory is important in everyday activities because if people know what they can remember and how much effort they will need to remember certain things, they can plan efficient and effective strategies for remembering. Because older adults tend to perceive themselves as less competent than younger adults or less competent than they actually are in many cognitive tasks, gerontologists emphasize the importance of addressing ageist attitudes that contribute to negative self-stereotypes about cognitive abilities (Hummert, 2011).

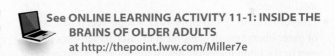

See ONLINE LEARNING ACTIVITY 11-1: INSIDE THE BRAINS OF OLDER ADULTS at http://thepoint.lww.com/Miller7e

> **Wellness Opportunity**
>
> Nurses can influence societal attitudes by conveying positive beliefs about the ability of older adults to improve memory skills.

Adult Psychological Development

Theories about psychological development postulate that the thinking of older adults becomes increasingly complex and shows progressive reorganization of intellectual skills (Labouvie-Vief & Blanchard-Fields, 1982). For example, a recent focus of these theories is on cognitive abilities associated with decision-making and **everyday problem solving**. Conclusions about decision-making skills are as follows (Peters et al., 2011):

- Older adults rely more on affective information when making decisions and judgments.
- Older adults require more time to make decisions, particularly if the information is new or complex.

- Older adults' life experiences can provide expertise that is beneficial for decision-making processes and may outweigh the cognitive deficits associated with age-related changes.
- Personality and motivation factors can exert a strong influence on decision-making processes in older adults.

Stage theories of adult cognitive development were first developed during the 1970s as an extension of Piaget's theory of intellectual development in children and adolescents. One such theory postulated that children and adolescents focus on acquiring knowledge, and adults focus on applying knowledge in the following stages (Schaie, 1977–1978):

- *Achieving stage* (early adulthood): adults apply acquired knowledge to demands and commitments, such as career and family; they use their intellectual abilities to establish their independence and develop goal-oriented behaviours.
- *Responsible stage* (late 30s to early 60s): adults integrate long-range goals and attend to the needs of their family and society.
- *Executive stage* (a subset of the responsible stage): applies to people who have high levels of social responsibilities.
- *Reintegration stage* (later adulthood): intellectual tasks are to simplify life and select only those responsibilities that have meaning and purpose; older adults ask "Why should I know?" rather than "What should I know?"

More recently, Cohen (2005) developed an **empowering model** on the basis of studies of more than 3,000 older adults. This model describes the following four phases of mature aging:

- *Midlife reevaluation* (early 40s to late 50s): people confront their sense of mortality; plans and actions are shaped by a quest or crisis; brain changes spur developmental intelligence.
- *Liberation* (late 50s to early 70s): people feel a new sense of inner liberation; development in information-processing part of the brain increases desire for novelty; plans and actions are shaped by personal freedom; retirement allows time for new experiences.
- *Summing up* (late 60s through 80s): people are motivated to share wisdom; plans and actions are shaped by a desire to find meaning; brain development improves capacity for autobiographical expression; people may feel compelled to attend to unfinished business and unresolved conflicts.
- *Encore* (late 70s to the end of life): plans and actions are shaped by the desire to restate and reaffirm major themes and to explore novel variations on those themes; brain changes promote positive emotions and morale; the desire to live well to the very end has a positive impact on others.

Gerontologists have also focused on the **paradox of well-being**, which describes the phenomenon of older adults suffering significant losses of health, cognition and social functioning but reporting high levels of well-being and positive emotions (Labouvie-Vief, 2009). The **socioemotional selectivity** theory addresses this question in the context of motivation. According to this theory, older adults recognize that time is limited, so they are motivated to pursue emotional satisfaction. Thus, they shift their focus from the pursuit of knowledge and information gathering and concentrate on relationships that are closer and more intimate (Labouvie-Vief, 2009).

Another focus is on **wisdom** as an aspect of cognitive function, which is viewed as "a multifaceted construct with elements of all the following: cognitive ability and insight, reflectivity, equanimity and compassionate concern for the welfare of others (Ardelt, 2011). A working definition of wisdom as an integral aspect of adult development includes the following (Knight & Laidlaw, 2009):

- An accumulation of "knowing how" expertise over "knowing what"
- A greater ability to integrate and balance emotion and reason
- An awareness of the many contexts of life and how they change over the years
- An acceptance of uncertainty in life and an understanding of how to handle this
- An understanding of the relativism of individual values and an increased tolerance for individual differences. (p. 684)

A similar concept is **developmental intelligence**, defined as "the maturing of cognition, emotional intelligence, judgment, social skills, life experience, and consciousness and their integration and synergy" (Cohen, 2005, p. 35). Cohen's view of cognitive aging, which is both optimistic and research based, emphasizes that many older adults display the age-dependent quality of wisdom because they integrate all the components of developmental intelligence (Box 11-1).

Box 11-1 Evidence-Informed Nursing Practice

Background: How do older adults age successfully and what does this mean to them? Researchers examined how Canadian seniors (including Anglophones and Francophones) live successfully.

Question: Older Canadians were asked, "What do you think makes people live long and keep well?"

Method: As part of the Canadian Study of Health and Aging, 2,783 older adults answered the above question, as well as other questions about healthy aging.

Findings: Many older Canadians mentioned that living long and keeping well involved being active, maintaining good nutrition, and living with motivation. Some noted the importance of relationships with family and others, as well as enjoying income security. Of note, physical illness was of less consequence to successful aging than the ability to adapt to illness and prevent further decline.

Implications for Nursing Practice: Although the researchers did not specifically discuss implications for nurses or other health care professionals, results of this study reveal the importance of asking older adults what successful aging means to them, what they are doing to maintain meaning in their lives, and what assistance would help them to continue to live well.

Source: Bassett, R., Bourbonnais, V., & McDowell, I. (2007). Living long and keeping well: Elderly Canadians account for success in aging. *Canadian Journal on Aging, 26*(2), 113–126.

RISK FACTORS THAT AFFECT COGNITIVE WELLNESS

A multitude of factors can affect cognitive function in people of all ages, but older adults are particularly vulnerable to these risk factors. As with other aspects of gerontological nursing, it is particularly important to identify the risk factors that can be addressed through health promotion interventions.

Personal, Social and Attitudinal Influences

Numerous personal, social and attitudinal factors affect cognitive abilities in people of any age, and researchers have tried to identify those that most significantly affect older adults. Quality and length of formal education is the factor most consistently associated with better cognitive performance and more cognitive reserve in older adults (Stine-Morrow & Chui, 2011). Other factors that affect cognitive function include occupation, social relations, socioeconomic status, hearing and vision problems, leisure and intellectual activities and lifestyle factors (e.g., nutrition, physical activity).

Ageism and diminished expectations of older adults in modern societies can negatively affect cognitive function. Studies indicate that older adults internalize stereotypes about memory decline as an inevitable outcome of aging and that these perceptions worsen their performance on tests of memory and other cognitive skills (Levy et al., 2011). Recent studies indicate that cognitive performance in older adults can be improved by providing positive stereotyping cues (Swift et al., 2013).

Health Factors and Health Behaviours

Many chronic conditions affect cognitive abilities in older adults to such a degree that gerontologists are emphasizing that researchers should view health conditions as the key explanatory variable in studies of cognitive aging (MacDonald et al., 2011; Spiro & Brady, 2011). Pathologic conditions that increase the risk for serious cognitive impairment due to dementia are discussed in Chapter 14, and this chapter discusses health factors that are associated with milder degrees of cognitive impairment. Examples of chronic conditions that are associated with impaired cognitive function (with or without dementia) include stroke, diabetes and cardiovascular disorders. For example, longitudinal studies confirm that overall cardiovascular health before older adulthood is associated with better verbal memory, **executive functions** (problem-solving skills, inhibition and flexibility) and psychomotor speed during later adulthood (Reis et al., 2013).

A major focus of current research is on the effects of inflammatory conditions that affect the immune, neurologic, and cardiovascular systems, with emphasis on how these pathologic processes can be a target for intervention (Barrientos et al., 2012; Rosano et al., 2012; Sartori et al., 2012). Specifically, one study concluded that higher infectious burden (i.e., the cumulative effects of pathogens such as *H. pylori* and herpes simplex virus) was an independent risk factor for cognitive impairment (Katan et al., 2013). Studies also found that cognitive impairment is common after lacunar strokes, which are associated with cerebral small vessel disease (Kloppenborg et al., 2012; Makin et al., 2013).

Nutritional status is widely recognized as a health factor that can affect cognitive function regardless of a person's age. For example, low levels of β-carotene, and vitamins B, C and D are associated with poor cognitive function. Researchers have focused much attention on nutritional factors that affect cognition because these can often be addressed through relatively simple interventions. The following conclusions are based on recent studies:

- Lower hemoglobin levels (i.e., anemia) are associated with cognitive decline in older adults (Shah et al., 2012).
- Studies have found that low serum vitamin D levels were associated with poorer cognitive function and a higher risk for Alzheimer disease (Annweiler et al., 2012; Balion et al., 2012; Peterson et al., 2012; Slinin et al., 2012).
- After conducting an extensive review of the literature, Health Quality Ontario (November, 2013) determined that among older adults, high levels of homocysteine (associated with low levels of vitamin B12) may be linked to dementia. However, they caution that this linkage cannot be made with confidence.
- Analysis of data from blood tests of 1,793 subjects in the Québec Longitudinal Study on Nutrition and Successful Aging found a positive correlation between low sodium intake and better cognitive function (Fiocco et al., 2012).
- Iron deficiency is associated with cognitive impairment, and its effect is independent from the presence of anemia (Yavuz et al., 2012).
- Dietary lutein and zeaxanthin can influence cognitive function in older adults (Johnson, 2012).

Sensory impairment is another aspect of health that affects cognitive processes because hearing or vision deficits limit the quantity and quality of information received from the environment. For example, studies have confirmed that hearing loss is independently associated with cognitive impairment and accelerated cognitive decline in community-dwelling older adults (Lin et al., 2013). Because sensory input significantly influences learning and other cognitive processes, nurses need to ensure optimal visual and hearing conditions when communicating with older adults (as discussed in Chapters 16 and 17).

Researchers are also focusing on mental health factors that can affect cognitive function. A review of literature related to stress and cognition found consistent evidence that stress is negatively associated with cognitive function in older adults (Almeida et al., 2011). Studies indicate that chronic stress is associated with cognitive impairment by increasing levels of cortisol (Kremen et al., 2012). Depression and even subclinical variations in depressive symptoms are strongly associated with impaired cognitive function (especially memory), as discussed in Chapter 15.

Some studies focus on a combination of health-related factors, with emphasis on health behaviours that promote good cognitive function. Data from a 17-year study of 5,100 men and women aged 42 to 63 years found an association between the number and duration of unhealthy behaviours and lower scores on measures of cognitive function in later life (Sabia, Singh-Manoux, et al., 2012). Smoking is a health-related behaviour that is a risk for cognitive decline (Sabia, Elbaz, et al., 2012). Many studies found that healthy lifestyle behaviours, such as physical activity and social engagement, are associated with maintaining good cognitive function (Gow et al., 2012; Lovden et al., 2013; Miller et al., 2012; Suzuki et al., 2012; Wang et al., 2013).

Medication Effects

Prescription and over-the-counter medications can interfere with memory and other cognitive functions in a variety of ways. For example, anticholinergic ingredients, contained in numerous prescription and over-the-counter medications, significantly affect memory and other cognitive functions and are a common cause of changes in mental status in older adults (Pasina et al., 2013). Because many medications have anticholinergic effects, researchers and clinicians have paid particular attention in recent years to the cumulative effects of these medications on acetylcholine, which is a neurotransmitter that directly affects cognitive function. Chapter 8 provides detailed information about anticholinergics and other types of medications that can interfere with cognitive function. Refer to Table 8-12 for information about specific medications and the modes of action that affect cognitive function.

Environmental Factors

Researchers are also examining risk factors related to long-term exposure to environmental toxins. Studies indicate that exposure to secondhand smoke is associated with increased risk of cognitive decline (Orsitto et al., 2012). Occupational and environmental exposure to lead can increase the risk for cognitive impairment, particularly through detrimental effects on neural processing speed (Grashow et al., 2013).

Wellness Opportunity

From a holistic perspective, nurses help older adults identify risk factors, such as nutrition and over-the-counter medications, that can be addressed through self-care actions.

FUNCTIONAL CONSEQUENCES AFFECTING COGNITION

Healthy older adults will not experience any significant cognitive impairment that interferes with daily life, but they will notice minor deficits in some aspects of cognitive function and improvements in other aspects. These changes can be summarized as follows (Stine-Morrow & Chui, 2011; Thinggaard et al., 2013):

- Age-related declines in some cognitive skills begin around the age of 40, but there are substantial individual variation in these changes.
- Earliest cognitive changes are due to decreased perceptual speed.
- Cognitive functions that depend on experience, accumulated knowledge and well-practiced tasks (e.g., vocabulary) do not decline in healthy older adults, and may even improve.
- Age-related cognitive changes generally occur at a slow linear rate; any major or rapid changes are due to pathologic processes.
- Many studies have found a protective effect of higher levels of education, which may be associated with the development of cognitive reserve.
- Many studies suggest that cognitive function is increasing in successive cohorts of older adults; this trend may continue, resulting in better cognition for people reaching older adulthood.
- Pathologic processes, such as those related to inflammatory processes and cardiovascular diseases, are associated with greater degrees of cognitive impairment.
- Health promotion interventions to protect and even improve cognitive abilities during older adulthood include activities that involve social engagement and cognitive stimulation and all actions that promote good overall health (e.g., optimal nutrition, physical activity, stress management, no smoking, healthy weight).

 See ONLINE LEARNING ACTIVITY 11-3: ARTICLE ABOUT EFFECTS OF CARDIORESPIRATORY FITNESS AND CEREBRAL BLOOD FLOW ON COGNITIVE OUTCOMES IN OLDER WOMEN at http://thepoint.lww.com/Miller7e

Although these conclusions about patterns of change are based on well-designed studies, gerontologists emphasize that there is a great deal of individual variation in cognitive changes, with some older adults showing no decline and others even showing improvement in cognitive abilities. Gerontologists also emphasize that studies focusing only on age-related cognitive changes do not address the strong interplay between cognition and other factors. In addition, many questions are emerging about confounding effects of undiagnosed pathologic conditions in apparently healthy older adults participating in studies.

Box 11-2 Cultural Considerations: Cultural Factors and Cognitive Function

- Recognize that the standards of intellectual performance used in Canada have been developed primarily for English-speaking white North Americans.
- Cognitive abilities are highly influenced by health, education, and socioeconomic status, and these factors and cultural factors are interrelated.
- Cultural and language factors may influence an older adult's perception and description of memory problems.
- Culture may impact how caregivers understand and respond to older adults with cognitive changes (e.g., some Canadian aboriginal cultures view cognitive decline as a normal part of aging).

Another important consideration is that conclusions about cognitive aging do not necessarily address cultural factors. For instance, older Aboriginal Canadians may view memory loss and behavioural changes of dementia as being a normal part of aging (Lanting et al., 2011). As such, culture influences how cognitive changes are viewed and how individuals within various cultures relate to individuals with cognitive changes (see factors cited in Box 11-2).

In summary, cognitive function in older adults must be considered in relation to social, emotional and other factors, as well as current limitations of research. This perspective is supported by studies that indicate that "healthy older brains are often as good as or better than younger brains in a wide variety of tasks" (Cohen, 2005, p. 4). Cohen cites the following evidence-based findings that support an optimistic view of cognitive aging:

- New brain cells form throughout life.
- Experience and learning enable the brain to "resculpt" itself.
- Emotional circuitry of the brain matures and becomes more balanced during older adulthood.
- Functions of the left and right hemispheres of the brain become more integrated in older adults.

Box 11-3 summarizes some of research-based conclusions about cognitive aging that are most relevant for identifying and implementing health education interventions for older adults.

See ONLINE LEARNING ACTIVITY 11-3: ARTICLE ABOUT NEUROPLASTICITY AND SUCCESSFUL COGNITIVE AGING
at http://thepoint.lww.com/Miller7e

Wellness Opportunity

Nurses promote wellness by encouraging older adults to identify ways in which their cognitive abilities have improved (e.g., wisdom based on experiences).

Box 11-3 Functional Consequences Affecting Cognition in Older Adults

Cognitive Abilities in Healthy Older Adults

- Skills that stay the same or improve: wisdom, creativity, common sense, coordination of facts and ideas, and breadth of knowledge and experience
- Skills that decline slightly and gradually: abstraction, calculation, word fluency, verbal comprehension, spatial orientation, inductive reasoning, and episodic memory
- Word finding may be more difficult (i.e., "tip-of-the-tongue" experiences), but total vocabulary increases.
- Remote memory remains intact and holds a large store of information about the past.
- Factors that can cause cognitive impairment: anxiety, depression, diminished sensory input, poor health, negative beliefs, ageist attitudes, pathologic processes (e.g., dementia)
- Factors that improve cognitive function: good nutrition, physical exercise, mental stimulation, challenging leisure activities, strong social networks, and activities that provide a sense of control and mastery

Learning Abilities

- Older adults are as capable of learning new things as younger people, but the speed with which they process information is slower.
- Older adults are more cautious in their responses and make more errors of omission.
- Potential barriers to learning in older adults include distractions, sensory deficits, lack of relevance, teacher–learner age differences, and values that are incongruent with new knowledge.

A PATHOLOGIC CONDITION AFFECTING COGNITION: MILD COGNITIVE IMPAIRMENT

Mild cognitive impairment (MCI) is widely recognized as a heterogeneous syndrome characterized by cognitive function that is impaired beyond "normal aging" but does not meet the criteria for mild dementia. Two subtypes of MCI are amnesic MCI, which involves memory loss, and nonamnesic MCI, which is the less common type and does not involve memory loss. During the early 1960s, symptoms that are now categorized as MCI were referred to as *benign senescent forgetfulness*. During the 1980s and 1990s, labels of *age-associated memory impairment, mild neurocognitive decline*, or *cognitive impairment no dementia* were commonly applied to this constellation of symptoms. By the early 2000s, MCI was viewed as a precursor to Alzheimer disease, but it is now considered a distinct syndrome with symptoms that can remain stable, resolve or progress (Patel & Holland, 2012). It is now known that MCI increases the risk for developing dementia, but it does not necessarily progress to dementia. Studies indicate that MCI improves significantly or reverts to baseline cognitive state in 15% to 40% of patients (Patel & Holland, 2012). In contrast to those who revert or improve, patients with MCI progress to Alzheimer disease at the rate of 10% to 15% per year compared with a rate of 1% to 2% in control groups (Freitas et al., 2013; Lopez, 2013).

Because MCI has only recently been defined as a distinct syndrome, diagnostic criteria are imprecise and current

TABLE 11-1 Distinguishing Characteristics of Normal Cognitive Aging and Mild Cognitive Impairment

Characteristic	Normal Cognitive Aging	Mild Cognitive Impairment (MCI)	Mild Dementia
Short-term memory changes	Preserved	Impaired in amnesic MCI, preserved in nonamnesic MCI	Noticeably impaired
Awareness of memory loss	Recognizes and remembers details about memory limitations	Little or no recognition and memory of details about limitations	Limited or absent awareness
Mental status assessment	No significant changes from baseline	Mild or no significant impairment	Measurable declines from baseline
Social skills	No significant changes	Usually unchanged from normal	Impaired
Activities of daily living	Preserved	Preserved	Impaired
Instrumental activities of daily living	No significant changes from baseline	Limited changes, apparent in complex tasks (e.g., managing finances, using appliances)	Impaired

Source: Patel, B. B., & Holland, N. W. (2012). Mild cognitive impairment: Hope for stability, plan for progression. *Cleveland Clinic Journal of Medicine, 79*(12), 857–864.

guidelines emphasize the need for a combination of clinical judgment, functional assessment and neuropsychological testing (Healey, 2012). Diagnosis of MCI depends on identifying declines in one or more cognitive domains (e.g., memory, attention, visuospatial abilities, executive functioning) without concurrent major effects on global cognition or daily functioning. Table 11.1 lists cognitive changes associated with normal aging and MCI. In addition to cognitive characteristics, behavioural symptoms, such as anxiety, depression and aggressiveness, have been identified in 13% of people with MCI, as compared with 39% of those with Alzheimer disease and 3% of controls (Van Der Mussele et al., 2013). Nurses can encourage older adults with noticeable cognitive deficits to obtain an appropriate evaluation, with emphasis on the importance of implementing interventions at a stage when progression to dementia could be delayed.

NURSING ASSESSMENT OF COGNITIVE FUNCTION

Formal assessment of intellectual performance involves neuropsychological testing, but nurses can assess cognitive skills by using evidence-based tools. In addition, it is important to assess for risk factors that are likely to interfere with cognitive function. Because nursing assessment of cognition is an integral part of the psychosocial assessment, it is addressed comprehensively in Chapter 13 rather than in this chapter. Nursing assessment of impaired cognitive function is addressed in Chapter 14.

NURSING DIAGNOSIS

Healthy older adults experience some changes in cognitive function, but, in the absence of pathologic conditions and other risk factors, these changes do not significantly affect their overall functioning. The nursing diagnosis of

Readiness for Enhanced Knowledge is appropriate for addressing normal cognitive aging because the focus is on health promotion interventions to maintain optimal cognitive functioning. Impaired memory may be appropriate for older adults with the amnesic type of MCI or memory limitations that affect daily functioning. Nursing diagnoses related to cognitive impairment associated with dementia, confusional states and other serious cognitive impairments are discussed in Chapter 14.

> ### Wellness Opportunity
>
> Recognize the detrimental influence of myths and negative attitudes about cognitive aging, and address these by using the nursing diagnosis of Readiness for Enhanced Knowledge.

PLANNING FOR WELLNESS OUTCOMES

A wellness-oriented outcome criterion related to cognitive function is that older adults take responsibility for addressing risk factors and compensating for age-related cognitive changes. The following are examples of outcomes that address risk factors: improved sensory function, control of cardiovascular diseases, smoking cessation, healthy lifestyle practices and social and intellectual engagement. Nurses can use the following Nursing Outcomes Classification (NOC) terminology related to cognitive wellness: Cognition, Concentration, Exercise Participation, Information Processing, Knowledge: Health Promotion, Stress Level, Leisure Participation, Hearing Compensation Behaviour and Vision Compensation Behaviour.

> ### Wellness Opportunity
>
> Address the detrimental influence of myths and negative attitudes about cognitive aging and address these by using the NOC of Health Beliefs in relation to the nursing diagnosis of Readiness for Enhanced Knowledge.

A Student's Perspective

At the beginning of the 5 weeks at Friendship Village, I didn't know what to expect. I assumed we would just be taking vital signs and making small talk with a few of the clients. I didn't realize I would learn so much by just listening to the life story of someone who is 96 years old. I realized that many of these individuals have had quite the amazing life and have a lot of wisdom and knowledge to pass down.

Needless to say, my expectations changed dramatically! They went from just getting the 5 weeks over with, to my not wanting to leave after the 5 weeks. Many of the residents were still "with it" and could remember a lot about their childhood and past experiences. This is the information that I did my best to take in. How did they get to live to be 96 years old and be able to look back on their life and be proud of their accomplishments. That's the life I want to live!!

Kim V.

NURSING INTERVENTIONS TO PROMOTE COGNITIVE WELLNESS

Nurses have key roles in teaching older adults about the following evidence-based strategies for cognitive health and vitality (Gow et al., 2012; Guiney & Machado, 2013; Miller et al., 2012; Stine-Morrow & Chui, 2011):

- Eat foods high in antioxidants (e.g., fruits and vegetables) and omega-3 fatty acids (e.g., fatty fish); limit salt, cholesterol and saturated fat.
- Maintain a healthy weight.
- Engage in regular physical activity, including aerobic activity, strengthening exercises and flexibility and balance exercises.
- Engage in new learning experiences that are appealing and challenging.
- Practice body–mind activities, such as tai chi and mindfulness-based meditation.
- Participate in leisure activities, such as dancing, playing board games, playing a musical instrument, doing crossword puzzles and reading.
- Choose activities in which there is a sense of control and mastery, such as playing computer games or learning a new skill.
- Maintain strong and frequent social relationships with family and friends.

Many of the health promotion interventions discussed throughout this book provide specific examples of these types of activities. For example, interventions for cardiovascular wellness (see Chapter 20) are particularly relevant to promoting optimal cognitive function. Also, because vision and hearing impairments can interfere with cognitive abilities, any interventions directed toward improving sensory function (discussed in Chapters 16 and 17) may also be effective in improving cognitive function.

See **ONLINE LEARNING ACTIVITY 11-4: EVIDENCE-BASED INTERVENTIONS FOR COGNITIVE WELLNESS** at http://thepoint.lww.com/Miller7e

The following Nursing Interventions Classification (NIC) terminologies identify interventions related to cognitive wellness: Cognitive Stimulation, Communication Enhancement: Hearing Deficit, Communication Enhancement: Visual Deficit, Exercise Promotion, Health Education, Learning Facilitation, Learning Readiness Enhancement, Meditation Facilitation, Progressive Muscle Relaxation, Role Enhancement, Self-Awareness Enhancement, Self-Responsibility Enhancement and Risk Identification.

Wellness Opportunity

Nurses promote personal responsibility for wellness by helping older adults identify ways of incorporating "brain fitness" activities into their daily lives.

Teaching About Memory and Cognition

Teaching older adults about techniques to maintain or improve cognitive skills is within the realm of nursing responsibilities, in the same way as is teaching about maintaining and improving physical function. The concept of metacognition suggests that an understanding of one's own cognitive processes can influence performance. For example, someone who wants to remember a list of names needs both the intent to remember and knowledge about techniques for remembering. Studies find that memory training can be effective in improving metamemory and other cognitive skills in older adults (Tullis & Benjamin, 2012).

In addition to addressing memory-training techniques, it is important to address beliefs about cognition and aging because these can significantly influence one's ability to learn. Thus, health education needs to include all of the following aspects:

- Correcting myths and misinformation
- Providing accurate information about age-related changes
- Communicating positive expectations
- Identifying goals for self-learning
- Providing information about techniques to enhance cognitive abilities
- Identifying the techniques that are most effective for the individual

In community and long-term care settings, group sessions can effectively and efficiently address many psychosocial aspects of aging, including cognitive function. The model developed by Turner Geriatric Services at the University of Michigan (Fogler & Stern, 2005) can be used to educate older adults about techniques for memory enhancement (see Box 11-4).

Box 11-4 Memory Training for Older Adults

Introduction

- Forgetting is a normal part of life for all people, but memory skills can be learned. The purposes of this program are to look at some reasons people forget things and to discuss ways of improving memory skills.
- When older adults are forgetful, they may blame it on old age, rather than seeing it as something that happens to everyone, regardless of age.
- Memory problems can be viewed as a challenge. Anyone can improve his or her memory, but as with any other skill, an effort must be made.

Stages of Memory

- *Sensory memory* lasts only a few seconds. It involves the awareness of information obtained through vision, hearing, smell, taste and touch.
- *Short-term memory* is your working memory, or what is in your conscious thoughts. This, too, is very brief and contains small amounts of information. For example, this type of memory allows you to recall a telephone number as you dial it.
- *Long-term memory* is the memory bank, or what you depend on whenever you need to retrieve information. This memory bank is almost limitless and contains information you just learned, as well as information from long ago.

Memory Changes and Aging

- Aging is blamed for a lot of memory problems, but very few changes occur solely because of aging.
- In older adulthood, the processes of learning new information and recalling old information slow down a little. The overall ability to learn and remember, however, is not significantly affected in healthy older people.

Factors That Interfere With Memory

As people grow older, an increasing number of factors may interfere with their ability to remember, including the following:

- Not being attentive to the situation. This might be attributable, for example, to the fact that the situation is not personally relevant.
- Being distracted can interfere with the ability to concentrate
- Feeling stressed, worried, or anxious
- Having a physical illness or being tired
- Having vision, hearing, or other functional impairments that interfere with the ability to obtain information
- Feeling sad or depressed, or coping with loss or grief
- Not being intellectually stimulated (principle of "use it or lose it!")
- Not having cues to prompt remembering
- Not organizing information for easy retention; not being organized in daily life
- Taking medications or alcohol that interfere with mental abilities
- Not being physically fit (e.g., as a result of poor nutrition or lack of exercise)

Ways of Improving Memory Skills

- Write things down (e.g., use lists, calendars and notebooks).
- Use auditory cues (e.g., timers, alarm clocks) combined with written cues.

- Use environmental cues. For instance, remove something from its usual place, then return it to its normal location after it has served its purpose.
- Assign specific places for specific items and keep the items in their proper place (e.g., keep keys on a hook near the door).
- Put reminders in appropriate places (e.g., place shoes that need to be repaired near the door).
- Use visual images. ("A picture is worth a thousand words.") Create a picture in your mind when you want to remember something; the more unusual the picture, the more likely it is that you will remember.
- Use active observation: pay attention to details of what is going on around you and be alert to the environment.
- Make associations between names and mental images (e.g., Carol and Christmas carol).
- Rehearse items you want to remember by repeating them aloud or writing the information on paper.
- Use self-instruction; say things aloud (e.g., "I'm putting my keys on the counter so I remember to turn off the stove before I leave.").
- Divide information into small parts that can be remembered easily (e.g., to remember an address or a postal code, divide it into groups [S4S, 4S2].).
- Organize information into logical categories (e.g., shampoo and hair spray, toothpaste and mouthwash, soap and deodorant).
- Use rhyming cues (e.g., "In 1492, Columbus sailed the ocean blue.").
- Use first-letter cues and make associations (e.g., to remember to buy soup, tea, oranges, rice, and eggs, remember the word STORE.).
- Make word associations (e.g., to remember the letters of your license plate, make a word, such as camel, out of the letters CML.).
- Search the alphabet while focusing on what you are trying to remember (e.g., to remember that someone's name is Martin, start with names that begin with A and continue naming names through the alphabet until your memory is jogged for the correct one.).
- Make up a story to connect things you want to remember (e.g., if you have to go to the cleaners and the post office, create a story about mailing a pair of pants.).

Conclusion

- Do not try to remember all of these techniques, but select a few techniques that you like, and use these whenever appropriate or needed.
- Minimize any distractions; pay attention to one thing at a time.
- Give yourself time to remember; forgetfulness is most likely to occur when you are in a hurry.
- Devise systems to organize routine tasks, such as taking medications.
- Carry a notepad or a calendar and do not rely entirely on mental cues.
- Relax and maintain a sense of humour. If you become anxious about your memory and are convinced you cannot remember, then you will create a self-fulfilling prophecy.

(Adapted with permission from Fogler, J., & Stern, L. [2005]. *Improving your memory: How to remember what you're starting to forget.* Baltimore, MD: Johns Hopkins University Press.)

Wellness Opportunity

Nurses holistically address learning needs of older adults by encouraging participation in group programs, which have the additional benefit of offering social support.

Improving Concentration and Attention

When one's ability to attend to the environment and concentrate on visual and auditory cues is limited, the ability to learn and remember is also impaired. Thus, techniques, such as relaxation, imagery and meditation, which enhance attention and concentration, may also improve memory and learning. Likewise, any method that reduces environmental distractions may also improve one's cognitive abilities. Mindfulness (also called *mindfulness meditation*), which is the practice of focused awareness of the environment and one's reactions to it, is a self-care practice that can improve attention and other cognitive skills. Many self-help books describe techniques for meditation, mindfulness and relaxation as ways of maintaining or improving cognitive function and opening the mind to new learning. Nurses can teach the relaxation technique outlined in Chapter 24 to older adults for a variety of uses, including the enhancement of mental skills.

Encouraging Participation in Mentally Stimulating Activities

Because there is much evidence that participation in mentally stimulating activities is effective for promoting cognitive wellness, nurses can encourage older adults to participate in adult learning activities. In some settings, nurses can address health-related concerns of older adults through group health education programs, which have the additional benefit of providing social support. A process for implementing a nurse-led health education group is described in Chapter 12.

Nurses can also promote the use of computers by older adults for mental stimulation and practical benefits, such as increased communication with others and the acquisition of information that is relevant to their health and daily functioning. Focus groups have found that older adults are interested in using computers and other technology to sustain and improve mental and physical abilities (Heinz et al., 2013). Studies also indicate that cognitive training interventions, such as computer-based brain exercises, are effective in improving cognitive abilities in older adults (Shatil, 2013). Increasingly, many cognitively stimulating and enjoyable brain games and brain exercises are available on the Internet, as described in Online Learning Activity 11-4.

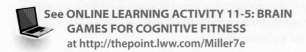

See **ONLINE LEARNING ACTIVITY 11-5: BRAIN GAMES FOR COGNITIVE FITNESS** at http://thepoint.lww.com/Miller7e

Another nursing intervention is to encourage older adults to participate in lifelong learning programs in local communities. Some universities and colleges offer reduced-rate or no-fee courses for students 60 years and older. Some programs also offer degrees, certification programs, or a general equivalency diploma (GED). The Canadian Network for Third Age Learning (http://dev.www.uregina.ca/catalist/eindex.html) is a community-based organization for retirement-age learners that develops and implements educational programs in affiliation with a college or university. These sessions typically involve homework and usually are held for a few hours weekly for several months. Less formal education programs often

are available through local senior centres and adult education programs affiliated with local school districts. Older adults can contact local colleges and obtain information on courses that are offered under this program.

Roadscholar is a nonprofit organization that was founded in 1975 (previously called Elderhostel) to provide opportunities for lifelong learning by combining travel and education at a reasonable cost. This program offers an extraordinary range of topics and formats in a wide range of accommodations throughout Canada and the world. Nurses can encourage older adults to obtain additional information about this and other programs that are identified in the resources listed in Online Learning Activity 11-5.

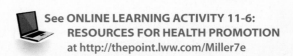

See **ONLINE LEARNING ACTIVITY 11-6: RESOURCES FOR HEALTH PROMOTION** at http://thepoint.lww.com/Miller7e

Wellness Opportunity

Nurses promote personal responsibility by helping older adults identify activities that address their unique learning needs on the basis of their life experiences and current interests.

Adapting Health Education Materials

Much of the research on cognitive aging has centred on factors that affect learning in older adulthood. Because many nursing interventions include patient teaching or health education, information about cognitive aging can be used to adapt educational methods and materials to older adults as summarized in Box 11-5. The suggestions presented in this text for communicating with older adults and compensating for hearing and vision deficit (see Chapters 13, 16 and 17) can be applied to health education.

Adaptations of health education materials may also be necessary to ensure they are culturally appropriate. For instance, many federal government sites provide health education materials that are available in either official language and other ethnic languages. Because there is growing emphasis on addressing needs of culturally diverse populations, it is important to check Internet resources periodically and explore the availability of teaching materials for specific ethnic/cultural groups. In addition, local community centres and senior centres often provide culturally specific health education materials related to culturally diverse populations in their service area. For example, organizations and provincial/territorial governments have developed advance directive forms and teaching tools that address learning needs of specific cultural groups, as discussed in Chapter 9. Chapter 2 further addresses the topic of culturally sensitive health education, and online learning activities in many chapters provide links to health education materials pertinent to topics in this book.

Box 11-5 Guidelines for Health Education for Older Adults

Environmental Conditions That Promote Learning

- Establish a warm, friendly environment.
- Eliminate distractions (e.g., noise, excessive visual stimulation).
- Provide good lighting and eliminate sources of glare as much as possible.
- Make sure older adults are using hearing aids and eyeglasses as appropriate.
- Use amplifying devices, such as microphones.

Teaching Strategies That Promote Learning

- Emphasize application of knowledge and experience, rather than the acquisition of irrelevant information.
- Use praise and positive feedback.
- Present one idea or small amounts of information at one time.

- Allow enough time for processing information.
- Use concrete rather than abstract teaching materials in all forms (verbal, written, audiovisual).
- Make sure that the information is personally relevant.
- Relate the information to the person's past experiences.
- As much as possible, adapt presentation to individualized rates of procession.
- Arrange for follow-up to reinforce teaching points.

Teaching Aids That Enhance Learning

- Use audio and visual aids that are relevant to older adults.
- Ensure that examples illustrate healthy aging and do not reinforce myths or stereotypes.
- Provide advance organizers, such as outlines and summaries.
- Explain how to use organizing aids.

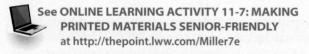 See **ONLINE LEARNING ACTIVITY 11-7: MAKING PRINTED MATERIALS SENIOR-FRIENDLY** at http://thepoint.lww.com/Miller7e

EVALUATING EFFECTIVENESS OF NURSING INTERVENTIONS

Effectiveness of nursing interventions is evaluated by the degree to which older adults who have mild memory impairments are able to use their cognitive abilities to meet their daily needs. For example, older adults who forget to keep appointments might learn to use a calendar or other organizational aids to remember the appointments. In these situations, the effectiveness of interventions is measured by how well these persons remember to keep appointments. Effectiveness of nursing interventions can also be measured subjectively, on the basis of the degree to which older adults express positive perceptions of their cognitive abilities and satisfaction with interventions, including self-care actions.

Unfolding Case Study

Part 1: Mrs. C. at 71 Years of Age

Mrs. C. is 71 years old and lives alone in her own home. She attends a local senior wellness clinic for blood pressure checks, health screenings (e.g., cholesterol levels) and her annual flu shot. During her monthly visit for a blood pressure check, she confides that she is embarrassed about missing a doctor's appointment last week. She says she has been noticing increased difficulties with memory, and one of her friends has told her that she probably has Alzheimer disease. She asks if there is a place where she can get a test for Alzheimer disease.

NURSING ASSESSMENT

Your nursing assessment indicates that Mrs. C. has missed a couple of health care appointments during the past year. She said she missed a dental appointment 6 months ago when she was very worried about her daughter, who was undergoing diagnostic tests for a lump in her breast. Last week, when she missed her doctor's appointment, she had been busy shopping for presents for her grandson's wedding. When you ask about additional problems with memory, Mrs. C. admits that she has more difficulty remembering people's names than she used to have. You do not identify any risk factors that might affect Mrs. C.'s cognitive abilities (e.g., depression, medication effects, poor nutrition). Mrs. C. has never used calendars, and she says she remembers her doctor's appointments by keeping the appointment cards in her desk drawer along with her bills and her checkbook. She says that she checks her appointment cards every month, but she had not noticed the cards for the two appointments she missed.

NURSING DIAGNOSIS

You use the nursing diagnosis of Health-Seeking Behaviours because Mrs. C. is interested in learning about memory-training skills to assist her in remembering appointments. Mrs. C. has a poor understanding of age-related cognitive changes, and she indicates that she is interested in learning about ways to improve her memory.

NURSING CARE PLAN FOR MRS. C.

Expected Outcome	Nursing Interventions	Nursing Evaluation
Mrs. C. will express an interest in improving her memory skills.	• Use information in Box 11-3 to teach Mrs. C. about age-related changes that affect cognitive abilities. • Discuss the characteristics of normal cognitive aging, mild cognitive impairment and dementia. • Emphasize that memory skills can be developed through memory-training techniques.	• Mrs. C. will agree to participate in a discussion of memory-training skills.
Mrs. C. will use memory-training techniques to improve her functional level.	• Give Mrs. C. a copy of Box 11-4 and review the information. • Assist Mrs. C. in identifying one or two strategies for remembering appointments (e.g., begin using a calendar). • Assist Mrs. C. in identifying one or two strategies for remembering the names of people she meets (e.g., using visual images).	• Mrs. C. will report success in using a method for remembering appointments. • Mrs. C. will report success in using a method for remembering names of people.
Mrs. C. will be aware of resources for assessment if memory does not improve.	• Provide information about local geriatric assessment program for cognitive assessment.	• Mrs. C. will follow up, as needed, with obtaining a comprehensive assessment of cognitive function.

THINKING POINTS

- What factors are likely to be contributing to Mrs. C.'s forgetting about her appointments?
- What is the most effective way of using information in Boxes 11-3 and 11-4 to facilitate learning for Mrs. C?
- What additional interventions would you suggest for Mrs. C?

QSEN APPLICATION

QSEN Competency	Knowledge/Skill/Attitude	Application to Mrs. C
Patient-centred care	(K) Integrate understanding of multiple dimensions of patient-centred care. (K) Describe strategies to empower patients in all aspects of the health care process. (S) Assess own level of communication skill in encounters with patients and families. (A) Value seeing health care situations "through patients' eyes."	Empower Mrs. C. to improve her memory skills by teaching her about normal cognitive aging and interventions to improve memory. Use good communication skills to express understanding of Mrs. C.'s concerns and at the same time dispel any myths about cognitive aging.
Teamwork and collaboration	(S) Integrate the contributions of others who play a role in helping the patient achieve health goals.	Provide information about obtaining a comprehensive geriatric assessment for cognitive function.
Evidence-based practice	(S) Base individualized care plan on patient values, clinical expertise and evidence. (S) Read original research and evidence reports related to clinical practice.	Use evidence-based information summarized in Table 11-1 to teach Mrs. C. about characteristics of normal cognitive aging, mild cognitive impairment and dementia.

Chapter Highlights

Age-Related Changes That Affect Cognition

- Central nervous system: degenerative changes in brain, slower reaction time
- Fluid intelligence (inductive reasoning, abstract thinking) declines, but crystallized intelligence (wisdom and judgment) improves.
- Some, but not all, memory functions decline in healthy older adults.
- Models of adult psychological development describe phases of mature aging.

Risk Factors That Affect Cognitive Wellness

- Personal and social influences: education, socioeconomic factors, ageism
- Physical health and functioning: chronic conditions, nutritional status, sensory impairment
- Mental health factors: stress, depression
- Health-related behaviours: physical activity, social engagement
- Adverse medication effects, especially from anticholinergics
- Exposure to environmental toxins

Functional Consequences Affecting Cognitive Function (Box 11-3)

- Cognitive skills that decline with age: perceptual speed, numerical ability, episodic memory, verbal ability, inductive reasoning, executive functions
- Cognitive skills that improve with age: word lexicon, general knowledge
- Rapid or significant declines are due to pathologic processes (e.g., strokes, dementia).
- Cultural factors and cognitive function (Box 11-2)

Pathologic Condition Affecting Cognition: Mild Cognitive Impairment

- Mild cognitive impairment (MCI) is a heterogeneous syndrome characterized by cognitive function that is impaired beyond "normal aging" but does not meet the criteria for mild dementia.
- Symptoms of MCI may improve or revert to prior level, but more often it progresses to Alzheimer disease.

Nursing Assessment of Cognitive Function

- Refer to Chapter 13

Nursing Diagnosis

- Readiness for Enhanced Knowledge
- Health-Seeking Behaviours

Planning for Wellness Outcomes

- Cognition
- Concentration
- Health Beliefs
- Health-Seeking Behaviour
- Information Processing
- Knowledge: Health Promotion
- Leisure Participation

Nursing Interventions to Promote Cognitive Wellness

- Evidence-based strategies for cognitive health: nutrition, mental exercise, physical exercise, challenging leisure activities, strong social networks, activities that foster a sense of control and mastery
- Teaching about memory and cognition for individuals and groups (Box 11-4)
- Improving concentration and attention (mindfulness, imagery, relaxation)
- Encouraging participation in mentally stimulating activities (e.g., computers, classes)
- Adapting health education materials (Box 11-5)

Evaluating Effectiveness of Nursing Interventions

- Expresses satisfaction with improved cognitive abilities
- Able to use cognitive skills in daily activities

Critical Thinking Exercises

1. Identify the factors in your own life that interfere with cognitive function.
2. What memory aids do you use in your life? Are they effective? Would you like to develop additional memory aids?
3. You are working in a senior centre and have suggested that the centre sponsor a series of classes on the memory problems of older adults. This suggestion is based on your observation that many of the older adults have asked you questions about memory problems and some are concerned about Alzheimer disease. Address each of the following issues:

   - The centre director is a firm believer in the adage, "You can't teach an old dog new tricks." How would you convince the director that the classes you wish to offer are worthwhile?
   - How would you structure the sessions (number and length of sessions, number of participants, and so forth)?
   - Describe the content you would cover and the approach you would use for each topic. Include information about normal cognitive aging, risk factors for impaired cognitive function and techniques for improving memory and other aspects of cognition.
   - What audiovisual aids, including written materials, would you use?
   - How would you adapt your teaching method and materials for the group?
   - How would you evaluate the sessions?

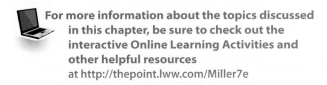

For more information about the topics discussed in this chapter, be sure to check out the interactive Online Learning Activities and other helpful resources
at http://thepoint.lww.com/Miller7e

REFERENCES

Aine, C. J., Sanfratello, L., Adair, J. C., et al. (2011). Development and decline of memory function in normal, pathological and healthy successful aging. *Brain Topography, 24*(3–4), 323–339.

Almeida, D. M., Piazza, J. R., Stawski, R. S., et al. (2011). The speedometer of life: Stress, health and aging. In K. W. Schaie & S. L. Willis (Eds.), *Handbook of the psychology of aging* (7th ed., pp. 191–206). New York, NY: Elsevier.

Annweiler, C., Rolland, Y., Schott, A. M., et al. (2012). Higher vitamin D dietary intake is associated with lower risk of Alzheimer's disease. *Journal of Gerontology: Medical Sciences, 67*(11), 1205–1211.

Ardelt, M. (2011). Wisdon, age, and well-being. In K. W. Schaie & S. L. Willis (Eds.), *Handbook of the psychology of aging* (7th ed., pp. 279–291). New York, NY: Elsevier.

Balion, C., Griffith, L. E., Strifler, L., et al. (2012). Vitamin D, cognition, and dementia. *Neurology, 79*, 1397–1405.

Barrientos, R. M., Frank, M. G., Watkins, L. R., et al. (2012). Aging-related changes in neuroimmune-endocrine function: Implications for hippocampal-dependent cognition. *Hormones and Behaviour, 62*, 219–227.

Bassett, R., Bourbonnais, V., & McDowell, I. (2007). Living long and keeping well: Elderly Canadians account for success in aging. *Canadian Journal on Aging, 26*(2), 113–126.

Bergman, I., & Almkvist, O. (2013). The effect of age on fluid intelligence is fully mediated by physical health. *Archives of Gerontology and Geriatrics, 57*(1), 100–109.

Botwinick, J. (1984). *Aging and behaviour* (3rd ed.). New York, NY: Springer.

Chou, Y., Chen, N., & Madden, D. J. (2013). Functional brain connectivity and cognition: Effects of adult age and task demands. *Neurobiology of Aging, 34*(8), 1925–1934.

Cohen, G. D. (2005). *The mature mind: The positive power of the aging brain*. New York, NY: Basic Books.

Farias, S. T., Mungas, D., Reed, B., et al. (2012). Maximal brain size remains and important predictor of cognition in old age, independent of current brain pathology. *Neurobiology of Aging, 22*(8), 1758–1768.

Fiocco, A. J., Shatenstein, B., Ferland, G., et al. (2012). Sodium intake and physical activity impact cognitive maintenance in older adults: The NuAge Study. *Neurobiology of Aging, 33*, 829.321–829.e28.

Fogler, J., & Stern, L. (2005). *Improving your memory: How to remember what you're starting to forget* (3rd ed.). Baltimore, MD: Johns Hopkins University Press.

Freitas, S., Simoes, M. R., Alves, L., et al. (2013). Montreal cognitive assessment. *Alzheimer's Disease and Associated Disorders, 27*, 38–43.

Geldmacher, D. S., Levin, B. E., & Wright, C. B. (2012, September 12). Characterizing healthy samples for studies of human cognitive aging. *Frontiers in Aging Neuroscience*. Advance online publication. doi:10.3389/fnagi.2012.00023

Goh, J. O. S. (2011). Functional dedifferentiation and altered connectivity in older adults. *Aging and Disease, 2*(1), 30–48.

Gow, A. J., Bastin, M. E., Munoz, M., et al. (2012). Neuroprotective lifestyles and the aging brain: Activity, atrophy, and white matter integrity. *Neurology, 79*(17), 1802–1808.

Grashow, R., Spiro, A., Taylor, K. M., et al. (2013). Cumulative lead exposure in community-dwelling adults and fine motor function. *Neurotoxicology, 35*, 154–161.

Gross, A. L., Rebok, G. W., Brandt, J., et al. (2013). Modelling learning and memory using verbal learning tests. *Journals of Gerontology: Psychological Sciences and Social Sciences, 68*(2), 153–167.

Guiney, H., & Machado, L. (2013). Benefits of regular aerobic exercise for executive functioning in healthy populations. *Psychonomic Bulletin & Review, 20*(1), 73–86.

Hasher, L., & Zacks, R. T. (1979). Autonomic and effortful processes in memory. *Journal of Experimental Psychology: General, 108*, 356–388.

Hayes, M. G., Kelly, A. J., & Smith, A. D. (2013). Working memory and the strategic control of attention in older and younger adults. *Journals of Gerontology: Psychological Sciences and Social Sciences, 68*(2), 176–183.

Healey, W. E. (2012). Mild cognitive impairment and aging. *Topics in Geriatric Rehabilitation, 28*(3), 157–162.

Health Quality Ontario. (2013, November). Vitamin B12 and cognitive function: An evidence-based analysis. *Ontario Health Technology Assessment Series, 13*(23), 1–45. Retrieved from http://www.hqontario.ca/evidence/publications-and-ohtac-recommendations/ontario-health-technology-assessment-series/B12-cognitive-function

Heinz, M., Martin, P., Margrett, J. A., et al. (2013). Perceptions of technology among older adults. *Journal of Gerontological Nursing, 39*(1), 42–51.

Hummert, M. L. (2011). Age stereotypes and aging. In K. W. Schaie & S. L. Willis (Eds.), *Handbook of the psychology of aging* (7th ed., pp. 249–277). New York, NY: Elsevier.

Johnson, E. J. (2012). A possible role for lutein and zeaxanthin in cognitive function in the elderly. *American Journal of Clinical Nutrition, 96*(5), 1161S–1165S.

Katan, M., Moon, Y. P., Paik, M. C., et al. (2013). Infectious burden and cognitive function: The Northern Manhattan study. *Neurology, 80*(13), 1209–1215.

Kloppenborg, R. P., Nederkoorn, P. J., Grool, A. M., et al. (2012). Cerebral small-vessel disease and progression of brain atrophy. *Neurology, 79*(20), 2029–2036.

Knight, B. G., & Laidlaw, K. (2009). Translations theory: A wisdom-based model for psychological interventions to enhance well-being in later life. In V. L. Bengston, M. Silverstein, N. M. Putnery et al. (Eds.), *Handbook of theories of aging* (2nd ed., pp. 693–705). New York, NY: Springer.

Kremen, W. S., Lachman, M. E., Pruessner, J. C., et al. (2012). Mechanisms of age-related cognitive change and targets for intervention. *Journals of Gerontology: Medical Sciences, 67*(7), 760–765.

Labouvie-Vief, G. (2009). Dynamic integration theory: Emotion, cognition, and equilibrium in later life. In V. L. Bengston, M. Silverstein, N. M. Putney, et al. (Eds.), *Handbook of theories of aging* (2nd ed., pp. 277–293). New York, NY: Springer.

Labouvie-Vief, G., & Blanchard-Fields, F. (1982). Cognitive aging and psychological growth. *Ageing and Society, 2*, 183–209.

Lanting, S., Crossley, M., Morgan, D., et al. (2011). Aboriginal experiences of aging and dementia in a context of sociocultural change: Qualitative analysis of key informant group interviews with aboriginal seniors. *Journal of Cross Cultural Gerontology, 26*(1), 103–117. doi:10.1007/s10823-010-9136-4

Levy, B. R., Zonderman, A. B., Slade, M. D., et al. (2011). Memory shaped by age stereotypes over time. *Journals of Gerontology: Psychological Sciences and Social Sciences, 67*(4), 432–436.

Lin, F. R., Yaffe, K., Xia, J., et al. (2013). Hearing loss and cognitive decline in older adults. *Journal of the American Medical Association, Internal Medicine, 173*(4), 293–299.

Lopez, O. L. (2013). Mild cognitive impairment. *Continuum, 19*(2), 411–424.

Lovden, M., Xu, W., & Wang, H. X. (2013). Lifestyle change and the prevention of cognitive decline and dementia: What is the evidence? *Current Opinions in Psychiatry, 26*(3), 239–243.

MacDonald, S., DeCarlo, C. A., & Dixon, R. A. (2011). Linking biological and cognitive aging. *Journals of Gerontology: Psychological Sciences and Social Sciences, 66B*(S1), i59–i70.

Makin, S., Turpin, S., Dennis, M. S., et al. (2013). Cognitive impairment after lacunar stroke: Systematic review and meta-analysis of incidence, prevalence and comparison with other stroke subtypes.

Journal of Neurology, Neurosurgery and Psychiatry, 84(8), 893–900. doi:10.1136/jnnp.2012.303645

Miller, K. J., Siddarth, P., Gaines, J. M., et al. (2012). The memory fitness program: Cognitive effects of a healthy aging intervention. *American Journal of Geriatric Psychiatry, 20,* 514–523.

Orsitto, G., Turi, V., Venezia, A., et al. (2012). Relation of secondhand smoking to mild cognitive impairment in older inpatients. *Scientific World Journal.* doi:10.1100/2012/726948

Park, D. C., & Bischof, G. N. (2011). Neuroplasticity, aging, and cognitive function. In K. W. Schaie & S. L. Willis (Eds.), *Handbook of the psychology of aging* (7th ed., pp. 109–119). New York, NY: Elsevier.

Pasina, L., Djade, C. D., Lucca, U., et al. (2013). Association of anticholinergic burden with cognitive and functional status in a cohort of hospitalized elderly. *Drugs and Aging, 30*(2), 103–112.

Patel, B. B., & Holland, N. W. (2012). Mild cognitive impairment: Hope for stability, plan for progression. *Cleveland Clinic Journal of Medicine, 79*(12), 857–864.

Peters, E., Dieckmann, N. F., & Weller, J. (2011). Age differences in complex decision making. In K. W. Schaie & S. L. Willis (Eds.), *Handbook of the psychology of aging* (7th ed., pp. 133–151). New York, NY: Elsevier.

Peterson, A., Mattek, N., Clemons, A., et al. (2012). Serum vitamin D concentrations are associated with falling and cognitive function in older adults. *Journal of Nutrition Health and Aging, 16*(10), 898–901.

Reis, J. P., Loria, C. M., Launer, L. J., et al. (2013). Cardiovascular health through young adulthood and cognitive functioning in midlife. *Annals of Neurology, 73*(2), 170–179.

Rosano, C., Marsland, A. L., & Gianaros, P. J. (2012). Maintaining brain health by monitoring inflammatory processes. *Aging and Disease, 3*(1), 16–33.

Sabia, S., Elbaz, A., Dugravot, A., et al. (2012). Impact of smoking on cognitive decline in early old age. *Archives of General Psychiatry, 69*(6), 627–635.

Sabia, S., Singh-Manoux, A., Hagger-Johnson, G., et al. (2012), Influence of individual and combined healthy behaviours on successful aging. *Canadian Medical Association Journal, 184*(18), 1985–1992.

Sartori, A. C., Vance, D. E., Slater, L. Z., et al. (2012). The impact of inflammation on cognitive function in older adults. *Journal of Neuroscience Nursing, 44*(4), 206–216.

Schaie, K. W. (1977–1978). Toward a stage theory of adult cognitive development. *Journal of Aging and Human Development, 8,* 129–138.

Shah, R. C., Schneider, J. A., Leurgans, S., et al. (2012). Association of lower hemoglobin level and neuropathology in community-dwelling older persons. *Journal of Alzheimer's Disease, 32*(3), 579–586.

Shatil, E. (2013). Does combined cognitive training and physical activity training enhance cognitive abilities more than either alone? *Frontiers in Aging Neuroscience, 5,* 8. doi:10.3389/fnagi.2013.00008

Slinin, Y., Paudel, M., Taylor, B. C., et al. (2012). Association between serum 25(OH) vitamin D and the risk of cognitive decline in older women. *Journals of Gerontology: Biological Sciences and Medical Sciences, 67*(10), 1092–1098.

Spiro, A., & Brady, C. B. (2011). Integrating health into cognitive aging. *Journals of Gerontology: Psychological Sciences and Social Sciences, 66*(S1), i17–i25.

Steffener, J., & Stern, Y. (2012). Exploring the neural basis of cognitive reserve in aging. *Biochim Biophys Acta, 1882*(3), 467–473.

Stern, Y. (2012). Cognitive reserve in ageing and Alzheimer's disease. *Lancet Neurology, 11*(11), 1006–1012.

Stine-Morrow, E., & Basak, C. (2011). Cognitive interventions. In K. W. Schaie & S. L. Willis. *Handbook of the psychology of aging* (7th ed., pp. 153–171). New York, NY: Elsevier.

Stine-Morrow, E., & Chui, H. (2011). Cognitive resilience in adulthood. In B. Hayslip & G. C. Smith (Eds.), *Annual review of gerontology and geriatrics* (Vol. 32, pp. 93–114). New York, NY: Springer.

Suzuki, T., Shimada, H., Makizako, H., et al. (2012). Effects of multicomponent exercise on cognitive function in older adults with amnesic mild cognitive impairment. *BMC Neurology, 12,* 128. Retrieved from www.biomedcentral.com/1471-2377/12/128

Swift, H. J., Abrams, D., & Marques, S. (2013). Threat or boost: Social comparison affects older people's performance differently depending on task domain. *Journals of Gerontology: Psychological Sciences and Social Sciences, 68*(1), 23–30.

Thinggaard, M., McGue, M., & Christensen, K. (2013). Age trajectory of high cognitive functioning among the oldest old. In J. Robine, C. Jagger, & E. M. Crimmins (Eds.), *Annual review of gerontology and geriatrics* (Vol. 33, pp. 35–59). New York, NY: Springer.

Tullis, J. G., & Benjamin, A. S. (2012). The effectiveness of updating metacognitive knowledge in the elderly. *Psychology and Aging, 27*(3), 683–690.

Van Der Mussele, S., Le Bastard, N., Vermeiren, Y., et al. (2013). Behavioural symptoms in mild cognitive impairment as compared with Alzheimer's disease and healthy older adults. *International Journal of Geriatric Psychiatry, 28*(3), 265–275.

Vance, D. E., Kaur, J., Fazeli, P. L., et al. (2012). Neuroplasticity and successful cognitive aging: A brief overview for nursing. *Journal of Neuroscience Nursing, 44*(4), 218–226.

Wang, H., Jin, Y., Hendrie, H. C., et al. (2013). Late life leisure activities and risk of cognitive decline. *Journals of Gerontology: Medical Sciences, 68*(2), 205–213.

Willis, K. J., & Hakim, A. M. (2013, March 21). Stroke preventions and cognitive reserve. *Frontiers in Neurology, 4.* doi:10.3389/fneur.2013.00013

Yavuz, B. B., Cankurtaran, M., Haznedaroglu, I. C., et al. (2012). Iron deficiency can cause cognitive impairment in geriatric patients. *Journal of Nutrition Health and Aging, 16*(3), 220–224.

chapter 12

Psychosocial Function

LEARNING OBJECTIVES

After reading this chapter, you will be able to:

1. Identify the life events that commonly occur in older adulthood.

2. Discuss theories related to stress and coping as they apply to older adults.

3. Identify the risk factors and cultural factors that influence psychosocial function in older adults.

4. Describe the functional consequences associated with psychosocial function in older adults.

5. Identify nursing interventions that promote psychosocial wellness in older adults.

6. Describe how to teach a "healthy aging class" for a small group of older adults.

KEY POINTS

anxiety

culture-bound syndromes

elderspeak

infantilization

late-life anxiety disorder

learned helplessness

religion

life events

life review

loneliness

reminiscence

resilience

self-esteem

spirituality

stress

stressors

Although the physiologic changes and chronic illnesses associated with older adulthood may affect a person's functional abilities, the psychosocial changes are often the most challenging and demanding in terms of coping energy. Of course, many psychosocial challenges are strongly associated with compromised health and functioning, but some are attributable to changes in roles, relationships and living environments. Because many of the psychosocial changes are inevitable and somewhat predictable, older adults can prepare for and respond to psychosocial challenges by developing and using effective coping strategies. Nurses promote psychosocial wellness by supporting effective coping mechanisms and assisting in the development of new coping strategies.

LIFE EVENTS: AGE-RELATED CHANGES AFFECTING PSYCHOSOCIAL FUNCTION

Life events are the major changes that occur at various times during the life cycle and significantly affect daily life. Certain events are commonly associated with different periods in one's life. For example, younger adults are likely to experience the following life events: establishing a career, moving away from the nuclear family, committing to a partner, creating a home and beginning a family. The major life events of younger adulthood are familiar to us through either personal experiences or the shared experiences of friends. People usually view these events as positive gains and choose them purposefully. By contrast, life events of older adulthood might be unknown, unexpected, inevitable and, in fact, unwanted or even feared. Thus, older adults may experience a greater loss of control or fear of losing control over their lives. In addition, life events during older adulthood are likely to involve losses of significant others and objects that have been part of life for many decades. Moreover, they tend to occur close together, with less time available to adjust to each event (Lane et al., 2013). Some life events evolve into chronic stresses. Dealing with ageist attitudes and behaviours of others is a life event that is specific to older adults.

Life events that are most likely to occur during older adulthood include retirement, relocation, chronic illness and functional impairments, decisions about driving a vehicle, widowhood, death of friends and family and confronting ageist attitudes. Figure 12-1 illustrates some of the major life events that are likely to occur in older adulthood, as well as the related consequences. Although most of the consequences are negative, some consequences can be positive. For example, because of these life events, older adults may focus on achieving integrity and meaning in life, and they may develop a greater acceptance of things that cannot be controlled. The illustration attempts to show the interrelatedness among the life events of older adulthood.

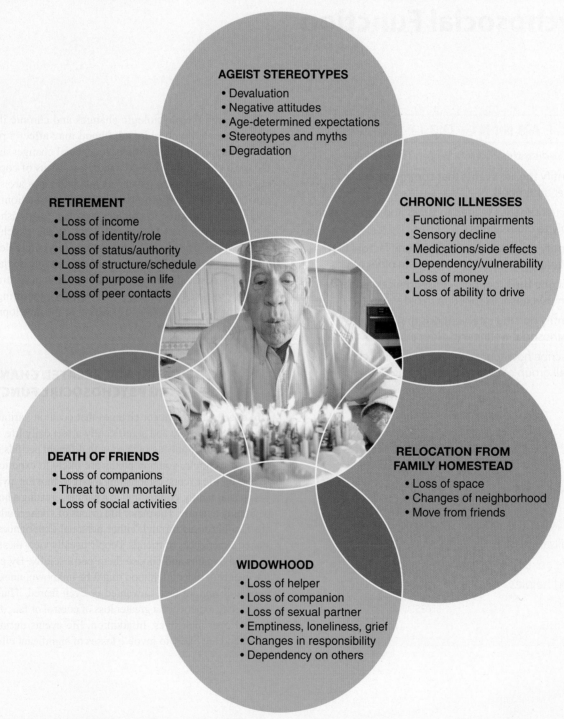

AGEIST STEREOTYPES
• Devaluation
• Negative attitudes
• Age-determined expectations
• Stereotypes and myths
• Degradation

CHRONIC ILLNESSES
• Functional impairments
• Sensory decline
• Medications/side effects
• Dependency/vulnerability
• Loss of money
• Loss of ability to drive

RETIREMENT
• Loss of income
• Loss of identity/role
• Loss of status/authority
• Loss of structure/schedule
• Loss of purpose in life
• Loss of peer contacts

DEATH OF FRIENDS
• Loss of companions
• Threat to own mortality
• Loss of social activities

RELOCATION FROM FAMILY HOMESTEAD
• Loss of space
• Changes of neighborhood
• Move from friends

WIDOWHOOD
• Loss of helper
• Loss of companion
• Loss of sexual partner
• Emptiness, loneliness, grief
• Changes in responsibility
• Dependency on others

FIGURE 12-1 Psychosocial challenges of older adulthood.

Retirement

Retirement from employment is often viewed as a milestone that marks the passage into older adulthood. The age of 65 years is the traditional retirement age; however, there is a growing movement toward "bridge employment" involving a gradual transition from full-time to part-time employment before full retirement. Current trends indicate that many older adults move into self-employment, change their occupation or become consultants as they phase into full retirement (Bowen et al., 2011; Rix, 2011). Delaying full retirement can be beneficial because studies demonstrate that maintaining work responsibilities is associated with improved physical and psychosocial functioning (Wickrama et al., 2013).

Societal attitudes can influence one's adjustment to retirement, particularly in societies with a strong work ethic. In these societies, working people have a higher status than do unemployed people and, among working people, status is based on the kind of job one holds and the salary one earns. Therefore, when people retire, they inevitably cope with a change in social status, and the psychosocial challenge may be the greatest for people whose **self-esteem** (the feelings one has about one's self) and self-concept are based on job status. The following factors commonly influence the decision to retire: health, financial assets, job conditions, pension availability, family circumstances (e.g., caregiving responsibilities), opportunities for continued employment and continued ability to perform job responsibilities. For married couples, both the worker and the spouse, or partner, must adjust to retirement. Sometimes the adjustment is more difficult for the partner who has not been employed.

Positive and negative outcomes of retirement vary significantly among older adults and are influenced by many factors, such as health, relationships with family and friends, and social and economic resources. A major determinant of the degree to which retirement is experienced as negative or positive is whether it is forced or voluntary. Studies reveal that involuntary retirement is linked to increased risk for depression, negative health effects and harmful health-related behaviours, including smoking, reduced physical activity and increased alcohol consumption among nondrinkers (Hershey & Henkens, 2014).

Relocation

Another common psychosocial adjustment for older adults is the decision to move from the family home because of factors such as loss of spouse, lack of available assistive services, lack of a kinship network or caregiver, chronic conditions and declining functional abilities, and cognitive impairment or psychiatric illness. Increased dependence on others because of health problems is a common reason for older adults to move to a facility where they can receive support services. Additional reasons for moving to another geographic location include being closer to younger family members, preferring a warmer climate or desiring a lower cost of living.

In addition to family and personal factors, many environmental conditions influence the decision to move. For example, older people in urban areas may find they are unsafe or socially isolated because the neighbourhood around them has changed gradually and they are no longer surrounded by people with whom they can easily relate. In rural areas, geographic distance and lack of support services can have serious consequences for older adults who are functionally impaired, especially if they have few social supports. Problems also arise for older homeowners who find it more difficult to physically and financially maintain their home and pay for utilities.

Relocation to a long-term care facility is a significant life event for some older adults, and these decisions have serious emotional and economic consequences. Because options for long-term care settings have been expanding significantly since the 1990s (discussed in Chapter 6), these decisions are complex. When older adults experience an abrupt or major change in health status, it is important to view these decisions as short-term rather than permanent. Nurses are in key positions to address these decisions holistically by ensuring that psychosocial issues are considered along with medical concerns. Also, nurses can ensure that older adults are involved as much as possible in decisions and that these decisions are periodically reviewed as the older adult's needs change.

Chronic Illness and Functional Impairments

Another major life adjustment for many older adults is coping with chronic illnesses and functional limitations, particularly limitations that curtail their independence. Although most older adults experience one or more chronic conditions that affect their daily functioning, 44% of older Canadians rated their health as excellent or very good and 70% reported that their mental health was excellent or good (Public Health Agency of Canada, 2010). Most functional limitations necessitate only minor adjustments in daily living, but some, such as considerable cognitive, mobility or visual impairments, are associated with consequences such as the following:

● Increased dependence on others
● Threats to self-esteem and altered self-concept
● Changes in lifestyle
● Unpredictability about one's ability to do what one wants
● Expenditures for assistance, medications and medical care
● Frequent trips to health care providers

- Adverse medication effects, which sometimes cause further functional impairments
- Increased vulnerability to personal crimes and fear of crime

Decisions About Driving a Vehicle

Decisions about driving a vehicle are often one of the most emotionally charged issues that older adults, their families and health care professionals face. In Canada, access to an automobile and the possession of a valid driver's license not only provide transportation but also serve as significant indicators of autonomy. In fact, for many older adults, the ability to drive is synonymous with independence, and the possession of a driver's license, even one that goes unused, is a symbol of one's ability to shield oneself from dependence on others. While cessation of driving is considered a normal transition of older adulthood, older Canadians tend to use other forms of transportation, such as taxis and public transit infrequently (Turcotte, 2012). As such, this transition can be very difficult for some older adults. Reviews of studies indicate that driving cessation is directly associated with serious negative consequences including depression, decreased social engagement, loss of personal identity and roles, increased mortality and accelerated declines in cognitive function and overall health (Boot et al., 2014; Choi et al., 2014; Liddle et al., 2014). In addition to increasing age, conditions associated with driving cessation are functional limitations, cognitive impairment, major illness (e.g., stroke, hip fracture) and sensory impairment (especially a combination of vision and hearing impairment) (Dugan & Lee, 2013; Green et al., 2013).

The loss of an independent means of transportation affects every aspect of an older person's life, from the acquisition of food and medicine to opportunities for social interaction. Because of this far-reaching impact, families of older persons may avoid dealing with driving-related issues. Family members may be reluctant to suggest that an older relative give up driving for a number of reasons. For example, family members may not want to assume an authority role, or they may lack acceptable alternatives for transportation. It is not surprising, then, that older adults and their families may avoid or resist the decision to stop driving. Neither is it surprising that when older adults give up or significantly curtail their driving, they face a difficult psychosocial challenge that may be viewed as a major life event. Implications for nursing assessment and interventions related to safe driving are discussed in Chapter 7 as an aspect of functional assessment.

Widowhood

The example of widowhood as a life event of older adulthood illustrates all of the characteristics discussed earlier. For most older couples, widowhood is inevitable, and the chances are greater that women become widowed more than men do. When widowhood occurs, additional consequences follow. Common additional consequences include the following:

- Loss of companionship and intimacy
- Loss of one's sexual partner
- Feelings of grief, loneliness and emptiness
- Increased responsibilities
- Increased dependence on others
- Loss of income and less efficient financial management
- Changes in relationships with children, married friends and other family members

When a marriage or partnership has lasted for many decades, as is common in people who are in their 70s and 80s, the impact of the loss can be tremendous, and the feelings of grief, loneliness and emptiness may be overwhelming. A review of studies emphasizes that psychological consequences of widowhood vary widely and are influenced by factors such as marital quality and whether the surviving partner had been a caregiver for the deceased one (Schaan, 2013). Research reviews also emphasize that patterns of bereavement during widowhood vary across a spectrum that includes common grief, chronic grief, chronic depression, improvement during bereavement and resilience (Whitbourne & Meeks, 2011). See Box 12-1 for the psychological impact of widowhood upon older adults, as well as the role of spirituality in processing grief.

Another characteristic of widowhood in older adulthood is that the chance of remarriage diminishes with advancing age. This is especially true for women because there are disproportionately fewer older men than older women due to greater longevity of women. Other reasons that older adults do not remarry include family issues, financial factors (e.g., decreased government benefits) and preference for their newly independent lifestyle. Even when widows or widowers do remarry, they need to adjust to entirely different roles with a new partner. If the married couple had clearly

---

Box 12-1 Evidence-Informed Nursing Practice

Background: Religious faith and spirituality are believed to assist older adults in dealing with the grief caused by the loss of a spouse. However, the role of spirituality in processing grief and moving through grief is less understood.

Question: How does spirituality assist older adults in processing and adjusting to the loss of a spouse?

Methods: Twenty-four Canadian seniors (ages 65 to 82) who had experienced the death of a spouse participated in therapy groups (6 adults per group). The groups ran for 14 weeks and were 1.5 hours in length. The groups were audiotaped for transcription. Although the groups did not focus on spirituality, themes were identified that demonstrated the role of spirituality in processing grief.

Findings: In the earlier stages of processing grief, spirituality was reflected in the conversations about loss of identity and life purpose in the remaining spouses. Older adults did, however, maintain the spiritual belief that their relationship with the deceased spouse endured. As time passed, older adults demonstrated spirituality in making meaning out of their spouses' death and in renewed sense of engaging with others and new purposes.

Implications for Nursing Practice: Nurses can explore with older adults the impact of their spouses' death upon their lives, as well as how they currently derive meaning and purpose in their lives.

Source: Damianakis, T., & Marziali, E. (2012). Older adults' response to the loss of a spouse: The function of spirituality in understanding the grieving process. *Aging & Mental Health, 16*(1), 57–66.

divided roles, as is common in the cohort of people who are old today, loss of the partner means an adjustment in important day-to-day tasks. For example, older couples often divide tasks so that only one of the two manages money, drives the vehicle, cleans the house, shops for groceries and does household repairs and maintenance. When the person responsible for a task no longer performs the role, the other person may be unable, unwilling or unprepared to assume this role. Two gender-specific strains during widowhood are financial strain for women and difficulty with household management for men (Schaan, 2013).

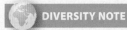

Wellness Opportunity

When applicable, nurses encourage older adults to talk about their experience of widowhood by opening the conversation with a question such as, "How is your life different since your partner passed away?"

Death of Friends and Family

Like other life events of older adulthood, the loss of friends and family becomes inevitable with increasing age. Many people who are in their 90s have outlived most, if not all, of their friends and many of their relatives. Indeed, people who are in their 90s may not even know anyone who is older than they are. Moreover, as people are confronted with the death of others who are younger than or similar to them in age, they become increasingly aware of their own mortality. Older people may read obituaries and death notices in the newspaper as a daily activity. Although families may view this activity as a morbid preoccupation, it may, in fact, be an effective way for older people to learn what is happening to their friends or acquaintances. Because meaningful social relationships are an important predictor of well-being for older adults, loss of family and friends is likely to have a negative impact on psychosocial wellness.

DIVERSITY NOTE

Experiences of grief are influenced by cultural and historical events that shaped a particular culture. For instance, aboriginal Canadians may be more at risk for complicated grief than their nonaboriginal counterparts, due to the historical colonization of their peoples, as well as the high rate of suicide within their culture (Spiwak et al., 2012).

Ageist Attitudes

A life adjustment that, by its nature, is unique to older adulthood is defending against negative ageist stereotypes and attitudes, which are pervasive in Western societies. Although stereotypes of older adults can be both positive (e.g., wise, respected, accomplished) or negative (e.g., slow, confused, incompetent), studies consistently find that negative ones far outweigh the positive ones in Western societies (Hummert, 2011). A recent content analysis of images of older individuals posted on Facebook by adults in their 20s found that

descriptors of older people excoriated (74%) or infantilized (27%) them and even advocated banning them from shopping and other public activities (37%) (Levy et al., 2014). Although these images may be discounted as harmless, negative stereotypes of aging can have subtle, but serious, detrimental effects on health and functioning of older adults. For example, studies indicate that negative stereotypes about aging can result in worse memory performance in older adults (Kotter-Gruhn & Hess, 2012; Levy et al., 2011; Mazerolle et al., 2012). In addition, a review of studies concluded that age stereotypes lead to negative attitudes and biased behaviour toward older people, even among older adults themselves (Hummert, 2011). Other studies find that positive age stereotypes can be beneficial for older adults. For example, longitudinal data from the home-based assessments performed every 18 months from 1998 through 2008 found that older people (i.e., age 70 years and older) with positive age stereotypes were 44% more likely to recover fully from severe disability than those with negative age stereotypes (Levy et al., 2012).

DIVERSITY NOTE

Many studies have linked Confucian values of filial piety and respect for ancestors in Asian cultures to enhanced self-esteem in elders and to better societal attitudes toward aging (Bonanno et al., 2012).

Wellness Opportunity

Nurses can promote positive attitudes about aging by talking about people who are examples of successful aging.

THEORIES ABOUT STRESS AND COPING IN OLDER ADULTS

Theories about stress and coping attempt to answer questions such as *How do life events affect older adults? Do coping patterns change in older adulthood?* and *How do stress and coping patterns affect health and functioning?* In keeping with the perspective of this text, these theories are discussed in relation to positive or negative functional consequences on psychosocial function. Additional psychological theories pertinent to older adults are discussed in Chapter 4.

Theories About Stress

Hans Selye, a Canadian, proposed the first major theory about stress in the mid-1950s. He defined **stress** as the sum of all the effects of factors that act on the body (Selye, 1956). According to Selye's theory, **stressors** include normal activities and disease states; all factors, whether pleasant or unpleasant, are equally important. Moreover, people respond to stressors in three stages: alarm, resistance and exhaustion. Limitations of this theory include the broad conceptualization of stress, the lack of distinction between pleasant and unpleasant stressors and the failure to address the meaning of events for the person.

Holmes and Rahe (1967) proposed that stress causes physical and psychological harm in proportion to the intensity of the impact on and duration of a disruption in one's usual life pattern. They developed the Social Readjustment Rating Scale as a tool for measuring the duration and intensity of 43 commonly experienced life events, with relative weights assigned to each according to the usual amount of adaptive effort required by each event. This rating scale has been criticized because it suggests that life events consistently have a negative impact for all people. Since the 1970s, researchers have developed stress scales that account for the meaning of life events for the individual or that measure effects of life events of particular age groups.

In addition to addressing the impact of major life events (e.g., acute stress), studies address the impact of chronic stressors, including those that evolve from a major life event. Scott and colleagues (2013) described types of chronic stressors as (1) role strains from ongoing problems with work, family, relationships and caregiving and (2) ambient stressors across life domains, such as health, finances, loneliness and neighbourhood. Daily hassles (i.e., relatively minor events arising from day-to-day living) are another source of stress that can negatively affect psychological well-being overall and cognitive function in particular (Stawski et al., 2013). Examples of hassles are misplacing or losing things and not having resources to meet demands (e.g., food, money, medications). When chronic stressors and daily hassles occur together—as is often the case—the negative effects are magnified, leading to declines in physical and cognitive functioning in older adults (Almeida et al., 2011). As summarized by Werner and colleagues (2012), "the level of stress experienced by individuals is dependent, in part, on all of the stressors they are currently experiencing and on their appraisal of any given situation" (p. 138).

A prominent current theme among gerontologists is expanding the "stress universe" to develop a more comprehensive approach to identifying many factors that affect the ways in which older adults experience and respond to stressors (George, 2011). In particular, researchers and clinicians focus attention on the connection between chronic stress and health. Currently, studies find that chronic stress increases the risk for all the following (Blume et al., 2011; Gouin & Kiecolt-Glaser, 2011; Lyon, 2012):

- Onset of major illnesses (e.g., cancer, cardiovascular conditions)
- Exacerbation of chronic conditions (e.g., diabetes, multiple sclerosis, respiratory disease, inflammatory bowel disease)
- Symptoms (e.g., pain, fatigue, insomnia, headache, gastrointestinal distress)
- Delayed wound healing
- Depression

Theories About Coping

Theories about age-related differences in coping address the following types of internal mechanisms that people use to deal with stressful situations: seeking information; reframing the situation; maintaining a hopeful outlook; using stress-reduction techniques; channelling energy into physical activity; creating fantasies about various outcomes; finding reassurance and emotional support; identifying limited and realistic goals; identifying a positive purpose for the event; getting involved in other activities, such as work and family; and expressing oneself creatively, for example, through music, art or writing. These coping styles are categorized as problem focused (i.e., directed toward altering the source of stress) or emotion focused (i.e., directed toward regulating one's response). Studies indicate that older adults are more likely to use coping mechanisms that involve management of thoughts and feelings, whereas younger adults are likely to take direct approaches to modify the events or challenging situations in their lives (Brennan et al., 2012; Mather, 2012). For example, a coping mechanism that promotes successful aging is the ability of older adults to compensate for a diminished sense of control by adjusting their personal expectations (Hayward & Krause, 2013a).

In recent years, gerontologists have focused on both the meaning of the event to the individual and the coping resources available to the individual. Studies consistently identify strong social supports, especially religious supports, as a way of facilitating coping in older adults (George, 2011; Underwood, 2012). Social resources include instrumental support (e.g., meals, transportation, personal care), informational support (e.g., information about resources and services) and emotional support (e.g., communication that provides comfort, companionship and other evidence that the person is loved, valued, esteemed and cared for).

Relevance for Nurses

Nurses can use theories about stress and coping to identify interventions that help older adults maintain optimal functioning and quality of life when faced with the many challenges of aging. A recent nursing study identified strategies used by older adults with chronic comorbid conditions to remain at home safely with optimal health and psychosocial well-being (Westra et al., 2013). The study identified two major themes related to coping with functional limitations: getting around at home and expanding life beyond self and home. Figure 12-2 provides an overview of strategies used by older adult for "getting on with living life," and Online Learning Activity 12-1 provides access to the article describing this study. Many of the significant stresses, such as decreasing eyesight and hearing, can be addressed through nursing interventions to improve functional abilities as discussed in all chapters of Part 4 in this text. Other significant stresses, such as losses of, or changes in, relationships, can be addressed through the psychosocial interventions discussed in the section on nursing interventions in this chapter.

 See ONLINE LEARNING ACTIVITY 12-1: EVIDENCE-BASED ARTICLE DESCRIBING STRATEGIES USED BY OLDER ADULTS WITH CHRONIC CONDITIONS TO REMAIN AT HOME SAFELY at http://thepoint.lww.com/Miller7e

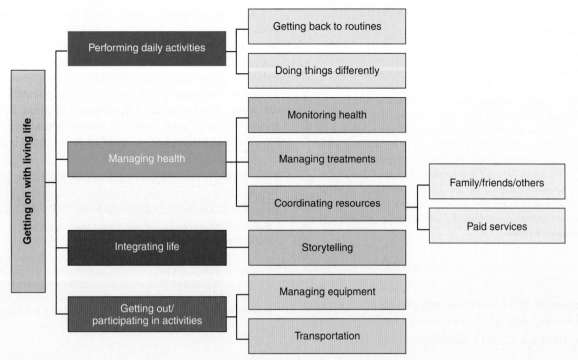

FIGURE 12-2 Strategies used by older adults to get on with living life. Adapted with permission from Westra, B. L., Paitich, N. Ekstrom, D., et al. (2013). Getting on with living life: Experiences of older adults after home care. *Home Health care Nurse, 31*(9), 493–501.

FACTORS THAT INFLUENCE PSYCHOSOCIAL FUNCTION IN OLDER ADULTS

Psychosocial function is influenced by numerous factors, including personality, experiences, physical and emotional health, and socioeconomic and environmental conditions. Because many of the factors are beyond the usual scope of nursing, this section focuses on two aspects that are particularly pertinent to usual nursing care of older adults: religion and spirituality and cultural considerations. Additional information about these topics is addressed in Chapter 13 (section on assessing religion and spirituality) and Chapter 2.

Religion and Spirituality

Religion and spirituality are widely recognized as major coping resources that have a positive effect on many aspects of psychosocial function for older adults. Religion and spirituality are closely related but distinct concepts. **Religion** and religiosity, which have a strong social component, refer to an organized system of beliefs and behaviours that are shared by a group of people who are associated with a defined faith community. Examples of religious practices are rituals, prayers, meditation, worship services, attendance at church, and adherence to certain dietary practices and style of clothing. Religious practices nurture spiritual development; however, spirituality is broader and less structured and does not necessarily include membership in a formal religious group. Gerontologists consistently find that religion becomes more important with age and that attendance at religious services is associated with many beneficial outcomes including better health and longer life expectancy (Fitchett et al., 2013; Hayward & Krause, 2013b; Pynnonen et al., 2012).

Florence Nightingale viewed **spirituality** as intrinsic to human nature and emphasized that it was an individual's deepest and the most potent resource for healing. Definitions of spirituality generally include the following concepts: healing; wholeness; social justice; personal growth; interpersonal relationships; a sense of meaning and purpose to life; a transcendent relationship with a higher being; an association with reverence, mystery and inspiration; connectedness with nature, other people and the universe; and feelings of and behaviours arising from love, faith, hope, trust and forgiveness. Current nursing references (e.g., Burkhardt & Nagai-Jacobson, 2013; Herdman, 2012) describe the following components of spirituality:

- Connectedness to self: joy, love, surrender, serenity, self-forgiveness, and meaning and purpose in life
- Connectedness with others: service, compassion, loving sexuality, forgiveness of others, shared genuine presence, meaningful interactions with significant others, reciprocal giving and receiving
- Connectedness with power greater than self: awe, prayer, ritual, reverence, meditation, reconciliation, mystical experiences
- Engagement in creative activities: art, music, nature, poetry, writing, singing, spiritual literature

Gerontologists describe these "everyday spiritual experiences" as effective coping resources that enhance well-being for older adults (Whitehead & Bergeman, 2011). Gerontologists

A Student's Perspective

When I interviewed one of the residents, I felt like I got a really good impression of the things he valued most and the exciting experiences in his life. I think the most significant part for me was when we talked about religion. When I asked Mr. E. if he was religious, he answered very politely saying that his parents tried to raise him Catholic but that it was never really him. I then asked if he saw himself as spiritual and he said that he is very spiritual and that he definitely thinks there is something "more" after death. He said that he didn't feel like he needed to go to a church to be a good person. I really connected with this because I was able to see that we have something in common. I also feel very spiritual even though I am not really affiliated with any particular religion.

Erika B.

also emphasize the importance of religious beliefs and spirituality in helping older adults make sense of challenges inherent in aging (Harris et al., 2013; Manning et al., 2012).

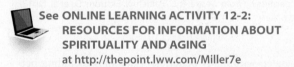

See **ONLINE LEARNING ACTIVITY 12-2: RESOURCES FOR INFORMATION ABOUT SPIRITUALITY AND AGING** at http://thepoint.lww.com/Miller7e

Wellness Opportunity

Nurses promote wellness by asking older adults about relationships that provide meaning in their lives.

Cultural Considerations

Cultural factors strongly influence the way a person defines and perceives all aspects of psychosocial function. In assessing psychosocial function in older adults, for example, it is essential to recognize that every society has guidelines for determining whether behaviours are healthy or unhealthy (Box 12-2). Many societies, however, do not have the rigid distinctions between health and illness that are part of Western cultures, and concepts, such as mental health, have little meaning in many non-Western societies (Ehrmin, 2012). Cultural perceptions determine all of the following aspects of psychosocial function:

- Definition of mental health and mental illness
- Belief about the causes of mental health and illness
- Expression of symptoms or clinical manifestations of mental health and illness
- Criteria for labelling or diagnosing someone as mentally ill
- Decisions concerning appropriate healer(s)
- Choice of treatment(s) to cure mental illness
- Determination that mental health has been restored after an illness episode
- Relative degree of tolerance for abnormal behaviour by other members of society

In some instances, people from diverse cultures may perceive or interpret physical symptoms and their related psychological or emotional components in a manner that is unfamiliar to professionals who do not share the same cultural background. This is likely to occur for **culture-bound syndromes**, which are specific manifestations that are unique to a particular cultural group (Ehrmin, 2012). In recent decades, more than 200 culture-bound syndromes have been identified, and many of these are listed in official

Box 12-2 Cultural Considerations: Cultural Influences on Psychosocial Function

Cultural Influences on Beliefs About the Cause of Mental Disorders

- In traditional Chinese culture, many diseases are attributed to an imbalance of yin and yang.
- Many Canadian aboriginals embrace a belief system in which balance and harmony are essential for mental and physical health.
- Some African Canadians, especially those of circum-Caribbean descent, may attribute the cause of mental illness to voodoo, sorcery or other spiritual forces.

Cultural Influences on the Manifestations of Mental Illness

- Cultural norms determine whether behaviours, such as any of the following, are viewed as either normal or abnormal: dreams, fainting, visions, trances, sorcery, delusions, hallucinations, intoxication, suicide, speaking in tongues, communicating with spirits and the use of certain substances (e.g., alcohol, tobacco, peyote, marijuana and other drugs).
- Posttraumatic stress disorders are relatively common in immigrants and refugees.
- Filipino Canadians consider forgetfulness and anger to be mental health problems.
- Hispanic, Chinese and other groups are likely to express psychological distress through physical symptoms.
- Depression may be expressed through physical symptoms, such as pain, headache or gastrointestinal symptoms.
- Although psychotic disorders (i.e., loss of contact with reality) occur in every society and are characterized by similar primary symptoms (e.g., delusions, hallucinations, flat affect, social or emotional withdrawal), the secondary features (e.g., content and focus) are highly influenced by cultural factors.
- In some groups, guilt and suicidal ideation do not accompany depression. For some Inuit communities in Canada, suicide rates are very high, despite a low self-reported rate of depression.

Cultural Influences on Stress and Coping

- Cultural factors often create barriers to the use of formal support services by ethnic elders, and these barriers may increase the feelings of burden experienced by caregivers.
- African Canadian families tend to use religion and spirituality to help them cope with caregiving stress, and religious organizations are a major source of social support for them.
- In Chinese families, cultural ideals promoting filial piety, family interdependence, veneration of elderly family members and acceptance of family caregiving roles may affect the way families experience and cope with stress related to their roles as caregivers.

Sources: Andrews, M. M., & Boyle, J. S., (2012). *Transcultural concepts in nursing care*. Philadelphia, PA: Wolters Kluwer/Lippincott, Williams, & Wilkins; Khan, S. (2008). Aboriginal mental health: The statistical report. Retrieved from http://www.heretohelp.bc.ca/visions/aboriginal-people-vol5/aboriginal-mental-health-the-statistical-report

diagnostic manuals, which are periodically updated. Examples of culture-bound syndromes that nurses in geriatric care settings may encounter include the following:

- *Dhat, Jiryan,* in people from India: dizziness, fatigue, weakness, loss of appetite, sexual dysfunction and feeling of guilt
- *Windigo (or Wendigo) Psychosis,* in some aboriginal tribes, such as the Ojibwe and Cree tribes living around the Great Lakes: During the cold winter months, some individuals began to see others as edible and developed an insatiable desire to eat human flesh (http://anthro.palomar.edu/medical/med_4.htm).
- *Nervios,* in Latino people: irritability, tearfulness, sleep disturbances, difficulty concentrating and feeling of vulnerability and emotional distress to stressful life experiences
- *Shenjing,* in Chinese people: depression, anxiety, dizziness, headaches, sleep and gastrointestinal disturbances

Professionals and folk or indigenous healers with the same cultural background usually are knowledgeable about interventions for culture-bound syndromes. Older adults may be reluctant to discuss culture-bound syndromes or folk treatments with health care professionals, especially if the care provider has a different cultural background. The reasons for withholding such information are complex and may include fears that the nurse or other health care provider will disapprove, ridicule or fail to understand their folk or indigenous healing system. Because of these factors, nurses may consider asking the person's permission to include folk or indigenous healers in discussions about health-related issues. These healers frequently have considerable insight into the cultural and psychosocial aspects of human behaviour, and they may be remarkably successful in treating culture-bound syndromes and other disorders that have psychological and emotional components. Because herbal remedies that are sometimes used to treat culture-bound syndromes may interact with prescription or over-the-counter medications, nurses need to make every effort to elicit information about such remedies as part of an assessment (see Chapter 8).

Case Study

Mrs. Y. is a 79-year-old native of the Philippines. She moved to an urban area in Ontario to be near her four children, who live in the same province. She had lived in the same town in the Philippines for her entire adult life and had stayed there to care for her husband and her sister, who both required care for chronic conditions. Although she was a much-needed and highly esteemed member of her household in the Philippines, Mrs. Y., like many other immigrants, experienced role reversal when she lost her once-dominant position in the family and became financially dependent on her adult children after her relocation.

Also like many older immigrants from the Philippines, Mrs. Y. had a more active social network before her relocation. As did many of her peers, Mrs. Y. spoke a dialect and did not speak Tagalog, the language spoken by many younger residents of the Philippines. After her relocation to Canada, her communication and interaction with others became restricted to her extended family because she did not feel confident using her limited English and could not find other speakers of her dialect. To buffer the disequilibrium she felt as a result of her migration, Mrs. Y. sought comfort through prayer and regular attendance at the local Roman Catholic church. She also began to care regularly for her two daughters' children.

You are the nurse at the local hospital who treated Mrs. Y. in the emergency department after she fractured her wrist. During your assessment, you note that Mrs. Y.'s injury would place a strain on the family because they would temporarily be without their child care provider.

THINKING POINTS

- How would you involve the family members in the discharge plan for Mrs. Y. so that her recovery could be ensured, she would not lose respect and she would not feel responsible to assume her usual duties until her injury healed and she felt better?
- What problems would you anticipate in communicating with Mrs. Y. in the emergency department? How would you handle these problems?
- What psychosocial repercussions did Mrs. Y.'s move to Canada have? Did she cope with these effectively? Would you have had any other suggestions for helping her to cope?
- How did Mrs. Y.'s culture influence her coping mechanisms?

Case example reprinted with permission from McKenna, M. A. (2012). Transcultural perspectives in the nursing care of older adults. In M. M. Andrews & J. S. Boyle. *Transcultural concepts in nursing care* (6th ed., pp. 182–207). Philadelphia, PA: Lippincott, Williams, & Wilkins. (Questions that follow the case example were written by Carol A. Miller.)

A Student's Perspective

While I was caring for my client, she asked if she could tell me a story. She proceeded to tell me that a few nights earlier, she was lying in bed unable to sleep because of various health issues. All of a sudden, she heard this calm yet intense chant moving down the hall. One of the residents is First Nations and recently received news that his nephew had passed away. He was performing a traditional chant in mourning for the loss of a loved one. My client said that the sound was peaceful and soothing as she lay awake in bed. She wished she could have recorded it to play every night. She felt it was special that this man was able to maintain his culture in a place far from home and that people respected his need to express himself in this way. She was very touched—and so was I—as she told me this story. I believe that maintaining one's culture is a part of the healing process and should be respected and upheld.

Eliza T.

RISK FACTORS THAT AFFECT PSYCHOSOCIAL FUNCTION

Theories about stress and coping and research about causes of impaired mental health in older adults provide information about risks that can affect psychosocial function. The following factors contribute to high levels of stress and poor coping in older adults:

- Poor physical health
- Impaired functional abilities
- Weak social supports
- Lack of economic resources
- An immature developmental level
- Narrow range of coping skills
- The occurrence of unanticipated events
- The occurrence of several daily hassles at the same time
- The occurrence of several major life events over a short time

In addition, because the ability to determine the potential for change influences one's response to a stressful situation, people who cannot realistically appraise a situation may have more difficulty coping effectively. This is particularly pertinent with regard to health and functioning because ageist attitudes and stereotypes may contribute to the false belief that health changes and functional decline are inevitable consequences of aging. Thus, nurses have important roles in teaching older adults about risk factors and potential interventions for health problems. For example, older adults who experience urinary incontinence or difficulties with sexual function may consider these changes to be inevitable consequences of age. Based on this appraisal, they may use passive, emotion-focused coping mechanisms, trying simply to accept the situation. In addition, they are more likely to experience an unnecessary and unfortunate functional impairment and a diminished quality of life. By contrast, if the situation is appraised more accurately as a potentially treatable condition, older adults are more likely to use active, problem-focused coping mechanisms. Even when older adults accurately appraise health problems as changeable, health care professionals also must understand the problem and attempt to find solutions. Thus, both older adults and health care professionals must accurately appraise the situation so they can initiate interventions and achieve wellness outcomes.

Learned helplessness is the experience of uncontrollable events that leads to expectations that future events will also be uncontrollable. Thus, actions that increase dependency or disempower older adults (e.g., providing assistance because this is more time-efficient rather than allowing the older person to function independently or with only a little assistance) are risk factors for diminished self-esteem and feelings of powerlessness. In addition, learned helplessness may contribute to depression, as discussed in Chapter 15. Studies indicate that older adults who have a reduced sense of control may be at increased risk for many negative consequences, such as stress, anxiety, depression, less engagement in health-promoting behaviours (e.g., exercise) and poorer health and memory functioning (Lachman et al., 2011).

FUNCTIONAL CONSEQUENCES ASSOCIATED WITH PSYCHOSOCIAL FUNCTION IN OLDER ADULTS

Although negative functional consequences are commonly associated with psychosocial function in older adults, positive functional consequences also occur in older adults. This section reviews anxiety and loneliness as two negative functional consequences that nurses can address. In addition, cognitive impairment and depression are serious negative functional consequences that are discussed in Chapters 14 and 15, respectively. Resilience in later life, which is a topic that is currently receiving much attention in gerontological literature, is discussed in this section as a positive functional consequence.

Anxiety is a feeling of distress, subjectively experienced as fear or worry and objectively expressed through autonomic and central nervous system responses. Prevalence of clinically significant anxiety symptoms in community-living older adults ranges from 15% to 52% (Yochim et al., 2011). Mild and moderate anxiety can be beneficial because it motivates protective behaviours, but excessive anxiety is detrimental because it channels personal energy into defensive behaviours. Currently increasing attention is paid to **late-life anxiety disorder,** a persistent condition of excessive anxiety characterized by uncontrollable worry that interferes with daily life and leads to serious physical and mental discomfort (Blay & Marinho, 2012). Serious consequences of anxiety disorders in older adults include sleep disturbances, diminished quality of life and increased morbidity (Brenes et al., 2012; Shrestha et al., 2011). Anxiety disorders are common in older adults and are often unrecognized and untreated (Lenze & Wetherell, 2011; Schuurmans & van Balkom, 2011). Information about nursing assessment of anxiety is discussed in Chapter 13. An important role for nurses is to facilitate referrals for professional interventions, such as medications or cognitive behavioural therapy, for older adults with anxiety disorders.

Older adults may experience feelings of loneliness. According to Statistics Canada, approximately 20% of older adults experience feelings of loneliness and dissatisfaction with life (Gilmour, 2012). **Loneliness** is defined as a feeling of emptiness or a lack of satisfying human relationships that is not alleviated by being around other people. Older adults are particularly vulnerable to experiencing loneliness because of the many losses associated with aging, including loss of health, spouse, friends and social status (Smith, 2012; Stessman et al., 2014). In addition to widowhood, life events of older adulthood that increase the risk for loneliness include retirement, death of friends, relocation to new environments and health-related problems (e.g., serious illness, significant vision or hearing impairment). Reviews of studies disclose that loneliness increases the risk for all the following: pain, anxiety, depression, cognitive decline, functional decline, impaired sleep, poor physical health and increased mortality (Park et al., 2013; Rote et al., 2012; Smith, 2012).

Resilience

During the early 2000s, gerontologists began studying the concept of **resilience** in older adults, and currently this topic is of great interest in relation to psychosocial wellness. Randall describes resilient older adults as follows: "Despite various adversities they've faced throughout their lives, certain people inspire us by their gift of keeping positive and open as the years advance: still learning and contributing—still *growing* old and not just getting old" (Randall, 2013, p. 9). A recent systematic review of 42 articles concluded that resilience in older adults is defined as the ability to bounce back and recover physical and psychological health in the face of adversity (van Kessel, 2013). Two key constructs identified in this review are (1) adversity, which is related to ongoing life experiences (e.g., aging, poor health) rather than distinct events, and (2) ability, which includes internal and external factors. Essential components of resilience include acceptance, meaningfulness, spirituality, caring for self, and social support and connectedness (van Kessel, 2013).

In addition to viewing resilience as a process of coping with adversity, resilience is discussed in the broader context of learning, growing and being positively transformed by adversity (Manning, 2013). As such, it is viewed as an outcome of increasing wisdom that is possible during later life. Examples of resilience of older adults in response to chronic illness include their ability to use coping mechanisms such as humour, acceptance, mindfulness, positive reframing, intellectual curiosity and realistic identification of the positive aspects in situations (Rybarcyk et al., 2012). Resilience is also closely linked to spirituality, a sense of hopefulness and finding meaning in life and losses (Ramsey, 2012). These concepts are pertinent to caring for older adults because nurses have many opportunities to support resilience through the interventions for promoting psychosocial wellness discussed in this chapter.

NURSING ASSESSMENT OF PSYCHOSOCIAL FUNCTION

Because psychosocial function encompasses a broad range of social, cognitive and emotional aspects of functioning that are intertwined, the assessment of psychosocial function is addressed comprehensively in a separate chapter. Readers are directed to Chapter 13 for a thorough review of nursing assessment of psychosocial function.

NURSING DIAGNOSIS

The nursing diagnoses of Situational Low Self-Esteem (or Risk for) are applicable in relation to some of the psychosocial adjustment issues of older adulthood. Situational Low Self-Esteem is defined as "development of a negative perception of self-worth in response to current situation" (Herdman, 2012, p. 287). Related factors might be the internalization of ageist attitudes, the loss of roles or financial security, the need for a change to a more dependent living arrangement and chronic illnesses that affect one's abilities and role identities.

If the nursing assessment identifies threats to the older person's sense of control, an appropriate nursing diagnosis is Powerlessness (or Risk for). This is defined as "the lived experience of lack of control over a situation, including a perception that one's actions do not significantly affect an outcome" (Herdman, 2012, p. 370). Common related factors for older adults are forced retirement, loss of the ability to drive a vehicle, lack of involvement in decision-making, chronic conditions that cause progressive functional declines (e.g., dementia) and institutional constraints, such as lack of privacy and the need to follow schedules, that do not meet the needs of the individual.

Social isolation is defined as "aloneness experienced by the individual and perceived as imposed by others and as a negative or threatening state" (Herdman, 2012, p. 480). A closely related nursing diagnosis is Impaired Social Interaction, defined as "insufficient or excessive quantity or ineffective quality of social exchange" (Herdman, 2012, p. 320). These nursing diagnoses can be used when making referrals for community resources to improve social supports for older adults.

Another nursing diagnosis that might be applied to the psychosocial needs of older adults is Ineffective Coping, which is defined as the "inability to form a valid appraisal of the stressors, inadequate choices of practiced responses, and/or inability to use available resources" (Herdman, 2012, p. 348). Other nursing diagnoses that might be applicable with regard to specific aspects of psychosocial function include Anxiety, Chronic Sorrow, Grieving, Relocation Stress Syndrome, Spiritual Distress and Stress Overload. The diagnosis of Readiness for Enhanced Spiritual Well-Being is applicable for addressing older adults' sense of meaning and purpose.

This wellness diagnosis is defined as "a pattern of experiencing and integrating meaning and purpose in life through connectedness with self, others, art, music, literature, nature, and/or a power greater than oneself that can be strengthened" (Herdman, 2012, p. 394).

> ### Wellness Opportunity
>
> Readiness for Enhanced Coping and Readiness for Enhanced Resilience are wellness nursing diagnoses that are applicable for many older adults who are experiencing psychosocial stress.

PLANNING FOR WELLNESS OUTCOMES

Wellness outcomes related to psychosocial function focus on stress reduction, enhanced coping skills and improved quality of life. When planning wellness outcomes pertinent to Situational Low Self-Esteem (or Risk for) or Readiness for Enhanced Self-Concept, nurses can apply any of the following Nursing Outcomes Classification (NOC) terminology: Psychosocial Adjustment: Life Change, Self-Esteem, Adaptation to Physical Disability, Body Image, Grief Resolution, Personal Autonomy, Depression Level and Quality of Life.

Outcomes for older adults who experience Powerlessness include Hope, Personal Autonomy and Participation in Health Care Decisions. Outcomes related to the nursing diagnosis of Social Isolation include Loneliness Severity, Social Support, Social Involvement, Leisure Participation and Personal Well-Being.

When nurses plan care for older adults with nursing diagnoses of Impaired Adjustment, Ineffective Coping or Readiness for Enhanced Coping, any of the following NOC terms may be pertinent: Psychosocial Adjustment: Life Change, Acceptance: Health Status, Adaptation to Physical Disability, Coping, Decision-Making, Knowledge: Health Resources, Personal Well-Being and Stress Level.

> ### Wellness Opportunity
>
> Hope and Quality of Life would be appropriate NOC terms when nurses direct care toward improving psychosocial wellness.

 ## NURSING INTERVENTIONS TO PROMOTE HEALTHY PSYCHOSOCIAL FUNCTION

Nurses have many opportunities to promote healthy psychosocial function during the usual course of caring for older adults. For example, they can incorporate communication techniques and other interventions to enhance self-esteem, promote a sense of control and address spiritual needs. They also can use life review and reminiscence interventions, especially in home and long-term care settings. In addition to incorporating interventions in usual care, nurses promote psychosocial wellness by facilitating referrals for social supports. In some settings, nurses can implement group interventions, such as healthy aging classes, to help older adults cope effectively with the life events of older adulthood.

The following Nursing Interventions Classification (NIC) terms relate to interventions discussed in this chapter: Active Listening, Anxiety Reduction, Coping Enhancement, Decision-Making Support, Emotional Support, Grief Work Facilitation, Hope Inspiration, Presence, Religious Ritual Enhancement, Reminiscence Therapy, Resiliency Promotion, Role Enhancement, Self-Esteem Enhancement, Socialization Enhancement, Spiritual Growth Facilitation, Spiritual Support, Support System Enhancement and Teaching: Group.

In addition to the interventions reviewed in this chapter, interventions that improve functional abilities promote psychosocial wellness because of the close relationship between physiologic and psychosocial aspects of health and function. A recent study emphasizes that interventions to improve "autonomy in activities of daily living" for older adults in long-term care settings are essential components of holistic nursing care (Candela et al., 2013). Nurses can apply information discussed in all chapters in Part 4 of this book to promote independent functioning of older adults, which in turn are interventions for improving many aspects of psychosocial function.

Enhancing Self-Esteem

Self-esteem enhancement is an essential component of nursing care for older adults because self-esteem is an important coping resource and a factor that influences well-being. Self-esteem is the emotional component of self-concept and is based on one's perceptions of other people's opinions about oneself. Good self-esteem is a characteristic that is associated with being happier, healthier, less anxious, more independent, more self-confident and more effective in meeting environmental demands than people with low self-esteem. Whereas this chapter focuses on nursing interventions that enhance self-esteem, with emphasis on addressing factors that threaten it (e.g., dependence, devaluation, depersonalization, powerlessness), Chapter 13 includes information on assessing self-esteem.

Many factors that are threats to self-esteem are associated with staff and environments of institutional settings and can be addressed through relatively simple nursing interventions. This is particularly important in environments such as long-term care settings where the caregiving environment affects virtually every aspect of daily life for the residents. For instance, in institutional settings, it is important to identify environmental or other factors that can be modified to promote a sense of control and minimize or eliminate a threat to self-esteem, as in the following examples:
- Ensuring easy access to usual assistive devices (walkers, eyeglasses, hearing aids)
- Providing as much privacy as possible
- Asking about food preferences and ensuring as much choice as possible

- Asking open-ended questions, such as, "What can we do to help you manage better while you're here?"
- Asking, "Is there anything you're worried about that I can help you with?"
- Ensuring that staff members address persons by their preferred names
- Involving older adults as much as possible in decisions that affect them

Threats to self-esteem also arise when caregivers promote unnecessary dependence for their own convenience. For example, using incontinence products in beds and telling a dependent person to wet the bed because it is easier to change the disposable pad than to assist with toileting is a tremendous blow to the person's self-esteem.

Because self-esteem depends to some extent on the perceived appraisal of significant others, it is important to avoid communicating even subtle messages that may be perceived as ageist. For example, a remark such as "You certainly look good for 85 years old," although said with good intentions, can reinforce ageist attitudes. Such a statement may subtly communicate the message that when you are old, you generally do not look good. In contrast, a statement such as the following might enhance an older person's self-esteem: "At 85 years old, you have acquired a lot of experiences in life. Can you share a bit of the wisdom that comes from those experiences with me?" Nonverbal communication also can influence the person's perception of self-worth. For example, a simple action like walking past an older person sitting in a hallway without acknowledging his or her presence may be perceived as an indicator that the nurse does not value the older person. Even though the nurse had not intended to communicate a negative message, this action may adversely affect that older person's self-esteem. Thus, nurses must keep in mind that the perception of their actions is often more important than their intent, and they must use verbal and nonverbal messages to communicate feelings of positive regard whenever possible.

For dependent older adults, the negative impact of disability and functional impairments on self-esteem is heightened by behaviours of others that convey attitudes of **infantilization** (i.e., treating an adult in a way that is similar to the way infants are treated). For example, remarks, such as "He acts just like a baby" or "Now, now, dear, let's be a good girl," convey infantilization. The term **elderspeak**—also called "baby talk"—describes speech that is modified when addressed to older adults, usually by younger adults. Elderspeak is characterized by short sentences, simplified vocabulary, exaggerated intonation, high and variable pitch and volume, and endearing or diminutive terms of endearment. This type of communication is demeaning and patronizing, and it can have serious negative consequences, such as resistance to care and negative vocalizations (e.g., crying, screaming, yelling) (Williams et al., 2009). Moreover, it can reflect ageist attitudes or negative and inaccurate stereotypes. Thus, nurses need to monitor their communication with older adults to ensure

Box 12-3 Nursing Interventions to Promote Self-Esteem

Communication Techniques
- Acknowledge person by using his or her preferred names and titles.
- When talking with older people, use the same tone of voice you use for your colleagues.
- Provide positive feedback for individual accomplishments, even in daily self-care tasks that require effort.
- Focus conversations on persons' strengths and positive attributes rather than on their limitations. (For example, for people who have physical impairments, focus on nonphysical attributes, such as personality characteristics or interpersonal relationships.)
- When negative functional consequences are attributed to old age, offer an alternative explanation and identify a contributing factor that is amenable to change. (For example, when older people attribute weakness "simply" to being old, remind them that they are recovering from hip surgery and should expect to improve with therapy.)
- Be cautious about communicating ageist attitudes, even inadvertently, in conversations.

Verbal Communication to Observe for and Avoid
- Do not use names or phrases that reflect ageist attitudes (e.g., "little old lady," "dirty old man"), even in jest.
- Do not raise your voice except when necessary to facilitate communication with someone who has impaired hearing.
- Do not use terms that are associated with babies (e.g., *diapers, baby food*).
- Do not use *we* or *us* unless the term is accurate. (For example, do not say "Let's take our medicine now.")
- Do not use the term *senile*.

Nonverbal Communication Techniques and Additional Nursing Actions
- When labelling clothing, put the person's name in an inconspicuous place.
- Use actions consciously to communicate positive regard (e.g., recognize the presence of someone as you walk past).

that they avoid inappropriate terminology and elderspeak. Box 12-3 summarizes nursing interventions for enhancing self-esteem in older adults.

Wellness Opportunity

Nurses can enhance self-esteem by pointing out an older adult's positive qualities during routine care activities.

Promoting a Sense of Control

Having a sense of control is a factor that significantly affects psychosocial wellness because many studies indicate that higher levels of perceived mastery are associated with benefits such as better physical, cognitive and psychological health (Mallers et al., 2014). Thus, nurses address psychosocial needs of older adults with interventions that promote a sense of control and that involve older adults in decisions. Nursing interventions to promote a sense of control for older adults include involving them as much as possible in organizing their care activities and providing information about their plan of care.

Many studies have confirmed the importance of modifying the way people perceive and explain events, shifting attention to factors that can be changed or controlled. In the classic study by Rodin and Langer (1980), whenever a nursing home resident attributed a problem to being old, the staff provided another explanation and identified a causative factor that was amenable to change. For instance, when residents attributed feelings of fatigue to being old, they were reminded that they were awakened at 5:30 AM (Rodin & Langer, 1980). Rodin and Langer's research laid the groundwork for the current emphasis on caring for older adults in ways that are compassionate, humanistic and empowering (Mallers et al., 2014). Nurses can find opportunities to challenge older adults' perceived lack of control and rephrase the situation in a context that is empowering. For example, they can help older adults develop problem-focused coping mechanisms rather than passively, and sometimes inaccurately, accepting the negative functional consequences of aging.

Nursing interventions also address factors that can threaten perceived control, such as lack of privacy and loss of individuality, which commonly occur in institutional settings. Nurses can show respect for privacy by knocking on bedroom doors and asking permission before entering, by closing doors when privacy is desired, by asking permission before pulling bed curtains open and by being careful about moving personal belongings without permission from the older person. Encouraging the person to have personal belongings and to arrange these belongings in whatever fashion is desired also shows concern for individuality.

Wellness Opportunity

Nurses show concern for individuality by asking an older adult about a family photograph or greeting card that is in view.

Involving Older Adults in Decision-Making

Older people are frequently left out of the decision-making process, even for those decisions that most profoundly affect their lives, such as moving to a long-term care facility. This lack of involvement occurs for a variety of reasons, related both to the older adult and to the decision makers. Some of the barriers within the older adult may be dementia, depression, long-term passivity regarding decisions, or hearing impairments or other communication barriers. Some of the barriers within the decision makers that may thwart the decision-making process include stereotypes of older people as incompetent, perceptions that the older adult is not interested in or capable of making decisions and an unwillingness to deal with the older person's anticipated resistance to the desired outcome.

Many of the reasons for excluding older adults from the decision-making process are related to the attitudes of the family and of professional caregivers, so one nursing intervention is to challenge these attitudes. For example, in acute care settings, nurses facilitate communication between older patients and their primary care provider to ensure that the older person is included in all decisions about medical treatment and discharge plans. In rehabilitation and long-term care settings, nurses have numerous opportunities to involve older adults in decisions about their daily care, medical interventions and discharge plans. In home settings, nurses can work with family members and older adults to ensure that the latter are involved in decisions about their care and that their rights are respected. In any setting, nurses may have to remind health care professionals, as well as family members and other caregivers, that although people may gain rights by virtue of being a certain age, they do not lose their rights just because they reach a certain age. For additional discussion of nurses' role in decisions regarding long-term care for people with dementia, refer to Chapter 9.

Other aspects of decision-making that can be addressed in nursing interventions are one's verbal interactions and choice of terminology. With regard to verbal communication, health care professionals often talk *about* older adults when in their presence rather than directing communication *to* them and focusing the conversation *on* them. This is especially common when family members or other caregivers are discussing situations with a nurse or other professional and the conversation takes place in the presence of the older person without directly involving him or her. Whenever appropriate, it is important to include older adults in conversations when the topic is directly related to them. However, if older adults cannot participate directly, make sure that the conversations takes place out of hearing distance. Another strategy is to ask the older person's permission to discuss his or her situation with family members or caregivers and then report back to the older person, in language that the person can understand, about any discussions that take place or decisions that are made or pending.

With regard to terminology, the phrase "nursing home placement" is commonly used in reference to an older adult's admission to a nursing home. This term denotes passivity on the part of the older adult—it is closer to the terminology used when objects are placed on a shelf than to words normally used in reference to human beings. An alternative approach that communicates a greater sense of control is to refer to an "admission" to a nursing home. This approach indicates that certain criteria have been met and that an active decision has been made to determine whether the person meets these criteria. Equally important, nurses must ensure that older adults are, in fact, actively involved in the decision-making process, rather than passively being "placed." Nurses can help older adults and their families with decisions about long-term care by helping them assess their situation and by correcting misinformation and providing accurate information about specific resources and the range of services available (as described in Chapter 6).

Addressing Role Loss

Meaningful roles (e.g., spouse, caregiver, volunteer) are important determinants of feelings of worth, efficacy and self-esteem. Participating in volunteer work is an excellent way of providing social interaction and a sense of purpose. Volunteer work that extends work-related roles is particularly rewarding and psychologically uplifting because it provides new fulfillment, life meaning and life direction (Cook, 2013). Research reviews have identified the following positive health effects associated with volunteering: improved functioning, longer life expectancy, increased social interaction, reduced pain and depression and increased life satisfaction and self-rated health (Jenkinson et al., 2013; Li et al., 2013; Okun et al., 2013). In addition to helping older adults develop new roles, nurses can focus on past and current achievements as an intervention for enhancing self-esteem. This is especially important for older adults who depend on others and who have limited opportunities for feeling a sense of accomplishment.

> **Wellness Opportunity**
>
> Nurses can ask older adults about their accomplishments in areas, such as work and family, and give positive feedback about meaningful roles.

Encouraging Life Review and Reminiscence

Life review and reminiscence are two closely related processes that are used to promote psychosocial health in older adults. Butler (2001) described **life review** as a progressive return to consciousness of past experiences, particularly unresolved conflicts, for reexamination and reintegration. If the reintegration process is successful, the process gives new significance and meaning to life and prepares the person for death by alleviating fear and anxiety (Butler, 2001). Positive effects of life review include accepting one's mortality, righting of old wrongs, taking pride in accomplishments, gaining a sense of serenity and feeling that one has done one's best (Butler, 2001). Nurses have used a life-story review group to improve mild to moderate depression in community-living older adults (Chan et al., 2014).

Reminiscence is based on the same theoretical framework as life review; however, it can be done outside the life-review process, and it is more informal and less intense. Another difference is that life review addresses both pleasant and unpleasant issues of the past, whereas reminiscence focuses primarily on pleasant and positive experiences. Reminiscence therapy as a nursing intervention is the recall of past events, feelings, images and memories that are associated with comfort, pleasure and pleasant experiences. As a group therapy, the reminiscence group is one of the most widely used interventions for older adults, including those with mild cognitive impairment and mild to moderate dementia. Nurses have many opportunities to incorporate principles of reminiscence during the usual course of care, for example, by asking about pleasant memories of holidays.

A Student's Perspective

Performing a life review on anyone from a time other than your own is an interesting experience. I found it to be an amazing opportunity to sit down with Mrs. B. and for her to open up to a 20-year-old girl that she had met only the week before. Within the first few minutes, she talked about her husband and I watched the tears roll down her face. This became the most significant part of our interview because I was able to understand how exposed she was allowing herself to be. It also made me realize how open the elderly can be in reminiscing about their lives and how important this topic is for them to share. It amazed me how just starting a conversation with an older person could bring so much emotion and joy at the exact same time.

The interview with Mrs. B. has affected my approach to older adults in clinical practice. I believe that a life review can be done on a daily basis while working with clients. This way, you can get to know each person on a personal level in order to provide individualized care. Each time you see a patient, you could continue the conversation and develop a relationship that benefits not only the client, but also yourself. I have learned that by showing interest in a person's life, you can allow them to discuss a significant part of who they have become, which is something they do not get to do on a daily basis.

Jillian B.

Fostering Social Supports

Nurses have many opportunities to foster the development of social networks for older adults, and this is an effective intervention for social isolation. Social isolation is likely to occur because of any of the following factors that commonly occur in older adulthood:

- Hearing impairments and other communication barriers
- Chronic illnesses that limit activity or energy
- Lack of social opportunities because of caregiving responsibilities
- Mobility limitations, including the inability to drive a vehicle
- Mental or psychosocial impairments that interfere with relationships
- Loss of spouse, friends or family through death, illness or physical distance

Thus, nursing interventions that address these risk factors (e.g., improved mobility or sensory function) are also likely to have the positive consequence of improved social supports.

In long-term care settings, nurses can foster positive social interactions in group settings, such as dining and activity rooms. Sometimes, a very simple intervention, such as positioning chairs (including wheelchairs) so that people can interact with each other, can significantly influence social contacts. Whenever possible, room assignments in long-term care settings should be directed toward facilitating positive social interactions. In addition, nurses can facilitate referrals for social and therapeutic activities in long-term care facilities.

In home settings, nurses can identify community resources, such as volunteer-friendly visitor and meal programs, to decrease social isolation. Support and education groups that primarily focus on coping with a chronic illness (e.g., stroke clubs, or better breathing groups) also provide excellent opportunities for social contact and the development of friendships with people who are in similar situations. For people who are socially isolated because of caregiving responsibility, caregiver support groups can enhance coping abilities and provide social support.

In any setting, nurses can encourage older adults to participate in structured group activities to enhance their well-being. A randomized control trial found that older adults who experienced loneliness showed significant health benefits, including improved cognitive function, from participation in weekly psychosocial groups for 3 months (Pitkala et al., 2011). Selected nursing interventions to promote psychosocial wellness are described in Box 12-4.

Wellness Opportunity

Nurses can talk with older adults about the benefits of support groups and provide a list of local resources that address specific needs of older adults and their caregivers.

Addressing Spiritual Needs

Addressing spiritual needs of patients is within the scope of nursing, as exemplified in the following interventions that are commonly included in nursing care:

- Intentionally communicating caring and compassion
- Facilitating reminiscence
- Honouring a person's integrity
- Providing active and passive listening
- Making referrals for spiritual care
- Caring for someone who feels hopeless
- Arranging for participation in religious services
- Encouraging or facilitating participation in activities such as prayer and meditation

Nursing interventions to address the spiritual needs of older adults need to be individualized and offered only if the person is receptive to the interventions. In addition, nurses need to be nonjudgmental about religion and spirituality and avoid imposing their personal beliefs. Moreover, because cultural factors significantly influence a person's spirituality and religious beliefs, interventions must be culturally sensitive.

In addition to addressing spiritual needs as a routine part of psychosocial nursing care, nurses often address spiritual

---

Box 12-4 Nursing Interventions to Promote Psychosocial Wellness

Facilitating Maximum Independence

- Make sure that the person has access to all necessary assistive devices and personal accessories (e.g., wigs, canes, dentures, walkers, hearing aids).
- Allow enough time for the person to perform tasks at her or his own pace, and avoid unnecessary dependence that results from an overemphasis on time efficiency.
- Make sure that the environment has been adapted as much as possible to compensate for sensory losses and other functional impairments.

Promoting a Sense of Control

- Make a conscious effort to involve older adults in decisions regarding their care, both in small daily matters and in major health care concerns.
- Ask about likes and dislikes and try to address personal preferences.
- Whenever possible, allow persons to choose between two alternatives, even if the options are in a very narrow range (e.g., "Would you prefer to wear the yellow sweater or the pink one today?").
- Ensure as much privacy, or perceived privacy, as possible.
- Knock on the door and ask for permission before entering a bedroom, even in institutional settings.
- Allow as much expression of individuality as possible in the personal environment (e.g., use personal furniture when possible and display family pictures in full view).
- Make sure that the call light is accessible for people who are confined.
- Do not talk about someone in his or her presence as if he or she does not exist.
- Avoid referring to nursing home *placement*. Refer instead to an *admission*, and include the person in the decision-making process.

Addressing Role Loss

- Identify new roles for people and acknowledge those past and present roles that are viewed positively.

- Encourage participation in reminiscence groups and other group therapies.
- Find opportunities to create meaningful roles, such as helper or assistant, by involving older adults in useful tasks, such as folding laundry.
- When older adults volunteer to assist others, acknowledge their contribution with a remark such as, "You certainly help us a lot when you help take Mrs. Smith to the dining room in her wheelchair."
- Acknowledge an older adult's nonphysical assets and attributes, such as family relationships or a good sense of humour.
- Focus on positive relationships by acknowledging or asking about the receipt of flowers, greeting cards and other visible signs of concern expressed by others.
- Ask older adults about their responsibilities as parents, grandparents or roommates and point out their positive contributions.
- Ask older adults about family photographs, initiate a discussion of positive relationships and remind them that others care about them (e.g., encourage them to talk about their grandchildren and great-grandchildren).
- Ask older adults about accomplishments in areas such as work, family, hobbies and volunteer activities.
- Respond with comments such as "You must be proud of your children" or "You certainly have accomplished a lot."

Fostering Social Supports

- Use interventions to address hearing impairments and other communication barriers (see Chapter 16).
- Encourage participation in group activities.
- For people in wheelchairs, especially those who cannot move independently, position the chair in a way that promotes social interaction.
- For residents in long-term care facilities, plan table and room arrangements in a way that fosters social relationships.

needs during times of spiritual distress. For example, older adults are likely to express spiritual needs when they are coping with the loss of a significant relationship or dealing with news about a serious or terminal illness. Older adults who are caregivers for others, especially a spouse, are likely to express spiritual needs in relation to decisions about the care of the other person. For example, they may experience feelings of guilt about not being able to meet the needs of a dependent loved one or feelings of "playing God" with regard to decisions about mentally incompetent loved ones. In these circumstances, the provision of support, information and reassurance from a nurse who has dealt with these decisions in professional experiences may be an effective counselling intervention. At times, information from the primary care provider may be helpful in alleviating spiritual distress associated with end-of-life decisions or decisions about long-term care. In these cases, the nurse may be able to facilitate communication between the primary care provider and the family to alleviate the spiritual distress. Some nursing interventions that address spiritual needs of older adults are listed in Box 12-5.

Teaching About Managing Stress in Daily Life

Nurses have important roles in teaching older adults, as well as caregivers, about managing stress in daily life as an intervention for promoting psychosocial wellness. Although stress management is often overlooked, it is an essential aspect of health promotion for people of all ages. Nurses can encourage and demonstrate the use of simple relaxation techniques, such as deep breathing, during the usual course of caring for older adults and talking with caregivers. Nurses can also encourage participation in individual and group activities that are effective for reducing stress, such as yoga, meditation and tai chi. Box 12-6 can be given to older adults and caregivers as a teaching tool.

Promoting Wellness Through Healthy Aging Classes

When older adults need assistance in coping with specific functional consequences or when they need education to clarify myths and misunderstandings about age-related changes, individual counselling may be the best intervention. When older adults need counselling about psychosocial adjustments, however, educational groups may be more effective. Nurses often are involved with establishing and leading support and educational groups for caregivers. Common themes that nurses can address in groups include use of resources, coping with losses and promoting optimal functioning.

An example of a nurse-led group intervention that allows for sharing of experiences among peers is the healthy aging class, developed by Carol Miller and used successfully during two decades in a variety of settings with older adults at various functional levels. This model is based on the belief that older adults who are beginning to recognize age-related physical and psychosocial changes or who are already dealing with such changes can benefit from sharing their experiences with their peers. Nurses can use this model, which is described in detail, to enhance the coping skills of older adults who are adjusting to any of the challenges of older adulthood.

Goals

Goals for older adults who participate in healthy aging classes follow:

- Recognize the impact of common age-related physical and psychosocial changes.
- Support and encourage any effective coping mechanisms already being used.

 Box 12-5 Nursing Interventions to Address Spiritual Needs

Therapeutic Communication Interventions

- Use verbal and nonverbal communication to establish trust and convey empathic caring.
- Use active supportive listening.
- Convey nonjudgmental attitudes.
- Communicate respect for individuality.
- Provide a supportive presence.
- Be open to expressions of feelings, such as fear, anger, loneliness and powerlessness.
- Honour a person's integrity.
- Support the person in his or her feeling of being loved by others and by a higher power (e.g., God, Allah, Jehovah).
- Encourage verbalization of feelings about meaning of illness.
- Provide positive feedback about faith, courage, sense of humour and other such feelings and experiences.
- Encourage discussion of events and relationships that provide spiritual support.

Actions to Foster Religious and Spiritual Activities

- Facilitate referrals for visits from religious care providers and sources of spiritual care (clergy, rabbis, church members, spiritual directors).
- Facilitate participation in religious services or activities (e.g., tapes, readings, videos, observations of "holy days").
- Assist with obtaining requested religious items (books, music, statues).
- Provide quiet and private time for individual spiritual or religious activities (e.g., prayer, reflection, meditation, guided imagery).
- Provide necessary support for religious rituals (e.g., lighting candles, receiving communion, praying the rosary, fasting during Ramadan).
- Encourage participation in relaxing and enjoyable activities (art, music, nature).

Interventions for Specific Circumstances

- Provide support and care during times of suffering.
- Emotionally assist the individual to cope with the process of dying.
- Assist a person who is fearful of the future.
- Provide care for the person who feels hopeless.
- Facilitate reconciliation among family members.
- Encourage participation in support groups.

Box 12-6 Tips on Managing Stress in Daily Life

Recognize the Different Types of Stressors

- Events are stressful according to the degree to which they have an emotional impact and are perceived as desirable and controllable.
- Even events that are desirable, such as holidays and births and weddings of grandchildren, can be stressful.
- When stress cannot be alleviated, it is important to manage your perception of, and emotional responses to, the situation.
- Use problem-focused strategies to cope with situations that can be changed.

Coping Strategies for Situations That Cannot Be Changed

- Develop an attitude of acceptance, reframe your perspective and focus on what you can learn from this.
- Acknowledge and express feelings, even those that are unpleasant, such as grief, anger and sadness.
- Talk with someone and accept their caring and understanding; communicate to them that you do not expect to change the situation but appreciate an opportunity to express feelings.
- Foster supports for social, emotional and spiritual enrichment (e.g., friends, family, pets, hobbies, groups).
- Identify and use healthy ways of releasing tension and expressing emotions (e.g., physical activity, actions that lead to a sense of accomplishment).
- Engage in distracting activities, especially those that are pleasurable, health enhancing and spiritually enriching.
- Use relaxation methods, such as meditation, yoga or progressive relaxation.
- Express feelings and develop insights through activities, such as journaling and self-talk.
- Seek guidance from counsellors or health care professionals.

Problem-Focused Coping Strategies

- Time pressures: evaluate demands, determine priorities and plan a schedule for the most important things; include time for activities that relieve stress.
- Set realistic limits and become comfortable telling others what the limits are.
- Seek advice and reliable information from friends, family or professionals who can assist with developing a problem-solving plan.
- Adapt to the environment so it is most conducive to your current needs.

Strategies to Avoid

- Smoking
- Excessive eating or drinking (including alcohol or caffeine)
- Inappropriate use of medications or recreational drugs
- Inaccurately or inappropriately directing anger or emotions toward others
- Actions that are harmful to people, animals or the environment

Adapted with permission from Miller, C. A. (2013). Wellness Activity Tool for stress management. In C. A. Miller (Ed.), *Fast facts for health promotion in nursing: Promoting wellness in a nutshell* (pp. 61–62). New York, NY: Springer.

- Develop new skills that could be effective for coping with current stressors.
- Obtain information that will facilitate problem-focused coping mechanisms for stressful situations that are amenable to change.
- Provide an opportunity for the sharing of similar experiences with peers.

Setting

Nurses in any setting can initiate healthy aging classes, but long-term care institutions are perhaps the most conducive setting for the following reasons:

- Nurses have many opportunities to establish and lead groups.
- Residents of long-term care facilities provide a captive audience from which to select group members.
- Residents of long-term care institutions usually are not acutely ill, and they are dealing with psychosocial adjustments that are readily identified.
- Residents of long-term care settings have in common at least one major life event, which is a temporary or permanent move to a more dependent setting.

Community settings also are conducive to successful healthy aging classes, but nurses may have to be more creative in gathering the group members. Nurses who provide health services or education programs for adults in senior centres or assisted-living facilities might be able to establish ongoing healthy aging classes as part of their responsibilities. In these settings, a healthy aging class may be an efficient, as well as effective, way of providing health education using a format that has the additional advantage of enhancing coping mechanisms.

In acute care settings, nurses usually do not plan and implement group therapies, but in rehabilitative settings, nurses may have the opportunity to initiate healthy aging classes. In psychiatric units, often there are enough older adults among the patient population to warrant the implementation of healthy aging classes as a form of group therapy.

Membership Criteria

The primary criteria for group membership are that the person be willing to acknowledge age-related changes and be capable of acquiring insight into his or her adjustment to these changes. Carol Miller has led groups ranging from highly functional older adults in community settings to seriously impaired older adults in a hospital-based medical geriatric mental health unit. Group members may be coping with similar psychosocial stresses, but this is not necessarily a criterion for participation. For example, a healthy aging class can comprise older adults who all have some degree of depression or who are coping with a particular stressful event, such as widowhood. An ideal group includes members who are coping with various life events commonly associated with older adulthood and who are motivated to learn effective coping styles.

The group works best if the membership is stable and closed, but this is not always possible. A disadvantage of an open group is that it is very difficult to develop cohesiveness. If the membership is open and changing, the leader must be more directive, and the group as a whole will not be able to establish ongoing priorities for discussion topics. In addition, with changing membership, the leader has to focus more attention on the exchange of information about group members at the beginning of each session.

Size of Group and Length, Duration and Frequency of Sessions

Although group size can range from 5 to 12 members, the ideal is about 8 members. Groups can be either ongoing or time limited. When the membership is changing, such as in acute or rehabilitative settings, sessions can be an ongoing mode of therapy. In long-term care or community settings, it is best to schedule group meetings for a predetermined length of time, such as 8 to 10 weeks, and allow for changes in membership at the end of each period. One-hour sessions are held at weekly intervals, at a consistent time and place. In community settings, it can be helpful to convene the groups in conjunction with a meal program because participants will already have social relationships. As in institutional settings, a community centre offers an audience from which to select the group members. Other potential community-based sites include assisted-living facilities and group settings, such as adult care homes (also called personal-and-care homes).

Criteria for and Responsibilities of Group Leaders

One nurse can lead group sessions, but it is often helpful to have a co-leader who has had education in working with individuals. An older adult who has made a positive psychosocial adjustment and who can serve as a role model also can be a good co-leader. The nurse must be able to clarify myths and misunderstandings about age-related changes and be skilled in group dynamics. As with the reminiscence group, the healthy aging class is not an intense psychotherapy session; therefore, the group leader is not required to be specially trained in mental health. To lead a healthy aging class, however, a good understanding of both the physiologic and psychosocial aspects of aging is essential.

The primary responsibilities of the group leaders are to facilitate the discussion of psychosocial adjustments of older adulthood and to provide feedback and clarification to the members. As with other groups, the leader must ensure that all members have an opportunity to participate and that the members attend to the identified topic. The leaders also must ensure that the group reaches some conclusions before the end of each session so that members leave with a feeling of accomplishment relating to at least one psychosocial challenge of older adulthood.

Format

As in all educational groups, the leader begins with an explanation of the purpose of the group and an introduction of the leaders and members. The leader also reviews the details of the sessions, such as their length, the duration of the group, the role of the leader and the expectations of the members. After addressing questions and introductory material, the leader introduces the concepts of life events and adjustments to the challenges of older adulthood. The leader can use a statement similar to the following:

> *Throughout life, certain events are likely to occur that affect us emotionally. These events may involve our health, our personal relationships, the place where we live, our job or career responsibilities and opportunities or other events that require an adjustment on our part. These are called major life events, and they often occur at certain points of life. To begin our discussion today, let's look at some of the major life events that are likely to occur in younger adulthood, around the age of 20 to 30 years.*

The group then identifies various life events, such as finding a job, moving from the family home, finding a partner and starting a family. The leader then asks members to identify life adjustments that are likely to occur between 30 and 50 years of age.

After the members have identified these life events, the leader emphasizes that one purpose of the healthy aging class is to identify effective ways of addressing the challenges inherent in the life events of older adulthood. The term *challenges* is used to communicate an active mode of addressing issues. The leader may want to discuss the phrase "challenges of older adulthood" and allow the group members to comment on what they see as challenges in their lives. As the members identify the life events of older adulthood, the leader writes the events on a board or paper so that all the members can see the list. The leader can then ask about life events that the members think they are likely to experience in the next few years. As events are identified, the members are also asked to identify the consequences of the events that require an adjustment. Examples of these life events and consequences have been discussed earlier in this chapter, and they are summarized in Figure 12-1. If group members do not identify all the life events, the leader may ask about a certain event, such as coping with one's own or a spouse's retirement. This discussion should continue until all the events and consequences in Figure 12-1 have been identified.

If the group is ongoing and has a stable membership, the leader may devote the majority of the first meeting to this discussion. The leader should emphasize that the rest of the meetings will be devoted to discussions of the identified issues, and that the first meeting will set the stage for future sessions. If the group is open and has a changing membership, the leader may need to be more directive during this first phase to limit the time spent on this topic. With changing membership, this initial identification of issues would be limited to the first 20 to 30 minutes. The group can then discuss coping mechanisms for one specific issue during the latter half of the meeting.

After the issues are identified, the leader summarizes the discussion, referring to the list of challenges written for the members to see. The members then share ideas about coping strategies that they have found to be helpful in adjusting to these changes. The leader may begin this part with a statement such as, "Now that we've identified the challenges of older adulthood, let's look at what things are helpful in responding to these challenges. I'd like each of you to share with the group one thing you do to help yourself face difficult challenges." After members have identified general coping mechanisms, the leader can suggest that the group choose one specific life event of older adulthood and discuss coping mechanisms that are helpful for addressing this challenge. Examples of coping strategies that might be discussed in relation to specific life events are summarized in Table 12-1. As these coping strategies are identified, they should be written on a surface for all to see, and members should be encouraged to relate their personal experiences.

As the cohesiveness and trust level among members increase, particularly in closed groups, the sharing of experiences may become very open and revealing. The task of the leader, then, is to keep the discussion focused on appropriate coping mechanisms. In cohesive groups with highly functional members, the leader might have an opportunity to discuss the difference between emotion-focused and problem-focused mechanisms. The depth of discussion will depend on the degree of group cohesiveness and trust, the functional level of the members and the comfort level and willingness of the leader to deal with the identified issues.

During the last 10 minutes of each session, the leader should attempt to bring the discussion to some closure on at least one issue. This may be accomplished by summarizing the issues and coping mechanisms that were identified. In open groups, the leader would end by encouraging those members who do not return to the group to look at coping mechanisms for their own specific issues, either by themselves or with a friend or confidant(e). For ongoing groups, the leader would end the session by facilitating agreement about the issues that will be discussed during the next session. The leader also can encourage members to think about the identified issues in the interim.

EVALUATING THE EFFECTIVENESS OF NURSING INTERVENTIONS

Nurses evaluate the effectiveness of interventions for older adults with Self-Concept Disturbance by determining the extent to which older adults express positive views of themselves. Another measure of effective nursing care is that older adults no longer verbalize ageist attitudes. Nursing care of older adults who express a sense of Powerlessness is evaluated by the extent to which they become involved in decisions that affect them and the degree to which they express feelings of control over their lives. Nurses evaluate care for older adults with Ineffective Individual Coping by observing behaviours that reflect the use of a variety of coping strategies (see Table 12-1). For example, an older adult might learn to use problem-focused coping strategies for a situation he or she previously viewed as hopeless and unchangeable.

TABLE 12-1 Coping Strategies for the Psychosocial Challenges of Older Adulthood

Psychosocial Adjustment	Coping Strategy
Ageist stereotypes	Develop a firm self-identity, challenge the myths, question any behaviours that are based on age-determined expectations
Retirement	Develop new skills, use time for hobbies and personal pursuits, become involved with meaningful volunteer activities
Reduced income	Take advantage of discounts for seniors
Declining physical condition	Maintain good health practices (nutrition, exercise, rest)
Functional limitations	Adapt to the environment to ensure safety and optimal functional status, take advantage of assistive devices and equipment, accept help when necessary
Changes in cognitive skills	Take advantage of educational opportunities, enrol in classes, keep mentally stimulated, join a discussion group, use the library, avoid dwelling on the things you cannot do and focus on your abilities. Take advantage of increased potential for wisdom and creativity
Death of spouse, friends and family members	Allow yourself to grieve appropriately, take advantage of opportunities for group or individual counselling and support, establish new relationships, renew old friendships, cherish the happy memories of the past, realize new freedoms
Relocation from family home	Look into the broad range of options for housing, appreciate the relief from the responsibilities of home ownership, take advantage of new services and opportunities for socialization
Other challenges to mental health	Maintain a sense of humour, use stress-reduction techniques, learn assertiveness skills, participate in support groups

Case Study

Mr. P. is 86 years old and was recently admitted to a long-term care facility. His medical diagnoses are diabetes, glaucoma, retinopathy and dementia of Alzheimer type. Mr. P. lived with his wife until 6 months ago, when she died after a brief illness. After her death, he needed help with all his activities of daily living, and his daughter arranged home care assistance for 6 hours a day. About 1 month ago, he started getting up and wandering outside at night. Once, he wandered off at 3:00 AM, and the police had to take him home. After this episode, he was afraid to be alone, and he agreed to go to a nursing facility because he could not afford to pay for 24-hour assistance at home.

During the first week in the long-term care facility, Mr. P. was cooperative with the staff and sociable with the other residents. He was resistant to the morning schedule of getting up at 6:00 AM and eating breakfast in the dining room at 7:30 AM, but he passively complied when the staff firmly directed him. His daughter visited him daily and accompanied him to social and recreational activities with other residents. Mr. P. has been in the facility for 10 days, and he is becoming very resistant to staff efforts to get him dressed for breakfast. When he attends group activities, he is disruptive, yelling about being a hostage in a monastery. Mr. P. tells other residents that he was tricked into coming to this place and that the only reason he has to stay is because his daughter has taken over his house and is living there with her family. He frequently paces up and down the corridors and says he has to find his daughter to take him home because his wife is sick and she needs him to take care of her. You walk with him in the hallway, and he says, "I don't know why they keep me locked up here. I can't do anything like I used to do at home. It's like a monastery where you have to get up in the middle of the night and they make you get cleaned up and eat breakfast when it's still dark out."

NURSING ASSESSMENT

Your nursing assessment shows that Mr. P. needs supervision in all activities of daily living because of poor vision and memory impairment. He needs some assistance with personal care, but he can dress himself if staff set his clothes out for him. When Mr. P. was admitted to the long-term care facility, he was assigned to the "night-shift wakers" group, which means that the night shift is responsible for waking him and getting him ready for breakfast by 7:30 AM. The night-shift nursing assistants help him with showering, shaving and dressing.

During the admission interview, Mr. P.'s daughter, Jane, said that his typical morning routine at home was to get up around 8:30 AM and get dressed independently, using the clothes that were set out for him by the home health aide. He would eat breakfast around 9:30 AM and then spend the day "working on his papers." Jane, who lives out of town, would call her father four times a week. When Jane talked with him on the phone, he always told her how busy he was working on his papers. Although Jane was paying all his bills from a joint bank account, Mr. P. would spend hours and hours with bill stubs, old bank statements and an inactive checking account, thinking he was paying his bills.

Jane was staying at her father's house for the 2 weeks before his admission and for 1 week after his admission to the facility. She plans to return to town for a couple of days every other month and will visit her father at those times. The only nearby relative is a sister-in-law who comes to visit Mr. P. every 2 weeks.

NURSING DIAGNOSIS

You use the nursing diagnosis of Powerlessness related to relocation to a long-term care facility and lack of control over activities of daily living. You select this diagnosis, rather than Impaired Adjustment or Ineffective Individual Coping, because Mr. P. focuses on a theme of loss of control. Your assessment identifies several factors that contribute to his powerlessness, and you address these factors in your nursing care plan.

NURSING CARE PLAN FOR MR. P.

Expected Outcome	Nursing Interventions	Nursing Evaluation
Mr. P. will feel he has greater control over his morning schedule	• Take Mr. P. off the "night-shift wakers" list and allow him to sleep until 8:00 AM • Allow Mr. P. to wear his pyjamas and robe to breakfast and to shower, bathe and dress after breakfast	• Mr. P. will no longer verbalize feelings of being locked up in a monastery or a prison
Mr. P. will function as independently as possible	• The staff will set out Mr. P.'s clothing and allow him to dress himself • The staff will give Mr. P. positive feedback for dressing himself	• Mr. P. will dress himself with minimal supervision • Mr. P. will perform his personal care activities at a pace that is comfortable for him

(continued)

Expected Outcome	Nursing Interventions	Nursing Evaluation
Mr. P. will engage in a familiar activity that gives him a meaningful role	• Ask Jane to send a set of bill stubs, old bank statements and the inactive checkbook so that Mr. P. can do his "work" • Encourage Mr. P. to "work with his papers" in the activity room, where he can interact with other residents • Give Mr. P. positive feedback when he interacts with other residents • Compliment Mr. P. about doing his paperwork	• Mr. P. will resume his former routine of working with his papers and will interact with other residents

Chapter Highlights

Life Events: Age-Related Changes Affecting Psychosocial Function (Fig. 12-1)

- Life events are the major changes that occur during the life cycle and significantly affect daily life.
- Life events commonly experienced by older adults are retirement, relocation, chronic illness and functional impairments, decisions about driving a vehicle, widowhood, death of family and friends and ageist attitudes.

Theories About Stress and Coping in Older Adults

- Sources of stress for older adults are major life events, daily hassles and chronic stressors.
- Older adults are more likely to use emotion-focused coping styles that involve management of thoughts and feelings.
- Social supports are an important resource for coping in older adults.
- Nurses facilitate effective coping in older adults through interventions that improve their functional abilities.

Factors That Influence Psychosocial Function in Older Adults

- Religion and spirituality are increasingly important resources for older adults.
- Cultural factors influence perceptions of all aspects of psychosocial functioning (Box 12-1).
- Culture-bound syndromes are culturally specific disorders associated with psychosocial characteristics of a particular group.

Risks Factors That Affect Psychosocial Function

- Physical, functional and psychosocial health significantly affect coping skills.
- The ability to accurately appraise a situation affects psychosocial function.
- Learned helplessness results when uncontrollable events reinforce the idea that future events will also be uncontrollable.

Functional Consequences Associated With Psychosocial Function in Older Adults

- Negative functional consequences include anxiety, loneliness, depression and cognitive impairment.

- Older adults also experience emotional well-being (e.g., joy, happiness, satisfaction, purpose in life, sense of mastery).
- Gerontologists are currently investigating the concept of resilience in older adults, which is defined as the ability to bounce back and recover physical and psychological health in the face of adversity.

Nursing Assessment of Psychosocial Function

- Refer to Chapter 13.

Nursing Diagnosis

- Situational Low Self-Esteem (or Risk for)
- Powerlessness
- Social Isolation
- Ineffective Coping
- Readiness for Enhanced Coping
- Readiness for Enhanced Resilience

Planning for Wellness Outcomes

- Psychosocial Adjustment: Life Change
- Adaptation to Physical Disability
- Personal Autonomy
- Self-Esteem
- Quality of Life

Nursing Interventions to Promote Healthy Psychosocial Function

- Enhancing self-esteem: improving functioning, using verbal and nonverbal communication, avoiding infantilization and elderspeak
- Promoting a sense of control: providing information, rephrasing events, addressing threats such as lack of privacy and loss of individuality
- Involving older adults in decision-making: challenging attitudes, facilitating communication, using verbal and nonverbal communication techniques
- Addressing role loss: identifying meaningful roles
- Encouraging life review and reminiscence
- Fostering social supports
- Addressing spiritual needs: communicating caring and compassion, instilling hope, referring for spiritual care, encouraging participation in religious activities
- Leading Healthy Aging classes

Evaluating the Effectiveness of Nursing Interventions

- Positive self-perceptions
- Involvement in decisions
- Effective coping strategies

Critical Thinking Exercises

1. Take a sheet of paper and draw two vertical lines to make three equal columns. Think of someone you know in your personal life or professional practice who is 80 years old or older. In the left column, list three or more life events that this person has experienced in later adulthood. In the centre column, describe the impact of the life event on the person's daily life. In the right column, list the coping mechanisms the person has used to deal with the life event. You can guess at the information, as needed, to complete the information in the centre and right columns.

2. Think of a recent life event in your own life and answer the following questions: How close in time was the life event to other stressful events in your life? What impact did the life event have, and what were the manifestations of stress in your life (e.g., in your work, your health, your personal life, your relationships with other people)? What coping mechanisms did you use? Were the coping mechanisms effective? What coping mechanisms would you like to develop to prepare yourself for older adulthood?

3. You are asked to lead a 1-hour discussion titled "Mental Health and Aging" for a group of 10 people at a senior citizen centre. Describe your approach to this topic. What would be your goals for the class? How would you involve the participants? What visual aids would you use?

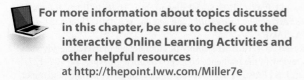

For more information about topics discussed in this chapter, be sure to check out the interactive Online Learning Activities and other helpful resources at http://thepoint.lww.com/Miller7e

REFERENCES

Almeida, D. M., Piazza, J. R., Stawski, R. S., et al. (2011). The speedometer of life: Stress, health and aging. In K. W. Schaie & S. L. Willis (Eds.), *Handbook of the psychology of aging* (7th ed., pp. 191–206). New York, NY: Elsevier.

Andrews, M. M., & Boyle, J. S. (2012). *Transcultural concepts in nursing care*. Philadelphia, PA: Wolters Kluwer/Lippincott Williams & Wilkins.

Blay, S. L., & Marinho, V. (2012). Anxiety disorders in old age. *Current Opinion in Psychiatry*, *25*(6), 462–467.

Blume, J., Douglas, S. D., & Evans, D. L. (2011). Immune suppression and immune activation in depression. *Brain Behavior & Immunology*, *25*(2), 221–229.

Bonanno, G. A., Westphal, M., & Mancini, A. D. (2012). Loss, trauma, and resilience in adulthood. *Annual Review of Gerontology and Geriatrics*, *32*, 189–210.

Boot, W. R., Stothart, C., & Charness, N. (2014). Improving the safety of aging road users: A mini-review. *Gerontology*, *60*(1), 90–96. doi:10.1159/000354212

Bowen, C. E., Noack, M. G., & Staudinger, U. M. (2011). Aging in the work context. In K. W. Schaie & S. L. Willis (Eds.), *Handbook of the psychology of aging* (7th ed., pp. 263–277). New York, NY: Elsevier.

Brenes, G. A., Miller, M. E., Williamson, J. D., et al. (2012). A randomized controlled trial of telephone-delivered cognitive-behavioral therapy for late-life anxiety disorders. *American Journal of Geriatric Psychiatry*, *20*(8), 707–716.

Brennan, P. L., Holland, J. M., Schutte, K. K., et al. (2012). Coping trajectories in later life: A 20-year predictive study. *Aging and Mental Health*, *16*(3), 305–316.

Burkhardt, M. A., & Nagai-Jacobson, M. G. (2013). Spirituality and health. In B. M. Dossey & L. Keegan (Eds.), *Holistic nursing: A handbook for practice* (5th ed., pp. 617–645). Boston, MA: Jones and Bartlett.

Butler, R. N. (2001). Life review. In M. D. Mezey (Ed.), *The encyclopedia of elder care* (pp. 401–402). New York, NY: Springer.

Candela, F., Zucchetti, G., & Magistro, D. (2013). Individual correlates of autonomy in activities of daily living in institutionalized elderly individuals. *Holistic Nursing Practice*, *27*(5), 284–291.

Chan, M. F., Leong, K. S., Heng, B. L., et al. (2014). Reducing depression among community-dwelling older adults using life-story review: A pilot study. *Geriatric Nursing*, *35*(2), 105–110. doi:10.1016/j.gerinurse.2013.10.011

Choi, M., Lohman, M. C., & Mezuk, B. (2014). Trajectories of cognitive decline by driving mobility: Evidence from Health and Retirement Study. *International Journal of Geriatric Psychiatry*, *29*(5), 447–453. doi:10.1002/gps.4024

Cook, S. L. (2013). Redirection: An extension of career during retirement. *The Gerontologist*, doi:10.1093/geront/gnt105

Dugan, E., & Lee, C. M. (2013, September 25). Biopsychosocial risk factors for driving cessation: Findings from the Health and Retirement Study. *Journal of Aging and Health*, *25*(8), 1313–1328.

Ehrmin, J. T. (2012). Transcultural perspectives in mental health nursing. In M. M. Andrews & J. S. Boyle (Eds.), *Transcultural concepts in nursing care* (6th ed., pp. 243–276). Philadelphia, PA: Lippincott Williams & Wilkins.

Fitchett, G., Benjamins, M. R., Skarupski, K. A., et al. (2013). Worship attendance and the disability process in community-dwelling older adults. *Journals of Gerontology: Psychological Sciences and Social Sciences*, *68*(2), 235–245.

George, L. K. (2011). Social factors, depression, and aging. In R. H. Binstock & L. K. George (Eds.), *Handbook of aging and the social sciences* (7th ed., pp. 149–162). New York, NY: Elsevier.

Gilmour, H. (2012). *Social participation and the health and well-being of Canadian seniors* (Catalogue no. 82-003-X). Ottawa, ON: Statistics Canada.

Gouin, J.-P., & Kiecolt-Glaser, J. K. (2011). The impact of psychological stress on wound healing: Methods and mechanisms. *Immunology and Allergy Clinics of North America*, *31*(1), 81–93.

Green, K. A., McGwin, F., & Owsley, C. (2013). Associations between visual, hearing, and dual sensory impairments and history of motor vehicle collision involvement of older drivers. *Journal of the American Geriatrics Society*, *61*(2), 252–257. doi:10.1111/jgs.12091

Harris, G. M., Allen, R. S., Dunn, L., et al. (2013). "Trouble won't last always": Religious coping and meaning in the stress process. *Qualitative Health Research*, *23*(6), 773–781.

Hayward, R. D., & Krause, N. (2013a). Trajectories of late-life change in God-mediated control. *Journals of Gerontology: Psychological and Social Sciences*, *68*(1), 49–58.

Hayward, R. D., & Krause, N. (2013b). Changes in church-based social support relationships during older adulthood. *Journals of Gerontology: Psychological and Social Sciences*, *68*(1), 85–96.

Herdman, T. H. (Ed.). (2012). *NANDA International Nursing Diagnoses: Definitions and classification 2012–1014.* Oxford, England: Wiley-Blackwell.

Hershey, D. A., & Henkens, K. (2014). Impact of different types of retirement transitions on perceived satisfaction with life. *The Gerontologist*, *54*(2), 232–244. doi:10.1093/geront/gnt006

Holmes, T. H., & Rahe, R. H. (1967). The social readjustment rating scale. *Journal of Psychosomatic Research*, *11*, 213–218.

Hummert, M. L. (2011). Age stereotypes and aging. In K. W. Schaie & S. L. Willis (Eds.), *Handbook of the psychology of aging* (7th ed., pp. 249–262). New York, NY: Elsevier.

Jenkinson, C. E., Dickens, A. P., Jones, K., et al. (2013). Is volunteering a public health intervention? A systematic review and meta-analysis of the health and survival of volunteers. *BioMed Central, 13*, 773. Retrieved from www.biomedcentral.com/1471-2458/13/773

Kotter-Gruhn, D., & Hess, T. M. (2012). The impact of age stereotypes on self-perceptions of aging across the adult lifespan. *Journals of Gerontology: Psychological Sciences and Social Sciences, 67*(5), 563–571.

Lachman, M. E., Neupert, S. D., & Agrigoroaei, S. (2011). The relevance of control beliefs for health and aging. In K. W. Schaie & S. L. Willis (Eds.), *Handbook of the psychology of aging* (7th ed., pp. 175–190). New York, NY: Elsevier.

Lane, A. M., Hirst, S. P., & Reed, M. B. (2013). *Older adults: Understanding and facilitating transitions.* Dubuque, IA: Kendall Hunt.

Lenze, E. J., & Wetherell, L. (2011). A lifespan view of anxiety disorders. *Dialogues in Clinical Neuroscience, 13*(4), 381–399.

Levy, B. R., Chung, P. H., Bedford, T., et al. (2014). Facebook as a site for negative age stereotypes. *Gerontologist, 54*(2), 172–176.

Levy, B. R., Slade, M. D., Murphy, T. E., et al. (2012). Association between positive age stereotypes and recovery from disability in older persons. *Journal of the American Medical Association, 308*(19), 1972–1973.

Levy, B. R., Zonderman, A. B., Slade, M. D., et al. (2011). Memory shaped by age stereotypes over time. *Journals of Gerontology: Psychological Sciences and Social Sciences, 67*(4), 432–436.

Li, Y.-P., Chen, Y.-M., & Chen, C.-H. (2013). Volunteer transitions and physical and psychological health among older adults in Taiwan. *Journals of Gerontology: Psychological Sciences and Social Sciences, 68*(6), 997–1008.

Liddle, J., Haynes, M., Pachana, N. A., et al. (2014). Effect of a group intervention to promote older adults' adjustment to driving cessation on community mobility: A randomized controlled trial. *The Gerontologist, 54*(3), 409–422. doi:10.1093/geront/gnt019

Lyon, B. L. (2012). Stress, coping, and health. In V. H. Rice, *Handbook of stress, coping, and health* (2nd ed., pp. 2–20). Thousand Oaks, CA: SAGE.

Mallers, M. H., Claver, M., & Lares, L. A. (2014). Perceived control in the lives of older adults: The influence of Langer and Rodin's work on gerontological theory, policy, and practice. *The Gerontologist, 54*(1), 67–74. doi:10.1093/geront/gnt051

Manning, L. K. (2013). Navigating hardships in old age: Exploring the relationship between spirituality and resilience in later life. *Qualitative Health Research, 23*(4), 568–575.

Manning, L. K., Leek, J. A., & Radina, M. E. (2012). Making sense of extreme longevity: Explorations into spiritual lives of centenarians. *Journal of Religion, Spirituality, and Aging, 24*(4), 345–359.

Mather, M. (2012). The emotion paradox in the aging brain. *Annals of the New York Academy of Science, 1251*(1), 33–49.

Mazerolle, M., Regner, I., Morisset, P., et al. (2012). Stereotype threat strengthens automatic recall and undermines controlled processes in older adults. *Psychological Science, 23*(7), 723–727.

McKenna, M. A. (2012). Transcultural perspectives in the nursing care of older adults. In M. M. Andrews & J. S. Boyle (Eds.), *Transcultural concepts in nursing care* (6th ed., pp. 182–207). Philadelphia, PA: Lippincott Williams & Wilkins.

Miller, C. A. (2013). Wellness Activity Tool for stress management. In C. A. Miller (Eds.), *Fast facts for health promotion in nursing: Promoting wellness in a nutshell* (pp. 61–62). New York, NY: Springer.

Okun, M. A., Yeung, E. W., & Brown, S. (2013). Volunteering by older adults and risk of mortality: A meta-analysis. *Psychology and Aging, 28*(2), 564–577.

Park, N. S., Jang, Y., Lee, B. S., et al. (2013). The mediating role of loneliness in the relation between social engagement and depressive symptoms among older Korean Americans: Do men and women differ? *Journals of Gerontology: Psychological Sciences and Social Sciences, 68*(2), 193–201.

Pitkala, K. H., Routasalo, P., Kautiainen, H., et al. (2011). Effects of socially stimulating group intervention on lonely, older people's cognition: A randomized, controlled trial. *American Journal of Geriatric Psychiatry, 19*(7), 654–663.

Public Health Agency of Canada. (2010). *The health and well-being of Canadian seniors.* Retrieved from http://www.phac-aspc.gc.ca/cphorsphc-respcacsp/2010/fr-rc/cphorsphc-respcacsp-06-eng.php

Pynnonen, K., Tormakangas, T., Heikkinen, R.-L., et al. (2012). Does social activity decrease risk for institutionalization and mortality in older

people? *Journals of Gerontology, Psychological Sciences and Social Sciences, 67*(6), 765–774.

Ramsey, J. L. (2012). Spirituality and aging. *Annual Review of Gerontology and Geriatrics, 32*, 131–151.

Randall, W. L. (2013). The importance of being ironic: Narrative openness and personal resilience in later life. *Gerontologist, 53*(1), 9–16.

Rix, S. E. (2011). Employment and aging. In R. H. Binstock & L. K. George (Eds.), *Handbook of aging and the social sciences* (7th ed., pp. 193–206). New York, NY: Elsevier.

Rodin, J., & Langer, E. (1980). Aging labels: The decline of control and the fall of self-esteem. *Journal of Social Issues, 36*(2), 12–29.

Rote, S., Hill, T. D., & Ellison, C. G. (2012). Religious attendance and loneliness in later life. *Gerontologist, 53*(1), 39–50.

Schaan, B. (2013). Widowhood and depression among older Europeans: The role of gender, caregiving, marital quality, and regional context. *Journals of Gerontology: Psychological Sciences and Social Sciences, 68*(3), 431–442.

Schuurmans, J., & van Balkom, A. (2011). Late-life anxiety disorders: A review. *Current Psychiatric Reports, 13*(4), 267–273.

Scott, S. B., Whitehead, B. R., Bergeman, C. S., et al. (2013). Combinations of stressors in midlife: Examining role and domain stressors using regression trees and random forests. *Journals of Gerontology, Psychological Sciences and Social Sciences, 68*(3), 464–475.

Selye, H. (1956). *The stress of life.* New York, NY: McGraw-Hill.

Shrestha, S., Robertson, S., & Stanley, M. A. (2011). Innovations in research for treatment of late-life anxiety. *Aging and Mental Health, 15*(7), 811–821.

Smith, J. M. (2012). Loneliness in older adults: An embodied experience. *Journal of Gerontological Nursing, 38*(8), 45–53.

Spiwak, R., Sareen, J., Elias, B., et al. (2012). Complicated grief in Aboriginal populations. *Dialogues in Clinical Neuroscience, 14*(2), 204–209.

Stawski, R. S., Mogle, J. A., & Sliwinski, M. J. (2013). Daily stressors and self-reported changes in memory in old age: The mediating effects of daily negative affect and cognitive interference. *Aging and Mental Health, 17*(2), 168–172.

Stessman, J., Rottenberg, Y., Shimshilashvili, I., et al. (2014). Loneliness, health, and longevity. *Journals of Gerontology: Biological Sciences and Medical Sciences, 69*(6), 744–750. doi:10.1093/gerona/glt147

Turcotte, M. (2012). *Profile of seniors' transportation habits* (Catalogue no. 11-008X). Ottawa, ON: Statistics Canada.

Underwood, P. W. (2012). Social support. In V. H. Rice (Eds.), *Handbook of stress, coping, and health* (2nd ed., pp. 355–380). Thousand Oaks, CA: SAGE.

Van Kessel, G. (2013). The ability of older people to overcome adversity: A review of the resilience concept. *Geriatric Nursing, 34*, 122–127.

Werner, J. S., Frost, M. H., Macnee, C. L., et al. (2012). Major and minor life stressors, measures, and health outcomes. In V. H. Rice (Eds.), *Handbook of stress, coping, and health* (2nd ed., pp. 126–154). Thousand Oaks, CA: SAGE.

Westra, B. L., Paitich, N., Ekstrom, D., et al. (2013). Getting on with living life: Experiences of older adults after home care. *Home Healthcare Nurse, 31*(9), 493–501.

Whitbourne, S. K., & Meeks, S. (2011). Psychopathology, bereavement, and aging. In K. W. Schaie & S. L. Willis (Eds.), *Handbook of the psychology of aging* (7th ed., pp. 311–324). New York, NY: Elsevier.

Whitehead, B. R., & Bergeman, C. S. (2011). Coping with daily stress: Differential role of spiritual experience on daily positive and negative affect. *Journals of Gerontology: Psychological Sciences and Social Sciences, 67*(4), 456–459.

Wickrama, K., O'Neal, C. W., Kwag, K. H., et al. (2013). Is working later in life good or bad for health? An investigation of multiple health outcomes. *Journals of Gerontology: Psychological Sciences and Social Sciences, 68*(5), 807–815.

Williams, K. N., Herman, R., Gajewsi, B., et al. (2009). Elderspeak communication: Impact on dementia care. *American Journal of Alzheimer's Disease and Other Dementias, 24*, 11–20.

Yochim, B. P., Mueller, A. E., June, A., et al. (2011). Psychometric properties of the Geriatric Anxiety Scale: Comparison to the Beck Anxiety Inventory and Geriatric Anxiety Inventory. *Clinical Gerontologist, 34*, 21–33.

Psychosocial Assessment

Geriatric Anxiety	memory
Inventory (GAI)	mental status
hallucinations	assessment
illusions	orientation
insight	social supports

LEARNING OBJECTIVES

After reading this chapter, you will be able to:

1. Describe the purpose, scope of and procedure for a psychosocial assessment of older adults.

2. Describe communication techniques that are helpful for conducting a psychosocial assessment.

3. Describe how to assess each of the following specific components of mental status: physical appearance, motor function, social skills, response to the interview, orientation, alertness, memory, and speech and language characteristics.

4. Explain how to perform a nursing assessment of skills involved with decision-making and executive function in older adults.

5. Describe how to assess each of the following components of affective function: mood, anxiety, self-esteem, depression, happiness and well-being.

6. Discuss distinguishing characteristics of delusions, hallucinations and illusions as they relate to the underlying conditions common in older adults.

7. Explain how to perform a nursing assessment of the following aspects of social supports: social network, barriers to services and economic resources.

8. Explain how to perform a nursing assessment of older adults' spiritual needs including factors that cause spiritual distress, as well as those that promote spiritual wellness.

KEY POINTS

affect	decision-making
circumstantiality	delusions
confabulation	executive function

Psychosocial assessment is a complex and challenging, but essential, aspect of nursing care for older adults. Although psychosocial impairments are often attributed to factors relating to normal aging or to untreatable conditions, a careful psychosocial assessment can identify the underlying cause(s) of mental changes, some of which can then be reversed or addressed through interventions. Thus, nurses can use assessment skills to improve quality of life for older adults by ensuring that psychosocial issues and underlying causes of mental status changes are identified and addressed. This chapter provides information on the assessment component of the nursing process related to cognitive and psychosocial function (Chapters 11 and 12). In addition, it supplements the assessment information in other chapters of this text, particularly the chapters on elder abuse (Chapter 10), delirium and dementia (Chapter 14) and depression (Chapter 15).

OVERVIEW OF PSYCHOSOCIAL ASSESSMENT OF OLDER ADULTS

In contrast to physical and functional assessment procedures, which are viewed as routine measures to identify the causes of troublesome symptoms, psychosocial assessment procedures tend to be perceived as formal psychological tests that analyse personality traits or identify the need for psychiatric treatment. Consequently, health care professionals may overlook the psychosocial component of assessment or relegate it to the realm of mental health professionals. However, an assessment of psychosocial function is an essential component of holistic nursing care, which addresses the body–mind–spirit needs of older adults.

This chapter focuses on those aspects of psychosocial function that are pertinent to caring for older adults from a wellness perspective. This comprehensive perspective is like the emergency cart that is available in every hospital unit. The cart stands ready at all times and is equipped with any items needed to handle medical emergencies. When a serious medical problem arises, health care professionals quickly pull the cart to the patient's bedside and select the needed items. Similarly, nurses must have access to an array of skills for assessing psychosocial function as the need arises. In a few situations, their entire array of skills will be called into play, but in most situations, only a few of the examination tools will be necessary. Nurses can use the material in this chapter to "fill their mental status assessment carts," so they can use appropriate tools for each situation.

The first sections of this chapter cover the purposes of, scope of and procedures for a psychosocial assessment and are applicable to nursing care of all older adults. The second major section reviews aspects of communication and cultural considerations in relation to a psychosocial assessment. Each of the following components, which nurses would selectively assess depending on the individual situation, are discussed in separate sections: mental status, decision-making and executive function, affective function, contact with reality and social supports.

Purposes of the Psychosocial Assessment

From a wellness perspective, the purposes of psychosocial assessment include the following:

- Detecting asymptomatic or unacknowledged health problems at an early stage
- Identifying signs or symptoms of psychosocial dysfunction (e.g., anxiety, depression, memory problems, depression, change in mental status)
- Identifying stressors and other risk factors that affect cognitive, emotional or social function
- Obtaining information about the person's usual personality, coping mechanisms and cognitive abilities
- Identifying social supports and other coping resources that could be supported or strengthened
- Identifying the older adult's personal goals for psychosocial wellness

As with other types of assessment, nurses use this information to plan interventions that are based on realistic expectations.

Older adults who experience a change in their mental status need a comprehensive assessment by an interprofessional team to assure that underlying causes are identified and addressed. A common mistake is to label the changes as "normal for the person's age." This is not only unfair to the older adult but can be detrimental, particularly if a treatable underlying condition is overlooked or appropriate interventions to improve functional abilities are neglected. As should be clear from the discussion of cognitive function in Chapter 11, age-related cognitive changes are rarely brought to the attention of health care professionals. For example, an older adult would be unlikely to make the following complaint: "I know I can learn new information, but I don't seem to be able to comprehend information as quickly as I used to." When older adults experience mental changes, every effort should be made to identify the underlying cause rather than simply attributing the changes to age.

Scope of the Psychosocial Assessment

An important part of a psychosocial assessment is identifying the unique meaning of life events, with particular attention on identifying any effects on health. Initial questions can focus on events that occurred many years ago, such as "What kind of work did you do?" may prompt a discussion of feelings about retirement. Because changes in living arrangements can precipitate feelings of loss, a nonthreatening question such as "What were the circumstances of your moving here?" might lead to further discussion of the meaning of the living arrangement for that person. People who have experienced the loss of a pet may be reluctant to acknowledge the depth of their feelings, and they need to know that they will not be judged. Because pets may be particularly significant for older adults, it is appropriate to include at least one question about pets in the psychosocial assessment of older adults.

Questions to assess the meaning of medical conditions and functional limitations are an essential component of the psychosocial assessment because coping with health changes is a common and challenging task for many older adults. Nurses also try to identify the person's concerns about the functional consequences that are likely to be associated with illness and disability. For example, older adults with diabetes may be less interested in knowing how the pancreas functions than in learning to cope with the attendant visual impairment or their fear of increasing dependence on others. Therefore, rather than focusing the assessment on medical diagnoses, ask a broader question such as "If you had to rate your health on a scale of 0% to 100%, what rating would you give it today?" After the person responds to this question, ask follow-up questions, such as "What would have to be changed for you to feel 25% more healthy?" or "What rating would you have given yourself a year ago?" Answers to these questions can assist in establishing realistic and person-centred goals for interventions.

During a psychosocial assessment, nurses might hear information that is contrary to their own values or cultural expectations, such as the following examples:

- Expressions of racial prejudice, including use of derogatory labels
- Attitudes of extreme passivity about decisions involving the patient's care
- Situations in which older adults are abused or exploited by friends, family or others
- Attitudes that are judgmental about women or other groups or not in accordance with the nurse's beliefs

When dealing with these types of situations, it helps to be aware of one's own feelings and to address them accordingly. Although it is essential to communicate a nonjudgmental attitude during interactions with patients and clients, it is also important to acknowledge their feelings. For instance, if the person describes an episode of extreme exploitation and expresses feelings of anger about the situation, the nurse can show empathy and understanding with a statement such as "That sounds like a terrible situation to have been in." Nurses also need to consider that some of the information they obtain may involve legal or ethical issues that require further action. For example, information about recent or ongoing abuse or exploitation may necessitate a referral for further investigation as discussed in Chapter 10.

Procedure for the Psychosocial Assessment

Nurses obtain psychosocial assessment information by interviewing older adults and their caregivers and by observing older adults in their environments. Opportunities for performing psychosocial assessments vary in different health care settings and much of the assessment information is obtained informally during the course of providing care. In acute care settings, nurses perform an assessment at the time of admission to establish a baseline for planning nursing care. Although the initial nursing assessment focuses on the patient's immediate physical needs, nurses should not overlook the psychosocial assessment because it often provides clues to the causes of existing medical problems. Thus, as soon as the patient's condition is medically stable, nurses assess psychosocial issues as an important component of holistic care and discharge planning. In long-term care settings, psychosocial assessment information is usually discussed during interprofessional care conferences. In home settings, nurses have unique opportunities to obtain valuable psychosocial assessment information by observing the older adult in his or her personal environment.

In addition to interviewing and observing older adults, it is often appropriate to obtain information from other sources. For example, when the older person's cognitive function is compromised, it is essential to obtain information from family members and others who can provide a reliable history of the mental changes. In long-term care settings, nursing assistants—the health care workers who spend the most time with residents—are an important source of psychosocial information. Although nursing assistants are not routinely included in team discussions when psychosocial problems are addressed, nurses can obtain information from them and incorporate it in the care plans.

The tools for an effective psychosocial assessment are a trusting relationship, a listening ear, an intuitive mind combined with a solid knowledge base about mental health issues in older adults, a sensitive heart and good communication skills. Because psychosocial issues may involve topics that are considered private, older adults may feel threatened by psychosocial assessment questions, particularly if they are trying to cover up cognitive deficits. Nurses,

Box 13-1 Self-Assessment of Attitudes About Psychosocial Aspects of Aging

What Is My Level of Comfort in Discussing Psychosocial Issues With Older Adults?

- How comfortable am I discussing emotional, cultural, spiritual, and psychosocial subjects?
- Are there certain topics with which I am uncomfortable (e.g., death, suicide, alcoholism, sexuality, spirituality, terminal illness, abusive relationships)?
- Does the person's age influence my degree of comfort (e.g., Am I more comfortable discussing certain topics with someone who is in their 30s than with someone who is in their 90s?)
- Does the person's gender influence my degree of comfort?
- To what groups of older adults do I find it easy or difficult to relate?
- How do I feel about older adults who are living in nontraditional relationships?

When I Was Growing up

- How were older adults in my family treated?
- What did I observe about the treatment of older adults in society?
- How were people with mental or emotional disorders viewed?
- What language was used to describe aging, old age, and older adults with altered mental function?
- What words did my family use, and what was the connotative meaning of the words used, to describe older adults? Was it positive, negative, or mixed?

What Experiences Have I Had with Older Adults

- From different racial, ethnic, religious, and socioeconomic backgrounds?
- With functional impairments or mental, psychological, or emotional disorders?

also, may be less comfortable with psychosocial aspects of the assessment process, so it is important to reflect on one's own attitudes and identify areas of discomfort, as described in Box 13-1.

A Student's Perspective

My experience interviewing Mr. M. was an amazing one. I learned a lot about older adults and also about my interview technique. I think several of my techniques helped Mr. M. feel more comfortable and at ease. I told him if he felt uncomfortable answering any questions, he should feel free to pass and that did not happen once. I started asking him easy questions about his job and things like that. Then I moved into more personal questions related to his childhood and whether he thought it had been easy or difficult. I thought he might not remember a lot of that time in his life, but he told me many stories from when he was younger. He also had a lot of pride in the work that he did as a middle-aged adult when he was foreman in a factory.

Another technique I used was to allow him to wander away from the "path" of the question that I had asked him, because I didn't want him to feel conformed to answer the specific question. By using this technique, I learned much more about him than the scope of my original question, and it also gave him time to tell me things at his own pace. I could also tell what information he valued as important and what he found more private.

Erin H.

Begin a psychosocial assessment by explaining the purpose in relation to a nursing goal, with a statement like one of the following:

- "I'd like to ask you some questions about your interests so we can plan for your care while you're here at the nursing facility."
- "I'd like to ask some questions so we can make the best plans for follow-up after you leave the hospital."
- "I'd like to ask some questions about how you've been managing things at home so we can identify any community services that may be helpful to you."

An effective approach is to ask social questions, such as where the person was born and grew up. Although health care professionals may believe that it is unprofessional to talk about themselves, offering a little information about their own family or pets, for instance, may help to establish a framework of mutual interest. Sharing information about ethnic background also can be an effective and nonthreatening way of obtaining information about possible cultural influences. Remember that some groups in Canada, for example, First Nations, may have different styles of communication from the general population.

If formal mental status assessment tools are to be used, they can be introduced after the older adult is more comfortable with discussing psychosocial issues. Because questions about memory can be very threatening, the topic might be introduced as follows: "I notice you have a hard time remembering dates. Have you noticed any other problems with your memory? Is it okay with you if I ask some questions about your memory?" If no evidence of cognitive impairment is evident, but other people have expressed concern about the person's memory, a statement such as the following might be used: "Your daughter is concerned that you don't remember to keep appointments. Have you noticed any problems with your memory? Is it okay with you if I ask some questions about your memory?"

COMMUNICATION SKILLS FOR PSYCHOSOCIAL ASSESSMENT

Just as nurses use a stethoscope and other tools for assessing physical function, nurses use communication techniques as an essential tool for establishing a trusting relationship and obtaining pertinent information about psychosocial function. Nurses frequently need to address communication barriers that arise from several sources: the older adult, the situation itself and the person who is communicating, as listed in Box 13-2. In addition, cultural differences can create communication barriers that are very challenging. For example, foreign-born people who have a condition that affects their cognitive function may revert to their first spoken language, even if they previously spoke English well. In these situations, family members may be able to facilitate communication, or it may be appropriate to use interpreters, as discussed in Chapter 2.

When discussing psychosocial issues, it is important to establish a private and comfortable environment and use

---

Box 13-2 Barriers to and Strategies for Effective Communication With Older Adults

Situational Barriers

- Different primary languages of speaker and listener.
- Too much information being exchanged at one time.
- More than one person communicating at one time.
- Environmental noise, particularly for people who have impaired hearing or use hearing aids.

Barriers Associated With the Older Adult

- Vision or hearing impairments.
- Neurologic conditions that affect skills related to concentration, language, information processing, language skills (e.g., anxiety, aphasia, dementia, mild cognitive impairment).
- Physical discomfort (e.g., pain, thirst, hunger, fatigue, bladder fullness, or uncomfortable temperatures).

Barriers Associated With the Person Who Is Communicating

- Rapid or inarticulate speech.
- Obstructive mannerisms (e.g., covering one's mouth or turning one's head away).
- Minimizing the person's feelings.
- Giving false reassurances.
- Offering trite responses (e.g., "Why cry over spilled milk?").
- Changing the subject to avoid sensitive issues.
- Jumping to conclusions.
- Using elderspeak or inappropriate titles (e.g., "dear," or "honey").

---

interventions to improve hearing and vision. Box 13-3 describes strategies for enhancing communication with older adults, with details specific to a psychosocial assessment.

Nurses have many opportunities to identify psychosocial issues by listening for pertinent concerns and asking appropriate

A Student's Perspective

When I conducted a functional assessment, I found some communication techniques were therapeutic, whereas others were not. One barrier that I encountered was the difficulty of understanding my client because he did not have any teeth, and, therefore, it was difficult for him to pronounce his words. Also, there was limited privacy, and the client seemed to be distracted by other people in the room. Another barrier was that I found myself looking down at the paper as opposed to maintaining consistent eye contact. To combat these barriers, it would be important to provide more privacy and to minimize distractions. Also, because the client was difficult to understand, it would be important to ask for clarification about anything that was unclear. In addition, it is important to remember that a lack of eye contact is nontherapeutic. In order to improve on communication techniques, it is important to realize any barriers, identify ways to combat them, and think about what to do differently in the next situation. A helpful way to combat barriers is to remember the communication model of SOLER: Sit facing the client, Observe an open posture, Lean toward the client, Establish and maintain intermittent eye contact, and Relax.

Brittany D.

Box 13-3 Strategies to Enhance Communication With Older Adults

General Strategies

- Arrange for face-to-face positioning.
- Ensure as much privacy as possible.
- Provide good lighting, and avoid background glare.
- Eliminate as much background noise as possible.
- Compensate as much as possible for vision or hearing impairments (e.g., make sure the person is using eyeglasses and hearing aids if appropriate).
- Address physical needs and concerns about comfort.
- Begin contact with an exchange of names and, if appropriate, a handshake.
- Use culturally appropriate titles of respect, such as Mr., Mrs., Ms., Monsieur, Madame, Dr., Reverend, Elder, Bishop, and so forth.
- Pronounce names correctly, and if in doubt, ask the older adult to say his or her name.
- Avoid linguistic messages that may convey bias or inequality.
- Avoid slang expressions and never use pejorative or derogatory terms to refer to ethnic, racial, religious, or any other group.
- Use touch purposefully and with awareness of individual preferences.
- Be aware of cultural differences that influence the perception and interpretation of verbal and nonverbal communication.

Strategies Specific to a Psychosocial Assessment

- Explain the purpose of the psychosocial assessment in relation to a nursing goal; then, begin with questions about remote, nonthreatening topics.
- Maintain good eye contact.
- Be comfortable using silence.
- Use attentive listening skills.
- Use open-ended questions.
- Encourage the person to elaborate on information with statements, such as "and then what happened?"
- Ask how the person felt about or responded to a situation.
- Periodically clarify the messages.
- Remain nonjudgmental in your responses, but show appropriate empathy.
- Ask formal mental status questions, or the most threatening questions, toward the end of the interview.
- Gain the person's permission before asking formal assessment questions regarding memory and other cognitive abilities.

questions to obtain further information. For example, consider the case of Mrs. P. who, during an admission interview, gave the following response to a question about where she lives:

I moved to Sunnybrook Retirement Village after my last stroke. I couldn't stay in my own home because the bedrooms were on the second floor. The doctor told me I had to live where I could get help, and my daughter didn't want me with her. Now that I've fallen and broken my wrist, I'm not sure what the doctor will tell me. My daughter doesn't want to be bothered with me.

This response gives clues to several potential issues, which the nurse can explore with any of the following questions:

- "What do you miss most since you moved?"
- "You mentioned that your daughter didn't want you living with her. Is that something you had hoped you could do?"
- "Do you worry that the doctor will suggest that you go to a nursing home?"
- "Do you see your daughter as often as you'd like?"

Answers to these questions might uncover psychosocial concerns that need to be addressed as a part of discharge planning.

When communicating about psychosocial issues, it is important to periodically clarify the messages. One clarification technique is to repeat part of a prior answer when asking further questions. For example, saying to Mrs. P., "You mentioned that your daughter doesn't want you living with her…," gives feedback about what the nurse heard and leads into further questions about underlying feelings. Feedback can also be helpful when discrepancies between verbal and nonverbal communication are observed. For example, Mrs. P. might begin to cry and clench her fists as she says, "My daughter has her own life to worry about. I can take care of myself. It doesn't bother me that I can't live with her." A statement such as "You look awfully sad. Are you sure it doesn't bother you?" might lead to an acknowledgment of feelings such as anger, rejection and loneliness.

Another important aspect is to consider the effects of nonverbal communication, which can be strongly influenced by cultural factors. For example, touch, hand shaking, eye contact and facial expressions can be used effectively to enhance communication, but they can also create barriers if they are misinterpreted. In addition, it is important to consider each person's "comfort zone," which is the physical space required for the person to feel at ease when communicating with others. This space is categorized as *intimate distance* (0–18 inches), *personal distance* (1.5–4 feet), and *social distance* (4–12 feet). Cultural factors can influence all these aspects of nonverbal communication, as described in Box 13-4.

A Student's Perspective

My communication with patients is something that I am always aware of. I have continued to learn something new each week. Silence during a conversation is something that is always uncomfortable for me. When talking with my client last week, I was trying to get a better sense of his level of family support. I began by asking him if he had any children. He indicated that he had two daughters, but they lived in Florida. Normally I would have had a follow-up question for this response, but I decided to give the client some time to see if he would expand on his original response. It was an awkward few minutes—okay, it was probably just a few seconds that seemed like minutes—but he did open up tremendously. He went on to explain to me that he felt like they have abandoned him since their mother passed away. He began to tear up as he went on to explain that he has grandchildren he has only seen in pictures in Christmas cards. I was able to talk with him about his feelings about these issues and offer him some encouragement. Had I chosen to guide the conversation I would have most likely never had this opportunity. I continue to enjoy confronting uncomfortable communication situations so that I can overcome them and foster better therapeutic communication between myself and clients.

Amanda A.

Box 13-4 Cultural Considerations: Cultural Influences on Communication

Touch

- Cultural groups that are likely to be most comfortable with physical touch are Jews, French, Spanish, Italians, Indonesian, and Latin Americans.
- Cultural groups that are likely to be uncomfortable with touch are British, Chinese, Germans, Hindus, and English-speaking Canadians.
- Asians may believe that it is disrespectful to touch the head, because it is thought to be a source of the person's strength.
- Vietnamese view the human head as the seat of life and highly personal; they may feel anxious if touched on their head or shoulders; if any orifice of the head is invaded, they may fear these procedures could provide an escape for the essence of life.
- Aboriginal Canadian women may be uncomfortable with male physicians, particularly with physical exams that involve touch in intimate areas.

Touch Between Men and Women

- Cultural groups that do not allow physical touch between men and women outside the home include the Inuit, Bosnians, Middle Easterners, Somalis.
- In many Middle Eastern cultures, male health care providers may be prohibited from touching or examining part or all of the female body.
- In some Asian cultures, touching between persons of the same sex (but not between those of the opposite sex) is common and acceptable.

Hand Shaking

- Middle Eastern women may not shake hands with men.
- Asian women may not shake hands with each other or with men.
- A soft handshake is acceptable for Aboriginal Canadians, but a firm handshake is not acceptable, as the handshake is not traditional in Aboriginal culture.

Eye Contact

- People from some Asian, Hispanic, Hindi, Hmong, Indochinese, Appalachian, Middle Eastern, and Aboriginal cultures may consider direct eye contact impolite, immodest, or aggressive, and they may avert their eyes when talking with health care professionals or, if female, when talking with men.
- As a sign of respect, some Aboriginal Canadians will not maintain prolonged eye contact with others, particularly those seen in positions of authority.
- Cultural groups that are likely to maintain steady eye contact during conversations include Arabs, European Americans, Greeks, and Turks.
- Some cultural groups (e.g., Bosnians) maintain eye contact between women but not between men and women.

Facial Expression

- Italians, Jews, and Black Canadians smile readily and use many facial expressions along with words and gestures to communicate pain, happiness, or displeasure.

Perception of Personal Space

- Cultural groups that are likely to have a closer range for personal distance include Arabs, Greeks, Japanese, Iranians, East Indian, Latin Americans, and Middle Easterners.
- Canadians, British, Irish, and European North Americans are likely to require the most personal space.
- Men usually like to have larger personal space than women.

Sources: Andrews, M. M., & Boyle, J. S. (2012). *Transcultural concepts in nursing care* (6th ed.). Philadelphia, PA: Lippincott Williams & Wilkins; Purnell, L. D. (2013). *Transcultural health care: A culturally competent approach* (4th ed.). Philadelphia, PA: F. A. Davis.

MENTAL STATUS ASSESSMENT

A **mental status assessment** is an organized approach to collecting data about a person's psychosocial function. The mental status assessment is very broad in scope, so this section focuses on cognitive abilities, and other aspects of psychosocial function (i.e., affective function, contact with reality and social supports) are discussed in the following sections. Indicators of psychosocial function that are addressed in this section on a mental status assessment are physical appearance, psychomotor behaviour, social skills, orientation, alertness, memory and speech characteristics. Mental status assessments are performed by various health care professionals, with each discipline specializing in various components. For example, psychiatrists are skilled in assessing affective and cognitive components, whereas social workers are skilled in assessing family relationship components. In the framework of this text, nurses assess the aspects of psychosocial function that most directly influence the day-to-day activities of older adults.

Mental Status Screening Tools

Screening tools are used in clinical settings to identify the need for further assessment. The Mini-Mental State Examination (MMSE) is a 30-point screening tool that has been widely used since the 1970s by many health care practitioners. In recent years, other easy-to-use tools have been developed and are commonly used to screen for cognitive impairment, as described in Table 13-1. A current trend in geriatric settings is to use the Montreal Cognitive Assessment (MoCA) tool because of its improved ability to screen for

TABLE 13-1 Tools Commonly Used to Screen for Cognitive Impairment

Tool	Features
Folstein Mini-Mental Status (MMSE)	Assesses orientation, memory, attention and abilities to name, follow verbal and written command, write a sentence spontaneously and copy a complex polygon. Maximum of 30 points
Mini-Cog with Clock Drawing Test	Assesses cognitive function, memory, language comprehension, visual-motor skills and executive function
AD8: The Washington University Dementia Screening Test	Uses eight items to assess changes in memory, orientation, judgment and function, as compared with previous levels
Montreal Cognitive Assessment (MoCA)	Includes 30 items assessing short-term memory recall, visuospatial abilities, 3-dimensional cube copy and executive functions
One-Minute Verbal Fluency for Animals	Tests ability to name as many animals as he/she can in 1 minute
Blessed Memory Test	Tests ability to recall 5-item name and address

mild cognitive impairment, as well as dementia (Freitas et al., 2013). Online Learning Activity 13-1 provides links to helpful information about using these screening tools in clinical settings with older adults. Keep in mind that the purpose of these tools is simply to identify indicators of altered mental status, but they do not provide a broad or in-depth perspective on psychosocial function, as is presented in this chapter. In addition, Chapters 14 and 15 provide information about screening tools for delirium and depression.

See **ONLINE LEARNING ACTIVITY 13-1: EVIDENCE-BASED INFORMATION ABOUT SCREENING TOOLS FOR IDENTIFYING COGNITIVE IMPAIRMENT IN OLDER ADULTS** at http://thepoint.lww.com/Miller7e

Physical Appearance

Physical appearance is readily observed and reveals many aspects of psychosocial function. Clothing, grooming, cosmetics and hygiene provide many clues to psychological function, but they are only clues, and questions must be asked before any conclusions are drawn. For example, the presence of body odour, poor hygiene and tattered clothing may be associated with any of the following conditions: depression, psychosis, incontinence, impaired cognitive abilities, limited financial resources, overwhelming caregiving responsibilities, impaired vision or sense of smell, or lack of access to or inability to use bathing facilities.

Motor Function, Body Language and Psychomotor Behaviours

Assessment of motor function, which includes posture, movement and body language, can provide clues to broader aspects of psychosocial function. For example, a shuffling, staggering or uncoordinated gait could indicate neurologic deficits secondary to a disease process or adverse effects from alcohol or medications. Gait disturbances, as well as other abnormal movements, are possible signs of tardive dyskinesia or extrapyramidal symptoms. Evidence of tardive dyskinesia raises the question of past or present use of psychotropic medications (discussed in Chapter 8) and may give clues to the individual's psychiatric history.

Body language also provides clues to affective illnesses. Slouching and head hanging are common manifestations of withdrawal and depression. Poor eye contact, particularly looking at the floor, may be indicative of depression. As with all aspects of assessment, it is important to consider that cultural factors can influence the type and amount of eye contact that is considered to be appropriate (refer to Box 13-4).

Psychomotor behaviours are part of the mental status assessment because the ability to purposefully carry out simple motor skills is highly influenced by cognitive status. For example, observations of how someone navigates and avoids obstacles in the environment provide clues to the person's judgment and awareness of the environment. Nurses can assess psychomotor behaviours by asking the person to perform a simple activity of daily living (e.g., combing hair) and observing the person's ability to comprehend and perform the request.

Another assessment component is observations related to abnormal psychomotor function, such as extreme slowness or agitation. Depression is usually associated with slowed psychomotor function, but excessive activity can be a symptom of agitated depression. Agitation also can be a symptom of an adverse medication effect or an indicator of a physiologic disturbance (e.g., dehydration, electrolyte imbalance) or a pathologic condition (e.g., pneumonia, urinary tract infection), particularly in older adults with dementia.

Social Skills

Assessment of social skills provides information about many aspects of psychosocial function. For example, friendly and cooperative people with good conversational skills may use social skills to hide their cognitive deficits, particularly if they are motivated to do so. By contrast, people with long-standing patterns of hostility, social isolation, poor social skills and a lack of ambition may be less motivated to perform well. In addition, people sometimes use the following social skills to cover up cognitive deficits: humour, evasiveness, leading the conversation and making up answers to questions. Some older adults with dementia maintain very good social skills, even in the middle stages of dementia when other skills have long since declined. Nurses also need to be aware of cultural factors that influence social skills and consider the cultural context of the relationship between the interviewer and the interviewee.

Response to the Interview

The older adult's initial response to the interview, as well as changes that occur during the interview, can provide important assessment information. For example, an older adult may initially be very receptive to the questions but may become defensive or sarcastic when he or she is uncomfortable with the line of questioning. In addition, nurses assess the amount of time and effort expended in answering questions. This is particularly important when trying to differentiate between dementia and depression because cognitively impaired people may exert great effort in responding to questions, but depressed people may lack energy or motivation to answer correctly. Thus, two people may score the same on a formal mental status questionnaire, but one may miss the questions because of dementia and the other may miss them because of depression. When nurses suspect that lack of motivation is a reason for incorrect or missing answers, they might clarify this by asking, "Is it that you don't know the answers or that you just don't feel like answering the questions?"

Nurses may encounter attitudes of resistance and defensiveness for a variety of reasons. A person who is depressed may be apathetic and may not want to expend the energy to answer the questions. A cognitively impaired person may be angry, hostile or defensive, particularly if he or she is trying to hide or deny cognitive deficits. A person who has always been reclusive or suspicious may be unwilling to answer questions or may feel very defensive. Assessing the person's underlying attitude is as important as assessing the accuracy of responses to questions.

Assessing for **confabulation**, which is the process of making up information, is difficult when the nurse does not know the correct information. For example, questions about the person's place of birth or childhood experiences are not effective for assessing cognitive function unless the accuracy of the answers can be confirmed. People with mild cognitive changes may use confabulation to conceal memory loss. **Circumstantiality** involves the use of excessive details and roundabout answers in responding to questions.

Finally, nurses assess all information in relation to the person's usual personality traits. For example, highly sociable people might always use humour, whereas talkative people might naturally use circumstantiality. The use of humour and circumstantiality by people who are normally quiet and serious might indicate a great effort to cover up cognitive deficits. On the other hand, people who are normally quiet and withdrawn may be perceived falsely as being depressed. Nurses can obtain information about a person's usual personality by asking a question such as "Would you describe what you were like when you were 40 years old?" Family members and caregivers who have known the person for a long time are good sources of information about lifelong personality characteristics. Box 13-5 summarizes guidelines for assessing physical appearance, motor function, social skills and responses to the interview in relation to the person's psychosocial function.

Orientation

Orientation to person, place and time is the indicator of mental status that is most routinely assessed and documented. Often, however, orientation is viewed as the primary indicator of cognitive function, rather than as one small piece of a larger picture. For example, the following questions are the gold standard for assessing orientation: "What is your name?" "Where are you?" and "What time is it?" Based on the accuracy of each answer, the person is then labelled as "oriented times one," "oriented times two" or "oriented times three." The superficial use of orientation questions and the subsequent labelling of the person as oriented times one, two or three ignores important considerations, such as the following:

- Are any environmental clues available to the person to orient him to the time or place?
- Has the person been at the institution long enough to have learned the name of the facility?
- If the person cannot state the exact name of the facility, can she describe the type of facility it is or its general location?
- Do sociocultural factors influence the person's response to these questions?

Box 13-5 Guidelines for Assessing Physical Appearance, Motor Function, Social Skills, and Response to the Interview

Observations Regarding Physical Appearance and Motor Function

- What is the person's apparent age in relation to his or her chronologic age?
- How do the following factors reflect psychological function: hygiene, grooming, clothing, cosmetics?
- Does the person's physical appearance provide clues to dementia or depression or to other impairments of psychosocial function?
- What do the person's gait, posture, and body language indicate about his or her psychological function?
- Is there any evidence of tardive dyskinesia or other adverse medication effects?
- How does the person manoeuvre in the environment, and what does this reflect regarding judgment, vision, and other skills?

Observations Regarding Social Skills and Response to the Interview

- What are the person's lifelong patterns of social skills, and how do these influence the assessment process?
- How do the person's social skills influence the interviewer's interpretation of other aspects of psychosocial function?
- Is the person motivated to answer questions?
- What is the person's attitude about the interview?
- If the person does not answer the questions, or gives incorrect answers, is it because of inability, cultural factors or lack of motivation?
- Does the person use any of the following in an attempt to hide possible cognitive deficits: humour, sarcasm, avoidance, evasiveness, confabulation, circumstantiality, or leading the conversation?
- Does the person manifest any of the following characteristics: anger, hostility, resistance, defensiveness, or suspiciousness?
- Do the person's underlying attitudes reflect his or her usual personality, or are they manifestations of cognitive or affective disturbances?

- Can the person name familiar people, such as a spouse or children, even if he cannot state his own name?
- If the person cannot give specific names of other people, can he describe the correct role of the other person?
- If the person cannot state the exact time, can she give the general time of day?
- Does the person have medical problems that interfere with cognition?
- Is the person taking medications that can influence mental function?

A good assessment extends beyond the three classic questions and describes levels of orientation that are meaningful for the person in a particular setting. For example, the following description is far more useful than simply noting that the person is "oriented times one":

Mrs. S. could state her name but did not remember the name of this hospital. She could not give her daughter's name but was able to introduce her daughter to me without stating her name. She thought that the month was December because of the Chanukah decorations in her room. She could not state the time because she did not have her watch with her, but she thought that it was afternoon because lunch had recently been served.

If the nurse had used only the standard questions of "What is your name?" "Where are you?" and "What time is it?" Mrs. S. would be judged to be "oriented times one." Most health care providers, after reading the results of that assessment, would have assumed that Mrs. S. had serious cognitive impairment, particularly if she were 85 years of age or older. Mrs. S.'s actual responses, however, reflected various cognitive skills involved in organizing information, making associations and using judgment. The more detailed description shows that Mrs. S. is probably quite a logical person who has not yet learned the name of the hospital and who might have some temporary memory impairment because of anxiety, medications or acute medical problems.

Alertness and Attention

Besides orientation, level of **alertness** is the mental status indicator that health care providers most frequently assess and document. Level of alertness is measured along a continuum, which includes stupor, drowsiness, somnolence, intermittent alertness/drowsiness and hyperalertness. An important aspect of assessing the person's level of alertness is the identification of any factors that can either increase or decrease alertness, with particular attention to those factors that can be addressed. For example, excessive daytime drowsiness can be associated with any of the following factors: medical problems, electrolyte imbalances, adverse medication effects (e.g., narcotics, anticholinergics, psychoactive medications), depression, dementia, excessive alcohol intake or lack of sleep at night because of a variety of reasons (e.g., caregiver responsibilities).

As a mental status indicator, **attention** describes the ability to focus on a task, filter out distractions and sustain focus as needed to complete a task. This is an essential, but often overlooked, indicator of altered mental status, particularly with regard to delirium (Steis & Fick, 2012). Kolanowski and colleagues (2012) described the following "everyday measures" that nurses can use in clinical settings to assess attention:

- Clap hands or ring a bell and have the person count the number of times you do this.
- Name the colours in the rainbow.
- Repeat a series of numbers forward and backward.
- State the days of the week or months of the year backward.
- Read a list of words and have the person signal when a certain word or letter is read.

As with other aspects of psychosocial assessment, attention skills are one piece of a large puzzle that is put together to provide a broader picture of mental status.

Memory

Formal memory testing assesses the person's **memory**, that is, recall of remote events, recent past events, and immediate memory, which is further divided into retention, recall, and recognition. Nurses can assess memory during regular conversations because all verbal communication depends to some degree on memory function. Nurses pay particular attention to assessing memory in relation to activities that are important in daily life, such as remembering to pay bills, take medications and shop for groceries. This assessment is made in relation to the expectations and demands of the person's usual environment. For example, if the person lives alone and manages finances independently, the ability to pay bills is quite important. By contrast, if the person lives with a daughter and her family, remembering the birth dates of grandchildren may be an important memory task.

Assessment of memory is particularly challenging because memory complaints are common among older adults, but they may not be based on actual deficits in memory function. For example, people who are depressed may perceive their memory skills as disproportionately impaired and may even exaggerate their deficits. In contrast to this situation, older adults with dementia (particularly in the middle stages) may have little or no awareness of their memory deficits, or they may deny memory problems as a self-protective response. Thus, the question, "Do you ever have trouble remembering things?" may elicit a positive response, but the response is likely to tell you more about the person's perception of memory than about his or her actual memory function. Although this question may be quite useful in identifying any concerns that the older adult might have, it does not conclusively demonstrate impaired memory function.

It is also important to assess the person's use of memory aids by posing a question such as "Is there anything you do to help you remember appointments or other things?" Assessment of the extent to which the person depends on memory aids is useful in setting goals and planning for improved memory function. For example, if the person's memory function is barely adequate and is based heavily on memory aids, then the potential for further improvement is minimal. By contrast, if the person has some memory deficits but does not use any memory aids, then the potential for improvement increases. Observations about the use of memory aids also may provide clues to unacknowledged memory deficits. For example, if the person denies problems with memory, but repeatedly refers to written notes during an interview, then he or she may be compensating for an impaired memory. In this situation, the person is quite willing to use memory aids but is unwilling to acknowledge the need for such help. Box 13-6 summarizes guidelines for nursing assessment of orientation, alertness and memory and includes examples of appropriate questions for assessing the different types of memory.

Speech and Language Characteristics

Speech and language characteristics provide important information about many aspects of psychosocial function, such as the ability to organize and communicate thoughts. In addition, a good assessment of language skills helps the nurse to identify words and language patterns that are most appropriate for use with an older person. Because speech and language skills are highly dependent on cultural, educational

Box 13-6 Guidelines for Assessing Orientation, Alertness and Memory

Interview Questions to Assess Orientation

Note: Examples of direct questions are identified by quotation marks to distinguish them from the questions that are answered indirectly through observations.

- *Person:* "What is your name?" "What is your wife's name?" If names can't be given, can the person describe roles?
- *Place:* "What is your address?" "What is the name of this place?" "What kind of place is this?" "What is the name of this city?" "What is the name of this state?"
- *Time:* "What time is it?" "What day of the week is today?" "What month and date is it today?" "What season is it?"

Observations to Assess Alertness

- What is the person's level of alertness on the following continuum: hyperalert, alert, drowsy, somnolent, stuporous?
- Does the person's level of alertness fluctuate? If so, is there any pattern to the fluctuations?
- Are there physiologic factors that might influence the person's level of alertness, such as medical conditions or effects of chemicals or medications?
- Are there psychosocial factors that might influence the person's level of alertness, such as anxiety, depression, nighttime caregiving responsibilities or any other factor that might disrupt nighttime sleep?

Interview Questions to Assess Memory

- *Remote events:* "Where were you born?" "Where did you go to grade school?" "What was your first job?" "When were you married?"
- *Recent past events:* "Do you live with anyone?" "Do you have any grandchildren?" "What are the names of your grandchildren?" "When was the last time you went to the doctor?"
- *Immediate memory, retention:* State three unrelated words and ask the person to repeat the information, both immediately and again after 5 minutes.
- *Immediate memory, general grasp and recall:* Ask the person to read a short story and then to summarize the information presented in the story.
- *Immediate memory, recognition:* Ask a multiple-choice question and then ask the person to choose the correct answer.

and socioeconomic factors, it is important to consider these influences, particularly when assessing foreign-born older adults.

During any verbal interaction, nurses can assess all of the following speech and language characteristics: pace, tone, volume, articulation, ability to organize and communicate thoughts, and any abnormal speech or language characteristics. The following examples describe some common speech variations and associated conditions:

- Rapid pace: anxiety, agitation or mental illness
- Slow-paced or excessively brief verbal communication: depression, cognitive impairment or simply cautiousness
- Tone of voice: indirectly expressed feelings such as anger, hostility and resentment
- Hypophonia (i.e., abnormally low speech volume): depression, physical illness, low self-esteem or long-standing speech habits

- Abnormally loud volume: impaired hearing or long-term experience communicating with someone who is hearing impaired
- Poor articulation or slurred speech: hearing impairment, ill-fitting dentures, lack of teeth or dentures, nervous system disorder, effects of alcohol or medications
- Phonemic errors (i.e., incorrect pronunciation): hearing impairment, cognitive deficits, educational and cultural influences
- Semantic errors (i.e., misinterpretation of the meaning of words): hearing impairment, cognitive deficits
- Neologisms (i.e., self-created and meaningless words): dementia, psychotic disorder (e.g., schizophrenia), repetition of a word that was not heard accurately
- Incoherent speech: dementia, aphasia, psychiatric disorders, alcohol or medication effects
- Perseveration (i.e., a repetitive or stuttering pattern of verbal or written communication) and agnosia (i.e., the inability to name an object accurately, particularly if it is unfamiliar): dementia

Aphasia is a communication disorder that is associated with neurologic conditions such as stroke or vascular dementia. Expressive aphasia occurs when comprehension abilities are not affected but word retrieval or word-finding abilities are impaired. Receptive aphasia occurs when verbal and comprehension abilities are impaired but some language skills are retained. Global aphasia, which is a combination of receptive and expressive aphasia, results from more extensive neurologic damage and is manifested by inconsistent and poorly controlled language skills.

Calculation and Higher Language Skills

Reading, writing, spelling and arithmetic are calculation and higher language skills that are assessed as indicators of cognition. As with assessments of other indicators, the person's education, occupation and other influencing factors must be considered. Nurses can informally assess these skills in relation to how the person performs important daily activities. For example, for an older adult who lives alone, an assessment of the ability to pay utility bills and use money to purchase groceries is more valuable than a measurement of mathematical skills using a psychometric test. Likewise, a person's ability to read the daily newspaper or the markings on a thermostat may be a more valid gauge of functional ability than a score on a formal reading test.

Nurses can use written health education materials to assess reading and comprehension skills informally, and this method serves a practical purpose. For example, when collecting a urine sample, the nurse can give the person a list of instructions and ask him or her to read the instructions aloud. An observation of how well the person comprehends the instructions provides an assessment of reading skills that are important in daily life. Another opportunity for assessing reading comprehension may arise if the nurse observes that an older adult has a newspaper nearby. A nonthreatening question such as "What's new in the paper today?" can provide information about the person's interests in outside events and his or her ability to comprehend and remember written information.

Nurses can assess writing and other higher language skills by observing older adults during interactions that pertain to their care. For example, nurses can observe the way an older adult signs his or her name on documents such as permission forms. Nurses can also observe the older adult during the performance of more complex tasks such as compiling a written medication list or a list of questions to discuss with the primary care provider. Difficulty with writing skills is a common sign of early stages of dementia. Of all the higher language skills, spelling is the least important in terms of daily function, but it is a good indicator of changes in mental abilities.

With traditional psychometric testing, calculation is measured with the "7s" test: the person is asked to subtract 7 from 100 and to continue subtracting 7s. Because this test is highly influenced by level of education, it is not necessarily the most appropriate test for older adults. It may be better to ask the older person to add 3 plus 3 and to continue adding 3s. Older adults who are depressed may not answer correctly because they do not want to expend the energy to calculate serial sevens. Older adults who have dementia may be able to perform well on this task if they try hard and if they previously had highly developed mathematical skills. Box 13-7 summarizes the considerations that are important in assessing speech characteristics and calculation and higher language skills.

Box 13-7 Guidelines for Assessing Speech Characteristics, Calculation and Higher Language Skills

Observations to Assess Speech Characteristics

- Is the pace of speech normal, slow or fast?
- Is the tone of voice suggestive of underlying feelings, such as anger, hostility or resentment?
- Is the volume abnormally soft or loud?
- Do the sentences flow coherently and smoothly?
- Is there evidence of any problem with integrating speech sounds into words (e.g., neologisms, or phonemic or semantic errors)?
- Do any of the following factors affect the person's speech: dry mouth, poorly fitting dentures, absence of teeth or dentures, alcohol or medication effects, or neurologic or other pathologic processes?
- Does the person exhibit any of the following: agnosia, perseveration or expressive, receptive or global aphasia?

Observations to Assess Calculation and Higher Language Skills

- What is the person's ability to comprehend written materials encountered in the course of routine activities, such as the daily newspaper or instructions for medications?
- What is the quality of the person's handwriting (e.g., his or her signature)?
- Is the person able to perform mathematical computations necessary for daily activities?

DECISION-MAKING AND EXECUTIVE FUNCTION

Decision-making—one of the most important and complex of all cognitive abilities—is an important aspect of psychosocial function because all legally competent older adults, including those with dementia, have the right to be involved in decisions about their care. Determination of competency is a complex issue with many implications not only for older adults and their families and caregivers, but also for health care professionals (as discussed in Chapter 9). As an integral part of psychosocial nursing care, nurses assess cognitive skills—including insight, learning, memory, reasoning, judgment, problem solving and abstract thinking—that are involved with decision-making. Although no one assessment tool focuses specifically on decision-making, nurses assess this aspect of psychosocial function by observing the abilities of older adults to solve problems during the course of daily activities and by asking pertinent assessment questions.

Abstract thinking is strongly influenced by other factors such as education, personality and affective state. People who are very anxious or depressed may lack the attention or motivation required to respond to the questions typically used for the assessment of abstract thinking patterns. Similarity questions such as "How are apples and oranges alike?" or "How are a table and chair alike?" are used to assess the person's ability to think abstractly.

During an interview, opportunities for assessing abstract thinking may arise, and the nurse listens for clues to the person's level of abstract versus concrete thinking. The following exchange is an example of an unsolicited opportunity that Carol Miller had to assess one older adult's concrete thinking pattern:

Nurse: How did you feel about having to move from your home in Texas to live with your daughter and her family here in Ohio?

Mr. L.: I don't know; how would you feel?

Nurse: I'm not sure how I'd feel; that's never happened to me. I'm not in your shoes.

Mr. L.: Well, here, put them on (stated emphatically while taking off his shoes to give to the nurse).

One interpretation of Mr. L.'s response is that his thinking pattern is very concrete, rather than abstract.

Nurses assess problem-solving abilities through observations about how older adults meet their needs in a particular situation. For instance, the nurse observes the way older adults use call lights to meet their needs when confined to a bed or the way in which they deal with complex decisions related to discharge planning. Similarly, a very important problem-solving task for an older adult who lives alone may be meeting basic safety needs. Therefore, questions such as "What would you do if you fell at home and could not get up?" or "What would you do if you woke up and smelled smoke?" might be an appropriate way of assessing judgment related to safety. For an older adult who lives in a nursing home, a very important but complex problem-solving task may involve dealing with a disruptive roommate. In this situation, the answer to a question such as "What would you do if your roommate started taking your belongings?" might provide the most pertinent information for assessing problem-solving skills.

Insight is the ability to understand the significance of the present situation. This skill is an important component of the problem-solving process because it establishes a basis for planning care. Level of insight is affected by pathologic changes in the brain and by psychosocial factors, such as feelings, personality and coping mechanisms. Lack of insight is sometimes labelled as *denial*, which is a defence mechanism that is often used to protect oneself from unpleasant realities. However, when insight is limited because of conditions, such as dementia, it is inappropriate and inaccurate to label this as denial; the more appropriate approach is to assess and document the person's level of insight.

Nursing assessment of insight concentrates on those areas of function that are pertinent to the care plan. For example, in assessing the insight of an older adult who has been brought to the hospital with malnutrition and uncontrolled hypertension, the nurse may ask questions such as the following:

- Why did your daughter bring you to the hospital?
- How do you manage with grocery shopping and getting your meals?
- Do you take any medications?
- What are the medications for?
- What kinds of things does your daughter do for you?
- What kind of help do you think you may need when you leave the hospital?

Answers to questions such as these facilitate care planning because they help the nurse assess the person's understanding of the present situation.

When the person has little or no understanding of his or her health situation, the nurse tries to identify the factors that interfere with insight. In the example just described, insight may be absent or limited because of one or more of the following conditions: dementia, depression, mild cognitive impairment, lack of information about the medication regimen, inability to remember information or fear of losing independence. An essential component of discharge planning is identifying both the level of insight and the factors that interfere with insight. In addition, the nurse attempts to identify factors that may improve the person's insight. If insight is lacking because of denial that stems from exaggerated fears, then alleviating the fears may facilitate insight.

In recent years, health care professionals have recognized the importance of assessing executive function abilities in conjunction with determining a patient's capacity to safely and reliably plan and carry out activities related to daily living. **Executive function** is multifaceted and involves an interrelated set of abilities that include cognitive flexibility, concept formation and self-monitoring; but it does not necessarily involve memory impairment (Kennedy, 2012). Executive function deficits, called executive dysfunction,

begin during the earliest stages of dementia and can be present even before memory problems are evident, particularly when the pathologic processes affect the frontal lobes. Indicators of executive function deficits include diminished mental flexibility, limited ability to think abstractly, difficulty with problem solving, decline in ability to conceptualize, diminished ability to adapt to new situations and difficulty shifting thought processes from one idea to another. People with executive cognitive dysfunction may perform well on the MMSE but still not be able to perform essential daily activities safely and independently. Online Learning Activity 13-2 provides additional information about screening tools nurses can use to identify executive dysfunction, as recommended by the Hartford Institute for Geriatric Nursing.

Because it is important to assess executive skills in relation to a previous level of function, it may be necessary to ask family members of the person being assessed if they have noticed changes in these abilities in recent years. When families or health care providers have serious questions about the decision-making abilities of an older person, or when a major decision must be made and there is disagreement about it, a more comprehensive assessment using neuropsychological tests may be warranted. For example, if a cognitively impaired older person expresses a strong desire to live alone but family members question the person's ability to function safely, a comprehensive geriatric assessment with emphasis on decision-making and executive function skills will provide useful information.

ONLINE LEARNING ACTIVITY 13-2 ADDITIONAL INFORMATION ABOUT EVIDENCE-BASED SCREENING TOOLS FOR ASSESSING EXECUTIVE FUNCTION AND DECISION-MAKING IN OLDER ADULTS at http://thepoint.lww.com/Miller7e

AFFECTIVE FUNCTION

Mood and affect are terms commonly used to describe individuals' affective function. Mood refers to an individual's emotional state, while a person's **affect** refers to his or her expressions of emotions, particularly facial expressions of underlying emotions. Happiness and sadness are common emotions, but all of the following can be used to describe emotions: joy, awe, hope, fear, pain, rage, pride, guilt, shame, anger, regret, relief, hatred, surprise, interest, boredom, elation, confusion, jealousy, depression, suspicion, frustration, anxiety, bewilderment, amorousness and lack of feelings.

The components of affective state that are reviewed in this section are general mood, anxiety, self-esteem, depression and happiness. These five aspects were selected for the following reasons:

- An assessment of general mood assists the nurse in determining appropriate goals based on the person's usual emotional state.
- Anxiety is a common factor in older adults that can often be alleviated or minimized through nursing interventions.

- Self-esteem is a major determinant of feelings, particularly depression and happiness.
- Self-esteem is particularly important because older adults face many conditions that threaten their self-esteem.
- Depression and happiness are two primary emotions that have been the target of much of the research regarding affective states in older people.

Nursing interventions are directed toward all of these components to improve the quality of life of older adults.

Guidelines for Assessing Affective Function

Affective function is assessed both quantitatively and qualitatively in relation to expectations about acceptable expressions of emotions. For example, people are expected to show some expression of sadness when talking about sad events. When the person's expression of feelings is not consistent with the external event, however, the affect is considered inappropriate. Affect is also assessed in relation to the personal meaning and the nearness in time of an event. People are expected to show greater feelings of sadness in response to tragic news than in response to neutral events. Likewise, people are expected to show a deeper emotional response soon after experiencing a sad event than they would years after the event occurred.

The depth and duration of emotion, which are important considerations in differentiating between dementia and depression in older adults, are also assessed. The affect of depressed people is generally sad and negativistic and is not influenced by external circumstances. By contrast, the affect of people who have dementia fluctuates more and changes in response to distractions. Emotional lability (i.e., emotional instability or fluctuation) occurs with strokes, vascular dementia, vascular depression and other pathologic conditions that affect certain areas of the brain.

Nonverbal behaviours, such as those indicating anxiety, sadness and happiness, provide important information about a person's emotional state that the person may not offer verbally. For example, despite a person's denial of feeling sad, he or she may exhibit the following nonverbal cues: crying, slouching over, looking at the ground, and having a mournful facial expression. The nurse uses this information as the basis for a leading comment such as "You look like you're feeling sad."

Expressions of emotions are strongly determined by cultural norms and personality characteristics. In most Western societies, crying is more acceptable for women and children than for men and older boys, and showing anger and rage is more acceptable for men than for women. Cultural expectations also influence the way a person expresses feelings in certain circumstances. For example, a person may be expected to cry and loudly proclaim mournful feelings at a funeral but may be prohibited from expressing any feelings in front of strangers or in a public place, such as a hospital. Because some emotions, such as anger or depression, are viewed as less acceptable than others, such as happiness,

people learn to deny and hide feelings that may be judged as unacceptable. Older adults, particularly, may have learned that certain feelings should not be expressed directly or verbally. Thus, it is particularly important to observe for any indirect or nonverbal clues of anger, depression and other less socially acceptable feelings.

In assessing the emotional state of older adults, it is important to identify the terminology that is most acceptable. Many people will not admit to feeling anxious or depressed because they associate these terms with a serious mental illness or with a socially unacceptable state. Therefore, the nurse begins the assessment of emotions by focusing on feelings that are viewed positively or neutrally. If the person initiates the topic of feeling anxious or depressed, the nurse responds to those feelings and pursues a related line of questioning. In most circumstances, however, it is best to begin with open-ended questions. A simple question such as "How are you feeling today?" asked with sincerity is a familiar and comfortable way of eliciting information.

Mood

Mood is closely associated with emotions but differs from them in that it is more pervasive, less intense and longer lasting. People are usually quite comfortable describing their mood as either bad or good and are more likely to offer information about their mood than their emotions. Thus, during a mental status examination, a question such as "How would you describe your usual mood?" may be perceived as less threatening than the question, "How do you feel most of the time?" Nonverbal behaviours provide many clues about a person's mood and may be more accurate than verbal responses as an indicator of affective state. Joy, anger, anxiety, sadness, happiness and depression are examples of moods that are expressed in nonverbal behaviours in everyday life by most people.

Anxiety

In assessing anxiety, nurses must identify the terminology that is most acceptable to the older adult. Words like "worries" and "concerns" are readily understood and usually elicit responses about sources of anxiety. Older adults may talk about "trouble with my nerves" in reference to anxiety. The **Geriatric Anxiety Inventory (GAI)** is an evidence-based screening tool used widely in research and clinical settings for measuring anxiety level in older adults (Pachana & Byrne, 2012). This tool has been translated into more than two dozen languages, with particular attention to cultural and language nuances. The version that is used in North America for English-speaking aging adults is shown in Figure 13-1. Although the GAI was developed for self-administration, nurses can ask older adults about each of the 20 items and score the tool. A positive response to 9 or more items indicates the need for further evaluation.

Nurses observe for nonverbal manifestations of anxiety to supplement the information obtained from verbal

	Agree	Disagree
* I worry a lot of the time.				
I find it difficult to make a decision.				
I often feel jumpy.				
I find it hard to relax.				
I often cannot enjoy things because of my worries.				
* Little things bother me a lot.				
I often feel like I have butterflies in my stomach.				
* I think of myself as a worrier.				
I can't help worrying about even trivial things.				
* I often feel nervous.				
* My own thoughts often make me anxious.				
I get an upset stomach due to my worrying.				
I think of myself as a nervous person.				
I always anticipate the worst will happen.				
I often feel shaky inside.				
I think that my worries interfere with my life.				
My worries often overwhelm me.				
I sometimes feel a great knot in my stomach.				
I miss out on things because I worry too much.				
I often feel upset.				

Please answer the items according to how you've felt in the past week.

Check the column under **Agree** if you mostly agree that the item describes you;
check the column under **Disagree** if you mostly disagree that the item describes you.

A score of 9 or more checks in the AGREE column indicates the need for further evaluation.

Items preceded by * are the ones most strongly associated with anxiety in older adults.

FIGURE 13-1 The Geriatric Anxiety Inventory. (Adapted with permission of UniQuest PtyLimited and the creators, Prof Nancy Pachana and Prof Gerard Byrne. Original GAI reference: Pachana, N. A., Byrne, G. J., Siddle, H., et al. (2007). Development and validation of the Geriatric Anxiety Inventory. *International Psychogeriatrics, 19,* 103–114.) © The University of Queensland 2010. Copyright in the Geriatric Anxiety Inventory is the property of The University of Queensland. All content is protected by Australian copyright law and, by virtue of international treaties, equivalent copyright laws in other countries. The Geriatric Anxiety Inventory may not be reproduced or copied without the prior written permission of UniQuest Pty Limited.

communication. In any adult, anxiety may be manifested in the following nonverbal ways: pacing, shakiness, restlessness, irritability, fidgeting, diaphoresis, tachycardia, hyperventilation, dry mouth, voice changes, smoking habits, urinary frequency, increased muscle tension, poor eye contact, poor attention span, inability to sit still, changes in eating patterns, rapid or disconnected speech or repetitive motions of facial muscles or any extremities. Although any of these indicators may be observed in older adults, the presence of mobility limitations or pathologic conditions can interfere with some of them. For example, older adults who

are confined to bed cannot pace but may experience subtle changes in eating or sleeping patterns because of anxiety. Older adults may be reluctant to report that they are worried or anxious; instead, they may focus on physiologic symptoms (e.g., pain, fatigue, anorexia, insomnia or stomach distress).

Because anxiety is always a response to real or perceived threats, the nurse tries to identify sources of anxiety, even though they may not be readily apparent. Potential sources of anxiety (i.e., real or perceived threats) include health, assets, values, environment, self-concept, role function, needs fulfillment, goal achievement, personal relationships and sense of security. People do not always recognize the source of their anxiety because it may arise from unconscious conflicts, unacknowledged fears, maturational crises or developmental challenges. Even when people recognize the source of anxiety, they may be reluctant to discuss it, or they may refer to the threat only indirectly. For example, an older adult may have the perception that other people have the power to "put him away" in a nursing home simply because of a slight memory impairment. If the person knows other older adults who have been admitted unwillingly to a nursing home, this fear may be exacerbated. Further anxiety may arise from the person's fear of discussing the subject because of the perception that initiating the topic might precipitate actions leading to nursing home admission. Rather than directly talking about the fears, the person may provide vague clues, for instance, "I felt so sorry for Mildred when her son put her in the nursing home."

Nurses must phrase questions aimed at identifying sources of anxiety in the least threatening way possible. When older adults express concerns about other older people, it may be appropriate to ask questions aimed at determining whether they have the same worries about themselves. For example, in response to the statement "I felt so sorry for Mildred," the nurse might ask, "Do you ever worry that you'll have to go to a nursing home?" Nurses use open-ended questions that allow for a wide range of answers to identify sources of anxiety that might not otherwise be revealed. For example, nurses in hospital settings can ask, "What is your biggest worry about going home?" or "Do you have any worries about how you'll manage at home after you leave here?" In home settings, the nurse might ask an even broader question such as "Do you have any concerns about the future?" or "What kinds of things do you worry about?" Answers to these questions are usually filled with clues to sources of anxiety and lead to many additional questions.

Anxiety can be caused or exacerbated by physiologic conditions arising from disease processes or the adverse effects of bioactive substances, as in the following examples:

- Herbs, caffeine, nicotine and medications (both prescription and over the counter) can cause anxiety reactions.
- Anxiety may be associated with withdrawal from nicotine or alcohol.
- Pathologic processes that diminish cerebral oxygen, such as pulmonary or cardiovascular diseases, can cause anxiety reactions.
- Endocrine disorders, such as hyperthyroidism, may be manifested primarily by anxiety or other psychosocial symptoms.
- People with dementia may show signs of excessive anxiety when they are experiencing pain or physical discomfort, particularly if their verbal communication skills are impaired.
- Pacing is a commonly observed manifestation of anxiety in ambulatory older adults who have dementia.

Therefore, information about medical conditions and the person's use of herbs, caffeine and medications is an essential component of the anxiety assessment.

Medications that affect the central or autonomic nervous systems may precipitate or exacerbate anxiety. *Akathisia* is a frequently reported extrapyramidal effect of some antipsychotic medications that may subjectively or objectively be interpreted as anxiety. Akathisia is defined as an inner sense of restlessness that is worsened by inactivity and is manifested by motor restlessness. It is more common in women and older adults, and it can occur any time during the course of treatment with psychotropic medications. Therefore, if an older adult who is taking antipsychotics complains of certain feelings, such as "shaking on the inside," the possibility of adverse medication effects must be considered as a cause.

In addition to identifying sources and manifestations of anxiety, it is important to identify appropriate methods for reducing anxiety. Even if the sources of anxiety are not identified or cannot be changed, the experience of anxiety can be addressed through self-care interventions that improve coping. To this end, the nurse asks questions about usual coping methods. Questions such as "What do you do when you have trouble with your nerves?" or "What do you find helpful when your nerves are bad?" can pave the way for a discussion about coping with anxiety. If the person cannot identify effective coping mechanisms, the nurse offers suggestions in a nonjudgmental way and assesses the person's response to them. For example, nurses can ask any of the following questions:

- "Does it help to talk to someone about your worries?"
- "Have you ever tried any relaxation methods when you're nervous?"
- "Do you find that taking a walk helps you when your nerves are bad?"

Box 13-8 summarizes guidelines on detection and assessment of late-life anxiety published by the University of Iowa, College of Nursing. See also http://www.anxietycanada.ca/english/pdf/ElderlyEn.pdf for more information on anxiety in older adults.

Self-Esteem

Self-esteem cannot be measured numerically, but nurses can observe for verbal and nonverbal indicators. For example, a statement such as "You're wasting your time on me; you have more important things to do," is a clue to poor self-esteem. Nonverbal indicators of self-esteem include the way people dress, care for themselves and present themselves to others. Although interpreting behaviours in relation to self-esteem must be done with caution, the following behaviours may be associated with low self-esteem: rigidity, procrastination, unnecessary apologies, lack of confidence, expectations of failure, exaggeration of deficits, disappointment in self, self-destructive behaviours, constant approval-seeking, overemphasis on weaknesses, inability to accept compliments, minimizing personal capabilities, disregarding one's

Box 13-8 Evidence-Based Practice: Detection and Assessment of Late-Life Anxiety

Statement of the Problem

- Anxiety, defined as apprehensive expectation and excessive worry, ranges from normal reactions to everyday stress to disabling levels, which are categorized as anxiety disorders.
- More than half of community-dwelling older adults report anxiety symptoms.
- Accurate assessment, referral, and treatment are necessary because anxiety is associated with functional disability, reduced quality of life, lower life satisfactions, impaired physical and social function and feelings of worthlessness.
- The following factors can interfere with recognition of anxiety in older adults: (1) stigma associated with mental illness, (2) older adults may focus on somatic symptoms and complaints, (3) manifestations may be considered normal consequences of aging, (4) underreporting and denial of problems are common among older adults, (5) inability to determine the degree to which worry is associated with realistic concerns.
- Factors consistently associated with increased risk of late-life anxiety include physical illness, psychosocial stress, depression, cognitive

impairment and personal characteristics (i.e., female gender, advanced age, lower socioeconomic status, external locus of control, family history of anxiety disorder, alcohol or drug use).

Recommendations for Nursing Assessment

- Nurses should assess for anxiety in any older adult who expresses worry or fear and who is at risk due to physical illness, recent psychosocial stress, depression, cognitive impairment, or somatic complaints that are not associated with an identifiable underlying cause.
- Nurses can use a screening tool, such as the Geriatric Anxiety Inventory, Short Anxiety Screening Test, Hospital Anxiety and Depression Scale, or the Rating Anxiety in Dementia Scale.

Source: Smith, M., Ingram, T., & Brighton, V. (2008). *Evidence-based practice guideline: Detection and assessment of late-life anxiety* Iowa City: University of Iowa Gerontological Nursing Interventions Research Centre. Available at National Guideline Clearinghouse, www.guideline.gov

---

own opinions, inability to form close relationships, inability to accept help from others and inability to say "no" when appropriate. It may be acceptable to ask some questions, however, particularly about the person's perception of positive qualities.

In addition to observing for indicators of self-esteem, nurses can ask questions that give insight into the older adult's self-perceptions. For example, a question such as "What is the quality in yourself that other people admire the most?" is nonthreatening. Moreover, this kind of question helps identify strengths that can be supported, and it provides clues to self-esteem. Nursing assessment is also directed toward identifying actual and potential threats to self-esteem, so they can be addressed through interventions, as discussed in Chapter 12.

Because self-esteem is influenced by the person's perception of the opinions held by significant others, it is important to identify who the significant others are for any particular person (e.g., peers, spouse or partner, authority figures, people in work, church and social environments). Culture often defines who adopts the role of the significant other. Some Chinese Canadian older adults, for example, expect their oldest son to look after their affairs and make key decisions about their health and well-being. Widows in some Middle Eastern and African cultures expect one of their husband's brothers to take care of them—an arrangement that fosters social and economic security for women who have lost a spouse. Being cared for by a family member (rather than by strangers) enhances self-esteem for older adults from all cultural backgrounds and increases the likelihood that their needs will be met as they age.

Depression

Depression is discussed as a general component of a psychosocial assessment in this chapter, and it is covered more comprehensively as an aspect of impaired psychosocial function in Chapter 15. Nurses can apply information in this chapter when assessing all older adults and use the information in

Chapter 15 as a guide to assessing and caring for older adults who are depressed. Also, because cultural factors strongly influence the ways in which emotions are expressed, cultural considerations related to assessment of depression as described in Chapter 15 (Box 15-7) are pertinent to assessing expressions of emotions.

Nurses assess for depression by identifying verbal and nonverbal cues. Direct questions such as "Are you depressed?" are usually not effective in drawing out information because people may associate the word "depressed" with states of overwhelming grief. Older adults may be more comfortable responding to questions about whether they feel "sad," "blue" or "down in the dumps." Therefore, unless the older adult uses the term "depressed" to describe his or her feelings, other terminology is more likely to elicit an accurate response. As with other aspects of the mental status assessment, it is best to start with open-ended questions, such as "How are you feeling right now?" or "How have you been feeling this week?"

One of the purposes of an assessment of depression is to identify the person's usual patterns of coping with losses. For this reason, the nurse encourages older adults to express their feelings about significant changes in their lives. For instance, when an older adult talks about a change that might be experienced as a loss, nurses can ask nonthreatening questions that might lead to a discussion of feelings, such as "What's it like to live alone after 50 years of being married?" "How is life different since your friend moved away?" "Are there people you miss seeing since you retired?" "Are there any activities you miss doing since you no longer drive?" If the questions do not generate information about feelings, the nurse can comment on specific feelings that the person is likely to be experiencing. For example, a remark such as "It seems like it would be pretty sad and lonely being here all by yourself after 55 years of marriage" allows the person to agree, disagree or offer an alternative to the suggested feelings.

Happiness and Well-Being

Happiness in relation to aging is often equated with morale, wellness, contentment, well-being, life satisfaction, successful aging, quality of life and "the good life." A literature review identified the following dimensions of well-being that can be addressed by health care professionals in relation to aging (Kiefer, 2008):

- Staying active
- Interacting with peers
- Feeling financially secure
- Having a sense of personal autonomy
- Setting personal goals and challenges
- Having positive social interactions
- Developing effective coping strategies
- Participating in exercise and sports activities
- Actively contributing to society through paid or volunteer work

Although nurses cannot address all these dimensions in a psychosocial assessment, they can include a few questions about happiness and well-being so they can identify ways of promoting wellness through nursing interventions. Psychologists sometimes use the following question to assess happiness: "Taking all things together, how would you say things are today—would you say you're very happy, pretty happy, or not too happy these days?" Nurses can ask a similar question such as "If you had to rate your present level of happiness on a scale of 0% to 100%, what rating would you give yourself?" Nurses can use the person's response as a base for additional questions such as "What would have to change to increase the rating by 10%?" "What kinds of things interfere with your happiness?" "If you could change one thing to be happier, what would it be?" Older adults will usually respond to these questions in a realistic manner, and their answers will provide information for establishing appropriate goals. Box 13-9 summarizes the considerations involved in assessing affective function in older adults.

CONTACT WITH REALITY

Although a certain amount of fantasy is acceptable in everyday patterns of thinking, people are expected to remain in contact with the world around them and to respond appropriately to the same realities that others perceive. People lose contact with reality for numerous reasons including dementia, delirium, psychotic disorders, and a transient denial of a threatening reality. Many of these underlying conditions are treatable; however, when older adults lose contact with reality, they are likely to be labelled as "senile." Thus, because of stereotypes about older people, as well as the broad array of potential causes for loss of contact with reality, the assessment of an older person's contact with reality is particularly challenging.

Loss of contact with reality includes a wide range of behaviours ranging from simple and harmless misperceptions of reality to unyielding delusions or disturbing hallucinations.

Box 13-9 Guidelines for Assessing Affective Function

General Affective Function

- Are the quantity and quality of emotions appropriate for the objective reality?
- What is the depth and duration of emotions regarding a particular event?
- What are the nonverbal cues to the person's affective state?
- How do sociocultural or environmental factors influence the person's expression of emotions?
- What terminology is acceptable to this person, particularly with regard to feelings such as anger, anxiety and depression?
- Does the person have any pets, or has he or she lost any pets?

Observations and Questions to Assess Mood

- What is the person's usual mood?
- What are the nonverbal indicators of the person's mood?

Observations and Questions to Assess Anxiety

- What are the nonverbal indicators of anxiety?
- What real or perceived threats are present that might be sources of anxiety for the person?
- Might any of the following factors be contributing to the person's anxiety: caffeine, pathologic conditions, medications, herbs or interventions by folk or indigenous healers that act on the central or autonomic nervous systems?
- What methods of coping has the person tried, and what have been the effects of these interventions?
- What kinds of things does the person worry about?
- Does the person have any worries that he or she would be willing to discuss with the nurse?
- Does the person ever have trouble with his or her nerves?

Observations and Questions to Assess Self-Esteem

- What verbal and nonverbal clues to self-esteem can be detected?
- What are the factors that influence self-esteem for this person?
- Does the environment present any real or potential threat to self-esteem?
- How are my actions as a nurse influencing the self-esteem of the older adults to whom I relate?
- Are caregiver attitudes and actions, such as infantilization or the promotion of unnecessary dependence, affecting the person's self-esteem?

Observations and Questions to Assess Depression

- What are the verbal and nonverbal clues to depression?
- Does the person ever feel blue or down in the dumps?
- How has the person's life changed since his or her spouse died?
- What does the person miss the most since he or she moved from his or her family home?

Observations and Questions to Assess Happiness and Life Satisfaction

- How is the person's happiness and life satisfaction influenced by the following: functional abilities, personal relationships and socioeconomic resources?
- On a scale of 0% to 100%, how happy would the person say he or she is right now?
- If the person could change one thing to increase his or her happiness rating, what would it be?

For example, people who are in the early stages of dementia may actively conceal or refuse to acknowledge memory deficits and those in later stages of dementia may experience delusions that lead to behaviours that are inappropriate or even dangerous. For instance, if someone believes that his belongings have been stolen, he may report the theft to the police or insist on going out to look for the robber. Three types of loss of contact with reality are delusions, hallucinations and illusions, which are defined as follows:

- **Delusions:** Fixed false beliefs that have little or no basis in reality and cannot be corrected by appealing to reason.
- **Hallucinations:** Sensory experiences that have no basis in an external stimulus. Visual and auditory hallucinations are most common, but tactile, olfactory and gustatory hallucinations also occur.
- **Illusions:** Misperceptions of an external stimulus. They may be mistaken for hallucinations, but differ in having some basis in reality, which is not the case in hallucinations.

Just as a fever is one manifestation of a physical illness, loss of contact with reality is one manifestation of an underlying disorder. For example, common manifestations of loss of contact with reality in people with dementia include delusions, hallucinations, misidentification and false accusations. Certain characteristics of delusions and hallucinations are associated with specific conditions such as delirium, dementia and depression. In addition, loss of contact with reality typically occurs in combination with other manifestations of an underlying condition. Thus, an astute nursing assessment of contact with reality can provide essential information for identifying underlying causes. Table 13-2 shows distinguishing features of delusions, hallucinations and illusions, and the following sections address these in relation to associated conditions that are most common in older adults.

Delusions

Delusions are a psychological mechanism that helps people preserve their egos, maintain control over threatening situations and organize information that is difficult to process. Paranoia (i.e., an extreme degree of suspiciousness) is a type of delusion that is common in older adults with dementia, as in the following examples:

- Accusing others of stealing their money or belongings
- Perceiving that they are being cheated, observed, attacked, persecuted or sexually harassed
- Believing that others are entering their rooms when they are not there and moving things or messing up their belongings

Although the terms *paranoia* and *delusions* are sometimes used interchangeably in geriatric practice and references, this is inaccurate because there are many types of delusions.

In older adults, delusions can arise from pathologic conditions, such as delirium, dementia, depression, and paranoid disorder. Delusions associated with each of these disorders are characterized in unique ways and occur in combination with other manifestations of the underlying condition, as discussed in the following sections. Additional information about psychotic symptoms of delirium and dementia is discussed in Chapter 14.

Delusions Associated With Pathophysiologic Conditions

Delusions arising from delirium are only one manifestation of a complex pathologic process that is further characterized by physiologic disturbances, diminished attention, a clouded state of consciousness and possibly hallucinations (described in Chapter 14) that subside once the delirium resolves. In addition to being associated with delirium, delusions may be

TABLE 13-2 Distinguishing Features of Delusions, Hallucinations and Illusions		
Underlying Cause	**Accompanying Manifestations**	**Characteristics**
Delirium	Diminished attention, a clouded state of consciousness and other typical manifestations of delirium; metabolic disturbance, adverse medication effect or other underlying cause	*Delusions:* poorly organized, persecutory *Hallucinations:* vivid, visual, colourful, threatening, accusatory, auditory hallucinations induced by alcohol withdrawal *Illusions:* brief, poorly organized
Dementia	Cognitive impairment (particularly memory deficits), alert level of consciousness. Agitation, anxiety or wandering may be associated with loss of contact with reality. Neurologic manifestations may accompany hallucinations, particularly when the underlying cause is vascular dementia	*Delusions:* not fixed, loosely organized, readily changed or forgotten. Themes may include theft, fears, misidentification of places or people and spousal infidelity *Illusions:* occur more commonly than hallucinations; may be partially attributable to environmental factors *Hallucinations:* more often visual than auditory; may be partially attributable to environmental factors
Depression	Typical depressive symptoms including anorexia, lack of energy, sleep disturbances and weight loss	*Delusions:* Themes may include death, guilt, money, illnesses, self-reproach, gloomy foreboding, diminished self-esteem and feelings of worthlessness. There may be some basis in reality, but perceptions are exaggerated *Hallucinations:* typically auditory and derogatory
Paranoid disorder	Absence of cognitive deficits or affective disorders; long-term social isolation or suspicious personality; may be well hidden for years	*Delusions:* fixed and well organized; may subside temporarily in different environments. Themes usually involve plots, noises, threats, obscenities or sexual assaults *Hallucinations:* If present, these are related to the delusional themes

TABLE 13-3 Physiologic Disorders Causing Delusions or Hallucinations

Type of Disorder	Specific Examples
Metabolic disorders	Uremia, dehydration, electrolyte imbalance
Endocrine disorders	Hypoglycemia, thyroid disorders
Neurologic disorders	Stroke, cerebral trauma, cortical ischemia
Infections	Septicemia, pneumonia, urinary tract infections, subacute bacterial endocarditis
Adverse medication effects	Anticholinergics, anticonvulsants, antidepressants, anti-Parkinson agents, benzodiazepines, corticosteroids, digitalis toxicity, narcotics
Drug or alcohol abuse or withdrawal	Alcohol, barbiturates, meprobamate

caused by pathologic conditions, such as strokes or dementia. Delusions can also be a result of adverse medication effects, as in the common occurrence of delusional jealousy associated with dopamine agonists for treatment of Parkinson disease (Perugi et al., 2013). They can also be caused by abuse of or withdrawal from alcohol or drugs. Some of the physiologic disorders that are likely to cause delusions or hallucinations in older adults are listed in Table 13-3.

Delusions Associated With Dementia

Delusions are a neuropsychiatric symptom of dementia, with a prevalence rate ranging from 16% to 70% in various studies (Cohen-Mansfield & Golander, 2011). Common delusional themes in people with dementia are theft, abandonment, suspiciousness, spousal infidelity, misidentification of familiar places or people and believing that loved ones who have died are still alive. Delusions in people with dementia can lead to problematic behaviours, which are often repetitive or even obsessive, as in the following examples:

- Accusing someone of being intent on harming the person
- Perceiving a family member as a stranger
- Believing that a family caregiver is intent on leaving (i.e., abandoning) the person
- Accusing others of stealing things
- Demanding that a family member leave the home that is shared by the person with dementia
- Refusing to let a caregiver or family member provide care because the person with dementia does not trust that person
- Insisting that a spouse or family member is not the person he or she claims to be
- Requesting to go home, even when the person is already at home
- Believing that one's spouse is having an affair
- Looking for a spouse or parent who has been deceased for many years, then grieving when informed that the person is dead
- Refusing to sleep in the same bed or room with spouse

- Believing that strangers are living in the house
- Insisting on leaving because "I need to go take care of the babies"

Studies suggest that certain delusional themes are associated with pathologic changes in specific brain regions, for example, delusions of theft, abandonment, infidelity and suspiciousness being associated with frontal and temporal regions (Nakatsuka et al., 2013; Nomura et al., 2012; Sultzer et al., 2013). Other studies have found associations between types of delusions and stages of dementia, with persecutory delusions occurring earlier and misidentification delusions occurring during later stages (Ismail et al., 2011; Reeves et al., 2012).

People with dementia will readily talk about delusions, whereas those who do not have dementia typically withhold or are secretive about information. The challenge in assessing these delusions, however, is to identify the possible reality of the situation. It is imperative to recognize that not all accusations are unfounded just because people have serious cognitive impairments. Before labelling ideas as delusional, assess for any basis in reality because even the most bizarre-sounding assertions may be totally or partially true.

Another consideration is that communication techniques differ for people with psychosis or dementia. For example, the usual psychiatric nursing approach for delusions associated with psychosis is to talk with the client about the delusional thoughts as a problem in his or her life. In contrast, for people with dementia, it is more appropriate to avoid arguing and provide distractions. In addition, it is essential to address underlying feelings of fear, anxiety and insecurity by providing reassurance. For example, it is usually effective to focus on the present with a reassuring statement, such as "I am staying here with you to make sure everything is OK, so let's have a little snack right now." This statement provides emotional reassurance and also attempts to distract the individual from the delusion.

Delusions Associated With Depression

Persecutory and other delusions can be a manifestation of a major depression, but they are often overlooked or attributed to other factors, particularly in older adults living in community or long-term care settings. For example, when dementia and depression coexist, delusional thoughts may be attributed to dementia rather than being identified as an indicator of an affective disorder. Likewise, when a person with a paranoid personality becomes depressed, the delusions may be falsely attributed to the personality, particularly if the delusions are persecutory in nature. When delusions arise from depression, other manifestations of depression are usually identified in a thorough assessment of depression, as discussed in Chapter 15.

Delusional themes may provide clues to a mood disorder, particularly if the focus is on a recent loss. Therefore, carefully listening to the content of the delusions is essential to an accurate assessment. In depressed older adults, delusional themes often revolve around an exaggerated emphasis on guilt, money, illnesses, self-reproach, gloomy foreboding, diminished self-esteem or feelings of worthlessness. Although some basis may exist in reality, the feelings of being persecuted and deserving of punishment are grossly exaggerated. The following are some examples of delusions arising from depression:

- Mrs. N. believes that she is responsible for her husband's death; therefore, she believes she does not deserve help for her own illness.
- Mr. A. believes that his Blue Cross health insurance has been cancelled as punishment for not helping his neighbour and insists that he cannot fill his medication prescription because he has no drug coverage.
- Ms. K. has an unshakable belief that she has undiagnosed cancer and begins to plan for her funeral, even though numerous doctors have not found any disease process.
- Mr. B., who recently had surgery for prostate cancer, is convinced that his house is going to explode from a gas leak and repeatedly calls the gas company to come check it.

Delusions Associated With Paranoid Disorder

Paranoid disorder—resulting in *paranoid ideation (or thoughts)*—refers to a delusional disorder that is not associated with schizophrenia and is characterized by the tendency to view individuals or agencies with suspicion or as having harmful intentions. Factors associated with an increased risk for developing a late-life paranoid disorder include depression, social isolation, pathologic conditions, sensory impairment and sense of loss of control over the environment. Common themes of paranoid delusions include spies, noises, threats, obscenities, lethal gases, bodily harm, stolen belongings, sexual infidelity or molestation, poisoned food or water and having people enter living quarters by mysterious means at night. The delusions may occur more often when the person is socially isolated or in a particular environment, such as the home. If the person takes action on the basis of the delusions, such as moving to another apartment or living with a family member, the delusions may subside temporarily.

Many people who have a paranoid disorder function well in the community, with the exception of one or two functional areas that are influenced by the delusions. Sometimes, a delusional state that was previously well hidden may surface when the person is admitted to a long-term care facility, and the staff may think that the problem is new. In other situations, nurses will identify a paranoid disorder upon making a home visit or interviewing an older person who has been admitted to the hospital. If the person also suffers from dementia, the delusions may be interpreted mistakenly as evidence of advancing dementia. When this occurs, a recommendation for long-term institutional care may be made when other recommendations might be more appropriate.

Identifying a paranoid disorder in the psychosocial assessment is important so that the symptoms can be alleviated with appropriate interventions. When left unattended or written off as eccentricities, these disorders may progress and seriously disrupt functional abilities. Therefore, when delusions and cognitive impairments coexist, it is essential to determine whether the delusions existed before the dementia and to what extent, if any, they interfered with daily activities. If the delusions are part of a long-term pattern that has not interfered with the person's ability to function in daily life, the person may be able to remain in the community with support services and treatment directed toward the cognitive impairment. When delusions interfere with daily activities, however, medical intervention (e.g., psychotropic medications) may be effective in eliminating the delusions or minimizing their effects so that the person can maintain an independent level of function. When interventions are directed toward both the delusions and the cognitive impairment, the older person may be able to remain independent.

Hallucinations

In older adults, hallucinations are associated with dementia, depression, social isolation, sensory impairment and physiologic disturbances, including adverse medication effects. Visual hallucinations are common in people with Parkinson disease and dementia with Lewy bodies and are related not only to the disease, but also to the medications (e.g., levodopa) used for treatment (Sawada et al., 2013; Svetel et al., 2012). As with delusions, it is important to identify the underlying cause of hallucinations because the selection of appropriate interventions depends on an accurate assessment.

Some older adults are aware of—and can describe—their hallucinatory experiences, particularly when hallucinations are caused by the adverse effects of medications (e.g., anticholinergics) or Parkinson disease. However, in many situations, identification of hallucinations is based on astute observations of behaviours such as the following:

- Reaching out for objects that are not there
- Stepping over objects on the ground that are not visible to others
- Conversing with people who are not there
- Reporting sounds that have no environmental source (e.g., knocking, ringing)

An appropriate assessment technique is to elicit information from family and caregivers with a statement such as "Sometimes people see or hear things that others don't perceive. Do you notice any evidence of that happening to your father?"

Because hallucinations are abnormal sensory experiences, it is essential to assess for environmental influences and to make sure that sensory deficits are compensated for as much as possible. This is especially important for people with dementia because they may have difficulty processing information. For example, an older adult who has dementia and is visually impaired may look at a chair and misperceive it as someone sitting. Similarly, auditory hallucinations are more common in people who have impaired hearing. In these situations, appropriate nursing interventions are implemented to compensate as much as possible for hearing and vision impairments and to facilitate referrals for hearing and vision evaluations.

Hallucinations Associated With Pathophysiologic Conditions

Hallucinations are a common manifestation of delirium and are assessed within the larger context of this complex condition. Hallucinations associated with delirium are characterized as brief, vivid, visual, colourful, threatening and poorly organized. Occasionally, hallucinations are the earliest sign of delirium, and they may be overlooked or attributed to another condition (e.g., dementia). Visual hallucinations are also symptoms of ophthalmic conditions, such as cataract, glaucoma or age-related macular degeneration (Hughes, 2013; Nguyen et al., 2013).

Hallucinations arising from drug or alcohol withdrawal may occur during the first days of admission to an acute care setting or in any circumstance in which the person suddenly does not have access to his or her usual drugs or alcohol. Auditory hallucinations associated with alcohol withdrawal are typically accusatory and threatening, and they are sometimes organized into a complete paranoid system. The detection of alcohol-induced delirium is particularly important in acute care settings because people who are dependent on alcohol are more likely to acknowledge the problem and agree to appropriate interventions when they are in a crisis. The following example illustrates such a situation.

Case Study

Mr. K. is 73 years old and has been caring for his wife, who has Alzheimer disease, for several years. He is a very proud man who has difficulty accepting help. One morning, Mr. K. began vomiting coffee-ground emesis and was admitted to an acute care setting with the diagnosis of gastrointestinal bleeding. On admission, Mr. K. is very pleasant and expresses concern about his wife's care. The next morning, Mr. K. complains angrily to the nurses about the bars on the windows and is belligerent about the fact that he has been put in jail. He develops additional manifestations of delirium and is treated for alcohol withdrawal.

When the delirium subsides, the nurse initiates a conversation about the care of his wife and asks him how he copes with the responsibility. Mr. K. admits that he has difficulty coping with his and his wife's declining health and his increasing loneliness and responsibilities. He has always been a social drinker, but he has gradually increased his consumption of alcohol to three six-packs of beer a day. As part of the discharge plan, Mr. K. agrees to talk with a sponsor from Alcoholics Anonymous.

Table 13-2 summarizes the physiologic disorders, including some adverse medication effects, which are most likely to cause hallucinations.

Hallucinations Associated With Dementia

Hallucinations and illusions may occur at any time in the course of a dementing illness and are also likely to occur during a transient ischemic attack—a condition associated with vascular dementia. Visual hallucinations are a key diagnostic indicator of Parkinson disease and dementia with Lewy bodies (Bertram & Williams, 2012; Hamilton et al., 2012). When illusions occur, they are often related to environmental conditions that can be modified. For example, poor lighting or reflections from glass or mirrors can cause visual illusions, and background noise can contribute to auditory illusions, particularly for people with hearing aids.

Psychiatric literature usually addresses illusions only with regard to misperceptions of visual or auditory stimuli, whereas an illusion, by definition, is a misinterpretation of any external stimulus. Nurses who care for people with dementia can cite numerous examples of behaviours that fit this broader definition of an illusion, such as the following:

- Mistaking the identity of caregivers, family members, or other familiar people
- Perceiving an object as something other than what it really is
- Taking an object under the mistaken belief that it belongs to them
- Refusing to believe that they are in their home when they really are

These experiences might be labelled as delusions or disorientation, but they are more accurately defined as illusions because they involve a misinterpretation of reality rather than a false perception that has no base in reality.

Hallucinations Associated With Depression

Severely depressed older adults are more likely to experience delusions rather than hallucinations, but visual and auditory hallucinations of deceased loved ones commonly occur during periods of bereavement. Hallucinations associated with depression are likely to be auditory and derogatory, or they may involve visual perceptions of dead people. The following examples are typical of hallucinations arising from depression:

- Ms. C. reports that at night she hears the people in the next apartment saying that she has cancer.
- Mr. T. reports hearing younger men say that he is sexually impotent and that he was not a good provider to his wife (who died within the past year).
- Ms. F. looks down from her second-floor window and sees a man, dressed in black, lying injured on the sidewalk.
- Mr. S. insists that there is a pervasive smell of skunk coming from his basement, and he believes he will be contaminated if he goes downstairs.

Hallucinations Associated With Paranoid Disorder

If hallucinations are a symptom of paranoid disorder, they are likely to be closely related to the theme of the delusions. The following examples are characteristic of hallucinations arising from paranoid states:

- Mr. J. says that he hears people in the next apartment talking about him. These are the same people whom he believes will come in and steal things when he leaves the apartment.

- Ms. J. reports seeing men observing her when she undresses or takes a bath. Moreover, when she goes to the grocery store, the man at the checkout always offers her money in exchange for sexual favours.

Table 13-3 summarizes the characteristics that distinguish delusions, hallucinations and illusions according to their underlying causes.

Special Considerations for Assessing Contact With Reality in Older Adults

Assessment of contact with reality presents a special assessment challenge for nurses for a variety of reasons:
- People often try to conceal delusions and hallucinations.
- When delusions and hallucinations arise from social isolation, opportunities for assessment are extremely limited.
- To determine whether a reported experience is delusional, the nurse needs information about the reality, which is difficult to obtain if a reliable and objective observer is not available.
- Even after delusions or hallucinations are identified as such, the underlying factors may be difficult to identify.
- Older adults often have more than one underlying condition, such as a delirium superimposed on a dementia.

Delusions are usually more readily acknowledged than hallucinations, and the most effective tools for assessing delusions are asking leading questions and listening attentively. Most older adults will confide their delusions to a nurse they perceive as interested, sympathetic and nonjudgmental, particularly if a trusting relationship has been established. Difficulty arises, however, when nurses hear information that may be interpreted as delusional but, in fact, is based wholly or partially in reality. For example, financial exploitation, violation of rights and other aspects of elder abuse are not uncommon, particularly in older adults who are cognitively impaired or who live with family members who are greatly stressed or have a history of conflict with their parent. When older adults who have cognitive impairments or a lifelong suspicious personality describe abusive or exploitative situations, they are likely to be considered delusional or not to be taken seriously. In these situations, the assessment challenge is to determine what is real, what is distorted and what is not based at all in reality.

Nurses also consider the potential effects of environmental and interpersonal factors in contributing to delusions, illusions or hallucinations. For example, the reflection of fluorescent lights on a highly polished floor can produce the illusion of water on the floor, and an older adult might walk around the reflection. Stressful interpersonal relationships may contribute to the development of paranoid ideations, particularly in the context of past or present exploitation or abuse. Another important assessment consideration is whether a lack of assistive devices, such as eyeglasses and hearing aids, is contributing to altered perceptions. For example, if someone usually depends on eyeglasses, contact lenses, or a hearing aid for adequate visual or auditory function, the absence of these items may contribute to the development of illusions or hallucinations.

Box 13-10 Guidelines for Assessing Contact With Reality

General Principles

- In assessing any loss of contact with reality, the effects of alcohol, medications and physiologic disturbances must always be considered as potential causative influences.
- People who are not cognitively impaired are usually more reluctant to talk about delusions and hallucinations than are people who have dementia.
- When people talk about things that might be delusional, it is important to determine, through information provided by a reliable and objective observer, whether their perceptions have any basis in reality.
- When delusions are initially identified, it is important to determine whether they are of recent onset or have been long-standing, but only recently discovered.
- When delusions are identified in someone who has dementia, it is particularly important to consider the influence of treatable causative factors, such as depression or physiologic disturbances.
- Some people who have dementia have illusions, rather than hallucinations.
- People who are socially isolated are usually quite successful in concealing hallucinations.
- In assessing hallucinations and illusions, it is particularly important to consider the influence of the environment.

Interview Questions to Assess Delusions, Hallucinations and Illusions

- "Do you have any thoughts that you can't seem to get rid of?"
- "People sometimes have thoughts that they're afraid to talk about because they believe others will think they're 'crazy.' Do you ever have thoughts like that?"
- "Do you sometimes hear voices when you're alone?"
- "Do you sometimes think you see things that other people don't see?"

Nonverbal Clues to Hallucinations

- Extreme withdrawal and isolation
- Contentment with social isolation, particularly if the person previously had many social contacts
- Gestures and other actions that normally occur in response to perceived stimuli

During the assessment, nurses consider cultural factors that are likely to influence perceptions of reality and manifestations of mental illness, as discussed in Chapter 12. Religious background is a common cultural factor that can influence the content of delusions or hallucinations. For example, delusions and hallucinations in Irish Catholics are likely to focus on Jesus, a saint, or the Virgin Mary. Similarly, Muslims with African, Near Eastern, or Middle Eastern cultural heritage may focus on the Prophet Mohammed. Box 13-10 summarizes guidelines for assessing an individual's contact with reality.

SOCIAL SUPPORTS

Social supports, which are categorized as *informal* and *formal*, refer to the services provided to address functional and psychosocial needs. Although even the most independent people receive social supports (e.g., emotional support from family and friends), social supports are usually discussed in relation to meeting the needs of people who depend on others in some way for assistance. While friends, family, clergy, neighbours, or coworkers provide informal social support, workers who are paid by the older person or his or her family or by health and social service agencies or institutions provide formal social support.

Social supports significantly influence psychosocial function in older adults because they affect one's ability to cope with stressful life experiences by acting as a buffer against harmful effects and improving one's physical and emotional well-being. Because the importance of social supports increases in relation to the degree of impairment of the older adult, it is essential to assess the social supports for any older adults who have conditions that affect their functional abilities. Nursing assessment of social supports identifies not only the resources that are needed, available or being used to support the highest level of functioning, but also the barriers to the use of appropriate resources. Specific aspects of social supports that nurses assess include social network, economic resources, and religion and spirituality. Box 13-11 summarizes important questions and considerations involved in assessing social supports.

Box 13-11 Guidelines for Assessing Social Supports

Interview Questions to Assess Social Supports

- "On whom do you rely for help?"
- "Is there anyone who helps you with grocery shopping? Getting to doctor appointments? Getting prescriptions filled? Managing your money and paying bills?"
- "Is there anyone you can talk to when you have worries or difficulties?"
- "Is there anything you would like help with that you don't have help with now?"
- "Is there anyone in the family who could help with grocery shopping?"
- "Have you ever received information about the transportation services (or meals or other services) that are available through the senior centre?"

Potential Barriers to the Use of Formal Supports

- Unwillingness to acknowledge, or lack of insight to recognize, the need for services
- Expectation that family members will provide the needed care
- Unwillingness to admit that family members cannot or will not provide the needed care
- Lack of financial resources to purchase services or unwillingness to spend money for services
- Perceived correlation between formal services and "welfare"
- Lack of transportation to access services
- Mistrust of service providers or an unwillingness to allow outsiders into the home
- Bad experiences with service providers or hearsay about the bad experiences of others
- Fear that the home situation will be judged as socially unacceptable, or embarrassment because it is socially unacceptable
- Fear that having outsiders in the house will lead to admission to a nursing home
- Lack of time, energy, or problem-solving ability to obtain information about and select the appropriate services
- Fear that the service will be provided by someone about whom the care recipient holds prejudices
- Language and cultural barriers

Interview Questions to Assess Financial Resources

- "Do you have any money worries?"
- "Do you have any concerns about paying for services that you might need?"
- "Would you like to talk to someone about any financial concerns?"
- "Do you think you can afford the kind of help that your doctor recommended?"
- "Have you received any advice about financial planning for nursing home care?"

Interview Questions to Assess Religious Affiliation

- "Do you belong to any church, synagogue or mosque?"
- "Are you aware of any programs available at your church, synagogue or mosque that might be helpful to you?"

Social Network

Nursing assessment of the social network addresses the social supports that are important for day-to-day functioning, as well as those that affect the person's quality of life. The nurse can initiate the assessment by asking a broad question such as "Whom do you rely on for help?" The nurse can then ask more specific questions about how the person accomplishes tasks that are most important for day-to-day function. For example, in discussing a follow-up appointment for medical care, the nurse may ask, "How do you get to your doctor appointments?" Because a relationship with a confidante is a significant predictor of quality of life for older adults, at least one question relating to this factor should be posed, such as "Is there anyone you can talk to about your worries?" The answer to this question may also be important if the nurse or health care team is assisting the older adult with a decision about long-term care because the older adult may want the confidante to be involved in the decision-making process. In addition, the response to this question may provide important information about whether the older person has recently experienced a loss or change in the availability of a confidante.

After identifying existing social networks, the nurse identifies the resources that might be helpful in addressing unmet needs. Such questions as "Do you have any grandchildren or neighbours who could help with shovelling the snow?" are aimed at identifying informal supports that are available but are not currently being used. A question such as "Are you aware that the senior centre has a van that takes people to doctor appointments?" is aimed at identifying the person's awareness of formal supports that may not be in use.

Barriers to Obtaining Social Supports

In addition to assessing the number and types of social supports available, nurses try to identify the barriers that interfere with the use of social supports. Many older adults who are eligible for service programs do not use these resources because they view them as costly, impersonal, overly structured and hard to arrange. Because older adults prefer

---

Box 13-12 Evidenced-Informed Nursing Practice

Background: Older adults from minority cultures have more difficulty accessing health care and supports due to age, gender, culture, etc. As such, these individuals may be more vulnerable than their younger counterparts.

Question: What is the impact of service barriers on the health of older South Asians living in Canada?

Methods: The researchers conducted a survey over the phone with 220 older adults originally from South Asia but now living in Canada. The mean age of the research participants was just above 65 years and just more than half of the participants were men. The participants had resided in Canada for more than 15 years (on average), and more than 75% had come from India.

Findings: The research participants reported the following barriers to receiving health services support: cultural incompatibility, personal attitudes (such as feeling uncomfortable asking for help), issues with administration of services (e.g., professionals too busy, bad experiences from others) and circumstantial experiences (such as expense of services, lack of transportation). Although personal attitudes of participants toward accessing services and supports were less common than other barriers, they were most significant in affecting physical and mental health.

Implications for Nursing Practice: Nurses need to inquire of older adults in general, as well as older adults from minority cultures in particular, about barriers to accessing supports and health services.

Source: Lai, D. W., & Surood, S. (2013). Effect of service barriers on health status of aging South Asian immigrants in Calgary, Canada. *Health & Social Work*, *38*(1), 41–50.

---

to receive help from family and friends, negative attitudes about the use of formal social supports may be a source of resistance to their use (see Box 13-12). Without adequate informal supports, or when conflicts exist between older adults and their informal supports, an increase in dependence can trigger less-effective coping mechanisms. The following example is typical of such a situation.

Case Study

Mr. and Mrs. D. are 81 and 79 years old, respectively. They always expected their children to care for them, but the children moved to other cities and visit several times a year. Mr. and Mrs. D. refuse to accept any of the formal services that are available because of their cost, and also because they expect their children to provide the services out of filial responsibility. Furthermore, Mrs. D. cared for her parents when they were old, so she expects her daughter to do the same for her.

Mr. and Mrs. D. frequently call their daughter and son-in-law to complain about their inability to get groceries and go to doctors' appointments. Rather than making use of transportation or other services available from the community, they neglect themselves. During a visit over the Christmas holiday, the children find that their parents have not been eating adequately and are not taking their prescribed medications. When they mention these observations to their parents, Mr. and Mrs. D. respond, "If you loved us, you'd be taking care of us, and this wouldn't be happening."

In addition to some older people's preference for obtaining services from families rather than outside agencies, there are many other barriers to the use of formal services. Fears about outsiders coming into the home rank high among the barriers to the provision of in-home services. Financial barriers also often exist, either because of an inability or an unwillingness to pay for services. Additional barriers include unwillingness to accept help, lack of knowledge about types of services available and not knowing where to go for specific services. The identification of these barriers is essential because counselling and educational interventions (e.g., providing information about services that are available) can address many of these issues. Issues that are not amenable to intervention may represent impenetrable barriers to the provision of social supports.

Assessing barriers to support services is particularly challenging because direct questions about these issues are often inappropriate and are usually very threatening. Rather, identification of these barriers is best accomplished by carefully listening to older people and their caregivers and by asking nonthreatening questions. For example, a caregiver might talk about a friend who had a home health aide who did nothing but watch television all day and got paid $18 an hour. In response to this, the nurse might ask, "Do you think that might happen if we arrange for a home health aide to care for your father?" Other attitudinal barriers, such as prejudices, may be identified through statements made by the caregiver about prior experiences.

Economic Resources

Financial issues are generally within the purview of social workers, and nurses usually prefer to avoid discussing money with older adults or their families. In planning for formal services for older adults, however, some assessment of financial assets is necessary, and the nurse is often the health care professional who obtains this information, particularly in home or other community settings. If no long-term care or community-based services are needed, the nurse can forgo the financial assessment.

Many older adults and their families are shocked to find out that provincial health care does not pay all the expenses of nursing home care, such as provision of razors, shampoo and other cleaning products and does not cover laundry services. Older adults and family members may also be upset when nursing homes do not reimburse family members for costs of lost personal items, such as clothing, eye glasses or dentures. Even if a social worker has explained these facts, it is usually the nurse who deals with the related anxiety and other emotional reactions of the older adults and their families. Because nurses are in a position to help older adults and their families address and cope with the financial issues of long-term care, they frequently become involved in assessing the financial resources of the person and family.

It is not always necessary to ask details about monthly income or the exact amount of savings and assets, but questions must be asked about the resources available for the purchase of services. Asking a question such as "Do you have any money worries?" might reveal some anxieties that can be dealt with or allayed through counselling or the provision of accurate information. When the nurse reviews with the older adult or caregiver the services that are available, information can also be provided about the cost of these services, at which time a question such as "Do you think you could afford this kind of help?" can be posed.

RELIGION AND SPIRITUALITY

As discussed in Chapter 12, religion and spirituality become more important in older adulthood, and they are resources that should be identified as a part of a comprehensive psychosocial assessment. The person's religious affiliation is assessed as a component of his or her social supports, whereas spirituality is assessed as a separate component of the psychosocial assessment. It is important to recognize that spirituality is an integral component of all humans, but not all people identify with a religious affiliation.

Identification of religious affiliation is a simple but important part of the psychosocial assessment because available religion-based programs for older adults may be perceived as more acceptable than those provided by a public or nonreligious agency. For example, an older Jewish person might be willing to go to the Jewish Community Centre for a senior meal program, and an older Roman Catholic adult might be willing to accept mental health services from Catholic Social Services, but these people might refuse to avail themselves of the same kinds of services when they are offered by another organization. Often, religion-based services are viewed by the older adult as services that they deserve as a reward for years of attendance at or service to a church or synagogue. Although most religion-based programs serve older adults, regardless of their religious affiliations, the programs are often perceived as more appropriate if the person is of the same faith.

In addition to being perceived as more appropriate, some religion-based services are not available elsewhere, and they are often provided by trained volunteers free of charge. Examples of programs or services that may be available to members of a particular church, synagogue or mosque include transportation, respite care, peer counselling, chore assistance, friendly visiting and telephone reassurance. Older adults can also take advantage of any church-, synagogue- or mosque-based program that is available for people of all ages. The Stephen Ministries, founded in 1975, is an example of a volunteer program that is available in many Christian denominations throughout Canada. This program offers peer counselling and other services, provided by volunteers with special training in ministering to older, depressed, shut-in and grieving persons.

Identification of a specific place of worship is also important because attendance at religious services may be a significant factor in the older adult's social life. For many older adults, particularly those with limited mobility or those who have full-time caregiving responsibilities, attendance at religious services is their only opportunity for social interaction

and personal support. Most people who are unable to attend religious services can arrange for home visits by a clergy person or lay minister; indeed, these visits may be the only source of outside contact and emotional support that is acceptable to a homebound older adult. Moreover, for people who are socially isolated, a visitor from their place of worship may be the only person monitoring the home situation. In these situations, health professionals who are concerned about homebound older adults may be able to monitor their status through these visitors, as in the following example.

Case Study

Mr. V. was admitted to the hospital after a syncopal episode that resulted in a minor car accident. On admission, Mr. V. was slightly unkempt and showed some memory deficits, but his self-care abilities improved during his 2-day hospitalisation. The nurse suggested that Mr. V. consider home-delivered meals and the use of other community resources, but he refused these services.

The nurse was concerned because Mr. V. lived alone and had no outside contacts other than Ms. C., a lay minister who had visited weekly for 2 years. The nurse asked for and received permission from Mr. V. to contact Ms. C. to inform her of available community services. Ms. C. was grateful for the information and said that she would contact the appropriate agencies if Mr. V.'s condition declined or if he agreed to accept help.

In this situation, information about the church affiliation enabled the nurse to implement a discharge plan that otherwise would not have been possible.

Spirituality is increasingly being recognized as an essential component of well-being for all humans, and for older adults in particular, as discussed in Chapter 12. The intent of a spiritual assessment is not to evaluate whether a person is more or less spiritual; rather the purpose is to identify indicators of spiritual distress so that these can be addressed in holistic care plans. Spiritual distress often occurs in the context of transitions that older adults face, such as needing to move from their homes or making decisions about treatments for serious conditions (Lane et al., 2013). Another purpose is to identify sources of strength and meaning in the older person's life so that these can be supported. An easy-to-use and evidence-based tool for four domains of spiritual assessment is the FICA, which is an acronym for **F**aith and belief, **I**mportance of beliefs, **C**ommunity for support, and concerns to **A**ddress in care. Online Learning Activity 13-3 provides links to this tool and additional information about how to use it in clinical settings.

Nurses, like many people, may not be comfortable discussing spirituality, but they can increase their comfort level by recognizing their own feelings and viewing spirituality as a universal human need. It is also helpful to recognize that many of the communication skills used in the course of providing nursing care are also effective for addressing spiritual needs. For example, active listening and expressions

Box 13-13 Guidelines for Assessing Spiritual Needs

Guidelines for Nursing Assessment

- Be aware of your own feelings about spirituality, so that you can recognize and respond to the spiritual needs of others.
- Recognize that spiritual needs are a universal human phenomenon. Although not all people experience spiritual distress, all people have spiritual needs and the potential for spiritual growth.
- Recognize that it is within the realm of holistic nursing care to identify and plan interventions for spiritual growth, as well as for spiritual distress.
- Convey a nonjudgmental, open-minded attitude when eliciting information about a person's spirituality and religious beliefs.

Questions to Assess Spiritual Health

- "What in your life is meaningful and important?"
- "What do you hope to accomplish in your life?"
- "What do you do that gives you pleasure and satisfaction?"
- "Who are the people you can turn to when you need someone to listen to you or to help you?"
- "Do you believe in a higher being?" (examples: God, the Transcendent) "How do you describe this being?"
- "Do you participate in any activities (rituals) that foster a connection with a higher being?" (examples: prayer or other religious activities)
- "What activities are helpful in bringing you inner peace and relieving stress?" (examples: meditation, walking in the woods)
- "What are your beliefs about death?"
- "Do you see a connection between your body, your mind, your emotions and your soul?"
- "Is there anything you need or would like to have to support your beliefs and your spiritual needs?" (example: Bible, sacred or revered object)
- "Would you like to arrange a visit from a spiritual leader?"
- "Are there any health practices that you would like to consider, even though our society may not consider them to be conventional?" (examples: an Aboriginal Smudging ceremony, therapeutic touch, guided imagery)

Observations/Questions to Assess Spiritual Distress

- During the psychosocial interview, listen for clues to spiritual distress, such as the following: suicidal ideation; anger toward God; inability to forgive others, or most commonly, inability to forgive one's self; feelings of hopelessness, uselessness or abandonment; questions about the meaning of life, losses or suffering.
- "Are there any conflicts between your beliefs or values and actions that you feel you should be taking?" (example: feeling entitled to some time to oneself, which may be in conflict with the demands of caregiving for a spouse)
- "Are there any conflicts between what you believe in and what society or health care professionals are encouraging or suggesting you to do?" (example: questioning the wisdom of using a feeding tube for a spouse who is chronically and severely impaired and unable to participate in the decision)
- "Do you have any special religious considerations that are not being addressed?" (examples: dietary practices, observance of religious holidays)
- *For people in institutional settings:* "Is there anything here that interferes with your spiritual needs?" (examples: noisy environment, lack of privacy)

a link to a nursing article describing a study pertinent to the topic of spiritual assessment.

ONLINE LEARNING ACTIVITY 13-3:
ADDITIONAL INFORMATION ABOUT ASSESSMENT OF SPIRITUALITY IN OLDER ADULTS AND AN ARTICLE DESCRIBING A STUDY ABOUT WAYS IN WHICH NURSES ADDRESS SPIRITUAL DISTRESS
at http://thepoint.lww.com/Miller7e

Chapter Highlights

Overview of Psychosocial Assessment of Older Adults

- Psychosocial assessment is a complex process that involves the use of good communication skills, appropriate interview questions, purposeful observations and relevant assessment tools.
- Nurses can assess their own attitudes to increase their comfort level in performing a psychosocial assessment of older adults (Box 13-1).

Communication Skills for Psychosocial Assessment (Boxes 13-2, 13-3 and 13-4)

- Barriers to communication are associated with the situation, the older adult and the person who is communicating.
- Establishing rapport, using touch if appropriate, listening, asking questions and giving feedback can enhance communication during psychosocial assessment.
- Nurses create an environment for effective communication by speaking face-to-face at eye level, respecting the person's comfort zone, ensuring privacy, eliminating distractions and facilitating optimal vision and hearing functioning.
- It is important to be aware of cultural influences on communication, particularly regarding nonverbal communication.

Mental Status Assessment (Boxes 13-5, 13-6 and 13-7, Table 13-1)

- An assessment of mental status involves an assessment of all of the following: physical appearance, motor function, social skills, response to the interview, orientation, alertness and attention, memory, speech characteristics, and calculation and higher language skills.

Decision-Making and Executive Function

- Assessment of cognitive skills, such as executive function, is particularly important for determining the ability of the older adult to participate in decision-making.
- Insight, learning, memory, reasoning, judgment, problem solving and abstract thinking are some of the cognitive skills that are involved with decision-making.

Affective Function (Boxes 13-8 and 13-9)

- An assessment of affective function includes consideration of mood, anxiety, self-esteem, depression, and happiness and well-being.

of empathy (as discussed in the section on communication skills) are effective for addressing spiritual distress (Taylor & Mamier, 2013). Box 13-13 presents guidelines for assessing spiritual needs, and Online Learning Activity 13-3 provides

Contact With Reality (Box 13-10, Tables 13-2 and 13-3)

- Nurses assess contact with reality within the context of behavioural indicators to identify potential underlying causes of any loss of contact with reality.
- Conditions associated with delusions and hallucinations in older adults include dementia, depression, paranoid disorder and pathophysiologic conditions.

Social Supports (Box 13-11)

- Psychosocial assessment identifies social supports and economic resources as well as barriers to obtaining services.

Religion and Spirituality (Box 13-13)

- A holistic nursing assessment addresses religious affiliation and spirituality.

For more information about topics discussed in this chapter, be sure to check out the interactive Online Learning Activities and other helpful resources at http://thepoint.lww.com/Miller7e

Critical Thinking Exercises

1. Complete the psychosocial self-assessment in Box 13-1.
2. Think of several different situations in the past few weeks in which you worked with older adults and answer the following questions:
   - What aspects of psychosocial function did you observe?
   - What questions did you ask that would give you information about their psychosocial function?
   - What information did you obtain about their social supports?
3. Name at least three things you would observe or determine in order to assess each of the following when you are working with older adults: physical appearance, social skills, orientation, alertness and attention, memory, speech characteristics, calculation and higher language skills, decision-making skills, anxiety, self-esteem, depression, and contact with reality.
4. What questions would you ask an older adult to identify social supports and barriers to the use of services?
5. What approach would you use to assess an older adult's spiritual health and identify spiritual distress?

For more information about the topics discussed in this chapter, be sure to check out the interactive Online Learning Activities and other helpful resources at http://thepoint.lww.com/Miller7e.

REFERENCES

Andrews, M. M., & Boyle, J. S. (2012). *Transcultural concepts in nursing care* (6th ed.). Philadelphia, PA: Lippincott Williams & Wilkins.

Bertram, K., & Williams, D. R. (2012). Visual hallucinations in the differential diagnosis of parkinsonism. *Journal of Neurology Neurosurgery and Psychiatry, 83*, 448–452.

Cohen-Mansfield, J., & Golander, H. (2011). The measurement of psychosis in dementia: A comparison of assessment tools. *Alzheimer Disease and Associated Disorders, 25*, 101–108.

Freitas, S., Simoes, M. R., Alves, L., et al. (2013). Montreal cognitive assessment: Validation study for mild cognitive impairment and Alzheimer disease. *Alzheimer Disease and Associated Disorders, 27*, 37–43.

Hamilton, J. M., Landy, K. M., Salmon, D. P., et al. (2012). Early visuospatial deficits predict the occurrence of visual hallucinations in autopsy-confirmed dementia with Lewy Bodies. *American Journal of Geriatric Psychiatry, 20*(9), 773–781.

Hughes, D. F. (2013). Charles Bonnet syndrome: A literature review into diagnostic criteria, treatment and implications for nursing practice. *Journal of Psychiatric and Mental Health Nursing, 20*(2), 169–175.

Ismail, A., Nguyen, M., Fischer, C. E., et al. (2011). Neurobiology of delusions in Alzheimer's disease. *Current Psychiatry Reports, 13*(3), 211–218.

Kennedy, G. J. (2012). Brief evaluation of executive dysfunction: An essential refinement in the assessment of cognitive impairment. *Try This: Best practices in Nursing Care to Older Adults*, Issue number D3. Retrieved from www.COncultGeriRn.org

Kiefer, R. A. (2008). An integrative review of the concept of well-being. *Holistic Nursing Practice, 22*, 244–252.

Kolanowski, A. M., Fick, D. M., Yevchak, A. M., et al. (2012). Pay attention! The critical importance of assessing attention in older adults with dementia. *Journal of Gerontological Nursing, 38*(11), 23–27.

Lane, A. M., Hirst, S. P., & Reed, M. B. (2013). *Older adults: Understanding and facilitating transitions*. Dubuque, IA: Kendall Hunt.

Nakatsuka, M., Meguro, K., Tsuboi, H., et al. (2013). Content of delusional thoughts in Alzheimer's disease and assessment of content-specific brain dysfunctions with BEHAVE-AD-FW and SPECT. *International Geropsychiatry, 25*(6), 939–948.

Nguyen, N. D., Osterweil, D., & Hoffman, J. (2013). Charles bonnet syndrome: Treating nonpsychiatric hallucinations. *Consults in Pharmacology, 28*(3), 184–188.

Nomura, K., Kazui, H., Wada, T., et al. (2012). Classification of delusions in Alzheimer's disease and their neural correlates. *Psychogeriatrics, 12*(3), 200–210.

Pachana, N.A., & Byrne, G.J. (2012). The Geriatric Anxiety Inventory: International use and future directions. *Australian Psychologist, 47*, 33–38. doi:10.1111/j.1742-9544.2011.00052.x

Perugi, G., Poletti, M., Logi, C., et al. (2013). Diagnosis, assessment, and management of delusional jealousy in Parkinson's disease with and without dementia. *Neurological Science, 34*(9), 1537–1541.

Purnell, L. D. (2013). *Transcultural health care: A culturally competent approach* (4th ed.). Philadelphia, PA: F. A. Davis.

Reeves, S. J., Gould, R. L., Powell, J. F., et al. (2012). Origins of delusions in Alzheimer's disease. *Neuroscience and Biobehavior Review, 36*(10), 2274–2287.

Sawada, H., Oeda, T., Yamamoto, K., et al. (2013). Trigger medications and patient-related risk factors for Parkinson disease psychosis requiring anti-psychotic drugs: A retrospective cohort study. *BMC Neurology, 13*, 145. doi:10.1186/1471-2377-13-145

Smith, M., Ingram, T., & Brighton, V. (2008). *Evidence-Based Practice Guideline: Detection and Assessment of Late-Life Anxiety*. University of Iowa Gerontological Nursing Interventions Research Centre. Retrieved from National Guideline Clearinghouse, www.guideline.gov

Steis, M. R., & Fick, D. M. (2012). Delirium superimposed on dementia: Accuracy of nurse documentation. *Journal of Gerontological Nursing, 38*(1), 32–42.

Sultzer, D. L., Leskin, L. P., Melrose, R. J., et al. (2013, September 7). Neurobiology of delusions, memory, and insight in Alzheimer disease. *American Journal of Geriatric Psychiatry, 22*(11), 1346–1355. doi:10.1016/j.jagp.2013.5.005

Svetel, M., Smilijkovic, T., Pekmezovic, T., et al. (2012). Hallucinations in Parkinson's disease: Cross-sectional study. *Acta Neurology Belgium, 112*(1), 33–37.

Taylor, E. J., & Mamier, I. (2013). Nurse responses to patient expressions of spiritual distress. *Holistic Nursing Practice, 27*(4), 217–224.

chapter 14

Impaired Cognitive Function: Delirium and Dementia (Neurocognitive Disorders)

LEARNING OBJECTIVES

After reading this chapter, you will be able to:

1. Describe delirium and discuss nursing assessment and interventions related to delirium.

2. Use appropriate terminology to describe impaired cognitive function in older adults.

3. Describe characteristics of Alzheimer disease, vascular dementia, Lewy body dementia, and frontotemporal degeneration.

4. List the factors that affect the risk for development of dementia.

5. Discuss the functional consequences of impaired cognitive function.

6. Describe guidelines for initial and ongoing assessment of cognitively impaired older adults.

7. Identify nonpharmacologic interventions for addressing dementia-related behaviours, including environmental modifications and communication techniques.

8. Discuss medications for slowing the progression of dementia and for managing dementia-related behaviours.

KEY POINTS

Alzheimer disease

anosognosia

behavioural and psychological symptoms of dementia (BPSD)

delirium

dementia (neurocognitive disorders)

excess disability

frontotemporal degeneration

Lewy body dementia

sundowning

vascular dementia

ealthy older adults experience only minor changes in cognitive abilities (as described in Chapter 11), but as people age, they are increasingly likely to experience pathologic conditions that have a major impact on cognitive function. Nurses in all settings frequently care for older adults who have dementia (now labelled neurocognitive disorders in the *Diagnostic and Statistical Manual of Mental Disorders,* 5th edition, published by the American Psychiatric Association [APA] in 2013) or delirium, which are the two main causes of significant cognitive impairment in older adults. Nurses are responsible for identifying factors that contribute to impaired cognitive functioning in older adults. In addition, nurses and others who care for people with dementia must meet the challenge of preserving as much of the person's dignity and quality of life as possible, despite the serious and progressive losses the person with dementia experiences.

DELIRIUM

Although delirium has been documented in patients for centuries, only in recent years have researchers and practitioners addressed delirium as a serious, preventable, treatable, commonly occurring and often unrecognized condition that disproportionately affects older adults. **Delirium** is a syndrome that develops over hours or days, fluctuates over the course of the day and can persist for months. Changes in mental status involve problems with attention and consciousness and several or many additional changes, including altered sleep–wake patterns.

Prevalence, Risk Factors and Functional Consequences of Delirium

Delirium results from an interaction between *predisposing factors*, which increase the person's vulnerability, and *precipitating factors*, which account for the immediate threat. The most commonly identified predisposing factors include advanced age, dementia, depression, functional dependency and number of medications. Common precipitating factors include surgery, infections, serious illness and physical restraints. The risk for developing delirium is highest for people with several predisposing factors in combination with one or more precipitating factors. Reviews of studies cite the following rates for delirium:

- 22% in community-living people with dementia
- 15% to 70% in long-term care residents
- 11% to 33% on admission to a hospital setting, with an additional 5% to 35% developing delirium after admission
- 80% or more in intensive care settings (Cole et al., 2013; de Lange et al., 2013; Godfrey et al., 2013; Popp, 2013).

Functional consequences include longer hospital stays, increased mortality, increased dependency, short- and long-term functional impairment and higher rates of permanent residency in long-term care facilities (Fong et al., 2012; Tullmann et al., 2012). A study of outcomes during 1 month following hospitalization found that those older adults who had dementia and were diagnosed as having delirium had a 25% short-term mortality rate, increased length of stay, and poorer function at discharge and greater functional decline at 1 month follow-up (Fick et al., 2013). Consistent evidence from longitudinal studies suggests that delirium strongly predicts development of dementia in the long term and acceleration of cognitive decline in people who already have dementia (Davis et al., 2012; Macluluch et al., 2013).

Nursing Assessment of Delirium

Because manifestations of delirium are wide ranging and can fluctuate quickly, frequent assessment is imperative for effective detection. Although nurses have essential roles in assessing delirium, studies indicate that they have difficulty identifying manifestations of delirium, particularly in the hypoactive form and in people with dementia (Gordon et al., 2013; Solberg et al., 2013; Steis & Fick, 2012). Because delirium occurs so commonly in hospitalized older adults and is often unrecognized, routine cognitive screening is recommended as a standard part of care (Wand et al., 2013). The Confusion Assessment Method (CAM), which was developed in 1990, is the most widely used screening tool in acute care units and long-term care facilities (Tullmann et al., 2012). According to the CAM model (Inouye et al., 1990), delirium is diagnosed on the basis of a four-point algorithm and confirming the presence of features in points one *and* two and *either* point three *or* point four of the following:

1. Acute onset or fluctuating course: change in mental status from baseline or onset of abnormal behaviours that tend to come and go or increase and decrease in severity.
2. Inattention: easy distractibility, difficulty focusing, diminished ability to keep track of conversations.
3. Disorganized thinking: incoherent, disorganized, rambling or illogical thinking or conversation.
4. Altered level of consciousness: alert (normal), vigilant, lethargic, stupor or coma.

An important consideration with regard to assessing the feature of inattention is that a lack of response or the response of "don't know" may indicate inattention (i.e., feature 2; Huang et al., 2012). Another consideration is that some people with delirium are aware of their cognitive deficits and can self-report. One study of 55 hospitalized adults with diagnosed delirium found that 31% recognized their delirium and this was associated with disorientation and acuity of onset (Ryan et al., 2013).

Another assessment consideration is that, in addition to mental status changes, delirium subtypes are categorized according to motor and behavioural manifestation. Three subtypes of delirium are characterized as follows:

- Hyperactive: restlessness, agitation, combativeness, anger, wandering, laughing, swearing, emotional lability and fast or loud speech
- Hypoactive: lethargy, staring, slowed movement, paucity of speech and unresponsiveness
- Mixed: fluctuations between hyperactive and hypoactive

The hypoactive type may occur more commonly in older adults; however, it is not as easily recognized, and manifestations may be dismissed as clinically unimportant (Blazer & van Nieuwenhuizen, 2012).

Nursing Diagnosis and Outcomes

The nursing diagnosis of Acute Confusion is defined as an "abrupt onset of reversible disturbances of consciousness, attention, cognition, and perception that develop over a short period of time" (Herdman, 2012, p. 262). Defining characteristics include fluctuation in cognition, consciousness or psychomotor activity; hallucinations or misperceptions; increased restlessness or agitation; and lack of motivation to initiate or follow through with purposeful or goal-directed behaviour.

To address this diagnosis, nurses can use the following Nursing Outcomes Classification (NOC) terms in their care plans: Anxiety Level, Cognition, Cognitive Orientation, Concentration, Comfort Status, Information Processing, Memory, Neurologic Status and Psychomotor Energy. In addition, the following NOC terms may be applicable to address causative factors: Electrolyte and Acid/Base Balance, Hydration, Infection Severity, Nutritional Status, Risk Control and Sensory Function.

> **Wellness Opportunity**
>
> Nurses can use the NOC Comfort Level in their care plans to holistically address the needs of older adults with delirium.

Nursing Interventions for Delirium

The complexity of delirium requires an interprofessional approach to management, with nurses having a key role in detection, ongoing assessment and management. Current emphasis is on prevention and early detection and treatment of delirium because outcomes are worse among those with more severe and persistent delirium. The importance of recognizing and intervening in delirium was emphasized in 2004 when the RNAO (Registered Nurses of Ontario) published Nursing Practice Guidelines for caring for older adults with delirium. Furthermore, the Canadian Coalition for Seniors' Mental Health published national guidelines for the assessment and treatment of delirium in 2006.

Essential components of a multifactorial approach to delirium are staff education, comprehensive geriatric assessment, treatment of all contributing factors (e.g., pain, medical conditions, sleep deprivation, adverse medication effects, fluid and electrolyte imbalances, vision or hearing impairments), orientation interventions, environmental modifications, physical and occupational therapies, nutritional interventions, measures for preventing complications (e.g., falls, injuries, sleep problems, pressure ulcers, aspiration), encouraging the presence of family and other support people, and comprehensive discharge planning. Examples of interventions that are pertinent to nursing care plans are as follows:

- Provision of aids to orientation (e.g., clock, watch, calendar) and aids to improve sensory function (e.g., eyeglasses, hearing aids)
- Frequent verbal orientation and reminders about daily events
- Environmental modification (e.g., noise reduction, familiar objects)
- Psychological support (e.g., cognitive and social stimulation)
- Identification of adverse medication effects and discussion of medication regimen with prescribing practitioners
- Promotion of physiologic stability (e.g., low-dose oxygenation, maintenance of fluid and electrolyte balance)
- Adequate pain management (refer to Chapter 28)
- Promotion of normal sleep–wake pattern (refer to Chapter 24)
- Maintenance of optimal bowel and bladder function (refer to Chapters 18 and 19)
- Physical activity (e.g., ambulation, physical therapy, occupational therapy)
- Provision of cognitively stimulating activities
- Encouragement of family and support people to be with the person

Figure 14-1 illustrates a flow chart for nursing care of older adults with delirium.

The following Nursing Interventions Classification (NIC) terms are examples of interventions that can be used in care plans for acute confusion: Anxiety Reduction, Behaviour Management, Cognitive Stimulation, Delirium Management, Energy Management, Environmental Management, Fluid/Electrolyte Management, Hallucination Management, Medication Management, Mood Management, Nutrition Management, Pain Management, Reality Orientation, Sedation Management and Surveillance: Safety.

Wellness Opportunity

Nursing interventions to holistically address the needs of older adults during confusional states include use of a Calming Technique, Emotional Support, Music Therapy, Presence and Touch.

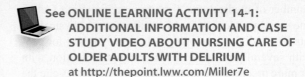
See **ONLINE LEARNING ACTIVITY 14-1: ADDITIONAL INFORMATION AND CASE STUDY VIDEO ABOUT NURSING CARE OF OLDER ADULTS WITH DELIRIUM** at http://thepoint.lww.com/Miller7e

OVERVIEW OF DEMENTIA

Dementia is one of the most multifaceted topics discussed in this book, with evidence-based information rapidly emerging from many clinical, scientific, social and ethical perspectives. This overview section provides background information that is relevant to current understanding of dementia, and the remainder of this chapter applies the information to clinical practice.

Two considerations need to be addressed in relation to evidence-based information about dementia. First, it is important to recognize that recent developments in neuro-imaging techniques have led to major improvements in the diagnosis of dementia, but these diagnostic methods are not widely available outside of research centres. Similarly, although many clinical trials of interventions for dementia are in progress, these are available only in research studies. Second, when reading results of studies of nonprescription products for the prevention of cognitive decline, it is crucial to pay close attention to the study design before drawing conclusions about effectiveness of the product. For example, some studies indicate that resveratrol, vitamin E and *Ginkgo biloba* may prevent cognitive decline in some people, but more studies are needed before these products can be recommended. Because media attention often highlights so-called breakthroughs in diagnosis of, or treatments for, dementia, nurses have important roles in teaching older adults and their care partners about diagnosis and management of declines in cognitive function. In addition to keeping current on research and focusing on the clinical application of evidence-based recommendations, nurses can teach older adults about obtaining information from reliable sources, as discussed in the section on nursing interventions.

Terminology to Describe Dementia

An understanding of impaired cognitive function is complicated by the many terms that are used interchangeably—and sometimes inaccurately—to describe dementia. Recent research has greatly improved the ability of clinicians to diagnose and treat different types of dementia, but it has also brought about a confusing proliferation of dementia-related terminology. Perhaps more than any other terms used in reference to older adults, those associated with cognitive impairment are the most misused, misunderstood and emotionally charged. The following are some of the terms commonly used in reference to cognitive impairment in older adults: confusion, dementia, senility, Alzheimer disease (AD), small strokes, memory problems and organic brain syndrome. Different terms are more or less acceptable to different people and the selection of a term is often based

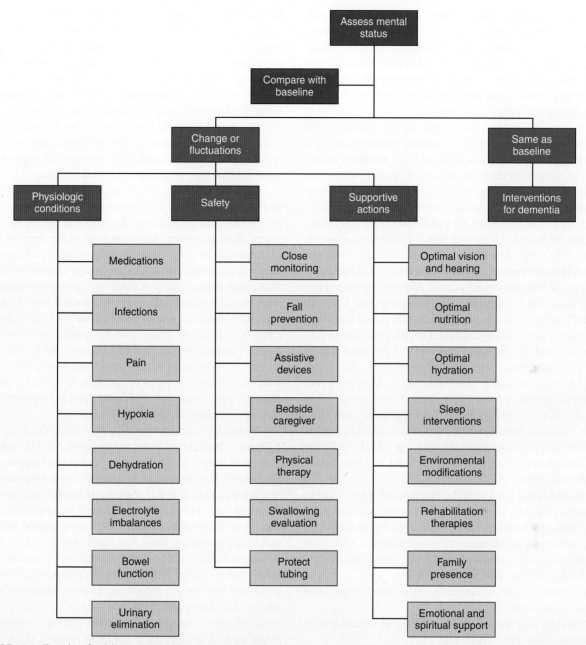

FIGURE 14-1 Flow chart for delirium. (From Miller, C. A. [2012]. *Fast facts for dementia care: What nurses need to know in a nutshell.* New York, NY: Springer. Used with permission from Springer Publishing Company.)

on emotional preferences or lack of accurate information. Because cognitive impairment is an emotionally charged subject, it is imperative to use the most appropriate term on the basis of an understanding of the underlying causes for the impairment and an assessment of what term is most acceptable to the older adult and his or her care partners.

Medical references to dementia can be traced back to 1906, when a German physician, Alois Alzheimer, described neuritic plaques in the autopsied brain of a woman who was 55 years old at the time of her death and had experienced cognitive and behaviour changes for about 5 years before her death. Building on earlier studies indicating that hardening of the arteries caused cognitive impairment in *older*

adults, Alzheimer concluded that neuritic plaques caused cognitive impairment in *younger* adults. By 1910, AD (i.e., presenile dementia) was considered a distinct disease differentiated from senile dementia by younger age at onset. This viewpoint was not challenged until the 1960s when autopsy studies indicated that many of the brain changes attributed to irreversible pathologic conditions were actually manifestations of treatable conditions. Landmark studies by Tomlinson et al. (1968, 1970) led to the conclusion that the neuropathologic changes of AD represent a single disease process, regardless of the age at onset. In 1974, another landmark study by Hachinski, Lassen and Marshall found that cerebral atherosclerosis was both a major cause of cognitive impairments and the most common medical *mis*diagnosis. Moreover, these scientists denounced the use of the phrase "hardening of the arteries" and introduced the term "multi-infarct dementia" to describe dementias of cerebrovascular origin. Based on recent research, the term vascular dementia is more appropriate than either of these terms, as discussed in the section on types of dementia.

In clinical settings, dementia is the medical term that includes a group of brain disorders characterized by a gradual decline in cognitive abilities (e.g., memory, understanding, judgment, decision-making, communication) and changes in personality and behaviour. Because AD is a type of dementia that occurs most commonly and has the longest history of recognition, *AD* and *dementia* are sometimes used interchangeably, although this is not always accurate. Because the term "dementia" is closely associated with the uncomplimentary use of the term "demented," a phrase, such as "a person with dementia," is more appropriate when referring to the medical syndrome of impaired cognitive function. Several leading gerontologists recently suggested that clinicians use the term "aging-associated cognitive challenges" to emphasize that this condition is something that can serve as a source of growth for older adults (George et al., 2012). Additionally, as noted earlier in this chapter, the *Diagnostic and Statistical Manual of Mental Disorders*, 5th edition (*DSM 5*; APA, 2013) now classifies dementias as "neurocognitive disorders." As such, for diagnostic purposes, AD is classified as major or mild neurocognitive disorder due to AD. Similarly, vascular dementia is termed major or mild vascular neurocognitive disorder.

An additional point must be emphasized with regard to the term *dementia*. Dementia is not a single disease but a group of diseases, and each type is associated with a different cause and unique combination of manifestations. Additional considerations that complicate the use of terms related to impaired cognitive function are as follows:

- Two or more types of dementia can develop at the same time or sequentially.
- Commonly available diagnostic techniques cannot always determine the type of dementia.
- Terms may be used inaccurately even by health care professionals.
- Because the ability to differentiate between types of dementia is still in early stages, many of the studies on AD have included subjects with other types of dementia.

In this chapter, the term *dementia* is used except when the information is pertinent to a particular type. The text refers to AD when a source used that term; however, it is important to recognize that many of the citations on AD refer to dementia in the broader sense.

TYPES OF DEMENTIA

The current approach to diagnosing dementia in usual clinical settings can be likened to the approach taken to diagnosing an infection. An infection is a generic diagnosis indicating the presence of a constellation of signs and symptoms (e.g., malaise, elevated temperature), but it does not indicate the causative factor. As additional information is collected, the specific type of infection is identified (e.g., pneumonia, urinary tract infection, bacterial, viral) and, sometimes, more than one infection is discovered. Until the specific causative agent is identified, generic measures are taken (e.g., antipyretics, broad-spectrum antibiotics). After the specific causative agent is identified (e.g., through culture and sensitivity tests), the infection is treated with very specific antimicrobial agents. At all stages, comfort measures are used.

Analogously, dementia is an umbrella diagnosis indicating a constellation of signs and symptoms (e.g., memory impairment, personality changes), but during the early stages there rarely are clear indicators of the specific types of dementia. In many cases, neuropsychological testing is required to distinguish patterns of change that are associated with either normal aging or pathologic processes during the early stages. As the condition progresses and more signs and symptoms develop, one or more causative factors may be identified. However, there is no diagnostic equivalent of a "culture and sensitivity" test for dementia, so it is difficult to distinguish between the different types of dementia. Thus, diagnosis of specific types of dementia is based on clinical observations, history of risk factors and information from currently available diagnostic methods.

Based on current scientific literature, the four most commonly recognized types of dementia are AD, vascular dementia, Lewy body dementia and frontotemporal degeneration. It is important to recognize that there are significant overlaps in manifestations of the different types of dementia, and during the early stage it is often difficult to determine if cognitive changes are due to normal aging or pathologic processes. Observations during the course of the dementia provide clues to the underlying pathologic processes, but it is often difficult, or even impossible, to distinguish one type of dementia from another. Moreover, older adults often have more than one type of dementia, which is called *mixed dementia*. Clinically relevant information about each of the four most common types of dementia is reviewed in this section, and the rest of this chapter presents information about functional consequences, assessment and interventions applicable to all types. Table 14-1 describes the distinguishing features of the four most common types of dementia.

Alzheimer Disease

Alzheimer disease accounts for 60% to 80% of the cases of dementia (Alzheimer's Association Report, 2013) and, as already discussed, is the type of dementia with the strongest research base. Hallmark pathologic characteristic of AD are as follows:

- Amyloid plaques in the spaces between the neurons: abnormal deposits of a protein fragment called b-amyloid, which is formed from the breakdown of a larger protein called amyloid precursor protein

TABLE 14-1 Distinguishing Features of Common Types of Dementia

Type	Onset and Course	Typical Manifestations
Alzheimer disease	Insidious onset; diagnosis often made retrospectively; slowly progressive over 5 to 10 years, with accelerated decline associated with concomitant conditions (e.g., heart failure, delirium)	Early cognitive changes, usually but not always involving memory loss. Gradual loss of other cognitive abilities (e.g., decision making, language) and communication skills. Gradual onset of behaviour and personality changes (e.g., depression, irritability, agitation, indifference)
Vascular dementia	Abrupt onset due to cumulative effects of small strokes *OR* sudden onset if related to major stroke. History of vascular risks (e.g., stroke, hypertension). Irregular course *OR* improvement is possible depending on causative factors	Manifestations consistent with area of brain that is affected: aphasia, memory impairment, apathy, depression, emotional lability and sensory–motor deficits (e.g., hemiparesis, gait disturbances, hemisensory loss, urinary incontinence)
Lewy body dementia	Insidious onset with a progressive decline in cognitive, behavioural and motor symptoms; manifestations similar to Parkinson disease	Significant cognitive impairment; fluctuating levels of cognition; parkinsonism; hallucinations; sleep disturbances; loss of postural stability; highly sensitive to neuroleptic medications
Frontotemporal degeneration	Gradual onset typically before the age of 65; family history common; progressive decline in functioning	Early and progressive changes in behaviour, motor abilities and/or speech-language skills. Memory impairments occur later during the course of the disease.

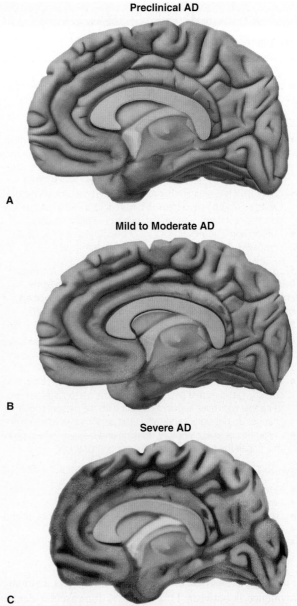

Preclinical AD

A

Mild to Moderate AD

B

Severe AD

C

FIGURE 14-2 (A) During preclinical Alzheimer disease, subtle degenerative changes begin to occur, and the person develops mild cognitive impairment. **(B)** In mild to moderate stages of Alzheimer disease, pathologic changes affect the areas of the brain that control memory, language and reasoning. **(C)** In the severe stage of Alzheimer disease, pathologic changes cause significant atrophy in many areas. (Courtesy of the National Institute on Aging/National Institutes of Health.)

- Neurofibrillary tangles inside the neurons: abnormal clusters of a protein called tau
- Loss of synaptic connections between neurons
- Cell death causing brain atrophy

The gradual progression of brain atrophy is correlated with stages of AD, from preclinical to severe, as illustrated in Figure 14-2.

In 2011, the National Institute on Aging and the Alzheimer's Association published the first major update on diagnostic guidelines for AD since 1984. These guidelines, which are similar to those published by the International Working Group on Alzheimer's Disease, define AD as a neurologic condition that begins with a preclinical stage and progresses to clinical diagnosis of dementia. The National Institute on Aging and Alzheimer's Association guidelines addressing the criteria for dementia, the criteria for probable

and possible AD and the criteria for mild cognitive impairment (MCI) were adopted at the 4th Canadian Consensus Conference on the Diagnosis and Treatment of Dementia in 2012 (Gauthier et al., 2012). Box 14-1 presents evidence-based information from these guidelines and additional pertinent research information about additional aspects of AD, on the basis of a major Alzheimer's Association report (2013).

Vascular Dementia

Vascular dementia refers to cognitive impairment, ranging from mild to severe, that is caused by the death of nerve cells

Box 14-1   Alzheimer Disease (AD) in Canada: Facts, Figures and Overview

Prevalence and Incidence of AD

- In 2011, 747,000 Canadians 65 years of age and older (almost 15% of the older adult population) were living with AD.
- It is estimated that by 2031, 1.4 million Canadians will suffer from AD (Alzheimer Society—Ontario, 2012).

Consequences of AD

- In 2009, AD was the 7th leading cause of death in Canadians of all ages. However, AD became the 6th leading cause of death for those between 75 and 84 and the 4th leading cause of death for Canadians 85 years of age and older in 2009 (Statistics Canada, 2012).
- Currently, it is estimated that AD and related dementias cost the Canadian health care system 15 billion dollars. Within one generation, this cost is projected to catapult to 153 billion dollars.
- Nursing home admission for 75% of people with AD by age 80, compared with only 4% of those without dementia.

Stages of AD as Proposed by 2011 Criteria of the National Institute on Aging and the Alzheimer Association (and endorsed by the 4th Canadian Consensus Conference on the Diagnosis and Treatment of Dementia [CCCDTD4]) (Gauthier et al., 2012)

- *Preclinical AD*: pathological changes begin 20 years or more before the onset of symptoms; this stage cannot be diagnosed in usual clinical settings, but is being used for research purposes.
- *Mild cognitive impairment (MCI) due to AD*: Measurable changes in cognitive abilities that are noticeable to the person affected and to people who have frequent contact with the person; cognitive changes do not significantly affect the person's everyday activities.
- *Dementia due to AD:* Memory, thinking and behavioural symptoms that impair the person's ability to function in daily life

Symptoms of AD

- Memory loss that disrupts daily life
- Challenges in planning or solving problems
- Difficulty completing familiar tasks at home, at work or at leisure
- Confusion with time and place
- Trouble understanding visual images and spatial relationships
- Changes in language or writing skills
- Misplacing things and losing the ability to retrace steps
- Impaired judgment
- Withdrawal from work or social activities
- Changes in mood and personality

Factors That Increase the Risk for AD

- Family history: increased risk in people who have first-degree relative with AD (i.e., parent or sibling)
- Inheriting the APOE-4 gene from one or both parents
- Diagnosis of MCI in combination with memory impairment
- Risks for cardiovascular disease: smoking, obesity, diabetes, hypertension, hypercholesterolemia
- Traumatic brain injury

Factors That Decrease the Risk for AD

- Physical activity
- Diet that is low in saturated fats and rich in vegetables and vegetable-based oils
- Higher levels of education, which help build a "cognitive reserve"
- Engaging in social and cognitive activities

Consequences for Families and Caregivers

- Significantly increased demands on caregivers, with AD caregivers providing an average of 21.9 hours of care per week
- In 2008, family and friends spent about 231 million hours in Canada providing care to individuals with AD and related dementias. These number of hours caregiving for family members with dementia is expected to triple by the year 2038.
- Increased length of time providing care: 32% of AD caregivers provided care for more than 5 years, compared with 28% of non-AD caregivers.
- Higher levels of stress and poor emotional health (e.g., 33% to 44% of AD caregivers reported depression, compared with 17% to 27% in non-AD caregivers).

Sources: Alzheimer's Association Report. (2013). *Alzheimer's & Dementia, 9,* 208–245; Alzheimer Society of Canada. (2010). *Rising tide report.* Retrieved from www.alzheimer.ca/~/media/Files/national/Advisory/ASC_Rising_Tide_Exec_summary_e.pdf.

---

in the regions nourished by the diseased vessels. Estimated prevalence is between 11% and 18% for vascular dementia alone and between 22% and 34% for a combination of vascular dementia and AD (Kling et al., 2013). Underlying pathologic processes include clinical stroke (e.g., hemorrhage or occlusion of blood vessels) or subclinical vascular brain injury (e.g., lacunar strokes of the small arteries). Although vascular dementia has been viewed as a distinct type of dementia, reviews of recent studies indicate that cerebrovascular damage most often occurs concurrently with the neuropathologic changes of other dementias (Gorelick & Nyenhuis, 2013; Kling et al., 2013). As with all types of dementia, manifestations range from mild to severe and fluctuations are associated with progression of the disease and the onset of concurrent conditions.

Factors that are strongly associated with increased risk for vascular dementia include stroke, hypertension, hypercholesterolemia, obesity, diabetes and atrial fibrillation. Table 14-1 provides information about the onset, course and typical manifestations of vascular dementia.

Lewy Body Dementia

Lewy body dementia is part of a group of disorders called Lewy body diseases, which also includes Parkinson disease and Parkinson disease with dementia. Lewy body dementia and Parkinson disease with dementia account for between 15% and 20% of dementia diagnoses (Gealogo, 2013). The hallmark pathologic characteristic of Lewy body disease is the presence of abnormal proteins (i.e., Lewy bodies) in the brain that eventually damage the neurons and affect all the following: cognitive abilities, motor function, sensory function, sleep patterns and autonomic function. Clinically it is difficult to differentiate between Lewy body dementia and AD because they have overlapping features and often occur together. Features that are more characteristic of dementia with Lewy bodies (compared with AD) include more pronounced cognitive fluctuations, spontaneous parkinsonism and visual hallucinations as an early and recurrent manifestation (Hanagasi et al., 2013; Huang & Halliday, 2013). Table 14-1 lists distinguishing features of Lewy body dementia.

People with Lewy body dementia are highly sensitive to medications with anticholinergic properties, and they can develop extreme, idiosyncratic or fatal reactions to even low doses of certain medications, such as phenothiazines and newer (atypical) antipsychotics (Kaur et al., 2012). For example, sedatives or antipsychotics may cause hallucinations, agitation or extreme somnolence. Thus, anticholinergic medications, including over-the-counter products, should be avoided, and if they are used, doses should be minimal and patients should be observed carefully for adverse effects. Another clinically important characteristic is that people with Lewy body dementia may decompensate rapidly and significantly when they have a medical condition (e.g., minor infection) or when their environment is changed. Also cognitive fluctuations commonly occur over minutes, hours or days. It is important to be alert to the possibility that people with Lewy body dementia may be misdiagnosed as having AD or they may have both types of dementia.

Frontotemporal Degeneration

Frontotemporal degeneration (also called frontotemporal disorders and formerly called frontotemporal dementia) describes a type of dementia cause by neurodegenerative conditions involving the frontal or temporal lobes or both, which collectively are referred to as frontotemporal degeneration. Pick disease was first identified as a type of frontotemporal dementia in 1892, and in recent years, frontotemporal degeneration is recognized as a major cause of young-onset dementia. Symptoms of frontotemporal degeneration typically begin during the sixth decade of life but may begin as early as the third decade (Warren et al., 2013).

Manifestations of frontotemporal degeneration vary widely according to the order in which the frontal or temporal lobes of the brain are affected. Types of frontotemporal degeneration as classified by symptoms are as follows:

- Progressive behavioural and personality decline: apathy, disinhibition, emotional lability, changes in behaviour and personality, and diminished concentration, attention, reasoning, judgment
- Progressive language decline: loss of abilities related to speaking, writing and language comprehension
- Progressive motor decline: falls, gait changes, movement disorders, muscle rigidity and difficulty with tasks involving fine-motor skills

Diagnosis of frontotemporal degeneration is difficult because manifestations vary widely and overlap with those of other types of dementia. People with frontotemporal degeneration are often misdiagnosed as having a psychiatric illness because they are younger in age, perform well on usual cognitive tests and lack insight. Because of its early onset and prominent and difficult-to-manage behavioural manifestations, frontotemporal degeneration is associated with significant stress and financial burden for spouses and other care partners (Massimo et al., 2013).

A consideration related to management is that usual medications for dementia (i.e., cholinesterase inhibitors or memantine) are not effective for frontotemporal degeneration; however, there is some evidence that trazodone at a dose of 100 mg three times a day may be helpful for managing symptoms (Chow & Alobaidy, 2013). In addition, because usual nonpharmacologic management strategies for dementia, such as redirecting the person, have limited effectiveness, nurses need to be creative in developing individualized care plans. For example, nurses can facilitate and coordinate an interprofessional team approach, including all the following: speech-language therapists to address speech, language and swallowing problems; physical and occupational therapists to address progressive motor decline; and social workers and mental health professionals to address behavioural and emotional components.

FACTORS ASSOCIATED WITH DEMENTIA

From a wellness perspective, it is important to recognize not only the factors that increase the risk for dementia but also those that protect against cognitive impairment. Researchers and policy makers are increasingly emphasizing the importance of addressing modifiable risk factors as an intervention for preventing dementia. In December 2013, 109 scientists from 36 countries issued a statement calling for international attention to making prevention of dementia a major health issue. Some highlights of the statement, which was published in the *Journal of Alzheimer's Disease* (Smith & Yaffe, 2014), are as follows:

- The same public health approach that has been effective for about half of the reduction in deaths from heart disease and stroke should be applied to dementia.
- About half of AD cases worldwide might be attributable to known risk factors. Taking immediate action on known risk factors could perhaps prevent up to one fifth of predicted new cases by 2025.
- There is already sufficient evidence to justify trials related to all the following: exercise, diabetes management, depression treatment, blood pressure control, B vitamins, omega-3 fatty acids, cognitive training and social activities.
- Public health policies should "tell people that adopting a healthy lifestyle may help ward off dementia as it does for other diseases."

A consistent conclusion of studies related to risks for dementia is that behaviours and interventions that are effective for preventing cardiovascular disease and promoting overall health (e.g., physical activity and healthy dietary practices) are also associated with improved cognitive function (Alzheimer's Association Report, 2013; Barnett et al., 2013; Justin et al., 2013; Mangialasche et al., 2012).

Wellness Opportunity

Nurses can teach all adults that engaging in social, mental and physical activity is a risk-free way of promoting cognitive wellness and may also prevent dementia.

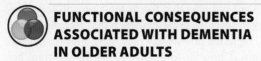

FUNCTIONAL CONSEQUENCES ASSOCIATED WITH DEMENTIA IN OLDER ADULTS

Functional consequences related to AD have been studied since the 1950s, but research on the unique manifestations of different dementias is in very early stages. Many functional consequences are common to all of the dementias, and as the disease progresses, manifestations of all types of dementia become more similar. It is important to recognize, however, that during all stages and in all types of dementia, functional consequences vary tremendously among individuals because of unique personality characteristics, coexisting conditions (e.g., depression, functional impairments) and other influences.

It is also imperative to acknowledge that the personhood of each individual who has dementia is always present and needs to be addressed in every interaction. Acknowledging personhood in people with dementia involves recognizing the needs, wants, emotions, personality, relationships, life story and need for connectedness of the individual (Palmer, 2013). Although dementia has long been associated with a "loss of self," a recent study stated that "personhood can be understood as increasingly concealed rather than lost" (Smebye & Kirkevold, 2013, p. 29). This perspective highlights the responsibility of nurses and all who provide care to acknowledge and discover the underlying personhood of each person who has dementia. In this and the following sections

of this chapter, the experiences of people with dementia are described in boxes to illustrate the unique ways in which dementia affects individuals and their care partners. In addition to the functional consequences that directly affect the person with dementia, caregivers and families of people with dementia also experience significant consequences.

Note that the term *care partners* is sometimes used in this chapter instead of *caregivers* to denote that the person with dementia is viewed as a *partner in the process* rather than a *passive recipient* especially during mild and even moderate stages. This phrase also emphasizes that care of people with dementia requires the *partnership* of many personal and professional support people working together to address this complex situation. The term *caregiver* is used in reference to the needs of family members and support people who are most directly affected, particularly during moderate or severe stages. The word "caregiver" is also used when citing a reference that uses that term.

Stages of Dementia

In the mid-1980s, an American psychiatrist, Reisberg, proposed a seven-stage model for describing the functional consequences of AD. Reisberg's staging schema, which has been updated and refined, is referred to as the Global Deterioration Scale/Functional Assessment Staging, or GDS/FAST. The GDS/FAST, as delineated in Table 14-2, is widely used as an evidence-based tool for determining the progression of AD from early to terminal stages. According to this framework, the

TABLE 14-2 Global Deterioration Scale/Functional Assessment Staging (GDS/FAST) of Alzheimer Disease	
Stage	**Effects on Functioning**
1: Normal adult	No deficits or complaints
2: Age-associated memory impairment	Deficits consistent with normal aging (i.e., no objective findings, difficulty with word finding, forgets location of objects)
3: Mild cognitive impairment	Some deficits in performing complex tasks, particularly in demanding social and employment settings; diminished organizational skills; deficits noted by others for the first time
4: Mild dementia	Diminished ability to perform complex tasks (e.g., meal planning, financial management); decreased knowledge of current and recent events; flattened affect and withdrawal from challenging situations
5: Moderate dementia	Obvious cognitive deficits; unable to manage complex daily tasks without some supervision or assistance; difficulty remembering names of familiar people
6: Moderately severe dementia	Increasingly obvious cognitive deficits (e.g., disorientation, significant short-term memory impairment); personality and emotional changes (e.g., anxiety, delusions) Loss of abilities in the following order: a. Difficulty putting clothing on properly without assistance b. Unable to bathe independently c. Unable to handle all aspects of toileting (e.g., does not wipe properly) d. Occasional or frequent urinary incontinence e. Occasional or frequent fecal incontinence
7: Severe dementia	Progressive loss of all verbal and psychomotor abilities: a. Verbal abilities limited to six or fewer different words b. Verbal abilities limited to a single intelligible word c. Unable to walk without assistance d. Unable to sit without assistance e. Unable to smile f. Unable to hold up head independently

Source: Reisberg, B. (1986). Dementia: A systematic approach to identifying reversible causes. *Geriatrics, 41*(4), 30–46.

diagnosis of AD is made retrospectively because it is based on a progression of manifestations. Although this staging system was developed three decades ago, it is consistent with current information confirming a preclinical stage and progressing to a terminal stage. In everyday practice, however, three staging categories—mild, moderate and late (or end)—are often used.

Self-awareness of People With Dementia

People with dementia are often perceived as having little or no awareness of, or insight into, their cognitive deficits and limitations. This perception has led to labelling people with dementia as being "in denial." It also underlies inaccurate statements about people with dementia, such as, "If they can ask if they have AD, then they don't have it." **Anosognosia**, which is the diagnostic term for lack of awareness, is assessed by having the person who is being evaluated and a family member or caregiver independently answer questions related to the person's behaviours and daily activities (e.g., repetitive talking, indicators of forgetfulness, lack of interest in usual activities) (Maki et al., 2013).

Although studies are just beginning to shed light on this multidimensional topic, research indicates that many people with dementia are aware of their deficits and that some level of awareness is retained as the dementia progresses (Clare et al., 2012, 2013; Mardh et al., 2013). Studies also indicate that a higher level of awareness is associated with greater levels of anxiety and depression (Horning et al., 2014; van Vliet et al., 2012; Verhulsdonk et al., 2013).

Programs emphasizing the provision of person-centred care are based on the premise that even when awareness of cognitive deficits is limited, people with dementia maintain emotional awareness and are capable of expressing their needs. Studies of the feelings and experiences of individuals with dementia provide important insight into their expressed needs as described in boxes throughout this chapter with direct quotes from people with dementia. Box 14-2 summarizes statements of people with dementia about how they are perceived by others.

Personal Experiences of Dementia

During the early stages, only the individual with dementia and people who live, work or have close contact with the person notice the initial changes, such as impaired judgment and short-term memory. When the changes are noticed, numerous explanations may be applicable and the deficits may be attributed to such factors as depression or the occurrence of a major life event (e.g., retirement, widowhood). People in the early stages of dementia may withdraw from complex tasks as a way of protecting themselves from the effects of diminishing cognitive abilities. For example, employed people may retire without acknowledging cognitive impairments as the reason. People who do not have to perform complex intellectual or psychomotor tasks may be able to conceal or compensate for the cognitive losses until the deficits seriously interfere with activities of daily living (ADLs). As the disease progresses, however, the person with dementia is less able to

---

Box 14-2 Lived Experiences: How People With Dementia Feel About Others' Perceptions

- It would be nice if a lot of people had more understanding and appreciate what you have got. I was in town, and this other lady started laughing because of the way I was trying to struggle to talk and that started to make me feel uncomfortable; I thought if only she understood, then perhaps she wouldn't stand there and laugh.
- If you say to someone, "Can you wait a couple of minutes; I've got dementia and I want to explain," they look at you and think there is nothing wrong with you; you should not be able to talk. Then again, you get someone who say "How-are-you?" and you think, "Grr, I'm not that bad."
- It's as though that's it, you are dribbling and nodding, and that's the picture of AD. But we are all sitting here and talking perfectly normally. We have got AD of some form; we are not nodding and dribbling.
- I'm trying to guard that I don't get looked down on. I don't want the feeling of being back in first grade or whatever ... of going in the other direction, of decreasing instead of improving, and I have inward anger.
- Everybody I have met has been absolutely amazed that (a) I can still talk and still think and (b) I have a diagnosis of dementia. They do not understand it.
- No one really understands how hard it is to live life like this, so people tend to trivialize how you feel, patronize you, and make out that they feel the same way.
- Written off as being devoid of feelings and needs, it was clear to me that my dementia negated the things that I said. It was very painful.
- It has been proven by thousands of early stage people with dementia to be capable and intelligent beings just moving a little slower.

Sources: Alzheimer's Society. (2008). *Dementia: Out of the shadows*. London, England: Author; Alzheimer's Society. (2010). *My name is not dementia: People with dementia discuss quality of life*. London, England: Author; Beard, R. L., & Fox, P. J. (2008). Resisting social disenfranchisement: Negotiating collective identities and everyday life with memory loss. *Social Science & Medicine, 66*, 1509–1520; Beard, R. L., Knauss, J., & Moyer, D. (2009). Managing disability and enjoying life: How we reframe dementia through personal narratives. *Journal of Aging Studies, 23*, 227–235; Clare, L., Rowlands, J. M., & Quin, R. (2008). Collective strength: The impact of developing a shared social identity in early-stage dementia. *Dementia, 7*(1), 9–30.

---

cover up the changes, and people with less intimate contact will begin to question the underlying cause of the deficits.

Common emotions and behaviours of people with dementia include loss, fear, shame, anger, sadness, anxiety, frustration, loneliness, depression, uncertainty, sense of uselessness, self-blame, diminished affect and withdrawal from challenging activities. Studies find that people with dementia want to understand their illness, maintain their personal identity, retain their functional independence and maintain their quality of life through health, relationships and positive coping (Dawson et al., 2013).

Even during the later stages of dementia when cognitive abilities are severely impaired and awareness is limited, emotional responses are directed toward preserving dignity and self-esteem (Mograbi et al., 2012). Dominant emotions during later stages of dementia include feelings of loss, anger, frustration, uncertainty, and lack of control or self-determination (Clare et al., 2008). It is imperative to recognize that emotional responses of people with dementia may be blunted or altered, but they are never absent. As dementia progresses, the person is likely to express emotions nonverbally and behaviourally. Thus, two important responsibilities

Box 14-3 Lived Experiences: Feelings About Earliest Dementia Changes

- I knew my brain wasn't what it used to be because I've always remembered that I gave birth to my girls and one time I thought, "I can't remember what their birthday is."
- To sing a song that I have sung 100 times before and the music I have heard 100 times before and I'm standing there thinking, "What the hell am I doing here and what am I going to sing?" This started to happen more and more, and when you are out on the stage on your own and you don't know what you are doing, it is a terrifying prospect.
- If I was getting dressed in the morning, I would put my clothes on, and I would guarantee you there was at least a pair of trousers, a shirt, or a hat and coat—and it had all gone on upside down, back to front.
- I'm still the same person I've always been. It's just that now I'm *me* with AD. I am still loving and caring, and I still have feelings, and I would like to think that I haven't changed in myself.
- Although I was expecting it by then, the words were still devastating to hear.
- I feel like I still have enough intelligence to be a person and not just someone you pat on the head as you go by. It's devastating, and it takes away your sense of self. I feel like I'm still a person and my wants and desires should at least be considered before decisions are made.
- The angst and anger that I went through during the diagnostic process—I could have actually gone and thumped people.
- It was as if the thunderclouds had been taken away because they had given an answer to me why I was treating my family so like a louse that I was.
- I was relieved really that what I was trying to convince people had been verified.
- I think the word *Alzheimer's* puts a fear in you, like cancer does.
- It is a really frightening thing when no one can tell you how fast you will deteriorate. It is hard to get across how that feels, but it gnaws at you continually, and each day you wonder what faculty will be lost next.
- It is quite strange because dementia seems to hit people in very different ways. There are little threads of commonality in it, but everyone is affected in a slightly different way.
- I think I have a very different view about how long I'll be around, or when life will come to an end, or when I'll be incompetent, than I did before the diagnosis. No question.
- I certainly think that it's important to let family be aware of one's problems. Not to the extent of complaining and complaining, but this is what it is, and I have to deal with that. I wouldn't deny it ever.

Sources: Alzheimer's Society. (2008). *Dementia: Out of the shadows.* London, England: Author; Alzheimer's Society. (2010). *My name is not dementia: People with dementia discuss quality of life.* London, England: Author; Beard, R. L., & Fox, P. J. (2008). Resisting social disenfranchisement: Negotiating collective identities and everyday life with memory loss. *Social Science & Medicine, 66,* 1509–1520; Beard, R. L., Knauss, J., & Moyer, D. (2009). Managing disability and enjoying life: How we reframe dementia through personal narratives. *Journal of Aging Studies, 23,* 227–235; Clare, L., Rowlands, J. M., & Quin, R. (2008). Collective strength: The impact of developing a shared social identity in early-stage dementia. *Dementia, 7*(1), 9–30.

of caregivers are to encourage and interpret nonverbal communication, which becomes the primary mode of communication during later stages of dementia. Box 14-3 describes the experiences and feelings of people with dementia about the earliest changes and their diagnoses.

Wellness Opportunity

Nurses holistically address psychosocial needs by recognizing that individuals vary significantly in their emotional responses, but people with dementia never lose the ability to respond to others.

A Student's Perspective

There is a woman at my nursing home who has severe dementia, to the point where she often is not very kind to the nurses, PTs, OTs and other staff. For most of our clinical rotation, I only heard reports of her being angry and sometimes insulting. This can be comical at times, and we all know not to take it personally because we know her attitude is a result of her disease. Understanding the chance I was taking, I went to talk to her during breakfast because she was just staring off into space. Kneeling at her eye level and placing my hand on her shoulder, I began by asking how her morning was. She complained about the cold weather and about how aggressive the OTs were in dressing her. I let her vent, I made some positive remarks and I complimented her on how beautiful she looked that day.

As I rose to my feet to leave her a few minutes later, she reached for my arm and said, "You're such a sweetheart; you're so kind." My first internal reaction was to be blown away! I had never heard of this woman delivering compliments! But throughout the rest of the day, I couldn't keep the smile off my face. This encounter helped me realize that this woman's beautiful personality is still with her and will always be a part of her. Yes, right now it's being masked most of the time by her dementia, but she still has feelings of kindness and a desire for happiness that fight past her disease every once in a while. I'm just glad I got to be part of that moment and discover that she's still there and needs to be treated like it always. One day she'll have the opportunity and power to express her thanks for those who showed her love and patience.

Shannon H.

Behavioural and Psychological Symptoms of Dementia

Significant behavioural disturbances, called **behavioural and psychological symptoms of dementia (BPSD)** (also called *neuropsychiatric symptoms*), occur at some point during the course of dementia in nearly all people with dementia (Burke et al., 2013; Selbaek et al., 2013). Some examples of BPSD are

- Agitation: abnormal level of verbal, vocal or motor activity (e.g., aggression, screaming)
- Psychiatric symptoms: delusions, hallucinations
- Personality changes, disinhibition
- Mood disturbances: apathy, depression, euphoria, emotional lability
- Aberrant motor movements: pacing, rummaging, wandering
- Changes in sleep, eating, appetite
- Hypersexual behaviour: inappropriate statements, sexually aggressive actions, masturbation in public places

When BPSD or increased confusion or restlessness occur only or primarily in the early evening, this is called **sundowning**. Factors associated with sundowning include fatigue, overstimulation, fear of darkness and altered circadian rhythm.

Aggression and agitation are types of BPSD that are strongly associated with serious functional consequences, including distress and reduced quality of life for the person with dementia and for those who are care partners and increased risk for being admitted to a hospital or long-term care setting (Ballard & Corbett, 2013; Toot et al., 2013). Conditions associated with physical and verbal aggressive behaviour include depression, psychosis, poor physical health, severe cognitive impairment and lack of environmental stimuli. Conditions associated with agitation include pain, overstimulation, social isolation, disruption of usual routines and unmet physical needs related to sleep, thirst, hunger, fatigue or elimination (Morgan et al., 2013).

Although BPSD occurs in almost all people with dementia, these symptoms vary widely and none of these behaviours occur in all people with dementia. Also, manifestations of BPSD change during the course of the illness in each person, and many resolve as dementia progresses. It is not unusual for one or more manifestation of BPSD to resolve at the same time that new ones develop. Because of the wide variability in these symptoms, many people, including health care professionals, hold stereotypes or misunderstandings about BPSD. Remarks such as "I know he doesn't have AD because he doesn't hallucinate" or "I know she doesn't have AD because she's not violent" reflect a false belief that certain difficult behaviours are an inevitable consequence of dementia. Similarly, a question such as "Can you tell if my mother will be the 'nice kind' or the 'mean kind' as her AD gets worse?" indicates the need for accurate information about BPSD. Another consideration is that spouses and other family members may have difficulty distinguishing between long-term personality patterns and behaviours arising from dementia. This is especially challenging when the person with dementia has a history of dysfunctional behaviours (e.g., alcohol abuse, anger management) or unhealthy relationships.

A serious consequence of these misunderstandings is that the symptoms are misinterpreted and causative factors are not addressed. Responsibilities of nurses include dispelling myths and misunderstandings and helping caregivers identify triggers. In addition, it is important to avoid terminology that perpetuates misunderstandings, such as the commonly used term "refuses to…." Table 14-3 summarizes some common misperceptions and related facts about dementia-associated behaviours.

A major nursing responsibility is to look for contributing causes and implement strategies to prevent BPSD or minimize the effects of these behaviours. Common contributing causes include pain, fatigue, physical discomfort, environmental conditions, changes in routine, overstimulation or lack of stimulation. It is also imperative to recognize that behavioural manifestations in people with dementia can be caused, at least in part, by delirium superimposed on dementia, as discussed in the Delirium section. Strategies for addressing behavioural symptoms are discussed in the section on nursing interventions.

Another nursing responsibility, which is consistent with a person-centred approach to care, is to identify the feelings and experiences that the person with dementia is attempting to communicate through his or her behaviour. Results of a study by Dupuis and colleagues (2012) suggest that professionals replace the concept of challenging behaviour with the term *responsive behaviour* in people with dementia. This approach emphasizes that behaviours are meaningful and "moves us away from judging behaviours to *understanding meaning in actions* and responses. It means moving away from a focus on dysfunction, deficit and decline, to recognizing, valuing and believing in the continued abilities of persons with dementia to express their experiences and act in purposeful, meaningful and even intentional ways" (Dupuis et al., 2012, p. 170).

NURSING ASSESSMENT OF DEMENTIA IN OLDER ADULTS

Dementia is a complex syndrome that usually involves a long and fluctuating course that progresses to a terminal phase. Thus, assessment is an ongoing process that focuses on identifying

TABLE 14-3 Misperceptions and Realities About Dementia-Associated Behaviours	
Misperceptions of Behaviours	**Realities**
"He refuses to …"	He has no idea about what is offered; needs to do something else before agreeing to the activity; wants to feel he has a choice; may not have ability to carry out the activity
"She fights me when I …"	She may be experiencing pain or discomfort, which is exacerbated by the activity; she may not understand the activity.
"He denies any problem."	The person may not have insight, awareness or ability to understand.
"There's no reason for him to act that way."	There is usually a triggering event or an unmet need and the behaviour is a way to cope, adapt, respond or express a need
Manipulative, deliberate actions to get attention	The person probably does not have enough insight or intent to be manipulative; may be the only way the person is able to express needs
Nothing to do to prevent the behaviour	Care partners can be proactive in identifying and addressing triggers.
Interventions that were effective in the past will be effective now	If usual interventions no longer work, be flexible, creative and try something else; use a "trial and error" approach by trying variations of interventions that worked

Adapted from Miller, C. A. (2012). *Fast Facts for Dementia Care: What Nurses Need to Know in a Nutshell.* Used with permission from Springer Publishing Company.

conditions that cause negative consequences during the course of dementia. It is also important to identify and address conditions that interfere with the assessment of dementia.

Factors That Influence the Assessment of Dementia

Attitudes, myths and lack of information are risk factors that can interfere with an appropriate assessment of, and interventions for, dementia. In recent years, tremendous progress has been made in understanding and identifying causes of impaired cognitive function; however, many older adults and their families and care partners still view serious cognitive impairments as an expected and normal concomitant of aging. When this happens, treatable conditions are likely to be overlooked, and older adults are denied the appropriate interventions for managing their conditions. Even in the absence of curative treatments, many interventions are effective in delaying the progression of the condition, managing symptoms, assisting with long-term planning and improving quality of life for the person with dementia and his or her care partners.

Cultural factors that influence perceptions about aging and illness can significantly affect both the evaluation and treatment of dementia. For example, some cultural groups accept cognitive impairment as "normal aging," whereas others view dementia-related behaviours as shameful. For example, in one study examining how South Asian Canadians came to a dementia diagnosis, researchers found that South Asian older adults and their caregivers viewed memory loss as normal initially and that caregivers described a longer process of coming to the point of seeking professional help (anywhere from 1 to 4 years after noticing signs of dementia) (McCleary et al., 2013).

Wellness Opportunity

Nurses have many opportunities to teach older adults and their care partners about the importance of evaluating any significant changes in cognitive function.

Initial Assessment

With the exception of delirium and poststroke dementia, manifestations of cognitive impairment develop and progress slowly and an assessment is often delayed until the changes significantly interfere with normal functioning. Because progressive cognitive impairment is a very complex phenomenon, the assessment process generally involves an interprofessional approach, requiring input from primary care providers, psychiatrists, nurses, social workers and rehabilitation therapists. Members of the assessment team must work with the family and other care partners to obtain information and determine the appropriate level of involvement of the cognitively impaired person with regard to discussing assessment results and planning care. The major nursing focus is to determine the person's level of function, to identify the factors that affect the person's level of function and to identify the person's response to his or her illness. Frequently,

the nurse serves as the team leader and is responsible for coordinating information and facilitating communication among team members and with the older adult and his or her family or other care partners. Nurses can use Box 14-4 as a guide for assessing progressive cognitive impairments in older adults.

Box 14-4 Assessing Progressive Cognitive Impairment in Older Adults

General Principles

- Assessment of impaired cognitive function is a long-term process.
- Even though the person with impaired cognitive function may not be a reliable reporter, his or her perceptions should be an integral part of the assessment and the accuracy of information should be validated.
  - The feelings of the person with cognitive impairment should be assessed and acknowledged.
- Health care professionals must respect the person's rights and ask permission before obtaining information from others, including family members.
- Do not assume that the family has drawn accurate conclusions about events of the past (e.g., family members may state that the person retired and then showed cognitive deficits when, in reality, the person retired because of an inability to cope with job demands).

Focus of the Assessment

- The primary purpose of the assessment is to identify the causes of the cognitive impairment.
- An assessment of a person with impaired cognitive function is an interprofessional approach and includes the following components: complete medical history and physical examination including a review of all medications, a functional assessment, a comprehensive psychosocial and formal mental status assessment, and an assessment of environmental and caregiver influences, with particular emphasis on those factors that affect safety and functional abilities.
- The assessment includes an interview with caregivers, family members and other people who can describe the progression of the manifestations of impairment.
- Information about lifelong patterns of personality, coping and performance characteristics is considered in relation to the person's current functional level.
- It may be necessary to ask probing questions to help family members recognize clues to cognitive deficits retrospectively.

Considerations in Assessing Risk Factors Contributing to Impaired Cognitive Function

- Never assume that all cognitive impairments and behavioural manifestations stem from a dementing illness.
- Because risk factors can either cause the initial cognitive impairments or develop later, causing additional impairments, they must be reassessed periodically.
- The following categories of risk factors must be assessed, both initially and on an ongoing basis: depression, physiologic alterations, functional impairments, adverse medication effects, and environmental and psychosocial influences.
- Early in the assessment, ensure that vision and hearing impairments are compensated for as much as possible and that the environment does not interfere with the person's performance (e.g., as possible, make sure the person is using eyeglasses and a hearing aid if needed, and make sure the lighting is optimal).
- A priority is to identify and treat those factors that are reversible before deciding on a long-term management plan.

Ongoing Assessment of Consequences

Because dementia is a progressive condition that commonly coexists with other conditions, all people with dementia require ongoing assessment of all of the following:

- Changes in cognitive and psychosocial function related to the dementia (e.g., a decline in cognitive abilities, the onset of anxiety or depression)
- Changes in mental status related to concurrent conditions (e.g., delirium due to a medical condition or adverse medication effects)
- Changes in functional abilities
- Causes of behavioural changes related to treatable conditions (e.g., anxiety, physical discomfort, environmental factors)

A major goal of ongoing assessment is to identify factors that interfere with the person's level of functioning or quality of life, so that interventions can be initiated to alleviate these contributing factors. Even though dementia is a progressive condition that gradually affects all levels of functioning, some of the changes that occur are caused by concurrent conditions rather than by the dementia itself. Thus, ongoing assessment to identify all factors that affect level of functioning is essential. Another goal of ongoing assessment is to identify the person's strengths and limitations in order to plan individualized interventions to improve the person's functioning and quality of life. One way of assessing strengths and weaknesses is to inquire about the ways in which dementia has affected daily living and how the person has coped with, or adjusted to, these changes. Box 14-5 summarizes some statements of people with dementia about ways of coping and daily living.

Nurses can use Table 14-2 as a guide to assessing the progression of dementia from early to later stages. In addition, the following nursing assessment guides are pertinent to aspects of functioning that are affected in people with dementia:

- Chapter 7, functioning and safety
- Chapter 8, medications Chapter 12, psychosocial function
- Chapter 15, depression
- Chapter 16, hearing
- Chapter 17, vision
- Chapter 18, pain Chapter 19, urinary function
- Chapter 22, fall risk
- Chapter 25, sleep and rest

Online Learning Activity 14-2 provides links to resources for assessing aspects of functioning in people with dementia.

See **ONLINE LEARNING ACTIVITY 14-2: EVIDENCE-BASED TOOLS FOR ASSESSING ASPECTS OF FUNCTIONING IN PEOPLE WITH DEMENTIA** at http://thepoint.lww.com/Miller7e

---

Box 14-5   Lived Experiences: Coping and Daily Living With Dementia

About Ways of Coping

- I think it is all right to allow yourself a bit of time to focus on the pain and fear. That is only human; but it is important to move away from the sad focus and not let it consume you.
- I try to be more patient with myself and forgive myself.
- Staying busy doing what I love to do really keeps me going and gets me through. I'm in two support groups; I have weekly mandolin lesions; I do a weekly men's meditation class with daily homework; I'm reading about consciousness and healing that supports my living in the now and taking care of my spirit.
- I think as long as I can make decisions, I can still go out and sail a boat. Sailing is all about making decisions. If you're racing a yacht, just about every 3 minutes you've got to make a decision, and I have some fantastic crew on my boat who are always going to guide me.
- We have this problem and we can't change that, but we can improve our lives by not letting it just bring us unhappiness 24 hours a day.
- Usually I just slow down and reset my expectations. Expecting that you can be who you used to be is just a recipe for pain and sadness.
- I need to have the knowledge that I'm doing what I can. Because oftentimes it's so subtle, and I curse it every now and then and that helps.
- I ask people not to expect me to remember to do things.
- Ahh! I have a great lack of ease with not remembering things. Oh God, it drives me crazy … but we have to accept what we cannot change.

About Day-to-Day Living

- Tomorrow I'll have little memory of today, and this makes living today like pushing the rock up the hill knowing it will roll back.
- Inertia is a serious problem with me, and sometimes I seem glued to my chair. Likely it's just that it's so much effort to get myself organized to do things, that I'm mentally exhausted before I even start.
- I streamline everything and get rid of everything I don't use very often. Keeping the house clutter-free helps to minimize the time necessary to find misplaced items.
- I try to find ways to compensate. For example, I now use a GPS to help me from getting lost when I drive.
- My brother-in-law removed all my cabinet doors in my kitchen so I can see all my food in my pantry when I walk into my kitchen.
- I do the shopping, and my wife does these beautiful lists and they're in order of where everything is in the shop.
- I think it would be better if I did not drive; and actually mentally, it is much better that I make that decision than somebody makes that decision for me. Psychologically, it is very good that I am actually in a position where they said, "OK you can drive," and just left it at that, and I turned around and said, "Well, thanks very much, but I am actually not going to drive."

Sources: Alzheimer's Society. (2008). *Dementia: Out of the shadows*. London, England: Author; Alzheimer's Society. (2010). *My name is not dementia: People with dementia discuss quality of life*. London, England: Author; Beard, R. L., & Fox, P. J. (2008). Resisting social disenfranchisement: Negotiating collective identities and everyday life with memory loss. *Social Science & Medicine, 66*, 1509–1520; Beard, R. L., Knauss, J., & Moyer, D. (2009). Managing disability and enjoying life: How we reframe dementia through personal narratives. *Journal of Aging Studies, 23*, 227–235; Clare, L., Rowlands, J. M., & Quin, R. (2008). Collective strength: The impact of developing a shared social identity in early-stage dementia. *Dementia, 7*(1), 9–30; Fetherstonhaugh, D., Tarzia, L., & Nay, R. (2013). Being central to decision making means I am still here!: The essence of decision making for people with dementia. *Journal of Aging Studies, 27*, 143–150.

Wellness Opportunity

Nurses promote wellness by identifying factors that support optimal functioning rather than focusing only on those that are problematic.

NURSING DIAGNOSIS

A nursing diagnosis commonly used for people with dementia is Chronic Confusion, defined as "irreversible, long-standing, and/or progressive deterioration of intellect and personality characterized by decreased ability to interpret environmental stimuli and decreased capacity for intellectual thought processes, and manifested by disturbances of memory, orientation, and behaviour" (Herdman, 2012, p. 265). Additional nursing diagnoses that are applicable to functional consequences associated with psychosocial responses to dementia include Fear, Anxiety, Risk for Compromised Human Dignity, Impaired Memory, Impaired Social Interaction, Self-Esteem Disturbance and Ineffective Coping. During the later stages when dementia affects the person's functional abilities, applicable nursing diagnoses include Wandering, Imbalanced Nutrition, Urinary Incontinence, Self-Care Deficit, Impaired Verbal communication, Risk for Falls, Risk for Injury, Disturbed Sensory Perception and Disturbed Sleep Pattern.

Nursing diagnoses also address the needs of caregivers because much of the care of people with dementia focuses on helping the family and other caregivers address the day-to-day needs and issues of the person with dementia. Nursing diagnoses that might be used to address caregiver needs include Stress Overload, Compromised Family Coping and Caregiver Role Strain (or Risk for Caregiver Role Strain). During all stages of dementia, but particularly the later stages of dementia, the nursing diagnosis Anticipatory Grieving may be appropriate, particularly for spousal caregivers.

> ### Wellness Opportunity
>
> Readiness for Enhanced Coping is a wellness nursing diagnosis that nurses can apply for people with dementia, as well as their caregivers.

PLANNING FOR WELLNESS OUTCOMES

During all stages of dementia, nursing care is directed toward promoting the highest level of functioning, while also supporting the highest quality of life. Nurses can apply the following NOC terminology to address the needs of people with dementia: Agitation Level, Cognition, Cognitive Orientation, Comfort Status, Communication, Coping, Leisure Participation, Memory, Mood Equilibrium, Nutritional Status, Quality of Life, Self-Care Status, Sleep, Social Interaction Skills and Symptom Control.

When friends, family members or paid caregivers care for the person with dementia, nurses plan outcomes to promote caregiver wellness. In the early stages of dementia, the foremost needs of care partners might be for information about the disease and about resources that address the changing needs of the person with dementia and all those involved. As the dementia progresses, caregivers are likely to need emotional support and practical assistance. That being said, caregivers often need emotional and informational

Box 14-6   Evidence-Informed Nursing Practice

Background: When families receive a diagnosis of AD, one or more family members assume the role of caregiver. This is a transition that requires learning and assuming new responsibilities.

Questions: What is the level of preparedness for caregiving, knowledge of formal support services, informal support and psychological distress experienced by new caregivers?

Method: The researchers conducted a multisite study examining the above questions with French-speaking caregivers in Quebec. Using standardized questionnaires, they interviewed 122 caregivers whose family members had received a diagnosis of AD in the past 9 months. Ninety-seven of the caregivers were women and 25 were men, and the mean age of the caregivers was 61 years.

Findings: Seventy percent of caregivers reported receiving low emotional support from family members. Furthermore, over 96% of caregivers stated that they received a low level of informational and instrumental support. Almost 40% of caregivers admitted to being not at all prepared or not very prepared for caregiving. While most caregivers denied experiencing psychological distress associated with caregiving, women were much more likely to report distress than were men.

Implications for Nursing Practice: Nurses should be particularly attuned to the emotional, informational and instrumental needs of caregivers in the early months following a diagnosis of AD in a family member. Addressing these needs may facilitate the transition to the caregiver role for family members of those with AD.

Source: Ducharme, F., Levesque, L., Lachance, L., et al. (2011). Challenges associated with transition to caregiver role following diagnostic disclosure of Alzheimer disease: A descriptive study. *International Journal of Nursing Studies, 48,* 1109–1119.

support at all stages of their family member's illness (see Box 14-6). Some NOC terms that are pertinent to caregivers include Anxiety Level, Caregiver Emotional Health, Caregiver Lifestyle Disruption, Caregiver–Patient Relationship, Caregiver Physical Health, Caregiver Role Endurance, Caregiver Stressors and Caregiver Well-Being.

> ### Wellness Opportunity
>
> Hope is an NOC that would be applicable when nurses plan wellness outcomes to address body–mind–spirit needs of both people with dementia and their caregivers.

NURSING INTERVENTIONS TO ADDRESS DEMENTIA

Information about interventions to address dementia is evolving at a rapid pace, and research by nurses and other health care professionals is shedding light on appropriate interventions for managing the functional consequences. Many interventions, such as reassurance for anxiety and confusion and redirection for unsafe or inappropriate behaviours, are applicable to all people with dementia and are individualized according to specific manifestations. Similarly, health promotion interventions, such as exercise and nutrition, are applicable for primary and secondary prevention in all people with dementia. Because a major focus of research is on identifying interventions specifically to address BPSD, information about interventions for dementia-related behaviours is presented in this section. In addition, because caregivers are an essential component of interventions at all stages of dementia, information about addressing needs of caregivers is also discussed.

Another major consideration about interventions for dementia is that nurses have key roles in planning and implementing interventions, but effective care for people with dementia requires consistent and significant input from many health care professionals and other care partners. Thus, it is imperative to address nursing interventions in the context of comprehensive, interprofessional and person-centred approach to the complex issues related to dementia. Because a comprehensive discussion of interventions for dementia is beyond the scope of this chapter, the topic is addressed by reviewing theoretical frameworks, applying general principles in different clinical settings, and giving an overview of nursing interventions that are applicable in all settings. Online Learning Activity 14-3 provides a link to a podcast related to nursing care of older adults with dementia.

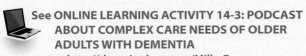

See **ONLINE LEARNING ACTIVITY 14-3: PODCAST ABOUT COMPLEX CARE NEEDS OF OLDER ADULTS WITH DEMENTIA** at http://thepoint.lww.com/Miller7e

Examples of NIC terminologies that may be applicable to caring for people with dementia include Active Listening, Activity Therapy, Anxiety Reduction, Behaviour Management, Calming Technique, Dementia Management, Elopement Precautions, Emotional Support, Environmental Management, Exercise Promotion, Fall Prevention, Humour, Memory Training, Milieu Therapy, Music Therapy, Presence, Reality Orientation, Reminiscence Therapy, Self-Care Assistance, Spiritual Support and Touch. Nurses can use the following NIC terms when they address caregiver needs: Anticipatory Guidance, Caregiver Support, Consultation, Coping Enhancement, Counselling, Decision-Making Support, Humour, Referral, Respite Care, Relaxation Therapy, Spiritual Growth Facilitation and Teaching.

Wellness Opportunity

Hope Inspiration is an NIC that nurses address when they help people with dementia and their caregivers to identify a positive meaning for their situation.

Teaching About Medications for Dementia

In 1993, the Food and Drug Administration (FDA) in the United States approved the first medication for the treatment of AD (Tacrine). However, it was never approved in Canada and, due to its hepatotoxicity, it is rarely given in westernized countries (Organization for Economic Co-operation and Development [OECD], 2004). By 2001, three additional cholinesterase inhibitors had been approved in Canada and the United States: donepezil (Aricept), rivastigmine (Exelon) and

galantamine (Razadyne, formerly called Reminyl) (OECD, 2004). These three cholinesterase inhibitors have become standard treatment for *mild to moderate* AD. In 2003, memantine (Namenda) became the first medication approved for treatment of *moderate to severe* AD. The physiologic action of this medication, which differs from that of cholinesterase inhibitors, blocks the neural toxicity associated with excess release of glutamate. These four drugs can reduce symptoms and slow the rate of decline in some patients with dementia, but they do not modify the underlying pathology. Reviews of research emphasize the importance of individualizing the selection and dose of medications, frequently assessing for adverse effects and including nonpharmacologic interventions as integral parts of care plans (Gomoll et al., 2014).

The usual pharmacologic approach is to begin a cholinesterase inhibitor before or during the moderate stage of dementia and to add memantine during the moderate or later stages. These drugs are usually started at a low dose, which is increased gradually if it is well tolerated. The most common adverse effects of cholinesterase inhibitors are nausea, vomiting, diarrhea, weight loss and loss of appetite. Cholinesterase inhibitors can also cause bradycardia and result in hospitalization (Park-Wyllie et al., 2009). Adverse effects of memantine include dizziness, headache, constipation and increased confusion.

It is important to recognize that in 2014 no disease-modifying drug was available in North America, despite intense and ongoing research related to the development of drugs for dementia during the past several decades (Anand et al., 2014). The Alzheimer Society of Canada (2014) emphasizes the importance of nonpharmacologic interventions for promoting wellness and enhancing quality of life for people with dementia, as discussed in the following sections.

Nonpharmaceutical Interventions for Promoting Wellness in People With Dementia

As anyone who has cared for a person with dementia knows, interventions must be highly individualized and frequently modified. An intervention that works for one person may not work for others, and interventions that are effective one day will not necessarily be effective the next day. A dominant theme of research and practice is the implementation of person-centred interventions that are based on a comprehensive and ongoing assessment of the person's unique and changing needs. These nonpharmaceutical interventions can enhance the lives of individuals with dementia. However, it should be noted that they do not "cure" dementia for those already affected, neither do they positively prevent dementia; for instance, while exercise and reading may reduce the risk of dementia in *some people*, others may live healthy lifestyles, remain active and engaged in life and still develop dementia (Alzheimer's Association, 2014).

One way in which nurses promote wellness for people with dementia is by addressing concerns that improve quality of life. Dementia can affect all the following aspects of quality of life for people with dementia: health, independence, self-determination, social interaction, financial security, psychological well-being, security and privacy, religion and spirituality, and being of use or giving meaning to life. An essential intervention for promoting wellness is to pay careful attention to the verbal and nonverbal ways in which the person with dementia communicates his or her needs and feelings. Box 14-7 provides statements of people with dementia about their needs and quality of life.

Another way of promoting wellness for people with dementia is through interventions that support the person's strengths and individuality during all stages of dementia by providing person-centred care, as described in the following sections. Nurses also promote wellness through interventions that support optimal levels of functioning because at least some of the functional decline associated with dementia can be categorized as **excess disability**, which is defined as limitations that are beyond what is to be expected. As an example, when caregivers provide unnecessary assistance with tasks such as eating or dressing, people with dementia may lose

their ability for self-care sooner than if they had performed the tasks with the necessary direction from caregivers. Environmental factors that do not support optimal functioning of people with dementia are another source of excess disability (Slaughter & Hayduk, 2012). Another major focus of current research is on nonpharmacologic interventions to improve functioning and quality of life for people with dementia and their care partners, as described in Table 14-4. Nurses can facilitate referrals for these interventions, which are particularly important during early and moderate stages of dementia. These interventions address aspects of functioning and quality of life, but they are not necessarily applicable to addressing dementia-related behaviours, which are discussed in a separate section.

Wellness Opportunity

Nurses holistically address behavioural symptoms by trying to identify nonpharmacologic interventions that improve quality of life for the person with dementia and his or her caregivers.

Box 14-7 Lived Experiences: Needs and Quality of Life

About Needs

- Just explain it a bit more, like when he said, "I will refer you to the memory clinic," you know, another two or three sentences. I just want to put you in the picture as to what will go on there, what it's for, what the setup is.
- My independence is really important to me, and I know if someone came in and started telling me how I should run things or do things, I would certainly retaliate and not conform to anything they would want to do.
- As you have been diagnosed, there should be a follow-up with information on what you have got, how you cope with it, what to look for and what's gonna happen.

About Quality of Life

- Quality of life is living with your family—your circle of friends and family.
- Friendship is good. It's very important to have friends.
- Oh there's nothing better than peace and quiet to be happy and comfortable, but if you ain't got peace, you're upset, and when you've got peace and quiet, you don't have anything in the mind.
- To feel safe. I've lived here for about 2 years and feel secure and safe. No accidents. This is important.
- I want to keep my own environment … because I am familiarized with it.
- It's not just the environment in the house, it's when you go out … in the bank, environment in the shops you go into, or restaurants is another environment, which you have got to overcome.
- I think your physical health is very important because even though I've got problems in myself, with my brain through my vascular dementia, I feel that if you have got your physical fitness then it still gives you that form of independence that you can still do things. Like I can still go to the bathroom and shave, where if you haven't got good health and you start having problems as well, it must be horrendous.

Sources: Alzheimer's Society. (2008). *Dementia: Out of the shadows*. London, England: Author; Alzheimer's Society. (2010). *My name is not dementia: People with dementia discuss quality of life*. London, England: Author; Fetherstonhaugh, D., Tarzia, L., & Nay, R. (2013). Being central to decision making means I am still here!: The essence of decision making for people with dementia. *Journal of Aging Studies, 27*, 143–150..

Improving Safety and Function Through Environmental Modifications

Environmental modifications are important interventions for people with dementia because environmental factors profoundly affect their safety, functioning and quality of life. Current emphasis is on the influence of all following aspects of the total physical and psychosocial environment:

- Noise
- Music
- Floor surfaces
- Colours and colour contrast
- Lighting (e.g., glare, shadows, brightness)
- Design and placement of exits and bathrooms
- Living things (e.g., plants, birds, fish, pets)
- Furniture (seating, placement, heights of tables and chairs)
- Safety devices (e.g., rails, grab bars)
- Provisions for privacy and social interaction
- Items that improve comfort and hominess (e.g., decorative items, textured items, meaningful personal belongings)
- Absence of potentially harmful items (e.g., clutter, obstacles, sharp knives, cleaning solutions and other potentially toxic products).

Box 14-8 summarizes environmental interventions and techniques to address safety and independence in ADLs.

Wellness Opportunity

Nurses promote emotional wellness by encouraging older adults with dementia to talk about happy memories of earlier years and by affirming the pleasant feelings the person experiences when recalling these events.

Communicating With Older Adults With Dementia

Verbal and nonverbal communication techniques are widely recognized as essential interventions for people with dementia throughout the entire course of the disease. Nurses need to

TABLE 14-4 Research on Nonpharmacologic Interventions for People With Dementia

Intervention	Results	References
Reviews of studies[a] related to exercise programs for people with dementia	Regular exercise interventions can improve mood, behaviour and functioning in people with dementia; some, but not all, studies show that participation in regular exercise is associated with improved cognitive function in people with dementia.	Amoyal and Fallon (2012), Forbes et al. (2013) and Kirk-Sanchez and McGough (2014)
Cochrane review[a] of studies of reality orientation as a form of cognitive stimulation	Consistent evidence shows that reality orientation is a beneficial form of cognitive stimulation for people with mild to moderate dementia	Woods et al. (2012)
Research reviews[a] on cognitive stimulation for mild cognitive impairment	Reviews of studies indicate that people with mild cognitive impairment and dementia can benefit from cognitive rehabilitation strategies such as memory aids and visual imagery.	Cotelli et al. (2012), Hopper et al. (2013) and Simon et al. (2012)
Meta-analysis review[a] of 23 studies on nonpharmacologic interventions for behavioural manifestations of dementia in community-living people with dementia	Support and educational sessions (in-person and by telephone) for caregivers using multiple components over 3 to 6 months are effective for addressing behaviours such as agitation, aggression, depression and repetitive behaviours	Brodaty and Arasaratnam (2012)
Learning Therapy: cognitive intervention using reading and arithmetic tasks carried out for 15 to 20 minutes 5 days weekly	Improved and sustained cognitive function after 6 months, compared with control group	Kawashima (2013)
Watermemories Swimming Club: 45-minute classes twice weekly for 12 weeks for people with dementia	Positive effects on quality of life, social interactions and functional abilities (no control group)	Neville et al. (2013)
Leisure activities 3 times per week for 12 weeks, 110 nursing home residents, with outcome measures at baseline and 3, 6 and 9 months	Residents in mah-jongg group (for cognitive stimulation) showed slower rate of global decline compared with control group.	Cheng et al. (2014)
Qualitative study of music-based interventions for residents of a care home	Music is important during all stages of dementia for reducing behavioural and psychological symptoms and promoting interpersonal connectedness.	McDermott et al. (2014)

[a]Italics differentiate research reviews from individual studies.

Box 14-8 Environmental Adaptations and Techniques for Improving Safety and Functioning in People With Dementia

General Environmental Modifications

- Modify the environment to compensate as much as possible for sensory deficits and other functional impairments. (Refer to interventions in Chapters 16 through 19 and 22.)
- Use clocks, calendars, daily newspapers and simple written cues for orientation (e.g., day, date, names, place, events).
- Use simple pictures, written cues or colour codes for identifying items and places (e.g., toilet, bedroom).
- Use simple written cues to clarify directions for operating radios, televisions, appliances and thermostats (e.g., on, off, directional arrows).
- Place pictures of familiar people in highly visible places, but use nonglossy pictures and nonglare glass in picture frames.
- Turn lights on as soon as, or before, it gets dark.
- Use nightlights, or leave dim lights on during the night.
- Provide adequate environmental stimuli while avoiding overstimulation.

Techniques to Ensure Safety

- Make sure the person carries some form of identification along with the phone number for someone to call.
- Adapt the environment for safety (e.g., use alarm devices on doors to prevent wandering).
- Keep the environment uncluttered.
- Keep medications, cleaning solutions and any poisonous chemicals in inaccessible places.

- Enrol the person in a protective program, such as the Safely Home—Alzheimer Wandering Registry Program through the Alzheimer Society of Canada and the RCMP.

Techniques to Facilitate Independent Performance of ADLs

- Keep all activities as simple and routine as possible.
- Establish routines that allow for maximum independence and the least amount of frustration.
- While keeping the routines as consistent as possible, recognize that they will have to be changed as the person's level of function changes.
- Lay out one set of clothing in the order in which the items are to be donned.
- If the person needs assistance with hygiene, use matter-of-fact statements such as "It's time for your bath."
- Arrange personal care items, such as grooming and hygiene aids, in a visible and uncluttered place, in the order in which the items are to be used.
- Leave a toothbrush on the bathroom sink with toothpaste already on it.
- Establish an individualized toileting plan that allows for maximum independence but minimal risk for incontinence episodes.
- Offer finger foods and nutritious snacks if the person will not sit at the table to eat a meal.

Box 14-9 Facilitating Communication With People Who Have Dementia

Verbal Communication

- Adapt your level of communication to the abilities of the person with dementia.
- Simplify sentences according to the person's ability to process information.
- Present only one idea at a time.
- Allow enough time for processing.
- Avoid infantilization (e.g., do not use baby talk or employ a demeaning or condescending tone of voice).
- Assist with word finding (e.g., supply missing words, repeat the person's sentence with the correct word).
- Avoid shaming the person (e.g., do not emphasize deficits).
- Paraphrase what the person says, and ask for clarification about the meaning.
- If the person does not understand a statement, repeat the statement using the same words, or simplify the wording.
- Do not argue with the person, unless it is a matter of safety.
- Avoid complex or sarcastic humour.
- Use positive statements (i.e., avoid using statements containing the word "don't" or other negative commands).
- Involve the person with decisions to the best of his or her ability by offering simple and concrete choices (e.g., "Do you want chicken or steak?" rather than "What do you want to eat?").
- Do not ask questions that you know the person cannot answer correctly.
- Do not test the person's memory unnecessarily.
- Listen to the feelings the person is trying to express and respond to the feelings, rather than the statement.
- When discussing activities of daily living (ADLs), avoid statements, such as "You need a bath now," which may be interpreted as judgmental.

Nonverbal Communication

- Attract and maintain the person's attention (e.g., through eye contact, pleasant facial expressions).
- Use a relaxed and smiling approach.
- Reinforce verbal communication with appropriate nonverbal communication (e.g., demonstrate what you are asking the person to do).
- Use simple pictures rather than written cues.
- Use appropriate touch for communication (e.g., to gain the person's attention or reinforce feelings of concern), unless the person responds negatively to touch.
- Be aware of your own nonverbal communication.
- Keep in mind that your nonverbal cues will probably communicate more than your spoken words and will not necessarily be interpreted correctly.
- Closely observe all nonverbal cues exhibited by the person, particularly those that express feelings.
- Assume that all nonverbal expressions of the person with dementia are attempts to communicate needs or feelings.

See **ONLINE LEARNING ACTIVITY 14-4: ARTICLE ABOUT IMPROVING COMMUNICATION WITH PATIENTS WITH DEMENTIA** at http://thepoint.lww.com/Miller7e

Interventions for Dementia-Related Behaviours

Health care professionals increasingly recognize that dementia-related behaviours reflect an attempt to communicate needs that the person may not consciously recognize and cannot express verbally. Thus, nurses must direct their interventions toward the underlying needs of the person with dementia. Hall and Buckwalter (1987) proposed a theoretical framework for addressing dementia-related behaviours called the *progressively lowered stress threshold* (PLST) model. Briefly stated, this model posits that dysfunctional behaviours indicate a progressive lowering of the stress threshold, which in turn, interferes with the person's functioning and ability to interact with the environment. Common stressors associated with dysfunctional episodes are fatigue; change of environment, routine or caregiver; misleading stimuli or inappropriate stimulus levels; internal or external demands that exceed functional capacity; physical stressors (e.g., pain, illness, depression) and affective response to loss. The goal of nursing care, then, is to maximize the person's function by relieving stressors that cause excess disability. The choice of interventions is based on an ongoing assessment of anxiety "as a barometer to determine how much activity and stimuli the anxious person can tolerate at any point during their illness. As anxious behaviours occur, activities and environmental stimuli are modified and simplified until the anxiety disappears" (Hall & Buckwalter, 1987, p. 403). This approach (summarized in Box 14-10) is highly individualized; from a nursing perspective, it is analogous to adjusting insulin doses for people with diabetes according to serum glucose levels. Box 14-11 summarizes statements of people

Box 14-10 Nursing Interventions for People With Dementia on the Basis of the Progressively Lowered Stress Threshold Model (PLST)

- Maximize safety by modifying the environment to compensate for cognitive losses.
- Control any factors that increase stress, such as fatigue; physical stressors; competing or overwhelming stimuli; changes in routine, caregiver or environment; and activities or demands that exceed the person's functional ability.
- Plan and maintain a consistent routine.
- Implement regular rest periods to compensate for fatigue and loss of reserve energy.
- Provide unconditional positive regard.
- Remain nonjudgmental about the appropriateness of all behaviours except those that present threats to safety.
- Recognize individual expressions of fatigue, anxiety and increasing stress and intervene to reduce stressors as soon as possible.
- Modify reality orientation and other therapeutic interventions to incorporate only that information needed for safe function.
- Use reassuring forms of therapy, such as music and reminiscence.

Source: Hall, G. R., & Buckwalter, K. C. (1987). Progressively lowered stress threshold: A conceptual model for care of adults with Alzheimer's disease. *Archives of Psychiatric Nursing, 1,* 399–406.

pay particular attention to the effects of touch, facial expressions, tone of voice and body language on communication. Box 14-9 summarizes techniques for facilitating communication with people with dementia. These techniques are general guidelines, and it is important to adapt communication to the particular needs of each person with dementia. Online Learning Activity 14-4 provides a link to an article about improving communication with patients with dementia.

Box 14-11 Lived Experiences: Experiences and Feelings About Needing Help From Others and Being Part of a Support Group

About Needing Help From Others

- When the day comes that I have got to start asking for help and if that independence is taken away, then I would like to think that I could still be consulted and still have some say in my independence.
- It is very beneficial, when I am unable to verbalize what I want, for my wife to display multiple options and allow me to choose one.
- If all else fails, I rely on my partner and my family to come up with solutions I cannot solve.
- I think it would be nice if people gave you the courtesy of time to finish what you are trying to say.
- You can't do what you want. You have to ask. So you have to adjust your schedule to someone else's. I guess the best word for it is that it is somewhat humiliating to be in that position when you're used to running your own life.
- I'm slower at making decisions, and I'm slower on purpose. And I talk to more people about it before I would do it. I'm quite dependent on my wife because I can't do most things independently any more.
- Before, I'd take a walk around the block rather than blow my stack. By the time I got back, my feet hurt so much that I quit worrying about what I was mad about. Now my husband will go with me, and that doesn't do it.

About Being Part of a Support Group

- Since it is difficult to maintain my old social networks, I reach out to others online through e-mail groups and chat rooms for people with dementia. These can be real life-savers some days.
- It is that bit of extra that you know these people are having the same problems and *really* understand.
- I commiserate with my friends going through the same things.
- When I've gotten real down, it seems as though my failure in things I do is exaggerated many times. I feel as though my power has been lost to do anything about it. I feel hopeless and helpless. Thank God for my chat group sticking with me to crawl out.
- I participate in the group in hopes that people with dementia will begin to be treated with more respect and dignity and to help others recognize how much coping we must do to accomplish even simple things throughout a normal day.
- I have always been a person who has wanted to make a difference in the world, and through the group, I feel I have been able to change a small part of the way some people think about early-stage dementia.
- Let's work together to change paradigms about what persons with dementia can and can't do. Don't limit us—help us push the envelopes of our new abilities.
- The benefits to me personally are so important, as I can still feel that I am a valuable contributing member of society, even though I'm "cognitively disabled."
- Today I have met people who are in very much the same boat as I am with things they can and can't do, so for me it's a relief to find that there are others in the same boat.

Sources: Alzheimer's Society. (2010). *My name is not dementia: People with dementia discuss quality of life.* London, England: Author; Beard, R. L., & Fox, P. J. (2008). Resisting social disenfranchisement: Negotiating collective identities and everyday life with memory loss. *Social Science & Medicine, 66,* 1509–1520; Beard, R. L., Knauss, J., & Moyer, D. (2009). Managing disability and enjoying life: How we reframe dementia through personal narratives. *Journal of Aging Studies, 23,* 227–235; Clare, L., Rowlands, J. M., & Quin, R. (2008). Collective strength: The impact of developing a shared social identity in early-stage dementia. *Dementia, 7*(1), 9–30; Fetherstonhaugh, D., Tarzia, L., & Nay, R. (2013). Being central to decision making means I am still here!: The essence of decision making for people with dementia. *Journal of Aging Studies, 27,* 143–150.

---

with dementia about their lived experiences related to needing help from others and being part of a support group.

Decisions about the use of psychotropic medications for dementia-related disruptive behaviours are complex for several reasons. First, because dementia-related behaviours are often precipitated by modifiable factors, including medical conditions, environmental influences and adverse medication effects (e.g., anticholinergic medications), initial interventions should always address any contributing factors. For example, if behaviours are due to the adverse effects of medications, initial interventions focus on eliminating or reducing the dose. Second, there is always a risk that medications will further interfere with function and perhaps even cause serious harm, such as further reduction in cognitive function or increased risk for falls. A third consideration is whether the behaviours justify the risks associated with medications. Bothersome or socially inappropriate behaviours may best be ignored or tolerated than treated with medications. However, if the behaviour is unsafe, uncomfortable or interferes with the function of the person with dementia or the rights or safety of others, then pharmaceutical intervention may be appropriate, but only if other interventions are not successful. In any situation, health care professionals should view behaviour-modifying medications as one component of a comprehensive management plan that addresses the complex nature of dementia-related behaviours.

Although antipsychotics have been used for the management of dementia-related behaviours for many decades, there is increasing concerns about serious adverse effects and lack of effectiveness in people with dementia. Concerns about safety of so-called first-generation antipsychotics (e.g., haloperidol) led to increased use of newer antipsychotics (called atypical antipsychotics), including olanzapine (Zyprexa), quetiapine (Seroquel) and risperidone (Risperdal). Current systematic reviews of studies conducted since 2000 indicate that all types of antipsychotics are associated with safety risks, including increased risk of death (e.g., Gareri et al., 2014; Langballe et al., 2013; Seitz et al., 2013). In fact, in 2005, Health Canada issued a warning about the use of atypical antipsychotics in older adults with dementia due to increased mortality rates. Because no medication is both safe and consistently more effective than nonpharmacologic interventions for BPSD, there is much support for nonpharmacologic approaches. Smith and colleagues (2013) described a major 3-year project funded by the Agency for Healthcare Research and Quality that culminated in the development of an evidence-based algorithm and guidelines related to treating problem behaviours in nursing home residents without the use of antipsychotic medications (see Box 14-12 for more information). Online Learning Activity 14-5 provides a link to additional evidence-based resources from this project and other major initiatives addressing problem behaviours in people with dementia.

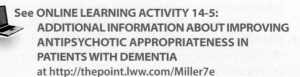

See ONLINE LEARNING ACTIVITY 14-5:
ADDITIONAL INFORMATION ABOUT IMPROVING ANTIPSYCHOTIC APPROPRIATENESS IN PATIENTS WITH DEMENTIA
at http://thepoint.lww.com/Miller7e

Box 14-12 Non-Drug Management of Problem Behaviors and Psychosis in Dementia

Step 1: Assess & Treat Contributing Factors

FOCUS on one behavior at a time

- Note how often, how bad, how long, & document specific details
- **Ask:** What is really going on? What is causing the problem behavior? What is making it worse?

IDENTIFY what leads to or triggers problems

- **Physical:** pain, infection, hunger/thirst, other needs?
- **Psychological:** loneliness, boredom, nothing to do?
- **Environment:** too much/too little going on; lost?
- **Psychiatric:** depression, anxiety, psychosis?

REDUCE, ELIMINATE things that lead to or trigger the problems

- Treat medical/physical problems
- Offer pain medications for comfort or to help cooperation
- Address emotional needs: reassure, encourage, engage
- Offer enjoyable activities to do alone, 1:1, small group
- Remove or disguise misleading objects
- Redirect away from people or areas that lead to problems
- Try another approach; try again later
- Find out what works for others; get someone to help

DOCUMENT outcomes

- If the behavior is reduced or manageable, go to Step 3
- If the behavior persists, go to Step 2

Step 2: Seleect & Apply Interventions

CONSIDER retained abilities, preferences, resources

- Cognitive level
- Physical functional level
- Long-standing personality, life history, interests
- Preferred personal routines, daily schedules
- Personal/family/facility resources

DEVELOP a Person-Centered plan

- Adjust caregiver approaches
- Adapt/change the environment
- Select/use best evidence-based interventions tailored to the person's unique needs/interests/abilities

ADJUST your approach to the person

- **Personal approach:** cue, prompt, remind, distract; focus on person's wishes, interests, concerns; use/avoid touch as indicated. Do not try to reason, teach new routines, or ask to "try harder."

- **Daily routines:** simplify tasks and put them in a regular order; offer limited choices; use long-standing patterns & preferences to guide routines & activities
- **Communication style:** simple words and phrases; speak in short sentences; speak clearly; wait for answers; make eye contact; monitor tone of voice and body language
- **Unconditional positive regard:** do not confront, challenge or explain misbeliefs (hallucinations, delusions, illusions); accept belief as real to the person; reassure, comfort, and distract

ADAPT or CHANGE the environment

- **Eliminate things that lead to confusion:** clutter, TV, radio, noise, people talking; reflections in mirrors/dark windows; misunderstood pictures or decor
- **Reduce things that cause stress:** caffeine; extra people; holiday decorations; public TV
- **Adjust stimulation:** if overstimulated–reduce noise, activity, and confusion; if under-stimulated (bored)–increase activity and involvement
- **Help with functioning:** signs, cues, pictures help way-finding; increase lighting to reduce misinterpretation
- **Involve in meaningful activities:** personalized program of 1:1 and small group or large group as needed
- **Change the setting:** secure outdoor areas; decorative objects; objects to touch and hold; homelike features; smaller, divided recreational and dining areas; natural and bright light; spa-like bathing facilities; signs to help way-finding

SELECT and USE evidence-based interventions

- Work with the team to fit the intervention to the person
- Check care plan for additional information
- Contact supervisor with problems/issues

Step 3: Monitor Outcomes & Adjust Course as Needed

- Track behavior problems using rating scale(s)
- Assure adequate "dose" (intensity, duration, frequency) of interventions
- Adapt/add interventions as needed to get the best possible outcomes
- Make sure all people working with the person understand and cooperate with the treatment plan and are trained as needed

Reprinted with permission from Carnahan, R., Smith, M., Reist, J., et al. (2012). *Improving antipsychotic appropriateness in dementia patients*. POGOe—Portal of Geriatrics Online Education. Available from: http://www.pogoe.org/productid/21209. Also available at: https://www.healthcare.uiowa.edu/igec/iaadapt/

Considerations for Non-Alzheimer Dementia

As already mentioned, more information is available for AD than for other types of dementia. However, information specific to other types of dementia is increasingly becoming available, particularly for Lewy body dementia, as in the following considerations that pertain to nursing care:

- Use anticholinergic medications (e.g., antipsychotics and benzodiazepines) with caution, and only in very low doses.
- Assess for physiologic disorders at the first sign of changes in behaviour because people with Lewy body dementia decompensate more when they have a medical condition.
- Assess for signs of autonomic nervous system dysfunction affecting swallowing, digestion, blood pressure, temperature regulation and bowel and bladder control.

- Consider referrals for occupational and physical therapy because movement and balance disorders occur early in the disease.

A consideration related to vascular dementia is that management of cardiovascular risk factors (e.g., lipids, blood pressure, lifestyle interventions) is an integral part of the treatment plan.

General Principles of Nursing Interventions in Different Settings

In recent years, there has been increasing implementation of multifaceted models of care for people with dementia in long-term care settings, including assisted living and nursing facilities. Some nursing facilities have specially designed dementia special care units (SCUs) and some assisted living facilities are designed specifically for the care of people with dementia. Essential features of these units for cognitively impaired residents include environmental modifications, family involvement, individualized care plans, dementia-specific activity programs and specially trained and selected staff. Some nursing homes incorporate these features into all nursing care units and address the individualized needs of the residents. Long-term residential facilities typically address the needs of people who are in moderate to severe stages of dementia, although some residents are in the early stages. Box 14-13 summarizes statements of people with moderate to severe dementia in a residential care home about their experiences.

Older adults with dementia are frequently admitted to acute care settings for evaluation and treatment of medical or behavioural problems that are superimposed on the dementia. Consequently, nurses in hospital settings usually deal not only with the acute illness but also with the dementia-related behaviours, which are exacerbated by the medical problem, the hospital environment, the unfamiliar caregivers and the change in routines. Thus, nurses in acute care settings face a tremendous challenge in caring for people with dementia.

One of the most important initial interventions is to involve at least one of the older adult's usual caregivers in planning and implementing care focused for the cognitively impaired person. Although the person with dementia is likely to exhibit different behaviours in the hospital than at home, it is crucial to identify interventions that were effective in the home environment. Because people with moderate to severe dementia may not be able to express their needs verbally, nurses need to obtain information from family caregivers who understand how the person expresses needs. During the admission process, nurses may save a lot of time and frustration by interviewing the caregivers about specific methods that help or hinder care. Figure 14-3 illustrates a form that can be used to obtain helpful information from family caregivers. Information about this form and additional information related to care of hospitalized patients with dementia is available through the link to Nurses Improving Care for Healthsystem Elders in Online Learning Activity 14-6.

Another strategy for addressing the needs of patients who have dementia is to involve the caregiver in care tasks such as feeding or to ask him or her to provide a familiar presence during the hospitalization. Despite a need for respite from caregiving responsibilities, family and other caregivers may be willing to provide assistance and guidance. This may be particularly helpful during the first few days of hospitalization, and with patients who are particularly difficult to manage. Assessment and intervention tools for addressing the needs of hospitalized people with dementia, including cost-free videos demonstrating the application of these tools, are available at the websites listed in Online Learning Activity 14-6.

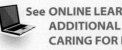

See **ONLINE LEARNING ACTIVITY 14-6:**
ADDITIONAL INFORMATION ABOUT
CARING FOR HOSPITALIZED PATIENTS WITH
DEMENTIA
at http://thepoint.lww.com/Miller7e

Box 14-13 Lived Experiences: People With Moderate to Severe Dementia in Residential Care Homes

I Still Am Somebody

- I can remember all those things, and they come back. And I know I can't do them now, but if I think about them, I'm sort of living them again, so that's really nice.
- Well, I ebb and flow a bit because I'm older and I've had heart trouble for years, so I think, really, I do ever so well. I've got no complaints at all.
- I used to do a lot. I may get back to it, and particularly if we get a nice spring sort of thing, it might be better for me.
- I'm thankful for what I can do, you know what I mean? I won't give in.

Nothing's Right Now

- Don't lose me, will you? Please don't lose me.
- Things you like to remember, you can't remember, and things that you can remember easily drift away in front of you.
- I don't know what's the matter with me and why people don't talk to me much. I feel to be an outsider.
- I don't know whether I'm stuck here for the rest of my life or what's happening really.
- I'm frightened; please help me to know.
- Nobody wants me. I mean, that's the case, nobody does. If I was wanted by anybody, I could be quite useful. But nobody knows that I want a job.

I'm All Right; I'll Manage

- I wouldn't say it was as good as home at a place like this. You're just one of a number—group—who are pretty well in a similar position, but you do your best and give as much help. I've been sorting books out all morning.
- It's not as nice as I'd like it to be, but I have to be satisfied with small things these days.
- I haven't got to do any shopping, I haven't got to cook any meals, and that's a lot, isn't it? You've gotta get used to it, haven't you?
- I never thought I'd come to a place like this, but I'm quite happy.
- I've got a pal; she helps me out.

It Drives Me Mad

- I'd rather be doing something, yes, although there's not a lot I can do ... I'm capable of doing.
- I get bored here. They go to sleep and I feel like throwing something at them, because they ... nobody talking or nobody goes walking. You've gotta do something, haven't you, to help you go through? Because it wasn't the things I've been used to. They just sit here; it drives me mad.
- I want to be free ... or die. I don't mind dying, but I don't want to be coddled here.

Sources: Clare, L., Rowlands, J. M., & Quin, R. (2008). Collective strength: The impact of developing a shared social identity in early-stage dementia. *Dementia, 7*(1), 9–30; Clare, L., Rowlands, J., Bruce, E., et al. (2008). The experience of living with dementia in residential care: An interpretative phenomenological analysis. *The Gerontologist, 48*(6), 711–720.

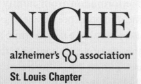

nicheprogram.org

Author: Maggie Murphy-White, MA, Alzheimer's Association St. Louis Chapter
Series Editor: Marie Boltz, PhD, RN, Managing Editor: Scott Bugg

NEED TO KNOW FOR PATIENTS & FAMILIES

Family Caregiver Report

Family Members, use this form to share information with staff about how your loved one is normally, when they are not sick or in crisis. Encourage patient involvement in the development of this information as much as possible. This information will help staff understand and provide for your loved one's needs.

Name: _____ What does he/she preferred to be called? _____

Where does he/she live? _____ Alone? Or with? _____

Does he/she become upset? Yes No How does he/she show this? _____

What triggers this? _____ What makes he/she feel comfortable? _____

In general, what helps he/she cope (for example, religion, music, certain people)? _____

What fluids or simple foods does he/she enjoy? _____

Would he/she like chaplain to visit? Yes No What other religious/spiritual activity would he/she desire? _____

What is his/her normal bedtime routine (for example, dentures in/out, call to family, a prayer, etc.)? _____
_____

What kind of work did he/she do? _____

What are his/her interests or hobbies? _____

What else can you tell us that will help us care for him/her? Strengths/Challenges? _____
_____

Does he/she normally need help...	Always	Sometimes	Never	Don't Know	Details
Understand where he/she is?					
Follow directions?					
Tell others what he/she needs?					
Tell others when he/she is in pain?					
Wear a hearing aid?					
Wear glasses?					
Have dentures?					
Using the bathroom?					
Walking?					
Getting out of bed?					
With bathing, brushing teeth, etc.?					
Dressing?					
Eating?					

Is there anything else you want the staff to know about him/her? _____

Name & relationship of person completing this form: _____

FIGURE 14-3 A form that can be used to obtain helpful information from family caregivers. (Used with permission from Murphy-White M. NICHE Need to Know: Dementia Transition Series. Nurses Improving Care for Healthsystem Elders & Alzheimer's Association St. Louis Chapter. 2013). © 2013 NICHE All rights reserved. The information contained in this tool is provided for informational purposes only.

Addressing Needs of Caregivers

In all settings, a major role of nurses is to work with family members or paid caregivers to provide appropriate interventions that focus on improving functioning for the person with dementia, alleviating the burden for the caregivers and improving quality of life for all. An intervention that might be most effective, as well as efficient, is to encourage caregivers' participation in educational or support groups, which often are led or co-led by nurses. The number of groups addressing the needs of caregivers is increasing rapidly, and information about these groups is available from the Alzheimer Society Canada, local Alzheimer Society chapters or local hospitals. Nurses can also encourage caregivers to purchase one of the many caregiver guides that are available in bookstores or through the Internet and other resources. Nurses should not assume that caregivers are receiving emotional support or instrumental support from family members or professionals, but should be proactive and specifically assess the needs of caregivers at every stage of their family member's illness (Ducharme et al., 2011).

In addition to educating caregivers about specific management problems, nurses in community settings must be ready to discuss resources for medical care, home services and other community-based services for people with dementia and their caregivers. As the number and range of services increase, it is becoming more and more difficult to keep up-to-date on the resources in one's own community. Although nurses cannot be expected to know all the details about all available community services, they should know generally about the services available. A good rule of thumb is to suggest that caregivers call the local Alzheimer Society chapter because these chapters are in a number of areas in Canada. Online Learning Activity 14-7 provides links to resources for caregivers of people with dementia.

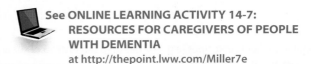

See **ONLINE LEARNING ACTIVITY 14-7:**
RESOURCES FOR CAREGIVERS OF PEOPLE
WITH DEMENTIA
at http://thepoint.lww.com/Miller7e

EVALUATING THE EFFECTIVENESS OF NURSING INTERVENTIONS

Nurses can evaluate the care of people with dementia according to the extent to which they receive necessary supports and maintain their dignity and quality of life. Because a decline in function is an inherent part of dementia, nursing care is evaluated on an ongoing basis as the person's condition changes and in relation to appropriate and changing goals. Nurses evaluate the degree to which quality of life is maintained by obtaining feedback about life satisfaction, which people in the early and middle stages of dementia usually can express verbally or nonverbally. For example, nurses can evaluate the extent to which the person enjoys or participates in meaningful activities and interactions. As dementia progresses, it becomes more difficult to obtain this kind of information, and nurses rely more on feedback from caregivers and their own judgment. During the later stages of dementia, measures of quality of life focus more on comfort and basic physical needs. Throughout the dementia course, care can be evaluated by the extent to which the person is free from pain, fear and anxiety.

Another evaluation consideration is the extent to which the needs of caregivers are met. One evaluation criterion is whether caregivers express satisfaction with their own quality of life, despite the demands of the situation. Other criteria may be a caregiver's attendance at support groups and his or her use of resources to assist with or guide care.

Case Study

Mrs. D. is 85 years old and lives with her 86-year-old husband in an apartment complex for the elderly. Two years ago, Mrs. D. was diagnosed with AD, but she was able to participate in her usual activities until the past year. Now she is neglecting her personal care and is unsafe during meal preparation.

When Mrs. D. wakes up several times nightly to go to the bathroom, she sometimes goes to the apartment door rather than returning to the bedroom. Mr. D. worries that she will leave in the middle of the night. This disrupts his sleep because he maintains a state of constant vigilance. Mr. D. has called Home Care requesting home health aide assistance, and you are the nurse responsible for the initial assessment about the need for home health aides.

NURSING ASSESSMENT

During your initial assessment, you find that Mrs. D. is pleasant and receptive but has little insight into her need for help. She acknowledges that her doctor told her she has "a memory problem" but reports that this problem doesn't affect her daily life, except that her husband has to remind her about things like turning the stove off after cooking meals. She acknowledges being lonely and says she misses being able to read books and talk to people. Mrs. D. takes donepezil (Aricept) and vitamin E and is otherwise physically healthy.

With regard to ADLs, Mrs. D. has not taken a bath or shower in several months, and she gets very angry if Mr. D. suggests that she take one. She gets confused about her clothing and sometimes wears her underwear over her regular clothes or wears a skirt and slacks at the same time. She insists on doing the meal preparation, but she is not safe while using the stove and gets confused

(continued)

Case Study (continued)

about ingredients in recipes (e.g., she has used salt instead of sugar). Mrs. D. has always done the laundry and housekeeping, but in the past months, she "made a lot of mistakes," such as using powdered milk for laundry detergent.

Mr. D. reports feeling very stressed about the full-time responsibilities of caring for his wife. This stress has escalated in the past month because he no longer feels he can leave her alone. Mrs. D. "shadows" him and feels very insecure if he is out of her sight for more than a few minutes. Mr. D. took her everywhere with him for the past year, but in the last few months, this has become increasingly difficult. For example, when they are grocery shopping, Mrs. D. gets very impatient and pushes the cart into other people. Then, while they are waiting in the checkout line, she insists on taking one of each of the nearby tabloids and magazines, and she creates a scene if Mr. D. doesn't buy them for her.

Mr. D. confides that he expected to be able to care for his wife at home "until the end," but now he has doubts about his ability to keep her at home. He perceives her as "senile" and feels he should be able to meet her needs. There are no nearby family members who can help with her care, but his son and daughter have offered to help pay for some services. Mr. D. is aware of support groups offered by the Alzheimer Society, but he has not attended any because he cannot leave his wife alone. When asked about his health, Mr. D. says, "I see the doctor for my arthritis and heart problems, but I get along okay, except that I'm supposed to have cataract surgery, and I don't know how I'll manage to get that done."

NURSING DIAGNOSIS

Your nursing diagnosis for Mrs. D. is Altered Thought Processes related to the effects of dementia. You use the nursing diagnosis of Caregiver Role Strain for Mr. D. because you recognize the need to address Mr. D.'s problems. Your immediate goal is to arrange for supportive services and assistance with Mrs. D.'s care because this will improve the quality of life for both Mr. and Mrs. D., and it will alleviate some of the caregiver stress for Mr. D. A long-term goal is to arrange for respite services, so Mr. D. can undergo cataract surgery. You also recognize the need for educational and support services for Mr. D.

NURSING CARE PLAN FOR MR. AND MRS. D.

Expected Outcome	Nursing Interventions	Nursing Evaluation
Mrs. D. will function at her highest level of independence.	• Work with Mr. D. to identify ways to improve Mrs. D.'s ability to function safely and independently in performing (ADLs). (For instance, Mr. D. can involve Mrs. D. in selecting an outfit to wear and can set out the clothing in the order in which it should be donned.) • Arrange for a home health aide (HHA) to work with Mrs. D. and assist her with complex tasks such as laundry, housekeeping and meal preparation. • Teach the HHA to assume an "assistant" and "friend" role by providing only subtle supervision and minimal direct help with activities such as laundry.	• Mrs. D. will perform ADLs and instrumental activities of daily living (IADLs) with minimal assistance.
Mrs. D.'s quality of life will be maintained.	• Work with Mr. D. and the HHA to identify activities that are interesting, satisfying, and intellectually stimulating (e.g., "word find" games). • Explore the possibility of Mrs. D.'s attending an adult day program for group activities. • Support Mrs. D. in carrying out familiar roles and meaningful activities.	• Mrs. D. will continue to engage in activities that are satisfying.
Mr. D. will use sources of support to alleviate caregiver-related stress.	• Arrange the HHA's schedule to enable Mr. D. to attend caregiver support groups and educational programs. • Help Mr. D. in identifying one activity per week that he could do to promote his own well-being (e.g., going to lunch with a friend). • Provide HHA assistance for 4-hour periods to allow Mr. D. time for grocery shopping and pursuing his own interests. • Provide Mr. D. with information about dementia telephone support (such as the telephone support line in Ontario instituted by the Alzheimer Society of Ontario and the Ontario Dementia Network).	• Mr. D. will verbalize feelings of being able to cope effectively with caregiver responsibilities. • Mr. D. will participate in one activity per week focused on his own needs and interests.

Case Study (continued)

THINKING POINTS

- Use the GDS/FAST in Table 14-2 to assess Mrs. D.'s stage of dementia.
- What would you identify as Mr. D.'s needs as a caregiver?
- What health education information would you plan for Mr. D.?

- What approaches would you suggest for Mr. D. and home care workers for communicating with Mrs. D.?
- What challenges would you anticipate having to address as you provide ongoing supervision of the HHA and continue to work with Mr. and Mrs. D.?

Chapter Highlights

Delirium

- Delirium is a serious, preventable, treatable, commonly occurring and often unrecognized in older adults.
- Delirium results from an interaction between predisposing factors, such as dementia and advanced age, and precipitating factors, such as surgery and infections.
- Functional consequences include decline in functioning, increased mortality and permanent residency in long-term care facilities.
- The CAM is an evidence-based tool for confirming the diagnosis of delirium on the basis of the following: acute onset or fluctuating course, inattention, disorganized thinking and altered level of consciousness.
- Interventions for delirium must be interprofessional and multifaceted to address the underlying factors (Fig. 14-1).

Overview of Dementia

- Dementia is a medical term that includes a group of brain disorders characterized by a gradual decline in cognitive abilities and changes in personality and behaviour.
- Many terms are used interchangeably—and not always accurately—to describe dementia.
- Current medical literature addresses four main types of dementia as AD, vascular dementia, Lewy body dementia and frontotemporal degeneration (Fig. 14-1 and Table 14-1).

Factors Associated With Dementia (Box 14-1 and Table 14-1)

- Risk factors for AD include family history, genetic factors, diagnosis of MCI and traumatic brain injury.
- Factors that decrease the risk for AD include physical activity, healthy diet, higher educational level and engagement in social and cognitive activities.

Functional Consequences Associated With Dementia

- Dementia progresses through stages involving cognitive and functional decline (Table 14-2).

- Self-awareness and personal experiences of people with dementia vary significantly (Boxes 14-2 and 14-3).
- Examples of behavioural and psychological symptoms of dementia include agitation, personality changes, mood disturbances, repetitive movements and changes in sleep and eating.
- Nurses need to recognize and address misperceptions about behaviours in people with dementia.

Nursing Assessment of Dementia

- The initial assessment of cognitive impairment is complex and based on an interprofessional assessment of all aspects of health and functioning (Box 14-4).
- Assessment is an ongoing process involving assessment of stages and all aspects of health and functioning (Table 14-2, many other chapters in this text).
- Ongoing assessment of consequences also includes attention to the emotional experiences of the person with dementia (Box 14-5).

Nursing Diagnosis

- Nursing diagnoses for the person with dementia include Chronic Confusion, Anxiety, Impaired Memory, Risk Falls, Self-Care Deficit, Disturbed Sleep Pattern, Imbalanced Nutrition, Wandering and Urinary Incontinence.
- Nursing diagnoses to address needs of caregivers include Family Coping and Caregiver Role Strain (or Risk for), and Anticipatory Grieving.

Planning for Wellness Outcomes

- Nursing Outcomes Classification for the person with dementia: Agitation Level, Cognition, Cognitive Orientation, Comfort Status, Communication, Memory, Mood Equilibrium, Nutritional Status, Self-Care Status, Sleep, Symptom Control.
- Nursing Outcomes Classification for caregivers: Anxiety Level, Caregiver Emotional Health, Caregiver Physical Health, Caregiver Stressors, Caregiving Endurance Potential.
- For both the person with dementia and his or her caregivers: Coping, Quality of life.

Nursing Interventions to Address Dementia

- Nurses have important roles in teaching older adults and their caregivers about medications for slowing the progression of dementia.
- Nurses use nonpharmacologic interventions to promote wellness and improve quality of life for people with dementia (Box 14-7 and Table 14-4).
- Environment modifications are effective for improving safety and functioning (Box 14-8).
- It is important to adapt communication techniques for people with dementia (Box 14-9).
- The PLST model is an evidence-based approach to addressing dementia-related behaviours (Box 14-10).
- It is important to recognize feelings of people with dementia about their lived experiences of needing help from others and being part of a support group (Box 14-11).
- Nonpharmacologic interventions can be used to address problem behaviours in people with dementia (Box 14-12).
- It is important to recognize the feelings of people with moderate to severe dementia about needing care in a residential or long-term care facilities (Box 14-13).

Evaluating the Effectiveness of Nursing Interventions

- Effectiveness of nursing interventions is evaluated as the person's condition changes and in relation to appropriate and changing goals.
- Nurses evaluate the degree to which quality of life is maintained by obtaining feedback about life satisfaction from people with dementia and their caregivers.

Critical Thinking Exercises

1. Define each of the following terms, and describe the relevance of each term according to our current understanding of impaired cognitive function: senility, organic brain syndrome, hardening of the arteries, delirium, dementia and AD.
2. Describe how you would explain the distinguishing features of AD, vascular dementia, Lewy body dementia and frontotemporal degeneration to the family of someone who asks about the types of dementia.
3. You are working in a nursing clinic at a senior centre. How would you respond to the following questions, posed by a 74-year-old woman: "I've been having memory problems lately, but I know it's not AD, because I haven't done anything really stupid. What do you think I should do? My friend says ginkgo helps her a lot, and I was thinking of trying that. Do you know how much of it I should take?"
4. You are planning an inservice program to nursing home staff about medications used in the treatment of dementia and the management of dementia-related behaviours. What information would you present?

 For more information about topics discussed in this chapter, be sure to check out the interactive Online Learning Activities and other helpful resources at http://thepoint.lww.com/Miller7e

REFERENCES

Alzheimer's Association. (2014). *Brain health*. Retrieved from http://www.alz.org/we_can_help_brain_health_maintain_your_brain.asp

Alzheimer's Association Report. (2013). 2013 Alzheimer's disease facts and figures. *Alzheimer's & Dementia, 9*, 208–245.

Alzheimer's Society. (2008). *Dementia: Out of the shadows*. London, England: Author.

Alzheimer's Society. (2010). *My name is not dementia: People with dementia discuss quality of life*. London, England: Author.

Alzheimer Society of Canada. (2014). *Living with dementia: Caring for someone*. Retrieved from www.alzheimer.ca/en/Living-with-dementia/Caring-for-someone.

Alzheimer Society—Ontario. (2012). *Facts about dementia*. Retrieved from http://www.alzheimer.ca/en/on/About-dementia/What-is-dementia/Facts-about-dementia

American Psychiatric Association. (2013). *Diagnostic and statistical manual of mental disorders* (5th ed.). Arlington, VA: Author.

Amoyal, N., & Fallon, E. (2012). Physical exercise and cognitive training clinical interventions used in slowing degeneration associated with mild cognitive impairment. *Topics in Geriatric Rehabilitation, 28*(3), 208–216.

Anand, R., Gill, K. D., & Mahdi, A. A. (2014). Therapeutics of Alzheimer's disease: Past, present and future. *Neuropharmacology, 76*(Part A), 27–50.

Ballard, C., & Corbett, A. (2013). Agitation and aggression in people with Alzheimer's disease. *Current Opinions in Psychiatry, 26*(3), 252–259.

Barnett, J. H., Hachinski, V., & Blackwell, A. D. (2013). Cognitive health begins at conception: Addressing dementia as a lifelong and preventable condition. *BioMed Central Medicine, 11*, 246. Retrieved from www.biomedcentral.com/1741-015/11/246

Blazer, D. G., & van Nieuwenhuizen, A. O. (2012). Evidence for the diagnostic criteria of delirium: An update. *Current Opinion in Psychiatry, 25*, 239–243.

Brodaty, H., & Arasaratnam, C. (2012). Meta-analysis of nonpharmacological interventions for neuropsychiatric symptoms of dementia. *American Journal of Psychiatry, 169*(9), 946–953.

Burke, A., Hall, G., & Tariot, P. N. (2013). The clinical problem of neuropsychiatric signs and symptoms in dementia. *Continuum, 19*(2 Dementia), 382–396.

Cheng, S. T., Chow, P. K., Song, Y. Q., et al. (2014). Can leisure activities slow dementia progression in nursing home residents? A cluster-randomized controlled trial. *International Psychogeriatrics, 26*(4), 637–643.

Chow, T., & Alobaidy, A. (2013). Incorporating new diagnostic schemas, genetics, and proteinopathy into evaluation of frontotemporal degeneration. *Continuum, 19*(2), 438–456.

Clare, L., Nelis, S. M., Martyr, A., et al. (2012). Longitudinal trajectories of awareness in early-stage dementia. *Alzheimer's Disease and Associated Disorders, 26*(2), 140–147.

Clare, L., Rowlands, J. M., & Quin, R. (2008). Collective strength: The impact of developing a shared social identity in early-stage dementia. *Dementia, 7*(1), 9–30.

Clare, L., Rowlands, J., Bruce, E., et al. (2008). The experience of living with dementia in residential care: An interpretative phenomenological analysis. *The Gerontologist, 48*(6), 711–720.

Clare, L., Whitaker, C. J., Roberts, S. M., et al. (2013). Memory awareness profiles differentiate mild cognitive impairment from early-stage dementia: Evidence from assessments of performance monitoring and evaluative judgment. *Dementia and Geriatric Cognitive Disorders*, *35*(5–6), 266–279.

Cole, M. G., McCusker, J., Voyer, P., et al. (2013). Symptoms of delirium predict incident delirium in older long-term care residents. *International Psychogeriatrics*, *25*(6), 887–894.

Cotelli, M., Manenti, R., Zanetti, O., et al. (2012). Non-pharmacological intervention for memory decline. *Frontiers in Human Neuroscience*, *6* [Article 46]. Retrieved from www.frontiersin.org

Davis, D. H. J., Terrera, G. M., Keage, H., et al. (2012). Delirium is a strong risk factor for dementia in the oldest-old: A population-based cohort study. *Brain: Journal of Neurology*, *135*, 2809–2816.

Dawson, N., T., Powers, S. M., Krestar, M., et al. (2013). Predictors of self-reported psychosocial outcomes in individuals with dementia. *The Gerontologist*, *53*(5), 748–759.

de Lange, E., Verhaak, P. F., & van der Meer, K. (2013). Prevalence, presentation and prognosis of delirium in older people in the population, at home and in long term care: A review. *International Journal of Geriatric Psychiatry*, *28*(2), 127–134.

Ducharme, F., Levesque, L., Lachance, L., et al. (2011). Challenges associated with transition to caregiver role following diagnostic disclosure of Alzheimer disease: A descriptive study. *International Journal of Nursing Studies*, *48*, 1109–1119.

Dupuis, S. L., Wiersma, E., & Loiselle, L. (2012). Pathologizing behaviour: Meanings of behaviours in dementia care. *Journal of Aging Studies*, *26*, 162–173.

Fick, D. M., Steis, M. R., Waller, J. L., et al. (2013). Delirium superimposed on dementia is associated with prolonged length of stay and poor outcomes in hospitalized older adults. *Journal of Hospital Medicine*, *8*(9), 500–505.

Fong, T. G., Jones, R. N., Marcantonio, E. R., et al. (2012). Adverse outcomes after hospitalization and delirium in persons with Alzheimer disease. *Annals of Internal Medicine*, *156*(12), 848–856.

Forbes, D., Thiessen, E. J., Blake, C. M., et al. (2013). Exercise programs for people with dementia. *Cochrane Database Systematic Review*, CD006489. doi:10.1002/14651858.CD006489.pub3

Gareri, P., De Fazio, P., Manfredi, V. G., et al. (2014). Use and safety of antipsychotics in behavioural disorders in elderly people with dementia. *Journal of Clinical Psychopharmacology*, *34*(1), 109–123.

Gauthier, S., Patterson, C., Chertkow, H., et al. (2012). Recommendations of the 4th Canadian Consensus Conference on the diagnosis and treatment of dementia. *Canadian Geriatrics Journal*, *15*(4), 120–126. doi:10.5770.cgj.15.49

Gealogo, G. A. (2013). Dementia with Lewy bodies: A comprehensive review for nurses. *Journal of Neuroscience Nursing*, *45*(6), 347–358.

George, D. R., Qualls, S. H., Camp, C. J., et al. (2012). Renovating Alzheimer's: "Constructive" reflections on the new clinical and research diagnostic guidelines. *The Gerontologist*, *53*(3), 378–387.

Godfrey, M., Smith, J., Green, J., et al. (2013). Developing and implementing an integrated delirium prevention system of care: A theory driven, participatory research study. *BioMed Central Health Services Research*, *13*, 341. Retrieved from www.biomedcentral.com

Gomoll, B. P., Sanders, B. D., & Caserta, M. T. (2014). Psychopharmacologic treatments for Alzheimer disease and related dementias. *Psychopharm Review*, *49*(1), 9–16.

Gordon, S. J., Melillo, K. D., Nannini, A., et al. (2013). Bedside coaching to improve nurses' recognition of delirium. *Journal of Neuroscience Nursing*, *45*(5), 288–293.

Gorelick, P. B., & Nyenhuis, D. (2013). Understanding and treating vascular cognitive impairment. *Continuum*, *19*(2), 425–437.

Hachinski, V. C., Lassen, N. A., & Marshall, J. (1974). Multi-infarct dementia: A cause of mental deterioration in elderly. *Lancet*, *2*, 207–209.

Hall, G. R., & Buckwalter, K. C. (1987). Progressively lowered threshold: A conceptual model for care of adults with Alzheimer's disease. *Archives of Psychiatric Nursing*, *1*, 399–406.

Hanagasi, H. A., Bilgic, B., & Emre, M. (2013). Neuroimaging, biomarkers, and management of dementia with Lewy bodies. *Frontiers in Neurology*, *4* [Article 151]. Retrieved from www.frontiersin.org

Herdman, T. H. (Ed.). (2012). *NANDA International Nursing Diagnoses: Definitions and classification 2012–1014*. Oxford, England: Wiley-Blackwell.

Hopper, T., Bourgeois, M., Pimentel, J., et al. (2013). An evidence-based systematic review on cognitive interventions for individuals with dementia. *American Journal of Speech Language Pathology*, *22*(1), 126–145.

Horning, S. M., Melrose, R., & Sultzer, D. (2014). Insight in Alzheimer's disease and its relation to psychiatric and behavioural disturbances. *International Journal of Geriatric Psychiatry*, *29*(1), 77–84.

Huang, L.-W., Inouye, S. K., Jones, R. N., et al. (2012). Identifying indicators of key diagnostic features of delirium. *Journal of the American Geriatrics Society*, *60*(6), 1044–1050.

Huang, Y., & Halliday, G. (2013). Can we clinically diagnose dementia with Lewy bodies yet? *Translational Neurodegeneration*, *2*, 4. Retrieved from www.translationalneurodegeneration.com/content/2/1/4

Inouye, S. K., van Dyck, C. H., Alessi, C. A., et al. (1990). Clarifying confusion: The confusion assessment method. A new method for detection of delirium. *Annals of Internal Medicine*, *113*(12), 941–948.

Justin, B. N., Turek, M., & Hakim, A. M. (2013). Heart disease as a risk factor for dementia. *Clinical Epidemiology*, *26*(5), 135–145.

Kaur, B., Harvey, D. J., DeCarli, C. S., et al. (2012). Extrapyramidal signs by dementia severity in Alzheimer disease and dementia with Lewy bodies. *Alzheimer's Disease and Associated Disorders*, *27*(3), 226–232.

Kawashima, R. (2013). Mental exercises for cognitive function: Clinical evidence. *Journal of Preventive Medicine & Public Health*, *46*, S22–S27.

Kirk-Sanchez, N., & McGough, E. L. (2014). Physical exercise and cognitive performance in the elderly: Current perspectives. *Clinical Interventions in Aging*, *9*, 51–62.

Kling, M. A., Trojanowski, J. Q., Wolk, D. A., et al. (2013). Vascular disease and dementias: Paradigm shifts to drive research in new directions. *Alzheimers and Dementia*, *9*(1), 76–92.

Langballe, E. M., Engdahl, B., Nordeng, H., et al. (2013). Short- and long-term mortality risk associated with the use of antipsychotics among 26,940 dementia outpatients: A population-based study. *American Journal of Geriatric Psychiatry*, *22*(4), 321–331. doi:10.1016/j/jagp.2013.06.007

Macluluch, A. M., Anand, A., Davis, D. H., et al. (2013). New horizons in the pathogenesis, assessment and management of delirium. *Age and Ageing*, *42*, 667–674.

Maki, Y., Yamaguchi, T., & Yamaguchi, H. (2013). Evaluation of anosognosia in Alzheimer's disease using the symptoms of early dementia-11 questionnaire (SED-11Q). *Dementia and Geriatric Cognitive Disorders*, *3*, 351–359.

Mangialasche, F., Kivipelto, M., Solomon, A., et al. (2012). Dementia prevention: Current epidemiological evidence and future perspective. *Alzheimer's Research & Therapy*, *4*, 6. Retrieved from http://alzres.com/content/4/1/6

Mardh, S., Karlsson, T., & Marcusson, J. (2013). Aspects of awareness in patients with Alzheimer's disease. *International Psychogeriatrics*, *25*(7), 1167–1179.

Massimo, L., Evans, L. K., & Benner, P. (2013). Caring for loved ones with frontotemporal degeneration: The lived experiences of spouses. *Geriatric Nursing*, *34*, 302–306.

McCleary, L., Persaud, M., Hum, S., et al. (2013). Pathways to dementia diagnosis among South Asian Canadians. *Dementia*, *12*(6), 769–789. doi:10.1177/1471301212444806

McDermott, O., Orrell, M., & Ridder, H. M. (2014). The importance of music for people with dementia: The perspectives of people with dementia, family carers, staff and music therapists. *Aging and Mental Health*, *18*(6), 706–716.

Mograbi, D. C., Brown, R. G., Salas, C., et al. (2012). Emotional reactivity and awareness of task performance in Alzheimer's disease. *Neuropsychologia*, *50*(8), 2075–2084.

Morgan, R. O., Sail, K. R., Snow, A. L., et al. (2013). Modelling causes of aggressive behaviour in patients with dementia. *The Gerontologist*, *53*(5), 738–747.

Neville, C., Clifton, K., Henwood, T., et al. (2013). Watermemories: A swimming club for adults with dementia. *Journal of Gerontological Nursing, 39*(2), 21–25.

Organization for Economic Co-operation and Development. (2004). *Dementia care in 9 OECD countries: A comparative analysis.* OECD Health Working Papers. Retrieved from http://www.oecd.org/health/health-systems/33661491.pdf

Palmer, J. L. (2013). Preserving personhood of individuals with advanced dementia: Lessons from family caregivers. *Geriatric Nursing, 34,* 224–229.

Park-Wyllie, L. Y., Mamdani, M. M., Li, P., et al. (2009). Cholinesterase inhibitors and hospitalization for bradycardia: A population-based study. *PLoS Medicine, 6*(9), 1–8.

Popp, J. (2013). Delirium and cognitive decline: More than a coincidence. *Current Opinion in Neurology, 26*(6), 634–639.

Ryan, D. J., O'Regan, N. A., Caoimh R. O., et al. (2013). Delirium in an adult acute hospital population: Predictors, prevalence and detection. *British Medical Journal Open Access, 3,* e001772. doi:10.1136/bmjopen-2012-001772

Seitz, D. P., Gill, S. S., Herrmann, N., et al. (2013). Pharmacological treatments for neuropsychiatric symptoms of dementia in long-term care: A systematic review. *International Psychogeriatrics, 25*(2), 185–203.

Selbaek, G., Engedal, K., & Bergh, S. (2013). The prevalence and course of neuropsychiatric symptoms in nursing home patients with dementia: A systematic review. *Journal of the American Medical Association, 14,* 161–169.

Simon, S. S., Yokomizo, J. E., & Bottino, C. (2012). Cognitive intervention in amnesic mild cognitive impairment: A systematic review. *Neuroscience and Biobehavioral Reviews, 36,* 1163–1178.

Slaughter, S. E., & Hayduk, L. A. (2012). Contributions of environment, comorbidity, and stage of dementia to the onset of walking and eating disability in long-term care residents. *Journal of the American Geriatrics Society, 60*(9), 1624–1631.

Smebye, K. L., & Kirkevold, M. (2013). The influence of relationships on personhood in dementia care: A qualitative, hermeneutic study. *BioMed Central Nursing, 12*(1), 29. doi:10.1186/1472-6955-12-29

Smith, A. D., & Yaffe, K. (2014). Dementia (including Alzheimer's disease) can be prevented: Statement supported by international experts. *Journal of Alzheimer's Disease, 38,* 699–703.

Smith, M., Schultz, S. K., Seydel, L. L., et al. (2013). Improving antipsychotic agent use in nursing homes: Development of an algorithm for treating problem behaviours in nursing homes. *Journal of Gerontological Nursing, 39*(5), 24–35.

Solberg, L. M., Plummer, C. E., May, K. N., et al. (2013). A quality improvement program to increase nurses' detection of delirium in an acute medical unit. *Geriatric Nursing, 34,* 75–79.

Statistics Canada. (2012). *Leading causes of death in Canada, 2009.* Retrieved from www.statcan.gc.ca/pub/84-215-x/2012001/hl-fs-eng.htm

Steis, M. R., & Fick, D. M. (2012). Delirium superimposed on dementia: Accuracy of nurse documentation. *Journal of Gerontological Nursing, 38*(1), 32–42.

Tomlinson, B. E., Blessed, G., & Roth, M. (1968). Observations on the brains of non-demented old people. *Journal of Neurological Science, 7,* 331–356.

Tomlinson, B. E., Blessed, G., & Roth, M. (1970). Observation on the brains of demented old people. *Journal of Neurological Science, 11,* 205–242.

Toot, S., Devine, M., Akporobaro, A., et al. (2013). Causes of hospital admission for people with dementia: A systematic review. *Journal of the American Medical Directors Association, 14*(7), 463–470.

Tullmann, D. F., Fletcher, K., & Foreman, M. D. (2012). Delirium. In M. Boltz, E. Capezuti, T. Fulmer, et al. (Eds.), *Evidence-based practice protocols for best practice* (4th ed., pp. 186–199). New York, NY: Springer.

van Vliet, D., de Vugt, M. E., Kohler, S., et al. (2012). Awareness and its association with affective symptoms in young-onset and late-onset Alzheimer disease. *Alzheimer's Disease and Associated Disorders, 27*(3), 265–271.

Verhulsdonk, S., Quack, R., Goft, B., et al. (2013). Anosognosia and depression in patients with Alzheimer's dementia. *Archives of Gerontology and Geriatrics, 57*(3), 282–287.

Wand, A., Thoo W., Ting, V., et al. (2013). Identification and rates of delirium in elderly medical inpatients from diverse language groups. *Geriatric Nursing, 34,* 355–360.

Warren, J. D., Rohrer, J. D., & Rossor, M. N. (2013). Frontotemporal dementia. *British Medical Journal Open Access, 347.* doi:10.1136/bmj.f4827

Woods, B., Aguirre, E., Spector, A. E., et al. (2012). Cognitive stimulation to improve cognitive functioning in people with dementia. *Cochrane Database Systematic Review,* CD005562. doi:10.1002/14651858.pub2

chapter 15

Impaired Affective Function: Depression

Despite the common occurrence of late-life depression as an impairment aspect of psychosocial function in older adults, this condition is often undetected and untreated. Theories to explain types of depression were first proposed during the 1970s, and theories to explain the complexity of late-life depression have been emerging more recently. Evidence-based recommendations related to late-life depression provide guidance for identifying and treating depression in older adults. Nurses have important roles in addressing late-life depression because there is a range of nursing interventions that can have a significant positive impact on the quality of life of older adults.

DEPRESSION IN OLDER ADULTS

Although psychiatric references describe many types of depression, which are also called *mood disorders*, the two types most commonly discussed in relation to older adults are major depression (also called major depressive disorder) or subthreshold (also called minor, subclinical, or nonmajor) depression. Diagnostic criterion for *major depression* include depressed mood and/or loss of interest or pleasure along with at least five of the following signs and symptoms: weight loss, appetite change, sleep disturbances, observable psychomotor agitation or retardation (i.e., slowness), fatigue or loss of energy, feeling worthless or excessively guilty, cognitive impairment, and recurrent thoughts of death or suicide (Snowden & Almeida, 2013). A defining characteristic of major depression is that it noticeably interferes with usual functioning and is associated with significantly diminished quality of life. Minor depression is characterized by these same signs and symptoms, but they are not as severe and their effects on functioning and quality of life are not as serious. Rather than defining types of depression in distinct categories, it should be viewed as a continuum of symptoms that should not be overlooked (Lee et al., 2013).

Late-life depression refers to the onset of depression after age 65. Although manifestations are similar to their

Addressing Depression in Older Adults

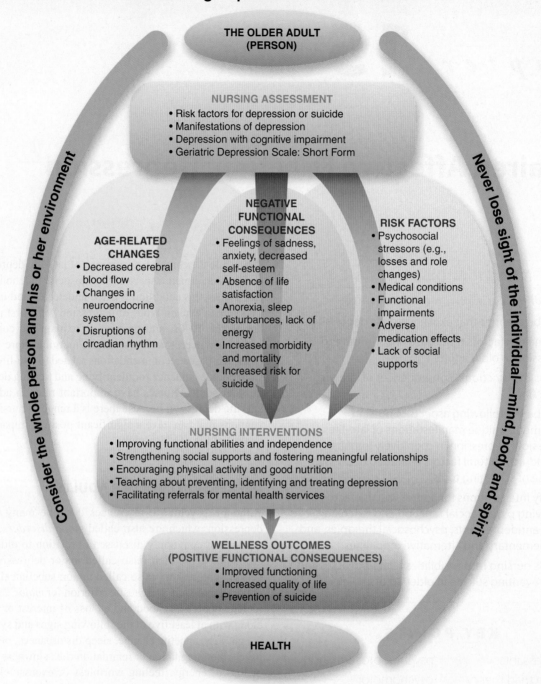

Consider the whole person and his or her environment

Never lose sight of the individual—mind, body and spirit

THE OLDER ADULT (PERSON)

NURSING ASSESSMENT
- Risk factors for depression or suicide
- Manifestations of depression
- Depression with cognitive impairment
- Geriatric Depression Scale: Short Form

AGE-RELATED CHANGES
- Decreased cerebral blood flow
- Changes in neuroendocrine system
- Disruptions of circadian rhythm

NEGATIVE FUNCTIONAL CONSEQUENCES
- Feelings of sadness, anxiety, decreased self-esteem
- Absence of life satisfaction
- Anorexia, sleep disturbances, lack of energy
- Increased morbidity and mortality
- Increased risk for suicide

RISK FACTORS
- Psychosocial stressors (e.g., losses and role changes)
- Medical conditions
- Functional impairments
- Adverse medication effects
- Lack of social supports

NURSING INTERVENTIONS
- Improving functional abilities and independence
- Strengthening social supports and fostering meaningful relationships
- Encouraging physical activity and good nutrition
- Teaching about preventing, identifying and treating depression
- Facilitating referrals for mental health services

WELLNESS OUTCOMES (POSITIVE FUNCTIONAL CONSEQUENCES)
- Improved functioning
- Increased quality of life
- Prevention of suicide

HEALTH

younger counterparts, older adults are less likely to admit to depression to health care professionals. Also, for older adults, causative factors are more complex and depression often occurs concomitantly with other conditions. In addition, late-life depression is associated with more serious consequences and it is often unrecognized and undertreated. Much of the current research focuses on the relationships between late-life depression and chronic conditions that are common in older adults, such as pain, strokes, dementia and cardiovascular disease. Estimates of prevalence of late-life depression in community settings range from 5% to 20% (Public Health

Agency of Canada, 2010) and, within nursing homes, at least 40% of older adults experience depression (Canadian Coalition on Seniors' Mental Health, 2009). See Figure 15-1 for percentages of older Canadians who self-identify as experiencing mood disorders (e.g., depression and bipolar disorder).

THEORIES ABOUT LATE-LIFE DEPRESSION

Late-life depression is multifaceted because it is associated with many interacting conditions and circumstances that commonly occur in or affect older adults. Although no

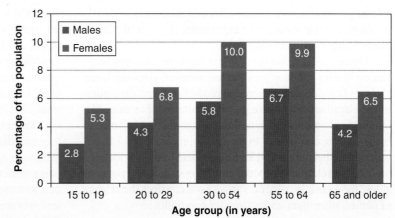

FIGURE 15-1 Self-reported percentages of Canadians experiencing mood disorders. (Public Health Agency of Canada [2012]. *The Chief Public Health Officer's Report on the state of public health in Canada, 2012—Chapter 1.* Retrieved from http://www.phac-aspc.gc.ca/cphorsphc-respcacsp/2012/chap-1-eng.php)

single theory can explain why older adults are likely to become depressed, psychosocial, cognitive and biologic theories help explain causative factors from various perspectives. Researchers currently are exploring the complex and bidirectional relationship between depression and concomitant conditions, including dementia, cardiovascular disease and cerebrovascular disease.

Psychosocial Theories

Psychosocial theories focus on the impact of loss, as well as the buffering effects of social supports and the social network in protecting against depression. Blazer (2002) reviewed psychosocial theories related to late-life depression and identified the following potential contributing factors:

- Ageism, loss of social roles and lower socioeconomic status
- Early experiences including impoverishment and childhood trauma
- Recent social stressors including stressful life events
- Inadequate social network (e.g., no spouse/partner, few friends, small family network)
- Diminished social interaction
- Poor social integration (e.g., unstable environment, lack of strong religious affiliation)
- A combination of the preceding factors

The **learned helplessness theory** has also been used to explain late-life depression. A cognitively oriented formulation of this theory describes depression as a deficit in the following four areas: cognitive, motivational, self-esteem and affective-somatic (Seligman, 1981). Depression occurs when people expect bad things to happen, believe they can do nothing to prevent them and perceive that the events result from internal, stable and global factors (Seligman, 1981). This theory would explain the occurrence of depression in older adults who are in situations over which they have little control. The learned helplessness theory supports the use of nursing interventions directed toward improving self-efficacy and a sense of control over one's environment.

Cognitive Triad Theory

Beck proposed the **cognitive triad theory** as a way of explaining depression in general and late-life depression in particular (Beck et al., 1979). According to this theory, people appraise themselves by the "cognitive triad" of their self-image, their environment or experiences, and their future. Depressed people judge these three realms as lacking some features that are necessary for happiness. Examples of negative appraisals are feelings of worthlessness, interpretations of neutral events as bad and unrealistic feelings of hopelessness. Beck postulates that depression is caused not by adverse events, but by distorted perceptions, which impair one's ability to appraise oneself and the event in a constructive manner. The second element of Beck's theory involves schemas, or consistent cognitive patterns. Schemas are assumptions, or unarticulated rules, that influence thoughts, feelings and behaviours. Depressed people typically hold negative assumptions that lead to faulty conclusions. For instance, a depressed person might believe, "I must not be important because the nurse didn't stop to see me." The third component of Beck's theory is the existence of certain logical errors such as personalization, minimization, magnification and overgeneralization. This theory underlies cognitive-behavioural therapy, which helps depressed people address their dysfunctional thought processes.

Biologic and Genetic Theories

Biologic theories about late-life depression investigate the relationships among aging, depression and changes in the brain, nervous system and neuroendocrine system. These theories focus on the changes in the neuroendocrine system that are associated with depression, such as alterations in cortisol levels and increased activity in the hypothalamic–pituitary–adrenal axis. A current focus of neurobiologic research is the potential role of inflammatory mechanisms as causative factors for depression (Catena-Dell'Osso et al., 2013). Studies are also addressing neurobiologic mechanisms that are associated with increased risk for suicide (Pandey, 2013). These theories are leading to a better understanding of the role of physical activity as an effective intervention for depression and depression-like behaviours (Eyre et al., 2013; Matta Mello Portugal et al., 2013).

Other biologic theories address anatomic changes (e.g., lesions in white or deep grey matter), neurophysiologic brain changes (e.g., decreased cerebral blood flow) and disruption of the circadian rhythms (e.g., sleep patterns). For example, longitudinal studies indicate that the age-related atrophy of brain volume contributes to the development of late-life depression (Ribeiz et al., 2013). Researchers have also focused on the interrelationship between biologic and genetic variables, for example, genetic variations that affect the release of neurotransmitters under stressful conditions.

Evolving Theories About Depression and Other Conditions

There is much current emphasis on the complex and bidirectional relationships between depression and pathologic conditions, such as dementia, cerebrovascular disease and cardiovascular disease. Although studies related to these topics are inconclusive about causative relationships, the co-occurrence of depression with medical conditions is cited as "the distinguishing feature of depression in late life" (Mezuk & Gallo, 2013). Studies consistently find that the co-occurrence of depression with chronic conditions in older adults is associated with more serious negative functional consequences, including all of the following: greater pain, diminished functioning, lower quality of life and increased risk for suicide (Byma et al., 2012).

Since the early 2000s, gerontologists have recognized a high correlation between depression and dementia, with cognitive deficits being both a predictor and consequence of depression (Diniz et al., 2013; Vilalta-Franch et al., 2013; Zeki Al Hazzouri et al., 2014). For instance, about 40% to 50% of individuals with dementia experience depression at some point in their illness (Alzheimer Society Canada, 2012). In addition, about 20% of people with mild cognitive impairment have symptoms of depression (Polyakova et al., 2014). Hypotheses about the relationship between depression and cognitive changes that are currently being investigated are (1) depression is a precursor or early manifestation of dementia; (2) depression occurs early in the course of dementia as a psychological reaction to eroding cognitive abilities; (3) depression and cognitive decline are associated with a common pathway of neurologic changes; and (4) depression causes neurologic and neuroendocrine changes that accelerate the rate of cognitive decline (Olazaran et al., 2013; Richard et al., 2013; van den Kommer et al., 2013). Distinguishing features of depression in people with dementia include increased manifestations related to motivation (e.g., apathy) and less overt mood complaints (Marano et al., 2013).

Another area of intense investigation is the common co-occurrence of depression and cerebrovascular disease caused by strokes or cumulative effects of ischemic episodes. **Poststroke depression** is the most common neuropsychiatric consequence of a stroke, with prevalence rates ranging from 9% to 34% during the first 6 months and up to 70% of all stroke survivors over the longer term (da Rocha e Silva et al., 2013; Flaster et al., 2013; Taylor-Piliae et al., 2013). Poststroke depression is most likely to occur in people with greater functional and cognitive impairment and it is associated with increased mortality and poor recovery (DeRyck et al., 2013; Hornsten et al., 2013).

Vascular depression occurs in the context of cerebrovascular disease without evidence or history of major stroke. Although research about vascular depression is in an early stage, studies indicate that the brain changes associated with cerebrovascular disease are strongly linked to the occurrence and worsening of depression in older adults (Taylor et al., 2013; Volk & Steffens, 2013). Vascular depression is characterized by apathy, functional impairment, psychomotor retardation and cognitive impairments, including poor insight and executive dysfunction.

The relationship between depression and cardiovascular disease is another current focus of intense investigation by cardiologists and gerontologists. During the past two decades, researchers have identified all the following links: (1) depression is an independent risk factor for cardiac disease; (2) depression is often chronic and recurrent in people with cardiovascular disease; (3) depression is an independent risk factor for adverse cardiovascular outcomes, including poor recovery and increased mortality (Huffman et al., 2013). Because depression occurs so frequently in people with cardiovascular disease, the American Heart Association recommends routine screening for depression in all people with coronary heart disease (Whooley & Wong, 2013). In response to this recommendation, researchers from Canada and the United States examined studies that addressed depression in coronary heart disease. They concluded that there is some evidence regarding the effectiveness of treating depression in individuals post–myocardial infarction or with coronary heart disease, but there is no evidence of the efficacy of depression treatment in those with heart failure (Thombs et al., 2013).

Wellness Opportunity

From a holistic nursing perspective, it is important to recognize that there are many types of depression, and in older adults particularly, depression is complex and likely to occur concomitantly with dementia and other conditions.

RISK FACTORS FOR DEPRESSION IN OLDER ADULTS

Risk factors that are likely to cause or contribute to depression in older adults include demographic factors and psychosocial influences, medical conditions and functional impairments, and effects of medications and alcohol. Although these factors can increase the risk for depression in people of any age, older adults are more likely than younger people to have one or more of these variables. The following sections discuss each category of risk in relation to older adults. Additional risk factors for depression include cognitive impairments and dementia, as discussed in other sections of this chapter.

Demographic Factors and Psychosocial Influences

Demographic factors and psychosocial influences that are associated with depression in older adults include

- Female sex
- Personal or family history of depression
- Bereavement, loss of significant relationships
- Loneliness
- Chronic stress
- Recent social stressors
- Stressful social environment
- Loss of meaningful social interaction
- Lack of social supports
- Loss of significant roles
- Current or previous experiences of abuse or neglect
- Being a caregiver (including assuming primary care of a grandchild).

Although losses and stress can be risk factors for depression, social supports (e.g., having at least one close relationship) and effective coping mechanisms can protect older adults from depression and improve recovery. Thus, the stressors alone are not the primary risk factor for depression; rather, it is the combination of stressors and the absence of social supports that increases the risk for depression. A review of studies identified social support, quality of relationships and presence of confidants as factors that are most significantly associated with depression (Schwarzbach et al., 2014).

Medical Conditions and Functional Impairments

The relationships between medical conditions, functional impairments and depression is complex and interactive, as in the following examples:

- Depression in medically ill older adults is associated with increased mortality, longer hospitalizations and extended recovery time.
- Medical illnesses can threaten survival, independence, self-concept, role functions, economic resources and sense of well-being.
- Disability leads to depression because it causes social isolation, low self-esteem, restricted social activity, strained interpersonal relationships and loss of perceived control.
- Depression in medically ill older adults can lead to other health problems, such as hip fractures and increased susceptibility to infection.
- Chronic pain is a common cause of depression, and it is sometimes a symptom of depression.
- Depression worsens pain, and pain worsens depression.
- Functional impairment is associated with depression as both a contributing factor and a consequence.
- Nutritional deficiencies can be both a risk factor for and effect of depression.

Box 15-1 lists medical conditions that are strongly linked to an increased risk for depression.

Box 15-1 Medical Conditions Associated With an Increased Risk for Depression

Central Nervous System Disorders

Dementia
Stroke
Parkinson disease
Tumours
Normal-pressure hydrocephalus

Cardiovascular Conditions

Myocardial infarction
Heart failure

Metabolic and Endocrine Disorders

Diabetes
Hypothyroidism/hyperthyroidism
Renal disease
Liver disease
Adrenal disease

Miscellaneous

Pain
Rheumatoid arthritis
Cancer
Nutritional deficiencies (e.g., iron, folate, vitamin D)

Gerontologists emphasize that depression is a treatable component of medical conditions that has a significant negative effect on health-related quality of life for older adults. For example, studies of people with Parkinson's disease consistently identify depression as a commonly occurring symptom that is the single strongest predictor of quality of life, even after accounting for effects on motor functioning (Zahodne et al., 2012). Current emphasis is on the importance of identifying and treating depression in people with functional impairments and pathologic conditions, such as cancer, chronic pain and neurologic disorders (Karp & McGovern, 2013; Steffens & Blazer, 2012; Wint & Cummings, 2013).

Effects of Medications and Alcohol

People of any age may experience depression as an adverse medication effect, but older adults are at higher risk because they are likely to take more medications. Medications may be risk factors for depression in the following ways:

- Adverse medication effects can cause a depressive syndrome that improves or disappears when the medication is stopped.
- Adverse medication effects can induce a depression that does not remit when the medications are stopped.
- Adverse medication effects can simulate a depressive syndrome by causing lethargy, insomnia and irritability.
- The withdrawal of certain medications, such as psychostimulants, can cause a depressive syndrome.

Depression, as an adverse effect of medications, is usually related to the use of medications, such as those prescribed for chronic conditions and listed in Box 15-2. However, depression

Box 15-2 Examples of Medications That Can Cause Depression

Analgesics
Indomethacin
Narcotics
Propoxyphene

Antihypertensives and Cardiovascular Agents
β-Blockers
Clonidine
Digitalis
Guanethidine
Hydralazine
Methyldopa
Reserpine

Antiparkinsonian Agents
Levodopa

Central Nervous System Agents
Alcohol
Barbiturates
Benzodiazepines
Fluphenazine
Haloperidol
Meprobamate

Histamine Blockers
Cimetidine

Steroids
Corticosteroids
Estrogen

Anticancer (Chemotherapeutic) Agents
Vinblastine

can also be an adverse effect of alcohol or drugs that are abused (e.g., benzodiazepines). Moreover, although people of any age may experience adverse effects from alcohol, older people are more sensitive to these adverse effects because of age-related changes. Alcohol and depression have a circular relationship: alcohol causes depression and depression leads to alcohol abuse, which in turn exacerbates the depression.

FUNCTIONAL CONSEQUENCES ASSOCIATED WITH DEPRESSION IN OLDER ADULTS

Depression has serious functional consequences for people of any age, but for frail and seriously depressed older adults, the effects can be life-threatening. Functional consequences range from a negative impact on well-being and quality of life to the most serious consequence, which is suicide, the intentional taking of one's own life. This section discusses the wide range of functional consequences that are associated with depression. Suicide is addressed as a separate topic at the end of this chapter because nurses need to address it

not only as the most serious consequence of depression, but also as an entity in itself.

Physical Health and Functioning

A decline in physical functioning is consistently identified as a serious functional consequence of depression in older adults (Barry et al., 2013). Additional functional consequences that affect health and functioning are a high number of physical complaints, perception of worse health and inability to carry out important life functions, such as managing money or medications. It is important to recognize that some of these consequences, such as the inability to manage money or medications, may be a central factor in preventing the person from living independently. Box 15-3 lists ways in which depression affects physical health and functioning.

Appetite disturbances, particularly anorexia, are among the most common physical complaints of depressed older adults. Sometimes, the depressed person does not complain of anorexia and may even deny the problem, but a caregiver or family member may note that the person is not interested in food and is losing weight. Other gastrointestinal complaints that may be functional consequences of depression include flatulence, constipation, early satiety and attention to bowels. Any of these disturbances may be attributed to or caused by other factors such as medical conditions or adverse medication effects; however, depression must be considered as a possible underlying factor. Chronic fatigue and diminished energy are additional functional consequences of late-life depression that are likely to be attributed to or caused by other conditions.

Box 15-3 Functional Consequences of Late-Life Depression

Impact on Physical Function
- Loss of appetite
- Weight loss
- Digestive system complaints, particularly dysphagia, flatulence, constipation, stomach distress or early satiety
- Insomnia, hypersomnia, frequent awakening, early-morning awakening and other sleep disturbances
- Fatigue, loss of energy
- Pain, discomfort, dyspnea, general malaise
- Slowed or increased psychomotor activities
- Loss of libido or other problems with sexual function

Impact on Psychosocial Function
- Affect: sad, low, "blue," worried, unhappy, "down in the dumps"

- Absence of feelings; feeling numb or empty
- Diminished life satisfaction
- Low self-esteem
- Loss of interest or pleasure
- Passivity, lack of motivation to do things
- Inattention to personal appearance
- Feelings of guilt, hopelessness, self-blame, unworthiness, uselessness, helplessness
- Anxiety, worry, irritability
- Slowed thinking, poor memory, inability to concentrate, poor attention span, inability to make decisions, exaggeration of any mental deficits
- Rumination about past and present problems and failures

Like weight loss and diminished appetite, sleep changes commonly occur in older adults, and they may or may not be caused by depression. Waking up more frequently during the night and early-morning awakening are two changes in sleep patterns that are characteristic of depression. Current research is exploring the bidirectional relationship between sleep changes and depression, with studies pointing toward insomnia being a risk factor for and a functional consequence of depression (Baglioni et al., 2013; Krystal et al., 2012).

Older adults, like seriously depressed people of any age, are likely to experience psychomotor agitation or retardation. **Psychomotor retardation** is manifested as slowed body movements and slowed verbal responses, sometimes to the point of muteness. A monotonous or whispering tone of voice might also be an indicator of psychomotor retardation. Affected people often complain of feeling extremely fatigued and having little or no energy. In contrast to people with psychomotor retardation, people with **psychomotor agitation** present an atypical picture of depression. These people manifest high levels of activity, such as pacing and hand wringing. They may be unable to sit still and may have verbal outbursts, such as shouting. Another activity associated with psychomotor agitation is compulsive behaviour, such as frequent toileting or handwashing.

In addition to direct functional consequences on health and functioning, late-life depression is associated with increased risk for developing medical conditions including cancer, coronary disease and type 2 diabetes (Park & Unutzer, 2013). Moreover, a review of studies concluded that there is strong evidence that depression increases morbidity and mortality (i.e., poor recovery, more complications and higher death rate) in people with all the following medical conditions: cancer, dementia, diabetes, osteoporosis, chronic pain, cardiovascular disease and cerebrovascular disease (Park & Unutzer, 2013).

Psychosocial Function and Quality of Life

Depression is inherently characterized by a depressed mood or sad affect, but older adults may not perceive or acknowledge these mood disturbances in themselves. Rather than acknowledging that they are depressed, older adults are more likely to talk about being "blue" or "down in the dumps." Or, depressed older adults may focus on physiological concerns, such as gastric problems. Depressed older people may feel like crying but may not be able to cry or identify the underlying reason for their sadness. Another psychosocial consequence of depression is the absence of life satisfaction, even when the person has reasons to feel satisfied.

Anxiety, irritability, diminished self-esteem and negative feelings about self are some of the more generalized affective consequences of depression. The absence of feelings, or a feeling of emptiness, can also be a functional consequence of depression. A loss of interest in social activities may be the depression-related psychosocial change that is most obvious to others. Similarly, other people are likely to observe that the depressed older person has little or no concern about personal appearance. In addition, the depressed person may be overly or unrealistically worried about illnesses, financial affairs and family issues.

Significantly slowed cognition can occur because of depression, and in older adults, these deficits are likely to be viewed as a primary problem rather than as a consequence of another problem. Depressed older adults may, in fact, exaggerate cognitive deficits and make statements about global deficits, such as, "I can't remember anything at all." In particular, they may emphasize memory deficits and attribute these to normal aging when the underlying problem is actually a depression-related difficulty in concentrating. See Box 15-3 for a list of functional consequences of depression that affect psychosocial function.

Late-life depression is strongly associated with diminished quality of life for older adults and their families. In fact, depression in older adults is associated with greater negative effects on quality of life than most chronic medical disorders, including diabetes and cancer (Park & Unutzer, 2013). Symptoms of depression that affect quality of life are fatigue, sad affect, excessive worry, sleep disturbances, a sense of hopelessness and loss of interest in social and productive relationships. Other consequences of depression that affect quality of life are unsatisfactory social functioning, lower levels of life satisfaction and poor perceptions of physical and mental health.

Wellness Opportunity

Because people who are depressed tend to have very low self-esteem, nurses can point out concrete examples of positive qualities that they see in the person.

NURSING ASSESSMENT OF DEPRESSION IN OLDER ADULTS

Whereas Chapter 13 addressed all aspects of psychosocial assessment, this section focuses on the following specific aspects of late-life depression: identifying the unique manifestations of depression in older adults, identifying depression in people with dementia and using screening tools to identify late-life depression. Assessing the suicide risk in older adults is discussed in the section on suicide. The assessment information in Chapter 13, particularly Box 13-9, can be used with the information in the following sections as a guide for assessing depression in older adults.

Wellness Opportunity

Nurses can ask a depressed older adult, "What is one thing that we can do to improve your quality of life today?"

Identifying the Unique Manifestations of Depression

Assessment of late-life depression is complicated by a wide array of possible manifestations, as reviewed in the

Functional Consequences section. Moreover, manifestations of depression in older adults may differ from those in younger adults. For example, older adults are less likely to show affective symptoms (e.g., sadness, crying spells, feeling fearful) and are more likely to have physical complaints (e.g., poor appetite, weight loss, gastrointestinal symptoms, loss of interest in sex) (Charlton et al., 2013; Hybels et al., 2012). Although it is difficult to generalize about manifestations of depression according to age categories, some conclusions about the differences in younger and older adults are summarized in Table 15-1.

In assessing depression in any cognitively impaired older adult, it is often difficult to distinguish between manifestations of depression and dementia. Table 15-2, which identifies specific features that are most likely to be associated with either dementia or depression, can be used as a guide for nursing assessment to differentiate between these two conditions. It is important to keep in mind that older adults with dementia frequently also have depression, so manifestations will not always be clearly distinguishable.

Cultural factors can influence one's perception of depression, and nurses must consider these, particularly during their assessments. Nurses can use the information in Box 15-4 to identify some of the cultural variations in expressions of depression. In addition, nurses need to be aware of and sensitive to the fact that many cultural groups attach a strong stigma to depression and other forms of mental illness. Thus, they need to use appropriate communication techniques when assessing for depression and discussing interventions with older adults and their caregivers.

> **Wellness Opportunity**
>
> Nurses respect individual preferences by listening carefully to identify acceptable terminology in older adults who do not want to acknowledge being "depressed."

TABLE 15-1 Comparison of Depression in Younger and Older Adults

Depressed Younger Adults	Depressed Older Adults
More likely to report emotional symptoms	Report more cognitive and physical symptoms
Sense of hopelessness, uselessness and helplessness	Apathy; exaggeration of personal helplessness
Negative feelings toward self	Sense of emptiness, loss of interest, withdrawal from social activities
Insomnia	Hypersomnia; early-morning awakening
Eating disorders	Anorexia, weight loss
More verbal expressions of suicidal ideation than successful attempts; more passive means of suicide	Less talk about suicide, but more successful attempts and more violent means of suicide

TABLE 15-2 Distinguishing Features of Dementia and Depression

Parameter	Dementia	Depression
Onset of symptoms	Gradual onset, recognized only by hindsight	Abrupt onset, possibly involving a triggering event
Presentation of symptoms	Unawareness of symptoms, or attribution to nonpathologic causes	Exaggeration of memory problems and other cognitive deficits
Memory and attention	Impaired memory, particularly for recent events; poor attention; strong attempts to perform well	Memory and attention deficits attributable to lack of motivation and inability to concentrate
Emotions	Labile affect that changes in response to suggestions; possible apathy owing to cognitive impairments	Consistent feelings of sadness and being "down in the dumps"; unresponsive to suggestions
Response to questions	Evasive, angry, sarcastic; use of humour, confabulation, or social skills to cover up deficits	Slowed, apathetic, frequent response of "I don't know," with no effort expended
Personal appearance	Inappropriate dress and actions owing to impaired perceptions and thought processes	Little or no concern about appearance because of lack of motivation or diminished self-esteem
Physical complaints	Vague fatigue and weakness; complaints are inconsistent and easily forgotten	Anorexia, weight loss, constipation, insomnia, decreased energy
Neurologic features	Aphasia, agnosia, agraphia, apraxia, perseveration	Complaints of dysphagia without any physical basis
Contact with reality	Denial of reality; illusions more predominant than hallucinations; if present, delusions are aimed at explaining deficits	Exaggerated sense of gloom; possible auditory hallucinations or self-derogatory delusions

Box 15-4 Cultural Considerations: Cultural Variations in Expressions of Depression

Cultural Group	Common Expressions of Depression
Aboriginal Canadians	Feelings of "heaviness" or "out of harmony"
African Canadians	Fatigue and somatic complaints
Arabs	Fatigue, sadness, restlessness, hypersomnia; talking about physical complaints protects the person from stigma associated with mental health problems
Chinese Canadians	Shameful to discuss; may be called "neurasthenia" (i.e., symptoms produced by social stressors or weak nerves)
Filipinos	Shameful to discuss; may refer to *Lungknot* (i.e., sadness)
Greeks	Emotional distress is likely to present with somatic complaints such as dizziness and paresthesias
Indians (South Asia)	Often focus on physical symptoms
Japanese Canadians	Because of shame and stigma, emotional distress may be expressed through physical symptoms and may become severe before help is sought
Koreans	Emotions are expressed as physical complaints, including headaches, insomnia, anorexia and lack of energy

Sources: Andrews, M. M., & Boyle, J. S. (2012). *Transcultural concepts in nursing care* (5th ed.). Philadelphia, PA: Lippincott Williams & Wilkins; Grover, S., Dutt, A., & Avasthi, A. (2010). An overview of Indian research in depression. Indian Journal of Psychiatry, 52, S178–S188; Lipson, J. G., & Dibble, S. L. (2005). *Culture and clinical care*. San Francisco, CA: UCSF Nursing Press; Purnell, L. D. (2013). *Transcultural health care: A culturally competent approach* (4th ed.). Philadelphia, PA: F.A. Davis.

Using Screening Tools

Concerns about depression being unrecognized and undertreated in older people have stimulated the development of very brief screening tools that health care professionals can use in a variety of settings. The Canadian Coalition for Seniors' Mental Health (2006a) proposed guidelines for the assessment and treatment of older adults with depression. They recommend that health care providers be aware of the risk factors for depression in older adults and assess their clients for these risk factors. If older individuals present with some of these risk factors (such as recent bereavement, social isolation, refusal to eat or neglect of self-care), health care providers should assess further with a formal depression scale.

The **Geriatric Depression Scale—Short Form** is a 15-question screening tool that is widely used across health care settings for older adults and can be administered in 5 to 7 minutes. The Canadian Coalition on Seniors' Mental Health (2006a) recommends the Geriatric Depression Scale (Fig. 15-2) as a screening tool to detect depression in older adults, and it can be used for older adults with cognitive impairment (Greenberg, 2012; Harvath & McKenzie, 2012). This tool and related scoring form can be downloaded free of cost in English and more than 30 other languages. Online Learning Activity 15-1 provides links to this tool and helpful resources related to this and other screening tools.

See **ONLINE LEARNING ACTIVITY 15-1: LINKS TO ADDITIONAL INFORMATION ABOUT ASSESSMENT OF DEPRESSION IN OLDER ADULTS**
at **http://thepoint.lww.com/Miller7e**

NURSING DIAGNOSIS

Because there is no specific nursing diagnosis for depression, the following nursing diagnoses may be applicable: Anxiety, Ineffective Coping, Grieving, Hopelessness, Powerlessness, Social Isolation, Caregiver Role Strain and Risk for Compromised Resilience. Related factors commonly found

---

Geriatric Depression Scale (Short Form)

1. Are you basically satisfied with your life?	Yes	No
2. Have you dropped many of your activities and interests?	Yes	No
3. Do you feel that your life is empty?	Yes	No
4. Do you often get bored?	Yes	No
5. Are you in good spririts most of the time?	Yes	No
6. Are you afraid that something bad is going to happen to you?	Yes	No
7. Do you feel happy most of the time?	Yes	No
8. Do you often feel helpless?	Yes	No
9. Do you prefer to stay at home rather than go out and do new things?	Yes	No
10. Do you feel you have more problems with memory than most?	Yes	No
11. Do you think it is wonderful to be alive now?	Yes	No
12. Do you feel pretty worthless the way you are now?	Yes	No
13. Do you feel full of energy?	Yes	No
14. Do you feel that your situation is hopeless?	Yes	No
15. Do you think that most people are better off than you are?	Yes	No

Score:___/15   One point for "No" to questions 1, 5, 7, 11, 13
One point for "Yes" to other questions

Normal	3 ± 2
Mildly depressed	7 ± 3
Very depressed	12 ± 2

FIGURE 15-2 Geriatric Depression Scale (Short Form). (Available at www.stanford.edu/~yesavage/GDS.html)

in older adults are chronic pain, cognitive impairment, medical conditions, functional limitations, financial concerns, social isolation, caregiving responsibilities, multiple social stressors and loss of significant roles or relationships.

> **Wellness Opportunity**
>
> Nurses can use the wellness nursing diagnosis of Readiness for Enhanced Coping for older adults who are interested in improving their coping skills to address depressive symptoms that are not severe.

PLANNING FOR WELLNESS OUTCOMES

When caring for older adults who are depressed, nurses identify outcomes as an essential part of the planning process. The following Nursing Outcomes Classification (NOC) terminology is applicable to depressed older adults: Caregiver Emotional Health, Coping, Depression Level, Hope, Knowledge: Depression Management, Self-Esteem, Social Support and Social Involvement. Suicide Self-Restraint is applicable when care plans address risks for suicide. Specific interventions to achieve outcomes related to depression and suicide are discussed in the following sections.

> **Wellness Opportunity**
>
> Quality of life is a wellness outcome that is achieved by addressing the functional and psychosocial consequences of depression.

 ## NURSING INTERVENTIONS TO ADDRESS DEPRESSION

Although all nurses are responsible for addressing depression in older adults, those who work in community-based and long-term care settings have the most ongoing opportunities to identify manifestations of depression and to request further evaluation and treatment. In recent years, primary care physicians and nurse practitioners have been the health care professionals evaluating and managing depression, and referrals to psychiatrists and other mental health professionals for depression have become less common. This trend is due to the emphasis on cost-effectiveness and the availability of safer and more effective antidepressant medications. Nursing protocols for depression in elderly patients emphasize the important responsibility of nurses in reducing the negative consequences of depression through early recognition, intervention and referral of patients with depression (Harvath & McKenzie, 2012).

Nursing Interventions Classification (NIC) terminologies pertinent to interventions for older adults who are depressed include the following: Caregiver Support, Coping Enhancement, Counselling, Crisis Intervention, Emotional Support, Exercise Promotion, Grief Work Facilitation, Hope Inspiration, Mood Management, Referral, Role

Enhancement, Self-Esteem Enhancement, Suicide Prevention and Teaching: Individual. The next sections review the role of the nurse in planning and implementing interventions for late-life depression.

Alleviating Risk Factors

Nurses promote wellness for depressed older adults by addressing the many risk factors that are well within the realm of nursing, such as functional impairments, adverse medication effects and excess alcohol use. Many nursing interventions that improve the level of functioning are also effective for alleviating or preventing depression. For example, dementia, sensory impairments, urinary incontinence and mobility impairments are examples of conditions that can contribute to depression and will respond to nursing interventions (refer to Chapters 14, 16, 17, 19 and 22), thereby positively affecting depression.

> **Wellness Opportunity**
>
> Nurses promote wellness by challenging ageist stereotypes that falsely attribute functional impairments to inevitable consequences of aging.

If adverse medication effects are a risk factor for depression, nurses can educate the person about this potential relationship and identify problem-solving strategies to address the adverse effects (as discussed in Chapter 8). For example, if the older person understands that there is a wide array of antihypertensive medications and that not all of them will cause depression, the person can use this information in discussing the problem with his or her primary care provider. Nurses can also reassure the older adult that it is acceptable to initiate this kind of problem-solving discussion with health care practitioners. When the nurse, rather than the patient, is the one who communicates with the primary care provider, the nurse can raise appropriate questions about depression as an adverse medication effect. This problem-solving approach is particularly important when the primary care provider is considering adding an antidepressant medication to a regimen that includes a depression-inducing medication. In these situations, the solution may be to change medications rather than to add another medication and increase the risk for adverse effects.

If excess alcohol use is a risk factor for depression, individual and group interventions can be effective, particularly when the alcohol abuse is a reaction to recent losses. Alcoholics Anonymous (AA) is the most widely used group program for alcoholics of any age, and in some areas, age-homogeneous groups have been established, including some for older adults. Nurses can encourage older adults to initiate contact with AA, or they might directly facilitate the referral if the person agrees to this. Individual and family counselling may also be effective, and nurses can suggest or facilitate referrals for these mental health services.

Improving Psychosocial Function

In any clinical setting, nurses can focus on interventions to promote autonomy, personal control, self-efficacy and decision making about daily care as an intervention for depression (Harvath & McKenzie, 2012). In addition, interventions to improve overall psychosocial function, as discussed in Chapter 12, are applicable for addressing risk factors for and symptoms of depression. For example, interventions to strengthen social supports and foster meaningful roles are particularly pertinent and relatively easy to implement. Nurses have many opportunities to encourage participation in group meals or social programs. Many communities in Canada have some social programs for older adults, and some provide transportation. Many churches and religious organizations also have programs designed to meet the social needs of isolated older adults. Volunteer visitor or phone call programs, for example, are sometimes available to address the needs of people who have difficulty with getting out of the house. Other programs, such as pet therapy or "Adopt-a-Grandparent," are available in some home, community-based, and long-term care settings, and they can be helpful in alleviating loneliness and depression. Nurses can also encourage older adults to maintain social contacts through simple measures such as phone calls.

Involvement in volunteer activities can enhance self-esteem and provide meaningful roles for older adults who are mildly depressed. Nurses can suggest that older adults explore opportunities for volunteer activities through Volunteer Canada (www.volunteer.ca). This site provides information salient to older adults who want to volunteer, as well as links to local volunteer agencies in specific provinces/territories.

Wellness Opportunity

Nurses promote quality of life by encouraging an older adult to engage in activities that are pleasant and meaningful to that person.

Promoting Health Through Physical Activity and Nutrition

The beneficial effects of exercise as an intervention for depression have been documented in research reviews (Cooney et al., 2013; Joutsenniemi et al., 2013). Older adults, however, may not view exercise as important, or they may be reluctant to participate in exercise programs because of chronic illnesses such as arthritis. If older adults understand the benefits of exercise for both their physical and mental health, and if an individually tailored program is developed for them, they may be more willing to become involved in exercise programs. In community and long-term care settings, nurses can facilitate the establishment of group exercise programs and encourage depressed older adults to participate in them. In addition to encouraging participation in exercise programs, nurses can encourage participation in many other

Box 15-5 Evidence-Informed Nursing Practice

Background: Physical activity is believed to improve physical health, but how it aids in improving mental health of older adults is less clear. Few studies have focused on walking as a predictor of the extent of depression in older adults.

Method: The researchers conducted a cross-sectional analysis of a 5-year longitudinal study. They examined data from 549 community-dwelling participants in Quebec aged 68 to 84 years (mean age = 74.6 years; approximately equal representation of males and females). Measures of analysis included the Geriatric Depression Scale (GDS) and the Physical Activity Scale for the Elderly (PASE).

Findings: The researchers discovered an inverse relationship between walking and depression; that is, participants who walked regularly outside of the home experienced significantly less depression than those who did not walk or rarely walked.

Implications for Nursing Practice: Unless contraindicated due to severe health challenges, nurses can educate older adults on the importance of walking as a protective factor against depression, as well as an important intervention to address depression.

Source: Julien, D., Gauvin, L., Richard, L., et al. (2013). The role of social participation and walking in depression among older adults: Results from the VoisiNuAge study. *Canadian Journal on Aging, 32*(1), 1–12. doi:10.1017/S071498081300007X

forms of physical activity (see Box 15-5 for research on the benefits of walking for older adults). Even in hospital settings, nurses can facilitate referrals to physical, occupational and recreational therapists as a psychosocial nursing intervention (Harvath & McKenzie, 2012).

Nutrition is an important consideration as an intervention for depression for three reasons. First, depression often negatively affects nutritional status, and this can cause additional negative consequences. Second, good nutrition has a positive effect on mental health and cognitive function. Third, constipation is both a consequence of depression and an adverse effect of some antidepressant medications, and nutritional interventions can be effective in alleviating it. During phases of serious depression, malnutrition can lead to medical problems, which may progress to the point of being life-threatening. When depression is severe enough to lead to malnutrition, the older person must be evaluated for in-patient psychiatric care. Interventions for less severely depressed older people are aimed at maintaining adequate hydration and nutrition and preventing or managing constipation (as discussed in Chapter 18).

Wellness Opportunity

Nurses address the body–mind–spirit interrelationship by incorporating interventions for optimal nutrition as an essential component of care for depressed older adults.

Providing Education and Counselling

Many types of individual and group **psychosocial therapies** are effective interventions for late-life depression. For example, when multiple stressors challenge the person's coping abilities and contribute to depression, individual or group therapy can be an important intervention for improving the person's psychosocial health and alleviating depression. In addition, nurses provide psychosocial support through holistic nursing interventions such as the following (Helming, 2013):

- Helping older adults identify nonverbalized fears and provide reality-based information to help them evaluate the fear
- Assisting older adults to verbalize emotions by identifying and labelling them so they can communicate more effectively about their emotions and fear
- Providing counselling on the basis of basic psychological theories and concepts
- Encouraging "storytelling" and helping older adults to acknowledge their strengths, as well as weaknesses, through the power of storytelling
- Facilitating referrals to appropriate mental health services

In addition, good communication skills, such as active listening and expressing empathy, can be effective for addressing sadness about losses. Nurses in home care settings are in a unique position to use psychosocial interventions for depression while they also are addressing needs related to functional impairment, and these can be especially effective for homebound older adults (Liebel & Powers, 2013; Madden-Baer et al., 2013).

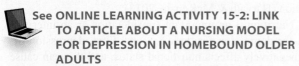

See ONLINE LEARNING ACTIVITY 15-2: LINK TO ARTICLE ABOUT A NURSING MODEL FOR DEPRESSION IN HOMEBOUND OLDER ADULTS
at http://thepoint.lww.com/Miller7e

A Student's Perspective

The life review interview with Mrs. R. enlightened me for one very simple reason: she loves the life she lived. She has no regrets about her life and said she would change nothing. She is a very positive person, and hearing her outlook at life really got me thinking about the way I want to continue to live my life. It was inspiring to hear her views, and it takes away some of my fears of growing older.

The most significant point in the life review interview is actually the same as the most difficult part. We were discussing family, and I wasn't sure if I should ask about her late husband because I didn't know how to bring him up. I finally found a way to ask about him and immediately her eyes filled with tears. She began to describe him and the things they used to do together. It was sad; yet hearing about how much she loved him was touching. She continued to cry as she said he was the best person she ever knew. Without even thinking, I grabbed her hand. As she squeezed my hand, I saw her become more at ease. With just that little action, I feel like I made her feel better. I had no idea that holding someone's hand could have such a powerful effect.

Molly D.

Nurses need to be sufficiently familiar with psychosocial therapies that are commonly used for depressed older adults, so they can encourage or facilitate referrals for these interventions. Types of psychosocial therapies that are effective for depression in older adults, either as individual or group therapies are as follows:

- Cognitive-behavioural therapy, which involves cognitive restructuring and behavioural activation
- Problem solving to address problems related to social engagement, relationships, mood and health
- Supportive therapy, which involves evaluating the person's strengths and weaknesses and facilitating choices that improve coping abilities
- Life review and reminiscence, which helps people reexperience meaningful events of their lives
- Bibliotherapy, which uses books and articles to enhance coping skills or assist the person in identifying and reducing dysfunctional thought processes (Arean, 2013; Lynch et al., 2012).

Support and self-help groups can also improve psychosocial function and alleviate depression in older adults who are coping with life events, such as caregiving, widowhood or grief reactions. Other group models used as interventions for late-life depression include relaxation, art therapy, focused imagery and creative movement. In addition to groups specifically targeted for depression, groups such as the "Healthy Aging Class" (described in Chapter 12), which are directed at developing coping skills, may be effective in alleviating depression.

Although adult day programs are not primarily a group therapy for depressed older adults, they are a commonly available resource for providing structured social and therapeutic activities. Similarly, many community-based senior programs provide opportunities for group meals, exercise and social interaction, and these can be quite effective in alleviating mild to moderate depression in older adults. Information about these and other group programs for older adults can be obtained from local seniors' centres, and nurses can encourage older adults or their caregivers to seek out and take advantage of these programs.

Facilitating Referrals for Psychosocial Therapies

Nurses have important roles in facilitating referrals for appropriate psychosocial therapies, particularly for older adults who are seriously depressed. In addition to facilitating referrals for mental health services, nurses often have opportunities to initiate discussion of psychosocial therapies during the course of their usual work with older adults. Interprofessional geriatric mental health and geriatric assessment offer assessment and treatment of late-life depression, and some community mental health centres have programs for depressed older adults. Nurses can either suggest or directly facilitate referrals to these programs. A major consideration with regard to referrals for depression interventions is that there is compelling evidence to support the effectiveness of many psychosocial therapies, as well as the use of antidepressant medications, either alone or in combination (Harvath & McKenzie, 2012; Trangle et al., 2012).

Teaching About and Managing Antidepressant Medications

Types of Antidepressant Medications

Nurses need to understand the types of antidepressants available in order to educate older adults about their medications. Major types of antidepressants are monoamine oxidase inhibitors, cyclic antidepressants, selective serotonin reuptake inhibitors (SSRIs), serotonin and norepinephrine reuptake inhibitors (SNRIs) and atypical antidepressants (i.e., those that do not fit any other category).

Monoamine oxidase inhibitors (e.g., phenelzine, isocarboxazid, tranylcypromine) were the first antidepressants developed during the 1960s. With increasing use of these medications, it became evident that they caused serious and even fatal adverse effects when they interacted with numerous other medications and with certain types of food. Another disadvantage is that monoamine oxidase inhibitors are associated with agitation and psychosis in older adults with dementia. Currently, these antidepressants are rarely used and only when other therapies have been ineffective and under the supervision of a psychiatrist.

Cyclic antidepressants are particularly effective in alleviating the following depression-related symptoms: loss of libido, sleep and appetite disturbances, and loss of interest and pleasure in activities. Cyclic antidepressants are usually categorized as tricyclic antidepressants, which were developed in the 1950s, and second-generation agents, which have been widely used since the mid-1980s. Because cyclic antidepressants affect several neurotransmitters, they are associated with a variety of anticholinergic and other detrimental effects. Two particular areas of concern in geriatric care are the potential for adverse cardiovascular and anticholinergic effects. The most likely cardiovascular effects are orthostatic hypotension and altered cardiac rate and rhythm. Serious anticholinergic effects include blurred vision, urinary retention and cognitive impairments. Additional common side effects are sedation, constipation, dry mouth and weight gain. Because of these side effects, people with glaucoma, prostatic hyperplasia or cardiac conduction abnormalities should not take cyclic antidepressants. In addition, cyclic antidepressants should be avoided in people with dementia or Parkinson disease because of the potential adverse effect of cognitive impairment. Anticholinergic potency varies among the tricyclic antidepressants, with amitriptyline having the strongest anticholinergic effects and desipramine having the weakest. As a rule of thumb for older adults, cyclic agents

with weaker anticholinergic effects should be prescribed over those with stronger anticholinergic effects. However, because of their side effects and lethality risk in situations of overdose, they are not the first line of treatment for older adults (Wiese, 2011).

During the late 1980s, pharmaceutical companies developed two classes of antidepressants that were chemically unrelated to and more selective in their action than the cyclic antidepressants. **Selective serotonin reuptake inhibitors (SSRIs)** relieve symptoms of depression by blocking the reuptake of serotonin, so the level of this neurotransmitter is increased in the brain cells. **Serotonin and norepinephrine reuptake inhibitors (SNRIs)** increase the levels of both serotonin and norepinephrine by inhibiting the reuptake of these neurotransmitters in the brain cells. This type of antidepressant is also called a dual reuptake inhibitor. The therapeutic effectiveness of SSRIs and SNRIs is similar to that of cyclic antidepressants, but they have minimal cholinergic, histaminic, dopaminergic and noradrenergic effects. Hyponatremia is an adverse effect of SSRIs and SNRIs that is common in older adults but rare in younger adults (Mulsant & Pollock, 2012). Because hyponatremia can develop rapidly and progress to serious consequences during antidepressant treatment, frequent monitoring of electrolytes is recommended (Giorlando et al., 2013).

Clinical guidelines recommend SSRIs as the first-line medications for depression because there is a strong base of evidence in support of their relative safety, high efficacy and broad spectrum of action (Mulsant & Pollock, 2012; Trangle et al., 2012). Although SSRIs are safer than other types of antidepressants, it is important to assess for adverse effects and drug interactions. For example, because SSRIs are metabolized in the liver and some of them are highly bound to plasma protein, SSRIs may interact with other drugs that are metabolized in the liver or are highly protein bound. In addition, it is important to observe for drug interactions, including interactions with over-the-counter products (e.g., nonsteroidal anti-inflammatory drugs or low-dose aspirin) or another drug or dietary supplement that increases serotonin levels in the brain (e.g., meperidine, dextromethorphan, L-tryptophan, St. John's wort). The general principle of treatment is to "start low and go slow." This means that half the adult dosage is usually given to older adults and if dosages need to be increased, incremental increases are given cautiously. Drug interactions may occur even after an SSRI with a long half-life (e.g., fluoxetine) has been discontinued. Common adverse effects of SSRIs include nausea, vomiting, diarrhea, headache, nervousness, insomnia, tremor, dry mouth and sexual dysfunction. Withdrawal effects of SSRIs include nausea, tremor, anxiety, dizziness, palpitations and paresthesias.

Antidepressants that are commonly used for older adults are listed in Table 15-3 according to their classifications. Special considerations in the use of some of these antidepressants are as follows: Venlafaxine may cause an increase in blood pressure (in particular, diastolic elevation); mirtazapine can be helpful for stimulating appetite, but it can

TABLE 15-3 Antidepressants Commonly Used for Older Adults

Category	Examples	Trade Names
Selective serotonin reuptake inhibitors (SSRIs)	Citalopram	Celexa
	Escitalopram	Cipralex
	Fluvoxamine	Luvox
	Paroxetine	Paxil
	Sertraline	Zoloft
Serotonin and norepinephrine reuptake inhibitors (SNRIs)	Desvenlafaxine	Pristiq
	Duloxetine	Cymbalta
	Venlafaxine	Effexor
Serotonin modulators	Nefazodone	Serzone
	Trazodone	Desyrel
Dopamine reuptake inhibitors	Bupropion	Wellbutrin
Cyclic antidepressants	Amoxapine	Asendin
	Desipramine	Norpramin
	Imipramine	Tofranil
	Nortriptyline	Pamelor
Tetracyclic antidepressants	Mirtazapine	Remeron

also be sedating; trazodone and nefazodone are very sedating and may be useful in the treatment of depression with sleep disturbances; bupropion has a stimulating effect, which can sometimes be therapeutic but is contraindicated in people with a seizure disorder; and bupropion and mirtazapine have the lowest rate of sexual side effects. Also, it is important to monitor serum sodium levels initially and periodically for older adults who are taking SSRIs.

Nurses also need to be aware that the following antidepressants that are contraindicated in older adults due to their adverse effects: amitriptyline (Elavil), doxepine (Sinequan) and fluoxetine daily dose (Prozac) (Wiese, 2011). Psychomotor stimulants (e.g., methylphenidate) have been used for decades for certain types of depression, but they are not commonly used for older adults.

Nursing Responsibilities Regarding Antidepressants

An important nursing responsibility regarding antidepressants is to educate older adults about the primary purpose of these medications, which is to alleviate depressive symptoms so that the person is able to respond to additional interventions such as psychosocial therapy. For older adults who have both depression and dementia, antidepressant medications may improve the affective symptoms so that overall abilities are improved and the person is able to function more effectively and independently.

Nursing responsibilities regarding antidepressant medication therapy include observing for both adverse and

therapeutic effects and educating the older adult about the unique aspects of these medication therapies. Another important responsibility is educating older adults about the need for ongoing evaluation and treatment of depression, including the monitoring of antidepressant medication use. Older adults who have been diagnosed with major depressive disorder are at high risk of recurrence, and this risk is increased if antidepressant medications are not maintained for at least 12 months (Frank, 2014). Older adults often want to discontinue medications when their depressive symptoms resolve, and nurses need to teach them about the importance of ongoing antidepressant therapy and periodic reevaluations after medications are discontinued. This is particularly important because a patient's beliefs about the use of medications affect adherence; therefore, beliefs need to be explored before and during medication therapy. Box 15-6 summarizes guidelines for the nursing responsibilities regarding antidepressant medications.

Teaching About Complementary and Alternative Interventions

There has been increasing interest in the use of herbs and other natural remedies for depression. **St. John's wort** (*Hypericum perforatum*) is widely used in Europe and is the most commonly used antidepressant in Germany. Recent reviews of studies concluded that St. John's wort may be effective for treating mild to moderate depression, but is not effective for serious depression (Merrill et al., 2013; National Centre on

Box 15-6 Health Education About Antidepressant Medications

Information to Be Shared With the Older Adult

- Immediate improvement will not be evident, but a fair trial must be given to the medication as long as serious adverse effects are not noticed.
- The fair trial may take as long as 12 weeks, but some positive effects should be noticed within 2 to 4 weeks.
- If one type of antidepressant is not effective, another type may be effective.
- Antidepressants cannot be used on an "as needed" basis.
- Antidepressants should be viewed as part of a comprehensive approach to treating depression, and psychosocial therapies should be considered along with antidepressants.
- Antidepressants can interact with alcohol, nicotine and other medications, including over-the-counter medications, possibly altering the effects of the medication or increasing the potential for adverse effects.
- It is important to have information about potential adverse effects and drug–drug or food–drug interactions.
- The prescribing health care practitioner should be consulted before discontinuing an antidepressant.
- If postural hypotension occurs, the effects can be minimized through such interventions as changing position slowly and maintaining adequate fluid intake.
- If monoamine oxidase inhibitors (MAOIs) are prescribed, certain medications must be avoided, and a low-tyramine diet must be followed (i.e., avoidance of beer, yogurt, red wine, fermented cheese and pickled foods, as well as excessive amounts of caffeine and chocolate).

Principles Regarding Dosage and Length of Treatment

- Older adults should be started at one-half to one-third the normal adult dose.
- Dosages can be increased gradually until maximal therapeutic levels are reached, while observing for adverse effects.
- Age-related changes may increase the time needed for medication to reach maximal effectiveness.
- A once-daily regimen usually is effective.
- Bedtime administration of an antidepressant may facilitate sleep as a result of the drug's hypnotic effects, but some antidepressants may be better taken in the morning because of side effects, such as agitation.
- The length of treatment is usually 9 to 12 months for a first-time depression, 1 to 2 years for people with a history of a prior depressive episode, and lifetime maintenance for people with a history of three or more depressive episodes.

Complementary and Alternative Medicine, 2013; Trangle et al., 2012). Common side effects include fatigue, headache, photosensitivity, dry mouth, and gastrointestinal effects. St. John's wort is relatively safe, but serious drug interactions can occur, for example, with antidepressants, digoxin and anticoagulants. This herb is widely available in Canada and inexpensive; however, not all preparations of St. John's wort are the same. They may have different standardized doses of hypericin (Health Link BC, 2011) (see Chapter 8).

Light therapy (also called bright-light therapy) is an evidence-based treatment of some types of depression, including those with seasonal patterns, both as a standalone intervention and to enhance the effects of antidepressants (Trangle et al., 2012). Light therapy involves exposure to 5,000 to 10,000 lux of bright light for 30 to 60 minutes daily. Nurses can use Box 15-7 as a guide to teaching older adults about interventions that may be helpful for preventing or alleviating depression.

Teaching About Electroconvulsive Therapy

Electroconvulsive therapy (ECT), which involves the electrical induction of seizures, is a treatment that is highly effective for treating severe depressive episodes. Studies consistently find that ECT is the most rapid and effective

Box 15-7 Interventions Commonly Used for Preventing or Alleviating Depression

Health Promotion Interventions

- Participate in enjoyable physical activity for a minimum of 30 minutes, five times weekly.
- Seek individual or group counselling to address stressful situations.
- If symptoms of depression affect daily functioning or quality of life, seek evaluation and treatment from a primary care practitioner.
- Use stress-reduction interventions, such as relaxation, meditation, yoga and tai chi.
- Use creative and expressive activities, such as dance, art, music and drama.

Nutritional Considerations

- Ensure adequate intake of (or use supplements of) the following nutrients: magnesium, selenium and vitamins B, C and D.

treatment for major depression in older adults and, in fact, has many potential advantages over antidepressants (McDonald & Vahabzadeh, 2013; Oudman, 2012; Weiner & Krystal, 2012). Evidence-based guidelines recommend consideration for ECT for older adults in any of the following circumstances (Frank, 2014):

- When antidepressants are ineffective, not tolerated or pose significant medical risk
- When any of the following conditions exist: catatonia, severe risk of suicide, depression with psychosis
- When the patient's health is significantly compromised due to depression (e.g. not eating, functional impairment)
- Combination of depression and Parkinson disease

Prevalent negative attitudes about ECT are attributable, in part, to the alleged inhumane use of this procedure when it was first developed a half century ago. In recent years, however, the technique for administering ECT has been refined, and the risks, discomfort and side effects are now quite minimal. Adverse effects include headache, nausea, disorientation, memory loss, impaired attention and decreased concentration. Adverse effects usually are transient; however, the adverse cognitive effects may be more extensive or even permanent, particularly after several courses of ECT. Studies are inconclusive with regard to increased vulnerability of older adults to adverse cognitive effects, but at least one study (Verwijk et al., 2013) found improvements in cognitive function at 6 months after ECT treatments in depressed patients aged 55 or older. After an initial course of ECT, antidepressants and maintenance treatments of ECT are effective for maintaining the positive results and preventing a relapse (Rapinesi et al., 2013; Weiner & Krystal, 2012).

With the exception of psychiatric settings, nurses will not be involved with the care of people who are undergoing ECT. Nurses caring for depressed people in any setting, however, need to be aware of evidence-based guidelines for the use of ECT and maintain an open mind about this therapy. In addition, nurses may be in a position to encourage older adults or their caregivers to seek advice about ECT from knowledgeable professionals.

EVALUATING THE EFFECTIVENESS OF NURSING INTERVENTIONS

Nurses evaluate their care of depressed older adults by documenting improved coping skills and diminished manifestations of depression. For example, the person may report diminished feelings of hopelessness and improved appetite and sleep. Another measure revealing improved quality of life would be the older adult's interest and participation in meaningful activities. Effectiveness of nursing interventions may also be evaluated by whether the older adult has begun taking antidepressant medications and participating in individual or group therapies. Box 15-8 summarizes evidence-based guidelines for nursing assessment and interventions related to depression in older adults.

Box 15-8 Evidence-Based Practice: Guidelines for Depression in Older Adults

Statement of the Problem

- Depression is highly prevalent in older adults and is not a natural part of aging.
- Depressive symptoms are associated with higher morbidity and mortality rates in older adults; specific consequences of depression include heightened pain and disability, delayed recovery from illness or surgery, worsening of medical conditions and suicide.
- Depressive symptoms are more common in older adults who have dementia or more severe or chronic disabling conditions.
  - In older adults who are cognitively impaired, depression may be expressed through the following behaviours: repetitive verbalizations, agitated vocalizations, expressions of unrealistic fears, repetitive statements about the occurrence of bad events, exaggerated concerns about health and verbal and/or physical aggression.
- Nurses are at the front line in the early recognition of depression and the facilitation of mental health services.

Recommendations for Nursing Assessment

- Depression may range in severity from mild symptoms to more severe forms, both of which can persist over longer periods and have serious negative consequences for the older adult.
- Depression can occur for the first time in late life or it can be part of a long-standing affective disorder.
- Recognition of depression in older adults is complicated by the coexistence of medical illnesses, disability, cognitive dysfunction and psychosocial adversity in older adults.
- The nursing standard of practice for depression in older adults includes the following assessment parameters: identifying risk factors and high-risk groups, using GDS-SF for screening, performing a focused depression assessment on all high-risk groups, obtaining and reviewing medical history and physical/neurologic examination, assessing for medications and medical conditions that may contribute to depression, assessing cognitive function and level of functioning.
- Risks for late-life suicide include depressive symptoms, perceived health status, sleep quality, absence of a confidant, disruption of social support, family conflict and loneliness.

Recommendations for Care

- For severe depression (e.g., GDS 11 or greater), refer for psychiatric evaluation and treatment with medication, psychosocial therapies, hospitalization or ECT.
- For less severe depression (e.g., GDS score between 6 and 10), refer to mental health services for psychosocial therapies and determination whether antidepressant therapy is warranted.
- For all levels of depression, develop an individualized plan integrating nursing interventions that address issues such as safety, nutrition, risk factors, health education, social support, pleasant reminiscence and relaxation therapies.

Recommendations for Patient Teaching

Teach older adults and caregivers about the following:
- Depression is common, treatable and not the depressed person's fault.
- Adherence to the prescribed treatment regimen, including medications, is imperative to prevent recurrence.
- It is important to be aware of the therapeutic and adverse effects of the prescribed antidepressant.

Source: Harvath, T. A., & McKenzie, G. (2012). Depression. In E. Capezuti, D. Zwicker, M. Mezey et al. (Eds.), *Evidence-based geriatric nursing protocols for best practice* (4th ed., pp. 135–162). New York, NY: Springer.

SUICIDE IN LATE LIFE

Suicide in late life is often overlooked because older adulthood is associated with passivity and nonviolence, whereas suicide is associated with aggressiveness and violence. In addition, there has been increasing media attention to suicide in teens and young adults, but less attention to suicide in older adults. Despite the lack of attention to suicide in older adults, this issue is a major public health concern that will likely increase in severity as indicated by the following statistics:

- Across groups by age and race, men age 85 years and older have the highest suicide rate in Canada (Public Health Agency of Canada, 2010).
- The rate of nonfatal attempt versus completed suicide is 4:1 for older adults, compared with 20:1 for younger adults who attempt suicide (Canadian Coalition for Seniors' Mental Health, 2006b; Centre for Suicide Prevention, 2012).
- There is particular concern about the cohort of adults born between 1946 and 1964 (i.e., "Baby Boomers") because this group has consistently had a high rate of suicide during their lifetime and continue to show high rates (Monette, 2012).

Official data about suicide do not include information about suicidal events that are unreported for reasons such as family efforts to conceal evidence and difficulty determining the true cause of death in medically ill people. Nor do these rates reflect the unrecognized suicidal acts that older adults indirectly or subtly use to take their own lives such as refusal to eat, failure to take medically necessary medications and other means of self-neglect. Suicide rates and mechanisms vary significantly by age groupings, as illustrated in Figure 15-3.

 DIVERSITY NOTE

At all ages, and by race and ethnicity, the suicide rates are consistently higher for males than for females.

Assessing the Risks for Suicide

Nursing assessment of suicide risk is particularly important because many older people give clues, sometimes to a number of people, about potential suicide. These clues, however, may be subtle, and the person who hears them may not associate them with suicide risk, particularly in older adults. By identifying risk factors, nurses can initiate interventions to prevent suicide. This is particularly important because approximately three quarters of older people who commit suicide visit their primary care provider within 1 month before the act, but they are not likely to directly express suicidal ideation. Thus, health care providers need to assess for risks and identify those older adults who may be contemplating

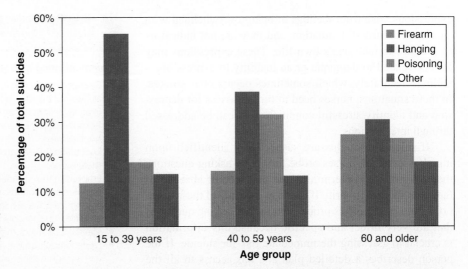

FIGURE 15-3 Percentage distribution of method used in suicide, by age group, Canada, 2000–2009 (10-year average). (Statistics Canada. [2012]. *Suicide rates: An overview.* Retrieved from http://www.statcan.gc.ca/pub/82-624-x/2012001/article/chart/11696-02-chart3-eng.htm)

suicide. The following are some of the more commonly identified risks for suicide in older adults:

- Depression, which may be masked by excessive focus on physical complaints
- Personal or family history of depression
- Past suicide attempts
- Loneliness, limited social support
- Family discord
- Feelings of abandonment
- Recent bereavement
- Presence of chronic or severe pain

Because depression is the factor most consistently identified across studies as a risk factor for suicide, it is important to assess for suicidal ideation in any depressed older adult. In addition to these factors that alert the nurse to risk for suicide, the factor that is most strongly predictive of actual suicide is current suicide ideation that includes a plan or evidence of preparation of a plan.

When risk factors or clues to potential suicide are identified, the nurse must further assess the actual risk for a suicide attempt. This assessment is multilevel, with each level of questions depending on the response to the previous level. Nurses begin the assessment with initial questions to determine the presence or absence of suicidal thoughts. Although health care professionals may be reluctant to initiate questions about suicide because they fear that this line of questioning may "put ideas in the person's head," this fear is unfounded. People who do not have suicidal thoughts usually respect the necessity of the questions but do not begin thinking about suicide just because the topic was broached. Even so, rather than beginning with a blunt question such as, "Do you ever think about committing suicide?" the nurse can phrase the question in such a way that the person will give clues to his or her intent if it exists, but will not be offended by the question if it does not (see Box 15-9 for examples).

Nurses need to recognize that older adults may express a loss of interest in living and may even state that they wish they were dead, but these verbalizations are not necessarily associated with suicidal thoughts. Many times these

---

Box 15-9 Guidelines for Assessing Suicide Risk

Risk Factors for Suicide in Older Adults

- Demographic factors: white race, male gender
- Depression, particularly when accompanied by insomnia, agitation and self-neglect
- Chronic illness with increasing dependence and helplessness; diagnosis of cancer or a terminal illness
- Poor social supports; social isolation, particularly recent isolation
- History of psychiatric illness, particularly major depression
- Onset of major depression within the past year
- Family history of suicide; personal or family history of suicide attempts
- Patterns of impulsive behaviour
- Alcohol abuse
- Poor communication skills

Verbal Clues to Suicide Intent

- "Pretty soon you won't have to worry about me."
- "I would be better off dead."
- "I'll make sure I won't be a burden to others."
- Expressions of hopelessness
- Remarks about life being unbearable
- Reflections on the worthlessness of life

Nonverbal Clues to Suicide Intent

- Making a will; giving belongings away; preparing for own funeral
- Serious self-neglect, particularly in people who have no cognitive impairments
- Frequent visits to primary care provider(s)
- Excessive use of medications or alcohol
- Accumulation of prescription medications
- Unusual preoccupation with self and withdrawal from others

Interview Questions to Assess the Immediate Risk of Suicide

- "Do you think that life is not worth living?"
- "Do you think about escaping from your problems?"
- "Do you wish you were dead?"
- "Do you think about harming yourself?"
- "Do you think about ending your life?"
- "Do you have a plan?"
- "What would you do to take your life?"
- "Have you ever started to act on a plan to harm yourself?"
- "Under what circumstances would you act on that plan?"
- "What prevents you from acting on the plan?"

expressions arise from feelings of being overwhelmed with an illness or stressful situation, and they are not indicators of a desire to take one's own life. These expressions may also be related to dementia or an inability to express one's feelings accurately, which sometimes occurs after strokes. In these situations, nurses need to further assess for depression and identify stressful conditions that can be addressed through interventions.

If suicidal thoughts are suspected or identified upon initial assessment, nurses probe further by asking questions that are aimed at determining the presence or absence of thoughts about self-harm. If the answer to any of these questions is positive, nurses probe even further, asking questions that are very direct and specific because this information is crucial to assessing the immediate risk for suicide. If the person describes a detailed plan and has access to all the necessary implements, the potential for suicide is extremely high. By contrast, if the person has a plan that is vague or that cannot possibly be carried out, the immediate potential for suicide is lower. For example, if the plan involves a gun, but the person does not have a gun and cannot get out of the house, then the chance of a successful suicide is low. By contrast, if the person threatens to consume the bottle of barbiturates that is readily available in the medicine cabinet, then the chance of a successful suicide is quite high. Nurses proceed to line of questions to assess the immediacy of the risk when the person has described a plan. When answers to questions about suicide plan and availability to the means to carry out that plan are positive (meaning that a person has a plan and access to that plan), the nurse must plan immediate interventions to deal with the suicide risk. An essential nursing responsibility with regard to questions is to ask what prevents the person from carrying out the plan because this information provides a base for supporting important patient-identified reasons for living.

Nursing Diagnosis and Outcomes

If the nursing assessment identifies risk factors for suicide, an applicable nursing diagnosis would be Risk for Suicide. Related factors would include any risk factors and verbal and nonverbal clues to suicide. An example is an 85-year-old widower who says his life is no longer worthwhile and who makes frequent visits to his doctor for complaints of weight loss and sleep disturbance. Outcomes for older adults at risk for suicide include Suicide Self-Restraint and Personal Safety Behaviour.

Nursing Interventions for Preventing Suicide

Nurses do not routinely encounter suicidal older adults, but they need to be prepared to implement immediate interventions whenever they identify a patient at risk. The most important intervention is to seek psychiatric resources and activate referrals to the appropriate protective service agency rather than attempting to deal with potentially suicidal people without the help of specialized resources. Most communities

Box 15-10 Nursing Interventions for People Who Are Potentially Suicidal

Communicating With Someone Who Is Potentially Suicidal

- Be direct and honest; do not be afraid to ask direct questions, such as, "Are you thinking of hurting yourself or taking your own life?"
- Express feelings of concern and confidence.
- Acknowledge the person's feelings of helplessness and hopelessness.
- Encourage the person to talk about the precipitating event, if there is one.
- Emphasize that suicide is only one of several options; then explore other options.
- Emphasize positive relationships; talk about the negative impact of suicide on survivors.
- Maintain a nonjudgmental attitude.
- Depending upon the health region within which you work, you may or may not make a contract for safety; that is, asking the person to agree to do certain things for limited amounts of time and to call for help if he or she cannot keep the agreement. (Some health regions in Canada have policies against "contracting around safety," as it is believed that health care professionals substitute this technique for careful suicide risk assessments.)
- Discuss reasons that the person identifies for not carrying out a suicide plan and find ways to support and strengthen these. You can ask, "What has made you choose life up to this point in time?"
- Discuss the problems openly with the family and caregivers.

Crisis Intervention

- Focus on the immediate precipitating event.
- Reduce the immediate danger by removing the implements, interfering with the plan and providing constant supervision.
- Obtain psychiatric help; call a suicide hot line, or activate emergency services (call 911 for police and ambulance) if necessary.

have some emergency psychiatric resources, and nurses can follow institutional policies regarding referrals for appropriate services. In any situation, nurses use appropriate communication techniques to address potentially suicidal older adults. Some guidelines for working with people who are potentially suicidal are listed in Box 15-10.

Evaluating the Effectiveness of Nursing Interventions

Nursing care of older adults who are at high risk for self-harm are evaluated by the prevention of harm. Another measure is the degree to which the older adult develops coping skills to deal with the issues that underlie his or her suicidal thoughts. Nurses can also find out whether the older adult obtained suggested mental health services and determine the effectiveness of any referrals that were made.

See **ONLINE LEARNING ACTIVITY 15-3: LINKS TO RESOURCES FOR FURTHER INFORMATION ABOUT LATE-LIFE DEPRESSION AND SUICIDE** at http://thepoint.lww.com/Miller7e

Case Study

Mrs. D. is 81 years old. Recently, she was diagnosed with vascular dementia. She lives with her husband, who has diabetes, macular degeneration, and severe arthritis. Mrs. D. had managed all household and financial responsibilities until approximately 1 year ago, when she began having trouble with her memory. Mrs. D. was evaluated at the geriatric assessment program where you work, and she was advised to stop driving and to arrange for some help with complex tasks, such as bill paying and grocery shopping. Two months after the initial evaluation, Mrs. D. returns for follow-up and informs you that she limits her driving to short, daytime trips in familiar areas. When asked about getting help with complex tasks, she states, "I just don't have any energy to make all those calls you suggested. Besides, I don't want anyone else looking at my finances or going to the store for me."

NURSING ASSESSMENT

A mental status assessment indicates that Mrs. D.'s level of cognitive impairment is unchanged since her initial evaluation. She has some deficits in calculation, short-term memory, abstract thinking, problem solving and language skills. Your psychosocial assessment reveals that Mrs. D. has a very sad affect and low self-esteem, and she expresses feelings of hopelessness and helplessness. She admits to being overwhelmed with feelings of responsibility for herself and her husband, and she says she feels "paralyzed because there's no light at the end of the tunnel." She scored 11 on the GDS-15.

When you ask about her daily life, Mrs. D. says she spends most of her time at home because she does not have the energy to go out. She admits that she has difficulty falling asleep at night, and she wakes up at around 4 AM and is unable to return to sleep. She naps for a couple of hours in the morning and in the afternoon because "I feel tired all the time, and I can't go out and do things anyway." Her appetite is poor, and in the past 2 months, her weight declined from 63.5 to 57 kg (her height is 167.6 cm). She complains of constipation and "heartburn."

When you ask about meaningful activities, she tells you she no longer goes to her weekly bowling club because it meets in the evening, and she does not want to drive at night. She has also given up her church activities (Thursday discussion club and Sunday service) because she does not want to inconvenience anyone by having them drive her. She feels it is "demeaning to have to tell my friends that I need a ride." She used to enjoy reading, but she has not felt like going to the library, and she is not interested in any of the books she has at home.

NURSING DIAGNOSIS

Expected Outcome	Nursing Interventions	Nursing Evaluation
Mrs. D. will be able to identify her coping patterns.	• Ask Mrs. D. to describe her prior experiences in dealing with her husband's illness. • Help Mrs. D. to identify coping strategies that have been helpful in the past.	• Mrs. D. will recognize and acknowledge the coping strategies that have been helpful in the past.
Mrs. D. will learn about depression and be encouraged to obtain further evaluation of her depression.	• Talk with Mrs. D. about her signs and symptoms of depression, emphasizing the fact that depression is a treatable condition. • Discuss the relationship between depression and the inability to cope effectively with stressful situations. • Ask Mrs. D. if she is willing to see a geriatric psychiatrist, or talk to her primary care practitioner for further evaluation and treatment. • Explain that antidepressant medications can be very effective when combined with counselling.	• Mrs. D. will follow through with an appointment with a geriatric psychiatrist or talk with her primary care practitioner.
Effective coping strategies for addressing Mrs. D.'s declining abilities will be identified.	• Discuss with Mrs. D. several options for ongoing support and counselling to assist her in coping with her declining abilities (e.g., support groups for individuals with dementia from local Alzheimer Society chapters or individual counselling sessions with the social worker who is affiliated with the geriatric assessment program).	• Mrs. D. will attend one support group on a trial basis and talk with you about the experience at her next appointment in 1 month. • Mrs. D. will make an appointment for counselling with the social worker.

(continued)

Case Study (continued)

Expected Outcome	Nursing Interventions	Nursing Evaluation
	• Emphasize the importance of developing short-term goals that can be addressed through problem solving (e.g., suggest that Mrs. D. begin to address her lack of meaningful activities by going to the library for reading material).	• Mrs. D. will participate in one meaningful activity each week for the next month.

THINKING POINTS

- What risk factors are likely contributing to Mrs. D.'s depression?
- What further assessment information would you obtain?
- What questions on the GDS-15 (Fig. 15-2) do you think would be indicative of depression for Mrs. D.?
- What additional interventions would you suggest for Mrs. D.?

Chapter Highlights

Depression in Older Adults

- Signs and symptoms of depression in older adults are on a continuum of severity from major depression to sub-threshold depression.
- Depression is characterized by depressed mood and/or loss of interest, along with additional manifestations, including weight loss, appetite change, sleep disturbances, psychomotor agitation or retardation, fatigue, cognitive impairment, feeling worthless or excessively guilty, and recurrent thoughts of death or suicide.
- Late-life depression refers to the onset of depression after the age of 65 years.

Theories About Late-Life Depression

- Psychosocial (impact of losses, learned helplessness)
- Cognitive triad (negative appraisals cause distorted perceptions and lead to faulty conclusions)
- Biologic and genetic (changes in the nervous system, genetic variables)
- Evolving theories about the interrelationship between depression and pathologic conditions (e.g., dementia, cerebrovascular disease, cardiovascular disease)

Risk Factors for Depression in Older Adults

- Demographic and psychosocial
- Medical conditions and functional impairment (Box 15-1)
- Effects of alcohol and medications (Box 15-2)

Functional Consequences Associated With Depression in Older Adults (Box 15-3)

- Physical health and functioning
- Psychosocial function and quality of life

Nursing Assessment of Depression in Older Adults

- Unique manifestations in older versus younger adults (Table 15-1)

- Differentiating between dementia and depression (Table 15-2)
- Cultural variations in expressions of depression (Box 15-4)
- Screening tools (Fig. 15-2)

Nursing Diagnosis

- Readiness for Enhanced Coping
- Ineffective Coping
- Hopelessness
- Caregiver Role Strain
- Risk for Compromised Resilience

Planning for Wellness Outcomes

- Coping
- Hope
- Caregiver Emotional Health
- Depression Level

Nursing Interventions to Address Depression (Boxes 15-6 and 15-7)

- Alleviating risk factors (addressing functional limitations, teaching about adverse effects of medications and excessive alcohol)
- Improving psychosocial function (social supports, meaningful activities)
- Promoting health through physical activity and nutrition
- Providing education and counselling (individual and group psychosocial interventions)
- Facilitating referrals for psychosocial therapies
- Teaching about antidepressant medications (Table 15-3)
- Teaching about ECT
- Teaching about alternative care practices (e.g., St. John's wort, bright-light therapy)

Evaluating the Effectiveness of Nursing Interventions (Box 15-8)

- Improved coping skills
- Fewer manifestations of depression
- Expressed feelings of improved quality of life
- Effective use of appropriate mental health services

Suicide in Late Life

- Suicide rates and mechanisms (Fig. 15-3)
- Nursing assessment of suicide risk (Box 15-9)
- Nursing diagnosis and outcomes
- Nursing interventions for preventing suicide (Box 15-10)
- Evaluating effectiveness of interventions

Critical Thinking Exercises

1. Think of an older adult in your personal life or professional practice who is or has been depressed. What are (were) the risk factors in that person's situation that might play (have played) a part in the depression?
2. Describe at least four cultural variations in the way depression might be expressed.
3. What assessment observations would you make and what questions would you ask to differentiate between dementia and depression in older adults?
4. Develop a case example of someone who is potentially suicidal and who would require all four levels of suicide assessment. Describe how you would phrase the questions for each of the levels.
5. Describe a teaching plan for an 84-year-old woman for whom Paxil, 10 mg daily, has been prescribed.

 For more information about the topics discussed in this chapter, be sure to check out the interactive Online Learning Activities and other helpful resources at http://thepoint.lww.com/Miller7e

REFERENCES

Alzheimer Society Canada. (2012). *Depression.* Retrieved from http://www.alzheimer.ca/en/About-dementia/Alzheimer-s-disease/Warning-signs-and-symptoms/Depression?gclid=CMStxurh6r8CFUKCMgodvGQArg

Arean, P. A. (2013). Psychotherapy. In H. Lavretsky, M. Sajatovic, & C. F. Reynolds, III (Eds.), *Late-life mood disorders* (pp. 390–405). Oxford, England: Oxford University Press.

Baglioni, C., Berger, M., & Riemann, D. (2013). Bidirectional relationships between sleep, insomnia, and depression. In H. Lavretsky, M. Sajatovic, & C. F. Reynolds, III (Eds.), *Late-life mood disorders* (pp. 347–360). Oxford, England: Oxford University Press.

Barry, L. C., Soulos, P. R., Murphy, S. V., et al. (2013). Association between indicators of disability burden and subsequent depression among older persons. *Journals of Gerontology: Biological Sciences and Medical Sciences, 68*(3), 286–292.

Beck, A. T., Rush, A. J., Shaw, B., et al. (1979). *Cognitive therapy of depression.* New York, NY: Guilford.

Blazer, D. G. (2002). *Depression in late life* (3rd ed.). New York, NY: Springer.

Byma, E. A., Given, C. W., & Given, B. A. (2012). Associations among indicators of depression in Medicaid-eligible community-dwelling older adults. *The Gerontologist, 53*(4), 608–617.

Canadian Coalition on Seniors' Mental Health. (2006a). *CCSMH national guidelines for seniors' mental health: The assessment and treatment of depression.* Retrieved from www.ccsmh.ca/en/projects/depression.cfm

Canadian Coalition on Seniors' Mental Health. (2006b). *CCSMH national guidelines for seniors' mental health: The assessment of suicide risk and prevention of suicide.* Retrieved from http://www.ccsmh.ca/en/projects/suicideAssessment.cfm

Canadian Coalition on Seniors' Mental Health. (2009). *Depression in older adults: A guide for seniors and their families.* Retrieved from http://www.ccsmh.ca/pdf/ccsmh_depressionBooklet.pdf

Catena-Dell'Osso, M., Rotella, F., Dell'Osso, A., et al. (2013). Inflammation, serotonin and major depression. *Current Drug Targets, 14*(5), 571–577.

Centre for Suicide Prevention. (2012). *Plus 65: At the end of the day.* Retrieved from http://suicideinfo.ca/LinkClick.aspx?fileticket=cmFwRL4DMJw%3d&tabid=563

Charlton, R. A., Lamar, M., Ajilore, O., et al. (2013). Preliminary analysis of age of illness onset effects on symptom profiles in major depressive disorder. *International Journal of Geriatric Psychiatry, 28*(11), 1166–1174.

Cooney, G. M., Dwan, K., Greig, C. A., et al. (2013). Exercise for depression. *Cochrane Database of Systematic Reviews, 19*(9), CD004366. doi:10.1002/14651858.CD004366.pub6

da Rocha e Silva, C. E., Alves Brasil, M. A., Matos do Nascimento, E., et al. (2013). Is poststroke depression a major depression? *Cerebrovascular Disease, 35*(4), 385–391.

DeRyck, A., Brouns, R., Fransen, M., et al. (2013). A prospective study on the prevalence and risk factors of poststroke depression. *Cerebrovascular Diseases, 3*(1–13). doi:10.1159/000345557

Diniz, B. S., Butters, M. A., Albert, S. M., et al. (2013). Late-life depression and risk of vascular dementia and Alzheimer's disease: Systematic review and meta-analysis of community-based cohort studies. *British Journal of Psychiatry, 202*(5), 329–335.

Eyre, H. A., Papps, E., & Baune, B. T. (2013). Treating depression and depression-like behavior with physical activity: An immune perspective. *Frontiers in Psychiatry, 4*(3). doi:10.3389/fpsycht.2013.00003.eCollection 2013

Flaster, M., Sharma, A., & Rao, M. (2013). Poststroke depression: A review emphasizing the role of prophylactic treatment and synergy with treatment for motor recovery. *Topics in Stroke Rehabilitation, 20*(2), 139–150.

Frank, C. (2014). Pharmacologic treatment of depression in the elderly. *Canadian Family Physician, 60*, 121–126.

Giorlando, F., Teister, J., Dodd, S., et al. (2013). Hyponatraemia: An audit of aged psychiatry patients taking SSRIs and SNRIs. *Current Drug Safety, 8*(3), 175–180.

Greenberg, S. A. (2012). *How to try this: The Geriatric Depression Scale: Short Form.* Retrieved from www.consultgerirn.org

Harvath, T. A., & McKenzie, G. (2012). Depression in older adults. In E. Capezuti, E. Zwicker, M. Mezey, et al. (Eds.), *Evidence-based geriatric nursing protocols for best practice* (4th ed., pp. 135–162). New York, NY: Springer.

Health Link BC. (2011). *St. John's Wort: Topic overview.* Retrieved from www.healthlinkbc.ca/kb/content/special/hw260538spec.html

Helming, M. B. (2013). Relationships. In B. M. Dossey & L. Keegan (Eds.), *Holistic nursing: A handbook for practice* (6th ed., pp. 439–462). Boston, MA: Jones and Bartlett.

Hornsten, C., Lovheim, H. J., & Gustafson, Y. (2013). The association between stroke, depression, and 5-year mortality among very old people. *Stroke, 44*(9), 2587–2589.

Huffman, J. C., Celano, C. M., Beach, S. R., et al. (2013). Depression and cardiac disease: Epidemiology, mechanisms, and diagnosis. *Cardiovascular Psychiatry and Neurology, 2013*, 1–14. doi:10.1155/2013/695925

Hybels, C. F., Landerman, L. R., & Blazer, D. G. (2012). Age differences in symptom expression in patients with major depression. *International Journal of Geriatric Psychiatry, 27*(6), 601–611.

Joutsenniemi, K., Tuulio-Henriksson, A., Elovainio, M., et al. (2013). Depressive symptoms, major depressive episodes and cognitive test performance: What is the role of physical activity? *Nordic Psychiatry, 67*(4), 265–273.

Karp, J. F., & McGovern, J. (2013). Comorbid pain disorders. In H. Lavretsky, M. Sajatovic, & C. F. Reynolds, III (Eds.), *Late-life mood disorders* (pp. 329–346). Oxford, England: Oxford University Press.

Krystal, A. D., Edinger, J. D., & Wohlgemuth, W. K. (2012). Sleep and circadian rhythm disorders. In D. G. Blazer & D. C. Steffens (Eds.), *Essentials of geriatric psychiatry* (2nd ed., pp. 209–221). Washington, DC: American Psychiatric Publishing.

Lee, M. J., Hasche, L. K., Choi, S., et al. (2013). Comparison of major depressive disorder and subthreshold depression among older adults in community long-term care. *Aging & Mental Health, 17*(4), 461–469.

Liebel, D. V., & Powers, B. A. (2013). Home health care nurse perceptions of geriatric depression and disability care management. *Gerontologist.* doi:10.1093/geront/gnt125

Lynch, T. R., Epstein, D. E., & Smoski, M. J. (2012). Individual and group psychotherapy. In D. G. Blazer & D. C. Steffens (Eds.), *Essentials of geriatric psychiatry* (2nd ed., pp. 319–336). Washington, DC: American Psychiatric Publishing.

Madden-Baer, R., McConnell, E., Rosati, R. J., et al. (2013). Implementation and evaluation of a depression care model for homebound elderly. *Journal of Nursing Care Quality, 28*(1), 33–42.

Marano, C. M., Rosenberg, P. B., & Lyketsos, C. G. (2013). Depression in dementia. In H. Lavretsky, M. Sajatovic, & C. F. Reynolds, III (Eds.), *Late-life mood disorders* (pp. 177–205). Oxford, England: Oxford University Press.

Matta Mello Portugal, E., Cevada, T., Sobral Monteiro, R., et al. (2013). Neuroscience of exercise: From neurobiology mechanisms to mental health. *Neuropsychology, 68*(1), 1–14.

McDonald, W. M., & Vahabzadeh, A. (2013). Electroconvulsive therapy and neuromodulation in the treatment of late-life mood disorders. In H. Lavretsky, M. Sajatovic, & C. F. Reynolds, III (Eds.), *Late-life mood disorders* (pp. 406–431). Oxford, England: Oxford University Press.

Merrill, D., Payne, M., & Lavretsky, H. (2013). Complementary and alternative medicine approaches for treatment and prevention of late-life mood disorders. In H. Lavretsky, M. Sajatovic, & C. F. Reynolds, III (Eds.), *Late-life mood disorders* (pp. 432–447). Oxford, England: Oxford University Press.

Mezuk, B., & Gallo, J. J. (2013). Depression and medical illness in late life. In H. Lavretsky, M. Sajatovic, & C. F. Reynolds, III (Eds.), *Late-life mood disorders* (pp. 270–294). Oxford, England: Oxford University Press.

Monette, M. (2012). Senior suicide: An overlooked problem. *CMAJ, 184*(17), E885–E886.

Mulsant, B. H., & Pollock, B. G. (2012). Psychopharmacology. In D. G. Blazer & D. C. Steffens (Eds.), *Essentials of geriatric psychiatry* (2nd ed., pp. 257–303). Washington, DC: American Psychiatric Publishing.

National Center for Complementary and Alternative Medicine. (2013). *Get the facts: St. John's wort and depression.* Retrieved from www.nccam.nih.gov

Olazaran, J., Trincado, R., & Bermejo-Pareja, F. (2013). Cumulative effect of depression on dementia risk. *International Journal of Alzheimer's Disease, 2013,* 1–6. doi:10.1155/2013/457175

Oudman, E. (2012). Is electroconvulsive therapy (ECT) effective and safe for treatment of depression in dementia? A short review. *Journal of ECT, 28*(1), 34–38.

Pandey, G. N. (2013). Biologic basis of suicide and suicidal behavior. *Bipolar disorders, 15*(5), 524–541.

Park, M., & Unutzer, J. (2013). Public health burden of late-life mood disorders. In H. Lavretsky, M. Sajatovic, & C. F. Reynolds, III (Eds.), *Late-life mood disorders* (pp. 42–60). Oxford, England: Oxford University Press.

Polyakova, M., Sonnabend, N., Sander, C., et al. (2014). Prevalence of minor depression in elderly persons with and without mild cognitive impairment: A systematic review. *Journal of Affective Disorders, 152–154,* 28–38. doi:10.1016/j.jad.2013.09.016

Public Health Agency of Canada. (2010). *The health and well-being of Canadian seniors.* Retrieved from http://www.phac-aspc.gc.ca/cphorsphc-respcacsp/2010/fr-rc/cphorsphc-respcacsp-06-eng.php

Rapinesi, C., Kotzalidis, G. D., Serata, D., et al. (2013). Prevention of relapse with maintenance electroconvulsive therapy in elderly patients with major depressive episodes. *Journal of ECT, 29*(1), 61–64.

Ribeiz, S., Duran, F., Oliveira, M., et al. (2013). Structural brain changes as biomarkers and outcome predictors in patients with late-life depression: A cross-sectional and prospective study. *PLOS One, 8*(11), e80049.

Richard, E., Reitz, C., Honig, L. H., et al. (2013). Late-life depression, mild cognitive impairment, and dementia. *Journal of the American Medical Society Neurology, 70*(3), 364–382.

Schwarzbach, M., Luppa, M., Forstmeier, S., et al. (2014). Social relations and depression in late life: A systematic review. *International Journal of Geriatric Psychiatry, 29*(1), 1–21. doi:10.1002/gps.3971

Seligman, M. E. P. (1981). A learned helplessness point of view. In L. P. Rehm (Ed.), *Behavior therapy for depression* (pp. 123–141). New York, NY: Academic Press.

Snowden, J., & Almeida, O. P. (2013). The diagnosis and treatment and unipolar depression in late life. In H. Lavretsky, M. Sajatovic, & C. F. Reynolds, III (Eds.), *Late-life mood disorders* (pp. 79–103). Oxford, England: Oxford University Press.

Steffens, D. C., & Blazer, D. G. (2012). Mood disorders. In D. G. Blazer & D. C. Steffens (Eds.), *Essentials of geriatric psychiatry* (2nd ed., pp. 125–148). Washington, DC: American Psychiatric Publishing.

Taylor, W. D., Aizenstein, H. J., & Alexopoulos, G. S. (2013). The vascular depression hypothesis: Mechanisms linking vascular disease with depression. *Molecular Psychiatry, 18*(9), 963–974.

Taylor-Piliae, R. E., Hepworth, J. T., & Coull, B. M. (2013). Predictors of depressive symptoms among community-dwelling stroke survivors. *Journal of Cardiovascular Nursing, 28*(5), 460–467.

Thombs, B. D., Roseman, M., Coyne, J. C., et al. (2013). Does evidence support the American Heart Association's recommendation to screen patients for depression in cardiovascular care? An updated systematic review. *PLOS One, 8*(1). Retrieved from http://share.eldoc.ub.rug.nl/FILES/root2/2013/Doesevsut/Thombs_2013_Plos_One.pdf

Trangle, M., Dieperink, B., Gabert, T., et al. (2012). *Institute for Clinical Systems Improvement: Health Care Guideline: Major depression in adults in primary care.* Bloomington, MN: ICSI. Retrieved from www.icsi.org

van den Kommer, T. N., Comijs, H. C., Aartsen, M. J., et al. (2013). Depression and cognition: How do they interrelate in old age? *American Journal of Geriatric Psychiatry, 21*(4), 398–410.

Verwijk, E., Comijs, H. C., Kok, R. M., et al. (2013, November). Short- and long-term neurocognitive functioning after electroconvulsive therapy in depressed elderly: A prospective naturalistic study. *International Psychogeriatrics, 26*(2), 315–324.

Vilalta-Franch, J., Lopez-Pousa, S., Llinas-Regla, J., et al. (2013). Depression subtypes and 5-year risk of dementia and Alzheimer disease in patients aged 70 years. *International Journal of Geriatric Psychiatry, 28*(4), 341–350.

Volk, S., & Steffens, D. C. (2013). Post-stroke depression and vascular depression. In H. Lavretsky, M. Sajatovic, & C. F. Reynolds, III (Eds.), *Late-life mood disorders* (pp. 254–269). Oxford, England: Oxford University Press.

Weiner, R. D., & Krystal, A. D. (2012). Electroconvulsive therapy. In D. G. Blazer & D. C. Steffens (Eds.), *Essentials of geriatric psychiatry* (2nd ed., pp. 305–318). Washington, DC: American Psychiatric Publishing.

Whooley, M. A., & Wong, J. M. (2013). Depression and cardiovascular disorders. *Annual Review of Clinical Psychology, 9,* 327–354.

Wiese, B. S. (2011). Geriatric depression: The use of antidepressants in the elderly. *BC Medical Journal, 53*(7), 341–347.

Wint, D., & Cummings, J. (2013). Comorbid neurological illness. In H. Lavretsky, M. Sajatovic, & C. F. Reynolds, III (Eds.), *Late-life mood disorders* (pp. 295–314). Oxford, England: Oxford University Press.

Zahodne, L. B., Marsiske, M., Okun, M. S., et al. (2012). Components of depression in Parkinson disease. *Journal of Geriatric Psychiatry and Neurology, 25*(3), 131–137.

Zeki Al Hazzouri, A., Vittinghoff, E., Byers, A., et al. (2014). Long-term cumulative depressive symptom burden and risk of cognitive decline and dementia among very old women. *Journals of Gerontology: Biological Sciences and Medical Sciences, 69*(5), 595–601.

Promoting Wellness in Physical Function

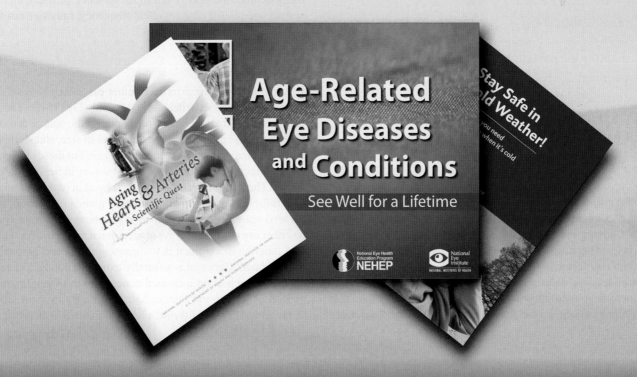

Hearing

LEARNING OBJECTIVES

After reading this chapter, you will be able to:

1. Describe age-related changes that affect hearing.
2. Identify risk factors that affect hearing wellness.
3. Discuss the functional consequences that affect hearing wellness.
4. Conduct a nursing assessment of hearing, with emphasis on identifying opportunities for health promotion.
5. Identify nursing interventions to promote hearing wellness for older adults by addressing risk factors that interfere with hearing.

KEY POINTS

assistive listening device

auditory rehabilitation

cerumen

cerumenolytics

conductive hearing loss

hearing aid

impacted cerumen

mixed hearing loss

noise-induced hearing loss (NIHL)

otosclerosis

presbycusis

sensorineural hearing loss

tinnitus

Performance of many important daily activities—including communicating, protecting oneself from danger and enjoying music, voices and sounds—is highly dependent on good hearing. In older adults, age-related changes combine with risk factors to affect hearing wellness. Nurses promote wellness for older adults when they use health promotion interventions to improve hearing and communication. This chapter addresses the functional consequences associated with hearing in older adults and provides guides for nursing assessment and interventions.

AGE-RELATED CHANGES THAT AFFECT HEARING

Auditory function depends on a sequence of processes, beginning in the three compartments of the ear and ending with the processing of information in the auditory cortex of the brain. Sounds are coded according to intensity and frequency. Intensity, or amplitude, reflects the loudness or softness of the sound and is measured in decibels (dB). Frequency, which is measured in cycles per second (cps) or hertz (Hz), determines whether the pitch is high or low. Sound intensity and frequency may be altered if certain risk factors come into play. Even in the absence of risk factors, normal age-related changes affect frequency, causing hearing problems for many older adults.

External Ear

Hearing begins in the external or outer ear, which consists of the pinna and the external auditory canal (Fig. 16-1). These cartilaginous structures localize sounds so the source can be identified. The pinna undergoes changes in size, shape, flexibility and hair growth with increasing age, but these changes do not affect the conduction of sound waves in healthy older adults. The auditory canal is covered by skin and lined with hair follicles and cerumen-producing glands. **Cerumen**, or earwax, is a natural substance that is genetically determined to be either dry (flaky and grey) or wet (moist and brown or tan). The function of cerumen is to cleanse, protect and lubricate the ear canal. Cerumen is naturally expelled, but age-related changes—such as an increased concentration of keratin, the growth of longer and thicker hair (especially in men), and thinning and drying of the skin lining the canal—can cause it

Promoting Hearing Wellness in Older Adults

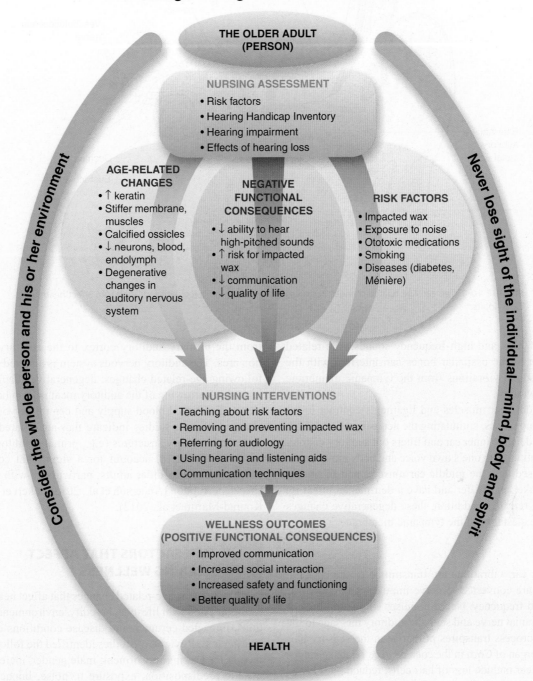

THE OLDER ADULT (PERSON)

NURSING ASSESSMENT
• Risk factors
• Hearing Handicap Inventory
• Hearing impairment
• Effects of hearing loss

AGE-RELATED CHANGES
• ↑ keratin
• Stiffer membrane, muscles
• Calcified ossicles
• ↓ neurons, blood, endolymph
• Degenerative changes in auditory nervous system

NEGATIVE FUNCTIONAL CONSEQUENCES
• ↓ ability to hear high-pitched sounds
• ↑ risk for impacted wax
• ↓ communication
• ↓ quality of life

RISK FACTORS
• Impacted wax
• Exposure to noise
• Ototoxic medications
• Smoking
• Diseases (diabetes, Ménière)

NURSING INTERVENTIONS
• Teaching about risk factors
• Removing and preventing impacted wax
• Referring for audiology
• Using hearing and listening aids
• Communication techniques

WELLNESS OUTCOMES (POSITIVE FUNCTIONAL CONSEQUENCES)
• Improved communication
• Increased social interaction
• Increased safety and functioning
• Better quality of life

HEALTH

Consider the whole person and his or her environment

Never lose sight of the individual—mind, body and spirit

---

to build up. An age-related diminution in sweat gland activity further increases the potential for cerumen to accumulate by making the cerumen drier and more difficult to remove.

Middle Ear

The tympanic membrane is a transparent, pearl-grey, slightly cone-shaped layer of flexible tissue, which separates the outer and middle ear. Its primary functions are to transmit sound energy and protect the middle and inner ear. With

increased age, collagenous tissue replaces the elastic tissue, resulting in a thinner and stiffer eardrum. Sound vibrations pass through the tympanic membrane to the three auditory ossicles: the malleus, incus and stapes. These bones are connected to each other but move independently, acting as a lever to amplify sound. Their primary function is to transmit vibrations across the air-filled middle ear, through the oval window and into the fluid-filled inner ear. Sound transmission depends on the frequency of each sound and is best for the middle-frequency range of normal voices and less

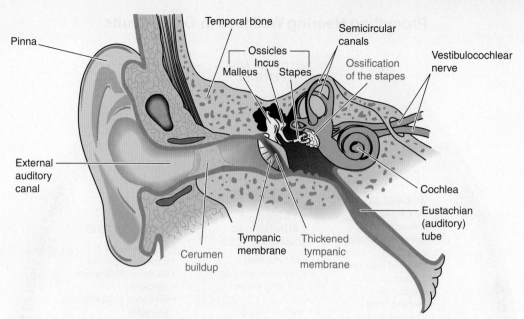

FIGURE 16-1 The ear. Age-related changes in structures of the ear, indicated with red labels, can affect hearing in older adults.

effective for low- and high-frequency sounds. Age-related calcification of the ossicular bones can interfere with the transfer of sound vibrations from the tympanic membrane to the oval window.

The middle ear muscles and ligaments contract in response to loud noises, stimulating the acoustic reflex, which protects the delicate inner ear and filters out auditory distractions originating from one's own voice and body movements. With increased age, the middle ear muscles and ligaments become weaker and stiffer and have a detrimental effect on the acoustic reflex. In addition, these degenerative changes diminish the elasticity of the tympanic membrane.

Inner Ear

In the inner ear, vibrations are transmitted to the cochlea, where they are converted to nerve impulses and coded for intensity and frequency. Nerve impulses stimulate fibres of the eighth cranial nerve and send the auditory message to the brain. This process transpires primarily in the sensory hair cells of the organ of Corti in the cochlea. Age-related changes of the inner ear include loss of hair cells, reduction of blood supply, diminution of endolymph production, decreased basilar membrane flexibility, degeneration of spiral ganglion cells and loss of neurons in the cochlear nuclei. These degenerative changes of the cochlea and other inner ear structures are the primary physiologic cause of the age-related hearing impairment that affects older adults (Lin et al., 2012).

Auditory Nervous System

From the inner ear, the auditory nerve fibres pass through the internal auditory meatus and enter the brain. Functions of the auditory nerve pathway include localizing sound direction, fine-tuning auditory stimuli and transferring information from the primary auditory cortex to the auditory association area. The auditory nervous system is affected by all the following age-related changes: degenerative changes in the inner ear, narrowing of the auditory meatus from bone apposition, diminished blood supply and central nervous system changes. Recent studies indicate that age-related changes in central auditory structures (e.g., primary auditory cortex, auditory brainstem) account for a significant component of hearing loss in older adults, particularly with regard to speech perception (Anderson et al., 2012; Eckert et al., 2012; Konrad-Martin et al., 2012).

 RISK FACTORS THAT AFFECT HEARING WELLNESS

In addition to the age-related changes that affect hearing, factors associated with lifestyle, heredity, environment, medications, impacted cerumen and disease conditions can cause hearing loss. Reviews of studies identified the following risk factors for hearing impairment: male gender, increased age, genetic predisposition, exposure to noise, impacted cerumen, smoking, exposure to secondhand smoke, use of ototoxic medications, education level less than or equal to high school diploma and certain medical conditions (e.g., stroke, diabetes, hypertension, cardiovascular disease) (Adobamen & Ogisi, 2012; Fabry et al., 2011; Kiely et al., 2012; Lin et al., 2012).

A major focus of research is on modifiable conditions, such as smoking and exposure to noise that can be addressed through health promotion interventions. Researchers also are exploring the potential interrelationship between two or more risk factors. For example, people who are genetically predisposed to hearing loss may be more susceptible to the damaging effects of noise exposure or ototoxic drugs. Because age-related changes increase the risk for hearing loss, it is especially important to identify modifiable risk factors in older adults so that those risks can be addressed. Most likely, some hearing loss attributed to age-related changes actually results from risk factors, such as exposure to noise or ototoxic substances. Box 16-1 summarizes some factors that interfere with hearing wellness, either alone or in combinations.

Exposure to Noise

A commonly occurring risk factor for impaired hearing is prolonged or intermittent exposure to noise, which can be viewed as both a lifestyle choice and an environmental factor. Although age-related changes account for a greater amount of hearing loss than occupational noise exposure, **noise-induced hearing loss (NIHL)** is an important preventable cause of hearing loss. A review of studies by Sliwinska-Kowalska and Davis (2012) found that prolonged exposure to high-intensity noise is associated with all of the following:

- Damage to sensory hair cells of the inner ear
- Permanent shift in hearing threshold
- Impaired speech discrimination
- Tinnitus

Studies have found an increased risk for NIHL associated with the occupations of the following people: farmers, miners, construction workers, musicians, bar employees and casting and forging industry workers (Kelly et al., 2012; Onder et al., 2012; Singh et al., 2012; Sliwinska-Kowalska & Davis, 2012; Yankaskas, 2013). Recreational

---

Box 16-1 Risk Factors for Impaired Hearing

Genetic predisposition
Increased age
White race
Recreational or occupational exposure to noise
Smoking of nicotine products
Secondhand smoke
Ototoxic medications
    Aminoglycosides (e.g., gentamicin, neomycin)
    Antifungals (e.g., amphotericin, flucytosine)
    Aspirin and other salicylates
    Cisplatin and other chemotherapeutic agents
    Hydroxychloroquine
    Loop diuretics (e.g., bumetanide, furosemide)
    Macrolides (e.g., erythromycin, clarithromycin)
    Nonsteroidal anti-inflammatory agents (NSAIDs)
    Quinine
    Quinolones (e.g., ciprofloxacin, ofloxacin)
Ototoxic environmental chemicals
    Carbon monoxide
    Fuels
    Lead
    Mercury
    Organophosphates
    Styrene
    Toluene

---

activities associated with increased risk for NIHL include using MP3 players and sound systems for music, hunting or target shooting, riding all-terrain vehicles or motorcycles and operating power tools (e.g., chain saws, leaf blowers, drills) (Humann et al., 2012; Neitzel et al., 2012). Exposure to toxic chemicals in the workplace or the environment is another risk factor for hearing loss that has been under investigation since the 1990s, with current research focusing on metals, solvents, asphyxiants and pesticides/herbicides. Studies also address synergistic effects of two risk factors, such as noise and ototoxic agents (Kirchner et al., 2012). Although the Canadian Centre for Occupational Health and Safety enforces safety standards for workplace noise, it is important to consider that many older adults were exposed to workplace noise before these standards were established. Because the effects of NIHL and age-related changes are cumulative, the hearing loss may not be noticed until later adulthood. Figure 16-2 illustrates the noise levels of various activities. Sounds louder than 80 dB are considered potentially ototoxic.

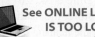

See ONLINE LEARNING ACTIVITY 16-1: HOW LOUD IS TOO LOUD?
at http://thepoint.lww.com/Miller7e

Impacted Cerumen

Impacted cerumen (also called impacted wax) is common in older adults as a leading cause of hearing loss, with up to 57% of older nursing home residents experiencing impacted cerumen (Roland et al., 2008). Age-related changes, which make the cerumen dryer and more concentrated, increase the risk of impaction. The use of hearing aids also increases the possibility of impacted cerumen, which can damage or interfere with the function of the hearing aid. In addition, impacted cerumen can cause pain, otitis, tinnitus, dizziness, fullness or coughing. Cerumen accumulation is preventable and treatable and, most important, it is readily amenable to nursing interventions (as discussed later in this chapter), which lead to improved hearing.

Ototoxic Medications

Adverse medication effects can cause or contribute to hearing impairments by damaging the cochlear and vestibular divisions of the auditory nerve. Despite the fact that quinine and salicylate ototoxicities were first observed more than a century ago, the ototoxic effects of medication have received little attention in clinical settings. Although age alone does not increase the risk for ototoxicity, older adults are more likely to be taking ototoxic medications, such as aspirin and furosemide. Other contributing factors that commonly occur in older adults and increase the risk for ototoxicity include renal failure, long-term use of ototoxic medications and potentiation between two ototoxic medications, such as furosemide and aminoglycoside antibiotics. Box 16-1 lists medications that are likely to be ototoxic. When ototoxicity is dose related, as with cisplatin, hearing loss can

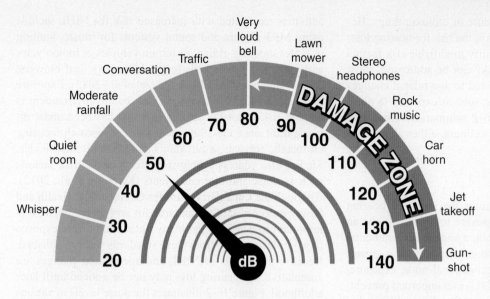

FIGURE 16-2 Noise levels associated with common activities are measured in decibels (dB). Sounds louder than 80 dB are potentially harmful to ears.

be prevented or alleviated if the medication dose is carefully monitored and altered accordingly (Dille et al., 2012). Although ototoxicity is potentially reversible, medications may be overlooked as a causative factor if the hearing loss is mistakenly ascribed to inevitable and irreversible degenerative changes.

Disease Processes

Otosclerosis is a hereditary disease of the auditory ossicles that causes ankylosis of the footplate of the stapes to the oval window. Although otosclerosis usually begins in youth or early adulthood, the hearing loss may not be detected until middle or later adulthood when age-related changes compound the disease-related changes. Otosclerosis primarily causes a conductive hearing loss, but some sensorineural loss may also occur. Initially, it is difficult to hear soft and low-pitched sounds; as the hearing loss worsens, the person is likely to experience dizziness, tinnitus or balance problems.

Ménière disease and acoustic neuromas are auditory system diseases that commonly cause hearing impairment. Medical conditions and systemic diseases that can cause or contribute to hearing impairment include diabetes, hypertension, meningitis, hypothyroidism, head injury, high fevers, Paget disease, renal failure, cardiovascular disease, radiation for head and neck cancers and viral infections (e.g., measles and mumps).

> ### Wellness Opportunity
>
> Modifiable and preventable risk factors for hearing loss include noise, medications and impacted cerumen.

Unfolding Case Study

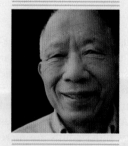

Part 1: Mr. H. at 60 Years of Age

Mr. H. is 60 years old and owns a small home-remodelling business. He has been a carpenter for 38 years, but in the past 9 years, he has spent most of his time in the office, managing his business. He enjoys hunting and fishing on weekends. He has smoked two packs of cigarettes a day since he was 16 years old. His wife has been telling him she thinks he hears only what he wants to hear. Mr. H. admits that he turns the television volume up louder than he used to but denies having any "real hearing problem."

THINKING POINTS

- What age-related changes and risk factors contribute to Mr. H.'s hearing loss?
- Describe the hearing loss that Mr. H. is likely to be experiencing.
- What environmental conditions will contribute to Mr. H.'s hearing difficulty?

FUNCTIONAL CONSEQUENCES AFFECTING HEARING WELLNESS

In 2006, according to Statistics Canada, more than 1 million Canadians reported having a hearing limitation. In the 65-to-74 age range, the prevalence was 11.9%, which rose to 25.9% in those above 75. Hearing impairment is most common in people who have one or more of the risk factors previously discussed.

Hearing impairment is categorized according to the site of impairment as follows:

- **Conductive hearing loss** results from abnormalities of the external and middle ear that interfere with sound conduction.
- **Sensorineural hearing loss** is caused by abnormalities of the sensory and neural structures of the inner ear, which usually are age related or noise induced.
- **Mixed hearing loss** involves both conductive and sensorineural impairments.

DIVERSITY NOTE

Studies have found that female gender, black race and darker skin decrease the risk for hearing loss (Lin et al., 2011, 2012). Veterans (of war) fare worse in their hearing than their age counterparts (Tansey et al., 2013).

Effects on Communication

Accurate comprehension of speech depends on speech pace, sound frequencies, environmental noise and internal auditory function. Hearing acuity for high-frequency tones normally begins to decline in early adulthood, and by the age of 30 years for men and 50 years for women, there is some decline in hearing sensitivity at all frequencies.

DIVERSITY NOTE

Because hearing loss in men begins at an earlier age and declines more rapidly, the cumulative effects are usually noticed by men in their 50s and by women in their 60s.

Speech comprehension is most directly influenced by the frequency of *phonemes*, the smallest units of sound. Each phoneme in a word has a different frequency; generally, vowels have lower frequencies and consonants have higher frequencies. Although most word phonemes have lower-range frequencies, sibilant consonants (those that have a whistling quality, such as *ch, f, g, s, sh, t, th* and *z*) have higher-range frequencies. Because the earliest and most universal age-related changes affect one's ability to code higher-frequency sounds, words rich in sibilants will be most affected by age-related changes of the auditory system. For example, studies confirm that older listeners are able to discern vowels in words better than consonants (Fogerty et al., 2012).

Presbycusis is the sensorineural hearing loss associated with an age-related degeneration of the auditory structures.

Presbycusis usually occurs in both ears, but the degree of impairment in each ear can vary. An early functional consequence of presbycusis is the loss of ability to hear high-pitched sounds and sibilant consonants. When high-pitched sounds are filtered out, words become distorted and jumbled, and sentences become incoherent. For example, someone with presbycusis might interpret a sentence like "I think she should go to the store" as "I wish we could go to the show." This characteristic, known as *diminished speech discrimination*, is influenced by the speaker's rate of speech: rapid, slow or slurred speech patterns make it increasingly difficult for the older person to discern words. As the hearing loss progresses, explosive consonants, such as *b, d, k, p* and *t*, also become distorted.

Background noise and environmental conditions, such as echoing or poor acoustics, compound the effects of sensorineural hearing loss and can interfere with the ability to recognize words, even in the absence of a significant hearing loss. Thus, older adults in a hospital or long-term care facility, for example, may be particularly sensitive to background noises to which the staff may have become accustomed. A related functional consequence is that sensorineural hearing loss interferes with the ability to identify the spatial location of the source of speech or noise (Glyde et al., 2013).

A conductive hearing loss is characterized by a reduced intensity of sounds and difficulty hearing vowels and low-pitched tones. In contrast to presbycusis, all sound frequencies are heard equally once the sound threshold is reached, and background noise does not interfere as much with speech comprehension. Often there is a history of otosclerosis, perforated eardrum or other ear disease. In older adults, impacted cerumen is a common contributing factor. Depending on the causative factor, conductive hearing loss occurs in one or both ears. See Table 16-1 for a summary of the functional consequences of age-related changes affecting hearing.

See ONLINE LEARNING ACTIVITY 16-2: THROUGH THE EARS OF OLDER ADULTS at http://thepoint.lww.com/Miller7e

Effects of Hearing Loss on Overall Wellness

Adequate hearing is a primary component of communication that enables people to enjoy humour, appreciate music, obtain information, relate to others and respond to threats. Thus, hearing deficits inevitably affect safety, functioning and quality of life in many ways. Reviews of studies have identified all the following effects of hearing loss on overall wellness and quality of life of older adults:

- Diminished physical and cognitive function
- Functional decline
- Perception of quality of life as excellent: only 39% of subjects with hearing loss compared with 68% of those without
- A source of loneliness, isolation, diminished participation in social activities
- Increased self-perception of poor social skills, which can result in diminished self-esteem

TABLE 16-1 Functional Consequences of Age-Related Changes Affecting Hearing

Structure	Change	Consequence
External ear	• Longer, thicker hair • Thinner, drier skin • Increased keratin	Potential for impacted cerumen and subsequent impaired sound conduction
Middle ear	• Diminished resiliency of tympanic membrane • Calcified, hardened ossicles • Weakened and stiff muscles and ligaments	Impaired sound conduction
Inner ear and nervous system	• Diminished neurons, endolymph, hair cells and blood supply • Degeneration of spiral ganglion and arterial blood vessels • Decreased flexibility of basilar membrane • Degeneration of central processing systems	*Presbycusis:* diminished ability to hear high-pitched sounds, especially in the presence of background noise

- Increased prevalence of depression
- Decreased autonomy
- Increased dependence on others (Ciorba et al., 2012; Li-Korotky, 2012; Mondelli & de Souza, 2012)

A study assessing the association between hearing impairment and activity limitation concluded that severely diminished hearing loss can make the difference between independent living and the need for formal support services or placement (Gopinath et al., 2012).

Although researchers have found a strong association between hearing loss and impaired cognitive function, many questions remain about the cause–effect relationship. Longitudinal data indicate that hearing loss is associated with both accelerated decline and increased incidence of cognitive impairment in community-dwelling older adults (Lin et al., 2013). A study of nursing home residents found that those with a more severe hearing loss also had poorer cognitive function (Jupiter, 2012).

It is important to consider the effect of hearing loss on cognitive function because any reduction in sensory stimuli can interfere with information perception and processing. Hearing loss may also affect performance on mental status assessments because people who cannot discriminate words may be reluctant to respond to questions and may refrain from answering rather than risk feeling foolish. Poor performance on tests of cognitive abilities can mistakenly lead to a perception that the person has cognitive impairments or dementia when, in fact, the person has a hearing loss. In addition, when hearing loss interferes with one's ability to perceive reality accurately, it can lead to suspiciousness, paranoia, and loss of contact with the reality. When only parts of a conversation are heard, a person is likely to believe that the conversation is about him or her, and persecutory delusions can develop.

In addition to having a negative influence on the quality of life, hearing deficits can affect the safety and functioning of older adults. For example, people with hearing impairments are likely to be less responsive when warning signals are sounded for fires, ambulances and other emergencies. Besides creating actual safety hazards, the hearing deficit can lead to fear and anxiety about personal safety (Box 16-2).

Box 16-2 Evidence-Informed Nursing Practice

Background: There is substantial evidence that baseline indicators (e.g., hearing) of overall quality of life predict subsequent health events.

Question: Is there an association between health-related quality of life attributes and mortality?

Method: Baseline data from the Canadian National Population Health Survey and 12 years of follow-up data were collected for 12,375 adults above 18 years of age. Deaths were confirmed from the Canadian Vital Statistics Database.

Findings: Hearing is statistically associated with an increased risk of mortality.

Implications for Nursing Practice: Nurses need to ensure that older adults are assessed for hearing difficulties and promote interventions that support quality of life.

Source: Feeny, D., Hugert, N., McFarland, B. H., et al. (2012). Hearing, mobility, and pain predict mortality: A longitudinal population based study. *Journal of Clinical Epidemiology, 65,* 764–777.

Negative societal attitudes about aging and hearing loss can result in a doubly negative effect on the person who is old as well as hard of hearing. The older person may be reluctant to acknowledge a hearing deficit, choosing to limit opportunities for communication rather than face the stigma associated with hearing impairments. These attitudes and accompanying behaviours can contribute to additional psychosocial consequences such as loneliness, depression and even more social isolation.

Wellness Opportunity

Nurses can initiate conversations that reflect positive and nonjudgmental attitudes about aging and hearing loss.

PATHOLOGIC CONDITION AFFECTING HEARING: TINNITUS

Tinnitus is the persistent sensation of ringing, roaring, blowing, buzzing or other types of noise that do not originate in the external environment. In Canada, approximately 360,000 people experience tinnitus (Tinnitus Association of Canada, 2010). Tinnitus is a symptom of an underlying condition, such as impacted cerumen, Ménière disease,

Unfolding Case Study

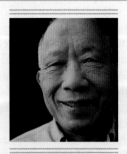

Part 2: Mr. H. at 69 Years of Age

Mr. H. is now 69 years old and has been retired for several years. He spends several days a week hunting and fishing seasonally. He also spends time in his basement making small pieces of furniture and doing other woodworking. He continues to smoke but has cut down to one pack per day. His wife and he attend the weekly "lunch bunch" group at the local senior centre where you are the nurse. They make an appointment to talk with you because Mrs. H. is concerned about her husband's hearing. Mr. H., who blames his problem on "old age," refuses to have an evaluation for a hearing aid because he does not think an aid would do any good and "besides, it would stick out like a sore thumb."

THINKING POINTS

- What factors contribute to Mr. H.'s hearing loss?
- What environmental and other conditions might make the hearing loss worse?

- What myths or misunderstandings are likely to influence Mr. H.'s perception of his hearing problem and potential interventions for it?

QSEN APPLICATION

QSEN Competency	Knowledge/Skill/Attitude	Application to Mr. H. When He Is 69 Years Old
Patient-centred care	(K) Integrate understanding of multiple dimensions of patient-centred care (K) Discuss principles of effective communication (S) Elicit patient values, preferences and expressed needs (A) Value seeing health care situations "through patients' eyes"	Identify Mr. H.'s misunderstandings about hearing loss and hearing aids and use a nonjudgmental approach to provide correct information Encourage Mrs. H. to verbalize her concerns directly to Mr. H. during your meeting so these can be addressed and misinformation can be corrected

traumatic brain injury or temporomandibular joint (TMJ) dysfunction. The two risk factors most commonly associated with tinnitus are the same ones associated with hearing loss: older age and increased exposure to noise. Similarly, ototoxic medications that are listed in Box 16-1 can cause tinnitus as well as hearing loss. Caffeine, alcohol or nicotine can exacerbate tinnitus.

A primary responsibility of nurses is to encourage people who have tinnitus to discuss this symptom with their primary care practitioners to identify reversible or serious causes. A referral to a specialist is especially important if tinnitus is unilateral or is accompanied by vertigo or the perception of pulsations in one ear (Agency for Health care Research and Quality, 2012). Nurses also can emphasize that the use of hearing aids may alleviate or at least improve symptoms of tinnitus, even if the underlying condition remains.

DIVERSITY NOTE

Tinnitus is more common in men than in women (Ruppert & Fay, 2012).

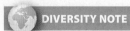
See ONLINE LEARNING ACTIVITY 16-3: THROUGH THE EARS OF SOMEONE WHO HAS TINNITUS at http://thepoint.lww.com/Miller7e

Wellness Opportunity

Nurses can teach people who have tinnitus about the exacerbating effects of conditions, including smoking cigarettes and drinking alcoholic or caffeinated beverages, that can be addressed through self-care actions.

 NURSING ASSESSMENT OF HEARING

Nursing assessment of hearing is aimed at identifying the following:
- Factors that interfere with hearing wellness
- Actual hearing deficit
- The impact of any hearing deficits on safety and quality of life
- Opportunities for improving hearing wellness
- Barriers to implementing interventions

Each of these factors is important in helping older adults and their caregivers compensate for hearing deficits. Assessment is accomplished through interviewing, observing behavioural cues and administering hearing tests.

Interviewing About Hearing Changes

Use interview questions, such as the ones in Box 16-3, to acquire information about (1) present and past risk factors,

Box 16-3 Guidelines for Assessing Hearing

Questions to Identify Risk Factors for Hearing Loss

- Do you have a family history of hearing loss or deafness?
- Have you been exposed to loud noises in your job or leisure activities?
- Do you have a history of any of the following: diabetes, hypothyroidism, Ménière disease or Paget disease?
- What medications do you take? (Refer to Box 16-1 to identify potentially ototoxic medications.)
- Have you ever had impacted wax in your ears?

Questions to Assess Awareness and Presence of Hearing Deficit

- Do you have any trouble with your hearing?
- Have you noticed any change in your ability to understand conversations or hear words?
- Are you bothered by any noises in your ears, such as ringing or buzzing?

Questions to Ask if Hearing Loss Is Acknowledged

- How long have you noticed a hearing loss?
- Do you notice differences in hearing in your left ear versus your right ear?
- Has there been a progressive loss, or did the hearing problem begin suddenly?
- Describe your hearing difficulty.
- Are there any conditions, such as noisy environments or particular voices or sounds, that especially interfere with your hearing?
- Does your hearing loss interfere with your ability to communicate with others, either individually or in groups?
- Are there any activities that you would like to do but feel you cannot because of hearing problems?
- Have you ever had, or thought about having, an evaluation for a hearing aid?
- Have you ever tried using a hearing aid?

Questions to Identify Opportunities for Education About Disease Prevention and Health Promotion

- Does the person engage in any activities that expose him or her to loud noises, such as woodworking or lawn mowing? If so, does he or she understand the importance of wearing ear protectors?
- If the person has a history of impacted wax, does he or she take preventive measures?
- Does the person smoke cigarettes or live in a household with a smoker? If so, does the person realize that this is a risk factor for hearing loss?
- What are the person's attitudes about hearing loss?
- Is hearing loss considered normal and untreatable?
- Is a hearing aid considered to be a stigma?
- If the person is resistant to an audiologic evaluation, what are the barriers? (E.g., are there financial or transportation limitations that interfere with obtaining a hearing aid?)
- Does the hearing loss contribute to a sense of isolation, depression, paranoia or low self-esteem?
- What are the person's usual communication opportunities, and how does the hearing loss influence these usual patterns? (For instance, does the person live in an environment where it is important to be able to use the phone?)
- Does the person live in a noisy environment and find relief in the hearing impairment?
- If the person lives in an environment where group activities are a large part of daily activities, does the person want to participate in these activities?

(2) the person's awareness and acknowledgment of a hearing impairment, (3) the psychosocial impact of any hearing deficit and (4) attitudes that might influence health promotion interventions. Begin with questions about family history of hearing impairments and a personal history of prolonged exposure to loud noises. Identification of ototoxic medications as a risk factor can be included as part of the hearing assessment or as part of the medication history.

If the older adult does not initiate a discussion of hearing problems, ask direct questions, such as "Do you think you have a hearing loss?" If the nursing assessment identifies behavioural cues indicative of a hearing deficit but the person denies having a hearing problem, attempt to elicit further information by asking questions such as "I notice you turn your left ear toward me. Is your hearing better in that ear?" If a hearing loss is present, assess related functional consequences by asking about changes in social activities or ability to function independently because of difficulty hearing.

Wellness Opportunity

Nurses address the whole person by including questions about the impact of a hearing loss on his or her quality of life.

Another assessment aspect for older adults with hearing loss is to identify their attitudes and perceptions about hearing aids and other interventions. Common barriers to use of hearing aids include all the following:

- Perception that hearing aids are of little use
- Concerns about cost
- Difficulty arranging for evaluations
- Lack of transportation for appointments
- Embarrassment about the visibility of hearing aids
- Lack of manual dexterity necessary for use of smaller hearing aids

Another assessment consideration is that the person may not be motivated toward improved communication and may even prefer social isolation or limited opportunities for communication. It is also important to consider whether a desire to avoid opportunities for communication may be associated with dementia, depression, close relationships or living arrangements.

The Hearing Handicap Inventory for the Elderly (HHIE-S) is a 10-item questionnaire that can be administered to older adults in approximately 5 minutes to assess the presence and functional consequences of hearing loss (Fig. 16-3). This tool has been widely used since the early 1980s in a variety of clinical settings and for research purposes. The Hartford Institute for Geriatric Nursing recommends it as a valid and reliable tool for measuring social and emotional effects of hearing loss (Greenberg, 2013).

Wellness Opportunity

Nurses promote self-care by asking an older adult to use the HHIE-S and then reviewing the results of this assessment to identify goals.

ITEM	YES (4 pts)	SOMETIMES (2 pts)	NO (0 pts)
Does a hearing problem cause you to feel embarrassed when you meet new people?	_____	_____	_____
Does a hearing problem cause you to feel frustrated when talking to members of your family?	_____	_____	_____
Do you have difficulty hearing when someone speaks in a whisper?	_____	_____	_____
Do you feel handicapped by a hearing problem?	_____	_____	_____
Does a hearing problem cause you difficulty when visiting friends, relatives or neighbors?	_____	_____	_____
Does a hearing problem cause you to attend religious services less often than you would like?	_____	_____	_____
Does a hearing problem cause you to have arguments with family members?	_____	_____	_____
Does a hearing problem cause you difficulty when listening to TV or radio?	_____	_____	_____
Do you feel that any difficulty with your hearing limits or hampers your personal or social life?	_____	_____	_____
Does a hearing problem cause you difficulty when in a restaurant with relatives or friends?	_____	_____	_____

RAW SCORE_____ (sum of the points assigned each of the items)

INTERPRETING THE RAW SCORE
0 to 8 = 13% probability of hearing impairment (no handicap/no referral)
10 to 24 = 50% probability of hearing impairment (mild-moderate handicap/refer)
26 to 40 = 84% probability of hearing impairment (severe handicap/refer)

FIGURE 16-3 The screening version of the Hearing Handicap Inventory for the Elderly (HHIE-S). (Reprinted with permission from Ventry, I., & Weinstein, B. [1983]. *Identification of elderly people with hearing problems* [pp. 37–42]. Rockville, MD: American Speech-Language-Hearing Association. Copyright, American Speech-Language-Hearing Association.)

Observing Behavioural Cues

Behavioural cues related to hearing loss provide important information about the presence of a hearing impairment, the psychosocial consequences of any such impairment and the person's attitudes about assistive devices. If the older adult denies a hearing deficit that has been noticed by others, behavioural cues can be an important source of assessment information. Denial of a hearing deficit can be rooted in lack of awareness of the impairment because of gradual onset or, if the older person is socially isolated, can be caused by a paucity of opportunities for communication. Feelings of embarrassment or misconceptions that the hearing loss is an inevitable and untreatable consequence of aging can also contribute to denial. Box 16-4 lists behavioural cues that the nurse should observe as part of the hearing assessment.

Using Hearing Assessment Tools

Nurses assess hearing by using an otoscope to examine the ear and a tuning fork to check hearing. The purpose of the otoscopic examination is to identify impacted cerumen and other factors that can interfere with hearing, whereas the purpose of the tuning fork test is to detect hearing impairments and to differentiate between conductive and sensorineural losses. Box 16-5 describes the procedure for performing a nursing assessment of hearing using the otoscope and tuning fork. A handheld audioscope is another assessment tool that is recommended in nursing guidelines; however, this tool is not as widely available as an otoscope or tuning fork. When a hearing deficit is identified, the nurse can recommend that further evaluation be conducted at a speech and hearing centre or by a specialized physician, such as an otolaryngologist.

See **ONLINE LEARNING ACTIVITY 16-4: ARTICLE AND VIDEO ABOUT NURSING ASSESSMENT AND INTERVENTIONS FOR HEARING LOSS**
at http://thepoint.lww.com/Miller7e

Box 16-4 Guidelines for Assessing Behavioural Cues Related to Hearing

Behavioural Cues to a Hearing Deficit

- Inappropriate or no response to questions, especially in the absence of opportunities for lip reading
- Inability to follow verbal directions without cues
- Short attention span, easy distractibility
- Frequent requests for repetition or clarification of verbal communication
- Intense observation of the speaker
- Mouthing of words spoken by the speaker
- Turning of one ear toward the speaker
- Unusual physical proximity to the speaker
- Lack of response to loud environmental noises
- Speech that is too loud or inarticulate
- Abnormal voice characteristics, such as monotony
- Misperception that others are talking about him or her

Behavioural Cues About Psychosocial Consequences

- Uncharacteristic avoidance of group settings
- Lack of interest in social activities, especially those requiring verbal communication or those that the person enjoyed in the past (e.g., bingo, card games)

Behavioural Cues About Assistive Devices

- Not using a hearing aid that has been purchased
- Failure to obtain batteries for a hearing aid
- Expression of embarrassment about using assistive devices

Box 16-5 Guidelines for Otoscopic and Tuning Fork Assessment

Using the Otoscope to Assess Factors That Could Interfere With Hearing

- Hold the otoscope upside down, resting your hand on the person's head to stabilize the instrument.
- Before inserting the speculum, pull the earlobe up and back, while tilting the person's head slightly back and toward the opposite shoulder.
- If cerumen has accumulated to the point of interfering with the examination or occluding the canal, follow the cerumen removal procedure described in the section on nursing interventions.
- Normal otoscopic findings in older adults include the following:
  Small amount of cerumen
  Pinkish-white epithelial lining, no redness or lesions
  Pearl-grey tympanic membrane, which is less translucent than in younger adults
  Light reflex anteroinferiorly from the umbo
  Visible landmarks

Using the Tuning Fork to Detect Hearing Impairment

- Use a tuning fork with frequencies of 512 to 1024 cps (Hz).
- Hold the tuning fork firmly at the stem.
- Strike the fork against the palm of your hand, or strike the fork with a rubber reflex hammer, to set it in motion.

Weber Test

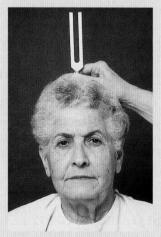

(Reprinted with permission from Bickley, L. S., & Szilagyi, P. G. [2009]. *Bates' guide to physical examination and history taking* (10th ed.). Philadelphia, PA: Lippincott Williams and Wilkins.)

Procedure: Place the tip of a vibrating tuning fork at the centre of the person's forehead or on the top of the person's head. Ask where they hear the sound and whether it is louder in one ear than in the other.
Normal finding: The sound from the tuning fork is heard equally in both ears.
Abnormal finding: The sound from the tuning fork is heard better in one ear, indicating a possible hearing loss.

Rinne Test

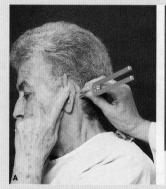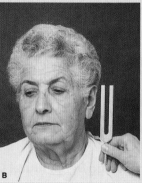

(Reprinted with permission from Bickley, L. S., & Szilagyi, P. G. [2009]. *Bates' guide to physical examination and history taking* (10th ed.). Philadelphia, PA: Lippincott Williams and Wilkins.)

Procedure: Mask one ear, then place a vibrating tuning fork on the mastoid process of the opposite ear until the person indicates that the sound from the vibrations can no longer be heard. Then, quickly place the tuning fork in front of the ear canal with the top near the ear canal.
Normal finding: The duration the tuning fork vibrations can be heard over the ear canal is approximately twice as long as the time it can be heard over the mastoid bone.
Abnormal finding: The length of time the tuning fork vibrations are heard in front of the ear is shorter than twice as long as the time it can be heard when placed on the mastoid process. In such a case, the person should undergo further tests for impaired hearing.

Unfolding Case Study

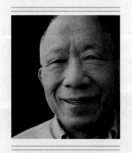

Part 2: Mr. H. at 69 Years of Age (continued)

Recall that Mr. H. is a 69-year-old participant in activities at the local senior centre where you are the nurse. You are meeting with Mr. and Mrs. H. to discuss Mrs. H.'s concerns about her husband's hearing problem.

THINKING POINTS

- Which of the questions and considerations in Boxes 16-3 and 16-4 would you use in assessing Mr. H.?
- Would you involve Mrs. H. in any part of the assessment? If so, how would you involve her?

- What health promotion advice would you give Mr. H. at this time?

NURSING DIAGNOSIS

A nursing assessment might identify an actual hearing deficit or risk factors for impaired hearing. To emphasize the goal of promoting wellness, use the diagnosis of Readiness for Enhanced Communication, defined as "a pattern of exchanging information and ideas with others that is sufficient for meeting one's needs and life's goals, and can be strengthened" (Herdman, 2012, p. 274). If psychosocial consequences are identified, pertinent nursing diagnoses might include Anxiety, Impaired Social Interaction, Ineffective Coping and Risk for Loneliness. When the hearing impairment is severe and uncompensated to the point that the person does not function safely, then Risk for Injury might be an applicable nursing diagnosis.

Wellness Opportunity

Nurses can use the wellness nursing diagnosis of Readiness for Enhanced Communication for older adults who are willing to explore possibilities for improving their hearing through health promotion interventions.

PLANNING FOR WELLNESS OUTCOMES

When risk factors for hearing loss are identified, an appropriate Nursing Outcomes Classification (NOC) label is Risk Control: Hearing Impairment, defined as "personal actions to understand, prevent, eliminate, or reduce threats, to hearing function" (Moorhead et al., 2013, p. 442). Two NOC labels applicable to older adults who are experiencing hearing loss or tinnitus are Hearing Compensation Behaviour and Sensory Function: Hearing. Additional NOC labels that are related to the functional consequences of hearing loss are Communication, Depression Level, Leisure Participation, Loneliness

Severity, Personal Safety Behaviour, Social Involvement and Social Interaction Skills. Nursing interventions to achieve these outcomes are discussed in the following section.

Wellness Opportunity

Quality of Life is a wellness outcome that is achieved through nursing interventions that improve communication for older adults with impaired hearing.

NURSING INTERVENTIONS FOR HEARING WELLNESS

Nursing interventions to promote hearing wellness for older adults focus on preventing hearing loss, helping older adults compensate for hearing deficits and using communication methods that facilitate optimal communication. Specific interventions to achieve these goals are discussed in detail in the following sections. Use any of the following pertinent Nursing Interventions Classification (NIC) labels in care plans: Communication Enhancement: Hearing Deficit, Ear Care, Environmental Management: Safety, Environmental Management: Risk Protection, Health Education, Health Screening, Health System Guidance or Risk Identification.

Wellness Opportunity

Nurses can emphasize that even though interventions to prevent hearing loss ideally begin early in life, it is never too late to begin protecting ears from noise.

Promoting Hearing Wellness for All Older Adults

For all older adults, it is important to correct the misperception that hearing loss is an inevitable and inconsequential effect of growing older. Emphasize that all people can take actions to protect their hearing and teach older adults about the exacerbating effects of two risk factors, such as noise and age-related changes. For example, many older adults engage in recreational or occupational activities that can cause NIHL and they may not realize that age-related changes increase their susceptibility to developing a hearing loss. Similarly, people who already experience a hearing loss and recognize that nicotine can be ototoxic may be more motivated to stop smoking. Encourage older adults who experience a hearing loss and take ototoxic medications (listed in Box 16-1) to discuss the risk with the prescribing health care practitioner, so effective alternatives can be considered. Use Box 16-6 to teach older adults about health promotion actions they can take to prevent or address hearing loss.

Nurses can also teach about the importance of having a hearing screening done by self-assessment (e.g., using the HHIE-S) or by audiometry. Group screenings are often available in community or residential settings for older adults, and these may be a helpful resource as long as sponsors of these programs do not have a vested interest in promoting a particular type of hearing aid. Whenever a nursing assessment identifies an actual or probable hearing loss, interventions focus on appropriate referrals for medical and audiology evaluations, as discussed in the section on compensating for hearing deficits.

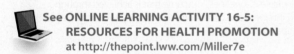

See ONLINE LEARNING ACTIVITY 16-5: RESOURCES FOR HEALTH PROMOTION at http://thepoint.lww.com/Miller7e

---

Box 16-6 Health Promotion Teaching About Hearing

Prevention of Hearing Loss
- Because exposure to loud noise is a major contributing factor to hearing loss, limit your exposure or use ear protectors that are appropriate to the task (e.g., when mowing the lawn, using equipment with gas or electric motors).
- Because smoking increases the risk of hearing loss, consider this as another reason to quit smoking.

Early Detection and Treatment of Hearing Loss
- Because some medications and medical conditions can cause hearing problems, ask your primary care practitioner to thoroughly evaluate for these conditions.
- Have your ears checked for impacted wax and talk with your primary health practitioner about preventing impacted wax if this has been a problem for you.
- Obtain evaluation at a speech and hearing centre for a hearing aid, assistive hearing device or auditory rehabilitation services.
- Consider using amplifying devices (e.g., for phones, radios, doorbells) or sound substitution devices (e.g., flashing lights, closed-captioned television) as needed for safety and improved quality of life.
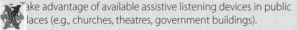
- Take advantage of available assistive listening devices in public places (e.g., churches, theatres, government buildings).

Preventing and Alleviating Impacted Cerumen

Nurses promote hearing wellness through interventions and health education aimed at alleviating or preventing hearing impairment caused by impacted cerumen. Over-the-counter **cerumenolytics** (i.e., eardrop solutions whose primary purpose is to soften cerumen) are commonly used to soften the cerumen before it can be removed. Bulechek and colleagues (2013) include the following nursing actions for ear care that are pertinent to preventing and alleviating impacted cerumen:
- Instructing patients how to cleanse ears
- Teaching patients not to use objects smaller than patient's fingertip for cerumen removal
- Monitoring for excessive cerumen accumulation
- Considering ear irrigation for removal of excessive cerumen if watchful waiting, manual, removal and cerumenolytic agents are ineffective
- Referring to ear care specialists as appropriate

Box 16-7 summarizes recommendations for patient teaching and direct interventions related to impacted cerumen. Keep in mind that monitoring and referrals are essential nursing interventions for older adults who have recurrent episodes of impacted cerumen, especially for those who use hearing aids.

Compensating for Hearing Deficits

Whenever a nursing assessment identifies a hearing impairment, the initial intervention is to ensure that a medical evaluation is performed by a qualified professional to identify treatable causes of the hearing loss. When teaching about evaluation of hearing loss, it may be helpful to review the qualifications of different ear care specialists, as described in Box 16-8. Interventions for hearing loss include sound amplification, surgical interventions and auditory rehabilitation. Nursing interventions should focus on a referral for medical and audiology evaluations. Sometimes the nursing interventions also need to address barriers to obtaining a hearing aid, as discussed in the section on hearing aids.

There are other assistive listening devices that may be helpful and are available commercially. These include text-messaging phones, closed-caption televisions, vibrating clocks and flashing door bells on the inside wall of a home. A program call Hearing Dogs of Canada, operated by the Lions Foundation of Canada, is also available.

Sound Amplification

Sound amplification is achieved by using hearing aids or assistive listening devices, often in combination. Hearing aids are individually prescribed and require audiology services, whereas assistive listening devices are not individualized and are available without professional assistance or recommendation.

Box 16-7 Evidence-Based Practice: Guidelines for Impacted Cerumen

Statement of the Problem

- Cerumen is normally expelled from the ear canal by a self-cleaning mechanism, but excessive or impacted cerumen occurs in high-risk populations, such as older adults, people who are cognitively impaired and people who use hearing aids.
- Impacted cerumen affects between 19% and 65% of patients above 65 years old and is often underdiagnosed and undertreated.
- Impacted cerumen can cause hearing loss, diminished cognitive function and symptoms such as pain, itching, tinnitus, cough, dizziness and sensation of fullness.
- Cerumen impaction may interfere with hearing aid performance by reducing the intensity of sound, changing the resonance properties of the ears, or causing feedback and poor fitting.
- Cerumen impaction is the cause of damage to 60% to 70% of hearing aids that are sent for repair.
- There are strong data indicating that removal of impacted cerumen can improve hearing.
- Older patients are often unaware that they have a cerumen impaction potentially impairing their hearing or that removal of the impaction may improve their hearing; they may even rate their hearing ability as good or fair.

Recommendations for Nursing Assessment

- Arrange for or perform an otoscopic examination whenever any of the following manifestations occur: hearing loss, ear pain, tinnitus, cough or vertigo.
- Arrange for or perform an otoscopic examination at intervals of 3 to 12 months for older adults who use hearing aids.

Recommendations for Patient Teaching

Teach older adults and caregivers about the following measures:
- Reduce the risk of developing impacted cerumen by using ceruminolytic agents prophylactically.
- Do not insert cotton-tipped applicators or any other foreign object in ear canals.
- Make sure that hearing aids are properly cleaned and cared for.
- If you have an increased risk for cerumen impaction, have your ears cleaned and checked by a qualified health care practitioner every 6 to 12 months.

Recommendations for Care

Ceruminolytic Agents

- Ceruminolytics are wax-softening agents that disperse the cerumen and reduce the need for other interventions.
- Three types of ceruminolytics are: water-based (e.g., water, saline, ducosate sodium, hydrogen peroxide, sodium bicarbonate); oil-based (e.g., almond oil, mineral oil, olive oil); and non-water-, non-oil-based (e.g., Debrox, Audax).
- Studies comparing two or more ceruminolytic agents indicate that any type of ceruminolytic is better than no treatment, but no particular agent is more effective than others.

Clearing the Cerumen

- The goal of clearing is to improve hearing and not as an attempt to remove all the cerumen.
- Impacted cerumen is removed cautiously by qualified professions by a variety of methods, including irrigation and manually with a specialized instrument .
- Instillation of ceruminolytic agents 15 minutes or for several days before the removal improves the success of the treatment.
- Ear irrigation should not be performed on patients with a history of ear surgery or those who have any abnormality of the ear canal or a nonintact tympanic membrane; it should be used cautiously in patients with diabetes.

Potentially Harmful Interventions

- Cotton-tipped swabs should not be used because they can cause further impaction and other complications; they may even be the cause of the original impaction.
- Home use of oral jet irrigators and cotton-tipped swabs are associated with increased risk of damage to the ear canal.
- Ear candling (also called ear coning or thermo-auricular therapy) is a commonly used alternative practice for cerumen removal. Research indicates that ear candling is not effective and is associated with considerable risks.

Sources: Ear wax removal interventions: A systematic review and economic evaluation. *British Journal of General Practice, 61*(591), 680–683. doi:10.3399/bjgp11X601497; Roland et al. (2008); Roth, Y., Oron, Y., & Goldfarb, A. (2011). Limited good-quality evidence available on earwax removal methods. *Evidence-Based Nursing, 14*(2), 60–61. doi:10.1136/ebn1132.

Box 16-8 Guide to Ear Care Professionals

ENT specialists, otolaryngolotists or *otorhinolaryngologists* (all terms used interchangeably) are licensed doctors of medicine who have received specialty training and are certified by the Royal College of Physicians and Surgeons of Canada. Services include the following:

- Diagnosis and management with medical or surgical interventions of conditions affecting the ear, nose, throat, areas of the neck, head and face
- Disorders of the ear that are diagnosed and treated: hearing loss, tinnitus, ear infections, ear pain and ear-related balance disorders
- Otologists are subspecialists within the specialty of ENT whose services include the following:
    - Diagnosis and treatment of ear disease
    - Surgical interventions for hearing loss: tympanoplasty, stapedectomy, and cochlear and middle-ear implants

Audiologists are certified professionals with a minimum of a master's degree in audiology. The profession is regulated in certain provinces. Audiology services include:

- Diagnosis and treatment of disorders of hearing and balance, including type and degree of hearing loss
- Prescribing and fitting hearing aids and assistive listening devices
- Counselling regarding communication strategies

Hearing instrument specialists conduct tests to determine the best type of hearing instrument for sale, lease or rental. They also provide ongoing care and adjustments for hearing aid users. Each province has specific guidelines for practicing in the hearing health care field.

Any device that amplifies or replaces sounds for individual or group communication without being individualized is categorized as an **assistive listening device**, as in the following examples:

- A stethoscope is an assistive listening device commonly used by health care workers.
- Megaphones and microphones are used for group communication.

- Closed-captioned televisions substitute visual cues for auditory cue.
- A personal listening system, which consists of a small, battery-powered amplifier and headphones, can be used easily in any setting.
- A small amplifying device can be attached to a telephone receiver.
- Some cell phones are designed to accommodate people who use hearing aids or need amplification. Visual stimuli, such as flashing lights, can be used as a signal for a doorbell.
- Vibratory stimuli can be used as a substitute for an alarm clock.

Advantages of assistive listening devices over hearing aids include lower cost (usually) and the ability to share a device among several people. In addition, these devices are less intrusive than hearing aids and they do not require as much manual dexterity. Assistive listening devices can be used alone or with hearing aids. Figure 16-4 shows several examples of devices that can be used to enhance communication with someone who is hard of hearing.

Nurses can teach older adults and their caregivers about using assistive listening devices as a substitute for or as an adjunct to hearing aids. For example, people may not realize that since 1990, all televisions with screens 13 inches

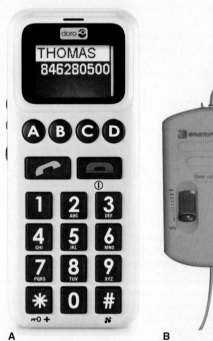

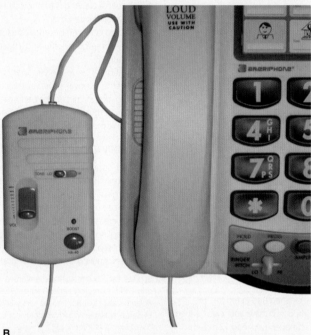

A   **B**

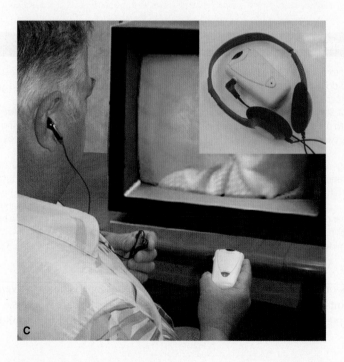

C

FIGURE 16-4 (A) Cell phone with amplification, large keypad, two-way speakerphone and vibrating ringer alert. **(B)** Easy-to-use in-line phone amplifier. **(C)** Personal sound amplifier with volume control, swivelling microphone and lightweight earbud headphones. (Reprinted with permission from ActiveForever.com)

or larger are required to include a closed-captioned option and this feature is available for many programs. Many public places, including churches, theatres and government buildings, provide portable assistive listening devices, and hearing-impaired people can ask about the availability of such a device.

A **hearing aid** is a battery-operated device that consists of an amplifier, a microphone and a receiver. Because of many recently evolving technological advances, selection of hearing aids has become increasingly complex. Figure 16-5 illustrates commonly available types according to style. Although it is impossible to know about all the available types of hearing aids, it is important to teach older adults about general principles related to selection of hearing aids. Thus, an essential teaching point is stressing the importance of obtaining an initial evaluation by a qualified hearing care professional, so reversible causes of hearing loss are identified and the most appropriate interventions are initiated.

Despite the major improvements in hearing aids in the last decade, fewer than 25% of people who could benefit from a hearing aid actually use one. Nurses can address negative attitudes and have a positive effect on the use of hearing aids by helping older adults to explore the many options for amplification, as described in Box 16-9. When working with older adults in residential or other institutional settings, teach about the most effective use of hearing aids in different circumstances. For example, encourage the older adult to use the aid for one-on-one conversations but to remove it

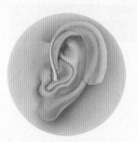
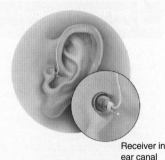

Behind-the-ear (BTE)   "Mini" BTE

Receiver in ear canal

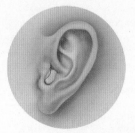
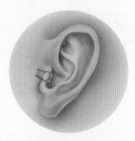

In-the-ear (ITE)   Completely-in-canal (CIC)

FIGURE 16-5 Examples of four types of hearing aids.

Box 16-9 Guide to the Selection and Care of Hearing Aids

Guidelines for Selecting a Hearing Aid

- Obtain a medical evaluation to identify treatable causes of hearing loss before being evaluated for a hearing aid.
- Obtain initial information about hearing aids from a speech and hearing centre or consumer organizations, rather than primarily from a hearing aid dealer who sells only one kind of device.
- Obtain an initial evaluation from that provides a range of hearing aids and services for people with hearing loss.
- Ask about audiology rehabilitation programs to improve communication skills and adjustment to hearing loss.
- If financial limitations are a concern, check with provincial or territorial health authorities to identify if subsidies are available, or federally with Workers' Compensation, Veterans Affairs Canada, Canada Pension Plan Disability Benefit, or First Nations and Inuit Health as each provides access to hearing aids and audiology care for people with limited incomes.
- Recognize that there are many types and styles of hearing aids, which vary significantly in their features and cost; it is important to consider more than one type:
  - Hearing aid styles include behind-the-ear, in-the-ear, in-the-canal, completely-in-the-canal, and mini-behind-the-ear.
  - Considerations for selection of style include features and cost of the aid and personal preferences related to aesthetics and manual dexterity.
  - Levels of technology, from simplest to most complex, are standard analogue, programmable analogue, entry-level digital, advanced digital and premium digital.
  - Available features of prescribed hearing aids include feedback cancellation, directional microphones, multiple channels, battery indicator and wax protection systems.
  - Disposable hearing aids are the least expensive (usually less than $100) and are designed as a one-size-fits-all; they are discarded after the built-in battery is exhausted. They also are the least individualized.

Guidelines for Care of a Hearing Aid

- Keep a fresh battery available but do not purchase batteries more than 1 month in advance.
- Turn off the hearing aid before changing the battery.
- Remove the battery or turn off the aid when not in use.
- Clean the aid weekly, using warm, soapy water for the earmold and a toothpick or pipe cleaner for the channel.
- Never use alcohol on the earmold because this will cause drying and cracking.
- Check the earmold for cracks or scratches.
- Avoid extreme heat, cold or moisture.
- Avoid exposure to chemicals, such as hairspray or permanent solutions.
- Avoid dropping the aid on a hard surface; when handling it, keep it over a soft or padded surface.

in the dining area or other large social areas where there is a lot of background noise. Promote realistic expectations with regard to hearing aids by explaining that hearing aids do not restore normal hearing but do improve communication and the quality of life.

Nurses must be familiar enough with hearing aids to assist older adults and their caregivers with their use and care. Although audiologists provide initial instructions about the use and care of hearing aids, these instructions may have to be reviewed or revamped as dependency needs and caregiver roles change. For example, when older adults are in a hospital or nursing home, nursing staff usually provide assistance with use of and care for hearing aids. Likewise, nurses in home settings may have to teach caregivers about hearing aids if the older adult's needs change. Use information in Box 16-9 as a guide to teaching about the selection and care of hearing aids.

Auditory Rehabilitation

Auditory rehabilitation (also called aural, hearing or audiologic rehab) refers to services that improve communication for people who are hearing impaired. Auditory rehabilitation programs provide the following services: counselling, education, amplification aids, communication methods and management of the environment. Studies indicate that although auditory rehabilitation programs can improve cognitive and social function in older adults, rates of utilization and compliance are very low (Li-Korotky, 2012; Parham et al., 2013). Nurses play an important role in discussing such programs with older adults and their caregivers and suggesting referrals for auditory rehabilitation. Speech and hearing centres, which are often affiliated with medical centres or universities, are good sources of information about auditory rehabilitation programs. Information is also available through Internet resources, such as the Canadian Association of Speech-Language Pathologists and Audiologists.

Surgical Interventions

Cochlear implants have been used for several decades, but criteria for this type of intervention have been narrow. In recent years, there have been remarkable developments with regard to types of inner- and middle-ear implants and bone-conduction hearing devices as interventions for hearing loss. These developments have been accompanied by expanded criteria for surgical interventions, which are increasingly being used for hearing-impaired older adults. A recent review of data from 12 years of cochlear implants in adults age 60 years and older found that this intervention consistently improved speech understanding scores. Older adults who were younger at implantation and had higher preoperative speech scores derived the greatest benefit (Lin et al., 2012). Based on current evidence, it is important to encourage older adults to explore options for surgical interventions when hearing loss is not adequately improved with other interventions.

When older adults have surgically implanted hearing devices, it is important to find out if an external component is attached to the body, inserted in the ear or kept close to the body. When this is the case, nurses document information in the patient's chart and assist with keeping track of all components. Another nursing implication is that some implanted hearing devices are affected by or interfere with magnetic resonance imaging (MRI), so it is essential to obtain information about compatibility if an MRI is being considered.

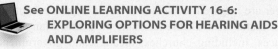

See ONLINE LEARNING ACTIVITY 16-6: EXPLORING OPTIONS FOR HEARING AIDS AND AMPLIFIERS at http://thepoint.lww.com/Miller7e

Communicating With Hearing-Impaired Older Adults

Good communication techniques are essential in assisting older adults to compensate for hearing deficits. The primary functional consequence of presbycusis is a diminished acuity for high-frequency sounds, which is exacerbated by fast-paced speech and environmental noise. Therefore, communication interventions are directed toward improving the clarity of words, slowing the rate of speech and eliminating environmental noise and distractions. Verbal techniques that enhance auditory communication should be augmented by nonverbal techniques, such as body language and written communication, as described in Box 16-10. Nurses can apply these techniques and use this box for teaching caregivers how to improve communication with hearing-impaired people. In recent years, increased attention has been directed toward planning or modifying environments to diminish background noise and to improve the ability of people to hear. Although some noise control modifications, such as using window draperies, are relatively simple and can be applied to many settings, other measures, such as selection of building materials, need to be implemented while environments are being designed.

 Box 16-10 Techniques for Communicating With Hearing-Impaired People

- Stand or sit directly in front of, and close to, the person.
- Talk toward the better ear, but make sure your lips can be seen.
- Make sure the person pays attention and looks at your face.
- Address the person by name, pause and then begin talking.
- Speak distinctly, slowly and directly to the person.
- Do not exaggerate lip movements because this will interfere with lip reading.
- Avoid chewing gum, covering your mouth or turning your head away.
- If the person does not understand, repeat the message by using different words.
- Avoid or eliminate any background noise.
- Avoid raising the volume of your voice; rather, try to lower the tone while still speaking in a moderately loud voice.
- Keep all instructions simple and ask for feedback to assess what the person heard.
- Avoid questions that elicit simple yes or no answers.
- Keep sentences short.
- Use body language that is congruent with what you are trying to communicate.
- Demonstrate what you are saying.
- Use large-print written communication and pictures to supplement verbal communication.
- Make sure only one person talks at a time; arrange for one-on-one communication whenever possible.
- If the hearing-impaired person normally wears eyeglasses to improve vision, make sure the eyeglasses are clean.
- Provide adequate lighting so that the person can see your lips; avoid settings in which there is glare behind or around you.

Unfolding Case Study

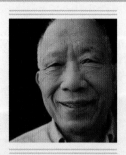

Part 3: Mr. H. at 83 Years of Age

Mr. H. is now 83 years old and has been a widower for 1 year. He has given up hunting and wood-working because he developed Parkinson disease 11 years ago and cannot manage the necessary fine motor movements. He continues to fish seasonally, play poker monthly and smoke one pack of cigarettes per day. In addition to Parkinson disease, he has hypertension and coronary artery disease. He still lives in his own home and attends the local senior centre for meals and social activities three times a week. His hearing loss has progressed to the point that he has difficulty with phone conversations and has to turn the television up loud. He cannot hear the doorbell. At the senior centre, participants avoid conversations with him because he has difficulty hearing.

You are the nurse at the senior centre, and you see him during the weekly "wellness clinic" for blood pressure checks. One week, he tells you that his daughter is upset with him because he never answers his phone when she calls, and she cannot have a decent phone conversation with him. She lives in another province and worries about him. She has offered to pay for a hearing aid evaluation for him, but he has told her, "Those things stick out like a sore thumb and they don't do any good anyway. I can hear anything I want to hear and there's a lot I don't care to hear, so why should you spend a lot of money for something that I won't use." He asks your opinion about this and is wondering whether he should at least get a checkup to pacify his daughter. He expects he will be told that nothing can be done and that his daughter will have to be satisfied with the situation.

THINKING POINTS

- Which information in Box 16-3 would be most pertinent to obtain at this time?
- What myths and misunderstandings influence Mr. H.?
- What nursing diagnosis would you apply to Mr. H.?
- Which information in Boxes 16-6 and 16-7 would be pertinent to this situation?

- What health promotion teaching would you do to address Mr. H.'s resistance to having his hearing evaluated?
- What additional health promotion advice would you give?
- Because you usually see Mr. H. weekly, you can develop a long-term teaching plan. How would you establish priorities for immediate and long-term goals?

QSEN APPLICATION

QSEN Competency	Knowledge/Skill/Attitude	Application to Mr. H.
Patient-centred care	(K) Examine common barriers to active involvement of patients in their own health care processes	Use assessment boxes and the HHIE-S (Fig. 16-3) to help identify and address Mr. H's resistance to obtaining a hearing evaluation
	(S) Elicit patient values, preferences and expressed needs	Emphasize the importance of obtaining a medical evaluation to identify reversible causes of hearing impairment
	(A) Value seeing health care situations "through patients' eyes"	
Evidence-based practice	(S) Base individualized care plan on patient values, clinical expertise and evidence	Provide a list of reliable and noncommercial sources of information about hearing loss (see Online Learning Activity 16-5 on the Point), and encourage him to obtain information and an evaluation

EVALUATING EFFECTIVENESS OF NURSING INTERVENTIONS

Nurses observe compensatory behaviours of hearing-impaired older adults to evaluate the effectiveness of interventions, as indicated by the following:
- Improved ability to communicate
- Effective use of hearing aids and amplification devices
- Increased participation in social activities
- Environmental modifications to eliminate background noise
- Participation in auditory rehabilitation program

Evaluation of effectiveness of interventions varies in different health care settings. For example, nurses in short-term settings provide health education as part of a discharge plan that includes information about resources for hearing evaluations. Evaluation of the effectiveness of this intervention is based on the patient's positive response to the nurse's suggestions, but the nurse is not likely to know whether the person followed through with the referral and had beneficial outcomes. In home, community and long-term care settings, nurses address long-term goals by facilitating referrals for audiology services. In these settings, the evaluation of interventions is based on the person's use of additional resources to improve communication abilities.

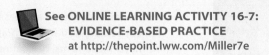

See ONLINE LEARNING ACTIVITY 16-7:
EVIDENCE-BASED PRACTICE
at http://thepoint.lww.com/Miller7e

Unfolding Case Study

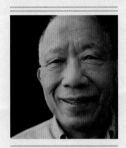

Part 4: Mr. H. at 89 Years of Age

Mr. H. is an 89-year-old widower who has had Parkinson disease for 17 years. Presbycusis is listed as an additional diagnosis on his medical record. He is being admitted to a nursing home because his condition has declined to the point that his daughter, Ms. D., can no longer manage his care in her home, where he has lived for several years. He is medically stable but needs assistance in all activities of daily living.

NURSING ASSESSMENT

During the admission interview, you notice that Mr. H. has difficulty hearing your questions and that he frequently asks his daughter to give the requested information. He shows no significant cognitive deficits, but he seems to have difficulty understanding verbal communication. When you ask about any hearing impairment, Ms. D. tells you that her father has used hearing aids for 5 years and has been re-evaluated periodically at a speech and hearing centre. Two months ago, he obtained new hearing aids, but wears them only for one-on-one conversations with her. Because of Mr. H.'s tremors and difficulty with fine motor movements, Ms. D. cares for his hearing aids and assists with their insertion and removal.

Ms. D. has encouraged her father to wear his hearing aids during family gatherings, but he says the noise from small children is too annoying. Except for family gatherings, Mr. H. has very few opportunities for social interaction, and he has become more and more withdrawn. He used to enjoy playing poker, but has not played in several years because all of his friends have died. Now he spends much of his time watching closed-captioned television programs. Ms. D. hopes that her father will respond to the opportunities for social interaction provided at the nursing home and that his quality of life will improve.

NURSING DIAGNOSIS

In addition to nursing diagnoses related to Mr. H.'s chronic illness and self-care deficits, you identify a nursing diagnosis of Impaired Social Interaction related to the effects of hearing loss. You select this as a nursing diagnosis because Mr. H.'s hearing impairment has already been evaluated and sound amplification devices are available to him.

NURSING CARE PLAN FOR MR. H.

In your care plan, you address the psychosocial consequences of Mr. H.'s hearing impairment. Your nursing care is directed toward improving his social interaction through the use of available devices and through other communication techniques that will enhance his social interaction skills.

Expected Outcome	Nursing Interventions	Nursing Evaluation
Mr. H. will develop effective communication techniques for resident–staff interactions.	• During the initial interview, talk with Mr. H. and Ms. D. about the importance of good verbal communication with staff; emphasize the need for the staff to get to know Mr. H so his needs can be addressed. • Ask Mr. H. to wear his hearing aids during all one-on-one interactions with staff.	• Mr. H. will wear his hearing aids during all one-on-one conversations with staff. • Mr. H. will report satisfactory verbal interactions with the staff.

Expected Outcome	Nursing Interventions	Nursing Evaluation
	• Use effective communication techniques when talking with Mr. H (as in Box 16-10). • Make sure all staff members provide appropriate assistance with insertion and removal of Mr. H.'s hearing aids. • Include hearing aid maintenance as part of the daily responsibilities of the nursing aide.	• Mr. H.'s hearing aids will be maintained in good operating condition.
Mr. H. will engage in social interaction with one other resident.	• During the initial care plan conference, identify several other residents who might converse with Mr. H. • Ask the staff to encourage one-on-one conversations between Mr. H. and the selected resident (e.g., suggest that they watch closed-captioned television programs together). • Ask Mr. H. to wear his hearing aids during one-on-one interactions with residents. • Provide assistance with inserting and removing hearing aids as needed. • Provide a quiet environment for one-on-one conversations with other residents.	• Mr. H. will wear his hearing aids at least once daily for a conversation with one other resident.
Mr. H. will engage in small group activities with other residents.	• During the first monthly care review conference, ask the activities staff to invite Mr. H. to a poker game with three other residents in the small-group room. • Make sure that environmental noise is controlled as much as possible.	• By the second month in this facility, Mr. H. will participate in weekly poker games with three other residents.

THINKING POINTS

- What nursing responsibilities would you have with regard to addressing Mr. H.'s hearing impairment? How would you work with other staff to implement the care plan described in the concluding case example?
- What are some of the advantages and disadvantages of hearing aids in a long-term care setting? How would you address the disadvantages?

- How would you involve Ms. D. in the care plan to address Mr. H.'s hearing impairment?
- If Mr. H. were in an acute care setting, how would you address his hearing problem?

Chapter Highlights

Age-Related Changes That Affect Hearing (Fig. 16-1 and Table 16-1)

- External ear: thicker hair, thinner skin, increased keratin
- Middle ear: less resilient tympanic membrane, calcified ossicles, stiffer muscles and ligaments
- Inner ear and auditory nervous system: fewer neurons and hair cells, diminished blood supply, degeneration of spiral ganglion and central processing systems
- Auditory nervous system: degenerative changes in the auditory nerve and central nervous system

Risk Factors That Affect Hearing Wellness (Fig. 16-2 and Box 16-1)

- Genetic predisposition to otosclerosis
- Exposure to noise
- Impacted cerumen

- Ototoxic medications: aminoglycosides, aspirin, loop diuretics, quinine
- Disease processes: otosclerosis, Paget disease, Ménière disease

Functional Consequences Affecting Hearing Wellness (Table 16-1)

- Presbycusis: diminished ability to hear high-pitched sounds, especially in the presence of background noise
- Predisposition to impacted cerumen
- Psychosocial consequences: depression, social isolation, declines in cognitive function, increased dependency, diminished quality of life

Pathologic Condition Affecting Hearing

- Tinnitus: persistent sensation of noises that do not originate in the external environment

Nursing Assessment of Hearing (Fig. 16-3; Boxes 16-3 to 16-5)

- Screening tool: The Hearing Handicap Inventory for the Elderly (HHEI-S)
- Past and present risk factors (e.g., use of ototoxic medications, noise exposure, family history of otosclerosis)
- Attitudes about hearing aids if impairment is present
- Impact of hearing impairment on communication and quality of life
- Behavioural cues to impaired hearing
- Otoscopic examination for impacted cerumen
- Tuning fork tests for hearing

Nursing Diagnosis

- Readiness for Enhanced Communication
- Additional diagnoses related to functional consequences of hearing loss: Anxiety, Impaired Social Interaction, Ineffective Coping, Risk for Injury, and Risk for Loneliness

Planning for Wellness Outcomes

- Improved communication
- Increased social interactions
- Improved quality of life
- Increased safety and functioning

Nursing Interventions for Hearing Wellness (Figs. 16-4 and 16-5; Boxes 16-6 to 16-9)

- Health promotion teaching to address modifiable risk factors: smoking, exposure to noise, use of ototoxic medications
- Removing and preventing impacted cerumen
- Promoting referrals for appropriate professional services
- Using assistive listening devices
- Teaching about the use and care of a hearing aid
- Communicating with hearing-impaired older adults
- Compensating for hearing deficits by using hearing devices and hearing aids

Evaluating Effectiveness of Nursing Interventions

- Improved communication
- Use of appropriate amplification aids
- Appropriate environmental modifications
- Increased participation in social activities

Critical Thinking Exercises

1. Describe presbycusis and explain the functional consequences of this condition as it affects the everyday life of an older adult.
2. What risk factors would you consider in an 83-year-old person who complains of recent problems with hearing?
3. What advice would you give to someone who asks you about a brochure she received from a hearing aid company that offers free hearing screenings describing a new high-powered hearing aid? The person has trouble hearing but has never had an evaluation.

4. Describe at least 10 ways in which you can adapt your communication for a hearing-impaired person.
5. Find at least one resource (*not* a hearing instrument specialist) in your community that you could recommend to an older adult who needs a hearing evaluation.
6. Visit at least three Internet sites that provide educational materials about hearing impairment, and choose the one you think would be best for obtaining health information brochures.

 For more information about the topics discussed in this chapter, be sure to check out the interactive Online Learning Activities and other helpful resources at http://thepoint.lww.com/Miller7e

REFERENCES

Adobamen, P. R., & Ogisi, F. O. (2012). Hearing loss due to wax impaction. *Nigerian Quarterly Journal of Hospital Medicine, 22*(2), 117–120.

Agency for Healthcare Research and Quality. (2012). *Evidence-based practice center systematic review protocol: Evaluation and treatment of tinnitus.* Retrieved from www.effectivehealthcare.ahrq.gov

Anderson, S., Parbery-Clark, A., White-Schwoch, T., et al. (2012). Aging affects neural precision of speech encoding. *Journal of Neuroscience, 32*(41), 14156–14164. doi:10.1523/JNEUROSCI.2176-12.2012

Bulechek, G. M., Butcher, H. K., Dochterman, J. M., et al. (2013). *Nursing Interventions Classification (NIC)* (6th ed.). St. Louis, MO: Elsevier.

Ciorba, A., Bianchini, C., Pelucchi, S., et al. (2012). The impact of hearing loss on quality of life of elderly adults. *Clinical Interventions in Aging, 7*, 159–163.

Dille, M. F., Wilmington, D., McMillan, G. P., et al. (2012). Development and validation of cisplatin dose-ototoxicity model. *Journal of the American Academy of Audiologists, 23*(7), 510–521.

Eckert, M. A., Cute, S. L., Vaden, K. I., et al. (2012). Auditory cortex signs of age-related hearing loss. *Journal of the Association of Researchers in Otolaryngology, 13*(5), 703–713.

Fabry, D. A., Davila, E. P., Arheart, K. L., et al. (2011). Secondhand smoke exposure and the risk of hearing loss. *Tobacco Control, 20*(1), 82–85.

Glyde, H., Cameron, S., Dillon, H., et al. (2013). The effects of hearing impairment and aging on spatial processing. *Ear and Hearing, 34*(1), 15–28.

Gopinath, B., Schneider, J., McMahon, C. M., et al. (2012). Severity of age-related hearing loss is associated with impaired activities of daily living. *Age and Ageing, 41*(2), 195–200.

Greenberg, H. S. (2013). Special Considerations. In T. M. Buttaro & K. A. Barba (Eds.), *Nursing care of the hospitalized older patient* (pp. 454–460). Oxford, England: Wiley-Blackwell.

Herdman, T. H. (Ed.). (2012). *NANDA International nursing diagnoses: Definitions and classification 2012–2014.* Oxford, England: Wiley-Blackwell.

Humann, M. J., Sanderson, W. T., Gerr, F., et al. (2012). Effects of common agricultural tasks on measures of hearing loss. *American Journal of Industrial Medicine, 55*(10), 904–916.

Jupiter, T. (2012). Cognition and screening for hearing loss in nursing home residents. *Journal of the American Medical Directors Association, 13*(8), 744–747.

Kelly, A. C., Boyd, S. M., Henehan, G. T., et al. (2012). Occupational noise exposure of nightclub bar employees in Ireland. *Noise and Health, 14*(59), 148–154.

Kiely, K. M., Gopinath, B., Mitchell, P., et al. (2012). Cognitive, health, and sociodemographic predictors of longitudinal decline in hearing acuity among older adults. *Journal of Gerontology: Medical Sciences, 67*(9), 997–1003.

Kirchner, D. B., Evenson, E., Dobie, R. A., et al. (2012). Occupational noise-induced hearing loss. *Journal of Occupational and Environmental Medicine, 54*(1), 106–108.

Konrad-Martin, D., Dille, M. F., McMillan, G., et al. (2012). Age-related changes in the auditory brainstem response. *Journal of the American Academy of Audiologists, 23*(1), 18–35.

Li-Korotky, H. S. (2012). Age-related hearing loss: Quality of care for quality of life. *The Gerontologist, 52*(2), 265–271.

Lin, F. R., Chien, W. W., Li, L., et al. (2012). Cochlear implantation in older adults. *Medicine, 91*(5), 229–241.

Lin, F. R., Maas, P., Chien, W., et al. (2011). Association of skin colour, race/ethnicity, and hearing loss among adults in the USA. *Journal of the Association for Research in Otolaryngology, 13*, 109–117.

Lin, F. R., Yaffe, K., Xia, J., et al. (2013). Hearing loss and cognitive decline in older adults. *Journal of the American Medical Association Internal Medicine, 21*, 1–7.

Loveman, E., Gospodarevskaya, E., Clegg, A., et al. (2011). Ear wax removal interventions: A systematic review and economic evaluation. *British Journal of General Practice, 61*(591), 680 -683. doi:10.3399/bjgp11X601497

Mondelli, M. F., & de Souza, P. J. (2012). Quality of life in elderly adults before and after hearing aid fitting. *Brazilian Journal of Otorhinolaryngology, 78*(3), 49–56.

Moorhead, S., Johnson, M., Maas, M. L., et al. (Eds.). (2013). *Nursing Outcomes Classification (NOC).* Philadelphia, PA: Elsevier.

Neitzel, R. L., Gershon, R. R., McAlexander, T. P., et al. (2012). Exposure to transit and other sources of noise among New York City residents. *Environment Science & Technology, 46*, 500–508.

Onder, M., Onder, S., & Mutlu, A. (2012). Determination of noise induced hearing loss in mining. *Environmental Monitoring and Assessment, 184*, 2443–2451.

Parham, K., Lin, F. R., Coelho, D. H., et al. (2013, February 8). Comprehensive management of presbycusis: Central and peripheral. *Otolaryngology Head and Neck Surgery, 148*(4), 537–539.

Roland, P. S., Smith, T. L., Schwartz, S. R., et al. (2008). Clinical practice guideline: Cerumen impaction. *Otolaryngology—Head and Neck Surgery, 139*, S1–S21.

Roth, Y., Oron, Y., & Goldfarb, A. (2011). Limited good-quality evidence available on earwax removal methods. *Evidence-Based Nursing, 14*(2), 60 -61. doi:10.1136/ebn1132

Ruppert, S. D., & Fay, V. P. (2012). Tinnitus evaluation in primary care. *The Nurse Practitioner, 37*(10), 20–26.

Singh, L. P., Bhardwaj, A., & Kumar, D. K. (2012). Prevalence of permanent hearing threshold shift among workers of Indian iron and steel small and medium enterprises: A study. *Noise & Health, 58*, 119–128.

Sliwinska-Kowalska, M., & Davis, A. (2012). Noise-induced hearing loss. *Noise & Health, 14*(61), 274–280.

Statistics Canada. (2006). *Participation and activity limitation survey* (Publication 89-628-X). Retrieved from http://www.statcan.gc.ca/pub/89-628-x/2009012/tab/tab1-eng.htm

Tansey, M., Raina, P., & Wolfson, C. (2013). Veterans' physical health. *Epidemiologic Reviews, 35*, 66–74. doi:10.1093/epirev/mxs005

Tinnitus Association of Canada. (2010). *What is Tinnitus?* Retrieved from http://www.canadianaudiology.ca/consumer/tinnitus.html

Yankaskas, K. (2013). Prelude: Noise-induced tinnitus and hearing loss in the military. *Hearing Research, 295*(1–2), 3–8.

chapter 17

Vision

LEARNING OBJECTIVES

After reading this chapter, you will be able to:

1. Describe age-related changes that affect vision.
2. Identify risk factors that can affect visual wellness.
3. Discuss the functional consequences that affect visual wellness.
4. Describe three pathologic conditions that cause vision impairments in older adults.
5. Conduct a nursing assessment of vision, with emphasis on identifying opportunities for health promotion.
6. Identify nursing interventions to facilitate visual wellness in older adults by addressing risk factors that interfere with vision.

KEY POINTS

accommodation

acuity

age-related macular degeneration (AMD)

arcus senilis

blepharochalasis

cataracts

colour perception

critical flicker fusion

depth perception

ectropion

enophthalmos

entropion

glare

glaucoma

low-vision aids

ophthalmologist

optician

optometrist

presbyopia

visual field

visual impairment

Because important daily activities—including communicating, enjoying visual images and manoeuvring in the environment—are highly dependent on eyesight, visual impairments can profoundly affect a person's safety, functioning and quality of life. Although age-related changes and risk factors affect visual wellness, nurses have an array of interventions to assist older adults in maintaining optimal visual function. This chapter addresses functional consequences affecting vision in older adults and focuses on the role of nurses in assessing vision and helping older adults achieve visual wellness.

AGE-RELATED CHANGES THAT AFFECT VISION

Visual function depends on a sequence of processes, beginning with the perception of an external stimulus and ending with the processing of neural impulses in the cerebral cortex. Age-related changes affect all of the structures involved in visual function; however, in the absence of disease processes, these gradual changes have only a subtle impact on the daily activities of the older person. Age-related changes in the structures of the eye are illustrated in Figure 17-1 and summarized in this section.

Eye Appearance and Tear Ducts

During early stages, age-related changes in the appearance of the eye and eyelids do not interfere with visual function, but they may progress to the point of requiring interventions. For example, drooping of the upper eyelid initially is a cosmetic issue, but if it progresses to the point of interfering with vision a minor surgical intervention might be appropriate. Table 17-1 summarizes age-related changes in appearance and tear ducts and the associated effects on visual function.

Promoting Visual Wellness in Older Adults

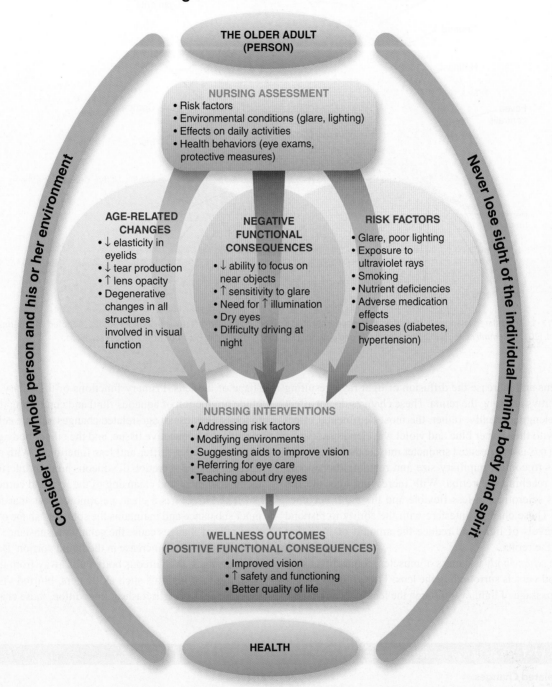

THE OLDER ADULT (PERSON)

NURSING ASSESSMENT
- Risk factors
- Environmental conditions (glare, lighting)
- Effects on daily activities
- Health behaviors (eye exams, protective measures)

AGE-RELATED CHANGES
- ↓ elasticity in eyelids
- ↓ tear production
- ↑ lens opacity
- Degenerative changes in all structures involved in visual function

NEGATIVE FUNCTIONAL CONSEQUENCES
- ↓ ability to focus on near objects
- ↑ sensitivity to glare
- Need for ↑ illumination
- Dry eyes
- Difficulty driving at night

RISK FACTORS
- Glare, poor lighting
- Exposure to ultraviolet rays
- Smoking
- Nutrient deficiencies
- Adverse medication effects
- Diseases (diabetes, hypertension)

NURSING INTERVENTIONS
- Addressing risk factors
- Modifying environments
- Suggesting aids to improve vision
- Referring for eye care
- Teaching about dry eyes

WELLNESS OUTCOMES (POSITIVE FUNCTIONAL CONSEQUENCES)
- Improved vision
- ↑ safety and functioning
- Better quality of life

HEALTH

Consider the whole person and his or her environment

Never lose sight of the individual—mind, body and spirit

The Eye

The *cornea* is a translucent covering over the eye that refracts light rays and provides 65% to 75% of the focusing power of the eye. As the eye ages, the cornea becomes opaque and yellow, interfering with the passage of light, especially ultraviolet (UV) rays, to the retina. Other corneal changes, such as the accumulation of lipid deposits, can cause an increased scattering of light rays and have a blurring effect on vision. In addition, age-related changes in the curvature of the cornea influence the refractive ability.

The *lens* consists of concentric and avascular layers of clear, crystalline protein. Because the lens has no blood supply, it depends on the aqueous humour for metabolic and support functions. New layers are continually formed peripherally and the old layers are compressed inward toward the centre, where they eventually become absorbed into the nucleus. This process gradually increases the size and density of the lens, causing a tripling of its mass by 70 years of age. Thus, the lens gradually becomes stiffer, denser and more opaque. These age-related changes decrease responsiveness

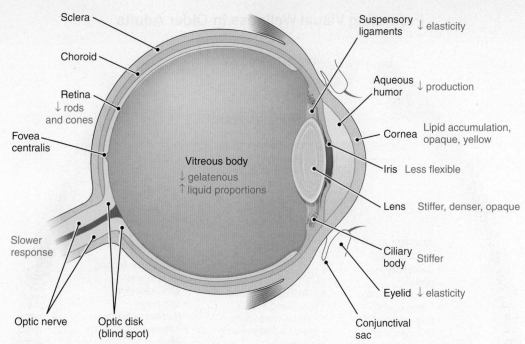

FIGURE 17-1 Age-related changes in structures of the eye, indicated with red labels, can affect vision in older adults. (Adapted with permission from Cohen, B. J. [2012]. *Memmler's The human body in health and disease* [12th ed.]. Philadelphia, PA: Lippincott Williams & Wilkins.)

of the lens and increase the diffusion of light rays, resulting in fewer rays reaching the retina. These changes do not affect all wavelengths equally; rather, the most detrimental effect occurs with the shorter blue and violet wavelengths.

The *iris* is a pigmented sphincter muscle that dilates and contracts to control pupillary size and regulate the amount of light reaching the retina. With increasing age, the iris becomes sclerotic and less flexible and the *pupil* becomes smaller. These changes interfere with the ability to respond to low levels of light and reduce the amount of light that reaches the retina.

The *ciliary body* is a mass of muscles, connective tissue and blood vessels surrounding the lens. These muscles regulate the passage of light rays through the lens by changing the

shape of the lens. Primary functions of the ciliary body include production of aqueous fluid and controlling the ability to focus. Because of age-related changes, muscle cells are replaced with connective tissue, and the ciliary body gradually becomes smaller, stiffer and less functional. With advanced age, diminished secretion of aqueous humour interferes with the nourishment and cleansing of the lens and cornea.

The *vitreous* is a clear, gelatinous mass that forms the inner substance and maintains the spherical shape of the eye. Age-related changes cause the gelatinous substance to shrink and a proportionate increase in the liquid portion. Because of these changes, the vitreous body pulls away from the retina, resulting in symptoms such as floaters, blurred vision, distorted images or light flashes. In addition, these changes can

TABLE 17-1 Effects of Age-Related Changes in Appearance and Tear Ducts	
Age-Related Changes	**Effect**
Loss of orbital fat, decreased elasticity of eyelid muscles, accumulation of dark pigment around the eyes	**Enophthalmos** = appearance of sunken eyes **Blepharochalasis** = drooping of upper eyelid, which can eventually impair vision
Relaxation of lower eyelid	**Ectropion** = lower eyelid falls away from conjunctiva, causing decreased lubrication **Entropion** = lower eyelid becomes inverted and eyelashes irritate the cornea
Accumulation of lipids in outer part of the cornea	**Arcus senilis** (also called corneal arcus) = development of yellow or grey-white ring around the iris
Narrowing of tear duct opening, reduced production of tears	**Dry eye syndrome** = excessive tearing, watery eyes, irritation and inflammation

cause light to scatter more diffusely through the vitreous, reducing the amount of light reaching the retina.

The process of transforming visual stimuli into neural impulses begins in the rods and cones in the *retina*. Rods do not perceive colours, but they are responsible for vision under low light. Cones require high levels of light to function effectively, and they are responsible for **colour perception** and **acuity**, which is the ability to detect details and discern objects. Rods are distributed throughout the peripheral retina, and cones are concentrated in the central and most sensitive part of the macula, called the *fovea*. Although both the rods and cones diminish with increasing age, the impact of these changes is minimal because loss of cones occurs primarily in the periphery of the retina, with only a minimal loss in the fovea. Also, although the number of rods declines in the central retina, the remaining rods increase in size and maintain their ability to capture light. Additional age-related changes in retinal structures include accumulation of lipofuscin and thinning and sclerosis of the blood vessels and pigment epithelium.

The Retinal–Neural Pathway

Photoreceptor cells converge in the ganglion cells of the optic nerve. Neurosensory information is passed from the optic nerve, through the thalamus, to the visual cortex. Age-related changes affecting these neurons result in slower processing of visual information.

EFFECTS OF AGE-RELATED CHANGES ON VISION

Best-corrected visual acuity begins to decrease in adults, after age 50, even in the absence of any other factors. However, despite the universal prevalence of age-related vision changes, most older adults can perform their usual activities by using low-vision aids and modifying their environment. **Visual impairment**, which is defined as vision loss that cannot be corrected by eyeglasses or contact lenses alone, ranges from mild impairment to blindness. Mild visual impairments are caused by normal age-related changes, but they are significantly exacerbated by environmental conditions such as glare and poor lighting. These mild visual impairments are illustrated in Figure 17-2 and discussed in the following sections; consequences of more significant visual impairments are discussed in the Pathologic Conditions Affecting Vision section.

Loss of Accommodation

Presbyopia is the loss of **accommodation**, which is the ability to focus clearly and quickly on objects at various distances. Presbyopia is an initial and universal age-related vision change, which begins in early adulthood and progresses through older adulthood at varying rates. This vision change is caused by degenerative changes in the lens and the ciliary body. Functionally, accommodative changes gradually extend the near point of vision, which is the closest point at which a small object can be seen clearly. A typical example of the effects of presbyopia is the need to hold reading materials farther from the eye to focus clearly on the print.

Diminished Acuity

Visual acuity, which is measured against a normal value of 20/20 is assessed by using a Snellen chart. Visual acuity is best around age 30, after which it gradually declines. Age-related ocular changes that affect acuity include decreased pupillary size, increased diffusion of light in the cornea and lens, opacification of the lens and vitreous and loss of photoreceptor cells in the retina. Because of these changes, between the ages of 20 and 60 years, there is a threefold reduction in the amount of light reaching the retina.

External conditions, such as size and movement of the object and the amount of light reflected off an object, also influence acuity. Because poor illumination compounds the effects of age-related ocular changes, older people require more illumination to see objects clearly. In addition, because visual acuity is more limited for moving objects, it becomes more impaired with increasing speed of the object. These changes in visual acuity can particularly affect night-driving competence.

Delayed Dark and Light Adaptation

The ability to respond to both dim and bright light begins to decline around the age of 20 years and diminishes more markedly after age 60. This decline is associated with decreased retinal illumination caused by age-related changes in the lens, pupil, retina and retinal–neural pathways. As a result, the older adult requires more time to adapt to dim lighting when moving from a brighter to a darker environment. For instance, when entering a darkened movie theatre, an older person needs extra time to adapt to the changes in lighting before proceeding to a seat. Another consequence is that an older person responds more slowly to lights, such as car or bus headlights, and requires more time to recover from exposure to glare and bright lights.

Increased Glare Sensitivity

Glare is experienced when light is reflected from shiny surfaces, when the light is excessively bright or inappropriately focused, or when bright light originates from several sources at once, as in the following examples:

- Bright fluorescent lights in a grocery store reflecting on the clear plastic covering over food products in a white case
- Glass-covered directories in brightly lit shopping malls, particularly when the contrast between the letters and the background is poor
- Facing into sun, especially at sunrise or sunset or in combination with snow
- Driving in rain

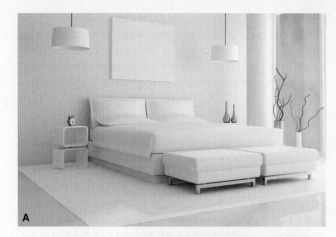

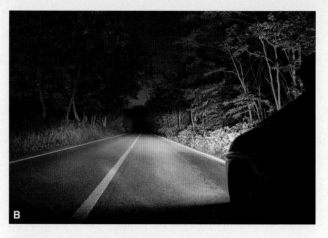

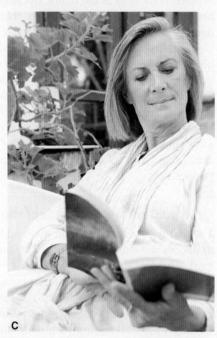

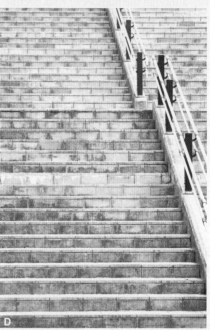

FIGURE 17-2 Mild visual impairments include (**A**) reduced contrast sensitivity, (**B**) increased sensitivity to glare and difficulty with night driving, (**C**) increased lighting requirements and decreased ability to focus close-up, (**D**) decreased ability to judge depth perception. (All images from shutterstock.com; copyrights: A—archideaphoto, B—ollyy, C—MJTH and D—Sakarin Sawasdinaka.)

Beginning in the fifth decade, age-related changes increase a person's sensitivity to glare and the time required to recover from glare. Glare sensitivity is influenced primarily by opacification of the lens; however, it is also affected by age-related changes in the pupil and vitreous. Effects on vision include diminished contrast of the viewed object, difficulty discerning details and blinding effects. In practical terms, these changes can significantly affect the person's ability to read signs, see objects, drive at night and manoeuvre safely in bright environments. In many modern buildings and shopping malls, the bright lights, large windows and highly reflective floors generate glare that can lead to accidents and inaccurate perceptions.

Reduced Visual Field

A **visual field** is an oval-shaped area encompassing the total view that people perceive while looking at a fixed point straight ahead. The scope of the visual field narrows slightly between the ages of 40 and 50 years and then declines steadily. Functionally, the visual field is important when people engage in tasks that require a broad perception of the environment and moving objects. Walking in crowded places and driving a vehicle are examples of activities that depend on the field of vision.

Diminished Depth Perception

Depth perception is the visual skill responsible for locating objects in three-dimensional space, judging differences in the depth of objects and observing relationships among objects in space. Factors that influence depth perception include age-related changes, prior perceptual experiences of the observer, movement of the observer's head or body and characteristics of the object, such as size, height, distance, texture, brightness and shading. Older adults experience diminished depth perception, making it more difficult to use objects effectively and manoeuvre safely in the environment.

Altered Colour Vision

Pigments in the retinal cones absorb light in the red, blue or yellow ranges of the spectrum. Because colour perception is influenced by the type and quantity of light waves reaching the retina, age-related changes that interfere with retinal illumination can influence accurate colour perception. Opacification and yellowing of the lens interferes most directly with shorter wavelengths, causing an altered perception of blues, greens and violets. Low levels of illumination and other environmental factors also interfere with colour perception.

Functionally, altered colour perception is manifested as a relative darkening of blue objects and a yellowed perception of white light. Accurate colour perception is not essential in all daily activities, but it is important, for instance, in differentiating between medications that are similar in colour or tone, especially those in the blue–green and yellow–white ranges. In addition, altered colour perception can interfere with the detection of spoiled food.

Diminished Critical Flicker Fusion

Critical flicker fusion is the point at which an intermittent light source is perceived as a continuous, rather than flashing, light. The ability to perceive flashing lights accurately is a function of the retinal receptors and is influenced by extraocular factors, such as the size, colour and luminance of the object. Age-related changes in the retina and retinal–neural pathway, as well as changes that decrease retinal illumination, interfere with critical flicker fusion. Low levels of illumination further exacerbate the effects of these changes. Functionally, diminished critical flicker fusion causes a flashing light to appear to be continuous and it can interfere with the discernment of emergency vehicles and road construction lights, especially at night.

Slower Visual Information Processing

Age-related changes of the retinal–neural pathway affect the accuracy and efficiency of visual information processing. Thus, older adults generally need more time to process visual information, but the effects are minimal or negligible when tasks are familiar. Table 17-2 summarizes age-related vision changes and their effects on vision.

See **ONLINE LEARNING ACTIVITY 17-1: THROUGH THE EYES OF OLDER ADULTS**
at http://thepoint.lww.com/Miller7e

RISK FACTORS THAT AFFECT VISUAL WELLNESS

Lifestyle, nutritional and environmental factors—including both immediate and long-term conditions—exacerbate age-related vision changes and interfere with visual wellness as in the following examples:

- Poor nutrition, cigarette smoking and exposure to sunlight are associated with the development of eye diseases.
- Older adults are more vulnerable to eye damage from sunlight because age-related changes alter the protective response to harmful UV light.
- Warmer environmental temperatures are associated with an earlier age of onset for presbyopia.
- Environmental conditions, such as wind, sunlight, low humidity and secondhand smoke, can cause dry eyes.
- Poor nutrition increases the risk for age-related macular degeneration (AMD).
- Environmental conditions, such as lighting and colour contrast, affect visual function in many ways.

Wellness Opportunity

Poor lighting and exposure to sunlight are risk factors that can readily be addressed through simple self-care practices.

Chronic conditions can adversely affect visual function in various ways. Vision impairments commonly occur in people with dementia or Parkinson disease, even during the early stages. Visuospatial changes and visual hallucinations are common with Lewy body dementia and are considered a distinguishing characteristic early in the course of the disease (Ferman et al., 2013; Hamilton et al., 2012; Yoshizawa et al.,

TABLE 17-2 Consequences of Age-Related Changes on Vision	
Changes	**Consequences**
• Corneal yellowing and increased opacity	• Diminished acuity
• Changes in the corneal curvature	• Slower response to changes in illumination
• Increase in lens size and density	• Increased sensitivity to glare
• Sclerosis and rigidity of the iris	• Narrowing of the visual field
• Decrease in pupillary size	• Diminished depth perception
• Atrophy of the ciliary muscle	• Altered colour perception
• Shrinkage of gelatinous substance in the vitreous	• Distorted perception of flashing lights
• Atrophy of photoreceptor cells	• Slower processing of visual information
• Thinning and sclerosis of retinal blood vessels	
• Degeneration of neurons in the visual cortex	

2013). People with diabetes are at increased risk for developing cataracts, glaucoma and diabetic retinopathy. People with hypertension or hypercholesterolemia are at higher risk for AMD. Malnutrition has been associated with cataract development, and vitamin A deficiency has been associated with dry eyes from reduced tear production.

The following medications are associated with potential adverse effects on vision: nonsteroidal anti-inflammatory agents (e.g., aspirin), anticholinergics, phenothiazines, amiodarone, sildenafil, α-blockers (e.g., doxazosin mesylate) and oral or inhaled corticosteroids. Medications that can cause or contribute to dry eyes include estrogen, diuretics, antihistamines, anticholinergics, phenothiazines, β-blockers and antiparkinson agents. Systemic anticoagulants can precipitate intraocular hemorrhage in people with preexisting macular degeneration.

DIVERSITY NOTE

Prevalence of diabetic retinopathy is higher in blacks and Hispanics than in whites and Chinese ancestry (Zambelli-Weiner et al., 2012).

FUNCTIONAL CONSEQUENCES AFFECTING VISUAL WELLNESS

Disease processes, as discussed in the section on pathologic changes affecting vision, are the most common cause of serious visual impairments in older adults. Visual impairments are categorized as "functional" when acuity is 20/50 or worse, as "low vision" when it is between 20/70 and 20/200 and as "blindness" when it is 20/400 or worse. The term "vision loss" refers to a significant decrease in vision that cannot be addressed by corrective lenses. According to the Canadian

Institute of the Blind (CNIB), vision loss affects one in 11 adults 65 years of age and one in 8 individuals 75 years of age and older (CNIB—Fast Facts About Vision Loss, n.d.). The following sections describe the functional consequences that are associated with the types of visual impairments that are most likely to occur in older adults.

Effects on Safety and Function

Because visual impairments are associated with many aspects of safety and functioning, people who are visually impaired are likely to be more dependent in their activities of daily living. Age-related vision changes most directly influence the following activities:

- Getting outside
- Driving a vehicle
- Shopping for groceries
- Going up and down stairs
- Getting in and out of bed or a chair
- Manoeuvring safely in dark or unfamiliar environments
- Seeing markings on clocks, radios, thermostats, appliances and televisions
- Reading newspapers, directories, small-print signs and posters, and labels on food items and medication containers

Most of these activities are affected not only by alterations in visual skills but also by environmental conditions, such as glare and lighting. A study of self-reported visual disability in older adults found that those who had glaucoma or AMD had significantly more difficulties with preparing meals, grocery shopping and out-of-home travel (Hochberg et al., 2012).

Low vision can affect self-management of chronic disease, with important implications for addressing health literacy (Warren, 2013), as discussed in Learning Activity 17-2.

Unfolding Case Study

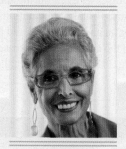

Part 1: Mrs. F. at 60 Years of Age

Mrs. F. is 60 years old and has used "readers" (reading glasses) for 15 years but has never needed glasses for anything other than reading and sewing. She recently noticed that she has trouble reading the glass-enclosed directory at the shopping mall. She works in an office building with an atrium that has skylights, and she has trouble reading the signs on the doors.

THINKING POINTS

- What age-related factors contribute to the vision changes that Mrs. F. notices?
- What environmental factors are likely to contribute to Mrs. F.'s difficulty when she is in the shopping mall or at work?

- When Mrs. F. is in her home environment, what tasks might be more difficult because of age-related vision changes?

ONLINE LEARNING ACTIVITY 17-2: ARTICLE ABOUT HEALTH LITERACY AND LOW VISION at http://thepoint.lww.com/Miller7e

Visual impairments threaten safe functioning because they can affect gait, balance and postural stability and they increase the risk of falls, fractures and other serious fall-related injuries. Visually impaired people enter nursing homes 3 years earlier, have twice the risk of fall and four times the risk of hip fractures (Eichenbaum, 2012). Studies have found that people with impaired vision not only have an increased risk of falls, but also experience greater fear of falling and activity limitation due to fear of falling (Ramulu et al., 2012; Tanabe et al., 2012; Wang et al., 2012).

Specific age-related vision changes that increase the risk for falls include diminished acuity, reduced visual field, diminished depth perception, reduced contrast sensitivity and increased sensitivity to glare. In addition, delayed processing of visual information can interfere with the quick responses necessary for avoiding falls.

Effects on Quality of Life

Age-related vision changes develop gradually and often go unnoticed for many years. As the changes progress and interfere with usual activities, older adults may withdraw from activities rather than acknowledge a vision problem or adjust to the changes. Studies find that visual impairments are associated with anxiety, depression and lower levels of psychological well-being (Mabuchi et al., 2012; Mathew et al., 2011; Popescu et al., 2012).

Of course, a person's usual lifestyle influences the extent of any psychosocial impact related to vision changes. For example, if the preferred leisure activities require good visual skills, the older adult is likely to become bored and even depressed when vision changes interfere with endeavours, such as reading, sewing or needlework. Similarly, when artistic pursuits and entertainment events are important activities, diminished visual function can interfere with the person's quality of life. By contrast, the effect of vision impairment on lifestyle may be minimal for people who prefer music or other activities that are less dependent on visual skills.

One's living environment and support systems are other determinants of the psychosocial consequences of vision changes. Good visual skills are more important for people who live alone or who provide care for others than they are for people who live with, or have frequent contact with, others who have good vision. Also, psychosocial consequences will be minimized if visually impaired people can modify their living environment to compensate for the impairments. By contrast, people who live in institutional settings may experience relatively greater negative consequences because of their inability to alter environmental conditions.

Some older adults who notice declines in vision develop fears that negatively affect their quality of life. For example, people may mistakenly fear going blind if they think they have a serious and progressive disease when, in reality, they have a treatable condition. Fear of blindness may be based on myths, inaccurate information or the experiences of friends who have serious visual impairments. Negative or hopeless attitudes about vision changes can deter the older person from acknowledging the problem or seeking help. Fear of falling is another source of anxiety associated with impaired vision. Inaccurate depth perception can lead to frequent bumping into objects, and the older adult may feel insecure and unsafe, even in familiar environments. If the person has experienced falls or tripping, or knows someone who suffered a fracture as a result of falling, the fears may be magnified.

Wellness Opportunity

Nurses assess the impact of vision impairment on the whole person so they can address fears, anxieties and other responses that affect quality of life.

Effects on Driving

Vision changes can significantly affect driving skills and exert a profound impact on older adults, their families and the society. Because driving is associated with considerable safety and independence concerns for drivers and their families—and because unsafe drivers place others at risk—there has been intense and increasing interest in the effects of vision changes on the driving skills of older adults. Visual dimensions that influence driving abilities are near vision, visual search, dynamic vision, contrast sensitivity and visual processing speed. Consequences of visual impairment with regard to driving include the following:

- Slower dark and light adaptation creates problems when driving in and out of tunnels and when driving at night on streets with variable lighting.
- Decreased peripheral vision interferes with the wide visual field that is important for avoiding collisions.
- Decreased acuity interferes with the perception of moving objects, especially fast-moving vehicles.
- Diminished accommodation and acuity create problems when the older adult tries to read dashboard indicators after focusing on the road.
- Glare interferes with the perception of objects and is heightened by rainy, snowy or sunny conditions.
- Bright sunlight shortly after sunrise or before sunset can significantly interfere with the perception of red and green traffic lights because of increased sensitivity to glare.
- If the car has tinted windows, the diminished illumination further interferes with visual skills.

In recent years, gerontologists and clinicians are focusing attention on identifying variables that affect driving in older adults, and many studies address visual skills as an important factor. Studies indicate that a combination of cognitive impairment and eye disease (i.e., cataract, glaucoma, AMD) can affect older driver safety, particularly at speeds above 60 mph (Andersen, 2012; Anstey et al., 2012;

Kaleem et al., 2012). One finding that is pertinent to teaching older adults is that having a cataract in one or both eyes is a common cause of driving difficulties, and the risk of driving-related accidents is significantly reduced after cataract surgery (Mennemeyer et al., 2013; Owsley et al., 2012).

Wellness Opportunity

Nurses need to be aware of the far-reaching implications of the ability to drive not only on safety of the individual and others but also on independence and the quality of life.

PATHOLOGIC CONDITIONS AFFECTING VISION

Chronic conditions that interfere with visual wellness occur very commonly in older adults, so nurses have important roles in detecting and managing these conditions. Health promotion interventions are particularly important with conditions such as glaucoma because interventions can prevent vision impairment. However, this condition is often undiagnosed so the interventions are not implemented in a timely manner. Among older adults, the three most common pathologic eye conditions are cataracts, AMD and glaucoma (Table 17-3).

Cataracts

Cataracts are a leading and reversible cause of visual impairment, affecting approximately 50% of people aged 80 years and older. It is estimated that 2.5 million Canadians are living with cataracts (http://www.eyesite.ca). Worldwide, cataract is the primary cause of avoidable blindness and significant visual loss, causing half of all blindness in low- and middle-income countries (Finger et al., 2012; Murthy et al., 2012). Cataracts are caused by the progression of age-related changes in the lens that begin in middle adulthood

and eventually can progress to total opacification. As cataracts develop, the normally transparent lens becomes cloudy, transmission of light to the retina is diminished and vision is impaired. In addition to being caused by age-related changes, risk factors include systemic disease, medications and environmental factors, as summarized in Table 17-3. Overall, the most modifiable and preventable risk factors for cataracts are cigarette smoking and exposure to sunlight.

Cataracts usually occur in both eyes, but they do not necessarily progress bilaterally at the same rate. Types of cataracts are listed below:

- *Nuclear:* most common type, begins in the centre of lens
- *Cortical:* begin in periphery and progress inward
- *Subcapsular:* begin in the posterior lens, progress more rapidly than other types

In their early stages, cataracts do not necessarily affect visual acuity, but as they progress, they cause difficulty performing activities such as reading and night driving (see Fig. 17-3 and Table 17-3).

When visual acuity declines to the point that it affects the person's safety or the quality of life and provides a reasonable likelihood of improved vision with intervention, cataract surgery is usually recommended. In recent years, major advances have been made in techniques for removal of cataracts as well as options for correction of presbyopia and other visual acuity problems during the surgery (Lichtinger & Rootman, 2012). An optometrist or an ophthalmologist can diagnose cataracts, but only an ophthalmologist can perform cataract surgery, which is the most commonly performed operation in Canada today. The surgical procedure is done with local anesthesia and takes less than 1 hour. Studies confirm that cataract surgery has a very low rate of complications and high rates of increased independence and improved visual function, including driving safety (Helbostad et al., 2013; Meuleners et al., 2012). People with both cataracts and

---

TABLE 17-3   Common Disease Conditions Affecting Vision

Condition	Risk Factors	Symptoms	Management
Cataract	Advanced age, exposure to sunlight, smoking, diabetes, malnutrition, trauma or radiation to the eye or head, adverse effect of medications (e.g., corticosteroids)	Dim or blurred vision, increased sensitivity to glare, decreased contrast sensitivity, double vision, seeing halos around bright lights, diminished colour perception	Initially managed with changes in correctives lenses Surgical removal of lens followed by implantation of an intraocular lens
Age-related macular degeneration (AMD)	Advanced age, family history of AMD, smoking, exposure to sunlight	Initial form: loss of central vision, faces or straight lines appear wavy, blurred vision Advanced form: progressive loss of vision	Smoking cessation, nutritional interventions, visual rehabilitation programs Medical or surgical treatments for wet type
Glaucoma	Advanced age; African, Latino and Asian descent; family history of glaucoma; diabetes; regular or long-term use of corticosteroids	**Chronic:** slow onset, diminished vision in dim light, increased sensitivity to glare, decreased contrast sensitivity, diminished peripheral vision	**Chronic:** medical therapy with prescription eye drops
		Acute: sudden onset, intense pain, blurred vision, halos around lights, nausea and vomiting	**Acute:** immediate treatment with medications, followed by surgery

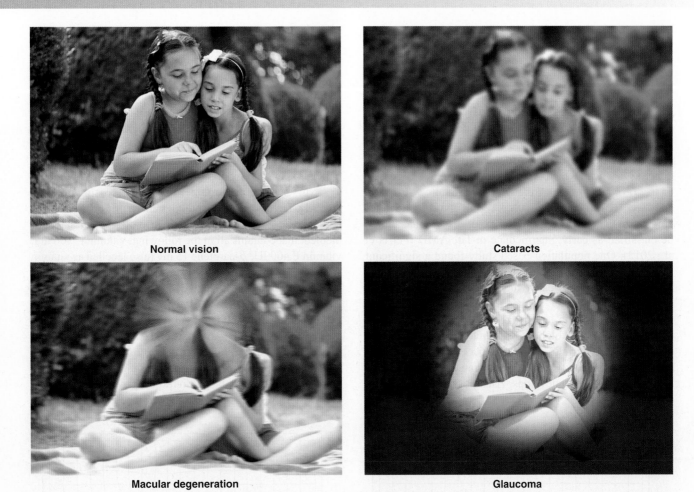

Normal vision

Cataracts

Macular degeneration

Glaucoma

FIGURE 17-3 Examples of normal vision, vision with cataracts, vision with age-related macular degeneration and vision with glaucoma (unmodified image from shutterstock.com; copyright: Olesya Feketa).

AMD have poorer long-term outcomes, but they can gain significant increases in visual function from cataract surgery (Monestam & Lundqvist, 2012). If the person needed corrective lenses before the surgery, the surgeon can insert an intraocular lens that mimics the natural focusing ability of the eye and results in improved vision, with little or no need for additional correction.

Nurses have an important role in dispelling myths and providing accurate information about cataract surgery. For example, older adults might think that cataract surgery is riskier or more complicated than it actually is because they are familiar with experiences of friends or relatives who had cataract surgery many years ago.

Important points to emphasize include the following:

- Advances in surgical techniques for cataract surgery have significantly improved both the process and the outcomes of cataract surgery.
- Cataract surgery has an extremely high success rate in significantly improving safety, functioning and the quality of life.
- People with dementia, depression or other conditions that affect information processing are particularly likely to benefit from improved vision.

- It is important to seek reliable information and obtain periodic evaluations from eye care professionals, rather than simply tolerating a loss of vision because of cataracts.

Wellness Opportunity

Nurses promote responsible decision making by encouraging older adults and their caregivers to find reliable information about cataract surgery.

Age-Related Macular Degeneration

Age-related macular degeneration (AMD) is the leading cause of severe vision loss and blindness in people 60 years and older in countries with high life expectancy, accounting for about half of all cases of central blindness in North America, Europe and Australia (Parmeggiani et al., 2012). In Canada, 1 million are living with AMD (Canadian National Institute for the Blind, 2010). Risk factors associated with AMD are listed in Table 17-3. Of particular relevance for health promotion, modifiable risk factors include smoking, obesity and exposure to sunlight (Parmeggiani et al., 2012; Sin et al., 2013).

Early in the disease, deposits of yellow by-products of retinal pigment, called *drusen*, build up in the macula, which is the area in the middle of the retina where visual acuity is the best. As the disease progresses, it is referred to as either as *dry type*, which accounts for 80% to 90% of cases, or *wet (exudative) type*. Although the terminology of "dry" and "wet" is still commonly used, recent clinical guidelines emphasize that AMD is a single type of disease that should be classified as early, intermediate or late AMD (Ferris et al., 2013). One population-based study found a significant age-associated increase in prevalence of late AMD between the ages of 70 and 90 years (Rudnicka et al., 2012). In early and intermediate AMD, damage is caused by the death of the photoreceptors; in late AMD, the damage is caused by the formation of new blood vessels in the choroid, followed by hemorrhage into the subretinal space. Early AMD usually progresses slowly and does not cause total blindness; however, if late AMD develops, visual loss can be rapid and severe.

As with most other eye conditions, AMD occurs in both eyes, but it can appear initially in only one eye, and its course may differ in each eye. During the early stages, vision loss is minimal, but as AMD progresses, it affects central vision and significantly interferes with activities such as reading, driving, watching television, recognizing people and performing many self-care activities (see Table 17-3 and Fig. 17-3). At all stages, the primary treatment goal is to reduce the risk of further vision loss, and all people with AMD require close follow-up by an ophthalmologist to monitor the progression of the condition.

Nurses have important roles in addressing modifiable risk factors, such as smoking and nutrition. A primary evidence-based intervention is the use of a nutritional supplement that contains all of the following: vitamin C 500 mg, vitamin E 400 IU, β-carotene 15 mg (also labelled as vitamin A 25,000 IU), zinc oxide 80 mg and cupric oxide 2 mg. This is often referred to as the AREDS formula, named after the Age-Related Eye Disease Study. Additional nursing interventions include teaching about the importance of ongoing evaluations by ophthalmologists and encouraging participation in vision rehabilitation programs to learn the most effective ways of compensating for declining vision. People with AMD are usually taught to test their eyes daily by using the Amsler grid (Fig. 17-4) so they will be aware of sudden

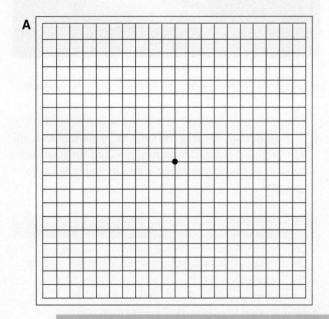
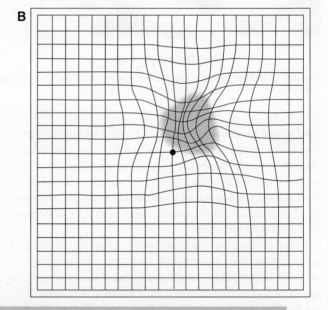

Instructions for Use

1. Tape this page at eye level where light is consistent and without glare.
2. Put on your reading glasses and cover one eye.
3. Fix your gaze on the center black dot.
4. Keeping your gaze fixed, try to see if any lines are distorted or missing.
5. Mark the defect on the chart.
6. TEST EACH EYE SEPARATELY.
7. If the distortion is new or has worsened, arrange to see your ophthalmologist at once.
8. **Always** keep the Amsler grid the **same distance** from your eyes each time you test.

FIGURE 17-4 Amsler grid. (**A**) People with age-related macular degeneration (AMD) use the Amsler grid to perform a simple daily test for sudden changes in their condition. (**B**) This is what the Amsler grid might look like to someone with AMD. (Part A: Reprinted with permission from American Macular Degeneration Foundation, 888-MACULAR, www.macular.org.)

changes. In long-term care settings and for older adults with memory problems, nurses may have to provide daily reminders or assistance with performing this task.

Wellness Opportunity

Nurses holistically address needs of people with AMD by encouraging them to explore support groups and educational services associated with a sight centre.

Glaucoma

The term **glaucoma** refers to a group of eye diseases in which the ganglion cells of the optic nerve are damaged by an abnormal buildup of aqueous humour in the eye. *Aqueous humour* is a clear fluid that is produced in the anterior chamber of the eye and normally maintains eye pressure between 10 and 20 mm Hg. If the fluid cannot flow out of the anterior chamber of the eye through the channel between the iris and the cornea, it accumulates and pushes the optic nerve into a cupped or concave shape. The resulting damage to the optic nerve causes a loss of peripheral vision. If left untreated, the damage can progress to blindness.

DIVERSITY NOTE

Older adults from higher socioeconomic groups have a lower risk for having moderate or advanced glaucoma at first presentation of the disease (Buys et al., 2013).

Chronic (open-angle) glaucoma, which accounts for as much as 90% of cases of glaucoma in Canada, occurs when the drainage canals become clogged. This condition has an insidious onset and affects vision when the optic nerve becomes damaged. Early signs include increased intraocular pressure, poor vision in dim lighting and increased sensitivity to glare. If the condition progresses, manifestations include headaches, "tired eyes," impaired peripheral vision, a fixed and dilated pupil, the perception of halos around lights and frequent changes in the prescription for corrective lenses. Chronic glaucoma usually occurs in both eyes, but it can begin in only one eye and does not necessarily progress at the same rate in both eyes. Because chronic glaucoma progresses slowly and causes little or no visual impairment in the early stage, annual assessments of intraocular pressure are necessary to detect the condition before visual impairments occur. Chronic glaucoma is most commonly managed with medications, but surgical treatment options include laser surgery and other types of eye surgery. Medication management commonly includes one or more of the following types of prescription eye drops: miotics, prostaglandins, β-blockers, adrenergic agonists and carbonic anhydrase inhibitors.

Normal-tension glaucoma is another type of glaucoma that occurs in older adults. With this type of glaucoma, the intraocular pressure is within the normal range, but the optic nerve is damaged and the visual field is narrowed (see Fig. 17-3). This condition is often managed with the same medications and surgical approaches that are used for chronic glaucoma.

Acute (closed-angle) glaucoma is caused by a sudden complete blockage of the flow of aqueous humour. This condition has an abrupt onset in one or both eyes and should be considered a medical emergency. People with acute glaucoma present with increased intraocular pressure, severe eye pain, clouded or blurred vision, dilation of the pupil, and nausea and vomiting. This condition can be precipitated by medications that cause pupil dilation, such as anticholinergics. Immediate treatment with medications is usually effective for acute attacks, but surgical intervention is often needed.

DIVERSITY NOTE

Older women are twice as likely as men to have glaucoma; African, Asian and Hispanic ancestry increases the risk of developing glaucoma (Glaucoma Research Society of Canada, n.d.).

Health education for older adults with glaucoma focuses on the importance of adhering to ongoing medication routines and regularly being evaluated by their eye care practitioner. If older adults with glaucoma are admitted for institutional care, nurses need to ensure that prescribed eye drops are administered as ordered. In home care situations, nurses may need to develop a plan for administering eye drops on a daily or more frequent basis. If an older adult has memory problems, establishing a routine for administering eye drops can be quite challenging. Many times, complicated eye drop regimens can be simplified by working with the eye care practitioner to decrease the number of eye drops that are necessary or to prescribe a longer-acting medication that can be administered less frequently.

Wellness Opportunity

Nurses promote self-care by teaching people with glaucoma to be aware of prescription and over-the-counter medications that can exacerbate glaucoma.

NURSING ASSESSMENT OF VISION

Nursing assessment of vision is aimed at identifying the following:

- Factors that interfere with visual wellness
- Vision problems
- The impact of vision changes on safety, independence or the quality of life
- Opportunities for promoting visual wellness
- Barriers to implementing interventions

Nursing assessment of visual function is not a substitute for an examination by an eye care specialist. Whereas the

Unfolding Case Study

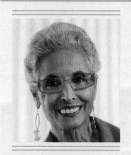

Part 2: Mrs. F. at 72 Years of Age

Mrs. F. is now 72 years old and has been retired for several years. You are the nurse at her local senior centre, and she makes an appointment to see you. Mrs. F.'s medical history indicates that she has smoked a pack of cigarettes a day for 40 years and has been taking medications for hypertension and arthritis for 5 years. During a recent medical checkup, her doctor said he thought she had early cataracts, but he told Mrs. F. that he felt it was too early to do anything about them. She has never had an eye examination, other than what her regular doctor does periodically. When asked about her symptoms, Mrs. F. tells you that she sometimes feels like there is a film over her eyes and she has trouble seeing when she is outside on sunny days. Mrs. F. says that she never liked wearing sunglasses and hopes she will not have to start wearing them now. She has recently purchased stronger reading glasses, and these help a little with reading and sewing.

THINKING POINTS

- What factors likely contributed to the development of Mrs. F.'s cataracts?
- When Mrs. F. is driving during the day, what difficulties might she notice because of vision changes? Because of environmental conditions?

- When Mrs. F. is driving at night, what difficulties might she notice because of vision changes? Because of environmental conditions?
- When Mrs. F. is in her home, what changes in visual abilities might she notice because of cataracts?

QSEN APPLICATION

QSEN Competency	Knowledge/Skill/Attitude	Application to Mrs. F.
Evidence-Based Practice.	(K) Describe how the strength and relevance of available evidence influence the choice of intervention.	Teach Mrs. F. about evidence-based interventions for preventing the development and progression of cataracts (i.e., quitting smoking and protecting eyes from sunlight).
	(S) Base individualized care plan on patient values, clinical expertise and evidence.	
	(A) Value evidence-based practice as integral to determining the best clinical practice.	Explore with Mrs. F. whether she is willing to wear broad-brimmed hats when out in the sun because she states that she doesn't like wearing sunglasses.

purpose of an examination by an eye care specialist is to detect and initiate appropriate treatment of vision problems, the goal of the nursing assessment is to assist the older adult in minimizing the negative consequences of vision changes.

Box 17-1 Evidence-Informed Nursing Practice

Background: Functional disability has numerous implications for public health, including increased demand for health care, reduced quality of life, increased cost of health care and higher mortality.

Question: What chronic conditions are independently associated with overall functional disability?

Method: Functional disability was measured by using ADL and IADLs for 9,008 community-dwelling adults above the age of 65 years from the Canadian Study of Heath and Aging.

Findings: Vision is one of the five chronic conditions that contribute to ADL- and IADL-related functional disabilities.

Implications for Nursing Practice: Attempts by registered nurses to reduce disability burden and promote wellness should target vision problems experienced by older adults.

Source: Griffith, L., Raina, P., Wu, H., et al. (2010). Population attributable risk for functional disability associated with chronic conditions in Canadian older adults. *Age and Ageing, 39,* 738–745.

Nursing assessment also aims at identifying modifiable risk factors that can be addressed through health promotion. Nurses assess visual abilities by interviewing the older adult (or caregivers of dependent older adults), by observing the older adult's ability to perform activities of daily living and by testing the older adult's visual skills (See Box 17-1).

Interviewing About Vision Changes

Nurses use interview questions to elicit the following information: past and present risk factors for vision impairment, the person's awareness of any vision changes, the impact of these changes on daily activities and the quality of life and the person's attitudes about interventions (Box 17-2). The interview begins with direct questions about the person's awareness of any changes in vision. If the person acknowledges a visual impairment, nurses elicit additional details about the onset and progression of vision changes. Nurses also ask about symptoms that cause discomfort or that indicate the possible presence of disease processes.

Nurses then ask about the impact of vision changes on the person's usual or desired activities. If the person

Box 17-2 Guidelines for Assessing Vision

Questions to Assess Awareness and Presence of Vision Impairment

- Have you noticed any changes in your vision during the past few years?
- Do you experience any uncomfortable symptoms, such as dry eyes?
- Do you have difficulty managing any of your usual activities because you have trouble seeing? (Consider asking about the following: sewing, reading, driving, grooming, hobbies, preparing meals, watching television, managing money, writing letters, using the telephone, using dials on appliances, shopping for groceries and going up and down stairs.)
- Have you ever tripped or fallen because you had trouble seeing?
- Have you stopped doing any activities because of vision problems? (For example, have you stopped driving at night because of difficulty seeing?)
- Are there things you would do if you could see better?

Questions to Ask if Vision Loss Is Acknowledged

- When did you first notice a loss of vision or a change in your ability to see?
- Have the changes been gradual, or did you notice sudden changes at any particular time?
- How would you describe the changes in your ability to see?
- Have you noticed pain, blurred vision, burning or itching, halos around lights, intolerance to bright light, a difference between day and night vision, or spots or flashing lights in front of your eyes?
- What kind of medical evaluation and care, if any, have you had for this problem?

Questions to Identify Opportunities for Education About Disease Prevention and Health Promotion

- When was the last time you had your eyes checked?
- Where do you go for eye care?
- Have you ever had your eyes checked for cataracts, glaucoma and other eye conditions?
- What do you think about going for regular checkups for glaucoma and other eye problems?

Questions to Identify Risk Factors for Vision Loss

- When you spend time outdoors in the sun, do you use sunglasses or a hat to protect your eyes from bright light?
- Do you smoke cigarettes?
- Do you have a history of diabetes or hypertension?
- Do you have a family history of glaucoma or macular degeneration?
- What medications do you take?

has acknowledged vision changes, nurses can ask specific questions about how these changes have influenced usual activities. If the person is not aware of vision changes, nurses inquire about any difficulties performing complex activities, such as driving, shopping and meal preparation. Questions about leisure interests are incorporated into the interview to obtain information about the psychosocial consequences of vision impairments. Although the older adult may not associate lifestyle changes with vision impairments, questions about changes in hobbies and leisure activities can help

nurses identify the need for interventions to improve visual wellness. Because poor vision increases the risk for falls, especially tripping-related falls, nurses ask about a history of tripping, falling and near-falling.

Wellness Opportunity

Nurses assess the impact of vision changes on the person's relationships with other people as one aspect of the quality of life.

Identifying Opportunities for Health Promotion

Nurses identify opportunities for health promotion by asking about the person's usual eye care practices and about factors that can interfere with visual wellness. Information about the source, frequency and dates of the person's eye examinations is particularly useful for planning health promotion interventions that address the early detection of eye disease. Nurses also listen for indicators of myths or misunderstandings that should be addressed through health education. If the person has cataracts, glaucoma or another chronic condition affecting vision, nurses ask questions to ascertain the person's self-care practices and attitude toward eye examinations and disease management. If no visual impairment is reported, nurses assess attitudes about early detection of treatable conditions.

Last, identification of modifiable risk factors provides an opportunity for health education. For example, it is especially important to ask about cigarette smoking if the person has cataracts, AMD or a family history of AMD. If the older person is likely to spend time outdoors in sunny climates, nurses ask about exposure to sunlight. Placing this question toward the end of the interview sets the stage for health education about protective measures, such as the use of sunglasses.

Wellness Opportunity

Nurses pave the way for teaching about self-care by assessing attitudes about preventive and protective activities, such as obtaining eye examinations and wearing sunglasses.

Observing Cues to Visual Function

Reliable information about a person's visual function can be obtained simply by being observant. For example, nurses can observe for any abnormalities of the eyelids, such as serious eyelid lag, that might interfere with visual wellness. Nurses can detect other, more subtle, indicators of impaired vision by observing the person's appearance and ability to perform daily activities. Finally, community-based nurses may have opportunities to observe older adults in their usual environments to assess their functioning and conditions that can affect visual abilities. When assessments cannot be performed in the person's usual environment, nurses can ask the older person and caregivers for information about the person's abilities in the home setting.

Box 17-3   Guidelines for Assessing Behavioural and Environmental Cues Related to Visual Performance

Behavioural Cues

- Is clothing spotted, soiled or mismatched, in contrast to a former pattern of neatness and sense of style?
- Is makeup applied in heavy quantities, in contrast to the usual manner of application?
- Does the person rely heavily on nonvisual cues in performing usual activities, especially manoeuvring in the environment (e.g., using the hands to find objects or to probe for obstacles)?

Environmental Cues

- What kind of lighting is used for various tasks? If the lighting is not adequate, can adjustments be made to improve the person's visual abilities?
- Does the person try to economize at home by using dim lights or no lights at all? If so, does this interfere with visual abilities or safe functioning?
- Where does the person usually sit in relation to light sources? Does glare from a window interfere with vision? Do shadows from lamps interfere with vision? Do overhead lights cause glare? Are light bulbs of sufficient wattage?
- What are the sources of light on stairways and hallways?
- Is there sufficient colour contrast in the following areas: walls and floors, stairs and landings, furniture, eating utensils and place settings, cooking utensils and counter tops, markings and background on appliance dials?
- Are nightlights used in hallways and bathrooms?

It is also important to identify environmental conditions that might influence visual performance, either positively or negatively. An example of a positive influence might be the presence of good lighting and colour contrast. Some negative influences, such as glare from fluorescent lights reflecting on highly polished floors, are more likely to exist in an institutional setting than a home setting. Another factor to consider is whether the person is using corrective lenses, which may not be available during the assessment. Box 17-3 summarizes behavioural and environmental cues related to visual function.

Using Standard Vision Tests

Nurses can assess vision by using both formal and informal tests. Before testing, however, eliminate sources of glare, make sure the testing materials have good colour contrast and place a light source above the person's head to provide good lighting while avoiding shadows. If the person normally wears corrective lenses, make sure that they are clean and in place. Test each eye separately, using an appropriate eye cover; avoid using a hand as a cover. Assessment Box 17-4 describes the Snellen chart for distance acuity and the Confrontation Test for peripheral vision, which nurses can use in clinical settings. Any of the following methods can be used as an informal test of vision:

- Ask the person to read a newspaper or other printed material of various type sizes.
- Ask the person to read a line or two of a form that needs to be signed and observe the person's ability to find the signature line.

Box 17-4   Guidelines for Using Vision Screening Tests

Using the Snellen Chart to Assess Distance Acuity

- Position the chart 20 feet away from the person, at eye level.
- If space does not permit a 20-foot distance, the distance between the person and the chart should be either 15 or 10 feet, with final measurements adjusted for distance. Alternatively, a scaled-down Snellen card can be used, if available.
- If the person usually wears corrective lenses, test the corrected vision.
- Ask the person to start reciting the letters in the line that can be read most easily; then ask him or her to read as many letters as possible in the lines directly below that line.
- Document the findings for each eye by noting the figure at the end of the last line on which at least half of the letters were read correctly.
- The upper figure denotes the distance of the person from the chart, whereas the lower figure denotes the distance from the chart at which a person with normal vision would be able to read the line. (That is, a vision measurement of 20/50 indicates that the person being tested can see things at a distance of 20 feet that a person with normal vision would be able to see at a distance of 50 feet.)
- Normal Snellen chart test results for older adults are as follows:
  - A corrected vision of 20/20 is considered to be normal.
  - If a distance of 10 feet is used, the corrected vision should be 10/10.
  - The average corrected vision for older adults ranges from 20/20 to 20/50.

Performing the Confrontation Test to Assess Peripheral Vision

- Sit directly across the older person, about 2 feet away.
- Cover your left eye and have the examinee cover his or her right eye.
- Instruct the examinee to focus on your right eye while you focus on the examinee's left eye.
- Fully extend your right arm midway between you and the examinee.
- While holding a pencil, slowly move your right hand, with the fingers wiggling, from the outer periphery toward the centre, testing visual fields from top to bottom.
- While maintaining continuous eye contact, ask the examinee to report the point at which the pencil is visualized.
- Repeat these steps, covering your right eye and the examinee's left eye and using your left arm.
- Normal confrontation test results for older adults: the pencil in your hand should be seen simultaneously by both you and the older person in all quadrants.

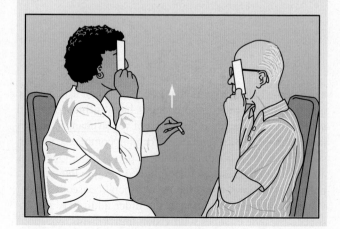

- Provide written educational materials and ask the person to read a specific part, such as a phone number.
- Have the person look out a window or down a hallway and describe certain details, such as the words on a sign.

These tests supplement information obtained through interviewing and observations, as described earlier. The purpose of nursing assessment of vision is to provide information that is useful for planning care and identifying the need for further evaluation, but it is not a substitute for a complete eye examination.

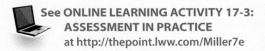

See ONLINE LEARNING ACTIVITY 17-3:
ASSESSMENT IN PRACTICE
at http://thepoint.lww.com/Miller7e

NURSING DIAGNOSIS

On the basis of the nursing assessment, the nurse might identify actual vision impairment or risk factors for impaired vision. The nursing diagnosis directly related to older adults with impaired vision is Disturbed Sensory Perception: Visual, which is applied to the care plan at the end of this chapter. Although this nursing diagnosis was retired for the 2012–2014 classification, it may be returned to the taxonomy in the future (Herdman, 2012). The nursing diagnosis of Readiness for Enhanced Knowledge: Improved Vision is appropriate for health promotion interventions. If the visual impairment interferes with the older adult's safety, quality of life or performance of activities of daily living, any of the following nursing diagnoses can be used to address these functional consequences: Anxiety, Self-Care Deficit, Risk for Injury, Impaired Social Interaction and Readiness for Enhanced Self-Care.

Wellness Opportunity

The wellness nursing diagnosis of Readiness for Enhanced Knowledge: Improved Vision would be applicable for older adults who are willing to explore interventions that improve their vision.

PLANNING FOR WELLNESS OUTCOMES

When older adults experience vision impairments or have risk factors that affect visual functioning, nurses identify wellness outcomes as an essential part of the planning process. The Nursing Outcomes Classifications (NOCs) that most directly relate to interventions to improve vision for older adults are Vision Compensation Behaviour, and Sensory Function: Vision. In addition, nurses can use any of the following NOCs to describe the effectiveness of interventions to improve vision: Coping, Self-Care: Activities of Daily Living, Self-Care: Instrumental Activities of Daily Living, Stress Level, Knowledge: Personal Safety, Fall Prevention Behaviour, and Risk Control: Visual Impairment. Specific interventions to achieve these outcomes are discussed in the following section.

Wellness Opportunity

Quality of Life is a wellness outcome that is achieved through nursing interventions that improve visual function.

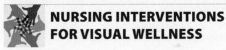

NURSING INTERVENTIONS FOR VISUAL WELLNESS

Nurses promote visual wellness through interventions directed toward preventing vision loss, promoting comfort measures for dry eyes and implementing or teaching about

Unfolding Case Study

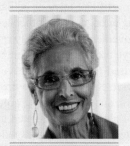

Part 2: Mrs. F. at 72 Years of Age (continued)

Recall that you are the nurse at the senior centre in Mrs. F.'s neighbourhood. During a recent visit, the 72-year-old Mrs. F. told you that she feels like there is a "film" over her eyes, and she has trouble seeing when she is outside on sunny days. Several months ago, Mrs. F.'s doctor told her that she has "early cataracts," but she has had no further evaluation.

THINKING POINTS

- Which questions from Box 17-2 would you ask Mrs. F. at this time?
- What sort of information might you be able to glean from behavioural or environmental cues about Mrs. F.'s ability to see? (See Box 17-3.)
- Would assessing Mrs. F.'s vision by using vision screening tests be appropriate? (See Box 17-4.) If so, which tests would you perform?
- What health promotion education would you give Mrs. F. at this time?

methods to foster optimal visual function. Interventions to achieve these goals are discussed in detail in the following sections. The following pertinent Nursing Interventions Classification (NIC) terminologies may be applicable to care plans: Communication Enhancement: Visual Deficit, Coping Enhancement, Dry Eye Prevention, Eye Care, Environmental Management, Environmental Management: Safety, Health Education, Health Screening, Health System Guidance, Risk Identification and Fall Prevention.

Health Promotion for Visual Wellness

Health promotion interventions focus on maintaining vision at an optimal level by compensating for any visual deficits and identifying any treatable conditions at an early stage. Another important aspect of health promotion is addressing modifiable risk factors, such as smoking and exposure to sunlight. In addition, nurses can teach about nutritional interventions to promote eye health. Box 17-5 summarizes teaching points related to promoting eye health.

In providing health education, it may be helpful to review the differences between opticians, optometrists and ophthalmologists and provide information about health insurance coverage for these services, as detailed in Box 17-6.

**See ONLINE LEARNING ACTIVITY 17-4:
RESOURCES FOR HEALTH EDUCATION**
at http://thepoint.lww.com/Miller7e

Wellness Opportunity

Nurses promote self-care by encouraging older adults and their families to obtain information from reliable resources.

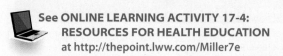

Box 17-5 Health Promotion Teaching About Visual Wellness

Prevention and Early Detection of Disease

- Minimize exposure to sunlight by using broad-brimmed hats and close-fitting sunglasses with UV-absorbing lenses.
- Have eyes examined annually or more frequently if you notice a change in vision; make sure the examination checks for glaucoma, cataracts and retinal disease.
- Use the appropriate eye care practitioner (ophthalmologist, optometrist and optician) as described in Box 17-6.
- Because smoking is a risk factor for many eye diseases, quit smoking.
- Maintain optimal control of hypertension, diabetes and other chronic conditions.

Nutritional Considerations

- Include foods high in lutein, such as fruits, corn, spinach, green leafy vegetables and egg yolks.
- Lutein supplements of 10 mg/day are safe and may be effective in preventing cataracts and age-related macular degeneration.
- People who have macular degeneration or risk factors for this condition are encouraged to take a daily supplement containing the following: 500 mg vitamin C, 400 IU vitamin E, 15 mg β-carotene (same as 25,000 IU of vitamin A), 80 mg zinc oxide and 2 mg cupric oxide (copper). However, people who smoke are advised to avoid β-carotene because it can increase the risk of developing lung cancer.

Box 17-6 Eye Care Practitioners

Ophthalmologist

An **ophthalmologist** is a licensed doctor of medicine (MD) who is trained to diagnose and treat diseases and conditions of the eye. Ophthalmologic services include the following:

- Comprehensive eye examinations
- Diagnosis of eye diseases and disorders of the eye
- Prescription medications for eye problems (e.g., glaucoma)
- Eye surgery and postoperative care (e.g., cataracts)
- Laser treatments (e.g., retinopathy)
- Prescriptions for eyeglasses and contact lenses
- Prescriptions for low-vision aids
- Referrals for low-vision aids and training
- Medical referrals for diseases of the body that affect the eyes

Optometrist

An **optometrist** is a licensed doctor of optometry (OD), not a physician, who is trained to examine eyes, screen for common eye problems and prescribe eye exercises or corrective lenses. Optometrists use diagnostic medications, and in some provinces, they can prescribe certain therapeutic drugs for eye diseases. Optometric services include the following:

- Comprehensive eye examinations
- Eye refractions to determine the need for corrective lenses
- Prescriptions for eyeglasses, contact lenses and low-vision aids
- Vision therapy to improve certain skills, such as tracking and focusing the eyes
- Referrals for low-vision aids and training
- Referrals to physicians for surgery, medication or further evaluation
- Diagnosis of eye disorders (in some provinces)
- Postoperative care (in some provinces)

Optician

An **optician** is an eye care practitioner who is trained to fit, adjust and dispense eyeglasses and contact lenses that have been prescribed by an optometrist or ophthalmologist. Opticians are licensed. They do not perform eye examinations or refractions, and they cannot prescribe corrective lenses or medications.

Comfort Measures for Dry Eyes

If pertinent, simple measures to relieve dry eyes can be discussed. Use of over-the-counter artificial tears or ocular lubricants, especially before reading or engaging in other activities that require frequent eye movements, will usually relieve symptoms. People who use eye drops more frequently than every 3 hours should be advised to use preservative-free solutions to prevent any adverse effects from the preservatives. Other comfort measures, such as applying cold compresses or wearing wraparound glasses, are designed to prevent evaporation of tears. Maintenance of adequate environmental humidity, especially during the winter months or in dry climates, also decreases evaporation of eye moisture and adds to eye comfort. People who experience discomfort from dry eyes should avoid irritants, such as smoke and hairspray, and adverse environmental conditions, such as hot rooms and high wind. People who are bothered by dry eyes and are taking a medication that might exacerbate the discomfort should be encouraged to discuss the problem with their primary care practitioner.

Environmental Modifications

Simple environmental modifications can improve the older person's safe performance of activities of daily living, thereby reducing risks of falls and accidents. Because older adults require more light for adequate vision, proper nonglare lighting is the single most important—as well as the easiest and the least costly—intervention to improve visual function (Box 17-7). Optimal illumination depends on both the quality and the quantity of lighting. For example, selection of broad-spectrum fluorescent lights and daylight-simulating lamps may be particularly beneficial in compensating for age-related vision changes.

Another important consideration in adapting the environment for optimal visual function is colour contrast. Appliances and other items, such as ovens, irons, radios, thermostats and televisions, may be difficult to use because of poor colour contrast around the control mechanisms. Modifications can easily be made to improve the older person's ability to use these items safely and accurately. For example, two dots of red nail polish can be used to mark a designated and commonly used temperature setting, and the older adult can be instructed to turn the dial above or below the matching dots for higher or lower settings.

Architectural designs and institutional constraints may limit the extent of environmental adaptations that nurses can implement, especially in institutional settings. In most settings, however, nurses can improve the visual abilities of older adults by using appropriate colours to enhance contrast, by using curtains to control light and glare and by placing chairs in positions that enhance illumination and avoid glare. Nurses have many opportunities to teach older adults and their caregivers about environmental modifications that can be used to compensate for deficits in visual skills and to improve safety, as described in Box 17-8. These environmental modifications can be implemented to improve visual function for all people.

Low-Vision Aids

People with visual impairments can improve their safety and quality of life by using **low-vision aids** to enhance contrast, improve focus, improve lighting or enlarge images (Box 17-9). Low-vision aids are most beneficial when used in conjunction with environmental modifications. For example, magnifiers are most effective when combined with measures that improve illumination and control glare. Low-vision aids

---

 Box 17-8 Environmental Adaptations for Improving Visual Performance

Illumination, Glare Control and Dark/Light Adaptation

- Position a 60- or 75-W soft-white light bulb above and close to the head of the older person.
- Use a clear plastic shower curtain, rather than solid colours or printed curtains, for the tub or shower.
- Use light-coloured, sheer curtains to eliminate glare from windows.
- Place nightlights in hallways and bathrooms, or keep a high-intensity flashlight at the bedside.
- Use illuminated light switches.
- Provide good lighting in stairways and hallways.
- Use illuminated or magnifying mirrors.

Colour Contrast

- Use brightly coloured tape or paint on the edges of stairs, especially on the top and bottom steps.
- Use light-coloured and dark-coloured cutting boards to contrast with dark and light foods.
- Use contrasting, rather than matching, colours for china, placemats and napkins.
- Use a toilet seat that contrasts with the bathroom walls and floor. Use coloured bars of soap on white sinks and tubs.
- Use utensils with brightly coloured handles.
- Place pillows of contrasting colours on stuffed furniture.
- Use decorative or lighted plates over light switches and wall sockets; avoid switch plates that blend in with the wallpaper or paint.
- Place decorative items of contrasting colours, such as plants and ceramics on tables, to provide cues to depth, especially on light-coloured furniture that is in a room with light-coloured walls.
- Use brightly coloured grooming utensils, such as combs, brushes and razors.
- Use pens with black ink rather than blue ink.

General Adaptive Measures and Environmental Modifications

- Do not rearrange furniture without informing or showing the older person.
- Advise older adults to pause in doorways when going from light to dark rooms (or vice versa) to allow time for their eyes to adjust to the light change.
- Teach older people to use their feet and hands as probes to feel for curbs, steps, edges of chairs and the like.
- When walking with an older person, stop when necessary to allow a change in focus from near to far and from light to dark.

Box 17-7 Considerations for Optimal Illumination

- Older adults need at least three times as much light as younger people do.
- Older adults function best in environments with bright, broad-spectrum, nonglaring, indirect sources of light.
- Sources of illumination should be placed 1 to 2 feet away from the object to be viewed.
- The amount of light decreases fourfold when the distance is doubled.
- Flickering light, such as that generated by a single fluorescent tube, will cause fatigue and decreased visual performance.
- Light bulbs should be kept clean.
- Increased illumination has a greater positive effect on impaired vision than it does on normal vision.
- A gradual decrease in illumination from foreground to background is better than sharp contrasts in lighting.
- Moderate overhead lighting can be used to enhance brighter foreground lighting and prevent sharp contrasts.
- To reduce glare from reading material, place the light source to the left side of right-handed readers and to the right side of left-handed readers.
- Avoid glossy paper for reading materials.

are widely available in stores, through catalogues or at local sight centres. In addition, everyday items if used advantageously, can serve as low-vision aids. For example, household lamps placed in the correct position and equipped with the right wattage bulb can also serve as low-vision aids. Nurses can use information presented in Boxes 17-7 and 17-10 to teach about effective use of lights and magnification. Low-vision aids in combination with a vision rehabilitation program are especially important for people with significant

---

Box 17-9 Low-Vision Aids for Improving Visual Performance

Enlargement Aids

- Microscopic spectacles
- Handheld or standing magnifiers

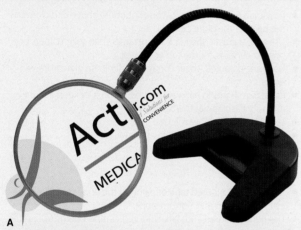

A

Examples of low-vision aids. **(A)** A combination of high-intensity lamp and magnifier.

- Binoculars and handheld or spectacle-mounted telescopes
- Magnifying sheets
- Field expanders for diminished peripheral vision
- Large-print books, magazines and newspapers
- Photocopy machines or printers to enlarge print
- Telephones with enlarged letters and numbers, or a pad with enlarged letters and numbers designed to fit over rotary-dial or push-button phones
- Large numbers on rulers, playing cards and other items
- Thermometers with good colour coding and enlarged numbers
- Large-eye sewing needles

Illumination Aids

- High-intensity lights
- Gooseneck lamps
- Floor or table lamps with three-way light bulbs

Contrast Aids

- Use of broad-tipped felt markers in dark, yet bright, colours and coloured construction paper for making signs
- Red print on a yellow background or white letters on a green background
- Reading and signature guides (typoscopes)
- Clip-on yellow lenses

Glare Control Aids

- Sunglasses with UV-absorbing lenses
- Sun visors and broad-brimmed hats
- Nonglare (antireflective) coating on eyeglasses
- Yellow and pink acetate sheets
- Pinhole occluders

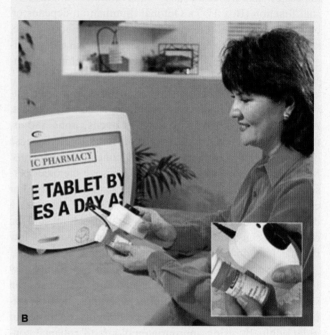

B

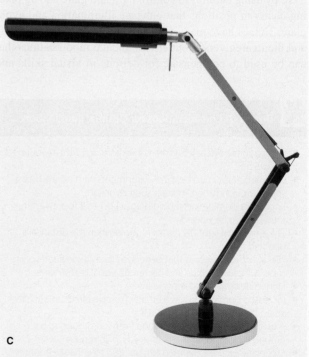

C

A handheld digital magnifier **(B)** that works with any television to magnify print. A versatile lamp **(C)** that uses an energy-efficient high-definition tube bulb for good contrast and brightness. (Photographs reprinted with permission from ActiveForever. com.)

Using a Handheld Magnifier

- Begin by holding the magnifier close to the reading material.
- Slowly move the magnifier toward the face until the image totally fills the lens.
- For optimal focus, move the magnifier back toward the print about a distance of 2 cm.

Using a Stand Magnifier

- Rest the stand flat against the reading material.
- Do not move the stand.

Using a Spectacle-Mounted Magnifier

- Begin with the reading material close to the nose.
- Slowly move the material away until it becomes clear.

visual impairment, for example, due to AMD. In addition to improving visual function, low-vision rehabilitation has a broader effect on quality of life and improved social functioning (Renieri et al., 2013).

See ONLINE LEARNING ACTIVITY 17-5: LIVING BETTER AT HOME: VIDEOS AND ARTICLES at http://thepoint.lww.com/Miller7e

Wellness Opportunity

Nurses promote self-care for people who are visually impaired by facilitating referrals to local vision rehabilitation services and encouraging older adults and their families to use these resources.

Providing Vision-Friendly Teaching Materials

Although written materials are often difficult to read—even for people who do not have significant visual impairment—there are many relatively simple ways to develop vision-friendly teaching materials, as in the following examples:

- Use a photocopy machine to convert regular-print materials into large-print materials.

- Use large font and plain text (e.g., Arial, Helvetica, Times New Roman).
- Avoid italics, underline and all-caps.
- Use strong contrast: black on white or pale coloured paper.
- Avoid yellow or pale colours on coloured background.
- Do not use glossy finished paper.
- Avoid placing text over graphics, photos or illustrations.
- Use generous spacing and margins.

See ONLINE LEARNING ACTIVITY 17-6: DEVELOPING VISION-FRIENDLY TEACHING MATERIALS at http://thepoint.lww.com/Miller7e

Maintaining and Improving the Quality of Life

As discussed earlier, the psychosocial consequences of impaired vision can be quite significant for older adults. Many of the interventions that help older adults compensate for visual deficits and function at their highest level will also improve their quality of life and address the psychosocial consequences of impaired vision. The use of appropriate reading glasses and good environmental lighting may enable the older adult to read books, newspapers and magazines. Subsequently, their quality of life may improve because they experience satisfying social interactions and increased intellectual stimulation. Nurses also encourage participation in support and educational groups because these interventions serve an important role in improving the quality of life for people with significant or progressive vision loss.

Promoting Caregiver Wellness

When caring for someone who is visually impaired, it is important to address the needs of the spouse, family and others who provide care and support. A primary intervention in these circumstances is to provide information about the many helpful resources available locally and through Internet sites. Caregivers of people who have dementia or other conditions that cause dependency may benefit from information about

Unfolding Case Study

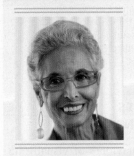

Part 3: Mrs. F. at 81 Years of Age

Mrs. F. is now 81 years old. She had cataract surgery and an intraocular lens implanted in her left eye when she was 76 years old, and in her right eye when she was 77. Her vision was good until a year ago, when she developed macular degeneration. She knows this condition will be progressive, but she continues to drive and live alone. Her current medical conditions are arthritis, hypertension and coronary artery disease. She quit smoking several years ago after she was hospitalized for coronary artery disease. You are the nurse at the senior care centre where Mrs. F. comes for lunch several times a week. During an appointment with you, Mrs. F. confides that she is terrified of becoming totally blind and of losing her independence. Her grandmother went blind several years before she died and she had to go to a long-term care facility.

THINKING POINTS

- Which nursing diagnosis or diagnoses would you apply to Mrs. F. at this time?
- Which information in Boxes 17-5 through 17-10 might be appropriate for Mrs. F.?
- What health promotion advice would you give?

- Would you suggest any referrals for information or community resources?
- What interventions would address Mrs. F.'s fear of becoming blind and losing her independence?

QSEN APPLICATION

QSEN Competency	Knowledge/Skill/Attitude	Application to Mrs. F.
Patient-centred care	(K) Integrate understanding of multiple dimensions of patient-centred care.	Take time to listen to Mrs. F. express her fears and concerns and help her identify her strengths and supports.
	(K) Describe strategies to empower patients in all aspects of the health care process.	Reassure Mrs. F. that there are many options available to help her remain as independent as possible, and these were not available when her grandmother had to move to a long-term care facility.
	(S) Provide patient-centred care with sensitivity and respect for diversity of the human experience.	
	(A) Value seeing health care situations "through patients' eyes."	
Teamwork and collaboration	(K) Recognize contributions of other individuals and groups in helping patient achieve health goals.	Encourage Mrs. F. to contact the local sight centre about their services and emphasize that their goal is to help people with vision loss to remain independent.
	(S) Integrate the contributions of others who play a role in helping patient achieve health goals.	

normal age-related vision changes, so they can take appropriate actions to detect eye disease and promote optimal vision. Nurses can use Box 17-11 for teaching caregivers and encouraging the use of helpful resources.

Box 17-11 Caregiver Wellness: Vision and Aging

Normal Vision Changes in Older Adults

- Difficulty focusing on near objects, such as small print
- Increased sensitivity to glare
- Decreased contrast sensitivity
- Slower adaptation to changes in lighting
- Diminished depth perception
- Altered colour perception
- Difficulty driving at night

Conditions Associated With Visual Impairment

- Lighting that is too dim or causes glare
- Eye diseases: cataracts, glaucoma, retinopathy, macular degeneration
- Conditions that increase the risk for eye disease: cigarette smoking, poor nutrition, exposure to sunlight, effects of some medications, family history of eye disease
- Chronic diseases that increase the risk for impaired vision: diabetes, hypertension, neurologic disease

Actions to Promote Vision Wellness

- Facilitate annual comprehensive eye examination, and immediately if a significant change in vision occurs.

- Seek timely, professional, and ongoing advice about medical or surgical interventions for eye diseases (e.g., cataracts, glaucoma, macular degeneration).
- Recognize the importance of interventions for vision impairments as essential actions to improve safety, functioning and quality of life.
- Assure good nutrition.
- Protect eyes from sunlight.
- Provide good nonglare lighting.
- Discuss concerns about driving with primary care practitioner and request appropriate professional evaluation.
- Facilitate the use of low-vision aids.

Resources for Support, Information and Low-Vision Aids

Canadian National Institute for the Blind, www.cnib.ca
Canadian Ophthalmological Society, www.cos-sco.ca
Health Canada, Seniors and Aging, Vision Care, http://hc-sc. gc.ca/hl-vs/iyh-vsv/life-vie/seniors-aines_vc-sv-eng.php
Lighthouse International, www.lighthouse.org
Lions Club International, www.lionsclubs.org
The Foundation Fighting Blindness, http://www.ffb.ca/ index.html

EVALUATING EFFECTIVENESS OF NURSING INTERVENTIONS

Nurses observe compensatory behaviours of visually impaired older adults to evaluate the effectiveness of interventions for Disturbed Sensory Perception: Visual. The following are indicators of successful interventions:

- Use of corrective lenses and low-vision aids to achieve the best possible visual function
- Adaptations of the environment for safety and improved visual function (e.g., bright, nonglare lighting, good colour contrast)
- Expressed feelings of safety in relation to visual function
- Maximum independence in activities such as dressing, personal care, using appliances and managing medications
- Expressed feelings of improved quality of life, despite visual impairments

Effectiveness of interventions to improve independence is evaluated by assessing and reassessing the older adult's abilities before and after interventions. When interventions address the psychosocial impact of visual impairment, observe the extent to which the person's quality of life and the ability to participate in enjoyable activities is improved. For example, better lighting and the use of audiobooks or large-print books may enable someone to enjoy reading again. Nurses evaluate the effectiveness of health education interventions according to the person's expressed intent to follow through with the recommended referral or course of action. In home, community, and long-term care settings, nurses may be able to facilitate referrals for vision screening or other vision care services. In these settings, effectiveness of interventions is evaluated by obtaining feedback from older adults or their caregivers about the actual use of suggested resources.

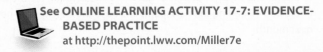

See **ONLINE LEARNING ACTIVITY 17-7: EVIDENCE-BASED PRACTICE** at http://thepoint.lww.com/Miller7e

Unfolding Case Study

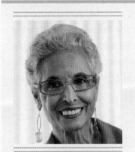

Part 4: Mrs. F. at 86 Years of Age

Mrs. F. is now 86 years old and is recovering from a recent fractured hip, which occurred when she fell while getting out of bed to go to the bathroom. After a brief hospitalization for surgical repair of the fractured hip and a 2-week period of skilled rehabilitation, Mrs. F. was referred to a home care agency for therapy, assessment, monitoring of her medical status and evaluation of her ability to manage at home.

In addition to AMD, Mrs. F.'s current medical diagnoses include arthritis, hypertension, coronary artery disease and heart failure. Mrs. F.'s medical conditions had been stable for several years, but during her hospitalization for the fractured hip, she was started on oxygen and her medications were changed. Current medications are furosemide 40 mg daily, digoxin 0.125 mg daily and enalapril 10 mg twice daily. A 2-g sodium diet has been prescribed, and she has been discharged with an order for oxygen per nasal cannula at a rate of 2 L/minute as needed.

Before her accident, despite the visual limitations from AMD, Mrs. F. had lived alone in her own home, but her daughter has become increasingly concerned about her mother's safety. Now Mrs. F.'s daughter is convinced that her mother should not remain in her own home but should instead move to an assisted-living facility. Mrs. F. is adamant in her desire to stay in her own home and says the only reason she fell and broke her hip was because she was rushing to get to the bathroom. She says she has learned a lesson and will not hurry when she gets up at night. Furthermore, she says, she gave up driving to satisfy her daughter last year—now she is to give up her home, too? Mrs. F.'s daughter is staying with her mother for a few weeks until her mother regains her mobility to the point of independence. The daughter hopes that in the interim, she will be able to convince her mother to move to an assisted-living facility. You are the home care nurse working with Mrs. F. in her home.

NURSING ASSESSMENT

During your initial nursing assessment, you determine that Mrs. F. is motivated to regain her mobility and manage her medical conditions, but she has difficulty reading small-print instructions because of poor vision. When you review Mrs. F.'s medications with her, you observe that she cannot read the labels on the bottles. You also observe that Mrs. F. keeps her medications on the shelf above the kitchen counter, where the lighting is very dim. When you review the proper use of the oxygen, you note that she has difficulty seeing the markings on the flow metre. Her daughter has been helping her with these regimens, but Mrs. F. hopes to perform these activities independently so she can remain in her own home.

Mrs. F. tells you that she is not concerned about falling because she walks slowly and carefully when she gets up during the night to go to the bathroom. She now uses a walker and says she feels safe. Her daughter expresses concern about her mother managing the oxygen and the walker when going to the bathroom. Mrs. F. uses the oxygen when she sleeps and her daughter is sceptical about her ability to get to the bathroom without rushing.

You observe that the hallway between the bedroom and bathroom is dark and that the bedroom has an overhead light but no bedside lamp. The bathroom has a narrow doorway, and the toilet is at the other side of the sink. You assess the home for safety and determine that the pathways are clear and there is good lighting on the stairway and in the living areas. You identify no additional risks (e.g., throw rugs) to Mrs. F.'s safe mobility, but you do have concerns about Mrs. F.'s ability to navigate safely to the toilet with a walker.

When questioned about her vision problems, Mrs. F. gives her history of successful cataract surgery and a diagnosis of AMD at the age of 80 years. Although her ophthalmologist has told her that her vision will get worse and that he can't do anything about it, she has talked with friends who say they are getting treatments. He had mentioned that the local sight centre provides some rehabilitation services for people with low vision, but he told her that those services are mostly for "younger blind people." She is also concerned that the sight centre will suggest she purchase items that cost a lot of money, which she would not be able to afford. She says her daughter got her a subscription for the large-print *Reader's Digest*, which she enjoys, and that she is not interested in reading the newspaper because she watches the news on television. She has an appointment to see her eye doctor next month.

NURSING DIAGNOSIS

In addition to the nursing diagnoses related to Mrs. F.'s medical condition, you identify a nursing diagnosis of Disturbed Sensory Perception: Visual, related to age-related changes, sensory organ alterations and environmental factors. Supporting evidence for this diagnosis can be found in Mrs. F.'s inability to read labels, instructions or the flow metre markings and the environmental factors that contribute to unsafe mobility. The nursing diagnoses of Anxiety, Self-Care Deficit and Risk for Injury might also be applicable. The diagnosis of Disturbed Sensory Perception: Visual, however, addresses the source of Mrs. F.'s anxiety, risk for injury and inability to perform her instrumental activities of daily living and, therefore, is probably the most comprehensive diagnosis. Also, this diagnosis prompts you to include a long-term goal of encouraging further evaluation and management of the visual impairments.

NURSING CARE PLAN FOR MRS. F.

Expected Outcome	Nursing Interventions	Nursing Evaluation
Mrs. F. will manage her medication regimen accurately and independently.	• Print simplified medication instructions on large index cards by using black felt-tip marker. • Use coloured dots to match pill bottles with instruction cards. • Establish a medication management system by using pill organizer boxes with markings that are bold and have good colour contrast. • Teach Mrs. F. how to fill the pill boxes weekly, using the index cards you prepared for her. • Suggest that Mrs. F. fill the pill boxes at the kitchen table during daylight hours while using overhead light.	• Mrs. F. will demonstrate that she can accurately fill the pill boxes. • Mrs. F. will take her medications correctly. • Mrs. F.'s daughter will observe that her mother follows the prescribed regimen.
Mrs. F. will self-administer oxygen as needed.	• Use a copy machine to enlarge the small-print instructions for the oxygen equipment. • Place a coloured dot at the 2-L mark on the flowmetre. • Keep the oxygen tank in a well-lit location and suggest using a flashlight to help illuminate the flowmetre setting.	• Mrs. F. will demonstrate a safe and independent operation of the oxygen equipment. • Mrs. F.'s daughter will observe that her mother administers her oxygen correctly.

Expected Outcome	Nursing Interventions	Nursing Evaluation
Mrs. F. will be able to use a commode safely and independently.	• Ask Mrs. F. to use a bedside commode during the night; emphasize the importance of preventing another fall. • Work with physical and occupational therapists to (1) evaluate the feasibility of installing grab bars or other devices that will assist Mrs. F. in safely using the toilet, (2) identify a safe way for Mrs. F. to use the bathroom during the daytime, (3) teach Mrs. F. to transfer between the bed and commode for nighttime use, (4) teach her to empty the bedside commode. • Place a lamp on the nightstand and make sure that Mrs. F. can turn it on easily while in bed. Teach Mrs. F. to turn the bedside lamp on and sit at the edge of the bed for a few minutes before getting up at night.	• Mrs. F. will demonstrate that she can safely use the bathroom during the day and a bedside commode at night. • Mrs. F. will be able to empty the commode independently. • Mrs. F. will have no further falls in the bathroom.
Mrs. F. will compensate as much as possible for her progressive visual loss.	• Educate Mrs. F. and her daughter about the services provided at the local sight centre (CNIB) for people with low vision; emphasize that these services address the needs of older adults and people with recent and progressive visual loss. The services are for anyone with low vision, and there are many low-vision aids available to improve the visual function of people with macular degeneration. • Suggest that Mrs. F. ask her eye doctor for a referral to the sight centre when she sees him next month. • Include Mrs. F.'s daughter in the discussion about these services, and ask her to assist with following through once a referral is obtained.	• Mrs. F. will make and keep an appointment for an initial evaluation at the sight centre. • Mrs. F. will use low-vision aids to improve visual function.

THINKING POINTS

- How would you address concerns about Mrs. F. living alone? What aspects of her safety and quality of life would you consider?
- How would you use any of the boxes in this chapter for health promotion teaching?
- What additional nursing diagnoses and outcomes would you identify for Mrs. F.?
- What additional interventions and referrals would you consider for Mrs. F.?
- Identify at least one resource in your community that might provide help or information for Mrs. F. Call that agency to obtain information about their services.

QSEN APPLICATION

QSEN Competency	Knowledge/Skill/Attitude	Application to Mrs. F.
Patient-centred care	(K) Integrate understanding of multiple dimensions of patient-centred care. (K) Examine nursing roles in assuring coordination, integration and continuity of care. (S) Elicit patient values, preferences and expressed needs. (S) Provide patient-centred care with sensitivity and respect for diversity of the human experience. (S) Assess own level of communication skill in encounters with patients and families. (A) Value seeing health care situations "through patients' eyes."	Recognize that the concerns and needs of Mrs. F. and her daughter are not the same and facilitate a conversation with both of them. Obtain permission from Mrs. F. and her daughter to have the social worker from your home care agency visit to talk with both of them about options for care (e.g., home care assistance, home-delivered meals). Emphasize that the social worker can assist them with making decisions about a plan of care that is mutually acceptable.

QSEN Competency	Knowledge/Skill/Attitude	Application to Mrs. F.
Teamwork and collaboration	(K) Recognize contributions of other individuals and groups in helping patient achieve health goals. (K) Describe impact of own communication style on others. (S) Integrate the contributions of others who play a role in helping patient achieve health goals.	Provide care coordination for all health care professionals involved with Mrs. F's care, including physical and occupational therapists, social workers and respiratory supply company. Encourage Mrs. F. and her daughter to call the sight centre and request that a low-vision specialist make a home visit to assess the need for low-vision aids and teaching about safe and independent functioning.

Chapter Highlights

Age-Related Changes That Affect Vision (Fig. 17-1, Tables 17-1 and 17-2)

- Changes in appearance include arcus senilis, loss of orbital fat and diminished elasticity of eyelid muscles.
- Diminished tear production
- Degenerative changes affect all structures of the eye, the retinal–neural pathway and the visual cortex of the brain.

Effects of Age-Related Changes on Vision (Fig. 17-2)

- Diminished ability to focus clearly on objects at various distances
- Diminished ability to detect details and discern objects
- Slower adaptive response to changes in lighting
- Increased sensitivity to glare
- Narrowed visual field
- Diminished depth perception
- Altered colour perception so objects look darker and whites appear more yellowed
- Diminished ability to perceive flashing lights
- Slower processing of visual information

Risks Factors That Affect Visual Wellness

- Environmental factors: glare, sunlight, poor lighting, low humidity
- Lifestyle factors: poor nutrition, cigarette smoking
- Chronic conditions: diabetes, hypertension, Alzheimer or Parkinson disease
- Adverse medication effects: estrogen, corticosteroids, anticholinergics, β-blockers, antiparkinson agents

Functional Consequences Affecting Visual Wellness

- Presbyopia (diminished ability to focus on near objects)
- Need for three to five times more light than previously
- Difficulty with night driving
- Increased risk for unsafe mobility and falls
- Increased difficulty in performing usual activities

Pathologic Conditions Affecting Vision (Figs. 17-3 and 17-4, Table 17-3)

- Cataracts
- AMD
- Glaucoma

Nursing Assessment of Vision (Boxes 17-2 through 17-4)

- Vision screening tests
- Risk factors that affect vision
- Influence of vision changes on performance of activities of daily living
- Attitudes about eye examinations and preventive measures
- Attitudes regarding use of low-vision aids

Nursing Diagnosis

- Readiness for Enhanced Knowledge: Improved Vision
- Diagnoses that address the functional consequences of visual impairment include the following: Anxiety, Ineffective Coping, Self-Care Deficit, Risk for Injury, Impaired Social Interaction, Readiness for Enhanced Coping and Readiness for Enhanced Self-Care.

Planning for Wellness Outcomes

- Improved visual function
- Increased safety
- Improved independence in activities of daily living
- Improved quality of life

Nursing Interventions for Visual Wellness (Boxes 17-5 through 17-10)

- Prevention and detection of eye disease
- Comfort measures for dry eyes
- Environmental modifications (e.g., optimal illumination)
- Low-vision aids

Evaluating Effectiveness of Nursing Interventions

- Use of corrective lenses and other aids that improve vision
- Environmental adaptations for optimal safety and visual function
- Improved independence in daily activities
- Expressed feelings of improved quality of life in relation to visual function

Critical Thinking Exercises

1. Describe presbyopia and explain the functional consequences of this condition in the everyday life of an older adult.
2. What environmental factors are likely to interfere with the visual function of older adults?

3. Describe the specific effects of glaucoma, cataracts or AMD on one's ability to see a television program.
4. How would you assess the visual abilities of an older adult?
5. Explain the differences between opticians, optometrists and ophthalmologists.
6. List at least 10 adaptations that might be implemented to improve the visual function of older adults.

 For more information about the topics discussed in this chapter, be sure to check out the interactive Online Learning Activities and other helpful resources at http://thepoint.lww.com/Miller7e

REFERENCES

Andersen, G. J. (2012). Aging and vision: Changes in function and performance from optics to perception. *Wiley Interdisciplinary Review of Cognitive Sciences, 3*(3), 403–410.

Anstey, K. J., Horswill, M. S., Wood, J. M., et al. (2012). The role of cognitive and visual abilities as predictors in the multifactorial model of driving safety. *Accident Analysis and Prevention, 45,* 766–774.

Buys, Y. M., Jin, Y. P., & Canadian Glaucoma Risk Factor Study Group. (2013). Socioeconomic status as a risk factor for late presentation of glaucoma in Canada. *Canadian Journal of Ophthalmology, 48*(2), 83–87.

Canadian National Institute for the Blind. (2010). *Eye connect: AMD.* Retrieved from http://www.cnib.ca/en/your-eyes/eye-conditions/eye-connect/amd/Pages/default.aspx

Canadian National Institute for the Blind. (2014). *Eye connect: AMD.* Retrieved from http://www.cnib.ca/en/your-eyes/eye-conditions/eye-connect/amd/Pages/default.aspx

Canadian National Institute for the Blind. (n.d.). *Fast facts about vision loss.* Retrieved from http://www.cnib.ca/en/about/media/vision-loss/Pages/default.aspx

Eichenbaum, J. W. (2012). Geriatric vision loss due to cataracts, macular degeneration, and glaucoma. *Mount Sinai Journal of Medicine, 79*(2), 276–294.

Ferman, T. J., Arvanitakis, Z., Fujishiro, H., et al. (2013). Pathology and temporal onset of visual hallucinations, misperceptions and family misidentification distinguishes dementia with Lewy bodies from Alzheimer's disease. *Parkinsonism and Related Disorders, 19*(2), 227–231.

Ferris, F. L., Wilkinson, C. P., Bird, A., et al. (2013). Clinical classification of age-related macular degeneration. *Ophthalmology, 120*(4), 844–851.

Finger, R. P., Kupitz, D. G., Fenwick, E., et al. (2012). The impact of successful cataract surgery on quality of life, household income and social status in South India. *PloS ONE, 7*(8), e44268. doi:10.1371/journal.pone.0044268

Glaucoma Research Society of Canada. (n.d.). *Learning about glaucoma.* Retrieved from http://www.glaucomaresearch.ca/en/about/about_glaucoma.shtml

Hamilton, J. M., Landy, K. M., Salmon, D. P., et al. (2012). Early visuospatial deficits predict the occurrence of visual hallucinations in autopsy-confirmed dementia with Lewy bodies. *American Journal of Geriatric Psychiatry, 20*(9), 773–781.

Helbostad, J. L., Oedegaard, M., Lamb, S. E., et al. (2013). Change in vision, visual disability, and health after cataract surgery. *Optometry & Vision Science, 90*(4), 392–399. doi:10.1097/OPX.0b013e3182843f16

Herdman, T. H. (Ed.). (2012). *NANDA International Nursing Diagnoses: Definitions and classification 2012–1014.* Oxford, England: Wiley-Blackwell.

Hochberg, C., Maul, E., Chan, E. S., et al. (2012). Association of vision loss in glaucoma and age-related macular degeneration with IADL disability. *Investigative Ophthalmology and Visual Science, 53,* 3201–3206.

Kaleem, M. A., Munoz, B. E., Munro, C. A., et al. (2012). Visual characteristics of elderly night drivers in the Salisbury Eye Evaluation Driving Study. *Investigative Ophthalmology and Visual Science, 53*(9), 5161–5167.

Lichtinger, A., & Rootman, D. S. (2012). Intraocular lenses for presbyopia correction: Past, present, and future. *Current Opinion in Ophthalmology, 23*(1), 40–46.

Mabuchi, F., Yoshimura, K., Kashiwagi, K., et al. (2012). Risk factors for anxiety and depression in patients with glaucoma. *British Journal of Ophthalmology, 96*(6), 821–825.

Mathew, R. S., Delbaere, K., Lord, S. R., et al. (2011). Depressive symptoms and quality of life in people with age-related macular degeneration. *Ophthalmic Physiological Optics, 31*(4), 375–380.

Mennemeyer, S. T., Owsley, C., & McGwin, G. (2013). Reducing older driver motor vehicle collisions via earlier cataract surgery. *Accident Analysis and Prevention, 61,* 203–211.

Meuleners, L. B., Hendrie, D., Lee, A. H., et al. (2012). The effectiveness of cataract surgery in reducing motor vehicle crashes. *Ophthalmic Epidemiology, 19*(1), 23–28.

Monestam, E., & Lundqvist, B. (2012). Long-term visual outcome after cataract surgery. *Journal of Cataract and Refractive Surgery, 38*(3), 409–414.

Murthy, G. V. S., John, N., Sharmanna, B. R., et al. (2012). Elimination of avoidable blindness due to cataract. *Indian Journal of Ophthalmology, 60*(5), 438–445.

Owsley, C., McGwin, G., & Searcey, K. (2012). A population-based examination of the visual and ophthalmological characteristics of licensed drivers aged 70 and older. *Journal of Gerontology: Biological Sciences, 68*(5), 567–573. doi:10.1093/gerona/gls185

Parmeggiani, F., Romano, M. R., Costagliola, C., et al. (2012). Mechanism of inflammation in age-related macular degeneration. *Mediators of Inflammation, 2012,* 1–16. doi:1155/2012/546786

Popescu, M. L., Boisjoly, H., Schmaltz, H., et al. (2012). Explaining the relationship between three eye diseases and depressive symptoms in older adults. *Investigative Ophthalmology and Visual Sciences, 53*(4), 2308–2313.

Ramulu, P. Y., van Landingham, S. W., Massof, R. W., et al. (2012). Fear of falling and visual field loss from glaucoma. *Ophthalmology, 119*(7), 1352–1358.

Renieri, G., Pitz, S., Pfeiffer, N., et al. (2013). Changes in quality of life in visually impaired patients after low-vision rehabilitation. *International Journal of Rehabilitation Research, 36*(1), 48–55.

Rudnicka, A. R., Jarrar, Z., Wormald, R., et al. (2012). Age and gender variations in age-related macular degeneration prevalence in populations of European ancestry: A meta-analysis. *Ophthalmology, 119*(3), 571–580.

Sin, H. P., Liu, D. T., & Lam, D. S. (2013). Lifestyle modification, nutritional and vitamins supplements for age-related macular degeneration. *Acta Ophthalmologica, 91*(1), 6–11.

Tanabe, S., Yuki, K., Ozeki, N., et al. (2012). The association between primary open-angle glaucoma and fall. *Clinical Ophthalmology, 6,* 327–331.

Wang, M. Y., Rousseau, J., Boisjoly, H., et al. (2012). Activity limitation due to fear of falling in older adults with eye disease. *Investigative Ophthalmology and Visual Sciences, 53*(13), 7967–7972.

Warren, M. (2013). Promoting health literacy in older adults with low vision. *Topics in Geriatric Rehabilitation, 29,* 107–115.

Yoshizawa, H., Vonsattel, J. P., & Honig, L. S. (2013). Early neuropsychological discriminants for Lewy Body disease. *Journal of Neurology and Neurosurgical Psychiatry, 84,* 1326–1330.

Zambelli-Weiner, A., Crews, J. E., & Friedman, D. S. (2012, December). Disparities in adult vision health in the United States. *American Journal of Ophthalmology, 154*(6 Suppl.), S23–S30.

chapter 18

Digestion and Nutrition

LEARNING OBJECTIVES

After reading this chapter, you will be able to:

1. Describe age-related changes that affect eating patterns and digestive processes.

2. List age-related changes in nutritional requirements.

3. Identify risk factors that affect the digestion and nutrition of older adults.

4. Explain the effects of age-related changes and risk factors on digestion and nutrition.

5. Assess aspects of nutrition, digestion, behaviours that affect eating and food preparation and oral care pertinent to care of older adults.

6. Identify nursing interventions to promote optimal nutrition, digestion and oral care.

KEY POINTS

body mass index (BMI)	Mini Nutritional Assessment (MNA)
constipation	olfaction
Dietary Reference Intakes (DRIs)	presbyphagia
dysphagia	protein-energy malnutrition
gustatory function	xerostomia

Digestion of food and maintenance of nutrition are influenced to a small degree by age-related gastrointestinal changes and to a large degree by risk factors that affect most older adults. Although older adults can easily compensate for age-related changes in the digestive tract, they have more difficulty compensating for the many factors that interfere with their ability to obtain, prepare and enjoy food.

This chapter discusses age-related changes and functional consequences in relation to digestion, eating patterns and nutritional requirements.

AGE-RELATED CHANGES THAT AFFECT DIGESTION AND EATING PATTERNS

Age-related changes affect the senses of smell and taste and all the organs of the digestive tract. These changes have very few functional consequences for healthy older adults, but they increase the vulnerability of older adults to risk factors.

Smell and Taste

The senses of taste and smell affect food enjoyment, and both these senses decline in older adults because of a combination of age-related changes and risk factors. **Olfaction** (i.e., the ability to smell odours) depends on the perception of odourants by the sensory cells in the nasal mucosa and on central nervous system processing of that information. The ability to detect and identify odours is best between the ages of 30 and 40 years; then it gradually declines, which is at least partly attributed to age-related changes. Prevalence rates for impaired sense of smell are between 1% and 5% in adults less than 35 years old and between 14% and 25% for those 50 years or older (Huttenbrink et al., 2013; Schubert et al., 2012). Currently, researchers are exploring the relationship between impaired sense of smell as an early diagnostic marker for neurodegenerative diseases, such as Parkinson disease and Alzheimer disease (Hummel et al., 2011). Additional conditions that can lead to impaired olfaction include smoking or chewing tobacco, viruses, poor oral health, periodontal disease, nasal sinus disease, trauma and medications. Medications that are associated with impaired olfactory function are angiotensin-converting enzyme (ACE) inhibitors, diuretics and antidepressants (Smoliner et al., 2013).

The ability to taste, called **gustatory function**, depends primarily on receptor cells in the taste buds, which are located on the tongue, palate and tonsils. Characteristics of

Promoting Digestive and Nutritional Wellness in Older Adults

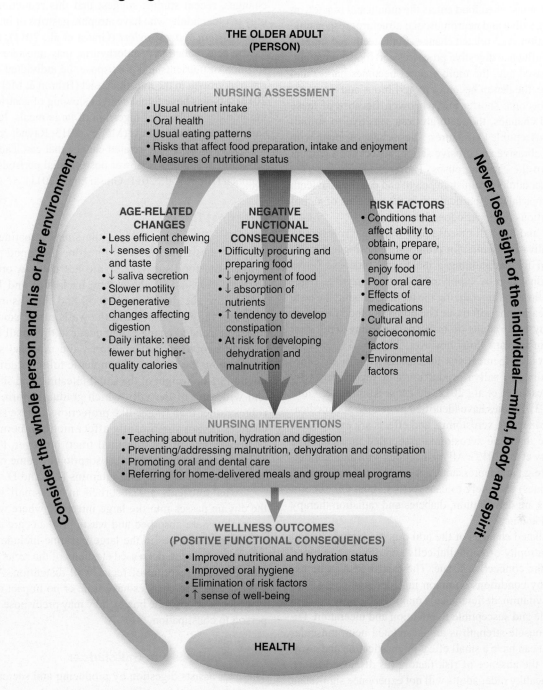

THE OLDER ADULT (PERSON)

Consider the whole person and his or her environment

Never lose sight of the individual—mind, body and spirit

NURSING ASSESSMENT
- Usual nutrient intake
- Oral health
- Usual eating patterns
- Risks that affect food preparation, intake and enjoyment
- Measures of nutritional status

AGE-RELATED CHANGES
- Less efficient chewing
- ↓ senses of smell and taste
- ↓ saliva secretion
- Slower motility
- Degenerative changes affecting digestion
- Daily intake: need fewer but higher-quality calories

NEGATIVE FUNCTIONAL CONSEQUENCES
- Difficulty procuring and preparing food
- ↓ enjoyment of food
- ↓ absorption of nutrients
- ↑ tendency to develop constipation
- At risk for developing dehydration and malnutrition

RISK FACTORS
- Conditions that affect ability to obtain, prepare, consume or enjoy food
- Poor oral care
- Effects of medications
- Cultural and socioeconomic factors
- Environmental factors

NURSING INTERVENTIONS
- Teaching about nutrition, hydration and digestion
- Preventing/addressing malnutrition, dehydration and constipation
- Promoting oral and dental care
- Referring for home-delivered meals and group meal programs

WELLNESS OUTCOMES (POSITIVE FUNCTIONAL CONSEQUENCES)
- Improved nutritional and hydration status
- Improved oral hygiene
- Elimination of risk factors
- ↑ sense of well-being

HEALTH

taste sensation are measured according to the ability to perceive the intensity of taste, which diminishes with aging, and the ability to identify different flavours. Although studies indicate that taste cells in the tongue papillae can regenerate and have a half-life of about 15 days, the sense of taste declines with increased age, but to a lesser degree than the sense of smell (Hummel et al., 2011). The most common causes of taste disorders are head trauma, radiation, upper respiratory tract infections and medical conditions such as diabetes or hypothyroidism. Medications that can cause taste disorders include antibiotics, antimycotics, antiepileptics, antihistamines, immunosuppressants, antirheumatic drugs, corticosteroids, diuretics, antidiabetics, antihypertensives, antiparkinson drugs and vasodilators (Hummel et al., 2011).

 DIVERSITY NOTE

Throughout life, the sense of smell is better in women than in men, particularly in aspects of smell detection and identification (Mullol et al., 2012). Similarly, gustatory function is better in women than in men (Hummel et al., 2011).

Oral Cavity

Digestion begins when food enters the mouth and is acted on by the teeth, saliva and neuromuscular structures responsible for mastication. Age-related changes in the teeth and support structures influence digestive processes and food enjoyment. With increased age, the tooth enamel becomes harder and more brittle, the dentin becomes more fibrous and the nerve chambers become shorter and narrower. Because of these age-related changes, the teeth are less sensitive to stimuli and more susceptible to fractures. These changes, along with decades of abrasive and erosive action, also cause a gradual flattening of the chewing cusps. The bones supporting the teeth of older adults diminish in height and density, and teeth may loosen or fall out, particularly in the presence of pathologic conditions (e.g., periodontal disease).

Saliva and the oral mucosa play important roles in digestion. Saliva is essential for promoting chewing and swallowing and for maintaining a moist oral mucosa. Saliva facilitates digestion by supplying digestive enzymes, regulating oral flora, remineralizing the teeth, cleansing the taste buds, lubricating the soft tissue and preparing food for chewing. Healthy older adults do not experience any significant decreases in salivary flow; however, 31% to 37% of older adults who take medications for chronic conditions experience diminished saliva production and **xerostomia** (dry mouth) (Desoutter et al., 2012; de Lima Saintrain & Goncalves, 2013). Studies have identified more than 500 medications that can cause xerostomia, and effects are exacerbated when more than one xerostomia-associated medication is used (Shetty et al., 2012). All medications with anticholinergic action (e.g., antidepressants, antipsychotics, antiemetics, antihistamines) are likely to cause xerostomia. Other common causes are dehydration, diabetes and radiation therapy to the head and neck.

Age-related changes of the oral mucosa include loss of elasticity, atrophy of epithelial cells and diminished blood supply to the connective tissue. These changes can be exacerbated by conditions common in older adults (e.g., xerostomia, vitamin deficiencies), making the oral mucosa more friable and susceptible to infection and ulceration. Diminished muscle strength is an age-related neuromuscular change that can have a small effect on mastication and swallowing. In the absence of risk factors (as discussed later), however, healthy older adults will not experience significant swallowing problems.

Esophagus and Stomach

The second phase of digestion occurs when a combination of propulsive and nonpropulsive waves propels food through the pharynx and esophagus into the stomach. In older adults, the esophagus stiffens, peristaltic waves decrease and **presbyphagia** (i.e., slowed swallowing) develops.

After passing through the esophageal sphincter, food enters the stomach, where gastric enzymes liquefy it and gastric action transforms it into chyme. Although reduced gastric acid secretions are sometimes attributed to age-related changes, recent studies suggest that this reduction occurs only in older adults who have atrophic gastritis or in the presence of *Helicobacter pylori* (Grassi et al., 2011). Reduced gastric acid, called hypochlorhydria, may interfere with absorption of nutrients and predispose the individual to bacterial overgrowth in the intestinal tract (Britton & McLaughlin, 2013). Studies have found a slight slowing of gastric emptying in older adults after ingestion of large meals, leading to early sensations of fullness (Morley, 2013; Rayner & Horowitz, 2013). Another age-related change that can lead to early sensation of fullness is slower postprandial peristalsis in the stomach (Bitar et al., 2011; Grassi et al., 2011).

Intestinal Tract

After the chyme passes into the small intestine, digestive enzymes from the small intestine, liver and pancreas convert the food substances into nutrients. A process of segmentation moves the chyme backward and forward, facilitating the digestion of food and the absorption of nutrients through the villi in the walls of the small intestine. Age-related changes that occur in the small intestine include atrophy of muscle fibres and mucosal surfaces, reduction in the number of lymphatic follicles, gradual reduction in the weight of the small intestine, and shortening and widening of the villi, which gradually form parallel ridges rather than finger-like projections. These structural changes do not significantly affect motility, permeability or transit time in the intestinal tract; however, they may affect immune function and absorption of some nutrients, such as folate, calcium and vitamins B_{12} and D.

After nutrients are absorbed in the small intestine, the chyme passes into the large intestine, where water and electrolytes are absorbed and waste products are expelled. Age-related changes in the large intestine include reduced secretion of mucus, decreased elasticity of the rectal wall and diminished perception of rectal wall distention. Although these age-related changes have little or no impact on motility of feces through the bowel, they may predispose the older person to constipation.

Liver, Pancreas and Gallbladder

The liver assists digestion by producing and secreting bile, which is essential for utilizing fats. It also plays an important role in metabolizing and storing medications and nutrients. With increasing age, the liver becomes smaller and more fibrous, lipofuscin (a brown pigment) accumulates and blood flow to the liver decreases by approximately one-third. However, some of these changes may be pathologic, rather than age related, in origin. Despite any age-related or pathologic changes, the liver has an enormous regenerative and reserve capacity, which allows it to compensate for such changes without significantly affecting digestive function.

A primary digestive function of the pancreas is the secretion of enzymes essential for neutralizing acids in the chyme and breaking down fats, proteins and carbohydrates in the small intestine. The pancreas also functions as an endocrine gland and produces insulin and glycogen, which are essential for glucose metabolism. Age-related changes in the pancreas include decreased weight, hyperplasia of the duct, fibrosis of the lobe and decreased responsiveness of pancreatic B cells to glucose. These changes do not directly affect digestive functioning; however, the effects on glucose metabolism can increase the susceptibility of older adults to the development of type 2 diabetes.

Age-related changes that affect the gallbladder and biliary tract include diminished bile acid synthesis, widening of the common bile duct and increased secretion of cholecystokinin, a peptide hormone that contracts the gallbladder and relaxes the biliary sphincter. These age-related changes can increase the susceptibility of older adults to the development of **cholelithiasis** (gallstones). In addition, a higher level of cholecystokinin can suppress the appetite.

AGE-RELATED CHANGES IN NUTRITIONAL REQUIREMENTS

In 2001, major organizations in Canada and the United States established **Dietary Reference Intakes (DRIs)** as the standards for meeting the basic nutrient needs of healthy adults according to specific age groups (e.g., adults aged 51–70 years and those 70 years and older). An important health promotion aspect is that DRIs include indicators for preventing chronic disease and avoiding the harmful effects of consuming too much of a nutrient. DRIs are adjusted to compensate for conditions such as aging, health problems, nutrient deficiencies and medication effects. DRIs that increase with aging are calcium (1,200 mg for those 50 years and older) and vitamin D (400 and 600 IU/day for those aged 51–70 years and those 70 years and older, respectively). The DRI for iron decreases to 8 mg/day in women 51 years and older as a result of menstruation cessation. Recent studies indicate that the intake of vitamin D should be increased to at least 800 IU daily, with emphasis on meeting the requirement for calcium through food sources rather than supplements (Gallagher, 2013).

Calories

The energy-producing potential of food is measured in units called *calories*. Caloric requirements are determined by a combination of factors, including height, weight, sex, body build, health–illness state and the usual level of physical activity. Energy requirements gradually decrease throughout adulthood because of decreased physical activity and the decline in basal metabolic rate that is associated with diminished muscle mass. Thus, nutritional guidelines recommend a gradual reduction in calories beginning between the ages of 40 and 50 years. This decrease in caloric intake requires a proportionate increase in the quality of calories (nutritional density) to meet minimal nutritional requirements. Thus,

nutritional deficiencies will occur unless a reduced caloric intake is accompanied by an increased intake of foods with a high nutritional value and a concomitant decrease in the intake of foods containing little or no nutrients.

Protein

Protein provides the essential components for new tissue growth in the human body. Age-related changes, such as decreased lean body mass and muscle tissue and decreased plasma albumin and total body albumin levels, may influence protein requirements in older adults. The recommended daily protein intake for all adults 19 years and older is 0.8 g/kg of body weight, which is less than the average intake for older adults. Because recent studies indicate that slightly higher levels (i.e., 1.0–1.6 g/kg daily) would be beneficial for preserving muscle function, many experts now recommend that older adults consume 25 to 30 g of high-quality protein at every meal (Academy of Nutrition and Dietetics, 2012).

Carbohydrates and Fibre

Carbohydrates provide an essential source of energy and fibre. Without an adequate intake of carbohydrates, the body will derive energy from fat and protein, causing an increase in serum cholesterol and triglyceride levels and a depletion of water, electrolytes and amino acids. Dietary fibre (i.e., the nondigestible carbohydrates and lignin in plants) has received much attention in recent years, primarily for its role in disease prevention, as an essential food component. Recent reviews conclude that most individuals need to double their consumption of fibre to meet the amounts of the 25 to 38 g/day for adults (Hornick et al., 2011). The following health benefits of dietary fibre that have been identified in studies: lower blood pressure, reduced cancer risk, improved weight management, improved serum lipid levels, maintenance of a healthy digestive system and improved glucose tolerance and insulin response (Hornick et al., 2011). Thus, dietary fibre may play a role in preventing and treating obesity, diabetes, cardiovascular disease and colorectal cancer. The Canada Food Guide suggests a daily intake of seven servings of fruits and vegetables for adults above the age of 50 years (Health Canada, 2011).

 DIVERSITY NOTE

Recognizing cultural and ethnic diversity, the Canada Food Guide has been modified for use with First Nations and other aboriginal groups, namely, Inuit and Métis people.

Fats

The primary functions of fat are to assist in temperature regulation, provide a reserve source of energy and facilitate the absorption of fat-soluble vitamins. Fats are also useful in providing a feeling of satiety and improving the taste of foods. Fats are categorized according to their source. Saturated fats are derived from animals, whereas unsaturated fats are found in vegetables. Although either type of fat can meet nutritional needs, only the saturated fats are associated with the detrimental accumulation of serum cholesterol. Adults in most industrialized societies consume far more calories in fats than is healthy or necessary. Because excessive fat intake is associated with harmful effects, such as hyperlipidemia, fat should constitute no more than 20% to 30% of a person's daily caloric intake (Dieticians of Canada, 2013a). Those fats that are consumed should be polyunsaturated and monounsaturated fatty acids, rather than cholesterol and saturated fats (see Chapter 20 for further discussion of types of fat).

Water

Although water is often overlooked as a nutritional requirement, adequate hydration is essential for all physiologic functions. Adequate hydration is essential for regulating body temperature, maintaining a suitable metabolic environment, diluting water-soluble medications and facilitating renal and bowel excretion. Potential consequences of reduced body water include decreased efficiency of thermoregulation, increased susceptibility to dehydration and increased concentrations of water-soluble medications in the body.

Throughout life, the proportion of total body water as a percentage of body weight gradually decreases from about 80% of a newborn infant's weight to less than half of an older adult's weight. This decrease in total body water is associated with a loss of lean body mass and is influenced by sex and the degree of leanness, with women and obese people having a lower percentage of body water than do men and lean, muscular people. Total body water may be further diminished by poor fluid intake, which is often caused by decreased thirst perception in older adults. The recommended amount of fluid intake (in beverages and drinking water) for adults of all ages is 3 L for men and 2.2 L for women daily (Dieticians of Canada, 2013b).

 ## RISK FACTORS THAT AFFECT DIGESTION AND NUTRITION

Certain behaviours and common disease processes are likely to interfere with nutrition and digestion in older adults. Some detrimental behaviours, such as limiting fluid intake and avoiding fresh fruit, may be based on myths and misconceptions. Although these conditions can create risks for people at any age, they occur more commonly in older adults, and the potential for harm is much greater than in other age groups because of the collective effects of risk factors and age-related changes. Risk factors affect every phase of digestion and nutrition, and they can significantly influence eating patterns and nutritional intake. Functional and cognitive impairment is the risk factor most closely associated with inadequate nutritional intake in older adults in community, acute-care and long-term care settings (Donini et al., 2013; Kiesswetter et al., 2013; Orsitto, 2012). Additional risks for poor nutritional status in older adults who live in

long-term care facilities include polypharmacy, depression, recent hospitalization and presence of a wound or pressure ulcer (Verbrugghe et al., 2012). Risks that can cause specific nutrient deficiencies are listed in Table 18-1, along with the related functional consequences.

Conditions Related to Oral Care

Oral health influences nutritional status because it affects chewing, eating, swallowing, speaking and social interaction. Until recently, being edentulous (i.e., having no natural teeth) was so common among older people that it has been inaccurately viewed as a normal consequence of aging. Although the percentage of older adults who are edentulous is gradually diminishing, 22% of men and 21% of women who are between the ages of 60 and 79 have no natural teeth (Statistics Canada, 2010).

Older adults who have natural teeth may have inadequate dental care, periodontal disease and other pathologic conditions that occur with increasing frequency in later years. In addition, because preventive dental care is a recent trend, older adults may falsely believe that they should visit a dentist only when a toothache does not respond to home remedies. Some factors that contribute to inadequate dental care include low income, less education, lack of transportation, lack of dental insurance, high cost of dental services, more pressing health concerns and inaccessibility of services as a result of distance or environmental barriers, such as stairs to dental offices.

Inadequate oral care is especially problematic for older adults who are cognitively impaired, dependent in activities of daily living or residing in long-term care settings. In particular for people with dementia, daily oral care, prevalence of dental problems and frequency of professional dental care are indicators that gradually worsen as the degree of cognitive impairment increases. Adverse effects of poor oral health include malnutrition, dehydration, periodontal disease, respiratory infections (e.g., pneumonia and aspiration pneumonia), joint infections, cardiovascular disease, poor glycemic control in diabetes and increased risk of stroke and heart attack (Johnson & Schoenfelder, 2012; O'Connor, 2012).

 See **ONLINE LEARNING ACTIVITY 18-1: EVIDENCE-BASED INFORMATION ABOUT ORAL CARE FOR OLDER ADULTS** at http://thepoint.lww.com/Miller7e

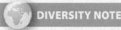 **DIVERSITY NOTE**

Older Canadians living in long-term care institution often receive poorer oral care than those living in the community (Stewart, 2013).

Wellness Opportunity

Nurses promote wellness by exploring reasons that older adults do not obtain dental care so that these barriers can be addressed.

TABLE 18-1 Causes and Consequences of Nutrient Deficiencies

Nutrient	Possible Causes of Deficiency	Functional Consequences of Deficiency
Calories	Anorexia, depression, mental or physical impairments	Weight loss, lethargy, edema, anemia
Protein	Lack of teeth or dentures, anorexia, depression, dementia, high alcohol or carbohydrate consumption	Poor tissue healing, hypoalbuminemia, reduced protein binding of drugs
Fat	Neomycin, phenytoin, laxatives, alcohol, colchicine, cholestyramine	Inability to absorb vitamins A, D, E and K
Vitamin A	Mineral oil, neomycin, alcohol, cholestyramine, aluminum antacids, liver disease	Dry skin and eyes, photophobia, night blindness, hyperkeratosis
Thiamine (B$_1$)	High consumption of alcohol or caffeinated tea, pernicious anemia, diuretics	Neuropathy, muscle weakness, heart disease, dementia, anorexia
Riboflavin (B$_2$)	Malabsorption syndromes, chronic diarrhea, laxative abuse, alcoholism, liver disease	Cheilitis, glossitis, photophobia, blepharitis, conjunctivitis
Niacin (B$_3$)	Poor dietary habits, diarrhea, cirrhosis, alcoholism	Dermatitis, stomatitis, diarrhea, dementia, depression
Pyridoxine (B$_6$)	Diuretics, hydralazine	Dermatitis, neuropathy
Folate (B$_9$)	Anticonvulsants, triamterene, sulfonamides, alcohol, smoking	Macrocytic anemia, elevated levels of homocysteine
Vitamin B$_{12}$	Malabsorption syndrome, H$_2$-receptor blockers, proton-pump inhibitors, colchicine, oral hypoglycemics, potassium supplements, vegetarian diet	Pernicious anemia, weakness, dyspnea, glossitis, numbness, dementia, depression
Vitamin C	Aspirin, tetracycline, lack of fruits and vegetables in diet	Lassitude, irritability, anemia, ecchymosis, impaired wound healing
Vitamin D	Phenytoin, mineral oil, phenobarbital, sunlight deprivation	Muscle weakness and atrophy, osteoporosis, fractures
Vitamin E	Malabsorption syndromes	Peripheral neuropathy, gait disturbance, retinopathy
Vitamin K	Mineral oil, warfarin sodium (Coumadin), antibiotics, cholestyramine, phenytoin	Ecchymosis; hemorrhage involving the gastrointestinal, urinary or central nervous system
Calcium	Phenytoin, aluminum-based antacids, laxatives, tetracycline, corticosteroids, furosemide, high intake of fibre or caffeine	Osteoporosis, fractures, low-back pain
Iron	Achlorhydria; neomycin; aspirin; antacids; low intake of animal protein; high consumption of fibre, caffeine or tannic acid (contained in some teas)	Anemia, weakness, lassitude, pallor
Magnesium	Alcohol, diuretics, diarrhea, bulk-forming laxatives	Cardiac arrhythmias, neuromuscular and central nervous system irritability, disorientation
Zinc	Penicillamine, aluminum-based antacids, bulk-forming laxatives, high consumption of fibre	Poor wound healing, hair loss
Potassium	Laxatives, furosemide, antibiotics, corticosteroids, diarrhea	Weakness, cardiac arrhythmias, digitalis toxicity
Water	Diuretics, laxatives, immobility, incontinence, diarrhea	Dry skin and mouth, dehydration, constipation
Fibre	Poor dietary habits	Constipation, hemorrhoids

Functional Impairments and Disease Processes

Functional impairments are strongly associated with poor nutrition, particularly with regard to dependence on others for assistance with eating. For example, mobility or visual impairments can interfere with the ability to procure and prepare food. In community settings, the extent to which functional impairments affect nutrition depends to a large degree on the availability of social supports, such as family, friends or agencies that assist with providing food.

Dysphagia (difficulty swallowing) is a functional impairment that can significantly affect chewing, nutrition and safe and effective swallowing (see Box 18-1).

According to the Canadian Association of Speech and Language Pathologists and Audiologists (CASLPA, 2013), approximately one in 10 adults above the age of 50 experience swallowing difficulties, and between 50% and 75% of nursing home residents have dysphagia, which most commonly is caused by neurologic and neuromuscular disorders (Gallagher, 2011). Because nurses caring for older adults are responsible for assessment and interventions related to this common problem, the topic is addressed in Box 18-2 and Online Learning Activity 18-2.

Pathological processes increase the risk for nutritional and digestive consequences in many ways. For example,

See ONLINE LEARNING ACTIVITY 18-2: EVIDENCE-BASED TOOL FOR PREVENTING ASPIRATION IN OLDER ADULTS WITH DYSPHAGIA
at http://thepoint.lww.com/Miller7e

vitamin B_{12} deficiency, which is more common with increasing age, can interfere with absorption of nutrients and may even be linked to some memory decline in older adults. Additionally, a deficiency in vitamin D may result in

---

Box 18-1 Evidence-Informed Nursing Practice

Background: Tube feeding of older adults with advanced-stage dementia is relatively common in Canada, despite being controversial.
Questions: Can a volitional breath-holding technique on swallowing assist older adults with distress and anxiety during meals caused by aspiration of food?
Method: The researcher—a specialist in swallowing and swallowing disorders—discussed a situation of a 77-year-old man who had moderate to severe dementia with problems swallowing and repeated aspiration of food when eating. His family decided against a tube feeding and agreed to participate in the behavioural swallowing treatment. The researcher taught the patient the preswallow breath-hold technique. He utilized the Swallowing Quality of Life Scale (SWAL-QOL) to test the effectiveness of this technique for his patient.

Findings: The researcher noted that the older client was able to learn this technique for reducing the risks of aspiration. After learning this technique, the client had no severe choking episodes and lungs remained clear of aspirate. The older client also reported decreased stress at times of eating.
Implications for Nursing Practice: The preswallow breath-holding technique may be a viable treatment for some older adults who have dysphagia and aspirate food and may be an alternative to the use of feeding tubes. Further research needs to be conducted.

Source: Cleary, S. (2013). Dysphagia treatment as an alternative to tube feeding in individuals with dementia: A case study. *Canadian Nursing Home*, *24*(1), 11–15.

E·B·P   Box 18-2 Evidence-Based Practice: Dysphagia

Statement of the Problem

- Dysphagia is defined as impairment of any part of the swallowing process.
- Aspiration, defined as the misdirection of oropharyngeal secretions or gastric content into the larynx and lower respiratory tract, is a common and serious consequence of dysphagia.
- Dysphagia is common in older adults with neurologic conditions, including stroke, dementia, multiple sclerosis and Parkinson disease.
- Up to 45% of people institutionalized with dementia and between 30% and 65% of people who have had strokes experience some degree of dysphagia.
- In addition to neurologic conditions, the following factors can increase the risk of dysphagia: absence of teeth, decreased saliva production, poorly fitting dentures, decreased level of consciousness and certain medications (e.g., anesthetics, anticholinergics, sedatives, psychotropics, antihistamines, amiodarone).
- Dysphagia increases the risk of malnutrition, aspiration and aspiration pneumonia.

Recommendations for Nursing Assessment

- Nursing assessment includes interview questions about difficulty with chewing or swallowing, avoidance of certain foods or beverages, sensation of food being stuck in throat, inability to handle secretions, voice changes and so forth.
- Nursing assessment of swallowing involves all the following: (1) examine the level of consciousness, posture, voluntary cough, voice quality and saliva control; (2) have the person drink 3 ounces of water without interruption; the person passes the test if he or she does not stop, choke or show a wet-hoarse vocal quality during the test or for 1 minute after.
- Signs and symptoms of dysphagia include drooling, coughing during meals, voice changes following meals, gurgling sounds in the throat, upper respiratory tract infection, wet lung sounds or packing food in the cheeks.
- Signs and symptoms of aspiration pneumonia include delirium, fever, chills, elevated respiratory rate, pleuritic chest pain and respiratory crackles.

Recommendations for Nursing Interventions

- Appropriate management of dysphagia requires an interprofessional team approach, which includes speech-language pathologists,

dietary professionals, primary care practitioners and all levels of nursing staff.
- Speech–language pathologists are the health care professionals who usually assume primary responsibility for recommendations, but nurses are responsible for initiating the referrals in a timely manner and implementing interventions.
- Interventions for prevention of aspiration are based on recommendations of the speech-language pathologist with regard to all the following compensatory strategies: postural adjustments (e.g., chin-down or chin-tuck manoeuvre), swallow manoeuvres and diet modification (e.g., appropriate food and liquid viscosity).
- Additional interventions include resting for 30 minutes before eating, sitting upright, avoid rushing or forced feeding, alternate small amounts of solid and liquid foods and minimize distractions.
- Interventions that may be appropriate based on recommendations of speech–language pathologist include the following: placement of food in one side of mouth, use of adaptive equipment and muscle-strengthening exercises.
- Recognize that individuals with dysphagia require approximately 30 minutes for eating/assisted feeding.
- Avoid medications that cause dry mouth (e.g., anticholinergics) or impair cough reflex and swallowing (e.g., sedatives and hypnotics).
- Good oral care is imperative for all patients with dysphagia because is it associated with a lower incidence of pneumonia.
- Provide referrals for regular and "as-needed" dental care.
- Be prepared to perform the Heimlich manoeuvre.

Additional Nursing Interventions for Preventing Aspiration During Tube Feeding

- Keep head of bed or chair elevated to at least 30 degrees during continuous feedings.
- Assess the following signs of gastrointestinal intolerance: nausea, feeling of fullness, abdominal pain or cramping.
- Measure gastric residual volumes every 4 to 6 hours during continuous feedings and immediately before each intermittent feeding.

Sources: Metheny, N. A. (2012). *Try this: Best practices in nursing care to older adults. Preventing aspiration in older adults with dysphagia* (No. 20). Retrieved from www.ConsultGeriRN.org; Nogueira, D., & Reis, E. (2013). Swallowing disorder in nursing home residents: How can the problem be explained? *Clinical Interventions in Aging*, *8*, 221–227; Sura, L., Madhavan, A., Carnaby, G., et al. (2012). Dysphagia in the elderly: Management and nutritional considerations. *Clinical Interventions in Aging*, *7*, 287–298.

osteoporosis, falls and fractures. Pathologic conditions also can interfere with appetite and enjoyment of food in many ways. For example, infections, hyperthyroidism, hypoadrenalism and heart failure are associated with anorexia, and rheumatoid conditions and chronic obstructive pulmonary disease (COPD) are associated with both decreased appetite and increased energy expenditure. Dementia and other neurodegenerative disorders often have serious negative effects on eating and nutrition related to procuring and preparing food, remembering to eat and chewing and swallowing food. Dysphagia, which leads to significant problems with chewing and swallowing, often occurs with dementia and other neurologic or neuromuscular conditions. A longitudinal study found that urinary tract infection during the preceding year was an independent risk for poor nutritional status in older nursing home residents (Carlsson et al., 2013).

Medication Effects

Medications, nutritional supplements and herbal preparations can create risk factors for impaired digestion and inadequate nutrition through their effects on digestion, eating patterns and utilization of nutrients. More than 250 medications have potential adverse effects on the absorption, metabolism and excretion of nutrients (Zadak et al., 2013). The following are examples:

- Broad-spectrum antibiotics can alter intestinal flora and impair nutrient synthesis.
- Medications and vitamins that are similar in chemical structure may compete at sites of action, thus altering their excretion pattern.
- Some medications bind to particular ions and form compounds that cannot be absorbed (e.g., tetracycline can bind to iron and calcium).
- Diuretics can interfere with the transport of water, sodium, glucose and amino acids.

Table 18-2 lists other examples of medications and the related adverse effects on digestion and nutrition. Additional food, herb and medication interactions are discussed in Chapter 8.

Lifestyle Factors

Alcohol and smoking can alter an older person's nutritional status in several ways. Alcohol has a high caloric content but low nutrient value, so it provides empty calories. In addition,

TABLE 18-2 Potential Effects of Medications on Digestion and Nutrition	
Medication Examples	**Potential Effect on Digestion and Nutrition**
Digoxin, theophylline, fluoxetine, antihistamines	Anorexia
Anticholinergics, narcotics, calcium-channel blockers, iron, aluminum- and calcium-based antacids	Constipation
Cimetidine, laxatives, antibiotics, cardiovascular drugs, cholinesterase inhibitors	Diarrhea, nausea, vomiting
Nonsteroidal anti-inflammatory drugs (NSAIDs), aspirin, corticosteroids	Gastric irritation
Phenytoin, nifedipine, diltiazem, cyclosporine	Gum hyperplasia
Anticholinergics, potassium-depleting medications	Paralytic ileus
Bulk-forming agents when taken before meals, anticholinergics	Early satiety
Potassium supplements, NSAIDs, bisphosphonates, prednisone	Dysphagia
Antihistamines, salicylates, hypoglycemics, antiparkinson drugs, psychoactive drugs	Altered smell and taste sensations
Mineral oil, cholestyramine	Diminished absorption of vitamins A, D, E and K
Anticonvulsants	Diminished storage of vitamin K, decreased absorption of calcium
Aluminum- or magnesium-based antacids	Diarrhea; decreased levels of calcium, fluoride and phosphorus
Ampicillin, amoxicillin, cephalosporins, clindamycin	*Clostridium difficile* diarrhea
Products containing sodium bicarbonate	Sodium overload, water retention
Gentamicin and penicillin	Hypokalemia
Tetracyclines	Diminished absorption of zinc, iron, calcium and magnesium
Neomycin	Diminished absorption of fat, iron, lactose, nitrogen, calcium, potassium and vitamin B_{12}
Aspirin	Gastrointestinal bleeding; decreased levels of iron, folate and vitamin C
Corticosteroids	Increased need for calcium, phosphorus, B vitamins and vitamins C and D
β-Carotene supplements	Vitamin E deficiency

it interferes with the absorption of the B-complex vitamins and vitamin C. Alcoholism is often unrecognized and under-treated in older adults and may be a common contributing factor to nutritional disorders. Smoking diminishes the ability to smell and taste food, and it also interferes with absorption of vitamin C and folic acid.

Psychosocial Factors

Psychosocial factors are likely to affect an older person's appetite and eating patterns. Any changes in mealtime companionship, as may occur through loss or disability of a spouse, are likely to have a negative impact on eating patterns. Studies have found that loneliness, which is common in older adults who live alone, is a significant predictor of and risk for malnutrition in older adults (Cousson et al., 2012; Wilson et al., 2011). When older adults have established a long-term pattern of preparing meals for family and spouse, it may be especially difficult for the older adult to adjust to purchasing, preparing and eating food for just one person. Similarly, older adults who have never participated in the purchase or preparation of foods may have great difficulty assuming these tasks after the loss of a spouse or other person who performed these tasks. If the older adult depends on others for assistance in procuring food, any factors that limit the availability of support resources may affect the older adult's ability to obtain food.

Stress and anxiety affect digestive processes through their influence on the autonomic nervous system. Although stress-related effects on digestion are not unique to older adults, any alteration of the autonomic nervous system may compound age-related effects that otherwise would not have much effect. Older adults who are depressed are likely to experience anorexia and loss of interest in food. Confusion, memory problems and other cognitive deficits may significantly interfere with eating patterns and the ability to prepare food.

Cultural and Socioeconomic Factors

Ethnic background, religious beliefs and other cultural factors strongly influence the way people define, select, prepare and eat food and beverages. Cultural factors also can influence eating patterns and selection of food in relation to health status. For example, some Asian people may classify foods, beverages and medicines as hot or cold, and they may select a particular food on the basis of their belief that their illness would respond to warm, hot, cool or cold types of remedies. According to this health belief model, illnesses are caused by an imbalance between hot and cold and so must be treated with substances that have the opposite characteristics. The characteristics of "hot" and "cold" are not related to temperature of the food but are culturally defined by different groups.

Cultural dietary customs usually are not detrimental for healthy older adults as long as the diet includes essential nutrients and avoids extremes. However, for older adults with medical conditions that require diet modification (e.g., diabetes or hypertension), cultural food patterns may aggravate the condition and create barriers to nutritional therapy. Box 18-3 summarizes some of the food habits that are associated with major cultural and religious groups in Canada. Nurses should remember, though, that individual older adults vary in their eating patterns and may not adhere to the patterns of their cultural group. It is usually not necessary to try to change culturally influenced eating patterns, but it is important to recognize any cultural factors that may affect older adults' nutritional status.

Wellness Opportunity

Nurses address cultural needs by identifying food preferences and finding reasonable ways to provide these foods.

A person's past and present economic status also influences food choices. If nutrient intake has been inadequate because of long-standing financial limitations, the progressive effects of poor nutrition may precipitate new problems

Box 18-3 Cultural Considerations: Cultural Influences on Eating Patterns

First Nations Canadians
- May be influenced by tribal culture
- May obtain foods from their natural environment (e.g., fish, roots, fruits, berries, wild greens, wild game) (if still living on the reserves)
- May have limited use of dairy products because of lactose intolerance

African Canadians
- Common main courses: wild game, fried fish and poultry, pork and all parts of the pig
- Common vegetables and side dishes: corn, rice, okra, greens, legumes, tomatoes, hot breads, sweet potatoes
- Methods of food preparation: stewing, barbecuing and frying with lard or salt pork
- Low consumption of milk (possibly owing to lactose intolerance)
- Low calcium dietary intake

Asian Canadians
- Common foods: rice, wheat, pork, eggs, chicken, soybean products and a variety of vegetables
- Methods of food preparation: stir-frying with lard, peanut oil, or sesame oil; seasoning with ginger, soy sauce, sesame seeds and monosodium glutamate
- Beverages: green tea; rare use of milk products because lactose intolerance is common

Religious Influences
- Some groups of Jews follow prescribed rules for preparing and serving foods (e.g., they eat only kosher meat and poultry and do not eat shellfish or any pork products).
- Mormons do not drink tea, coffee or alcohol.
- Hindus may be vegetarians.
- Seventh-Day Adventists may be lacto-ovo-vegetarians.
- Some Catholics do not eat meat on Ash Wednesday or Good Friday.

in older adults, especially in combination with age-related changes in nutrient intake and utilization. People with limited finances usually have a narrower selection of foods than do people with higher incomes. Lower socioeconomic status, including educational level, is associated also with lack of dental care and more tooth loss. According to the 2011 Canadian Community Health Survey, 6.3% of all older Canadians living alone experienced food insecurity (severe, moderate or minimal). The highest rates of food insecurity occur in Nunavut and the Maritime provinces (Tarasuk et al., 2013).

Environmental Factors

Environmental factors affect the enjoyment of food and the ability to obtain and prepare it. Many barriers to food enjoyment have been identified in the dining environments of long-term care facilities and other institutional settings. Older adults in congregate housing and long-term care facilities may find it difficult to adjust to unfamiliar environments. Moreover, they may not desire the mealtime social interaction that is part of the institutional environment. A noisy or crowded dining room may have a negative impact on food enjoyment and consumption. Such an environment may be particularly stressful for older adults who use hearing aids or who are accustomed to eating alone. The potential outcomes of a move to a new environment include poor nutrition and loss of interest in eating, particularly during the initial adjustment period.

Environmental influences, such as inclement weather conditions, can affect functionally impaired older adults who live in their own homes. For example, older persons who walk to the store or depend on public transportation may be unable or unwilling to obtain groceries in snowy or rainy weather. Likewise, older adults may not be able to tolerate hot or humid conditions, especially if transportation is not readily available. People who depend on others for transportation or who have difficulty manoeuvring in adverse weather conditions are likely to shop for groceries less frequently and to purchase their groceries at smaller convenience stores, where prices are higher and selection is limited. The additional cost and limited selection may interfere with food intake and lead to nutrient deficiencies. Finally, environmental conditions and packaging trends in the grocery store may create additional difficulties for older people, especially those who are functionally impaired. For example, the combined glare of fluorescent lights; highly polished floors; shiny, clear wrappers; and white freezer cases often make it extremely difficult, if not impossible, for older adults with vision changes to read labels, especially when the print is small and contrasts poorly against the background.

Behaviours Based on Myths and Misunderstandings

Myths and misunderstandings may be detrimental to a person's food intake and behaviours related to bowel function. For example, during the 1950s and 1960s, a widely held belief was that roughage and raw fruits or vegetables were harmful to the older person. It is now known that lack of roughage in the diet and consumption of only cooked fruits and vegetables are eating patterns that contribute to constipation by slowing the transit time of feces through the large intestine. Another commonly held belief is that a daily bowel movement is the norm for good digestive function. Rigid adherence to this standard may, in fact, lead to the unnecessary and detrimental use of laxatives. Advertisements have further reinforced this false belief by implying that daily bowel movements should be attained through medication. Although recent advertising trends emphasize the achievement of healthy bowel patterns through the ingestion of high-fibre food items, the negative impact of long-term beliefs may be difficult to overcome.

Misunderstandings about fluid intake may also interfere with digestion and nutrition. Many older adults reduce the amount of liquids they consume in an attempt to decrease the incidence of urinary incontinence. Fluid intake may also be restricted if functional limitations, such as impaired mobility or manual dexterity, interfere with either the ability to obtain liquids or the ease of urinary elimination. Reduced fluid intake can have a number of detrimental consequences, such as constipation, xerostomia and diminished food enjoyment.

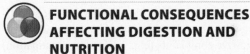

Wellness Opportunity

Nurses identify myths and misunderstandings about constipation and teach older adults about habits that promote healthy elimination patterns.

FUNCTIONAL CONSEQUENCES AFFECTING DIGESTION AND NUTRITION

Functional consequences affect the following aspects of digestion and nutrition of older adults:
- Procurement, preparation and enjoyment of food
- Mastication and digestion of food
- Nutritional status
- Psychosocial function

Negative functional consequences occur primarily because of the many risk factors that affect older adults, rather than because of age-related changes alone.

Ability to Procure, Prepare and Enjoy Food

Activities involved in procuring, preparing, consuming and enjoying food depend on the skills of cognition, balance, mobility and manual dexterity, as well as on the five senses. Food procurement depends on getting to the grocery store, pushing a shopping cart, reaching for food items on high shelves, reading the small print on shelves and food packages for cost and nutrition information and coping with the glare of bright lights, especially in the frozen-food sections. Age-related changes and conditions that may interfere with these activities include vision impairments and any illness, such as arthritis, that limits mobility, balance or manual dexterity.

Food preparation activities that are likely to be more difficult for older adults include cutting food items, measuring ingredients accurately, carrying food and liquid without spilling, standing for long periods in the kitchen, reaching for items on high shelves and in cupboards, safely using the oven or stove and reading the temperature controls correctly. Impairments of vision, balance, cognition, mobility or manual dexterity are likely to cause difficulties in performing these tasks.

Diminished sensory function can affect food enjoyment in all the following ways:

- Inaccurate perception of colour, taste or smell can interfere with appetite and food appeal.
- Diminished gustatory and olfactory sensitivity may lead to excessive use of condiments and seasonings, such as salt and sugar.
- Visual, olfactory and gustatory impairments may make it difficult to detect spoiled food.

Moreover, food choices are influenced by the condition of the oral cavity and teeth, as well as by the quantity and the quality of natural or replacement teeth.

> **Wellness Opportunity**
>
> Nurses promote wellness through interventions that improve the older adult's independence in procuring and preparing satisfying meals.

Changes in Oral Function

Digestive processes in healthy older adults are not significantly affected by age-related changes, but older adults often have digestive complaints (e.g., heartburn, constipation) caused by commonly occurring risk factors. For example, many negative functional consequences are associated with medications (see Table 18-2). Xerostomia causes negative functional consequences because it can interfere with oral comfort, food enjoyment and taste sensitivity. In addition, diminished saliva production makes it more difficult to chew food and increases the susceptibility of the teeth and tongue to bacterial action. Poor oral care increases the risk for gingivitis, oral lesions, dental caries, excessive plaque, periodontal disease and impaired taste. The functional consequences of being edentulous or using dentures include avoidance of certain foods, decreased chewing efficiency and increased risk for malnutrition (Cousson et al., 2012). Studies find that a combination of complete well-fitting dentures and dietary counselling improve the nutritional status of edentulous people (Prakash et al., 2012).

Poor Nutritional Status and Weight Changes

Because older adults need fewer calories, a deficiency of essential minerals or vitamins is likely to occur if the quantity of calories is reduced without a corresponding increase in the quality of the food consumed. In addition, risk factors (e.g., medications and pathologic processes) that commonly occur in older adults often cause nutrient deficiencies. For example, iron deficiency is associated with chronic diseases and low socioeconomic status. Specific nutrients that are likely to be deficient in older adults in Canada include fibre, calcium, zinc, magnesium and vitamins A and D (Health Canada, 2012). These nutrient deficiencies are due to the Canadian diet, which is often rich in calories and fat content, but deficient in fibre, fish, milk and vegetable intake. See Table 18-1 for examples of nutrient deficiencies and associated risk factors and functional consequences that are likely to affect older adults.

A type of malnutrition that is common in frail older adults is **protein-energy malnutrition** (also called *protein-calorie malnutrition*), which occurs when the intake of calories and protein is less than the amount required to meet daily needs. Studies indicate that between 20% and 85% of nursing home residents meet the criteria for malnutrition and half of nursing home residents have risk factors for malnutrition (Bocock & Keller, 2009; Torma et al., 2013). There is also a high prevalence of malnutrition in hospitalized older Canadians, ranging between 40% and 69% (Allard, 2012); yet, malnutrition is often not diagnosed in hospitals (Bocock & Keller, 2009). This condition is associated with a high-carbohydrate, low-protein diet, in combination with one or several of the risk factors already discussed. A systematic review of studies identified the following conditions that were most consistently associated with malnutrition among nursing home residents: depression, immobility, poor oral intake, cognitive or functional impairment, dependency in eating and problems with chewing and swallowing (Stange et al., 2013; Tamura et al., 2013).

Characteristics of mild or moderate protein-energy malnutrition include weakness, lethargy, unintentional weight loss, diminished muscle mass, decrease in subcutaneous fat and impaired ability to respond to physiologic stresses (e.g., surgery, infection). If the condition progresses, functional consequences of malnutrition include frailty, marked cognitive and functional impairment, increased risk of falls and shorter life expectancy. A study of nutritional risk among older cognitively intact Canadians revealed that women were more likely to be nutritionally at risk than were men, particularly those aged 75 years and older. Furthermore, older Canadians who moderately to severely physically disabled were more likely to be nutritionally at risk (44% as compared with 27%), and seniors who were depressed were almost double the likelihood to be nutritionally at risk than those who were not (66% compared with 33%) (Ramage-Morin & Garriguet, 2013).

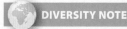 **DIVERSITY NOTE**

A nutritional screening study of nonagenarians in the community and nursing homes found a significant risk of malnutrition in women (Vandewoude & Van Gossum, 2013).

Age-related changes in body composition and carbohydrate metabolism contribute to gradual weight gains. The proportion of body fat to lean tissue begins to increase around 30 years of age and leads to disproportionately increased abdominal fat during later adulthood. This pattern of fat distribution is associated with increased risk for diabetes, cardiovascular disease and other chronic conditions. The gradually increasing prevalence of obesity is a major public health concern for all population groups, and continues to be prevalent among older adults between the ages of 65–74, as illustrated in Figure 18-1. Even though there is some evidence that the **body mass index (BMI)** standards should be increased for older adults, abdominal obesity as measured by waist circumference is an independent risk factor for many serious chronic conditions.

See ONLINE LEARNING ACTIVITY 18-3: ADDITIONAL INFORMATION AND CASE STUDY ABOUT NUTRITIONAL DEFICIENCIES AND UNINTENTIONAL WEIGHT LOSS at http://thepoint.lww.com/Miller7e

Quality of Life

Good food and nutrition are important components of health-related quality of life in many ways. Food-related activities are often a focal point of celebrations, religious rituals or gatherings to share significant events. In addition, mealtimes are typically associated with caring, comfort, nurturing and social interaction. Thus, when mealtime enjoyment is diminished, the psychosocial aspects of eating are also affected. Older adults who enjoyed participating in family meals or eating in restaurants may withdraw from these activities if food is no longer enjoyable. Similarly, when these events are no longer part of life for older adults, they may lose interest in eating.

> **Wellness Opportunity**
>
> Nurses can work with older adults to identify ways of promoting positive social interaction during mealtimes.

Perhaps even more detrimental than the psychosocial consequences of diminished food enjoyment are the psychosocial effects of inadequate nutrition. When fluid or nutrient intake is inadequate, older adults are likely to develop malnutrition and dehydration because of impaired homeostatic mechanisms. Changes in mental status, including memory impairment, are among the early signs of malnutrition, dehydration and electrolyte imbalance in older adults. Sometimes these mental changes are attributed incorrectly to irreversible conditions (e.g., dementia) rather than to a treatable and reversible nutritional deficiency (e.g., vitamins B_{12} or D).

PATHOLOGIC CONDITIONS AFFECTING DIGESTIVE WELLNESS: CONSTIPATION

Constipation, which is defined as "decrease in normal frequency of defecation accompanied by difficult or incomplete passage of stool and/or passage of excessively hard, dry

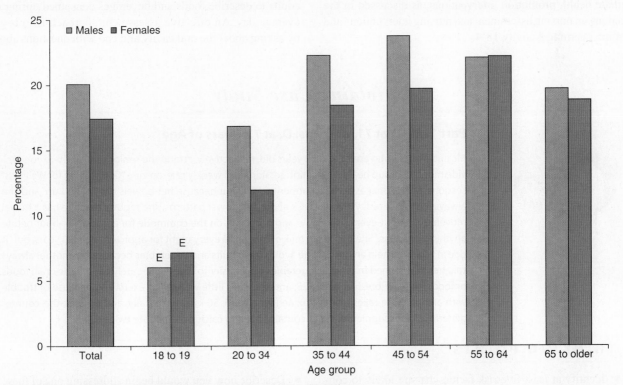

Note: E: Use with caution (coefficient of variation 16.6% to 33.3%)

FIGURE 18-1 Percentage who were obese (self-reported), by age group and sex, household population aged 18 or older, Canada 2013

stool" (Herdman, 2012, p. 203), is one of the most common pathologic conditions associated with digestion. The normal frequency for bowel movements, which shows significant individual variation but does not necessarily change with aging, ranges from three times daily to once or twice weekly. Another characteristic is that persons experience a feeling of incomplete evacuation after a bowel movement. Prevalence of constipation in older adults within North America is anywhere between 2% and 27% of individuals living in the community (depending upon how constipation is defined) (Pinto Sanchez & Bercik, 2011) and is considered to be higher within the older adult population. For those livening in institutional settings, the prevalence rate is as high as 75% to 80% (McKay et al., 2012).

Although constipation is a common complaint of older adults, it is caused by risk factors rather than age-related changes alone. A small slowing of food transit through the gastrointestinal tract may predispose older adults to constipation, but dietary patterns that include adequate fibre and fluid will compensate for this age-related change. Risk factors common in older adults include functional impairments (e.g., diminished mobility), pathologic conditions (e.g., hypothyroidism), adverse medication effects (including long-term laxative abuse) and poor dietary habits (e.g., inadequate intake of bulk, fibre and fluid). Risk factors associated with constipation include female sex, older age, higher BMI, limited physical activity, inadequate diet, lower socioeconomic status and history of chronic constipation (McKay et al., 2012; Mugie et al., 2011). Because constipation occurs so commonly in older adults, nurses assess for risk factors and initiate health promotion interventions, as discussed in the sections on nursing assessment and nursing interventions and Online Learning Activity 18-4.

 See **ONLINE LEARNING ACTIVITY 18-4: EVIDENCE-BASED INFORMATION AND MANAGEMENT OF CONSTIPATION** at http://thepoint.lww.com/Miller7e

NURSING ASSESSMENT OF DIGESTION AND NUTRITION

Nurses assess digestion and nutrition to identify (1) effects of age-related changes on digestion, nutrition and eating patterns; (2) risk factors that interfere with optimal nutrition; (3) cultural factors that influence eating patterns; (4) nutritional status and usual eating patterns and (5) negative functional consequences of altered digestion or inadequate nutrition. This nursing assessment is used to identify opportunities for health promotion interventions.

Interviewing About Digestion and Nutrition

Opportunities for health promotion are identified by asking about the following:
- Usual eating patterns and nutrient intake
- Health behaviours associated with oral care
- Age-related changes and risk factors that affect nutritional needs or digestive processes
- Environmental or social support factors that affect the procurement, preparation and enjoyment of food
- Symptoms of gastrointestinal dysfunction

Assess the adequacy of nutrient intake by asking older adults to describe foods and beverages consumed during an average day. An effective assessment approach is to begin by asking about the oral cavity and end with questions about

Unfolding Case Study

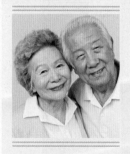

Part 1: Mr. D at 71, and Mrs. D. at 72, Years of Age

Mr. and Mrs. D., who are 71 and 72 years old, respectively, attend the senior centre where you provide monthly group health education sessions and weekly one-on-one "Counselling for Wellness" sessions. Mrs. D. makes an appointment to see you because her bowels get "bound up" and she always feels "bloated." When you ask about her bowel patterns, she reports that she has a bowel movement "about every other day" and has to "sit on the commode for a good half-hour before anything happens." She has taken milk of magnesia every night for approximately 20 years, but "it doesn't seem to help anymore." She avoids fresh fruits and vegetables because her mother always told her that canned fruits and vegetables were easier to digest. She rarely eats whole grain foods or foods high in fibre. Her BMI is 25, and she does little walking or exercising because of trouble with arthritis. She takes levothyroxine (Synthroid), 50 mcg once daily, and an over-the-counter generic calcium supplement that contains 500 mg calcium carbonate twice daily.

THINKING POINTS

- Identify at least five risk factors that are likely to contribute to Mrs. D.'s constipation.

- Describe how you would begin addressing one of these risk factors in health education.

bowel elimination, including questions related to risks for constipation and poor nutrition. Box 18-4 summarizes interview questions for a nursing assessment of nutrition and digestion in older adults.

Wellness Opportunity

Nurses promote personal responsibility by asking older adults to keep a 7-day diary of food and beverage intake and eating patterns and reviewing this to identify strengths and weaknesses of their diet.

Using Physical Assessment and Laboratory Information

Physical assessment and laboratory data provide important additional information for assessing the older adult's nutritional and hydration status. Height, weight and BMI provide important clues to nutritional status. The BMI—a measure of body composition related to body fat—is commonly used as an indicator of malnutrition (when it is low) and risk for disease (when it is high). Healthy BMI is between 18.5 and 24.9 kg/m² for adults. Although there is no benefit to severe obesity, studies indicate that a BMI of 30 or more may be healthy for adults older than age 65 (Bahat et al., 2012; Veronese et al., 2013). One review of studies found that optimal BMI for longer life expectancy in people older than age 70 is in the range of 25 to 30; however, this is higher than the ideal BMI associated with optimal function and lack of disability (Soenen & Chapman, 2013). Thus it is imperative to consider the BMI in relation to overall health and risk factors, additional assessment findings and long-term patterns. Also, keep in mind that a high BMI does not eliminate the possibility of risk for malnutrition. For example, one study of community-living adults aged 75 and above found that one third of those identified as at risk for malnutrition had a BMI of 25 or more and only 13% had a BMI in the underweight category (Winter et al., 2013).

Nurses need to consider individual circumstances in relation to ideal body weight because standardized tables do not necessarily provide the most realistic or appropriate goal for older adults. Rather, for many older adults, maintenance of a stable weight may be more important because patterns of weight loss and gain are important indicators of overall health condition. Weight loss is considered in relation to percentage of loss, which is calculated by subtracting current weight from usual weight and dividing that by the usual weight—for example, (72.5 kg − 54.4 kg) / 72.5 kg = 18.1 kg / 72.5 kg, or a 25% weight loss. An unintentional weight loss of more than 5% of body weight in 1 month or more than 10% in 6 months is considered a significant indicator of poor nutrition. In long-term care facilities, unintentional weight loss is an indicator of quality of care provided by the facility.

Assessment of hydration status is based on physical assessment observations and blood and urine tests. Physical indicators of dehydration include muscle weakness, speech difficulties, dry tongue with longitudinal furrows and dry

Box 18-4 Guidelines for Assessing Digestion and Nutrition

Assessing Oral Comfort and Chewing Ability

- Do you have any difficulty with soreness or bleeding in your mouth?
- Do you have any teeth that hurt, are loose or are sensitive to hot or cold temperatures?
- Do your gums bleed?
- Do you have any problems chewing or swallowing food or liquids? *If yes, ask about particular types of food or liquids that are problematic.*
- Are there foods you avoid because of problems with chewing or swallowing?
- Does your mouth or tongue ever feel dry?

Assessing Dental Habits and Attitudes Toward Dental Care

- How often do you see a dentist?
- When is the last time you had dental care?
- Where do you go for dental care?
- If the person does not seek dental care at least once per year: What prevents you from seeing the dentist?
- How do you care for your teeth?
- Do you use dental floss? If yes: How often? If no: Have you ever been taught to use dental floss?

Assessing Nutritional Needs

- Do you have diabetes, heart disease or any condition that requires dietary modifications?
- Do you have any food allergies?
- What medications do you take?
- What is your usual daily activity pattern?

Identifying Patterns of Food Procurement

- How do you get your grocery shopping done?
- Do you have any help getting to the store?
- Where and how often do you do your grocery shopping?
- What is your usual food budget?
- Do you have any difficulty getting food because of problems with vision, walking or transportation?

Identifying Patterns of Food Preparation and Consumption

- Where do you eat your meals?
- With whom do you eat?
- Does anyone help you prepare your meals?
- Do you have any trouble fixing your meals (e.g., difficulty opening containers)?
- Do you have any difficulties getting around your kitchen, using appliances or reaching the cupboards?
- Have there been recent changes in your eating or food preparation patterns (e.g., loss of eating companion or change in caregiver situation)?

Assessing Patterns of Bowel Elimination

- How often do you have a bowel movement?
- Have you noticed any recent changes in your pattern of bowel movements?
- Do you have any difficulty with your bowel movements? (e.g., Do you strain with bowel movements? or Is the stool hard, dry or difficult to pass?)
- Do you ever have problems with loose stools or diarrhea?
- Do you take laxatives or any other products to help you move your bowels?
- Do you ever have pain or bleeding when you move your bowels?

and pale oral mucous membranes (Mentes & Kang, 2013). Dark coloured, scant amounts of, and highly concentrated urine (i.e., specific gravity above 1.029) are other indicators of dehydration. Blood values that may be elevated in dehydration include sodium, hematocrit, hemoglobin, creatinine, osmolality and blood urea nitrogen. Laboratory data can provide clues to nutritional deficiencies, even before any clinical signs are evident; however, test results must be evaluated in relation to persons' overall health status. For instance, low serum albumin is an indicator of poor nutrition, but it also occurs with trauma, edema, infection and neoplasm. Box 18-5 summarizes information about physical assessment indicators and laboratory values that are especially important in assessing the nutritional status of older adults. Additional

Box 18-5 Physical Assessment and Laboratory Data

Examination of the Oral Cavity

- Inspect the oral cavity by using a tongue depressor and a light.
- Observe for evidence of oral disease, including pain, lumps, soreness, bleeding, swelling, loose teeth and abraded areas.
- Note the presence or absence of teeth, dentures and partial bridges.

Normal Findings

- Lips: pink, moist, symmetrical
- Teeth: intact, without cavities or tartar
- Gums: pink, no bleeding
- Mucous membranes: pink, moist
- Tongue: pink, moist, presence of numerous varicosities on undersurface
- Pharynx: soft palate rises slightly when "ahh" is vocalized.

Indicators of Nutritional Deficiency

- Lips: dry, fissured, cracked at corners
- Teeth: decayed or missing
- Gums: red, swollen, recessed, spongy or prone to bleeding
- Mucous membranes: dry, ulcerated, inflamed, bleeding, white patches
- Tongue: dry, swollen, reddened or very smooth

Examination of the Abdomen and Rectum

- Examine the abdomen with the person lying comfortably in the supine position.
- Perform a rectal examination with the person in the side-lying position.

Normal Findings

- Symmetrical, soft abdomen that moves with respirations
- Audible bowel sounds (heard through the diaphragm of a stethoscope) occurring at irregular intervals (5 to 15 seconds apart)
- Smooth skin around anus; no evidence of hemorrhoids, fissures, inflammation or rectal prolapse
- Soft, brown stool that tests negative for occult blood

Indicators of Nutritional Deficiency

- Swollen abdomen
- Stool that tests positive for occult blood

General Physical Assessment Indicators of Malnutrition

- Weight loss
- Lack of subcutaneous fat
- Diminished size and strength of muscles
- Skin that is dry, rough or tissue thin
- Abnormal pulse or blood pressure
- Edema, especially in the face or lower extremities
- Hair that is dry, dull, thin, brittle or sparse
- Dry or dull-looking eyes
- Listless, apathetic or depressed mood
- Difficulty with walking or maintaining balance

Laboratory Data

- Biochemical data that will provide information about nutritional status: serum ferritin, complete blood count, vitamin B_{12}, vitamin D [25(OH)D], complete lipid profile, and serum albumin, glucose, sodium, magnesium and potassium levels
- Urinalysis results should be within the normal adult range, except for a slight decrease in the upper limit for specific gravity.

Indicators of Nutritional Deficiency

- Anemia
- Lymphocytopenia
  - Serum 25-hydroxyvitamin D level <30 nmol/L
- Serum albumin level of <35 g/L
- Cholesterol levels of <4.14 mmol/L
- Total iron-binding capacity <44.75 μmol/L

indicators of nutrient deficiencies are listed in Table 18-1 in the column describing functional consequences.

See ONLINE LEARNING ACTIVITY 18-5: EVIDENCE-BASED INFORMATION AND CASE STUDY ABOUT DEHYDRATION AND HYDRATION MANAGEMENT at http://thepoint.lww.com/Miller7e

Observing Cues to Digestion and Nutrition

Assess oral health by observing all components of the mouth and oral cavity and pay particular attention to indicators of oral hygiene and the need for dental care, as described in Box 18-6. Observe eating patterns and environments for cues to digestion and nutrition, and consider social and cultural factors that influence eating and nutrition. Box 18-7 summarizes observations and cultural considerations that are pertinent to the nursing assessment of digestion and nutrition. Nursing assessment of chewing and swallowing is especially important for older adults at risk for dysphagia, as discussed previously and described in Box 18-7.

Wellness Opportunity

Nurses observe environmental conditions to identify positive or negative effects on eating patterns.

Using Assessment Tools

Nutrition assessment tools are used for identifying individuals at risk for dehydration and nutritional problems so

Box 18-6 Evidence-Based Practice: Oral Health Care for Older Adults

Statement of the Problem

- Oral health is essential for promoting overall health, preventing disease, maintaining speech and alimentary functioning, and preserving quality of life.
- Even though regular oral care is essential for good health, it is often neglected as an aspect of care for older adults.
- Oral hygiene declines as older adults experience cognitive and functional impairments and become increasingly dependent in daily activities.
- Oral problems are not the direct result of aging and can be prevented or at least detected at an early stage.
- Medications and medical conditions can increase the risk for oral problems, even when good oral care is provided.
- Dental caries and periodontal disease are plaque-related and preventable oral diseases that are likely to develop from poor oral hygiene.
- When untreated, poor oral health leads to malnutrition, dehydration, pneumonia, cardiovascular disease, joint infections and poor diabetic control.

Recommendations for Nursing Assessment

- Make use of the 10-item Kayser-Jones Brief Oral Health Status Examination, an evidence-based tool for assessing and rating the following aspects of oral health in older adults: lymph nodes, lips, tongue, mouth and cheek tissue, gums, saliva, condition of natural and artificial teeth, chewing position of teeth and oral cleanliness (available at http://consultgerirn.org).
- Recognize assessment findings that indicate the need for a dental evaluation and follow-up immediately including enlarged and tender lymph nodes; lips red at corners; discoloration, break in integrity, or an abnormality of any oral tissue that has been present for 2 weeks or more; more than 1 loose, broken, or missing tooth; redness at borders around teeth; redness or soreness under artificial teeth; fewer than 4 teeth in either jaw; 7 or fewer pairs of teeth in chewing position; and dentures missing, not being worn or damaged.
- Assess self-care ability of older adults related to effective oral care, and involve occupational therapy services as appropriate.

Recommendations for Nursing Interventions

- Use toothbrush with soft nylon bristles and a toothpaste with fluoride.
- Provide oral care (for teeth and dentures) morning, evening and as needed.
- Brush teeth, dentures and tongue.
- Plain foam swabs can be used for cleaning oral mucous membrane of an edentulous adult, but they are not as effective as toothbrushes for cleaning teeth.
- Never use lemon-glycerin swabs because they dry the mucous membrane and erode tooth enamel.
- Mouth rinses that contain alcohol dry the mucous membrane and should be diluted in half with water if they are used.
- Use chlorhexidine (e.g., Peridex) only if it is prescribed by a dentist.
- Brush dentures before placing them in a denture cup.
- Arrange for at least annual dental evaluations and more frequent evaluations if problems are identified.

Additional Recommendations for Nursing Interventions for People With Dementia

- If the person resists oral care, consider that oral pain is the cause of the resistance.
- Develop an individualized oral care plan that includes specific communication techniques (e.g., avoid elderspeak, approach person at eye level) and care strategies (e.g., demonstrating, task segmentation) for each person.
- Teach all nursing staff about the individualized care plan and involve family caregivers as appropriate.
- Arrange for more frequent dental examinations if it is difficult to provide adequate oral hygiene.

Sources: Johnson and Schoenfelder (2012); Legg, T. J. (2012). Oral care in older adults with dementia: Challenges and approaches. *Journal of Gerontological Nursing*, 38(8), 10–13.; O'Connor (2012); Taub, L.-F. (2012). *Try this: Best practices in nursing care to older adults, Oral Health Assessment of Older Adults: The Kayser Jones Brief Oral Health Status Examination (BOHSE)* (No. 18). Retrieved from www.ConsultGeriRN.org.

 Box 18-7 Behavioural Cues to Nutrition and Digestion

Observations to Assess Oral Health

- What is the condition of lips, teeth, gums, tongue and oral mucous membrane?
- Does the person have a sufficient number of teeth and/or use of full or partial dentures?
- How well do dentures fit?
- What are the features of oral care items, for example, condition of toothbrush, type of toothbrush or denture cleaning supplies, use of floss?

Observations to Assess Eating Patterns

- Does the person seem to enjoy eating meals with others, or does the presence of other people seem to interfere with mealtime enjoyment?
- If the person has dentures, are they worn at meals? If not, why not?
- What are the person's between-meal food and fluid consumption patterns?
- Are enjoyable noncaffeinated liquids readily available for between-meal fluid intake?
- What cultural influences affect the person's food preferences and preparation?

Observations to Assess the Eating Environment

- Do environmental or social influences negatively affect mealtime enjoyment (e.g., a noisy dining room or disruptive mealtime companions)?
- If the person eats alone, is this the best arrangement or should consideration be given to providing mealtime social interaction?

Cultural Considerations That May Influence Nutrition and Eating Patterns

- What are the usual patterns of meals eaten (e.g., content, frequency, timing)? What is the usual social context of meals?
- Are there any culturally influenced food taboos or preferences? (Refer to Cultural Considerations 18-3.)
- Are there any special foods that are important because of religious or cultural factors? (If yes, are they accessible to the older adult?)
- Are certain foods or beverages avoided or preferred in relation to an illness or chronic condition (e.g., foods or beverages that are considered yin-and-yang foods)?
- Is there a preference for the temperature of beverages (e.g., use of iced or heated beverages)?
- Is the person's ethnic background likely to increase his or her chance of being lactose intolerant? (Prevalence is highest among Asians, First Nations people and African Canadians and lowest among whites of northern European descent.)

that preventive and therapeutic interventions can be implemented. The **Mini Nutritional Assessment (MNA)** is an evidence-based tool that has been widely used since 1990 in a variety of settings. A revised short-form, called the MNA-SF, was validated in 2009 as a standalone screening tool with six questions to identify individuals as malnourished, at risk for malnourishment or normally nourished. The MNA-SF is now widely used in clinical and research settings because of its validation, reliability, ease of use, low cost, acceptability, effectiveness and availability in many languages (Dent et al., 2012; Skates & Anthony, 2012). This tool is illustrated in Figure 18-2 and additional information and resources are described in Online Learning Activity 18-6. Because of the high prevalence and serious consequences of nutritional deficits in older adults, routine screening for malnutrition or risks for malnutrition is recommended for all older adults in long-term care facilities (Volkert, 2013).

See **ONLINE LEARNING ACTIVITY 18-6: ASSESSING NUTRITIONAL STATUS IN OLDER ADULTS** at http://thepoint.lww.com/Miller7e

NURSING DIAGNOSIS

The nursing assessment may identify problems related to nutrition, digestion or oral health. If nutritional deficits are identified, a pertinent nursing diagnosis is Imbalanced Nutrition: Less Than Body Requirements, defined as "intake of nutrients insufficient to meet metabolic needs" (Herdman, 2012, p. 174). Related factors that may affect older adults include cognitive or functional impairments, medications, anorexia, depression, chewing or swallowing difficulties, social isolation and inability to procure or prepare food.

If the nursing assessment identifies constipation or risks for constipation, the applicable nursing diagnosis is Constipation. The nursing assessment may also identify certain oral health problems that are common in older adults. These include xerostomia, medication effects, chewing difficulties, periodontal disease, diminished taste sensation, ill-fitting dentures, inadequate oral hygiene and broken or missing teeth. A relevant nursing diagnosis to address these problems would be Impaired Oral Mucous Membrane. Risk for Aspiration is an appropriate nursing diagnosis for older adults who have any difficulty chewing or swallowing.

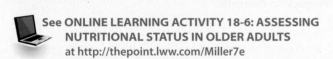

Unfolding Case Study

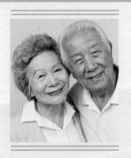

Part 2: Mr. D. at 75, and Mrs. D. at 76, Years of Age

Recall that you are the nurse at the senior centre attended by Mr. and Mrs. D., who now are 75 and 76 years old, respectively. During a "Counselling for Health" session, Mrs. D. asks your advice about her gradual unintended weight loss over the past few months. Although Mrs. D. continues to cook meals because her husband enjoys eating, she states that food no longer appeals to her. You notice that her mouth is very dry and her teeth are in poor condition. She had a stroke 2 years ago and recovered well except for some dysphagia and right-sided weakness. Her BMI is 18. She takes an antidepressant and two blood pressure medications but does not know the names of the pills. She asks what she can do about the weight loss.

THINKING POINTS

- What risk factors are likely to be contributing to Mrs. D.'s weight loss?
- Make a list of assessment questions you would use with Mrs. D. Select applicable questions from Box 18-4 and list any additional questions that you would use for further assessment.

- What would you ask Mrs. D. to do to provide additional assessment information so that you can plan some teaching interventions?

QSEN APPLICATION

QSEN Competency	Knowledge/Skill/Attitude	Application to Mrs. D. When She is 76 Years of Age
Patient-centred care	(K) Integrate understanding of multiple dimensions of patient-centred care. (S) Elicit patient values, preferences and expressed needs. (S) Provide patient-centred care with sensitivity and respect for diversity of the human experience.	Identify the many interacting factors (including physical and psychosocial conditions) that are likely to contribute to Mrs. D.'s unintentional weight loss. Use a nonjudgmental approach to explore potential reasons for Mrs. D.'s poor oral care and depression.

Mini Nutritional Assessment
MNA®

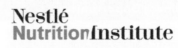

Last name: _____   First name: _____

Sex: _____ Age: _____ Weight, kg: _____ Height, cm: _____ Date: _____

Complete the screen by filling in the boxes with the appropriate numbers. Total the numbers for the final screening score.

Screening

A Has food intake declined over the past 3 months due to loss of appetitie, digestive problems, chewing or swallowing difficulties?
0 = severe decrease in food intake
1 = moderate decrease in food intake
2 = no decrease in food intake   ☐

B Weight loss during the last 3 months
0 = weight loss greater than 3 kg (6.6 lbs)
1 = does not know
2 = weight loss between 1 and 3 kg (2.2 and 6.6 lbs)
3 = no weight loss   ☐

C Mobility
0 = bed or chair bound
1 = able to get out of bed / chair but does not go out
2 = goes out   ☐

D Has suffered psychological stress or acute disease in the past 3 months?
0 = yes   2 = no   ☐

E Neuropsychological problems
0 = severe dementia or depression
1 = mild dementia
2 = no psychological problems   ☐

F1 Body Mass Index (BMI) (weight in kg) / (height in m²)
0 = BMI less than 19
1 = BMI 19 to less than 21
2 = BMI 21 to less than 23
3 = BMI 23 or greater   ☐

IF BMI IS NOT AVAILABLE, REPLACE QUESTION F1 WITH QUESTION F2.
DO NOT ANSWER QUESTION F2 IF QUESTION F1 IS ALREADY COMPLETED.

F2 Calf circumference (CC) in cm
0 = CC less than 31
3 = CC 31 or greater   ☐

Screening score (max. 14 points)

12 – 14 points: Normal nutritional status
8 – 11 points: At risk of malnutrition
0 – 7 points: Malnourished   ☐☐

References
1. Vellas B, Villars H, Abellan G, *et al*. Overview of MNA®—Its History and Challenges. *J Nutr Health Aging.* 2006;**10**:456-465.
2. Rubenstein LZ, Harker JO, Salva A, Guigoz Y, Vellas B. Screening for Undernutrition in Geriatric Practice: Developing the Short-Form Mini Nutritional Assessment (MNA-SF). *J Geront.* 2001;**56A**:M366-377.
3. Guigoz Y. The Mini-Nutritional Assessment (MNA®) Review of the Literature—What does it tell us? *J Nutr Health Aging.* 2006;**10**:466-487.
4. Kaiser MJ, Bauer JM, Ramsch C, et al. Validation of the Mini Nutritional Assessment Short-Form (MNA®-SF): A practical tool for identification of nutritional status. *J Nutr Health Aging.* 2009;**13**:782-788.
® Société des Produits Nestlé, S.A., Vevey, Switzerland, Trademark Owners © Nestlé, 1994, Revision 2009. N67200 12/99 10M
For more information: www.mna-elderly.com

FIGURE 18-2 The Mini Nutritional Assessment-Short Form (MNA-SF). (From Nestlé Nutrition Services. Copyright Nestlé, 1994, Revision 2009. Retrieved from www.mna-elderly.com)

PLANNING FOR WELLNESS OUTCOMES

Nurses can apply the following Nursing Outcomes Classification (NOC) terms to address risk factors and promote improved nutrition in older adults: Appetite, Bowel Elimination, Knowledge: Diet, Nutritional Status, Oral Health, Self-Care: Oral Hygiene, Sensory Function: Taste and Smell, Swallowing Status, Weight: Body Mass. NOCs related to Constipation include Hydration, Bowel Elimination, Medication Response and Symptom Control.

NURSING INTERVENTIONS TO PROMOTE HEALTHY DIGESTION AND NUTRITION

Nurses can apply the following Nursing Interventions Classification (NIC) terminologies in care plans: Bowel Management, Health Education, Nutrition Management, Nutritional Counselling, Nutritional Monitoring, Oral Health Maintenance, Oral Health Promotion, Referral, Self-Care Assistance and Weight Management. Nursing interventions to promote healthy digestion and nutrition in older adults include health education about optimal nutrition and disease prevention and direct interventions to eliminate risk factors that interfere with digestion, nutrition and oral health.

Addressing Risk Factors That Interfere With Digestion and Nutrition

Nursing interventions address functional consequences of age-related changes that affect digestion and nutrition in all older adults. For example, if older adults experience early satiety during meals, they may benefit from eating five smaller meals a day, rather than the customary three meals a day. Similarly, teach older adults to maintain a sitting or upright position during eating and for ½ to 1 hour after eating to compensate for any effects of slowed swallowing.

When functional limitations interfere with the activities involved in procuring, preparing and enjoying food, interventions focus on improving the persons' access to palatable and nutritious meals. For the community-living older adults, this may involve identifying resources that offer assistance in obtaining food. An approach that has been used

to improve functioning in frail older adults living in their homes is to provide a commercially available protein-energy supplement containing 400 kcal of energy, 25 g of protein, 9.4 g of essential amino acids and 400 mL of water daily (Kim & Lee, 2013).

Home-delivered meal programs are widely available to older adults at minimal cost, and group meal programs are available in many cities within Canada. These programs are effective in reducing nutritional risk for community-living older adults (Institute of Medicine, 2012). In addition to providing inexpensive and nutritionally balanced meals, these programs provide opportunities for social interaction. Local agencies for older adults may provide assistance with transportation or grocery shopping and are an excellent source of information about group and home-delivered meal programs.

When environmental barriers, such as high cupboards, interfere with older adults' ability to prepare meals safely, environmental modifications can be made. Nurses can apply many of the environmental adaptations suggested in the chapters on vision (see Chapter 17) and mobility (see Chapter 22) to improve the ability of older persons to prepare meals. When older adults have functional impairments, nurses can suggest specially adapted items for improving independence in eating and food preparation, such as the ones illustrated in Figure 18-3.

In long-term care settings, the following interventions address risk factors related to eating:

- Plan seating arrangements in the dining area to improve social interaction and to minimize the negative effects of disruptive people.
- Use low- or no-sodium flavour enhancers (e.g., herbs and lemon).
- Provide good oral hygiene before meals.
- Provide easy access to fluids and nutritious snacks.

Provision of liquid nutritional supplements containing protein and essential micro-nutrients is an effective intervention for improving nutritional status in nursing home residents at risk for undernourishment (Lee et al., 2013).

When older adults need accurate information about preventing constipation, or when other risk factors (e.g., a low-fibre diet) interfere with good bowel function, nursing interventions are directed toward education. Daily use of bran cereals or bran mixed with other foods is a common and effective strategy for preventing constipation. Box 18-8 identifies some of the foods and other interventions that aid in preventing constipation.

When medications affect nutrition and digestion, nurses, caregivers or older adults can discuss this problem

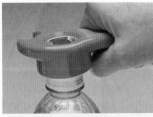
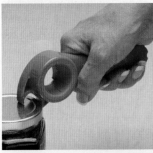
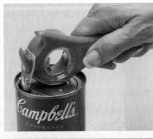

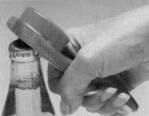
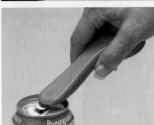

FIGURE 18-3 Adaptive devices. (Reprinted with permission of www.activeforever.com)

with prescribing health care practitioners to identify ways of alleviating this risk or addressing the consequences. If over-the-counter medications have a detrimental effect on nutrition or digestion, nurses educate older adults about medication–nutrient interactions and discuss ways of addressing the negative effects. Pharmacists help by suggesting interventions that will compensate for, or minimize, the effects of both prescription and over-the-counter medications on nutrition and digestion.

 Box 18-8   Health Education Regarding Constipation

- A bowel movement every day is not necessarily the norm for every adult.
- Each adult has an individual pattern of bowel regularity, with the normal range varying from 3 times a day to 2 times a week.
- Include several portions of the following high-fibre foods in your daily diet: fresh, uncooked fruits and vegetables; bran and other cereal products made from whole grains.
- Drink 8 to 10 glasses of noncaffeinated liquid, including fruit juices, every day.
- Avoid laxatives and enemas; instead, use dietary measures to promote good bowel functioning.
- If medication is needed to promote bowel regularity, a bulk-forming agent (e.g., psyllium or methylcellulose) is least likely to have detrimental effects, especially if fluid intake is adequate.
- Do not ignore the urge to defecate; try to respond as soon as you feel the urge.
- Exercise regularly.

When alcohol consumption interferes with nutrition, interventions might address the potential problem of alcoholism, or they may be aimed at compensating for the detrimental effects on nutrition. Nurses can recommend vitamin supplementation for people with a history of alcoholism after a medical evaluation has been performed to identify any underlying conditions, such as pernicious anemia.

See **ONLINE LEARNING ACTIVITY 18-7 ADDITIONAL INFORMATION ON CARE OF OLDER ADULTS AT RISK FOR MALNUTRITION** at http://thepoint.lww.com/Miller7e

Promoting Oral and Dental Health

Nurses have important responsibilities in implementing interventions to promote oral and dental health. If older adults have avoided dental care because of resignation to poor oral health or a poor understanding of the need for preventive dental care, nurses attempt to change these attitudes through education. Nurses also emphasize the importance of obtaining dental care every 6 months and, if appropriate, facilitate referrals for dental care. For homebound older adults, home dental services are often available, especially in large urban communities. There are also some mobile dental services for older adults living in long-term care facilities. In addition, low-cost dental services and dentures may be available through schools of dentistry. Nurses need to be familiar with local resources, so that they can inform older adults and their caregivers about the dental services that are available in their community. In long-term care settings, nurses are usually responsible for facilitating referrals for professional dental care every 6 to 12 months. For older adults in any setting, if xerostomia interferes with digestion or nutrition, nurses may suggest or facilitate a referral for a medical evaluation to identify disease processes or medication effects that may be contributing factors.

Good oral care is an essential, but often overlooked, component of daily nursing care for dependent older adults. In institutional settings, staff education about oral care, including information about the myths related to oral health and aging, is imperative (O'Connor, 2012). Evidence-based recommendations related to oral care are described in Box 18-6.

For independent older adults, nurses provide health education about oral care, including alleviation of dry mouth if this is pertinent, as described in Box 18-9. Older adults who have any impairment of manual dexterity can adapt handles of toothbrushes for ease of use or obtain specially designed brushes to increase the self-care abilities. Nurses can also suggest the use of battery-operated brushes, which are effective, easy to use and relatively inexpensive. Child-size toothbrushes (manual or automatic) may be easier to use for dependent older adults, especially if access to all their teeth is limited.

Wellness Opportunity

Nurses promote independence and self-care in oral hygiene by facilitating referrals for occupational therapy for older adults with functional impairments.

Box 18-9 Health Education Regarding Oral and Dental Care

Health Education Regarding Care of the Teeth and Gums

- Oral care should include daily use of dental floss and twice-daily brushing of all tooth surfaces.
- Use a soft-bristled toothbrush and fluoridated toothpaste.
- If you have any limitations that interfere with your ability to use a regular toothbrush, you may benefit from using an electric or battery-powered brush or a brush with a specially designed handle (available where medical supplies are sold).
- Easy-to-use floss aids are inexpensive and widely available for facilitating dental flossing; they are especially helpful for people with any limitations in manual strength or dexterity or limited range of motion in the upper extremities.
- Some mouth rinses have cleansing, antimicrobial and moisturizing effect, but they are used in conjunction with, not instead of, brushing.
- Avoid using alcohol-containing mouthwashes because of their drying effect.
- Because sugar is a major contributing factor to tooth decay, it is important to limit the intake of sugary substances, especially substances that are kept in the mouth for long periods (e.g., gum, hard candy).
- After eating sugar-containing foods, rinse your mouth or brush your teeth.
- Visit a dentist every 6 months for regular oral care.
- If partial or complete dentures are worn, remove them at night, keep them in water and clean them before placing them back in your mouth.

Health Education Regarding Dry Mouth

- Excessive dry mouth may be caused by medical conditions or medication effects and should be evaluated before symptomatic treatment is initiated.
- Drink at least 10 eight-ounce glasses of noncaffeinated fluid during the day, and drink sips of water at frequent intervals.
- Suck on xylitol-flavoured fluoride tablets or sugar-free hard candies to stimulate saliva flow.
- Chew sugar-free gum with xylitol for 15 minutes after meals to stimulate saliva flow and promote oral hygiene.
- Try using one of the many brands of saliva substitutes available at drugstores, but avoid those that contain sorbitol because this can worsen the condition.
- Avoid sucking lozenges containing citric acid because of their detrimental effects on tooth enamel.
- Avoid alcohol, alcohol-containing mouthwashes, and highly acidic drinks (e.g., orange or grapefruit juice) because these tend to exacerbate the condition.
- Avoid smoking because this exacerbates the symptoms and further irritates the oral mucous membranes.
- Pay particular attention to oral hygiene because a dry mouth increases the risk for gum and dental diseases.
- Maintain optimal room humidity, especially at night.

Promoting Optimal Nutrition and Preventing Disease

Therapeutic diets have long been recognized as essential interventions for diseases, such as diabetes and cardiovascular conditions, and in recent years, there is increasing recognition of the role nutrients play in preventing disease. For example, nutritional strategies are an essential component of improving wound healing and preventing pressure ulcers in frail older adults (Posthauer et al., 2013). Nutritional interventions for healthy aging emphasize the inclusion of foods containing antioxidants and other nutrients that may play a protective and preventive role. For example, diets rich in antioxidants and omega-3 fatty acids can prevent age-related macular degeneration (Sin et al., 2012). In analysing information about nutrients as preventive interventions, distinctions must be made between nutrients obtained from foods and those that are found in supplements. For example, a high dietary intake of a particular nutrient (e.g., carotenoids) may be beneficial in health promotion or disease prevention, but a dietary supplement product with the same nutrient may not necessarily have the same beneficial effects. Thus, nurses need to educate older adults about the importance of obtaining nutrients from food sources rather than relying primarily on dietary supplements.

Nurses teach older adults about basic nutritional requirements, using easy-to-understand educational materials. Recommendations for older adults, based on national dietary guidelines published, emphasize that older adults need to do the following:

- Increase intake of whole grains, dried peas and beans, all types of fruits and vegetables (especially dark green and orange vegetables).
- Consume fat-free or low-fat dairy products.
- Replace solid fats with oils, including those in fish, nuts and seeds.
- Consume less sodium and saturated fat.
- Consume less food and beverages with added sugar, solid fats and alcohol.
- Reduce caloric intake to maintain healthy weight (Eat Right Ontario, 2012).

Healthy older adults generally maintain optimal nutritional status through the daily intake of the foods listed in Box 18-10 and illustrated in Figure 18-4. If older adults have any illness or take any medications or chemicals that interfere with homeostasis, digestion or nutrition, the daily diet will have to be modified to compensate for these effects. If, for any reason, the food intake is inadequate to meet daily nutritional requirements, a broad-spectrum vitamin and mineral supplement may be used as necessary.

Wellness Opportunity

Nurses promote personal responsibility by suggesting that older adults use MyPlate, as shown in Figure 18-4, to identify beneficial and detrimental eating patterns.

Nutrition education can be provided on an individual basis or in group settings, perhaps with registered dietitians. In acute care settings, registered dietitians are usually available, but their services are often limited to people who have special dietary needs or an identified nutritional problem. In long-term care settings, a registered dietitian generally assesses the nutritional needs and usual eating patterns of older adults and establishes a plan of care aimed at attaining

Box 18-10 Guidelines for Daily Food Intake for Older Adults

- Because older adults need fewer calories but the same amount of nutrients, it is important to select a variety of high-quality foods and avoid "empty calories."
- Use salt, sugar and sodium only in moderation.
- Avoid saturated fats and replace solid fats with oils, including those in fish, nuts and seeds.
- Choose fibre-rich foods.
- Drink plenty of liquids without added sugars.

Servings and Food Group

Basic nutritional requirements will be met if the daily diet includes at least the minimum number of servings from each food group listed below and if it includes complex carbohydrates and high-fibre foods. Basic nutritional requirements are as follows:

- 6–7 Grain products, including bread, rice, pasta and cereal
- 7 Vegetables and fruits
- 2–3 Meat, fish, poultry or legumes (dried peas and beans, lentils, nut butters, soy products)
- 3 Nonfat or low-fat milk, cheese, yogurt and dairy desserts 8 or more 8-ounce glasses of water or other fluids that are low in added sugars

and maintaining optimal nutrition. In community settings, nurses sometimes provide nutrition education to groups of older adults. Nurses making home visits include nutrition education in their health teaching, make referrals for registered dietitian assessment and recommendations and use available community resources to supplement these interventions. Models of health promotion discussed in Chapter 5 can be applied to working with older adults toward improved nutrition and changes in eating patterns.

 See **ONLINE LEARNING ACTIVITY 18-8: RESOURCES FOR HEALTH PROMOTION RELATED TO NUTRITION IN OLDER ADULTS** at http://thepoint.lww.com/Miller7e

EVALUATING EFFECTIVENESS OF NURSING INTERVENTIONS

Nursing care for older adults with Imbalanced Nutrition: Less Than Body Requirements is evaluated by determining whether older adults have a daily nutrient intake that

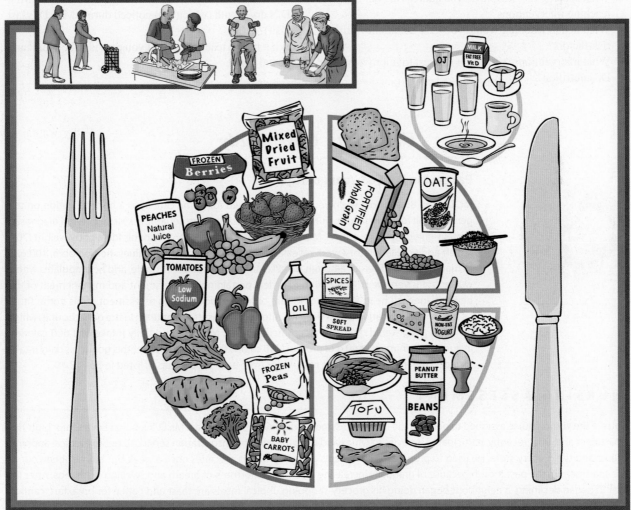

2011© TUFTS UNIVERSITY

FIGURE 18-4 MyPlate for older adults. (Reprinted with permission from Tufts University.)

corresponds with metabolic needs and by older adults' achieving a body weight within 110% of their ideal body weight. For older adults with constipation, or risks for constipation, evaluation criteria would depend on their verbalizing accurate information about constipation, identifying the factors that contribute to constipation and reporting that they pass soft stools on a regular basis without any straining or discomfort.

Unfolding Case Study

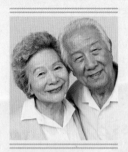

Part 3: Mrs. D. at 76 Years of Age

Mrs. D. returns for a "Counselling for Health" follow-up session with a 7-day diet history and a list of her medications, as you requested. You review the diet history and find that in response to your previous health education about constipation, Mrs. D. now uses whole-wheat bread instead of white and eats more fresh fruits and vegetables. You assess that her daily intake is only approximately 800 calories, of which pastries account for a high percentage. She rarely eats meat, perhaps because of the poor condition of her teeth. Her medications include levothyroxine (Synthroid) 50 mcg daily, citalopram (Celexa) 20 mg daily, clonidine (Catapres) 0.2 mg daily, triamterene 37.5 mg/hydrochlorothiazide 25 mg (Dyazide) daily and 500 mg calcium carbonate twice daily.

THINKING POINTS

- What specific risk factors do you address in your health teaching interventions?
- What health teaching would you give about alleviating risk factors?
- What interventions would you suggest to improve Mrs. D.'s nutrition?

- What interventions would you suggest to address Mrs. D.'s dry mouth (which you noticed during Mrs. D.'s last visit)?
- What health teaching would you provide about oral and dental care?

Unfolding Case Study

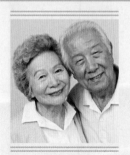

Part 4: Mr. D. at 85 Years of Age

Mr. D. is an 85-year-old widower who was referred for home care after a hospitalization on the geriatric unit for heart failure. During the hospitalization, the geriatric assessment team diagnosed protein-energy undernutrition. Mr. D.'s weight (52.6 kg) is only 75% of his ideal body weight (70.5 kg). In addition, laboratory work revealed the following abnormal values: hemoglobin, 100 g/L; hematocrit, .33 and serum albumin, 32 g/L. Mr. D.'s heart failure is stable, and he ambulates with a walker but is very weak. In addition to orders pertaining to assessment and management of the newly diagnosed heart failure, home care orders include nursing assessment of his home situation, nutrition education and weight monitoring. The assessment team in the geriatric unit, which included a registered dietitian, recommended that Mr. D. have a daily intake of 1,600 calories, including a minimum of 60 g of protein (240 calories). Mr. D. could meet this goal if his daily intake included the minimum number of servings from each food group as listed in Box 18-10.

NURSING ASSESSMENT

You are the visiting nurse assigned to perform the initial assessment and develop a care plan. Mr. D. lives alone in a senior high-rise apartment and, until recently, participated in social activities and used the senior transportation service to get to medical appointments and the grocery store. He used to prepare his own meals and shop for his groceries once a week but has not been out of his apartment in the past month because of gradually increasing weakness, shortness of breath and swelling in his legs. After his health began declining, a neighbour began doing his grocery shopping. Typical meals are toast and coffee for breakfast; canned soup, a deli meat sandwich and cookies for lunch; and a Budget Gourmet entrée for supper. Mr. D. says that he never really learned to cook very well but that he got along "well enough for a man my age." He says that he does not particularly enjoy the convenience foods that he eats but states, "They sure are easy to fix, even if they are boring." Mr. D. acknowledges that he has thought about going to the daily noon meal offered at a nearby church but has not followed through because "the senior van doesn't go there, but it does go to the grocery store. Besides, I'm never very hungry because food just doesn't interest me the way it used to when I had Magda's good Hungarian cooking." Mr. D. reports a gradual weight loss of approximately 22.7 kg since his wife died 2 years ago. He says that he was too heavy when his wife used to do the cooking, so he is not concerned about his weight loss. He has full dentures but has not used them for the past year because they are loose and uncomfortable. He has not done anything about his dentures because he manages to chew soft foods and his dentist retired several years ago.

NURSING DIAGNOSIS

One of the nursing diagnoses that you address in your home care plan is Altered Nutrition: Less Than Body Requirements, related to social isolation, declining health, ill-fitting dentures and lack of enjoyment of food. You also question whether depression may be a contributing factor. Evidence comes from his low body weight, laboratory data consistent with poor nutritional status and his descriptions of his eating and food preparation patterns.

NURSING CARE PLAN FOR MR. D.

Expected Outcome	Nursing Interventions	Nursing Evaluation
Mr. D. will state what his daily needs are for each food group.	• Give Mr. D. a copy of Box 18-10 and use it as a basis for teaching about daily nutrient requirements. • Review Canada's Food Guide with Mr. D.	• Mr. D. will describe an eating pattern that meets his daily nutritional needs. • Mr. D. will describe how his daily food intake meets Canada's Food Guide.
Mr. D. will identify a method for meeting his nutrient needs.	• Gain Mr. D.'s permission to arrange for home health aide assistance three times weekly for meal preparation and grocery shopping. • Teach about eating smaller meals more frequently. • Explore with Mr. D. various options for broadening his food selection to improve his nutritional intake (e.g., including dairy products and more fruits and vegetables). • Develop a meal plan with Mr. D. that includes foods that he enjoys but are not currently part of his diet. • Discuss the nutritional value of these foods and suggest that he add new food items in each of the food group categories in which he is deficient.	• Mr. D. will describe an acceptable plan for meeting his nutritional needs. • Mr. D. will gain between 0.22 and 0.45 kg weekly until he reaches the goal of 68 kg.
Mr. D. will have his dentures evaluated and modified or replaced.	• Discuss with Mr. D. the importance of dentures in chewing efficiency and food enjoyment. • Discuss the long-term detrimental effects of lack of dentures. • Explore ways of obtaining a dental evaluation.	• Mr. D. will chew his food with dentures that fit properly.

THINKING POINTS

• What risk factors are likely to be contributing to Mr. D.'s gradual weight loss during the past?

• What further assessment information would you want to have?

QSEN APPLICATION

QSEN Competency	Knowledge/Skill/Attitude	Application to Mr. D. When He is 85 Years of Age
Patient-centred care	(K) Integrate understanding of multiple dimensions of patient-centred care.	Develop individualized plan for improving nutritional intake, as described in care plan.
	(K) Examine common barriers to active involvement in patients.	Identify barriers to obtaining dentures and address these in care plan.
	(S) Elicit patient values, preferences and expressed needs.	
Teamwork and collaboration	(K) Recognize contributions of other individuals and groups in helping patient achieve health goals.	Integrate the services of a home health aide to provide assistance with meal preparation, grocery shopping and transportation for dental appointments.
	(S) Integrate the contributions of others who play a role in helping patient achieve health goals.	Consider a referral for a registered dietitian consultation to reinforce and support nutrition teaching.
		Develop plan for Mr. D. to obtain dentures.
Evidence-Based Practice	(S) Base individualized care plan on patient values, clinical expertise and evidence.	Discuss information in Box 18-10 in the context of Mr. D.'s food preferences and individualized dietary needs.
	(A) Value evidence-based practice as integral to determining the best clinical practice.	

Chapter Highlights

Age-Related Changes That Affect Digestion and Eating Patterns

- Diminished senses of smell and taste
- Less efficient chewing
- Decreased saliva secretion
- Degenerative changes in all structures of the gastrointestinal tract

Age-Related Changes in Nutritional Requirements

- Calories: need less quantity, better quality
- Protein: minimum daily intake of 1.0 to 1.6 g/kg of body weight (i.e., 25 to 30 g of high-quality protein at every meal)
- Fibre: 25 to 38 g/day
- Fat: no more than 10% to 30% of daily caloric intake

Risk Factors That Affect Digestion and Nutrition

- Conditions that can lead to nutritional deficiencies (Table 18-1)
- Poor oral care (Box 18-1)
- Functional impairments and disease processes
- Dysphagia (Box 18-2)
- Effects of medications (Table 18-2)
- Effects of alcohol and smoking
- Psychosocial factors (e.g., dementia, depression, loneliness)
- Cultural and socioeconomic factors (Box 18-3)

- Environmental factors related to institutional or home settings
- Behaviours based on myths and misunderstandings (e.g., overuse of laxatives)

Functional Consequences Affecting Digestion and Nutrition

- Limited ability to procure, prepare and enjoy food
- Changes in oral function
- Nutritional deficiencies, weight changes, unintentional weight loss (Fig. 18-1)
- Effects on quality of life

Pathologic Condition Affecting Digestive Wellness

- Constipation: two or fewer bowel movements weekly, or hard, dry feces

Nursing Assessment of Digestion and Nutrition (Boxes 18-4 through 18-7)

- Usual nutrient intake and eating patterns
- Risks that interfere with any aspect of obtaining, preparing, eating and enjoying food
- Physical examination and laboratory data regarding nutritional status
- The Mini Nutritional Assessment (MNA) tool (Fig. 18-2)

Nursing Diagnosis

- Readiness for Enhanced Nutrition

- Imbalanced Nutrition: Less Than Body Requirements
- Constipation
- Impaired Oral Mucous Membrane

Planning for Wellness Outcomes

- Improved appetite, nutritional status, oral health, depression level
- Increased knowledge about diet, improved health beliefs about constipation

Nursing Interventions to Promote Healthy Digestion and Nutrition (Figs. 18-2 and 18-4, Boxes 18-8 through 18-10)

- Addressing risk factors: functional limitation, environmental factors, medications, alcohol consumption
- Promoting oral and dental health
- Teaching about optimal nutrition

Evaluating Effectiveness of Nursing Interventions

- Daily nutrient intake that corresponds to metabolic needs
- Achieving/maintaining body weight within 110% of ideal body weight for the individual
- Achieving/maintaining regular bowel elimination

Critical Thinking Exercises

1. Discuss specific ways in which each of the following factors might influence the eating patterns of older adults: depression, medications, sensory changes, cognitive impairments, functional impairments, economic factors, social circumstances and oral health factors.
2. Describe at least three characteristics of eating patterns for each of the following cultural groups: First Nations peoples, Asian Canadians and African Canadians.
3. How would you assess digestion and nutrition for an older adult in each of the following settings: home, long-term care facility and acute care facility?
4. Outline a health education plan for teaching older adults about constipation. Include the following points: definition of constipation, risk factors for constipation and interventions to prevent and address constipation.
5. Outline a health education plan for teaching older adults about oral hygiene and dental care.

For more information about the topics discussed in this chapter, be sure to check out the interactive Online Learning Activities and other helpful resources at http://thepoint.lww.com/Miller7e

REFERENCES

Academy of Nutrition and Dietetics. (2012). Position of the Academy of Nutrition and Dietetics: Food and nutrition for older adults: Promoting Health and Wellness. *Journal of the Academy of Nutrition and Dietetics, 112*(8), 1255–1277.

Allard, J. (2012). *Malnutrition is a big problem in Canadian hospitals.* Retrieved December 07, 2014 from http://nutritioncareincanada.ca/wp-content/uploads/2014/03/CMTF-Brochure-ENG.pdf

Bahat, G., Tufan, F., Saka, B., et al. (2012). Which body mass index (BMI) is better in the elderly for functional status? *Archives of Gerontology and Geriatrics, 54*(1), 78–81.

Bitar, K., Greenwood-Van Meerveld, B., Saad, R., et al. (2011). Aging and gastrointestinal neuromuscular function. *Neurogastrointestinal Motility, 23*(6), 490–501. doi:10.1111/j.1365-2982.2011.01678.x

Bocock, M. A., & Keller, H. H. (2009). Hospital diagnosis of malnutrition: A call for action. *Canadian Journal of Dietetic Practice and Research, 70*(1), 37–41.

Britton, E., & McLaughlin, J. T. (2013). Ageing and the gut. *Proceedings of Nutrition Society, 72*(1), 173–177.

Carlsson, M., Haglin, L., Rosendahl, E., et al. (2013). Poor nutritional status is associated with urinary tract infection among older people living in residential care facilities. *Journal of Nutrition, Health and Aging, 17*(2), 186–191.

Canadian Association of Speech and Language Pathologists and Audiologists. (2013). *Swallowing awareness day: May 8, 2013.* Retrieved from http://maymonth.ca/wp-content/uploads/2012/04/Swallowing-Awareness-Day-Media-Kit.pdf

Cousson, P. Y., Bessadet, M., Nicolas, E., et al. (2012). Nutritional status, dietary intake and oral quality of life in elderly complete denture wearers. *Gerodontology, 29*(2), e685–e692.

de Lima Saintrain, M. V., & Goncalves, R. D. (2013). Salivary tests associated with elderly people's oral health. *Gerodontology, 30*(2), 91–97.

Dent, E., Visvanathan, R., Piantadosi, C., et al. (2012). Use of the mini nutritional assessment to detect frailty in hospitalized older people. *Journal of Nutrition, Health & Aging, 16*(9), 764–767.

Desoutter, A., Soudain-Pineau, M., Munsch, F., et al. (2012). Xerostomia and medication: A cross-sectional study in long-term geriatric wards. *Journal of Nutrition, Health & Aging, 16*(6), 575–579.

Dieticians of Canada. (2013a). *Fat.* Retrieved December 07, 2014 from http://www.dietitians.ca/Your-Health/Nutrition-A-Z/Fat.aspx?categoryID=19

Dieticians of Canada. (2013b). *Guidelines for staying hydrated.* Retrieved from http://www.dieticians.ca/Nutrition-Resources-A-Z/Factsheets/Miscellaneous/Why-is-water-so-important-for-my-body-Know-when.aspx

Donini, L. M., Scardella, P., Piombo, L., et al. (2013). Malnutrition in the elderly: Social and economic determinants. *Journal of Nutrition, Health & Aging, 17*(1), 9–15.

Eat Right Ontario. (2012). *A guide to healthy eating for older adults.* Retrieved from http://www.eatrightontario.ca/EatRightOntario/media/ERO_PDF/en/Seniors/Older-Adult-Guide.pdf

Gallagher, J. C. (2013). Vitamin D and aging. *Endocrinology and Metabolism Clinics of North America, 42*(2), 319–332. doi:10.1016/j.ecl.2013.02.004

Gallagher, R. (2011). Swallowing difficulties. *Canadian Family Physician, 57*(12), 1407–1409.

Grassi, M., Petraccia, L., Mennuni, G., et al. (2011). Changes, functional disorders, and diseases in the gastrointestinal tract of elderly. *Nutricion Hospialiaria, 26*(4), 659–668.

Health Canada. (2011). *Canada's food guide.* Ottawa, ON, Canada: Minister of Health.

Health Canada. (2012). *Do Canadian adults meet their nutrient requirements through food intake alone?* Retrieved from http://www.hc-sc.gc.ca/fn-an/surveill/nutrition/commun/art-nutr-adult-eng.php

Herdman, T. H. (Ed.). (2012). *NANDA International Nursing Diagnoses: Definitions and classification 2012–2014.* Oxford, England: Wiley-Blackwell.

Hornick, B., Liska, D., Dolven, C., et al. (2011). The fibre deficit, Part I: Whole grain contributions to health and fibre intake. *Nutrition Today, 46*(6), 293–298.

Hummel, T., Landis, B., & Huttenbrink, K.-B. (2011). Smell and taste disorders. *GMS Current Topics in Otorhinolaryngology*, 10, ISSN 1865-1011.

Huttenbrink, K.-B., Hummel, T., Berg, D., et al. (2013). Olfactory dysfunction: Common in later life and early warning of neurodegenerative disease. *Deutsches Arzteblatt International, 110*(1–2), 1–7.

Institute of Medicine. (2012). *Nutrition and healthy aging in the community: Workshop summary.* Washington, DC: National Academies Press.

Johnson, V. B., & Schoenfelder, D. P. (2012). Evidence-based practice guideline: Oral hygiene care for functionally dependent and cognitively impaired older adults. *Journal of Gerontological Nursing, 38*(11), 11–19.

Kiesswetter, E., Pohlhausen, S., Uhlig, K., et al. (2013). Malnutrition is related to functional impairment in older adults receiving home care. *Journal of Nutrition, Health & Aging, 17*(4), 345–350.

Kim, C.-O., & Lee, K.-R. (2013). Preventive effect of protein-energy supplementation on the functional decline of frail older adults with low socioeconomic status: A community-based randomized controlled study. *Journals of Gerontology: Medical Sciences, 68*(3), 300–316.

Lee, L. C., Tsai, A. C., Wang, J. Y., et al. (2013). Need-based intervention is an effective strategy for improving the nutritional status of older people living in a nursing home: A randomized controlled trial. *International Journal of Nursing Studies, 50*(12), 1580–1588. doi:10.1016/j.ijnurstu.2013.04.004

McKay, S. L., Fravel, M., & Scanlon, C. (2012). Evidence-based practice guideline: Management of constipation. *Journal of Gerontological Nursing, 38*(7), 9–15.

Mentes, J. C., & Kang, S. (2013). Evidence-based practice guideline: Hydration management. *Journal of Gerontological Nursing, 39*(2), 11–19.

Morley, J. E. (2013). Pathophysiology of the anorexia of aging. *Current Opinions in Nutrition and Metabolism Care, 16*, 27–32.

Mugie, S. M., Bennings, M. A., & DiLorenzo, C. (2011). Epidemiology of constipation in children and adults: A systematic review. *Best Practice & Research in Clinical Gastroenterology, 25*, 3–18. doi:10.1016/j.bpg.2010.12.010

Mullol, J., Alobid, I., Marino-Sanchez, F., et al. (2012). Furthering the understanding of olfaction, prevalence of loss of smell and risk factors. *British Medical Journal Open, 2*, e001256. doi:10.1136/bmjopen-2012-001256

O'Connor, L. J. (2012). Oral health care. In M. Boltz, E. Capezuti, T. Fulmer, et al. (Eds.), *Evidence-based practice protocols for best practice* (4th ed., pp. 409–418). New York, NY: Springer.

Orsitto, G. (2012). Different components of nutritional status in older inpatients with cognitive impairment. *Journal of Nutrition, Health & Aging, 16*(5), 468–471.

Pinto Sanchez, M. I., & Bercik, P. (2011). Epidemiology and burden of chronic constipation. *Canadian Journal of Gastroenterology, 25*(Suppl. B), 11B–15B.

Posthauer, M. E., Collins, N., Dorner, B., et al. (2013). Nutritional strategies for frail older adults. *Advances in Skin and Wound Care, 26*(3), 128–140.

Prakash, N., Kalavathy, N., Sridevi, J., et al. (2012). Nutritional status assessment in complete denture wearers. *Gerodontology, 29*(3), 224–230.

Ramage-Morin, P. L., & Garriguet, D. (2013). *Nutritional risk among older Canadians* (Statistics Canada Catalogue no. 82-003-X). Ottawa, ON: Statistics Canada.

Rayner, C. K., & Horowitz, M. (2013). Physiology of the ageing gut. *Current Opinion in Clinical Nutrition and Metabolism Care, 16*, 33–38.

Schubert, C. R., Cruikshanks, K. J., Fischer, M. E., et al. (2012). Olfactory impairment in an adult population. *Chemical Senses, 37*(4), 325–334.

Shetty, S., Bhowmick, S, Castelino, R., et al. (2012). Drug induced xerostomia in elderly individuals. *Contemporary Clinical Dentistry, 3*(2), 173–175.

Sin, H. P., Liu, D. T., & Lam, D. S. (2013). Lifestyle modification, nutritional and vitamins supplements for age-related macular degeneration. *Acta Ophthalmology, 91*(1), 6–11. doi:10.1111/j.1755-3768.2011.02357.x

Skates, J. J., & Anthony, P. S. (2012). Identifying geriatric malnutrition in nursing practice. *Journal of Gerontological Nursing, 38*(3), 18–25.

Smoliner, C., Fischedick, A., Sieber, C., et al. (2013). Olfactory function and malnutrition in geriatric patients. *Journals of Gerontology: Medical Sciences, 68*(12), 1582–1588.

Soenen, S., & Chapman, I. M. (2013). Body weight, anorexia, and undernutrition in older people. *Journal of the American Medical Directors Association, 14*(9), 642–648. doi:10.1016/jamda.2013.02.004

Stange, I., Poeschl, K., Stehle, P., et al. (2013). Screening for malnutrition in nursing home residents: comparison of different risk markers and their association to functional impairment. *Journal of Nutrition, Health & Aging, 17*(4), 357–363.

Statistics Canada. (2010). *Older teeth, stronger bite.* Retrieved from http://www.statcan.gc.ca/pub/11-402-x/2010000/chap/h-s/h-s01-eng.htm

Stewart, S. L. (2013). Daily oral hygiene in residential care. *Canadian Journal of Dental Hygiene, 47*(1), 25–30.

Tamura, B. K., Bell, C. L., Masaki, K., et al. (2013). Prevalence and measures of weight loss, low BMI, malnutrition, and feeding dependency among nursing home patients: A systematic literature review. *Journal of the American Medical Directors Association, 14*, 94–100.

Tarasuk, V., Mitchell, A., & Dachner, N. (2013). *Household food insecurity in Canada, 2011.* Retrieved from http://nutritionalsciences.lamp.utoronto.ca/

Torma, J., Winblad, U., Cederholm, T., et al. (2013). Does undernutrition still prevail among nursing home residents? *Clinical Nutrition, 32*(4), 562–568. doi:10.1016/j.clinu.2012.10.007

Vandewoude, M., & Van Gossum, A. (2013). Nutritional screening strategy in nonagenarians: The value of the MNA-SF in NutriAction. *Journal of Nutrition, Health & Aging, 17*(5), 310–314.

Verbrugghe, M., Beeckman, D., Van Hecke, A., et al. (2012). Malnutrition and associated factors in nursing home residents. *Clinical Nutrition, 32*(3), 438–443. doi:10.1016/j.clnu.2012.09.008

Veronese, N., De Rui, M., Toffanello, E. D., et al. (2013). Body mass index as a predictor of all-cause mortality in nursing home residents during a 5-year follow-up. *Journal of the American Medical Directors Association, 14*, 53–57.

Volkert, D. (2013). Malnutrition in older adults—Urgent need for action. *Gerontology.* Retrieved from www.nhlbi.nlm.nih/gov/pubmed/23406648

Wilson, D. M., Harris, A., Hollis, V., et al. (2011). Upstream thinking and health promotion planning for older adults at risk of social isolation. *International Journal of Older People Nursing, 6*, 282–288. doi:10.1111/j.1748-3743.2010.00259.x

Winter, J., Flanagan, D., McNaughton, S. A., et al. (2013). Nutrition screening of older people in a community general practice using the MNA-SF. *Journal of Nutrition, Health & Aging, 17*(4), 322–325.

Zadak, Z., Hyspler, R., Ticha, A., et al. (2013). Polypharmacy and malnutrition. *Current Opinion in Clinical Nutrition and Metabolism Care, 16*(1), 50–55.

chapter 19

Urinary Function

The primary function of urinary elimination is the excretion of water and chemical wastes, such as metabolic and pharmacologic by-products that would become toxic if allowed to accumulate. Efficient urinary excretion depends on renal blood flow, filtering activities within the kidneys, good functioning of the urinary tract muscles and nervous system control over voluntary and involuntary mechanisms of elimination. Control of urinary elimination also depends on cognitive, sensory and ambulatory abilities and on social, emotional and environmental factors.

Healthy older adults do not experience major functional consequences affecting urinary elimination, but when risk factors are present, which is very common, negative functional consequences are likely to occur. For example, **urinary incontinence**, which is defined as any involuntary leakage of urine, is common among older adults. A risk factor that is especially pertinent to health promotion for older adults is the widely held perception that urinary incontinence is an inevitable and untreatable consequence of normal aging. Nurses have many opportunities to improve quality of life for older adults by addressing the risk factors that contribute to urinary incontinence.

 AGE-RELATED CHANGES THAT AFFECT URINARY WELLNESS

Age-related changes in the kidneys, bladder, urethra and control mechanisms in the nervous and other body systems affect the physiologic processes that control urinary elimination. In addition, any age-related change that interferes with the skills involved in socially appropriate urinary elimination can interfere with urinary control. The next two sections review age-related changes that directly or indirectly affect urinary function and control.

Promoting Urinary Wellness in Older Adults

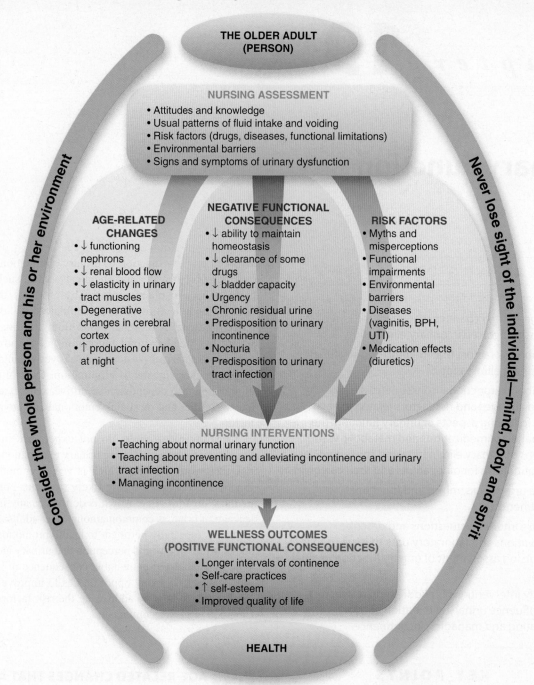

THE OLDER ADULT
(PERSON)

Consider the whole person and his or her environment

Never lose sight of the individual—mind, body and spirit

NURSING ASSESSMENT
- Attitudes and knowledge
- Usual patterns of fluid intake and voiding
- Risk factors (drugs, diseases, functional limitations)
- Environmental barriers
- Signs and symptoms of urinary dysfunction

AGE-RELATED CHANGES
- ↓ functioning nephrons
- ↓ renal blood flow
- ↓ elasticity in urinary tract muscles
- Degenerative changes in cerebral cortex
- ↑ production of urine at night

NEGATIVE FUNCTIONAL CONSEQUENCES
- ↓ ability to maintain homeostasis
- ↓ clearance of some drugs
- ↓ bladder capacity
- Urgency
- Chronic residual urine
- Predisposition to urinary incontinence
- Nocturia
- Predisposition to urinary tract infection

RISK FACTORS
- Myths and misperceptions
- Functional impairments
- Environmental barriers
- Diseases (vaginitis, BPH, UTI)
- Medication effects (diuretics)

NURSING INTERVENTIONS
- Teaching about normal urinary function
- Teaching about preventing and alleviating incontinence and urinary tract infection
- Managing incontinence

WELLNESS OUTCOMES (POSITIVE FUNCTIONAL CONSEQUENCES)
- Longer intervals of continence
- Self-care practices
- ↑ self-esteem
- Improved quality of life

HEALTH

Changes in the Kidneys

The complex process of urinary excretion begins in the kidneys with the filtering and removal of chemical wastes from the blood. Blood circulates through the glomeruli, where liquid wastes, called *glomerular filtrate*, pass through Bowman capsule and the renal tubules to the collecting ducts. During this process, substances needed by the body (such as water, glucose and sodium) are retained and waste products are excreted in the urine. These functions are important for

maintaining homeostasis and excreting many medications. Excretory function, which is measured by the glomerular filtration rate (GFR), depends on the number and efficiency of nephrons and on the amount and rate of renal blood flow.

The kidney increases in weight and mass from birth until early adulthood, when the number of functioning nephrons begins to decline, particularly in the cortex, where the glomeruli are located. This decline continues throughout life, resulting in an approximately 25% decrease in kidney mass by the age of 80 years. Glomerulosclerosis is present in 70% of people aged 40 years and older, with a gradual age-related increase in prevalence and extent (Wiggins, 2012). Beginning in the fourth decade, renal blood flow gradually diminishes, particularly in the cortex, at a rate of 10% per decade.

An average decline in renal function of 1% per year has been widely accepted since the 1970s as a hallmark of aging that begins between the ages of 30 and 40 years. However, these changes vary widely and any *substantial* decline in renal function is associated with other factors, such as physiologic stress due to pathologic conditions (Striker, 2012).

Renal tubules regulate the dilution and concentration of urine, and subsequent excretion of water from the body, in a diurnal rhythm. The physiologic processes responsible for urine concentration and water excretion are influenced by the following factors:

- The amount of fluid in the body
- Resorption of water through, and transport of substances across, the tubular membrane
- Osmoreceptors in the hypothalamus, which regulate the level of circulating antidiuretic hormone (ADH) according to plasma–water concentration
- Substances and activities that influence ADH secretion, such as caffeine, medications, alcohol, pain, stress and exercise
- The concentration of sodium in the glomerular filtrate

Many age-related changes affect the renal tubules and thereby affect the dilution and concentration of urine. These changes include fatty degeneration, diverticula, a loss of convoluted cells and alterations in the composition of the basement membranes. Functionally, the renal tubules in older adults are less efficient in the exchange of substances, the conservation of water and the suppression of ADH secretion in the presence of hypo-osmolality. Age-related changes also decrease the ability of the older kidney to conserve sodium in response to salt restriction. These age-related changes predispose healthy older adults to hyponatremia and other fluid and electrolyte imbalances, particularly in the presence of any condition that alters renal circulation, water or sodium balance, or plasma volume or osmolality.

Changes in the Bladder and Urinary Tract

After being filtered by the kidneys, liquid wastes pass through the ureters into the bladder for temporary storage. The bladder is a balloon-like structure composed of collagen, smooth muscle (called *detrusor*) and elastic tissue. Liquid wastes are eliminated from the bladder through a complex physiologic process involving the following mechanisms, which are affected by age-related changes:

- The ability of the bladder to expand for adequate storage and to contract for complete expulsion of liquid wastes
- The maintenance of higher urethral pressure relative to intravesicular pressure
- Regulation of the lower urinary tract through autonomic and somatic nerves
- Voluntary control of urination (micturition) through the cerebral centres

As urine flows into the bladder, the smooth muscle expands without increasing intravesical pressure, and the urethral pressure increases to the point that it is slightly higher than the intravesical pressure. This balance is maintained and urination can be controlled as long as the volume of urine does not rise above about 450 mL in younger adults or about 350 mL in older adults. If the volume rises above this level, or if the detrusor muscle contracts involuntarily, the intravesical pressure will exceed the urethral pressure, and leakage of urine is likely to occur. In addition to the amount of urine in the bladder, the following factors influence the balance between intravesical and urethral pressure:

- Abdominal pressure
- Thickness of the urethral mucosa
- Tone of the pelvic, detrusor, urethral and bladder neck muscles
- Replacement of the smooth muscle tissue in the bladder and urethra with less elastic connective tissue

Internal and external sphincters regulate urine storage and bladder emptying. The internal sphincter is part of the base of the bladder and is controlled by autonomic nerves. The external sphincter is part of the pelvic floor musculature and is controlled by the pudendal nerve. When urination takes place, the detrusor and abdominal muscles contract, and the perineal and external sphincter muscles relax. When necessary, the external sphincter contracts to inhibit or interrupt voiding and to compensate for sudden surges in abdominal pressure. Age-related changes involving the loss of smooth muscle in the urethra and the relaxation of the pelvic floor muscles reduce the urethral resistance and diminish the tone of the sphincters.

Additional Age-Related Changes That Affect Urinary Function

Changes in the nervous system and other regulatory systems affect urinary function. For example, motor impulses in the spinal cord control urination, but higher centres in the brain are responsible for detecting the sensation of bladder fullness, for inhibiting bladder emptying when necessary and for stimulating bladder contractions for complete emptying. As the bladder fills, sensory receptors in the bladder wall send a signal to the sacral spinal cord. In older adults, degenerative changes in the cerebral cortex may alter both the sensation of bladder fullness and the ability to empty the bladder completely. Younger adults perceive a sensation of fullness when the bladder is about half full, but this occurs at a later point for older adults.

Many urinary tract structures contain estrogen receptors and are affected by hormonal changes, particularly those that occur at menopause. For example, diminished estrogen causes a loss of tone, strength and collagen support in the urogenital tissues and can predispose the urinary system to leakage problems. Also, diminished estrogen can increase bladder sensitivity and lead to an increased urge to void. Diminished thirst perception is another age-related change that can affect urinary function because underhydration or dehydration can interfere with maintenance of homeostasis, which is necessary for optimal urinary function.

▶ RISK FACTORS THAT AFFECT URINARY WELLNESS

As with many other areas of functioning, risk factors play a significant role in causing negative functional consequences related to urinary wellness. Because urinary incontinence is a fundamental aspect of urinary wellness for older adults—and an aspect that is affected by many risk factors—this section discusses risks in relation to both overall urinary wellness and urinary incontinence.

Fluid Intake and Dietary Factors

Limited fluid intake, which often is perceived as a method of maintaining continence, can unintentionally have the opposite effect and lead to lower urinary tract symptoms (Lukacz et al., 2011). Inadequate fluid intake causes urine to be more concentrated, and this leads to increased bladder irritability and subsequent difficulty maintaining continence. In addition, limited fluid intake is a risk factor for urinary incontinence because perception of the need to void depends on adequate bladder fullness. Inadequate fluid intake is also important for clearance of pathologic organisms from the bladder and prevention of bacteriuria (Lin, 2013).

Dietary factors can affect urinary wellness, particularly with regard to foods and beverages that irritate the bladder or increase the risk for urinary incontinence. The following relationships between dietary factors and urinary wellness have been identified in studies:

- Caffeine, carbonated beverages and artificial sweeteners stimulate diuresis and cause urinary urgency or other symptoms (Lukacz et al., 2011).
- Tea, coffee, soda, alcohol, artificial sweeteners, citrus products, sugar, chocolate and hot peppers are common bladder irritants (Canadian Cancer Society, n.d.; Health Canada, 2006; Lukacz et al., 2011).
- Consumption of green tea is associated with lower risk of urinary incontinence in middle-aged and older women (Hirayama & Lee, 2011).

Medication Effects

Medications influence urinary function in a number of ways and are common risk factors in the development of urinary incontinence. Examples of medications that increase the risk for urinary incontinence include antihistamines, atypical antipsychotics and antihypertensive agents, particularly diuretics, calcium-channel blockers and angiotensin II receptor blockers (Hall, Chiu, et al., 2012; Hall, Maserejian, et al., 2012; Hall, Yang, et al., 2012). A longitudinal study of the effects of antihypertensive medications found that independent older women taking a peripheral α-blocker agent (e.g., prazosin, terazosin, doxazosin) had four times the risk of developing urinary incontinence; this risk nearly doubled in those who also were taking a loop diuretic (Peron et al., 2012). Findings from this study are pertinent to older men because this class of drugs is often prescribed for benign prostatic hyperplasia, but the mechanism of action can cause urethral relaxation and stress incontinence. Older adults with a urinary tract condition or risk for urinary incontinence may be particularly susceptible to adverse medication effects. Organist and Engberg (2013) describe an unfolding case example of a 69-year-old man who had benign prostatic hyperplasia and developed acute urinary retention after he started using an anticholinergic inhaler to improve symptoms of his chronic obstructive pulmonary disease (COPD).

In addition to causing incontinence through their direct effects on the urinary tract, medications can increase the risk for urinary incontinence through their effects on functional abilities. Anticholinergics (including those in over-the-counter agents) can cause cognitive and other functional impairments, which can interfere with voluntary control over urination. Many medications cause constipation, which is a causative factor for incontinence. This adverse effect may be particularly detrimental in the presence of prostatic hyperplasia or weakened pelvic floor muscles. Table 19-1 lists types and examples of medications that can cause incontinence in older adults through various mechanisms of action.

TABLE 19-1 Medications That Can Cause Urinary Incontinence

Medication Type	Examples	Mechanism of Action
Diuretics	Furosemide, bumetanide	Increased diuresis can cause urinary urgency, frequency and polyuria.
Anticholinergic agents	Antihistamines, antipsychotics, antidepressants, antispasmodics, anti-Parkinsonian agents	Decreased bladder contractility and relaxed bladder muscle can cause urinary retention, frequency and incontinence.
Adrenergics (α-adrenergic agonists)	Decongestants	Decreased bladder contractility and increased sphincter tone can cause urinary retention, frequency and incontinence.
α-Adrenergic blockers	Prazosin, terazosin, doxazosin	Decreased urethral and internal sphincter tone can cause leakage and stress incontinence.
Calcium-channel blockers	Nifedipine, nicardipine, isradipine, felodipine, nimodipine	Decreased bladder contractility can cause urinary retention, frequency, nocturia and incontinence.
Angiotensin-converting enzyme inhibitors	Captopril, enalapril, lisinopril	Can cause chronic cough, which precipitates or exacerbates stress incontinence
Hypnotics and antianxiety agents	Benzodiazepines	Can interfere with voluntary control over urination by causing sedation, delirium and cognitive impairments
Alcohol	Wine, beer, liquor	Can interfere with voluntary control over urination by causing sedation, delirium, increased diuresis and cognitive impairments

Myths and Misunderstandings

Attitudes based on myths or lack of knowledge about urinary function can have a detrimental effect on the behaviour of older adults and their caregivers. Despite the fact that increased age is a risk factor for urinary incontinence, it is a major mistake to perceive incontinence as an inevitable consequence of aging that cannot be reversed. This commonly held misperception can lead to underdiagnosis and mismanagement of urinary incontinence, which causes serious functional consequences. Studies in Canada and other countries consistently find that assessment of urinary incontinence is often delayed until symptoms progress to the point that they significantly affect quality of life, and at least some of the delay is caused by myths about aging (Adedokun et al., 2012; Rios et al., 2011; Welch et al., 2011).

Influence of Caregivers

Behaviours of caregivers based on misperceptions or lack of information can affect the care of older adults. For instance, if an episode of incontinence occurs soon after an older adult is admitted to an acute care or long-term care facility, nursing staff may falsely assume that this has been an ongoing symptom. Subsequent behaviours of nursing staff, such as using absorbent products rather than initiating an appropriate care plan, may give the message that voluntary control over urination is not expected. Similarly, caregivers in institutional and home care settings may promote the use of absorbent products as a substitute for more time-consuming interventions, such as providing assistance with toileting. When incontinence products are used for ease or convenience, incontinence is likely to develop unnecessarily (Zisberg et al., 2011).

Wellness Opportunity

It is important to identify one's own misperceptions or ageist perspectives that can interfere with providing evidence-based nursing care to promote urinary wellness.

Functional Impairments and Environmental Conditions

Control over urination is affected not only by age-related changes that directly affect urinary function but also by many conditions that affect socially appropriate urinary elimination. All the following conditions can affect one's ability to identify and use appropriate toilet facilities in a timely manner:

- Cognition, balance, mobility, coordination, visual function and manual dexterity
- Identification of a designated receptacle in a private area
- Accessibility and acceptability of toilet facilities
- Ability to get to and use a suitable receptacle
- Amount of time between the perception of the urge to void and the actual need to empty the bladder
- Ability to voluntarily control the urge to void

Box 19-1 Environmental Factors That Can Contribute to Urinary Incontinence

- Stairways between the bathroom level and the living or sleeping areas
- A distance to the bathroom that is more than 40 feet
- Living arrangements where several or many people share a bathroom
- Small bathrooms and narrow doors and hallways that do not accommodate walkers or wheelchairs
- Chair designs and bed heights that hinder mobility
- Poor colour contrast, as between a white toilet and seat and light-coloured floor or walls
- Public settings with poorly visible or poorly colour-contrasted signs designating gender-specific bathroom facilities
- Public settings with dim lighting and out-of-the-way bathroom facilities
- Very bright environments, where glare interferes with the perception of signs for bathrooms
- Mirrored walls, which reflect bright lights and create glare

Functional impairments are a major risk factor for the development of incontinence because they can interfere with the ability to recognize and respond to the urge to void in a timely manner. Because older adults have a shorter interval between the perception of the urge to void and the actual need to empty the bladder, any delay in reaching an appropriate receptacle can result in incontinence. Thus, dependency in performing activities of daily living (ADLs) for any reason is strongly associated with incontinence. Conditions, such as arthritis or Parkinson disease, may slow the ambulation of older adults, as well as their ability to manipulate clothing. Likewise, dementia and other conditions that impair cognitive abilities can interfere with the timely processing of information that is necessary for maintaining voluntary control over urination. Finally, restraints can cause significant functional limitations and increase the risk for developing incontinence.

People with limited mobility or impaired vision encounter many environmental factors that can interfere with their ability to get to accessible toileting facilities in home, public and institutional settings. Examples of environmental obstacles include stairs, inadequate signage, lack of grab bars and toilet seats that are too low. Box 19-1 summarizes some environmental risk factors that may contribute to the incidence of incontinence in older adults.

Pathologic and Other Factors

An increased risk for urinary incontinence is associated with many pathologic conditions including all the following: stroke, arthritis, dementia, delirium, depression, diabetes mellitus, metabolic syndrome, Parkinson disease, fecal impaction and chronic obstructive pulmonary disease (COPD) (Devore et al., 2012; Dowling-Castronovo & Bradway, 2012; Kupelian et al., 2013). In addition, any acute illness or surgical intervention that temporarily limits mobility or compromises mental abilities also represents a risk factor for urinary incontinence. Constipation and low stool frequency (i.e., fewer than three bowel movements weekly) are other conditions that increase the risk for urinary incontinence and other urinary tract symptoms in men and women (Carter & Beer-Gabel, 2012; Thurmon et al., 2012).

Although dementia is strongly associated with urinary incontinence, the relationship between these two conditions is complex and episodes of incontinence can often be prevented or minimized particularly during early and middle stages. For example, older adults with dementia may lack the perceptual abilities that are necessary for finding and using appropriate facilities, but they may be able to maintain continence when given appropriate cues and reminders.

Obesity and smoking are conditions that are strongly associated with urinary incontinence and urinary tract symptoms (Tahtinen et al., 2011; Vaughan et al., 2012). Other risk factors associated with urinary incontinence that commonly occur in older adults include hearing and/or vision impairment, radiation or surgical treatments for prostate cancer and residence in a long-term care facility (Dowling-Castronovo & Bradway, 2012). Researchers also are investigating a potential link between vitamin D and urinary incontinence, with emphasis on its influence on pelvic floor muscle functioning (Parker-Autry et al., 2012).

Wellness Opportunity

Nurses holistically assess older adults by recognizing that urinary incontinence can be an indicator of physiologic disturbances (e.g., urinary tract infection [UTI]), conditions that affect cognition or mood (e.g., dementia or depression), or a combination of functional limitations and environmental barriers.

Gender-Specific Conditions

Gender-specific conditions of the genitourinary tract commonly occur in older adults and increase the risk for urinary incontinence and other lower urinary tract symptoms, including pain and infection. Although these conditions are generally addressed by a gynecologist or urologist, they are discussed in relation to urinary wellness because of their direct effects on control over urination in older men and women.

The term **pelvic floor disorders** (also called pelvic support problems) refers to a group of medical conditions in which a pelvic organ prolapses into the vagina due to weakness or injury involving muscles and connective tissue of the pelvic floor and related structures. These conditions, which sometimes occur together, can involve any of the following structures:

- Urinary bladder (cystocele)
- Bladder and urethra (cystourethrocele)
- Bladder neck (urethrocele)
- Uterus (uterine prolapse)
- Part of the small bowel and peritoneum (enterocele)
- Rectum (rectocele or rectal prolapse)

Sometimes, terms such as "dropped," "sagging" or "fallen" are used in reference to the involved structure (e.g., "dropped bladder").

In addition to increased age and postmenopausal status, factors that increase the risk for pelvic floor disorders include smoking, obesity, surgery, pelvic radiation, genetic predisposition, chronic constipation, high number of vaginal births and fractures of the pelvis or lower vertebrae. Pelvic floor disorders can lead to urinary frequency and incontinence because these conditions interfere with the complete emptying of the bladder, resulting in residual urine and an increased risk of bacteriuria. Atrophy of the vaginal and trigonal tissue with subsequent diminished resistance to pathogens is another condition that can affect urinary wellness in older women because vaginitis and trigonitis can cause urinary urgency, frequency and incontinence.

DIVERSITY NOTE

Caucasian women are more likely than black Canadian women to have pelvic organ prolapse. It may be that the strength of bones, muscles and connective tissue are influenced by one's genes and ethnicity background.

Benign prostatic hyperplasia (also called benign prostatic hypertrophy) is a common cause of voiding problems in older men because the enlarged prostate compresses the urethra, which leads to obstruction of the vesical neck. As the condition progresses, the bladder wall becomes thinner and less elastic and urinary retention occurs, increasing the risk of bacteriuria and infection. Men with prostatic hyperplasia may experience decreased urine flow, incomplete bladder emptying and urinary urgency and frequency. Eventually, the ureters and kidneys are affected, and hydroureter, hydronephrosis, diminished glomerular filtration rate (GFR) and uremia may develop.

See **ONLINE LEARNING ACTIVITY 19-1: CASE STUDY VIDEO DISCUSSING TRANSIENT URINARY INCONTINENCE THAT DEVELOPS DURING HOSPITALIZATION** at http://thepoint.lww.com/Miller7e

FUNCTIONAL CONSEQUENCES AFFECTING URINARY WELLNESS

Despite the many age-related changes in the urinary tract, the elimination of wastes is not significantly affected in healthy, nonmedicated older adults. However, with any unusual physiologic demands, such as those that occur with medications or disease conditions, older adults are likely to experience functional consequences affecting homeostatic mechanisms and urinary control. The most significant functional consequences are those that affect patterns of urinary elimination and predispose older adults to incontinence. When incontinence occurs, additional functional consequences, particularly psychosocial effects, can be quite serious. This section reviews functional consequences that are related to overall renal function and to control over urination.

Effects on Renal Function

Functional consequences related to renal function in healthy older adults include impaired absorption of calcium, a predisposition to hyponatremia and hyperkalemia, and a diminished ability to maintain fluid and electrolyte balance and to correct pH imbalances. In addition, urine is more concentrated because the kidneys become less responsive to antidiuretic hormone (ADH). Because of these changes, older adults will more readily develop dehydration, volume depletion, and other fluid and electrolyte imbalances under conditions of physiologic stress (e.g., surgery, infection, fever-producing illness, excessive fluid loss).

Diminished renal function contributes to the increased incidence of drug interactions and adverse medication reactions in older adults. These age-related changes are most likely to affect water-soluble medications that are highly dependent on GFR (e.g., digoxin, cimetidine, aminoglycoside antibiotics) or renal tubular function (e.g., penicillin, procainamide). Unless medication doses are adjusted to account for age-related changes in GFR and renal tubular function, excretion may be delayed and toxic substances are likely to accumulate. These adverse medication effects can significantly impair physical and mental abilities and have profound functional consequences, as discussed in Chapter 8.

Effects on Voiding Patterns

Because of age-related changes, the bladder of the older adult has a smaller capacity, empties incompletely and contracts during filling. Thus, older adults experience shorter intervals between voiding, and they have less time between the perception of the urge to void and the actual need to empty the bladder. Older adults often describe this by saying, "When you gotta go, you gotta go." Another consequence is that the bladder retains residual urine after voiding, causing symptomatic or asymptomatic bacteriuria and predisposing older adults to UTIs.

Age-related changes in the diurnal production of urine cause a shift in voiding pattern to more urinary output at night than during the day. Prevalence of **nocturia** (i.e., frequent urination at night) increases with age, with up to 60% of older adults voiding two or more times nightly (Bosch & Weiss, 2013). Nocturia is a common symptom of many urinary tract disorders and it also occurs with conditions that affect ADH secretion, including endocrine disorders, heart failure, renal insufficiency and certain medication such as diuretics (Van Kerrebroeck, 2011). Functional consequences of nocturia include disturbed sleep, increased risk for nighttime falls and decreased quality of life.

Urinary Incontinence

As already emphasized, urinary incontinence is not inevitable with aging, but it occurs more commonly in older adults due to a combination of age-related changes and risk factors. Estimated prevalence of incontinence for older adults varies widely due to many factors, including underreporting and inconsistent definitions. A study, released in October 2013 (Ramage-Morin & Gilmour), used data from the 2008/2009

Box 19-2 Characteristics of Types of Incontinence

Stress: sudden leakage of urine as a result of an activity that increases abdominal pressure, such as lifting, coughing, sneezing, laughing or exercise

Urge: involuntary urinary leakage soon after perceiving the urge to void

Mixed: involuntary leakage of urine with both the sensation of urgency and activities such as coughing, sneezing or exertion

Overflow: involuntary loss of urine due to overdistention of the bladder associated with underactive detrusor muscle or outlet obstruction

Functional: involuntary loss of control over urination due to inability to reach appropriate toileting facility

Reflex: involuntary release of urine at predictable intervals when bladder fullness is reached

---

Canadian Community Health Survey—Healthy Aging to examine the prevalence of urinary incontinence among seniors. An estimated 512,000 older adults, about 12% of the population aged 65 or older, reported urinary incontinence. Women were more likely than men to have the condition (14% vs. 9%), and older adults 85 or older were more prone to urinary incontinence. In another study that involved self-reported prevalence and knowledge of urinary incontinence among 93 Canadian women living in the community, 36.5% admitted to having incontinence, of which one third did not know the causes of urinary incontinence (Taylor et al., 2013).

Urinary incontinence is categorized according to potential for reversibility as transient (also called acute) or established (also called chronic or persistent). Transient urinary incontinence is characterized by recent and sudden onset and is associated with resolvable causes, such as delirium, UTI, medications, constipation, limited mobility or lack of appropriate assistance with toileting. Types of established urinary incontinence include stress, urge, mixed, overflow, functional and reflex, as described in Box 19-2. **Overactive bladder (OAB)** is a syndrome that is closely associated with urinary incontinence and is now widely recognized due to increasing media attention. OAB is characterized by bothersome urgency, usually accompanied by day and night frequency and *sometimes* accompanied by urge urinary incontinence.

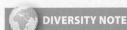 **DIVERSITY NOTE**

In Canada, research shows that almost one third of Canadian women of all ages experience urinary incontinence (Taylor et al., 2013) a rate higher than men. Rates are higher for both men and women living in long-term care facilities.

Urinary incontinence can negatively affect quality of life through both physical and psychosocial consequences. Physical consequences of incontinence include a predisposition to falls, fractures, pressure ulcers, UTIs & limitation of functional status (Dowling-Castronovo & Bradway, 2012). In recent years, health care professionals have drawn attention to incontinence-associated dermatitis, which is an inflammatory condition of the skin that differs clinically and pathologically from pressure ulcers and other skin disorders (Doughty et al., 2012; Zulkowski, 2012). Psychosocial consequences associated with urinary incontinence include significantly decreased quality of life, shame or embarrassment, anxiety, depression, social isolation and loss of self-confidence (Aguilar-Navarro et al., 2012; de Vries et al., 2012; Felde et al., 2012; Yip et al., 2013). Urinary incontinence has significant negative effects on sexuality and intimacy that extend to existing and new partners (Hayder, 2012). Another consequence is that people who have experienced episodes of incontinence may become preoccupied with covering up any evidence of wetness or urinary odours, so they can avoid social stigma.

DIVERSITY NOTE

The chances of being lonely are significantly higher for older Canadians who reports UI than for those who do not (Ramage-Morin & Gilmour, 2013).

Negative psychosocial consequences can arise when caregivers communicate infantilizing attitudes and behaviours, such as unnecessarily using incontinence products rather than providing assistance with toileting. These attitudes and behaviours can have a devastating effect on the older adult's dignity and self-esteem (See Box 19-3). In addition, older adults who do not understand age-related changes may have exaggerated fears of progressive incontinence, triggered by the onset of urgency or frequency. Even in older adults who are not incontinent, the experience of urinary urgency and frequency can cause psychosocial consequences, such as anxiety, restricted activity, feelings of insecurity and powerlessness, and embarrassment about frequent trips to the bathroom.

See ONLINE LEARNING ACTIVITY 19-2:
EVIDENCE-BASED INFORMATION ABOUT URINARY INCONTINENCE
at http://thepoint.lww.com/Miller7e

A Student's Perspective

One morning, I was caring for a client who had a Foley catheter. While preparing her to go to breakfast, I noticed there was no cover on her catheter bag and asked her if she had one. My client explained that she once had a cover, but the nurses did not know where it went. I decided to do some searching, which only required my asking the laundry lady, and I discovered that several covers were stored in the linen closet. When I came back to the client's room with the cover, my client was so grateful. She said she had been asking for a long time if she could get another one, but the nurses and aides never cared to search for one. She explained that she doesn't like everyone to be able to see her catheter bag as she rides around the nursing home in her wheelchair. My finding the cover for her catheter bag was a very simple act requiring very little effort, but it showed me the importance of putting a little extra time into the client's care. Although this seemed like a miniscule problem to the nurses, it was a real concern to my client. I hope that as we continue in our nursing careers, we remember to do these simple acts because a seemingly insignificant thing to us can mean the world to a client.

Katrina D.

Wellness Opportunity

Nurses address the person's relationships with others by being sensitive to the psychosocial responses of family caregivers who are dealing with incontinence.

Unfolding Case Study

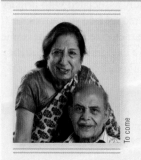

Part 1: Mr. and Mrs. U. at 69 and 68 Years of Age

Mr. and Mrs. U., who are 69 and 68 years old, respectively, attend the senior centre where you provide monthly group health education sessions, weekly blood pressure checks and one-on-one "Counselling for Wellness" sessions. During a recent health counselling session, Mrs. U. confided that she does not know what to do about her husband's "smelly dribbling" and that she worries that he has prostate problems. She has perceived a strong odour of urine and has noticed yellow stains on his clothing when she does the laundry. Even their children have mentioned the odour to her, but when she tries to discuss it with her husband, he changes the subject. She says that he will not talk with his doctor about it because he "hears so much about prostate cancer, and he's afraid that he has an untreatable condition." She seeks your advice about this and asks if you would talk with him when he comes to see you next week. Your next group health education session is titled "Control of Urine: What's Normal With Aging?" and you plan to have separate group discussions for the men and women. Since Mr. and Mrs. U. usually attend these sessions, you see this as an opportunity to initiate health education about this sensitive topic.

THINKING POINTS

Decide what information you would include in the group session about each of the following topics:

- What can older men (women) expect of their urinary tract?

- What factors increase the risk of having problems with urinary control in older men (women)?

PATHOLOGIC CONDITION AFFECTING URINARY FUNCTION: UTIs

Urinary tract infections (UTIs) are common in older adults, particularly in long-term care settings. Incidence of UTI in older adults is between 12% and 29% for those in community settings and 44% to 58% for residents of long-term care facilities (Caljouw et al., 2011). Risk factors include increased age, urinary incontinence and impaired functional or cognitive status. In institutional settings, the use of indwelling catheters increases the risk of infection and is time dependent and reaching almost 100% by 30 days (Andreessen et al., 2012). Since 2008, there has been increasing attention to catheter-associated urinary tract infections (CAUTIs), which is the single-most common cause of preventable health care–associated infections.

Box 19-4 summarizes current evidence-based guidelines for prevention, diagnosis and management of CAUTI.

In any setting, assessment of UTI is complicated by the fact that symptoms in older adults are likely to be subtle and generalized, rather than specific to the urinary tract. A change in behaviour or mental status may be the primary presenting manifestation in older adults, particularly in those who have dementia.

 See **ONLINE LEARNING ACTIVITY 19-3: CASE STUDY VIDEO DISCUSSING URINARY TRACT INFECTIONS** at http://thepoint.lww.com/Miller7e

 ## NURSING ASSESSMENT OF URINARY FUNCTION

Nurses can identify opportunities for health promotion interventions by assessing all of the following aspects of urinary function:

- Risk factors that influence overall urinary function
- Risk factors that increase the potential for incontinence
- Signs and symptoms of any dysfunction involving urinary elimination
- Fears and attitudes about urinary dysfunction
- Psychosocial consequences of incontinence

Assessment information is obtained by reviewing urinalysis results, interviewing older adults and caregivers when appropriate, and observing behaviours and environmental influences.

E B P   **Box 19-4 Evidence-Based Practice: Prevention of Catheter-Associated Urinary Tract Infections**

Statement of the Problem

- Catheter-associated urinary tract infections (CAUTIs) account for 34% to 40% of healthcare-associated infections, which are considered largely preventable adverse events that occur during hospitalization.
- Between 21% and 54% of indwelling urinary catheters (IUCs) (also called Foley catheters) are used inappropriately when they are not medically necessary.
- IUCs are frequently left in patients longer than necessary.
- IUCs significantly increase the risk for urinary tract infection, delirium, local trauma and encrustation.
- The risk for developing a CAUTI is directly related to the duration of IUC use, beginning at 48 hours after insertion and increasing at the rate of 5% per day and reaching almost 100% by day 30.
- Adherence to recommended infection control measures (as described in the section on recommendations for care) would prevent 17% to 69% of CAUTI.

Recommendations for Nursing Assessment

- Identify appropriate indications for use of an IUC: perioperative care, prolonged surgery, operative patients with urinary incontinence, monitoring during surgery or critical illness, major trauma patients, urinary retention or obstruction, pressure ulcer management and comfort care during terminal illness.
- Recognize the definition of a CAUTI, which is a UTI that occurs while a patient has an IUC or within 48 hours of its removal.

- Assess for the following indicators of CAUTI: suprapubic tenderness, costovertebral angle pain or tenderness, fever above 38 °C without another identifiable cause, positive blood culture with the same organisms as in the urine.
- Recognize the definition of a positive urine culture as: (1) 10^5 or more microorganisms/cc of urine with no more than two species of microorganisms, OR (2) 10^3 microorganisms/cc of urine with no more than two species of microorganisms AND a positive urinalysis involving dipstick, pyuria and organisms seen on Gram stain of unspun urine.

Recommendations for Nursing Care

- Avoid use of IUC: adhere to criteria and protocols for medically necessary use; incorporate alternative methods for urinary elimination in the care plan (e.g., toileting program, collecting devices, absorbent products, intermittent straight catheterization).
- Recommended care strategies for IUC: smallest effective size for catheter, use aseptic technique for insertion, provide routine mental care, prevent reflux, maintain closed system, keep catheter secure in place.
- Nurses have essential roles in ensuring the timely removal of IUCs by frequently reassessing the need for keeping the catheter inserted.

Sources: Andreessen, L., Wilde, M. H., & Herendeen, P. (2012). Preventing catheter-associated urinary tract infections in acute care: The bundle approach. *Journal of Nursing Care Quarterly, 27*(3), 209–217; Wald, H. L., Fink, R. M., Makic, M. B. F. et al. (2012). Catheter-associated urinary tract infection prevention. In M. Boltz, E. Capezuti, R. Fulmer, et al. (Eds.), *Evidence-based geriatric nursing protocols for best practice* (4th ed., pp. 388–408). New York, NY: Springer. Modified version is available online at: http://consultgerirn.org

Talking With Older Adults About Urinary Function

Because urinary elimination is associated with certain social expectations, discussion of this topic may be particularly influenced by a person's attitudes and feelings. People with urinary incontinence often experience stigma, discomfort and embarrassment. Factors that contribute to the challenge of discussing urinary function include age, gender or cultural differences; communication barriers such as hearing impairment; and the misperception that urinary problems are an inevitable and untreatable consequence of aging.

Terminology related to urinary elimination presents further difficulties in interviewing older adults. In social settings, people commonly use euphemisms to avoid directly discussing urination (e.g., "I'm going to the powder room," "I'm going to take a leak"). Even the sounds associated with urinary elimination may be viewed as embarrassing, so people may run the faucet or flush the toilet to disguise the sound of urination when others are present. Because of this social context, successful interviewing about urinary elimination and incontinence depends on identifying the terms that are least embarrassing and most understandable to the older adult. If any hearing impairment is present, a term such as "urinate," which is not used in everyday social language or a one-syllable word like "pee" may be difficult to understand or may be misinterpreted. Although phrases like "use the toilet" and "go to the bathroom" are not specific to urinary elimination, they may prove to be acceptable, particularly if additional questions are asked in order to distinguish between urinary and bowel elimination. Similarly, the term "incontinence" may be problematic for people who may not be familiar with this term. Older adults are likely to use any of the following words and phrases when referring to urinary incontinence: "accidents," "leaking," "weak kidneys," "bladder trouble" or "trouble holding my water."

Wellness Opportunity

Show respect for older adults by using terms such as "briefs" rather than terms such as diapers, which are associated with infants.

Identifying Opportunities for Health Promotion

Begin a nursing assessment by asking about risk factors and observing the person's responses. If the older adults acknowledge incontinence, ask about any actions they have taken and about any effects on their daily activities and social life. Box 19-5 presents interview questions related to urinary elimination. Check other parts of patient records for pertinent information (e.g., medication use and medical history) and incorporate it into the assessment of urinary elimination. Supplement the assessment interview by obtaining information about the person's patterns of urinary elimination and by assessing environmental factors that may interfere with control over urinary elimination. A **bladder diary** (also called a bladder record, or voiding or urinary diary) can be used to obtain information about fluid intake, the times of urination and other factors that can affect continence (Fig. 19-1). Use the information from the bladder diary to identify potential causes of and interventions for incontinence, particularly with regard to identifying

Box 19-5 Guidelines for Assessing Urinary Elimination

Interview Questions to Assess Risk Factors Influencing Urinary Elimination

- (Men) Have you had any surgery for prostate or bladder problems?
- (Men) Have you ever been told you had prostate problems? (or Do you think you have prostate problems?)
- (Women) Have you had any children? (If yes, ask about the number of pregnancies and any problems with childbirth.)
- (Women) Have you had any surgery for pelvic, bladder or uterine disorders?
- (Women) Have you had any infections in your vaginal area?
- Do you have any pain, burning or discomfort when you urinate (pass water)?
- Have you had any urinary tract infections?
- Do you have any chronic illnesses?
- Do you have any problems with your bowels?
- How much water and other liquids do you drink during the day? (Ask for details about timing and the amount of alcoholic, carbonated and caffeinated beverages consumed.)

Interview Questions to Assess Risk Factors for Socially Appropriate Urinary Elimination

- Do you have any trouble walking or any difficulty with balance?
- Do you have any trouble reading signs or finding restrooms when you are in public places?

Interview Questions to Assess Signs and Symptoms of Urinary Dysfunction

- Do you ever leak urine?
- Do you ever wear pads or protective garments to protect your clothing from wetness?
- Do you ever have difficulty holding your urine (water) long enough to get to the toilet? (or How long can you hold your urine after you first feel the need to go to the bathroom?)
- Do you have trouble holding your urine (water) when you cough, laugh or make sudden movements?
- Do you wake up at night because you have to go to the bathroom to urinate (pass water)? (If the response is affirmative, try to differentiate between this symptom and the habit of going to the bathroom after waking up for some other reason.)
- Immediately after urinating (passing your water), does it feel like you have not emptied your bladder completely?
- Do you have to exert pressure during urination to feel like your bladder is being completely emptied?
- (Men) When you urinate (pass water), do you have any difficulty starting the stream or keeping the stream going?

Interview Questions if Incontinence Has Been Acknowledged

- When did your incontinence begin?
- What have you done to manage the problem? (Have you cut down on the amount of liquids you drink? Do you empty your bladder at frequent intervals as a precautionary measure?)
- Are there certain things that make the problem worse or better?
- Does it happen all the time, or just at certain times?
- Do you have any pain when you urinate (pass water)?
- (Women) Do you feel any pressure in your pelvic area?

Interview Questions to Assess Fears, Attitudes and Psychosocial Consequences of Incontinence

- Have you ever sought help or talked to a primary care provider or other health care professional about this problem?
- Have you changed any of your activities because you need to stay near a toilet?
- Do you avoid going to certain places because of difficulty holding your urine (water)?

Your Daily Bladder Diary

This diary will help you and your health care team figure out the causes of your bladder control trouble. The "sample" line shows you how to use the diary.

Your name: _____

Date: _____

Time	Drinks		Trips to the bathroom		Accidental leaks	Did you feel a strong urge to go?	What were you doing at the time?
	What kind?	How much?	How many times?	How much urine? (circle one)	How much? (circle one)	Circle one	Sneezing, exercising, having sex, lifting, etc.
Sample	Coffee	2 cups	✓✓	sm med lg	sm med lg	Yes No	Running
6–7 AM				sm med lg	sm med lg	Yes No	
7–8 AM				sm med lg	sm med lg	Yes No	
8–9 AM				sm med lg	sm med lg	Yes No	
9–10 AM				sm med lg	sm med lg	Yes No	
10–11 AM				sm med lg	sm med lg	Yes No	
11–12 noon				sm med lg	sm med lg	Yes No	
12–1 PM				sm med lg	sm med lg	Yes No	
1–2 PM				sm med lg	sm med lg	Yes No	
2–3 PM				sm med lg	sm med lg	Yes No	
3–4 PM				sm med lg	sm med lg	Yes No	
4–5 PM				sm med lg	sm med lg	Yes No	
5–6 PM				sm med lg	sm med lg	Yes No	
6–7 PM				sm med lg	sm med lg	Yes No	
7–8 PM				sm med lg	sm med lg	Yes No	
8–9 PM				sm med lg	sm med lg	Yes No	
9–10 PM				sm med lg	sm med lg	Yes No	
10–11 PM				sm med lg	sm med lg	Yes No	
11–12 midnight				sm med lg	sm med lg	Yes No	
12–1 AM				sm med lg	sm med lg	Yes No	
1–2 AM				sm med lg	sm med lg	Yes No	
2–3 AM				sm med lg	sm med lg	Yes No	

Type and amount of incontinence products used today: _____

_____

Questions to ask my health care team:

_____

_____

FIGURE 19-1 Example of a bladder diary. (Adapted from *Let's Talk About Bladder Control for Women*, National Kidney and Urologic Diseases Information Clearinghouse. www.kidney.niddk.nih.gov)

Box 19-6 Guidelines for Assessing Behavioural Cues to and Environmental Influences on Incontinence

Behavioural Cues

- Does the older adult use disposable or washable pads or products?
- Is there an odour of urine on clothing, floor coverings or furniture (particularly couches and stuffed chairs)?
- Has the older adult withdrawn from social activities, particularly those held away from home?

Environmental Influences

- Where are the bathroom facilities located in relation to the older adult's usual daytime and nighttime activities?
- Does the person have to go up or down stairs to use the toilet at night or during the day?
- Are there any grab bars or other aids in, near or on the way to the bathroom?
- Is lighting adequate and the pathway uncluttered for safety?
- Would the person benefit from using an elevated toilet seat?
- Does the person use a urinal or other aid to cut down on the number of trips to the bathroom?
- How many people share the same bathroom facilities?
- Is privacy ensured?

Wellness Opportunity

Nurses promote self-care by encouraging older adults to assess their patterns of urinary elimination in relation to factors such as food and fluid intake.

Assess home environments for conditions that affect timely access to bathrooms, particularly for people who have a functional impairment or use assistive devices, such as walkers (refer to Box 19-1). Also, assess the environment for safety and assistive devices or their potential benefit to the individual. For instance, an elevated toilet seat, grab bars near the toilet and grab bars on the walls leading to the toilet may improve the person's safety and ability to maintain urinary continence.

Using Laboratory Information

Data from urinalysis and blood chemistry tests contribute valuable assessment information. A midstream or second-void specimen is the best type of sample for a urinalysis. At the age of 80, the normal upper limit for specific gravity is 1.024, and slight proteinuria is normal in older adults. Other than these two variations, the urinalysis results should be within the normal range for healthy older adults. Diagnosis of a UTI is based on results from a dipstick or microscopic examination of a clean-catch urine specimen.

An important assessment consideration is distinguishing between UTI and asymptomatic bacteriuria, which is characterized by urinalysis results of 10^5 or more colony-forming units but a lack of localized symptoms, such as dysuria. Asymptomatic bacteriuria is very common in older adults, particularly in long-term care settings and in those with indwelling catheters. An important nursing consideration is that even though the urinalysis shows bacteriuria, concerns have been raised about the use of antibiotics as a

opportunities for health education. Older adults who are cognitively impaired or dependent on others for their care may not be able to keep a bladder diary. In these situations, it is important to obtain information from nursing staff in institutional settings and from caregivers in community-based settings. Box 19-6 summarizes specific observations that may yield important assessment information.

**See ONLINE LEARNING ACTIVITY 19-4:
CASE STUDY VIDEO DISCUSSING THE USE OF A BLADDER RECORD FOR ASSESSING URINARY INCONTINENCE**
at http://thepoint.lww.com/Miller7e

Unfolding Case Study

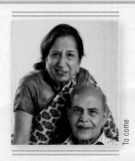

Part 1: Mr. and Mrs. U. at 69 and 68 Years of Age (continued)

Recall that you are the nurse at the senior centre attended by Mr. and Mrs. U. After your class ("Control of Urine: What's Normal With Aging?"), Mr. U. schedules an appointment for a Counselling for Wellness session. He tells you that he has a "little dribbling" problem but has ignored it because it did not bother him very much. He has not talked with any doctor about this because he thought it was "to be expected," but now that he attended your session, he thinks that maybe he should have the problem evaluated and wants further information from you. During other health counselling sessions with Mr. U., he has told you that he is taking medications for hypertension and Parkinson disease.

THINKING POINTS

- What risk factors are likely to be contributing to Mr. U.'s problems with urinary control?
- Make a list of assessment questions that you would use with Mr. U. (Use applicable questions from Box 19-5 and any additional questions that might be appropriate.)
- What observations would you make as part of your assessment?
- What would you teach Mr. U. about filling out the bladder diary (see Fig. 19-1)?

potentially harmful medical intervention that is not evidence based (Phillips et al., 2012).

Blood chemistry values that are pertinent to assessment of renal function include the following: electrolyte level, creatinine level, creatinine clearance, nonprotein nitrogen level and blood urea nitrogen level. In older adults, the serum creatinine may not be an accurate indicator of the GFR, but a 24-hour urine collection for creatinine clearance may have greater value as an indicator of renal functioning.

NURSING DIAGNOSIS

Impaired Urinary Elimination is an appropriate nursing diagnosis in that the assessment identifies any risk factors for, any complaints about or evidence of incontinence. Defining characteristics commonly found in older adults include urgency, frequency, nocturia, hesitancy and incontinence. The following nursing diagnoses might be applicable for negative consequences of urinary incontinence: Anxiety, Social Isolation, Disturbed Sleep Pattern, Impaired Skin Integrity or Caregiver Role Strain (or Risk for).

> **Wellness Opportunity**
>
> Nurses can use the wellness nursing diagnosis of Readiness for Enhanced Urinary Elimination for older adults who are interested in learning self-care practices, such as pelvic floor muscle exercises.

PLANNING FOR WELLNESS OUTCOMES

Nursing care plans are directed toward preventing, minimizing or compensating for the negative functional consequences that affect urinary elimination. Specific outcomes related to promoting urinary wellness are Fluid Balance, Kidney Function or Risk Detection. Outcomes for older adults who have urinary incontinence include achieving continence and preventing negative consequences; initial outcomes focus on controlling and alleviating, rather than simply managing, incontinence. The following NOC terminology is pertinent to older adults who experience urinary incontinence and related consequences: Urinary Continence, Symptom Severity, Urinary Elimination, Self-Care: Toileting, Health Beliefs: Perceived Control; Immobility Consequences: Physiologic and Tissue Integrity: Skin.

In addition, any of the following NOCs may be pertinent to caregivers, particularly family members, who are caring for someone with urinary incontinence: Caregiver Stressors; Caregiver Well-Being; Caregiver Performance: Direct Care; Caregiver Lifestyle Disruption; Caregiver Emotional Health and Caregiver Endurance Potential.

> **Wellness Opportunity**
>
> Quality of life is an outcome that can be achieved for older adults and their caregivers through nursing interventions that are effective in alleviating or managing urinary incontinence.

 ## NURSING INTERVENTIONS TO PROMOTE URINARY WELLNESS

Nurses have numerous opportunities to promote wellness in relation to urinary function, particularly for older adults who have difficulty maintaining urinary control. For example, nurses can challenge myths about urinary incontinence, address attitudes of resignation and teach self-care interventions. The following NIC terminology is pertinent to promoting urinary continence and addressing the associated psychosocial consequences: Biofeedback, Emotional Support, Environmental Management, Fluid Management, Health Education, Pelvic Muscle Exercise, Prompted Voiding, Referral, Self-Esteem Enhancement, Urinary Bladder Training, Urinary Elimination Management, Urinary Habit Training and Urinary Incontinence Care.

Teaching About Overall Urinary Wellness

Healthy older adults are not significantly affected by age-related kidney changes during normal activities; however, under conditions of physiologic stress, such as exercise, homeostasis can be affected unless the older adult initiates compensatory actions. Thus, an important aspect of health promotion is to teach older adults about self-care actions, such as drinking adequate fluid before exercise and avoiding strenuous physical activity in hot or humid conditions. Teach older adults about measures to protect themselves in very hot and humid environments by using fans and air conditioners, maintaining good fluid intake and avoiding alcoholic, carbonated and caffeinated beverages. Because older adults with diminished renal function are at increased risk for adverse effects when taking one or more water-soluble medications, dose adjustments may be necessary, as discussed in Chapter 8.

A risk factor that can be alleviated through health education is the false perception of incontinence as an inevitable and irreversible effect of aging. Nurses have important roles in addressing risks for urinary incontinence as an integral aspect of health promotion. For example, interventions for preventing constipation, as discussed in Chapter 18, may improve control over urination. Similarly, health education about the rationale for maintaining adequate fluid intake as a means of preventing incontinence and maintaining good urinary function is a simple but important intervention. Also explain that because the sensation of thirst diminishes or is absent in older adults, this is not a good indicator of the need for fluids. Box 19-7 summarizes teaching points about health promotion actions for maintaining optimal urinary function and continence.

> **Wellness Opportunity**
>
> Nurses promote personal responsibility by encouraging older adults to talk with their health care practitioner about identifying risk factors for urinary incontinence that can be addressed through self-care measures.

Box 19-7   Health Education to Promote Urinary Wellness

Facts About Urinary Control

- Incontinence is not an inevitable age-related change, but it occurs more commonly in older adults due to risk factors.
- Older adults may experience urinary urgency, which means there is a shorter duration between the perception of the urge to void and the actual need to empty the bladder.
- It is normal for older adults to urinate once or twice during the night.
- Conditions that interfere with good urinary control include restricted fluid intake and consuming foods and beverages that irritate the bladder or cause increase urine production.
- If incontinence occurs, a pathologic condition or other influencing factor can usually be identified through a comprehensive evaluation.

Actions to Promote Good Urinary Control

- Avoid foods and beverages that can irritate the bladder (e.g., caffeine, alcohol, artificial sweeteners and spicy and acidic foods).
- Avoid smoking.
- Maintain ideal body weight and good physical fitness.
- Take steps to prevent constipation (refer to Chapter 18, Box 18-6).
- Practice pelvic muscle exercises (refer to Box 19-9).

Interventions for Urinary Incontinence

Interventions for urinary incontinence are initially directed toward resolution of any conditions that affect control over urination. Nursing interventions directly related to this goal are as follows:

- Facilitating referrals to appropriate professionals
- Teaching about pelvic floor muscle exercises (PFME)
- Initiating continence training programs
- Suggesting environmental modifications

When incontinence cannot be alleviated, nursing responsibilities include using appropriate continence aids, being knowledgeable about commonly used medications and medical and surgical interventions, and promoting wellness for caregivers of dependent older adults in home settings.

Facilitating Referrals

Nurses facilitate referrals for medical professionals and specialized advance practice nurses who can perform comprehensive evaluations and prescribe medications or medical devices or perform surgical procedures. An important nursing role is to encourage older adults who experience urinary incontinence to explore options for treatment rather than only self-managing their symptoms. Studies consistently find that lack of knowledge about available options is a major barrier to obtaining treatment for urinary incontinence (Berger et al., 2011).

A resource that is available in some health care settings is a wound, ostomy and continence (WOC) nurse. WOC nurses have specialized training and certification and are able to provide expert assessment and management of patients with ostomies, wounds, and urinary and fecal incontinence. WOC nurses are effective in achieving important health outcomes, including improved resolution and prevention of urinary incontinence and UTI (Bliss et al., 2013).

Nurses are not usually involved with medical or surgical interventions for urinary incontinence, but it is important to be knowledgeable about safe and effective options for treatment. A variety of intravaginal or intraurethral devices are available for resolving stress incontinence. For many decades, pessaries have been used as an inexpensive, low-risk and conservative treatment for pelvic organ prolapse in women. These simple devices are placed in the vagina to support the bladder, compress the urethra or both. They are available in many sizes and shapes and are individually fitted by a health care practitioner (Fig. 19-2). Pessaries need to be removed and reinserted at intervals ranging from nightly to once every few months, depending on the type that is used.

In recent years, many urinary control devices have become available or are used in clinical trials for self-insertion

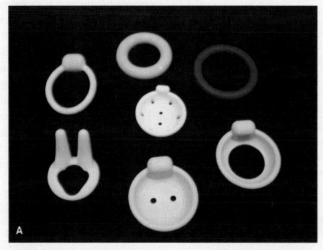

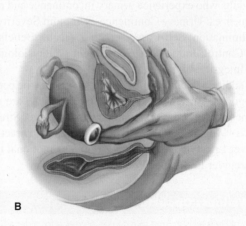

FIGURE 19-2 Examples of pessaries. Various shapes and sizes of pessaries available **(A)**, insertion of one type of pessary **(B)**. (**A**, reprinted with permission from Berek, J. S. [2012]. *Novak's gynecology* [15th ed.]. Philadelphia, PA: Lippincott Williams & Wilkins; **B**, reprinted with permission from Ricci, S. S. [2008]. *Essentials of maternity, newborn, and women's health nursing* [2nd ed.]. Philadelphia, PA: Lippincott Williams & Wilkins.)

into the urethra. For example, one type of device controls urination through the inflation and deflation of a small balloon that rests at the bladder neck. Other currently available devices for women include urethral plugs; intraurethral catheters with unidirectional valves; and external occlusive devices, which cover the external urinary meatus and provide a watertight seal to prevent leakage. For men, foam-cushioned penile clamps with compression mechanisms are available. Interventions for urinary incontinence are developing rapidly and evidence-based and up-to-date information is available at websites listed in Online Learning Activity 19-5. Use Box 19-8 to teach about types of options that patients can discuss with a health care professional.

Indwelling catheters are an intervention that until recently was commonly used for long-term management of urinary incontinence. However, because they are associated with a high rate of serious UTIs (as discussed in Box 19-4 about CAUTI), their use is limited primarily to short term. Medicare and other major health care organizations consider indwelling catheters

as an indicator of quality of care, with lower numbers of indwelling catheters being associated with better quality of care. The only acceptable indications for the use of indwelling catheters are stage III or IV pressure sores when urine impedes healing, urinary retention that cannot be treated medically or surgically, or for comfort during terminal illness. Intermittent clean catheterization is sometimes used as a self-care or caregiver-administered intervention for some types of incontinence.

See **ONLINE LEARNING ACTIVITY 19-5:**
RESOURCES FOR ADDITIONAL INFORMATION ABOUT URINARY WELLNESS AND INCONTINENCE
at http://thepoint.lww.com/Miller7e

Wellness Opportunity

Nurses promote self-care by encouraging older adults to seek further evaluation by qualified health care professionals rather than relying solely on the reported experiences of friends.

Box 19-8 Evidence-Based Interventions for Urinary Incontinence

Nonpharmacologic Interventions Effective for Men and Women

- Pelvic floor muscle exercises
- Achieving and maintaining healthy weight
- Behavioural techniques: fluid management (i.e., intake of adequate amounts of fluids until several hours before bedtime, timed voiding (i.e., gradually lengthening the interval between urination)

Medical and Surgical Treatment for Men and Women

- Antimuscarinic medications for overactive bladder (pills, patch, gel): darifenacin (Enablex), festoterodine (Toviaz), oxybutinin (Ditropan, Gelnique, Oxytrol), solifenacin (Vesicare), tolterodine (Detrol), tropsium (Sanctura)
- Biofeedback to enhance performance of pelvic floor muscle exercises through the use of a simple probe placed in the vagina (women) or rectum (men) to measure physiologic processes involving pelvic muscle contractions
- Neuromodulation (i.e., stimulation of nerves through the use of an implantable device)
- Injection of bulking agent (e.g., collagen, carbon spheres) into tissues around the bladder neck and urethra

Specific for Women

- Vaginal estrogen (cream or intravaginal ring)
- Pessary (i.e., ring or other inserted into the vagina to place pressure on the urethra)
- Surgery for pelvic floor disorders (e.g., retropubic suspension or sling procedure)

Specific for Men

- α-Blockers or 5-α reductase inhibitors for prostate enlargement and bladder outlet obstruction: alfuzosin (Uroxatral), doxasosin (Cardura), dutaseride (Avodart), finasteride (Proscar), tamsulosin (Flomax), terazosin (Hytrin)
- Surgical implantation of an artificial urinary sphincter to keep the urethra closed
- Male sling surgery to provide support for the urethra
- Urinary diversion surgery

Teaching About PFME

Pelvic floor muscle exercise (PFME) is an evidence-based practice that is effective as a first-line intervention for men and women with stress, urge and mixed incontinence and in women with pelvic organ prolapse (Bø & Hilde, 2013; Hagen & Stark, 2011; Hay-Smith et al., 2012; Tienforti et al., 2012). These exercises were first promoted for postpartum therapy by an American gynecologist named A. H. Kegel, and they are now widely used for control of urinary incontinence. Other terms used interchangeably with PFME include Kegels, pelvic muscle exercise, pelvic floor training and pelvic muscle rehabilitation. The goal of PFME is the improvement of urethral resistance through active exercise of the pubococcygeal muscle. There are no contraindications to or negative effects of these exercises, which can be initiated by any motivated person who is able to learn the technique. Nurses can use the information in Box 19-9 to teach older men and women to perform PFME, which is a nursing intervention recognized by NANDA. A related nursing intervention is to facilitate referrals to physical therapists who are skilled in teaching about these exercises.

See **ONLINE LEARNING ACTIVITY 19-6:**
ARTICLE ON UNDERSTANDING STRESS URINARY INCONTINENCE
at http://thepoint.lww.com/Miller7e

Initiating Continence Training Programs

Continence training is a nursing intervention that can be categorized as (1) methods that are self-directed by motivated and cognitively intact people or (2) methods that are directed by motivated caregivers of cognitively impaired people. The goal of continence training is to achieve a continent interval of 2 to 4 hours between voiding. These intervals will not necessarily be equal and will usually be longer during the night. In self-directed programs, the person hopes to regain voluntary urinary control, whereas in caregiver-directed programs, the caregiver hopes to reduce the episodes of incontinence. Self-directed

Box 19-9 Instructions for Performing Pelvic Muscle Exercises

Purpose: To prevent the involuntary loss of urine by strengthening the pelvic floor muscles

Frequency: Minimum of 3 sets of 10 contractions/relaxations daily, continued indefinitely

Position: Lying, sitting, walking or standing with the muscles of your thighs, buttocks and abdomen relaxed

Results: Most people begin to notice an improvement in urinary control after 3 to 6 weeks, but some will not notice the improvement until several months later.

Techniques to Identify the Pubococcygeal Muscle

- Contract the muscle that stops the flow of urine. Do NOT do this regularly when urinating.
- (*Women*) Imagine that you are sitting on a marble and trying to suck it up into your vagina.
- (*Women*) Lie down and insert a finger about three quarters of the way up your vagina. Squeeze the vaginal wall so you feel pressure on your finger and a sensation in your vagina.
- (*Men*) Stand in front of a mirror and try to make the base of your penis move up and down without moving the rest of your body.
- Biofeedback, weighted vaginal cones or a perineometer (a balloon-like device that is placed in the vagina) can be used to assist in identifying the pubococcygeal muscle and in measuring the strength of the contraction.

Method

- Tighten your pubococcygeal muscle and hold for a period of at least 3 seconds; gradually increase the contraction time by 1 second per week until you can do a 10-second squeeze.
- Relax this muscle for an equal period; rest and take deep breaths between contractions.
- Do 10 sets of a contraction–relaxation cycle (one exercise) 3 times daily.
- Breathe normally during these exercises and do NOT tighten other muscles at the same time. Be careful not to contract your legs, buttocks or abdominal muscles while you are contracting your pubococcygeal muscle.
- For each of the daily sessions, vary your position (e.g., perform the exercise while lying down in the morning, standing in the afternoon and sitting in the evening).

Additional information: You can ask your primary care practitioner for a referral to a physical therapist or continence advisor who can teach you to do these exercises.

continence training, alone or in combination with biofeedback or medications, is most successful with urge incontinence.

Although specific techniques vary, essential elements of any continence training program include motivation, an assessment of voiding patterns, an individualized and carefully timed intake of approximately 1,500 to 2,000 mL of fluid per day, timed voiding in the most appropriate place, methods of reinforcing expected behaviours and ongoing monitoring. During the initial assessment, diaries are used to record times and circumstances of toileting, as well as times of and reasons for any episode of incontinence. After the usual voiding pattern is identified, the older adult is encouraged to resist the sensation of urgency and to postpone voiding rather than responding immediately to an urge.

With caregiver-directed methods—often referred to as **prompted voiding** programs—the caregiver uses the initial assessment of voiding patterns to establish a schedule for assisting

Box 19-10 Continence Training Programs

Goal of Programs

To achieve voluntary control over urination at intervals of 2 to 4 hours

Terminology

Terms used for self-directed programs: bladder drill, bladder training, bladder retraining, bladder exercise, bladder retention exercise

Terms used for caregiver-directed programs: scheduled toileting, routine toileting, prompted voiding, timed voiding, habit training

Method

Step 1: Identify the usual voiding pattern, noting the times of incontinence and information about fluid intake. During the first few days, keep a diary to record the following information at hourly intervals: dry or wet, amount voided, place of voiding, fluid intake and sensation and awareness of need to void.

Step 2: Using information from the voiding diary, establish a schedule that allows for emptying of the bladder before incontinence is likely to occur.

Step 3: Provide the equipment and assistance necessary for optimal voiding at scheduled times.

Step 4: Provide 2,000 mL of noncaffeinated liquids per day for liquid intake. Consume the largest amounts during the early part of the day, and limit fluid intake at about 2 to 4 hours before bedtime.

Step 5: Gradually increase the length of time between voidings until the interval is 2 to 4 hours long.

with voiding. The caregiver gradually increases the interval between voidings until the person can maintain continence for 2 to 4 hours. These methods are most successful when the timed intervals are flexible and are adjusted on the basis of a good assessment of the person's needs and voiding patterns. Caregiver-directed programs include the use of behaviour modification techniques, such as praising the person for staying dry between scheduled trips to the bathroom and self-initiating requests to use the toilet. Box 19-10 identifies some of the terms used for and the general principles of continence training programs.

Suggesting Environmental Modifications

When incontinence is associated with the inability to reach an appropriate receptacle after perceiving the need to void, interventions are directed toward modifying the environment and improving functional abilities. If environmental adaptations cannot be made, as in public places, older adults are encouraged to become familiar with the location and arrangement of the bathroom facilities before the need to urinate is imminent. In home and institutional settings, the provision of bedside commodes and privacy can be an effective intervention. If space is limited or privacy cannot be assured, however, bedside commodes may not be acceptable. Box 19-11 lists environmental modifications that are for preventing incontinence when functional limitations are a contributing factor. Interventions discussed in chapters on vision (Chapter 17) and mobility (Chapter 22) can address functional limitations that can contribute to incontinence.

Wellness Opportunity

Nurses promote self-care by helping older adults to identify ways of improving their functional abilities that can affect urinary control.

Box 19-11 Environmental Modifications for Preventing Incontinence

Modifications to Enhance Visibility of Facilities

- Use contrasting colours for the toilet seat and surroundings.
- Provide adequate lighting in and near toilet areas, but avoid creating glare.
- Use nightlights in the pathway between the bedroom and bathroom.

Modifications to Improve the Ability to Use the Toilet in Time

- Encourage the use of chairs or beds that are designed to help the person arise unaided after sitting or lying.
- Install handrails in the hallway(s) leading to the bathroom.
- Make sure the pathway to the bathroom is safe and uncluttered.

Modifications to Improve the Ability to Use the Toilet

- Place grab bars at appropriate places to facilitate getting on and off the toilet and to assist men in maintaining their balance when standing at the toilet.
- Use elevated toilet seats or an over-the-toilet chair to compensate for any functional limitations of the lower extremities.
- If the person has functional limitations involving the upper extremities, clothing for the lower body should feature easy-open closures such as Velcro or elastic waistbands.

Box 19-12 Considerations Regarding Continence Aids and Equipment

Assessment Considerations

- What are the costs of various disposable and washable products, both initially and over a period of time? (Include the time and expense of laundry when considering costs of washable products.)
- What are the person's preferences? (e.g., Is a "brief" or "pull-up" style garment more acceptable than a "diaper" style product?)
- What level of absorbency is appropriate for different circumstances?
- What are the needs and abilities of the caregivers of dependent older adults in home settings? (Can the caregiver manage the tasks involved in toileting?)
- What are the consequences if the incontinence cannot be managed in the home setting? (e.g., will the older adult need to be in a long-term care setting?)

Teaching Related to Aids and Equipment

- Many types of external collecting devices are available for men and women (e.g., male or female urinals, condom catheters, retracted penis pouches, and bedside urinals with attached drainage bags).
- An elevated toilet seat with rails can be used to increase safety and transfer mobility.
- Commodes are useful in diminishing the distance between the place of usual activities and toilet facilities.
- A variety of commodes are available and can be selected according to needs and preferences of the dependent person.
- Measures can be taken to ensure privacy and increase social acceptability of commodes (e.g., by placing an attractive screen around the commode).
- Some commodes are attractively designed to resemble normal furniture items.
- A bedpan can be placed on a regular chair, particularly in the bedroom, and removed when not in use.

Using Appropriate Continence Aids

When incontinence cannot be alleviated, it can be managed with the use of various aids and equipment, such as incontinence products and collecting devices. When used in conjunction with environmental modifications to increase the accessibility of toilet facilities, such equipment usually has beneficial effects; however, when aids and equipment are used by caregivers as substitutes for other methods of promoting continence, they are beneficial only to the caregiver and are detrimental to the older adult. For example, if protective products are used to manage incontinence, the positive effect for the caregiver may be the ease of care; however, the negative effects for the older adult include the likelihood of skin breakdown and decreased self-esteem. Because continence aids can be beneficial as well as detrimental, they should be used only after careful evaluation of all contributing factors, including needs of family caregivers in home settings.

Selection of the most appropriate products for managing incontinence depends on factors such as cost, convenience, preference and effectiveness. Economic considerations are particularly important because disposable incontinence products can be quite expensive, particularly if used daily. The initial and periodic cost of reusable products also needs to be considered, as does the time and expense of laundering. Many products are designed specifically for either male or female incontinence. Product absorbency is affected by variables such as size, shape, depth and location and type of absorbent material (e.g., gel, pulp, polymer). Keep in mind that someone may need several types of products for different activities (e.g., light protection during the day and heavy protection during the night). Ease of use is a major consideration, particularly for people who are independent and can manage incontinence with little or no supervision. "Pull-ups" now provide a convenient alternative to the products with tabs that cannot be easily

removed before and reapplied after toileting. Box 19-12 lists factors to be considered in selecting and using various types of aids and equipment for managing urinary incontinence. Use Online Learning Activity 19-7 to find information about various products for managing urinary incontinence.

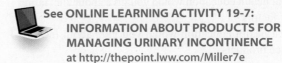

See **ONLINE LEARNING ACTIVITY 19-7: INFORMATION ABOUT PRODUCTS FOR MANAGING URINARY INCONTINENCE** at http://thepoint.lww.com/Miller7e

Being Knowledgeable About Medications for Urinary Incontinence

Medications have varying degrees of success for treating incontinence, but their effectiveness depends greatly on identifying and addressing the specific type of incontinence. Medications can also effectively treat an underlying condition that contributes to incontinence (e.g., OAB, vaginitis, benign prostatic hyperplasia). When medications are prescribed, nurses are responsible for knowing their expected positive effects as well as their potential adverse effects. Nurses also have important roles in teaching about medications, including over-the-counter ones that became available for OAB (e.g., Oxytrol patches) beginning in 2013.

Medications that act on the autonomic nervous system are most often used for the control of incontinence. α-Adrenergic agents control stress incontinence by increasing bladder outlet resistance through stimulating receptors at the trigone and internal sphincter. α-Adrenergic blocking agents, used either alone or in combination with cholinergic agents, can treat incontinence by decreasing bladder outlet resistance. Antimuscarinic agents are used for urge urinary incontinence and OAB because they control the uninhibited or unstable bladder by blocking the transmission of nerve impulses.

In recent years, geriatricians have expressed concern about the adverse effects of antimuscarinic agents because they have the potential to cross the blood–brain barrier and cause adverse effects on the central nervous system. Oxybutinin is the medication most commonly associated with cognitive impairment, but all antimuscarinic agents need to be used with caution in older adults with preexisting dementia (Chancellor & Boone, 2012; Pagoria et al., 2011). These medications have the same adverse effect profile as other anticholinergics, such as dry mouth, constipation, blurred vision and mental changes. People who have glaucoma need to

Unfolding Case Study

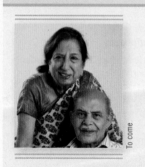

To come

Part 2: Mr. and Mrs. U. at 73 and 72 Years of Age

Mr. and Mrs. U. are now 73 and 72 years old, respectively, and continue to attend the senior centre where you are the nurse.

Mr. U.

Mr. U. has been under the care of a urologist for 3 years and has been taking terazosin for prostatic hyperplasia. Until recently, he was able to maintain urinary continence, but lately his Parkinson disease has worsened. Then, 1 month ago, he started taking 80 mg of furosemide daily for congestive heart failure. He makes an appointment to seek your advice about incontinence products that would be best for him because "it's just hopeless to get to the toilet on time because our only bathroom is upstairs, and I like to be downstairs during the day." He reports that he limits his fluid intake to four cups of liquid daily, which includes two cups of black coffee. Because of his Parkinson disease, he has trouble standing at the toilet and usually sits down; however, he is "slow and clumsy" in managing his clothing. His son bought him some "jogging" outfits with elastic waists, but he does not wear them because he prefers to "dress up" when he goes to the senior centre, so he wears trousers with belts.

THINKING POINTS WITH REGARD TO MR. U.

- What risk factors are likely to be contributing to Mr. U.'s incontinence, and which factors might be alleviated with interventions?
- What environmental modifications might be helpful in addressing the incontinence?
- What health education would you give about alleviating risk factors?
- What health education would you give about incontinence products?

Mrs. U.

Mrs. U. also makes an appointment to see you to discuss her recent problem with incontinence. She tells you that for several years she has been wearing "light-days pads" because "I have trouble holding my water whenever I sneeze or cough." In the past few months, she notices that she has to go to the bathroom every hour or two and is reluctant to be away from her house for more than an hour at a time. Her health has been good overall, but her arthritis has been getting worse, and she is very slow moving, particularly when she needs to go up and down stairs. She drinks about six cups of liquid daily, consisting mostly of tea and coffee. She has heard some of her friends talking about "those Kegel exercises we had to do when we had our babies."

THINKING POINTS WITH REGARD TO MRS. U.

- What risk factors are likely to be contributing to Mrs. U.'s incontinence?
- What environmental modifications might be helpful in addressing the incontinence?
- What health education would you give about alleviating risk factors?

- What health education would you give about Kegel exercises?
- What health education would you give about incontinence products?

ask their ophthalmologist if they can safely take these drugs. Another nursing implication is that it is important to raise questions about a potential relationship between the onset and worsening of mental changes in anyone taking medications with antimuscarinic action, particularly if the person has dementia or takes other anticholinergic agents.

Promoting Caregiver Wellness

For caregivers of dependent older adults in home settings, the onset of urinary incontinence often is associated with significant additional stress, particularly in combination with environmental barriers that cannot be modified. Tasks related to incontinence are some of the most difficult, stressful and time-consuming aspects of caregiving. Caregivers in home settings are likely to feel angry, guilty, frustrated or inadequate when dealing with incontinence on a daily basis. Lifelong attitudes about control over urination may contribute to feelings of disgust about the care demands, which may be further compounded by feelings of guilt about this initial reaction to

caregiving tasks. If the caregiver perceives intentionality on the part of the dependent person in his or her failure to control urination, these feelings will likely be intensified.

Nurses have key roles in promoting caregiver wellness by teaching caregivers about the importance of addressing all treatable contributing conditions. In addition to applying the information already discussed in the Nursing Interventions sections, Box 19-13 can be used to teach caregivers of older adults who have urinary incontinence.

EVALUATING EFFECTIVENESS OF NURSING INTERVENTIONS

Nursing care for older adults with urinary incontinence is evaluated by measuring the extent to which the person can achieve periods of continence that are as long as possible. When older adults attribute incontinence to aging processes, nurses evaluate the effectiveness of their teaching by the degree to which the person verbalizes accurate information and

---

Box 19-13 Caregiver Wellness: Facts About Urinary Incontinence

- Healthy older adults normally experience the following changes affecting urinary control: diminished bladder capacity, urgency (i.e., shorter interval for maintaining control after perceiving the need to void) and frequency (e.g., voiding once or twice during the night).
- Urinary incontinence (i.e., involuntary loss of urine) occurs more often in older adults, but it is NOT an inevitable or untreatable condition.
- Urinary incontinence ranges from periodic episodes of "leakage" (especially when coughing or laughing) to total inability to maintain control over urination, but causes and treatments for each type differ.
- Stress incontinence is the involuntary loss of small amounts of urine due to activities that increase pressure on the lower abdominal wall, such as coughing, laughing, sneezing or exercising.
- Urge incontinence is the sudden loss of large amounts of urine soon after feeling the need to urinate.
- Overactive bladder (OAB) occurs when the bladder muscles contract due to abnormal signals, causing urgency and frequency, and sometimes causing incontinence.
- Never assume that urinary incontinence is irreversible or untreatable—it is not necessarily a condition that should just be tolerated and managed as well as possible.

Conditions That Increase the Risk for Urinary Incontinence

Diseases: dementia, stroke, diabetes, urinary tract infections, Parkinson's disease, multiple sclerosis, spinal cord injury
- Conditions: constipation, obesity, limited mobility, cognitive impairment
- Conditions specific to women: pelvic floor disorders, such as prolapsed ("dropped") bladder or uterus, history of vaginal childbirths
- Conditions specific to men: benign prostatic hypertrophy (BPH), radiation or surgery for prostate cancer
- Adverse effects of the following types of medications: diuretics, drugs that act on the autonomic nervous system
- Environmental conditions that interfere with ability to use toileting facility in timely manner (e.g., inaccessible toilets, toilet seats that are too low, lack of handrails)

Actions to Take to Identify Causes and Treatments for Urinary Incontinence

- Recognize that there are many types of medical, surgical and minimally invasive treatments for urinary incontinence (see Box 19-8).
- Keep a voiding diary for a few days with information about fluids intake, voiding pattern and episodes of involuntary loss of urine.
- Talk with your primary care practitioner about a referral for specialized health care professionals, such as a urologist, urogynecologist (for women) or specialized nurse or physical therapist.

Actions to Promote Good Control Over Urination

- Maintain good fluid intake, with the largest amounts being consumed at least several hours before bedtime.
- Avoid or limit the following foods and fluids that irritate the bladder or cause urinary incontinence: caffeine, carbonated beverages, citrus products, alcohol, artificial sweeteners, spicy foods.
- In addition to using self-management strategies (e.g., pads or briefs for incontinence), it is imperative to obtain a medical evaluation to identify causes and appropriate treatments.
- Practice pelvic floor muscle exercises (also called Kegel exercises), which can be effective for alleviating or reducing episodes of urinary incontinence (see Box 19-9).

Resources for Support, Information and Continence Aids

- *Canadian Foundation for Women's Heath,* http://cfwh.org/index.php?page=incontinence-awareness-month&hl=en_CA
- *Canadian Urological Association,* http://www.cua.org/
- *Continence Product Advisor,* www.continenceproductadvisor.org
- *Health Canada,* Seniors and aging, bladder control problems, http://www.hc-sc.gc.ca/hl-vs/iyh-vsv/med/incont-eng.php
- *RNAO,* Promoting continence through using promoted voiding, http://rnao.ca/bpg/guidelines/promoting-continence-using-prompted-voiding
- *The Canadian Continence Foundation,* http://www.canadiancontinence.ca/index.html

understands the importance of identifying treatable causes. Another measure of the effectiveness of nursing interventions in such cases would be that the person seeks evaluation for his or her incontinence, rather than accepting this condition as inevitable.

If incontinence cannot be resolved, nursing care is directed toward managing urinary elimination in such a way as to maintain the dignity of the older adult and to prevent negative consequences. In these situations, the effectiveness of nursing interventions might be measured by the extent to which the person maintains daily activities. For example, if older adults restrict their social activities because of incontinence, a measure of the success of nursing interventions might be that they begin using incontinence products to permit them to be away from their home for 4 hours at a time. For people with total incontinence, a measure of the effectiveness of nursing interventions would be the absence of skin irritation and breakdown.

Unfolding Case Study

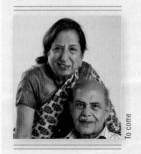

Part 3: Mrs. U. at 79 Years of Age

Mrs. U., who is now 79 years old, is being transferred to a rehabilitation facility after sustaining a hip fracture. An indwelling catheter was inserted before her hip surgery 7 days ago, and it was removed yesterday. She is ambulating with a walker but needs one-person assistance. The discharge summary describes her as incontinent of urine. Mrs. U. hopes to regain her independence in performing ADLs so that she can return to her own home, where she lives with her husband.

NURSING ASSESSMENT

During your functional assessment, Mrs. U. tells you she has had "trouble holding her water" since they removed the catheter yesterday. She is quite embarrassed about this and has not discussed it with any other health care practitioner. She says that she had too many other questions to discuss with her orthopedic surgeon and states that the nurses kept a large absorbent pad on her bed so that she would not have to walk to the bathroom. When she went to physical therapy, she used sanitary napkins, which her friend brought to her. She limited her fluid intake to a cup of coffee with each meal and a few sips of water with her pills.

Further assessment of Mrs. U's incontinence reveals that, for many years, she has had difficulty with "leaking," particularly when she coughs, sneezes or exercises. Also, she gets up to urinate about four to five times nightly. It was during one of these trips to the bathroom that she tripped and fractured her hip. She says that she wakes up a lot during the night and goes to the bathroom because she is afraid of wetting the bed. She does not feel the need to urinate every time she wakes up but goes to the bathroom to prevent any leakage. She limits her fluid intake to six glasses per day and does not drink anything after 5 PM. Mrs. U says, "A few years ago, I started doing Kegel exercises and that helped for a while but I don't bother to do them anymore." She tearfully confides that she thinks that the orthopedic surgeon damaged a nerve in her bladder, which she believes is the reason she has had such little control over urination since the surgery. She thinks that the hospital staff inserted the catheter because she has "weak kidneys." She states, "Before I had this fractured hip, I just had the usual problems holding water like all my friends have, but now it's really bad and I'll probably never be able to hold my water again. I wish you'd just put that tube back in me, so I can go home again and not worry about accidents."

NURSING DIAGNOSIS

In addition to the nursing diagnoses related to Mrs. U.'s impaired mobility, you address her problem with urinary incontinence. In deciding which type of urinary incontinence to include in your nursing diagnosis, you conclude that both Stress Incontinence and Functional Incontinence are appropriate because of the combination of long-term and recent factors that contribute to her incontinence. Your nursing diagnosis is Stress/Functional Incontinence related to limited mobility, recent indwelling catheter, and insufficient knowledge of normal urinary function and pelvic muscle exercises. Evidence for this diagnosis can be found in Mrs. U.'s statements reflecting misconceptions and lack of information and in her description of current and past problems with incontinence. Evidence is also derived from your observations that she needs one-person assistance for walking and that she uses sanitary napkins and bed pads for urinary incontinence.

(continued)

Unfolding Case Study (continued)

Nursing Care Plan for Mrs. U.

Expected Outcome	N Nursing Interventions	N Nursing Education
Mrs. U.'s knowledge of normal urinary function will increase.	• Discuss normal urinary function using a balloon partially filled with water and a simple illustration of the female urinary tract. • Emphasize the relationship between adequate fluid intake and continence.	• Mrs. U. will be able to describe normal urinary function and the mechanisms involved in maintaining continence.
Mrs. U.'s knowledge about causative factors for incontinence will increase.	• Describe age-related changes that contribute to incontinence using the information in Box 19-6. • Discuss the effects of frequent bladder emptying and limited fluid intake on the maintenance of continence. • Discuss the relationship between limited mobility and urinary incontinence.	• Mrs. U. will describe age-related changes that influence urinary elimination. • Mrs. U. will identify risk factors that contribute to her incontinence.
Mrs. U.'s misconceptions about her urinary incontinence will be corrected.	• Emphasize that as Mrs. U. regains her mobility, she will regain continence. • Emphasize that urinary incontinence is not an inevitable consequence of aging. • Explain that the orthopedic surgeon was not operating on or near her bladder or urinary tract. • Explain that the Foley catheter probably contributed to her current incontinence, but that this is a temporary situation that will resolve with proper interventions. • Emphasize that the nursing home staff will work with her to improve or alleviate her incontinence.	• Mrs. U. will state correct information about the relationship between her hip surgery and her incontinence. • Mrs. U. will express confidence in regaining urinary control.
The factors that contribute to Mrs. U.'s functional incontinence will be eliminated.	• Provide a bedside commode for Mrs. U.'s use until she is able to walk to the bathroom without assistance. • Work with the physical therapy staff to teach Mrs. U. a proper technique for independent transfer to the commode. • The nursing and dietary staff will provide 2,000 mL of fluids per day taking into consideration Mrs. U.'s preferences. • The nursing and dietary staff will work with Mrs. U. to schedule her fluid intake at acceptable times of the day with minimal intake in the evening. • Talk with Mrs. U. about eliminating the bed pads as soon as she feels confident about maintaining continence.	• Mrs. U. will be continent of urine, except for stress incontinence.
Mrs. U. will regain full control over urination.	• Suggest that Mrs. U. seek a comprehensive assessment of her urinary incontinence. • Give Mrs. U. a copy of Box 19-7 as a guide for performing PFME. • Emphasize the need to perform PFME on an ongoing basis for the alleviation of stress incontinence. • Give Mrs. U. information about health education that may be helpful for her.	• Mrs. U. will report a reduction in or elimination of her stress incontinence.

THINKING POINTS

- What myths and misunderstandings affect Mrs. U.'s attitude about urinary incontinence?
- What risk factors are contributing to Mrs. U's urinary incontinence?
- What additional assessment information would you want to obtain?

Unfolding Case Study (continued)

QSEN APPLICATION

QSEN Competency	Knowledge/Skill/Attitude	Application to Mrs. U.
Patient-centred care	(K) Integrate understanding of multiple dimensions of patient-centred care.	Identify the many factors that interact to contribute to Mrs. U's current difficulty maintaining urinary continence.
	(K) Describe how diverse backgrounds function as a source of values.	
	(K) Describe strategies to empower patients in all aspects of the health care process.	Provide accurate information to dispel myths and misunderstandings and improve Mrs. U's self-efficacy related to urinary control.
	(K) Examine common barriers to active involvement of patients in their own health care processes.	
	(S) Provide patient-centred care with sensitivity and respect for diversity of the human experience.	Use good communication skills to address this sensitive topic.
	(S) Assess own level of communication skill in encounters with patients and families.	
	(S) Communicate care provided and needed at each transition in care.	Address Mrs. U's concerns about being able to return to her own home.
	(A) Value seeing health care situations "through patients' eyes."	
Teamwork and collaboration	(K) Describe scopes of practice and role of health care team members.	Work closely with nursing assistants, dietary staff and physical and occupational therapists to implement interprofessional care plan to address issues that affect Mrs. U's ability to maintain urinary continence.
	(K) Recognize contributions of other individuals and groups in helping patient achieve health goals.	
	(S) Integrate the contributions of others who play a role in helping patient achieve health goals.	
Evidence-based practice	(K) Describe how the strength and relevance of available evidence influence the choice of intervention.	Base care plan on evidence-based information discussed in this chapter and in Online Learning Activities 19-2 and 19-5.
	(S) Base individualized care plan on patient values, clinical expertise and evidence.	
	(S) Read original research and evidence reports related to clinical practice.	
	(A) Value evidence-based practice as integral to determining the best clinical practice.	

Chapter Highlights

Age-Related Changes That Affect Urinary Wellness

- *Kidney:* degenerative changes, decreased blood flow, decreased number of functioning nephrons
- *Urinary tract muscles:* hypertrophy of bladder muscle, replacement of smooth muscle with connective tissue, relaxation of pelvic floor muscles (Fig. 19-3)
- *Voluntary control mechanisms:* central nervous system, urinary tract, age-related changes of other systems (e.g., increased postural sway)

Risk Factors That Affect Urinary Wellness

- Limited fluid intake promoting other dietary factors
- Medication effects (Table 19-1)

- Misperceptions and misunderstandings (e.g., resignation, viewing urinary incontinence as "normal," staff and caregiver attitudes that interfere with maintaining continence)
- Influence of caregivers
- Functional impairments and environmental factors (Box 19-1)
- Pathologic and other conditions (e.g., dementia, risk factors associated with urinary incontinence)
- Gender-specific conditions (e.g., pelvic floor disorders, benign prostatic hyperplasia)

Functional Consequences Affecting Urinary Wellness

- Effects on renal function: diminished ability to maintain homeostasis, delayed excretion of water-soluble medications and increased risk of drug interactions and adverse effects

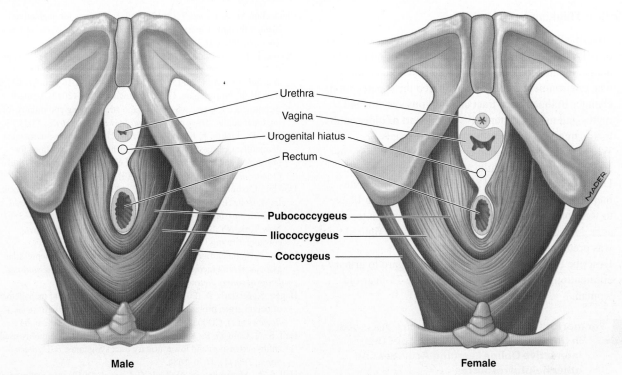

FIGURE 19-3 Illustration of male and female pelvic floor anatomy and the muscles that affect control over urination.(Reprinted with permission from Moore, K. L., Agur, A. M., & Dalley, A. F. [2013]. *Clinically oriented anatomy* [7th ed.]. Philadelphia, PA: Lippincott Williams & Wilkins.)

- Effects on voiding patterns: changes in diurnal pattern of urine production
- Urinary incontinence (Box 19-2)
- Psychosocial consequences of urinary incontinence

Pathologic Condition Affecting Urinary Function: Urinary Tract Infections

- Urinary tract infections are common and sometimes overlooked because the symptoms are subtle and generalized (Table 10-1 and Box 19-4)

Nursing Assessment of Urinary Function (Fig. 19-3, Boxes 19-5 and 19-6)

- Talk with older adults about urinary function (finding appropriate terminology)
- Assess usual voiding patterns and influencing factors (Fig. 19-1)
- Identify risk factors for urinary incontinence
- Identify risk factors that influence renal function and homeostasis
- Assess symptoms of impaired urinary elimination
- Be alert to misunderstandings about urinary elimination
- Assess psychosocial consequences of incontinence (e.g., anxiety, depression, social isolation)

Nursing Diagnosis

- Readiness for Enhanced Urinary Elimination
- Impaired Urinary Elimination

- Social Isolation
- Caregiver Role Strain (or Risk for)

Planning for Wellness Outcomes

- Urinary Continence
- Urinary Elimination
- Health Beliefs: Perceived Control
- Caregiver Stressors
- Caregiver Endurance Potential

Nursing Interventions to Promote Healthy Urinary Function (Boxes 19-7 through 19-13)

- Teaching older adults about age-related changes and preventing urinary incontinence
- Promoting continence and alleviating incontinence (pelvic floor muscle training, urinary control devices, continence training, environmental modifications, medications, and surgical or minimally invasive procedures)
- Managing urinary incontinence

Evaluating Effectiveness of Nursing Interventions

- Longer intervals of continence
- Accurate understanding of normal urinary function and risks for incontinence
- Self-care practices to promote continence and urinary wellness
- Use of resources for further evaluation of incontinence when appropriate

Critical Thinking Exercises

1. Describe how each of the following age-related changes or risk factors might influence urinary function in older adults: medications, renal function, functional abilities, environmental conditions, altered thirst perception, changes in the urinary tract and nervous system, and myths and misunderstandings on the part of older adults, their caregivers and health care professionals.
2. What are the psychosocial consequences of urinary incontinence for older adults and their caregivers?
3. Describe how you would address the following statement made by a 74-year-old woman: "Of course I have to wear pads all the time, just like when I was a teenager. I haven't talked to the doctor because I figured this was pretty normal at my age."
4. Describe the nursing assessment, with regard to urinary elimination, for a 75-year-old man and a 75-year-old woman.

For more information about the topics discussed in this chapter, be sure to check out the interactive Online Learning Activities and other helpful resources at http://thepoint.lww.com/Miller7e

REFERENCES

Adedokun, B. O., Morhason-Bello, I. O., Ojengbede, O. A., et al. (2012). Help-seeking behavior among women currently leaking urine in Nigeria. *Patient Preference and Adherence*, 6, 815–819.

Aguilar-Navarro, S., Navarrete-Reyes, A. P., Grados-Chavarria, B. H., et al. (2012). The severity of urinary incontinence decreases health-related quality of life among community-dwelling elderly. *Journal of Gerontology: Biological Sciences & Medical Sciences*, 67(11), 1266–1271.

Andreessen, L., Wilde, M. H., & Herendeen, P. (2012). Preventing catheter-associated urinary tract infections in acute care: The bundle approach. *Journal of Nursing Care Quarterly*, 27(3), 209–217.

Berger, M. B., Patel, J. M., Miller, J. M., et al. (2011). Racial differences in self-reported healthcare seeking and treatment for urinary incontinence in community-dwelling women from the EPI study. *Neurology Urodynamics*, 30(8), 1442–1447.

Bliss, D. Z., Westra, B. L., Savik, K., et al. (2013). Effectiveness of wound, ostomy and continence-certified nurses on individual patient outcomes in home health care. *Journal of Wound Ostomy and Continence Nursing*, 40(2), 135–142.

Bø, K., & Hilde, G. (2013). A systematic review on pelvic floor muscle training for female stress urinary incontinence. *Neurological Urodynamics*, 32(3), 215–223. doi:10.1002/nau.22292

Bosch, J. L., & Weiss, J. P. (2013). The prevalence and cause of nocturia. *Journal of Urology*, 189(1 Suppl.), S86–S92.

Caljouw, M. A., den Elzen, W., Cools, H., et al. (2011). Predictive factors of urinary tract infections among the oldest old in the general population. *BioMedCentral Medicine*, 9(1), 57. Retrieved from www.biomedcentral.com/1741-7015/9/57

Canadian Cancer Society. (n.d.). *Urinary incontinence*. Retrieved from http://www.cancer.ca/en/cancer-information/diagnosis-and-treatment/managing-side-effects/urinary-incontinence/?region=on

Carter, D., & Beer-Gabel, M. (2012). Lower urinary tract symptoms in chronically constipated women. *International Urogynecology Journal*, 23(12), 1785–1789.

Chancellor, M., & Boone, T. (2012). Anticholinergics for overactive bladder therapy: Central nervous system effects. *CNS Neuroscience Therapy*, 18(2), 167–174.

Devore, E. E., Townsend, M. K., Resnick, N. M., et al. (2012). The epidemiology of urinary incontinence in women with type 2 diabetes. *Journal of Urology*, 188(5), 1816–1821. doi:10.1016/juro.2012.07.027

de Vries, H. F., Northington, G. M., & Bogner, H. R. (2012). Urinary incontinence and new psychological distress among community dwelling older adults. *Archives of Gerontology and Geriatrics*, 55(1), 49–54.

Doughty, D., Junkin, J., Kurz, P., et al. (2012). Incontinence-associated dermatitis: Consensus statements, evidence-based guidelines for prevention and treatment, and current challenges. *Journal of Wound Ostomy and Continence Nursing*, 39(3), 303–315.

Dowling-Castronovo, A., & Bradway, C. (2012). Urinary incontinence. In M. Boltz, E. Capezuti, R. Fulmer, et al. (Eds.), *Evidence-based geriatric nursing protocols for best practice* (4th ed., pp. 363–386). New York, NY: Springer. Modified version available at http://consultgerirn.org

Felde, G., Bjelland, I., & Hunskaar, S. (2012). Anxiety and depression associated with incontinence in middle-aged women. *International Urogynecology Journal*, 23(3), 299–306.

Hagen, S., & Stark, D. (2011). Conservative prevention and management of pelvic organ prolapse in women. *Cochrane Database Systematic Reviews* (12), CD003882. doi:1002/14651858.CD003882.pub4

Hall, S. A., Chiu, G. R., Kaufman, D. W., et al. (2012). Commonly used antihypertensives and lower urinary tract symptoms. *BJU International*, 109(11), 1676–1684.

Hall, S. A., Maserejian, N. N., Link, C. L., et al. (2012). Are commonly used psychoactive medications associated with lower urinary tract symptoms? *European Journal of Clinical Pharmacology*, 68(5), 783–791.

Hall, S. A., Yang, M., Gates, M. A., et al. (2012). Associations of commonly used medications with urinary incontinence in a community based sample. *Journal of Urology*, 188(1), 183–189.

Hayder, D. (2012). The effects of urinary incontinence on sexuality. *Journal of Wound Ostomy and Continence Nursing*, 39(5), 539–544.

Hay-Smith, J., Herderschee, R., Dumoulin, C., et al. (2012). Comparison of approaches to pelvic floor muscle training for urinary incontinence in women. *European Journal of Physical Rehabilitation Medicine*, 48(4), 689–705.

Health Canada. (2006). *Seniors and aging: Bladder control problems*. Retrieved from http://www.hc-sc.gc.ca/hl-vs/alt_formats/pacrb-dgapcr/pdf/iyh-vsv/med/incont-eng.pdf

Hirayama, F., & Lee, A. H. (2011). Green tea drinking is inversely associated with urinary incontinence in middle-aged and older women. *Neurourology Urodynamics*, 30(7), 1262–1265.

Kupelian, V., McVary, K. T., Kaplan, S. A., et al. (2013). Association of lower urinary tract symptoms and the metabolic syndrome. *Journal of Urology*, 189(1 Suppl.), S107–S114.

Lin, S. Y. (2013). A pilot study: Fluid intake and bacteriuria in nursing home residents in southern Taiwan. *Nursing Research*, 62(1), 66–72.

Lukacz, E. S., Sampselle, C., Gray, M., et al. (2011). A healthy bladder: Consensus statement. *The International Journal of Clinical Practice*, 65(10), 1026–1036.

Organist, L., & Engberg, S. (2013). WOC nurse consult: Difficulty voiding. *Journal of Wound Ostomy and Continence Nursing*, 40(1), 97–100.

Pagoria, D., O'Connor, R. C., & Guralnick, M. L. (2011). Antimuscarinic drugs: Review of the cognitive impact when used to treat overactive bladder in elderly patients. *Current Urology Reports*, 12(5), 351–357.

Parker-Autry, C. Y., Markland, A. D., Ballard, A. C., et al. (2012). Vitamin D status in women with pelvic floor disorder symptoms. *International Urogynecology Journal*, 23(12), 1699–1705.

Peron, E. P., Zheng, Y., Perera, S., et al. (2012). Antihypertensive drug class use and differential risk of urinary incontinence in community-dwelling older women. *Journal of Gerontology: Biological Sciences and Medical Sciences*, 67A(12), 1373–1378.

Phillips, C. D., Adepoju, O., Stone, N., et al. (2012). Asymptomatic bacteriuria, antibiotic use, and suspected urinary tract infections in four nursing homes. *BioMed Central Geriatrics, 12,* 73.

Ramage-Morin, P., & Gilmour, H. (2013). Urinary incontinence and loneliness in Canadian seniors. *Health Reports* (Components of Statistics Canada no 82-0003-X). Ottawa, ON: Statistics Canada.

Rios, A. A., Cardosa, J. R., Rodriques, M. A., et al. (2011). The help-seeking by women with urinary incontinence in Brazil. *International Urogynecology Journal, 22*(7), 879–884.

Striker, G. (2012). Introduction to the aging kidney. *Journals of Gerontology: Biological Sciences, 67,* 1341–1342.

Tahtinen, R. M., Auvinen, A., Cartwright, R., et al. (2011). Smoking and bladder symptoms in women. *Obstetrics and Gynecology, 118*(3), 643–648.

Taylor, D. W., Weir, M., Cahill, J. J. et al. (2013). The self-reported prevalence and knowledge of urinary incontinence and barriers to health care-seeking in a community sample of Canadian women. *American Journal of Medicine and Medical Sciences, 3*(5), 97–102.

Tienforti, D., Sacco, E., Marangi, F., et al. (2012). Efficacy of an assisted low-density programme of perioperative pelvic floor muscle training in improving recovery after radical prostatectomy. *BJU International, 110*(7), 1004–1010.

Thurmon, K. L., Breyer, B. N., & Erickson, B. A. (2012). Association of bowel habits with lower urinary tract symptoms in men. *Journal of Urology.* doi:10.1016/juro.2012.10.008

Van Kerrebroeck, P. (2011). Nocturia: Current status and future perspectives. *Current Opinion in Obstetrics and Gynecology, 23,* 376–385.

Vaughan, C. P., Auvinen, A., Cartwright, R., et al. (2012). Impact of obesity on urinary storage symptoms. *Journal of Urology, 24,* doi:10.j.juro.2012.10.058

Welch, L. C., Taubenberger, S., & Tennstedt, S. L. (2011). Patients' experiences of seeking health care for lower urinary tract symptoms. *Research in Nursing and Health, 34*(6), 496–507.

Wiggins, J. E. (2012). Aging in the glomerulus. *Journals of Gerontology: Biological Sciences, 67A*(12), 1358–1364.

Yip, S. O., Dick, M. A., McPencow, A. M., et al. (2013). The association between urinary and fecal incontinence and social isolation in older women. *American Journal of Obstetrics and Gynecology, 208*(2), 146. e1–146.e7. doi:10.1016/j.ajog.11.010

Zisberg, A., Sinoff, G., Gur-Yaish, N., et al. (2011). In-hospital use of continence aids and new-onset urinary incontinence in adults aged 70 and older. *Journal of the American Geriatric Society, 59,* 1099–1104. doi:10.1111/j.1532-5415.2011.03413.x

Zulkowski, K. (2012). Diagnosing and treating moisture-associated skin damage. *Advances in Skin and Wound Care, 25*(5), 231–236.

Cardiovascular Function

The cardiovascular system helps maintain homeostasis by bringing oxygen and nutrients to organs and tissues and by transporting carbon dioxide and other waste products to other body systems for removal. Because the cardiovascular system has a tremendous adaptive capacity, healthy older adults will not experience any significant change in cardiovascular performance because of age-related changes alone. In the presence of risk factors, however, the cardiovascular system is less efficient in performing life-sustaining activities and serious negative functional consequences can occur. The high prevalence of risk factors among older adults—and the fact that most risk factors can be reduced by lifestyle and medical interventions—provides numerous opportunities for health promotion. Thus, a major focus of this chapter is on the essential role of nurses in addressing risks for cardiovascular disease.

AGE-RELATED CHANGES THAT AFFECT CARDIOVASCULAR FUNCTION

As with many aspects of physiologic function, it is difficult to determine whether cardiovascular changes are attributable to normal aging or other factors. Knowledge about distinct age- or disease-related changes in cardiovascular function is confounded by the fact that, until recently, there was no technology to detect asymptomatic pathologic cardiovascular processes. Because some conclusions from earlier studies may have attributed pathologic changes to normal aging, current emphasis is on longitudinal studies of subjects who have been carefully screened for asymptomatic cardiovascular disease.

Another confounding factor is the inability to separate sociocultural factors that can affect cardiovascular function in large groups of people. Systolic blood pressure, for example, increases gradually in adults who live in Western societies but not in those from less industrialized societies.

Promoting Cardiovascular Wellness in Older Adults

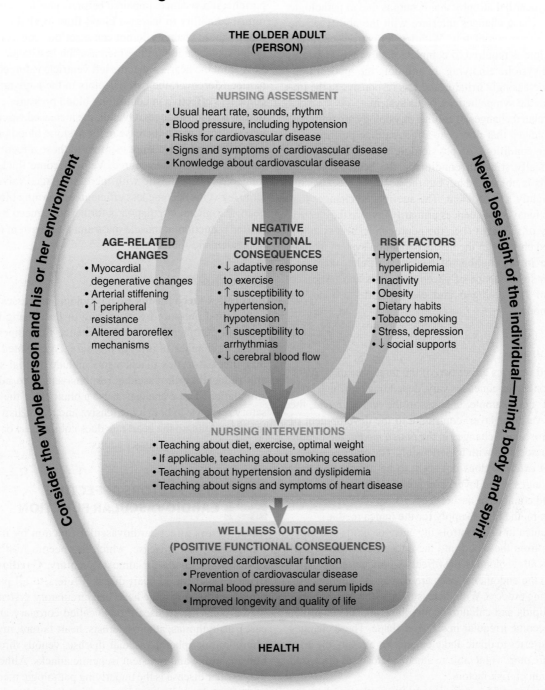

THE OLDER ADULT (PERSON)

NURSING ASSESSMENT
- Usual heart rate, sounds, rhythm
- Blood pressure, including hypotension
- Risks for cardiovascular disease
- Signs and symptoms of cardiovascular disease
- Knowledge about cardiovascular disease

AGE-RELATED CHANGES
- Myocardial degenerative changes
- Arterial stiffening
- ↑ peripheral resistance
- Altered baroreflex mechanisms

NEGATIVE FUNCTIONAL CONSEQUENCES
- ↓ adaptive response to exercise
- ↑ susceptibility to hypertension, hypotension
- ↑ susceptibility to arrhythmias
- ↓ cerebral blood flow

RISK FACTORS
- Hypertension, hyperlipidemia
- Inactivity
- Obesity
- Dietary habits
- Tobacco smoking
- Stress, depression
- ↓ social supports

NURSING INTERVENTIONS
- Teaching about diet, exercise, optimal weight
- If applicable, teaching about smoking cessation
- Teaching about hypertension and dyslipidemia
- Teaching about signs and symptoms of heart disease

WELLNESS OUTCOMES (POSITIVE FUNCTIONAL CONSEQUENCES)
- Improved cardiovascular function
- Prevention of cardiovascular disease
- Normal blood pressure and serum lipids
- Improved longevity and quality of life

HEALTH

Consider the whole person and his or her environment

Never lose sight of the individual—mind, body and spirit

Therefore, changes that have been attributed to increased age may, in fact, be related to lifestyle, sociocultural factors or pathologic conditions. Cross-cultural studies are now being used to identify the effects of lifestyle and other sociocultural factors that affect cardiovascular function. A major focus of research is on identifying those risk factors that are most amenable to interventions so that evidence-based interventions can be recommended. For example, Heart and Stroke Canada emphasizes the importance of heart-healthy nutrition and physical activity behaviours as interventions for all adults who are at risk for cardiovascular disease.

Myocardium and Neuroconduction Mechanisms

Age-related changes of the myocardium include amyloid deposits, lipofuscin accumulation, basophilic degeneration, myocardial atrophy or hypertrophy, valvular thickening and stiffening, and increased amounts of connective tissue. The left atrium and ventricular wall enlarge slightly but any significant myocardial atrophy that occurs is due to pathologic processes. These changes interfere with the ability of the heart to contract completely. With less effective contractility, more time is required to complete the cycle of diastolic filling and systolic emptying. In addition, the myocardium becomes increasingly irritable and less responsive to the impulses from the sympathetic nervous system.

Age-related changes in cardiac physiology are minimal, and the changes that do occur affect cardiac performance only under conditions of physiologic stress. Even under physiologically stressful conditions, the heart in healthy older adults is able to adapt, but the adaptive mechanisms may be slightly less efficient. The age-related changes that cause functional consequences primarily involve the electrophysiology of the heart (i.e., the neuroconduction system). Age-related changes in the neuroconduction system include a decrease in the number of pacemaker cells, increased irregularity in the shape of pacemaker cells and increased deposits of fat, collagen and elastic fibres around the sinoatrial node.

Vasculature

Age-related changes affect two of the three vascular layers, and functional consequences vary, depending on which layer is affected. For example, changes in the *tunica intima*, the innermost vascular layer, contribute to the development of atherosclerosis, and changes in the *tunica media,* the middle layer, are associated with hypertension. The outermost layer (*the tunica externa*) does not seem to be affected by age-related changes. This layer, composed of loosely meshed adipose and connective tissue, supports nerve fibres and the vasa vasorum, the blood supply for the tunica media.

The tunica intima controls the entry of lipids and other substances from the blood into the artery wall. Intact endothelial cells allow blood to flow freely without clotting; however, when the endothelial cells are damaged, they function in the clotting process. With increasing age, the tunica intima thickens, lipids and calcium accumulate, and the endothelial cells become irregular in size and shape. These changes cause the arteries to dilate and elongate. As a result, the arterial walls are more vulnerable to atherosclerosis, as discussed in the section on risk factors.

The tunica media is composed of smooth muscle cells, which are involved in producing collagen, proteoglycans and elastic fibres. This layer provides structural support and controls arterial expansion and contraction. Age-related changes that affect the tunica media include an increase in collagen and a thinning and calcification of elastin fibres, resulting in stiffened blood vessels. These changes are particularly pronounced in the aorta, where the diameter of the lumen increases to compensate for the age-related arterial stiffening. Although these changes are viewed as age related, recent studies indicate that lifestyle variables exert a significant influence on arterial stiffness (Go et al., 2014).

Age-related changes in the tunica media cause increased peripheral resistance, impaired baroreceptor function and diminished ability to increase blood flow to vital organs. Although these changes do not cause serious consequences in healthy older adults, they increase the resistance to blood flow from the heart so that the left ventricle is forced to work harder. Moreover, the baroreceptors in the large arteries become less effective in controlling blood pressure, especially during postural changes. Overall, the increased vascular stiffness causes a slight increase in the systolic blood pressure.

Veins undergo changes similar to those affecting the arteries, but to a lesser degree. Veins become thicker, more dilated and less elastic with increasing age. Valves of the large leg veins become less efficient in returning blood to the heart. Peripheral circulation is further influenced by an age-related reduction in muscle mass and a concurrent reduction in the demand for oxygen.

Baroreflex Mechanisms

Baroreflex mechanisms are physiologic processes that regulate blood pressure by increasing or decreasing the heart rate and peripheral vascular resistance to compensate for transient changes in arterial pressure. Age-related changes that alter baroreflex mechanisms include arterial stiffening and reduced cardiovascular responsiveness to adrenergic stimulation. These changes cause a blunting of the compensatory response to both hypertensive and hypotensive stimuli in older adults, so the heart rate does not increase or decrease as efficiently as in younger adults.

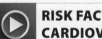

RISK FACTORS AFFECTING CARDIOVASCULAR FUNCTION

Many factors affect cardiovascular function by increasing the risk for heart disease, which has been a leading cause of death in Canada for almost a century. **Cardiovascular disease** (also called heart disease) refers to all pathologic processes that affect the heart and circulatory system including coronary heart disease (also called coronary artery disease), arrhythmias, atherosclerosis, heart failure, myocardial infarction, peripheral vascular disease, venous thromboembolism, stroke and transient ischemic attacks. Although cardiovascular disease is the underlying pathologic mechanisms of stroke (also called cerebrovascular disease) and transient ischemic attacks, they are considered neurologic conditions in clinical practice because of their effects. Chapter 27 discusses heart failure as a common cardiovascular disease, and this chapter focuses on conditions that can be addressed through health promotion interventions to reduce all types of cardiovascular disease.

Researchers, health planners and health care providers are concerned about risks for cardiovascular disease not only because of its significant prevalence and mortality rate but also because it poses a heavy economic burden. Heart disease and stroke costs the Canadian economy more than

$20.9 billion annually in physician services, hospital costs, lost wages and decreased productivity (Conference Board of Canada, 2010). Most importantly from a wellness perspective, there is mounting evidence that most cardiovascular disease is preventable through interventions to reduce risk factors. Thus, prevention is a major focus of health promotion efforts, including patient education and motivation for behaviour change.

Modifiable conditions associated with the highest risk for cardiovascular disease include physical inactivity, elevated blood pressure, obesity, tobacco smoking, dyslipidemia and excessive alcohol consumption (Smith et al., 2012). These conditions can be addressed through medical management and health promotion interventions, as discussed in this chapter and in Chapters 21 (smoking cessation) and 27 (diabetes). In addition, evidence-based dietary measures include limited intake of foods with sodium or saturated fats and increased intake of fruits, vegetables and all plant-based foods.

Some risk factors, such as age, race, gender and heredity, cannot be modified, but it is important to consider their influence on the overall risk profile. In recent years, there is increasing recognition that race and gender can affect both the risk for developing cardiovascular disease and the chance of having adverse outcomes. For example, there is strong evidence of health disparities associated with increased prevalence and poorer management of heart disease and related risk factors in women (Go et al., 2014). Similarly, current emphasis is on developing evidence-based guidelines for risk assessment in blacks and women (Goff et al., 2014). Socioeconomic and psychosocial factors, which are particularly relevant to a holistic health promotion approach to care of older adults, also affect the risk profile for heart disease.

 DIVERSITY NOTE

Smoking rates are over two times higher among the three Aboriginal groups than the non-Aboriginal population. Aboriginal people were also twice as likely to be exposed to secondhand smoke in the home (Gionet & Roshanafshar, 2013).

Atherosclerosis

Atherosclerosis is a disorder of the medium and small arteries in which patchy deposits of lipids and *atherosclerotic plaques* reduce or obstruct blood flow. The development of sophisticated imaging techniques has improved our understanding about the pathophysiology of atherosclerosis since the first theories were proposed during the mid-1970s. It is now understood that atherosclerosis is a pathologic condition that begins during childhood with asymptomatic but identifiable changes and progresses through adulthood.

Atherosclerosis involves a continuum of changes in the arterial wall that develop in the following sequence:

1. During childhood and adolescence: low-density lipoprotein (LDL) cholesterol particles accumulate in the arterial intima and initiate an inflammatory response.

2. During teens and 20s: (a) inflammatory cells accumulate, (b) protective responses are initiated but necrotic debris causes further inflammation, (c) extracellular lipids accumulate in the arterial walls and (d) a fibrous cap, called a plaque, forms over the necrotic core under the endothelium.

3. After mid-50s: (a) the plaque in a few sites becomes thin and weakened; (b) the plaque is susceptible to rupturing and causing a life-threatening thrombosis; (c) if the plaque does not rupture, it may enlarge and further reduce the arterial lumen; (d) if the plaque occupies more than 40% of the lumen it causes symptoms (e.g., angina) and (e) the pathologic processes within the arterial wall can provoke further plaque formation.

In summary, atherosclerotic changes begin in childhood and can progress to plaque formation. Atherosclerosis is systemic disease process that develops in many arteries but may be more concentrated in some parts of the body, such as the coronary or carotid arteries (Go et al., 2014). Plaque lesions, which can rupture, remain stable or continue to grow, are the underlying cause of most cardiovascular disease. When coronary arteries are affected, sudden death is the primary consequence in 50% of men and 64% of women (Castellon & Bogdanova, 2013). Thus, it is important to identify and address risk factors before patients experience symptoms. All the risk factors described in this section increase the risk for the development and progression of atherosclerosis and consequent cardiovascular disease.

Physical Inactivity

Physical inactivity (also called physical deconditioning) is a factor that compromises cardiovascular function and interferes with the ability of older adults to adapt to age-related cardiovascular changes. Evidence-based guidelines state that the risk for cardiovascular disease is increased in people who have fewer than 30 minutes of moderate physical activity at least 5 days weekly or 20 minutes of vigorous physical activity at least 3 days weekly. National data indicate that level of inactivity increases with increased age (Statistics Canada, 2012). Although older adults are likely to have conditions that make it difficult to obtain adequate physical activity, even 75 minutes a week of light physical activity can reduce cardiovascular risk by as much as 14% (Barnes, 2012). Conditions that often occur in older adults and contribute to physical deconditioning include acute illness, a sedentary lifestyle, mobility limitations, any chronic condition that interferes with physical activity and psychosocial influences, such as depression or lack of motivation.

 DIVERSITY NOTE

Physical inactivity increases with increased age and is higher in women than in men and in black adults than in white adults (Go et al., 2014).

Tobacco Smoking and Secondhand Smoke

Tobacco smoking is a major avoidable cause of cardiovascular disease, and there is indisputable evidence that all forms of tobacco (i.e., smoking tobacco, using smokeless tobacco products, exposure to secondhand smoke) increase the risk for cardiovascular disease and mortality, as illustrated by the following research findings (Go et al., 2014; Statistics Canada, 2011):

- Each day, 100 Canadians die of a smoking-related illness.
- There is a dose-dependent relationship between increased risk for cardiovascular disease and exposure to cigarette smoke.
- Current smokers have a 2 to 4 times increased risk of stroke compared with nonsmokers or those who have quit for more than 10 years.
- Relative risk ratio for smokers to nonsmokers for developing coronary heart disease was 25% higher in women than in men.
- Nonsmokers exposed to secondhand smoke at home or work increase their risk of developing coronary heart disease by 25% to 30%.
- On average, male and female smokers shorten their life expectancy by 13.2 and 14.5 years, respectively, compared with nonsmokers.

Effects of smoking on the cardiovascular system include acceleration of atherosclerotic processes, increased systolic blood pressure, elevated LDL cholesterol level and decreased high-density lipoprotein (HDL) cholesterol level. Even short exposures to secondhand smoke increase the risk of a heart attack because of immediate adverse effects on the heart, blood and vascular systems. These cardiovascular effects are in addition to the effects of nicotine on respiratory function (see Chapter 21) and other aspects of health (as discussed in other chapters).

Dietary Habits

Randomized controlled trials confirm that dietary habits can increase many risk factors for cardiovascular disease, including weight, blood pressure, glucose levels, and lipoprotein and triglyceride levels. A review of studies summarized the following findings related to dietary habits and cardiovascular health (Go et al., 2014):

- Replacing saturated fat with polyunsaturated fat reduced cardiovascular risk by 10% for each 5% reduction in energy exchange.
- Each 2% of calories from trans fats was associated with a 23% higher risk of coronary heart disease.
- Intake of 2.5 servings daily of whole grains was associated with a 21% lower risk of cardiovascular disease when compared with 0.2 servings daily.
- When compared with little or no consumption of fish or fish oil, consumption of one to two servings per week of oily fish was associated with a 36% lower risk of cardiovascular mortality.
- Each daily serving of fruits or vegetables was associated with a 4% lower risk of coronary heart disease and 5% lower risk of stroke.

- Low-sodium interventions were associated with a 25% lower risk of cardiovascular disease after 10 to 15 years of follow-up.

The section on nursing interventions provides teaching information about dietary patterns that are most effective for preventing cardiovascular disease.

Obesity

Obesity, which is defined by body mass index (BMI) 30 kg/m² or more, is associated with increased risk for many pathologic conditions including stroke, diabetes, lipid disorders, atherosclerosis, hypertension and coronary heart disease. In recent years, increasing attention is being paid to abdominal obesity as an independent risk factor for cardiovascular disease. **Abdominal obesity**, defined as a waist circumference of more than 102 and 88 cm or waist-to-hip ratio of 0.95 and 0.88 for men and women, respectively, can occur even in people with normal BMI. Because abdominal adipose tissue is biologically and metabolically different from subcutaneous fat, it is a risk factor for mortality from cardiovascular disease even among normal-weight women.

 DIVERSITY NOTE

Inuit living in Arctic Canada are undergoing a lifestyle transition leading toward decreased physical activity and increased body mass (BMI) (Hopping et al., 2010).

Hypertension

Hypertension is a disease of the cardiovascular system, and it is also an independent risk factor for additional cardiovascular diseases, including coronary artery disease, ischemic stroke, peripheral arterial disease and congestive heart failure. The Canadian Hypertension Education Program (CHEP) provides annually updated standardized evidence-based recommendations and clinical practice guidelines to detect, treat and control hypertension. The recommendations are developed through discussion of the clinical implications via a systematic review of the literature. Research on treatment thresholds for adults older than 80 years are limited, but reviews of studies suggest a target of 150/90 mm Hg or less (Oliva & Bakris, 2012; Weber et al., 2014).

Risk factors for the development of hypertension include age, ethnicity, genetic factors, overweight, physical inactivity, sleep apnea, psychosocial stressors, and lower education and socioeconomic status. In addition, dietary patterns that increase the risk for hypertension include higher intake of fats and sodium, lower potassium intake and excessive alcohol consumption (Go et al., 2014).

 DIVERSITY NOTE

Black Canadians are significantly more likely than Asian, South Asian and white Canadians to report hypertension (Veenstra, 2012).

Lipid Disorders

Lipid disorders (also called *dyslipidemias* or *hyperlipidemias*) is a broad term that encompasses all abnormalities of lipoprotein metabolism, including low levels of HDL (often referred to as "good cholesterol") and elevated levels of total cholesterol, triglycerides or LDL (often referred to as "bad cholesterol"). Public awareness of the importance of testing for lipid disorders has increased since the early 1980s, when *cholesterol* and *saturated fat* became household words. By the 1990s, numerous studies began confirming a positive association between lipoprotein levels and coronary heart disease, and there was widespread support for cholesterol screening for all adults. In 2012, the Canadian Cardiovascular Society published guidelines for the diagnosis and treatment of dyslipidemia for the prevention of cardiovascular disease in the adult.

Although there is much scientific support for addressing lipid disorders as a risk for cardiovascular disease, questions have been raised about the value of cholesterol screening and treatment for adults after age 80. Current emphasis is on clinical judgment based on the older person's overall health and risk factors (Felix-Redondo et al., 2013). Box 20-1 summarizes pertinent evidence about preventing cardiovascular disease.

Metabolic Syndrome

Metabolic syndrome (also called *insulin resistance syndrome*) refers to a group of clinically identifiable conditions that doubles the risk of cardiovascular and increases the risk of diabetes by fivefold regardless of ethnic diversity (Setayeshgar et al., 2013). The presence of at least three of the following five metabolic risk factors constitutes the diagnosis of metabolic syndrome:

- Abdominal obesity, defined as waist circumference of 90 cm in men or 80 cm in women
- Blood pressure equal to or higher than 130/85 mm Hg
- HDL cholesterol level less than 1.03 mmol/L in men or equal to or lower than 1.3 mmol/L in women, or drug treatment for a lipid disorder
- Triglyceride levels higher than 1.7 mmol/L, or specific treatment for hypertriglyceridemia
- Fasting blood glucose level higher than 5.6 mmol/L or more, or drug treatment for increased glucose levels (HealthLink BC, 2012)

This combination of conditions is a "call to action" to address underlying lifestyle-related risks factors and manage all contributing factors (Go et al., 2014).

Psychosocial Factors

Psychosocial factors that are associated with increased risk for developing cardiovascular disease include stress, anxiety, depression, social isolation, poor social supports and personality characteristics, such as higher anger and hostility indices. A review of studies found that one third of the attributable risk of acute myocardial infarction is associated with psychosocial factors, such as major life events, depression or stress related to work, family or finances (Prata et al., 2014). Studies have identified the following associations between psychosocial factors and risk for cardiovascular disease:

- Stress, anger, anxiety and depressed mood are modifiable risk factors for both acute and chronic cardiovascular conditions (Kim & Cho, 2013; Thurston et al., 2013).

Box 20-1 Evidence-Based Practice: Prevention of Cardiovascular Disease

Statement of the Problem

- Although significant advances have been made in preventing and treating cardiovascular disease through medical and surgical interventions, diet and lifestyle interventions are the foundation of clinical intervention for prevention.

Recommendations for Nursing Assessment

- Assess health-related behaviours pertinent to cardiovascular health: dietary patterns, weight, level of physical activity and smoking.

Recommendations for Nursing Care

- Calculate BMI and discuss with patients.
- Advocate a healthy dietary pattern consistent with American Heart Association recommendations.
- Encourage regular physical activity.
- Discourage smoking among nonsmokers and encourage smoking cessation among patients who do smoke.

Teaching Points for Older Adults and Caregivers

- Consume an overall healthful diet: variety of fruits, vegetables and grains, especially whole grains; choose fat-free and low-fat dairy products, legumes, poultry and lean meats; eat fish, preferably oily fish, at least twice weekly; limit intake of saturated and trans fats and cholesterol; limit intake of foods and beverages that have added sugar; select nutrient-dense foods.
- Aim for a healthy BMI of 18.5 to 24.9 kg/m².
- Aim for optimal lipid profile: LDL levels below 100 mg/dL, HDL levels above 50 mg/dL in women and above 40 mg/dL in men, and triglyceride levels below 150 mg/dL.
- Aim for normal blood pressure: systolic blood pressure below 120 mm Hg and diastolic blood pressure below 80 mm Hg.
- Adopt dietary modifications that lower blood pressure: reduced salt intake, increased potassium intake, caloric deficit to induce weight loss, moderation of alcohol intake for those who drink.
- Aim for fasting blood glucose level of 100 mg/dL or less.
- Be physically active: accumulate 30 or more minutes of physical activity most days of the week and at least 60 minutes most days of the week for people attempting to lose weight or maintain weight loss.
- Avoid use of and exposure to tobacco products.

- Loneliness, depression, social isolation and work-related stress are specific stressors that are linked to increased risk of coronary heart disease (Neylon et al., 2013; Steptoe & Kivimaki, 2013).
- Chronic feelings of anger, cynical distrust and antagonistic behaviour may increase the risk of onset and progression of cardiovascular disease (Suls, 2013).
- Poor social support increases the risk for depression in patients with heart failure, which affects up to 50% of these patients (Friedmann et al., 2013; Graven & Grant, 2013).

Researchers have explored the relationship between depression and cardiovascular disease but the cause–effect relationship remains unclear, particularly with regard to whether depression is a risk for first-time coronary events. Many studies show that there is a high prevalence of depression in patients with symptomatic cardiovascular disease and that it is an independent risk for recurrent cardiovascular events and poorer prognosis after the first coronary event (Colquhoun et al., 2013). For example, prevalence of depression in patients hospitalized with acute coronary syndrome is three times higher than the general population (Frazier et al., 2014). Moreover, depression after cardiac surgery is a major cause of death and decreased functional status and its effects are long lasting, with deaths increasing for up to 10 years after surgery (Doering et al., 2013). Because of the close association between depression and chronic cardiovascular disease (e.g., heart failure) or a history of a major cardiovascular event (e.g., myocardial infarction), it is important to routinely screen for depression in this population.

 DIVERSITY NOTE

Studies find that depressive symptoms are associated with a higher prevalence of cardiovascular risk factors in the black population compared with the white (Mody et al., 2012).

Heredity and Socioeconomic Factors

Heredity plays a significant role in the risk for developing cardiovascular disease. Large population-based studies show a strong link between reported history of premature parental coronary heart disease and cardiovascular disease, including atherosclerosis and myocardial infarction, in offspring (Go et al., 2014). Although inherited conditions cannot be changed, people who are aware of having these risk factors may be more motivated to address modifiable risks.

The relationship between socioeconomic status and cardiovascular disease has been a focus of research for several decades. The 2013 Canadian Institute for Health Information report indicates that improved population health and health equity are strategic priorities for many regional health authorities across Canada. Although income and education are not easily modified, it is important to recognize that these conditions influence not only the risk for cardiovascular disease but also the use of preventive and interventional measures. From a holistic perspective, nurses need to consider these factors when planning health education interventions to address individualized needs of older adults.

Risk for Cardiovascular Disease in Women and Minority Groups

Because cardiovascular disease had long been viewed as a disease of middle-aged men, early research focused almost exclusively on men. This perspective began changing during the 1990s when studies showed that although the prevalence of cardiovascular disease is lower in younger women than in younger men, it increases dramatically after the age of 50 years in women. The Heart and Stroke Foundation identifies that most Canadian women have at least one risk factor for cardiovascular disease. Women who have diabetes, come from certain ethnic backgrounds or are menopausal are even more at risk.

The following statistics reflect the extent of cardiovascular morbidity and mortality among women in Canada (Mosca et al., 2011; Statistics Canada, 2011):

- Since 1952, the cardiovascular death rate in Canada has declined by more than 75% and almost 40% in the last decade.
- Every 7 minutes in Canada, someone dies from heart disease or stroke.
- Heart disease and stroke are two of the three leading causes of death in Canada.
- In 2008, cardiovascular disease accounted for 29% of all deaths in Canada (28% of all male deaths; 29.7% of all female deaths).
- Cardiovascular disease causes more deaths among women in Canada than cancer, chronic lower respiratory disease, Alzheimer disease and accidents combined.
- Ninety percent of women have one or more risk factors for heart disease.
- Symptoms of heart disease differ in women and men and are often unrecognized in women.

Along with the growing recognition of unique aspects of cardiovascular disease in women, there has been increasing focus on the disproportionate burden of cardiovascular-related death and disability among minority populations. Data from the Canadian Community Health Survey reveals that compared with white people, people from visible minorities (i.e., neither white nor Aboriginal) had a lower prevalence of diabetes mellitus, hypertension, smoking and obesity but a higher prevalence of physical inactivity. In addition, after adjustment for sociodemographic characteristics, people from most visible minorities, in comparison with the white population, were less likely to smoke; were more likely to be physically inactive, with the exception of people of Korean, Japanese and Latin ethnicity; and were less likely to be obese, with the exception of people of black, Latin, Arab or West Asian ethnicity. However, relative to white people, hypertension was more prevalent among those of Filipino or South East Asian background and those of black ancestry (Liu et al., 2010).

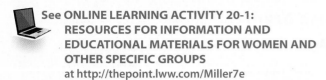

See **ONLINE LEARNING ACTIVITY 20-1:**
RESOURCES FOR INFORMATION AND
EDUCATIONAL MATERIALS FOR WOMEN AND
OTHER SPECIFIC GROUPS
at http://thepoint.lww.com/Miller7e

Online Learning Activity 20-1 provides links to information about cardiovascular disease in women and minority groups, including links to educational materials developed for non-English- and French-speaking people in Canada.

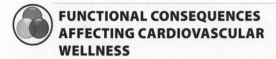

FUNCTIONAL CONSEQUENCES AFFECTING CARDIOVASCULAR WELLNESS

Healthy older adults experience no significant cardiovascular effects when they are resting, but, when they engage in exercise, their cardiovascular function is less efficient. However, older adults who have risk factors for cardiovascular disease are likely to experience negative functional consequences associated with pathologic processes. This section reviews the functional consequences in older adults who have no risk factors, and the sections on nursing assessment and interventions focus on risk factors that can be addressed to prevent pathologic processes that commonly affect cardiovascular function.

Effects on Cardiac Function

Cardiac output, the amount of blood pumped by the heart per minute, is an important measure of cardiac performance because it represents the heart's ability to meet the oxygen requirements of the body. Although reduced cardiac output is common in older adults, it is associated primarily with pathologic, rather than age-related, conditions. With the exception of a slight decrease in cardiac output at rest in older women, healthy older adults do not experience any decline in cardiac output.

Effects on Pulse and Blood Pressure

Normal pulse rate for healthy older adults is slightly lower than that for younger adults, but older adults are likely to have harmless ventricular and supraventricular arrhythmias because of age-related changes that affect cardiac conduction mechanisms. Atrial fibrillation—a more serious arrhythmia—commonly occurs in older adults, but this is associated with pathologic conditions (e.g., hypertension, coronary artery disease) rather than with age-related changes. In most populations across the world, there is an age-related linear increase in systolic blood pressure from ages 30 to 40 years, and this change is steeper for women than for men.

Effects on the Response to Exercise

A negative functional consequence that affects cardiovascular performance in healthy older adults is a blunted adaptive response to physical exercise. Physiologic stress, such as

that associated with exercise, increases the demands on the cardiovascular system by four to five times the basal level. The adaptive response involves many aspects of physiologic function, including the respiratory, cardiovascular, musculoskeletal and autonomic nervous systems. The maximum heart rate achieved during exercise is markedly decreased, and the peak exercise capacity and oxygen consumption decline in older adults. Most of this decline is attributable to physical deconditioning and other risk factors, rather than to age-related changes alone.

Effects on Circulation

Functional consequences also affect circulation to the brain and the lower extremities. For example, age-related changes in cardiovascular and baroreflex mechanisms can reduce cerebral blood flow to some extent in healthy older adults and to a greater extent in older adults who have diabetes, hypertension, lipid disorders and heart disease. In addition, increased tortuosity and dilation of the veins, along with decreased efficiency of the valves, lead to impaired venous return from the lower extremities. Consequently, older adults are prone to developing stasis edema of the feet and ankles, and they are more likely to develop venous stasis ulcers.

PATHOLOGIC CONDITIONS AFFECTING CARDIOVASCULAR WELLNESS: ORTHOSTATIC AND POSTPRANDIAL HYPOTENSION

Orthostatic and postprandial hypotension are conditions that occur in older adults due to a combination of age-related changes (e.g., decreased baroreflex sensitivity) and risk factors (e.g., hypertension and antihypertensive medications). These conditions may be symptomatic or asymptomatic and it clearly is within the realm of nursing to identify hypotension in older adults by assessing lying and standing blood pressure as discussed in the section on nursing assessment. Assessing for these conditions is important because orthostatic and postprandial hypotension occur more frequently in older adults and they can lead to serious consequences, including falls and fall-related injuries.

Orthostatic hypotension (also called *postural hypotension*) is a reduction in systolic blood pressure and diastolic blood pressure of at least 20 or 10 mm Hg, respectively, within 3 minutes of standing after being recumbent for at least 5 minutes. Prevalence of orthostatic hypotension ranges from 6% in healthy older adults to 68% of hospitalized older adults (Aung et al., 2012; Pepersack et al., 2013). Orthostatic hypotension is often associated with the risk factors listed in Box 20-2, with an underlying impairment in autonomic response being the most likely common denominator (Aung et al., 2012; Lagro et al., 2013). The risk can be increased by a combination of conditions, such as Parkinson disease and anti-Parkinson medications.

unfolding Case Study

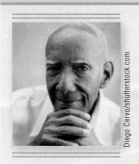

Diego Cervo/shutterstock.com

Part 1: Mr. C. at 64 Years of Age

Mr. C. is a 64-year-old Black Canadian who frequently comes to your senior wellness clinic to have you check his blood pressure. He has been taking hydrochlorothiazide, 25 mg, and verapamil, 120 mg, every morning, and his blood pressures ranges between 128/84 and 136/88 mm Hg. Mr. C. sees his primary care provider once a year and obtains additional health care through community resources, such as health fairs. Mr. C.'s 86-year-old mother recently died of a cerebrovascular accident, and his father died in his early 50s of a heart attack. Mr. C. has had hypertension since he was 24, and both of his daughters have high blood pressure as well. Neither Mr. C. nor anyone in the household smokes tobacco. He has low levels of daily physical activity and weighs 95 kg. At a height of 1.7 m, his BMI is 32, which is 21 kg above ideal weight. He reports that he "gets winded easily" when walking up or down a flight of steps or when he has to walk "a long distance" (which he defines as the distance across the parking lot to the senior centre). He attributes this to "getting old."

THINKING POINTS

- What age-related changes in cardiovascular function is Mr. C. likely to be experiencing?
- What risk factors are likely to be contributing to Mr. C.'s experience of "getting winded?"

- What risk factors does Mr. C. have for cardiovascular disease?
- What further information would you want to obtain for assessing his risk for cardiovascular disease?

Box 20-2 Risk Factors for Hypotension

Risks for Orthostatic Hypotension

Pathologic Processes

- Hypertension, including isolated systolic hypertension
- Parkinson disease
- Cerebrovascular disorders
- Diabetes
- Anemia
- Autonomic dysfunction
- Arrhythmias
- Volume depletion (e.g., dehydration)
- Electrolyte imbalances (e.g., hyponatremia, hypokalemia)

Medications

- Antihypertensives
- Anticholinergics
- Phenothiazines
- Antidepressants
- Anti-Parkinson agents
- Vasodilators
- Diuretics
- Alcohol

Risks for Postprandial Hypotension

Pathologic Processes

- Systolic hypertension
- Diabetes mellitus
- Parkinson disease
- Multisystem atrophy

Medications

- Diuretics
- Antihypertensive medications ingested before meals

Orthostatic hypotension can be asymptomatic (i.e., identified by physical assessment) or it can be accompanied by symptoms such as fatigue, lightheadedness, blurred vision or syncope upon standing. Whether orthostatic hypotension is symptomatic or asymptomatic, it can affect the safety and quality of life and lead to serious negative functional consequences, such as increased risk for falls and the development of cardiovascular problems, such as congestive heart failure (van Hateren et al., 2012; Xin et al., 2013).

Postprandial hypotension, defined as a systolic blood pressure reduction of 20 mm Hg or more within 2 hours of eating a meal, affects up to two thirds of older adults and as many as 72.8% of older adults with hypertension (Zanasi et al., 2012). Impaired autonomic function is the pathophysiologic mechanism that is responsible for postprandial hypotension. Contributing factors include gastrointestinal vasoactive peptides and impaired glucose metabolism, which is often associated with diabetes (Abdel-Rahman, 2012; Fukushima et al., 2013). It is recommended that nurses assess for postprandial hypotension, even in older adults who are in bed, as an important intervention for reducing the incidence of falls, syncope, strokes and other complications (Son & Lee, 2012, 2013).

NURSING ASSESSMENT OF CARDIOVASCULAR FUNCTION

From a wellness perspective, nursing assessment of cardiovascular function focuses on identifying risks for cardiovascular disease and the older adult's knowledge about his or her risk profile because many risks can be addressed through health education interventions. Moreover, when older adults would benefit from improving their health-related behaviours (e.g., nutrition, physical activity), it is important to assess their readiness for changing behaviours, as discussed in Chapter 5. Although assessment of blood pressure does not differ in older and younger adults, it is essential to assess for hypotension in older adults. In addition, nursing assessment needs to consider that older adults may have atypical manifestations of cardiovascular disease (e.g., a heart attack) and they may have risk factors that are unrecognized.

Wellness Opportunity

Nurses address body–mind–spirit interconnectedness by identifying stress-related factors that increase the risk for cardiovascular disease and encouraging the use of stress management methods, such as meditation.

Assessing Baseline Cardiovascular Function

Physical assessment indicators of cardiovascular function (e.g., peripheral pulses and heart rhythm and sounds) are the same for all healthy adults. Keep in mind, however, that older adults are more likely to have chronic conditions that affect cardiovascular function. The following findings are common in older adults, but in the absence of symptoms or other abnormal findings, they usually are not indicative of any serious pathologic process:

- Auscultation of a fourth heart sound
- Auscultation of short systolic ejection murmurs
- Difficulty percussing heart borders
- Diminished or distant-sounding heart sounds
- Electrocardiographic changes such as arrhythmias, left axis deviation, bundle branch blocks, ST-T wave changes and prolongation of the P-R interval

If a murmur, arrhythmia or any other unusual finding is detected, it is important to determine whether it reflects a new development, a preexisting but previously unidentified condition or a preexisting condition that has already been evaluated. The nurse asks questions to determine the person's awareness of such abnormal findings. Older adults may use any of the following terms to describe arrhythmias: fluttering, palpitations, skipped beats, extra beats or flip-flops. During the assessment, ask the older person about a history of arrhythmias before listening to the heart because asking immediately after auscultation could cause undue concern.

Arrhythmias may be caused by cardiac diseases, electrolyte imbalances, physiologic disturbances or adverse medication effects; alternatively, they may be harmless manifestations of age-related changes. Likewise, murmurs may be caused by age- or disease-related conditions. Therefore, when murmurs or arrhythmias are detected, their significance is assessed in relation to the person's history as well as in relation to the potential underlying causes. It is also important to find out the date of the person's last electrocardiogram

because this may provide baseline information regarding the duration of asymptomatic or unrecognized changes.

Assessing Blood Pressure

Most nurses do not have primary responsibility for medical management of blood pressure, but all nurses are responsible for accurate assessment of blood pressure and for decisions regarding the implications of these findings. Thus, it is important to be familiar with the most current guidelines for detecting hypertension so that health promotion efforts can be directed toward interventions. Despite mounting medical evidence that the identification and management of hypertension has important health benefits, only 46% of people with hypertension achieve good control in community settings (Pearson et al., 2013). Nurses are in a key position to detect hypertension, provide health education and refer older adults for further medical evaluation and treatment.

Accurately assessing blood pressure in older adults may be more difficult than in younger adults for several reasons. First, blood pressure in older adults is more variable and has an increased tendency to fluctuate in response to postural changes and other factors. In addition, older adults commonly have **pseudohypertension**, which is the phenomenon of elevated systolic blood pressure readings that result from the inability of the external cuff to compress the arteries in older people with arteriosclerosis. This phenomenon explains the finding of extremely elevated systolic blood pressure readings in people without any evidence of end-organ damage and with normal diastolic blood pressure readings. Another assessment consideration is the common occurrence of **white coat hypertension** (also called *isolated office hypertension*), which is the phenomenon of blood pressure readings being high only when checked by a health care practitioner.

In recent years, **home blood pressure monitoring**, which is the practice of self-measurement of blood pressure, has been endorsed by national and international guidelines including those posted by Hypertension Canada and the Public Health Agency of Canada. Extensive evidence from randomized controlled studies concludes that home blood pressure monitoring by patients with hypertension is feasible and is associated with improved outcomes (Cacciolati et al., 2013; Omboni et al., 2013). Self-monitoring is particularly important for older adults because they are more susceptible to white coat hypertension and their systolic readings are more variable (Noguchi et al., 2013; Weber et al., 2014). Moreover, self-measurement of blood pressure can also be used to detect orthostatic or postprandial hypotension if readings are taken in both sitting and standing positions. Assessment of blood pressure in older adults is aimed at detecting not only hypertension but also orthostatic and postprandial hypotension, as summarized in Box 20-3.

Identifying Risks for Cardiovascular Disease

The assessment of risks for cardiovascular disease, with emphasis on identifying modifiable risk factors, provides a

Box 20-3 Guidelines for Assessing for Hypotension

For Assessment of Orthostatic Hypotension

- Maintain the person's arm in the same position (either parallel or perpendicular to the torso) during supine and standing positions.
- Obtain initial blood pressure reading after the person has been in a sitting or lying position for at least 5 minutes.
- Obtain second blood pressure reading after the person has been standing for 1 to 3 minutes.

For Assessment of Postprandial Hypotension

- Obtain initial blood pressure reading before a meal.
- Obtain second and third reading at 15-minute intervals after the meal is completed.

Normal Findings

- The normal difference between lying/sitting and standing systolic blood pressure is 20 mm Hg or less after standing for 1 minute.
- The normal difference between lying/sitting and standing diastolic blood pressure is 10 mm Hg or less after standing for 1 minute.

Box 20-4 Guidelines for Assessing Risks for Cardiovascular Disease in Older Adults

Questions to Identify Risk Factors for Cardiovascular Disease

- Do you have, or have you ever had, any heart or circulation problems (e.g., stroke, angina, heart attack, blood clots or peripheral vascular disease)? *If yes, ask the usual questions about type of therapy, and so on.*
- When was the last time you had an electrocardiogram?
- What is your normal blood pressure? Have you ever been told that you have high blood pressure, or borderline high blood pressure?
- Do you take, or have you ever taken, medications for heart problems or blood pressure? *If yes, ask the usual questions about type, dose, duration of therapy and the like.*
- Do you smoke, or have you ever smoked? *If yes, ask additional questions, such as those appropriate for assessing respiratory function; see Chapter 21.*
- Do you know what your cholesterol levels are? When was the last time you had your cholesterol checked?
- Do you have diabetes? When was the last time you had your blood sugar (glucose) level checked and what was the result?
- What is your usual pattern of exercise?

Additional Considerations Regarding Risk Factors

- Calculate BMI and compare the person's ideal weight to his or her present weight.
- Determine usual dietary habits, paying particular attention to the person's intake of sodium, fibre and types of fat. (This information is usually obtained during the nutritional assessment.)

basis for health promotion interventions. Hypertension, lipid disorders and smoking cessation (discussed in Chapter 21) are important remediable conditions for older adults who have these risks. In addition, obesity, physical inactivity and certain dietary habits are risk factors that can be addressed through improved health-related behaviours. It is especially important to identify older adults who have several risk factors because the co-occurrence of several risks can amplify the effect of individual risk factors (Berry et al., 2012; Kariuki et al., 2013).

Figure 20-1 is an example of an easy-to-use assessment tool based on Framingham Risk Score, which is recommended to identify high-risk asymptomatic adults who may benefit from preventive interventions (Canadian Cardiovascular Society). Additional tests, including electrocardiogram, exercise-stress testing and ankle-brachial index are not currently recommended for routine screening; however, a one-time screening for abdominal aortic aneurysm is recommended for men aged 65 to 75 years who are current or past smokers (Lim et al., 2011). It is recommended that C-reactive protein (CRP) levels be tested in people with moderate risk for cardiovascular disease. In recent years, questions have been raised about this recommendation and a recent review of studies indicate that it may be useful in men, but not in women (Emerging Risk Factors Collaboration, 2012). Nurses can use Box 20-4 as a guide for nursing assessment of risks.

Wellness Opportunity

Nurses promote personal responsibility and self-awareness by teaching older adults to use self-assessment tools (e.g., Fig. 20-1) to identify their risks for heart disease.

Assessing Signs and Symptoms of Heart Disease

Assessment of older adults for heart disease is complicated by the fact that the symptoms often differ from the expected manifestations. Congestive heart failure, for example, often begins very subtly, and the early manifestations may be mental changes secondary to the physiologic stress. Thus, older adults are likely to be in more advanced stages of heart failure before an accurate diagnosis is made. Likewise, older people with angina and acute myocardial infarctions are likely to have subtle and unusual manifestations, called **atypical presentation**, rather than the classic symptom of chest pain. Between one fourth and two thirds of all myocardial infarctions are not clinically recognized as such, with women and older adults having a higher rate of atypical presentation. Atypical signs and symptoms include fatigue, nausea, anxiety, headache, cough, visual disturbance, shortness of breath and pain in the jaw, neck or throat.

An important nursing assessment consideration is that older adults, as well as health care professionals, are likely

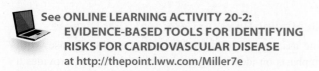

See ONLINE LEARNING ACTIVITY 20-2:
EVIDENCE-BASED TOOLS FOR IDENTIFYING RISKS FOR CARDIOVASCULAR DISEASE
at http://thepoint.lww.com/Miller7e

What Is Your Risk of Developing Heart Disease or Having a Heart Attack?

In general, the higher your LDL level and the more risk factors you have (other than LDL), the greater your chances of developing heart disease or having a heart attack. Some people are at high risk for a heart attack because they already have heart disease. Other people are at high risk for developing heart disease because they have diabetes (which is a strong risk factor) or a combination of risk factors for heart disease. Follow these steps to find out your risk for developing heart disease.

Step 1   **Check the table below to see how many of the listed risk factors you have; these are the risk factors that affect your LDL goal.**

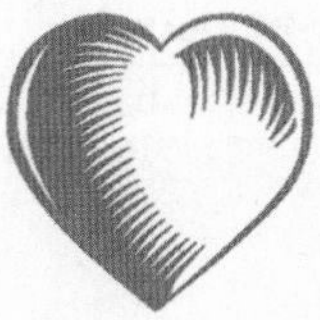

Major Risk Factors That Affect Your LDL Goal

- ○ Cigarette smoking
- ○ High blood pressure (140/90 mm Hg or higher or on blood pressure medication)
- ○ Low HDL cholesterol (less than 40 mg/dL)*
- ○ Family history of early heart disease (heart disease in father or brother before age 55; heart disease in mother or sister before age 65)
- ○ Age (men 45 years or older; women 55 years or older)

If your HDL cholesterol is 60 mg/dL or higher, subtract 1 from your total count.

Even though obesity and physical inactivity are not counted in this list, they are conditions that need to be corrected.

Step 2   **How many major risk factors do you have? If you have 2 or more risk factors in the table above, use the risk scoring tables on the opposite page (which include your cholesterol levels) to find your risk score. Risk score refers to the chance of having a heart attack in the next 10 years, given as a percentage.** 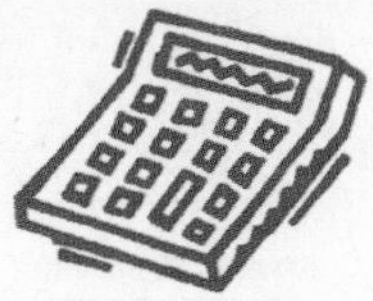
(Use the Framingham Point Scores on the opposite page.)

| My 10-year risk score is _____%. |

Step 3   **Use your medical history, number of risk factors and risk score to find your risk of developing heart disease or having a heart attack in the table below.**

If You Have	You Are in Category
Heart disease, diabetes or risk score more than 20%*	I. Highest Risk
2 or more risk factors and risk score 10%–20%	II. Next Highest Risk
2 or more risk factors and risk score less than 10%	III. Moderate Risk
0 or 1 risk factor	IV. Low-to-Moderate Risk

Means that more than 20 of 100 people in this category will have a heart attack within 10 years.

| My risk category is _____. |

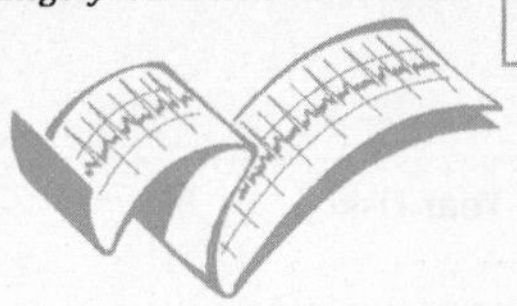

FIGURE 20.1 Example of an easy-to-use assessment tool for identifying risk factors for cardiovascular disease. An interactive tool for assessing risk factors is available at http://www.nhlbi.nih.gov. (Reprinted from U.S. Department of Health and Human Services, Public Health Service, National Institutes of Health, National Heart, Lung, and Blood Institute. [May 2001]. What is your risk of developing heart disease or having a heart attack? NIH publication no. 01–3290. Rockville, MD: Author.)

Estimate of 10-Year Risk for Men

(Framingham Point Scores)

Age	Points
20–34	–9
35–39	–4
40–44	0
45–49	3
50–54	6
55–59	8
60–64	10
65–69	11
70–74	12
75–79	13

Total Cholesterol	Points				
	Age 20–39	Age 40–49	Age 50–59	Age 60–69	Age 70–79
<160	0	0	0	0	0
160–199	4	3	2	1	0
200–239	7	5	3	1	0
240–279	9	6	4	2	1
≥280	11	8	5	3	1

	Points				
	Age 20–39	Age 40–49	Age 50–59	Age 60–69	Age 70–79
Nonsmoker	0	0	0	0	0
Smoker	8	5	3	1	1

HDL (mg/dL)	Points
≥60	–1
50–59	0
40–49	1
<40	2

Systolic BP (mmHg)	If Untreated	If Treated
<120	0	0
120–129	0	1
130–139	1	2
140–159	1	2
≥160	2	3

Point Total	10-Year Risk %
<0	<1
0	1
1	1
2	1
3	1
4	1
5	2
6	2
7	3
8	4
9	5
10	6
11	8
12	10
13	12
14	16
15	20
16	25
≥17	≥30

10-Year risk _____ %

Estimate of 10-Year Risk for Women

(Framingham Point Scores)

Age	Points
20–34	–7
35–39	–3
40–44	0
45–49	3
50–54	6
55–59	8
60–64	10
65–69	12
70–74	14
75–79	16

Total Cholesterol	Points				
	Age 20–39	Age 40–49	Age 50–59	Age 60–69	Age 70–79
<160	0	0	0	0	0
160–199	4	3	2	1	1
200–239	8	6	4	2	1
240–279	11	8	5	3	2
≥280	13	10	7	4	2

	Points				
	Age 20–39	Age 40–49	Age 50–59	Age 60–69	Age 70–79
Nonsmoker	0	0	0	0	0
Smoker	9	7	4	2	1

HDL (mg/dL)	Points
≥60	–1
50–59	0
40–49	1
<40	2

Systolic BP (mmHg)	If Untreated	If Treated
<120	0	0
120–129	1	3
130–139	2	4
140–159	3	5
≥160	4	6

Point Total	10-Year Risk %
<9	<1
9	1
10	1
11	1
12	1
13	2
14	2
15	3
16	4
17	5
18	6
19	8
20	11
21	14
22	17
23	22
24	27
≥25	≥30

10-Year risk _____ %

U.S. DEPARTMENT OF HEALTH AND HUMAN SERVICES
Public Health Service
National Institutes of Health
National Heart, Lung, and Blood Institute

NIH Publication No. 01-3290
May 2001

to attribute atypical symptoms to other conditions, such as arthritis or indigestion, or even to "normal aging." Therefore, it is important to recognize that complaints about fatigue, digestion, respiration or musculoskeletal pain in the upper body can be indicators of cardiac disease. Assessment is further complicated by the fact that older adults often have more than one underlying condition that could be responsible for these symptoms. It is not unusual, for example, for an older person to have an esophageal reflux disorder, as well as a history of ischemic heart disease. Another consideration is that older adults with functional impairments or limited mobility may not be active enough to experience exertion-related symptoms. Therefore, in addition to focusing on the usual manifestations of cardiovascular function, information about other systems and overall functioning provides pertinent assessment information. In addition, a baseline electrocardiogram is helpful in establishing the possibility of silent or atypical myocardial ischemia.

Assessing Knowledge About Heart Disease

In addition to assessing signs and symptoms, nurses assess the older adult's knowledge about manifestations of heart disease. This is particularly important because immediate medical attention is a major factor in determining outcomes of heart attacks, and all people need to be aware of the warning signs so that they can initiate appropriate help-seeking actions. Thus, it is important to ask at least one question to assess the older adult's knowledge about the signs and symptoms of a heart attack. In addition, include a question about what the person would do and whom he or she would call if experiencing symptoms of a heart attack. Box 20-5 summarizes the guidelines for assessing cardiovascular function and detecting cardiovascular disease in older adults, emphasizes the assessment components that are unique to older adults and refers to additional assessment components that apply to adults in general.

DIVERSITY NOTE

Knowledge of heart attack and stroke symptoms is lacking among adults in Canada and is lowest among older adults, racial minorities and other groups who are at highest risk for cardiovascular disease.

NURSING DIAGNOSIS

If the nursing assessment identifies risks for cardiovascular disease, a nursing diagnosis of Ineffective Health Maintenance may be applicable. This diagnosis is defined as "inability to identify, manage, and/or seek out help to maintain health" (Herdman, 2012, p. 157). Related factors common in older adults include lack of physical activity and insufficient knowledge about preventive measures. For older adults with impaired cardiovascular function, applicable nursing diagnoses include Activity Intolerance and Decreased Cardiac

Box 20-5 Guidelines for Assessing Cardiovascular Function in Older Adults

Questions to Assess for Cardiovascular Disease

- Do you ever have chest pain or tightness in your chest? *If yes, ask the usual questions to explore the type, onset, duration and other characteristics.*
- Do you ever have difficulty breathing? *If yes, ask the usual questions regarding onset and other characteristics.*
- Do you ever feel lightheaded or dizzy? *If yes, ask about specific circumstances, medical evaluation and methods of dealing with symptoms and ensuring safety.*
- Do you ever feel like your heart is racing, is irregular or has extra or skipped beats? *If yes, ask about any prior medical evaluation.*
- Have you ever been told that you had a heart murmur? *If yes, ask about any prior medical evaluation.*

Information Obtained During Other Portions of an Assessment That May Be Useful in Assessing Cardiovascular Function

- Do you tire easily or feel that you need more rest than is ordinarily required?
- Do you have any problems with indigestion?
- Do your feet or ankles ever get swollen?
- Do you wake up at night because of difficulty breathing or because of any other discomfort? Have you made any adjustments in your sleeping habits because of difficulty breathing (e.g., do you use more than one pillow or sleep in a chair)?
- Do you have any pain in your upper back or shoulders?

Interview Questions to Assess for Postural Hypotension

- Do you ever feel lightheaded or dizzy, especially when you get up in the morning or after you've been lying down?
  If yes: Is this feeling accompanied by any additional symptoms, such as sweating, nausea or confusion?
  If yes: Do any of the risks listed in Box 20-2 apply to you? If yes, ask about any prior medical evaluation.

Output. The nursing diagnosis of Risk for Injury may be appropriate for older adults with orthostatic or postprandial hypotension, particularly in the presence of additional risk factors for falls and fractures (e.g., osteoporosis, neurologic disorders, medication side effects).

Wellness Opportunity

Nurses can use the wellness nursing diagnoses, Readiness for Enhanced Nutrition or Readiness for Enhanced Knowledge, for older adults who are interested in developing heart-healthy dietary habits or learning about health-promoting behaviours to prevent heart disease.

PLANNING FOR WELLNESS OUTCOMES

When older adults have risks for cardiovascular disease, nurses can apply any of the following Nursing Outcomes Classification (NOC) terminologies to identify wellness outcomes in their care plans: Health Orientation, Health-Promoting Behaviour, Knowledge: Healthy Diet, Knowledge: Lipid

Disorder Management, Risk Control: Tobacco Use, and Weight Loss Behaviour. Wellness outcomes for older adults with cardiovascular disease include Self-Management: Cardiac Disease, Circulation Status, Health Seeking Behaviour, and Knowledge: Cardiac Disease Management. Additional outcomes include maintaining blood pressure within the normal range and preventing negative consequences of orthostatic or postprandial hypotension (e.g., falls and fractures).

Wellness Opportunity

Nurses address body–mind–spirit interconnectedness by including stress level as an outcome directed toward reducing the risk for cardiovascular disease.

NURSING INTERVENTIONS TO PROMOTE HEALTHY CARDIOVASCULAR FUNCTION

From a wellness perspective, nursing interventions to promote healthy cardiovascular function focus on primary and secondary prevention of cardiovascular disease. These interventions address specific risk factors, such as smoking, hypertension, obesity and lipid disorders as well as preventive measures, such as optimal levels of physical activity, heart-healthy dietary patterns and stress-reduction actions. Although pharmacologic and medical interventions are often used to reduce risk factors, teaching about health promotion actions is a nursing intervention that is appropriate in almost all situations. In addition to addressing risks for cardiovascular disease, nurses can address orthostatic or postprandial hypotension and the related functional consequences, such as falls and fractures.

Nurses can use the following Nursing Interventions Classification (NIC) terminologies in care plans to promote cardiovascular wellness: Cardiac Risk Management, Coping Enhancement, Counselling, Exercise Promotion, Guided Imagery, Health Education, Meditation Facilitation, Nutritional Counselling, Relaxation Therapy, Self-Responsibility Facilitation and Teaching: Individual.

Role of Nurses in Teaching About Cardiovascular Disease

In recent years, there is increasing emphasis on the importance of health promotion for prevention of cardiovascular disease, with particular attention to teaching women and members of minority groups about this leading cause of morbidity and mortality. One major recent initiative is the Heart and Stroke Foundation's "The Heart Truth" campaign, which calls on women to put their own health first by assessing their risk for heart disease and stroke, talking to their doctor and making heart-healthy lifestyle choices. Nurses are taking leading roles in health promotion related to cardiovascular diseases through organizations such as the

Canadian Council of Cardiovascular Nurses. For example, Peterson (2012) describes how nurses can apply the PRECEDE-PROCEED model to guide nursing interventions for cardiovascular disease prevention for women. Online Learning Activity 20-3 provides a link to this article and links to many resources for health promotion in relation to cardiovascular disease. Box 20-6 can be used for health promotion to teach older adults about steps they can take to reduce their risk for cardiovascular disease. See Box 20-7 for a research study revealing the effectiveness of a cardiovascular health awareness program on older adults' blood pressure.

See ONLINE LEARNING ACTIVITY 20-3: JOURNAL ARTICLE AND RESOURCES RELATED TO HEALTH PROMOTION AND CARDIOVASCULAR DISEASE at http://thepoint.lww.com/Miller7e

 Box 20-6 Health Promotion Activities to Reduce the Risks for Cardiovascular Disease

Detection of Risks
- Have blood pressure checked annually.
- Talk with your primary care practitioner about tests that identify risks for cardiovascular disease.
- If the total serum cholesterol level is less than 200 mg/dL, have it rechecked every 5 years. If the total serum cholesterol level is between 200 and 239 mg/dL, follow dietary measures to reduce it and have it rechecked annually. If the total serum cholesterol level is 240 mg/dL or more, obtain a further medical evaluation.
- Ask your primary care provider about the use of low-dose aspirin as a preventive measure, particularly if there is any history of coronary artery disease or cerebrovascular events.

Reduction of Risks
- Do not smoke.
- Engage in moderate physical activity for 30 minutes at least 5 days a week.
- Maintain weight within normal limits.
- Avoid breathing secondary smoke and other air pollutants whenever possible.
- Engage in stress management activities such as meditation and yoga.
- Eat heart-healthy foods, as described in the next section.

Heart-Healthy Eating Pattern
- Consume at least 3 to 5 servings of fruits daily, especially the deeply coloured ones.
- Consume at least 3 to 5 servings of vegetables daily, especially the deeply coloured ones.
- Include 2 to 3 servings of low-fat or nonfat dairy products.
- Choose whole-grain products as sources of carbohydrates and fibre (e.g., rye, barley, oats, whole wheat).
- Aim for at least 25 g of fibre daily.
- Choose only the leanest meats, poultry, fish and shellfish.
- Avoid foods that are high in calories, trans fats or refined sugars.
- Use oils that are least saturated (e.g., canola, safflower, sunflower, corn, olive, soybean, peanut oils; use margarine that is soft and free of trans fats).
- Limit salt intake to no more than 1,500 mg daily.

Box 20-7 Evidence-Informed Nursing Practice

Background: Hypertension is a modifiable cardiovascular risk factor for older Canadians.

Question: What is the effectiveness of a community-based cardiovascular health awareness program on participants' blood pressure?

Method: The researchers followed a cohort of community residing adults in 22 Ontario communities over an 18-month period. Participants' baseline risk factors (e.g., blood pressure) were recorded. Participants attended at least two cardiovascular health awareness program sessions.

Findings: Repeat participants had a significant reduction in systolic and diastolic blood pressure readings.

Implications for Nursing Practice: Nurses need to actively encourage older adults to be aware of their blood pressure readings and to promote self-care through education and other risk-reduction activities.

Source: Ye, C., Foster, G., Kaczorowski, J., et al. (2013). The impact of a cardiovascular health awareness program (CHAP) on reducing blood pressure: A prospective cohort study. *BMC Public Health, 13,* 1230.

Addressing Risks Through Nutritional Interventions

Nutritional interventions are particularly important for prevention or management of obesity, hypertension and lipid disorders. Research reviews related to dietary influences on cardiovascular disease support the following evidence-based recommendations (Go et al., 2014; Miller et al., 2011; Miuri et al., 2013; Scholl, 2012; Weihua et al., 2013):

- Type and quality of fats consumed is more important than total fat content or relative percentage of fat, with polyunsaturated and monounsaturated fatty acids (e.g., olive oil, oleic acid from vegetable sources) being the most beneficial and trans fats and saturated fats being the most detrimental.
- Heart-healthy diets includes high intake of nuts, fish, fruits, vegetables and fibre-rich whole grains; less than 1,500 mg of sodium a day; and no more than 36 ounces of sugar-sweetened beverages a week.
- Although one alcoholic beverage a day for women and two for men may reduce the risk for cardiovascular disease, excessive use increases the risk and alcohol consumption is contraindicated in some conditions (e.g., cardiomyopathy, risk for alcoholism).
- Current evidence does not support the use of dietary supplements, but diets should include fruits and vegetables that are rich in essential nutrients, including antioxidants.

Many studies have looked at the effects of a **Mediterranean dietary pattern**, which is characterized by higher intakes of fish, poultry, nuts, fruits, legumes, vegetables and lower intake of red and processed meats (Go et al., 2014). Overall, the Mediterranean dietary pattern involves lower intake of saturated and trans fats, higher intake of monounsaturated and polyunsaturated fats, and complex carbohydrates as the main type of carbohydrates. There is much evidence-based support for benefits of this dietary pattern

both for primary prevention of coronary heart disease in the general population and for secondary prevention for people who already have pathologic changes (e.g., Estruch et al., 2013; Rees et al., 2013).

The **DASH dietary pattern**, which refers to the *Dietary Approaches to Stop Hypertension*, is an evidence-based eating plan that is promoted by many organizations including the Heart & Stroke Foundation and the Public Health Agency of Canada. This dietary pattern is characterized by high intake of fruits, vegetables and plant proteins from grains, nuts and legumes; moderate intake of low-fat or nonfat dairy foods; and low intakes of sodium and animal protein and is widely recognized as a primary and secondary preventive intervention for hypertension. Beneficial effects of DASH-type diets include lowered blood pressure, decreased LDL and triglyceride levels, and lower morality rates. Studies have confirmed a strong association between a DASH-like diet and reduced incidence of cardiovascular diseases by at least 20% (Fitzgerald et al., 2012; Go et al., 2014; Salehi-Abargouei et al., 2013).

Another focus of nutrition-related research is on the potential benefits of commonly consumed foods and beverages that are rich in polyphenols. Although there is increasing evidence that cocoa and dark chocolate have cardioprotective effects (e.g., antioxidant, anti-inflammatory, antiplatelet and vasodilatation actions), larger randomized trials are required to establish a cause–effect relationship (Arranz et al., 2013; Ellam & Williamson, 2013). Similarly, although there is increasing evidence that both green and black tea may reduce the risk for cardiovascular disease, research is not sufficient to support an evidence-based recommendation (Hartley et al., 2013).

Addressing Risks Through Lifestyle Interventions

Lifestyle interventions that are a mainstay of interventions for preventing cardiovascular disease include remaining physically active, managing stress, refraining from smoking and maintaining ideal body weight. There is strong evidence supporting the importance of physical activity as an intervention for preventing cardiovascular disease and improving life expectancy. For example, a meta-analysis of studies concluded that high levels of leisure-time physical activity reduced the risk of cardiovascular disease by 20% to 30%, whereas moderate leisure or occupational physical activity reduced the risk by 10% to 20% (Li & Siegrist, 2012). Specific positive effects on cardiovascular function include weight loss; reduced blood pressure; improved overall cardiac function; lower rates of cardiovascular disease; improved lipid, glucose and triglyceride levels; and decreased risk of developing diabetes and cardiovascular disease. There is also abundant evidence that aerobic exercise is a "decisive factor in reducing cardiovascular morbidity and mortality" (Nilsson et al., 2013). Positive effects of exercise on other aspects of health are noted throughout this book, and nurses can incorporate this information when they teach about the many positive functional consequences of regular physical exercise.

Smoking is a major risk factor for cardiovascular disease, and quitting smoking is beneficial for people at any age. A longitudinal study found that smoking cessation was the most important independent predictor of mortality in patients who had coronary artery bypass graft surgery, with a 30-year survival rate of 29% in patients who quit smoking and 14% in those who continued to smoke (de Boer et al., 2013). Benefits of smoking cessation as a secondary prevention intervention begin immediately and are as effective in older adults as they are in younger people. An important nursing responsibility is to provide health education regarding smoking cessation, as discussed in Chapter 21.

Teaching about stress reduction is an important health promotion intervention for reducing risks related to cardiovascular disease. An evidence-based review found that mind–body therapies have positive effects on cardiovascular function by improving stress management and coping skills and influencing physiologic stress mechanisms (Rabito & Kaye, 2013). For example, many studies indicate that yoga can reduce cardiovascular risk factors, including obesity, hypertension, high cholesterol and high blood glucose (e.g., Hagins et al., 2013; Okonta, 2012). Studies have also found that tai chi may prevent and reverse the progression of cardiovascular disease (Dalusung-Angosta, 2011; Lo et al., 2012; Ng et al., 2012). Nurses can encourage older adults to participate in mind–body activities, which community- or hospital-based senior centres offer.

Secondary Prevention

When nurses care for older adults who have cardiovascular disease, referrals for secondary prevention programs, such as cardiac rehabilitation, are an important part of care. Evidence-based guideline recommend cardiac rehabilitation programs as a comprehensive approach to reducing mortality by nearly 25% and restoring individuals to their optimal physiologic, psychosocial, nutritional and functional status (Arena et al., 2012). Despite this evidence of efficacy and cost-effectiveness, referral and participation rates for cardiac rehabilitation programs are low. Although referrals need to be initiated by primary care practitioners, nurses have important roles in encouraging participation when referrals are made. Nurses can also suggest referrals for additional preventive services that address stress management, smoking cessation or exercise counselling.

DIVERSITY NOTE

Very low rates of participation in cardiac rehabilitation are associated with the following conditions: rural areas, lower socioeconomic status, limited education, advanced age and female sex (Arena et al., 2012).

Wellness Opportunity

Nurses communicate positive attitudes about aging by talking with older adults about personal responsibility for addressing risks for cardiovascular disease and communicating that it's never too late to incorporate healthy behaviours into daily life.

Addressing Risks Through Pharmacologic Interventions

Before and during the 1990s, hormonal replacement therapy was recommended for menopausal women as an intervention for preventing cardiovascular disease. This recommendation was based on epidemiologic studies, but it was reversed in 2002 when longitudinal and large-scale investigations concluded that risks outweighed the benefits as a preventive intervention. The use of low-dose aspirin is another pharmacologic intervention that has been investigated for the prevention of cardiovascular disease, with emphasis on determining whether the potential benefits outweigh the increased risks for gastrointestinal bleeding and hemorrhagic stroke. In the early 2000s, studies concluded that the balance of benefit and harm is most favourable in people with a high risk for, or a history of, cardiovascular disease. In 2012, the U.S. Preventive Services Task Force [USPTF] (2012) published updated evidence-based guidelines with the following recommendations:

- Men aged 45 to 79 years and women aged 55 to 79 years: encourage aspirin use when potential cardiovascular benefit outweighs potential harm of gastrointestinal hemorrhage or ischemic strokes.
- Men less than age 45 and women less than age 55 years: do not encourage aspirin use.
- Men and women aged 80 years and older: no recommendation due to insufficient evidence.

Preventing and Managing Hypertension

Although relatively few nurses prescribe medications for hypertension, all nurses need to apply current guidelines and recommendations for management of hypertension when caring for older adults. Nursing interventions for people with hypertension include evaluating a patient's response to prescribed medications and teaching about interventions for hypertension. In addition, nurses can promote wellness by teaching about self-care measures for preventing and treating hypertension. This is particularly important because lifestyle interventions—including diet, weight loss, physical activity, stress-reduction techniques and moderation of alcohol—are an integral component of effective hypertension management (Brook et al., 2013).

The **stepped-care approach** to management of hypertension was introduced in the first Joint National Committee (JNC) report, and it has been consistently recommended in subsequent reports. This approach recommends that lifestyle modifications be tried initially, followed by pharmacologic interventions to achieve target blood pressure. Lifestyle interventions that have the most significant impact on hypertension are substantial weight loss and a dietary pattern that includes low-sodium and high-potassium foods. Guidelines from major organizations, such as the American Heart Association and the American College of Cardiology emphasize that sodium intake of 1,500 mg/day or less is associated with greater reductions in blood pressure (Eckel et al., 2014). Although recommendations for lower sodium intake apply to about 70% of U.S. adults, daily sodium intake for most adults is between 3,000 and more than 4,000 mg/day (Whelton et al., 2012). Thus, nurses have important responsibilities with regard to teaching older adults and their caregivers about sodium intake.

Many medications are used for treating hypertension, and selection of the best medication is based on variables such as therapeutic effectiveness, the presence of concomitant conditions and avoidance of adverse effects. Table 20-1 includes information about classes of medications recommended in the 2014 Evidence-Based Guideline for the Management of High Blood Pressure in Adults (JNC 8). Current emphasis is on the need for individualized treatment options, particularly for certain groups, such as African Americans

and people with chronic kidney disease. This attention is warranted because people of African ancestry respond better to calcium-channel blockers and diuretics and are less responsive to β-blockers and ACE inhibitors (Brewster & Seedat, 2013). Box 20-8 summarizes guidelines for interventions for hypertension and includes health education information about nutrition and lifestyle interventions. Figure 20-2 illustrates examples of some of the culturally specific health education materials that are available at the National Institutes of Health.

Wellness Opportunity

Nurses promote personal responsibility for managing hypertension by talking with older adults about self-monitoring of blood pressure.

 Box 20-8 Guidelines for Nursing Management of Hypertension

Health Promotion Interventions

The following lifestyle modifications are recommended for all people with hypertension:

- Avoidance of tobacco
- Weight reduction when appropriate (i.e., when the person weighs more than 110% of his or her ideal weight)
- 30 to 45 minutes of exercise, such as brisk walking, at least five times weekly
- Limitation of alcohol intake to one drink per day (e.g., 2 ounces of 100-proof whiskey, 8 ounces of wine or 24 ounces of beer).
   The following nutritional interventions are recommended for all people with hypertension:
- Sodium intake limited to 1.5 g daily
- Avoidance of processed foods
- Daily intake of 7 to 8 servings of grains and grain products and 8 to 10 servings of fruits and vegetables

Considerations Regarding the Treatment of Hypertension

- Risks from and definitions of hypertension apply to all age categories (refer to Table 20-1 for criteria).
- A person's blood pressure should be measured at least three times before making any decisions about treatment.
- Home blood pressure monitoring is recommended for initial and ongoing assessment.
- The safety of antihypertensive agents is improved by carefully selecting the medication, starting with low doses and changing the medication regimen gradually, in small increments, if necessary.
- The goals of hypertensive treatment are to control blood pressure by the least intrusive means and to prevent cardiovascular morbidity and mortality.
- Treatment is directed toward achieving and maintaining a systolic blood pressure of <130/80 mm Hg if this can be achieved without compromising cardiovascular function.
- For older adults with isolated systolic hypertension or systolic blood pressure levels of 140 to 160 mm Hg, lifestyle modifications should be the first treatment step.

TABLE 20-1 2014 Evidence-Based Guidelines for the Management of High Blood Pressure in Adults Aged 60 Years or Older	
Group	**Recommendation**
General population aged 60 years or older	Pharmacologic treatment to reach a goal of 150 or lower mm Hg systolic BP and 90 mm Hg or lower diastolic BP; if pharmacologic treatment can achieve a lower systolic BP (e.g., 140 mm Hg) and is not associated with adverse effects, continue treating
All adults with diabetes or chronic kidney disease	Pharmacologic treatment to reach a goal of 140 mm Hg or lower systolic BP and 90 mm Hg or lower diastolic BP
General population of nonblack adults	Initial antihypertensive treatment with a thiazide-type diuretic, calcium-channel blocker, angiotensin-converting enzyme inhibitor or angiotensin-receptor blocker
General population of black adults	Initial antihypertensive treatment with a thiazide-type diuretic or calcium-channel blocker
Adults with chronic kidney disease, regardless of race or diabetes status	Initial antihypertensive treatment should include angiotensin-converting enzyme inhibitor, or angiotensin-receptor blocker to improve kidney outcomes

Source: James P. A., Oparil, S., Carter, B. L., et al. (2013). 2014 Evidence-Based Guideline for the Management of High Blood Pressure in Adults: Report from the Panel Members Appointed to the Eighth Joint National Committee (JNC 8). *Journal of the American Medical Association.* doi:10.1001/jama.2013.284427

Unfolding Case Study

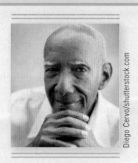

Part 2: Mr. C. at 70 Years of Age

Mr. C. is now 70 years old and his blood pressure fluctuates between 136/88 and 146/94 mm Hg. He continues to take hydrochlorothiazide, 25 mg, and verapamil, 120 mg, every morning. Mr. C. and his wife live with their daughter and her teenage children. Mr. and Mrs. C. usually do the family grocery shopping, and his wife and daughter prepare the family meals. A diet history reveals that the family usually eats fried fish or chicken about four times a week and pig's feet or ham hocks for the other main meals. Common side dishes are corn, okra, grits, cornbread, sweet potatoes, black-eyed peas and fried greens. For cooking, the family uses lard, salt pork or bacon drippings. Their usual beverage is decaffeinated coffee with sugar and cream. The family generally has cereal and toast for breakfast, but they have bacon and eggs on Saturdays and Sundays. Mr. and Mrs. C. eat their noon meal at the senior centre 5 days a week. Mr. C.'s BMI is still in the obesity range, and he has gradually gained a few pounds. For the past several years, he has participated in the exercise program at the senior centre, but gets little additional exercise and continues to complain of "getting winded" when he walks across the parking lot.

THINKING POINTS

- What additional information would you obtain for further assessment of Mr. C.'s cardiovascular status?
- What nutritional and lifestyle interventions would you discuss with Mr. C. regarding his hypertension?
- What teaching materials would you use for health education with Mr. C.?

QSEN APPLICATION

QSEN Competency	Knowledge/Skill/Attitude	Application to Mr. C.
Patient-centred care	(K) Integrate understanding of multiple dimensions of patient-centred care.	Assess sociocultural factors that influence Mr. C.'s dietary patterns.
	(K) Describe how diverse backgrounds function as a source of values.	Discuss benefits of weight loss that would have measurable positive effects during daily activities (e.g., improved breathing during mild exertion or walking).
	(K) Describe strategies to empower patients in all aspects of the health care process.	
	(S) Elicit patient values, preferences and expressed needs.	
	(S) Provide patient-centred care with sensitivity and respect for diversity of the human experience.	

Preventing and Managing Lipid Disorders

Although nurses usually do not prescribe medications for treatment of lipid disorders, they are responsible for teaching about preventing and managing lipid disorders. Recent guidelines developed jointly by the American College of Cardiology and the American Heart Association recommend the initiation of statin therapy based on assessment of risks for individuals with any of the following conditions (Stone et al., 2013):

- Clinical evidence of cardiovascular disease
- Primary elevations of LDL-C 190 mg/dL or above
- Diabetes and aged 40 to 75 years with LDL-C 70 to 189 mg/dL and without clinical evidence of cardiovascular disease

Although there is some controversy about the prescription of statins for primary prevention for older adults without cardiovascular disease or other clearly identified risk factors, reviews of studies find that the benefits of statins outweigh the risk of adverse effects (Savarese et al., 2013; Taylor et al., 2013).

As with treatment of hypertension, nutrition and lifestyle interventions are the first-line approaches, and medications (e.g., statins) are prescribed if goals are not achieved with nonpharmacologic interventions. Essential nutrition and lifestyle interventions for lipid disorders include dietary modifications, maintenance of ideal body weight and incorporation of regular exercise in one's daily routine. Nutritional interventions focus on dietary fat intake, with emphasis on

中風的徵兆

如果您有以下任何一項中風的徵兆，應立即撥打 **9-1-1** 或當地緊急求救電話，或請他人代您致電求助。

 虛弱無力 – 突然感到周身乏力，或臉部、手臂或腳出現麻痺，即使這情況只是短暫出現。

 說話困難 – 突然出現說話或理解語言有困難，或突然感到混亂，即使這情況只是短暫出現。

 視力問題 – 視力突然出現問題，即使這情況只是短暫出現。

 頭痛 – 突發性嚴重及不尋常的頭痛。

 眩暈 – 突然失去平衡，特別是同時出現上述任何一種徵兆。

heartandstroke.ca/Chinese

ਸਟਰੋਕ (ਦਿਮਾਗ਼ ਨੂੰ ਆਕਸੀਜਨ ਨਾ ਪਹੁੰਚਣ ਕਾਰਨ ਬੇਹੋਸ਼ੀ) ਦੀ ਚਿਤਾਵਨੀ ਦੀਆਂ ਨਿਸ਼ਾਨੀਆਂ

ਜੇ ਇਨ੍ਹਾਂ ਵਿੱਚੋਂ ਤੁਹਾਨੂੰ ਕੋਈ ਵੀ ਨਿਸ਼ਾਨੀ ਮਹਿਸਸ ਹੁੰਦੀ ਹੋਵੇ ਤਾਂ ਤੁਰੰਤ ਹੀ **9-1-1** ਨੂੰ ਜਾਂ ਆਪਣੇ ਸਥਾਨਕ ਐਮਰਜੰਸੀ ਨੰਬਰ 'ਤੇ ਫੋਨ ਕਰੋ

 ਕਮਜ਼ੋਰੀ – ਅਚਾਨਕ ਤਾਕਤ ਘਟ ਜਾਣੀ ਜਾਂ ਚਿਹਰੇ, ਬਾਂਹ ਜਾਂ ਲੱਤ ਵਿੱਚ ਅਚਾਨਕ ਸਿਥਲਤਾ ਆਉਣੀ, ਭਾਵੇਂ ਥੋੜ੍ਹੇ ਸਮੇਂ ਲਈ ਹੀ ਹੋਵੇ।

 ਬੋਲਣ ਵਿੱਚ ਮੁਸ਼ਕਲ ਆਉਣੀ – ਬੋਲਣ ਜਾਂ ਸਮਝਣ ਵਿੱਚ ਅਚਾਨਕ ਮੁਸ਼ਕਲ ਆਉਣੀ ਜਾਂ ਅਚਾਨਕ ਘਬਰਾਹਟ ਹੋਣੀ, ਭਾਵੇਂ ਥੋੜ੍ਹੇ ਸਮੇਂ ਲਈ ਹੀ ਹੋਵੇ।

 ਨਿਗ੍ਹਾ ਦੀਆਂ ਸਮਿੱਸਆਵਾਂ – ਨਿਗ੍ਹਾ ਵਿੱਚ ਅਚਾਨਕ ਮੁਸ਼ਕਲ ਆਉਣੀ, ਭਾਵੇਂ ਇਹ ਥੋੜ੍ਹੇ ਸਮੇਂ ਲਈ ਹੀ ਹੋਵੇ।

 ਸਿਰ ਦਰਦ – ਅਚਾਨਕ ਸਖ਼ਤ ਅਤੇ ਅਸ਼ਧਾਰਨ ਸਿਰ ਦਰਦ।

 ਚੱਕਰ ਆਉਣੇ – ਅਚਾਨਕ ਸੰਤੁਲਨ ਖੋ ਬੈਠਣਾ, ਖ਼ਾਸ ਕਰ ਉਕਤ ਨਿਸ਼ਾਨੀਆਂ ਵਿੱਚੋਂ ਕਿਸੇ ਦੇ ਵੀ ਨਾਲ।

heartandstroke.ca/SouthAsian

FIGURE 20-2 Examples of culturally specific health education materials that are available from the National Institutes of Health.

Box 20-9 Nutritional Interventions for People With High Cholesterol

Dietary Measures to Promote a Healthy Lipid Profile

- Include foods that are high in fibre content in your daily diet (e.g., whole grains).
- Include soy proteins in your daily diet (e.g., tofu, soy milk).
- Eat a minimum of two servings of fatty fish weekly.
- Limit total fat intake to less than 30% of your total daily calorie intake.
- Limit total daily cholesterol intake to 200 mg.
- Use nonfat or low-fat dairy desserts.

- Limit consumption of butter or margarine, but margarines that contain stanols are beneficial (e.g., Becanol).
- Use egg whites, omega-3 eggs or egg substitutes.
- Limit consumption of lean meats to five or fewer 3- to 5-ounce servings per week. Trim fat off meats and the skin off poultry.
- Avoid eating processed meats (e.g., bacon, bologna, sausage, hot dogs).
- Avoid gravies, fried foods and organ meats.

Guide to Types of Fats

Type of Fat	Sources	Examples	Effect on Lipid Profile
Saturated fatty acids	Animal fats and some vegetable oils (usually solid at room temperatures)	Meat, poultry, butter and lauric and palm oils	Negative: increases LDL and total cholesterol levels
Trans fatty acids	Vegetable oils that are processed into margarine or shortening	Dairy products, baked goods, snack foods	Negative: increases LDL cholesterol and lowers cholesterol levels
Monounsaturated fatty acids	Vegetable oils (usually liquid at room temperatures)	Olive, peanut and canola oils	Positive: decreases LDL level
Polyunsaturated fatty acids	Seafood and vegetable oils (soft or liquid at room temperatures)	Corn, sunflower, safflower, canola and linoleic oils	Positive: decreases LDL level
Omega-3 fatty acids	Fatty fish	Tuna, salmon, herring, mackerel	Positive: decreases LDL cholesterol and triglyceride levels

limiting foods containing saturated fats and trans-fatty acids and increasing foods that are high in polyunsaturated and monounsaturated fats. Box 20-9 summarizes health education interventions for prevention and management of lipid disorders in older adults.

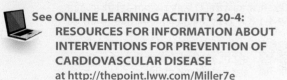

See ONLINE LEARNING ACTIVITY 20-4: RESOURCES FOR INFORMATION ABOUT INTERVENTIONS FOR PREVENTION OF CARDIOVASCULAR DISEASE at http://thepoint.lww.com/Miller7e

Preventing and Managing Orthostatic or Postprandial Hypotension

Interventions aimed at preventing orthostatic and postprandial hypotension can be initiated as health measures for older adults who have any of the risk factors listed in Box 20-2. For older adults with symptomatic orthostatic hypotension, interventions to alleviate the problem are important for maintaining quality of life and preventing serious consequences. In addition, nurses address safety issues by implementing interventions that are directed toward preventing falls and fractures, as discussed in Chapter 22.

For older adults with postprandial hypotension, interventions can be implemented around mealtimes. In institutional or home care settings, registered dietitians may be helpful in developing a plan for addressing postprandial hypotension, but in any setting, nurses assume responsibility for health education about interventions. Some interventions that may be effective in reducing postprandial hypotension are low-carbohydrate meals, acarbose, green tea and agents that delay gastric emptying (e.g., xylose and the natural food supplement guar gum). Additional interventions are summarized in Box 20-10, which can be used as a tool for educating older adults about orthostatic and postprandial hypotension.

EVALUATING EFFECTIVENESS OF NURSING INTERVENTIONS

One measure of the effectiveness of health promotion interventions is the extent to which the older adult verbalizes correct information about the risks. Also, the older adult may verbalize intent to change or eliminate the lifestyle factors that increase the risk of impaired cardiovascular function. For example, the older adult may agree to join an exercise program and follow dietary measures to reduce serum cholesterol levels. Effectiveness of interventions can also be measured by determining the actual reduction in risk factors. For example, the person's serum cholesterol level may decrease from 238 to 198 mg/dL after 6 months of regular exercise and dietary modifications. For older adults with

impaired cardiovascular function, nurses evaluate the extent to which the signs and symptoms are alleviated and the extent to which older adults verbalize correct information about managing their condition.

Box 20-10 Education Regarding Orthostatic and Postprandial Hypotension

Preventing and Managing Orthostatic and Postprandial Hypotension

- Maintain adequate fluid intake (i.e., eight glasses of noncaffeinated beverages daily).
- Eat five or six smaller meals daily, rather than large meals.
- Avoid excessive alcohol consumption.
- Avoid sitting or standing still for prolonged periods, especially after meals.

Health Promotion Measures Specific to Orthostatic Hypotension

- Change your position slowly, especially when moving from a sitting or lying position to a standing position.
- Before standing up, sit at the side of the bed for several minutes after rising from a lying position.
- Maintain good physical fitness, especially good muscle tone, and engage in regular, but not excessive, exercise. (Swimming is an excellent form of exercise because the hydrostatic pressure prevents blood from pooling in the legs.)
- Wear a waist-high elastic support garment or thigh-high elastic stockings during the day, and put them on before getting out of bed in the morning.
- Sleep with the head of the bed elevated on blocks.
- During the day, rest in a recliner chair with your legs elevated.
- Take measures to prevent constipation and avoid straining during bowel movements.
- Avoid medications that increase the risk for orthostatic hypotension, particularly if additional risk factors are present (refer to Box 20-2).
- Avoid sources of intense heat (e.g., direct sun, electric blankets, hot baths and showers) because these cause peripheral vasodilation.
- If taking nitroglycerin, do not take it while standing.

Health Promotion Measures Specific to Postprandial Hypotension

- Minimize the risk for postprandial hypotension by taking antihypertensive medications (if prescribed) 1 hour after meals rather than before meals.
- Eat small, low-carbohydrate meals.
- Avoid alcohol consumption.
- Avoid strenuous exercise, especially for 2 hours after meals.

Safety Precautions if Hypotension Cannot Be Prevented

- Reduce the potential for falls and other negative functional consequences of postprandial hypotension by remaining seated (or by lying down) after meals.
- Call for assistance if help is needed with walking.
- Adapt the environment to minimize the risk and consequences of falling (e.g., ensure good lighting, install grab bars, keep pathways clear).

Unfolding Case Study

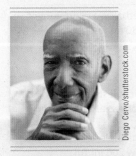

Diego Cervo/shutterstock.com

Part 3: Mr. C. at 74 Years of Age

Mr. C. is now 74 years old and continues to come to the senior wellness clinic for monthly blood pressure checks. He reports that his doctor recently started him on a medication for high cholesterol and told him to "watch my diet," but gave no further information or educational materials about what to do about his cholesterol.

NURSING ASSESSMENT

Mr. C. has no knowledge about the effects of various types of fat on cholesterol and triglyceride levels, and he is unaware that his diet, which he terms "soul food," increases the risk for cardiovascular disease. Although he says that he has heard a lot about "good and bad cholesterol" in the news, he does not know which foods are good or bad. He tries to buy foods that say "no cholesterol" on the label, but says that the labels are too confusing about the different kinds of fats.

NURSING DIAGNOSIS

Your nursing diagnosis is Ineffective Health Maintenance related to lack of regular exercise, dietary habits that contribute to hyperlipidemia and insufficient information about lifestyle factors that increase the risk of cardiovascular disease. Evidence of these risk factors comes from Mr. C.'s inactivity, eating patterns, history of hypertension and family history of cardiovascular disease. Also, Mr. C. has verbalized insufficient information about the relationship between exercise and cardiovascular function and about dietary measures to control cholesterol.

NURSING CARE PLAN FOR Mr. C.

Expected Outcome	Nursing Interventions	Nursing Evaluation
Mr. C.'s knowledge of risk factors for cardiovascular impairment will increase.	• Discuss the risk factors for impaired cardiovascular function, using Figure 20-1 and information from Box 20-4. • Emphasize the risk factors that can be addressed through lifestyle modifications (e.g., exercise, weight loss, dietary measures to control cholesterol levels).	• Mr. C. will be able to describe his risk factors for cardiovascular disease. • Mr. C. will identify those risk factors that he can address through lifestyle changes.
Mr. C.'s knowledge of the relationship between diet and serum cholesterol levels will increase.	• Use teaching materials obtained from the Heart and Stroke Foundation to illustrate the relationship between diet and serum cholesterol levels. Provide a copy of this information for Mr. C. to take home. • Suggest that Mr. C. discuss the information in the printouts with his wife and daughter. • Ask Mr. C. to bring his wife to the nursing clinic next month so that you can talk with both of them about dietary measures to control cholesterol.	• Mr. C. will accurately describe the relationship between food intake and cholesterol levels. • Mr. C. will identify family eating habits that contribute to his elevated serum cholesterol level.
Mr. C. will modify one dietary habit that contributes to his high cholesterol level.	• Work with Mr. C. to make a list of the foods associated with high cholesterol levels (e.g., fried foods, ham hocks, lard, bacon, eggs). • Give Mr. C. a copy of Box 20-9 and use it to discuss dietary measures to reduce cholesterol. • Ask Mr. C. to select one change in dietary habits that will have a positive effect on his cholesterol level (e.g., switching from lard to vegetable oil for frying foods).	• Mr. C. will state that he is willing to change one eating habit that contributes to his high cholesterol level. • Next month, Mr. C. will report that he has changed one eating pattern that contributes to high cholesterol levels.
Mr. C. will increase his knowledge about the relationship between exercise and cardiovascular function.	• Use information from the Heart and Stroke Foundation to teach about the effects of aerobic exercise on cardiovascular function. • Review information about the relationship between exercise and weight.	• Mr. C. will describe the beneficial effects of regular aerobic exercise.

Expected Outcome	Nursing Interventions	Nursing Evaluation
Mr. C. will begin exercising on a regular basis.	• Discuss ways in which Mr. C. can incorporate regular exercise into his daily activities. • Invite Mr. C. and his wife to participate in the daily Eldercise program that is offered following the noon meal at the senior centre.	• Mr. C. will verbalize a commitment to perform 30 minutes of exercise 3 days a week.
Mr. C. will eliminate lifestyle factors that increase the risk for cardiovascular disease.	• Ask Mr. C. to invite his wife to your monthly appointments so that she can also receive important health education. • Identify a plan that will enable Mr. and Mrs. C. to gradually incorporate additional dietary measures aimed at reducing cholesterol into the family meal plans. • Identify a plan that will enable Mr. and Mrs. C. to include 30 minutes of exercise five times a week. • Discuss weight reduction with Mr. C. and emphasize that dietary modifications and regular exercise are interventions that should facilitate weight loss.	• Mr. C.'s total cholesterol level will be 200 mg/dL or less at the end of 6 months. • Mr. C.'s serum cholesterol level will remain below 200 mg/dL. • Mr. C. will report that he engages in 30 minutes of exercise five times weekly. • Mr. C. will report that he follows the dietary measures presented in Box 20-9. • Mr. C.'s weight will decrease to between 82 and 86 kg, and he will maintain that weight.

THINKING POINTS

- What factors affect Mr. C.'s ability to manage his cardiovascular condition and address his risk factors, and how would you address these factors in your interventions?

- Explore some of the health education listed at the end of this chapter to find teaching tools that would be appropriate for Mr. C.

QSEN APPLICATION

QSEN Competency	Knowledge/Skill/Attitude	Application to Mr. C.
Patient-centred care	(K) Integrate understanding of multiple dimensions of patient-centred care. (K) Describe strategies to empower patients in all aspects of the health care process. (K) Examine common barriers to active involvement in patients. (S) Elicit patient values, preferences and expressed needs. (S) Provide patient-centred care with sensitivity and respect for diversity of the human experience.	Help Mr. C. identify one lifestyle change he is willing to address to reduce his risk for cardiovascular disease. Talk with Mr. C. about participating with his wife in daily Eldercise after they eat lunch at the senior centre. Ask Mr. C. to invite his wife the next time he comes to the Senior Wellness Clinic, so she can be included in discussions about reducing his risk for cardiovascular disease.
Teamwork and collaboration	(K) Recognize contributions of other individuals and groups in helping patient achieve health goals. (S) Integrate the contributions of others who play a role in helping patient achieve health goals.	Use teaching materials from the American Heart Association and the National Institutes of Health, including materials designed specifically for black Canadians (will be referred to as African Americans in the United States).
Evidence-based practice	(S) Base individualized care plan on patient values, clinical expertise and evidence. (A) Value evidence-based practice as integral to determining the best clinical practice.	Use evidence-based information in Box 20-9 to teach about nutritional interventions for people with high cholesterol.

Chapter Highlights

Age-Related Changes That Affect Cardiovascular Function

- Degenerative changes of myocardium and neuroconduction mechanisms
- Degenerative changes of the arteries and veins
- Altered baroreflex mechanisms

Risk Factors That Affect Cardiovascular Function (Box 20-1)

- Atherosclerosis involves pathologic changes of the arteries that begin in childhood and progress through adulthood and predispose older adults to cardiovascular diseases
- Physical inactivity
- Tobacco smoking and secondhand smoke
- Dietary habits
- Prevalence of obesity (i.e., BMI 30 kg/m² or more)
- Hypertension (i.e., blood pressure of 140/90 or higher)
- Lipid disorders
- Metabolic syndrome
- Psychosocial factors
- Heredity and socioeconomic factors
- Special considerations for women and minority groups

Functional Consequences Affecting Cardiovascular Wellness

- Effects on cardiac function
- Effects on pulse and blood pressure
- Effects on response to exercise
- Effects on circulation

Pathologic Condition Affecting Cardiovascular Function

- Orthostatic and postprandial hypotension

Nursing Assessment of Cardiovascular Function (Fig. 20-1; Table 20-1; Boxes 20-3 through 20-5)

- Baseline cardiovascular function (heart rate, sounds and rhythm)
- Blood pressure, including hypertension and orthostatic or postprandial hypotension
- Risks for cardiovascular disease, with emphasis on modifiable conditions
- Signs and symptoms of heart disease
- Knowledge about heart disease

Nursing Diagnosis

- Ineffective Health Maintenance
- Decreased Cardiac Output
- Readiness for Enhanced Nutrition
- Readiness for Enhanced Knowledge

Planning for Wellness Outcomes

- Health-Promoting Behaviours
- Risk Control: Cardiovascular Health
- Risk Control: Tobacco Use
- Cardiac Disease Self-Management

Nursing Interventions to Promote Healthy Cardiovascular Function (Box 20-1; Boxes 20-7 through 20-10)

- Addressing risks through nutritional interventions
- Addressing risks through lifestyle interventions (exercise, heart-healthy diet, optimal body weight, cessation of smoking if applicable)
- Secondary prevention programs for older adults who have cardiovascular disease
- Pharmacologic interventions for prevention of cardiovascular disease
- Preventing and managing hypertension
- Preventing and managing lipid disorders
- Prevention and management of orthostatic and postprandial hypotension

Evaluating Effectiveness of Nursing Interventions

- Verbalization of correct information about risks
- Reported participation in health promotion interventions (e.g., heart-healthy diet, regular exercise, weight reduction and smoking cessation when applicable)
- Indicators of cardiovascular function within normal range (e.g., blood pressure, serum lipids)
- If applicable, alleviation of signs and symptoms of cardiovascular disease

Critical Thinking Exercises

1. Discuss how each of the following factors influences cardiovascular function, including orthostatic hypotension, lifestyle, medications, age-related changes and pathologic conditions.
2. Demonstrate how you would teach a home health aide to assess blood pressure and orthostatic hypotension correctly.
3. Describe the questions and considerations that you would include in an assessment of cardiovascular function in an older adult who has no complaints of heart problems, but who has a history of falling twice in the past month and who has not been evaluated by a primary care provider in the past year.
4. You are asked to give a health education talk titled "Keeping Your Heart Healthy" at a senior centre. What information would you include in the presentation? What local resources (i.e., specific contact information for agencies or organizations in your area) would you suggest your audience contact for further information?

What audiovisual aids would you use? How would you involve the participants in the discussion?

5. You are working in an assisted-living facility in which several of the residents have orthostatic hypotension. What would you include in your health education regarding management of orthostatic hypotension?

For more information about the topics discussed in this chapter, be sure to check out the interactive Online Learning Activities and other helpful resources
at http://thepoint.lww.com/Miller7e

REFERENCES

Abdel-Rahman, T. A. (2012). Orthostatic hypotension before and after meal intake in diabetic patients and healthy elderly people. *Journal of Family and Community Medicine, 19*(1), 20–25.

Arena, R., Williams, M., Forman, D. E., et al. (2012). Increasing referral and participation rates to outpatient cardiac rehabilitation: The valuable role of health care professionals in inpatient and home health settings. *Circulation, 125*, 1321–1329.

Arranz, S., Valderas-Martinez, P., Chiva-Blanch, G., et al. (2013). Cardioprotective effects of cocoa: Clinical evidence from randomized clinical intervention trials in humans. *Molecular Nutrition and Food Research, 57*(6), 936–947.

Aung, A. K., Corcoran, S. J., Nagalingam, V., et al. (2012). Prevalence, associations, and risk factors for orthostatic hypotension in medical, surgical, and trauma patients. *The Ochsner Journal, 12*(1), 35–41.

Barnes, A. S. (2012). Obesity and sedentary lifestyles risk for cardiovascular disease in women. *The Texas Heart Institute Journal, 39*(2), 224–227.

Berry, J. D., Dyer, A., Cai, X., et al. (2012). Lifetime risks of cardiovascular disease. *New England Journal of Medicine, 366*(4), 321–329.

Brewster, L. M., & Seedat, Y. K. (2013). Why do hypertensive patients of African ancestry respond better to calcium blockers and diuretics than to ACE inhibitors and beta-adrenergic blockers? A systematic review. *BioMed Central Medicine, 11*(1), 141. Retrieved from www.biomedcentral.cm/1741-7015/11/141

Brook, R. D., Appel, L. J., Rubenfire, M., et al. (2013). Beyond medications and diet:alternative approaches to lowering blood pressure: A scientific statement from the American Heart Association. *Hypertension, 61*(6), 1360–1383.

Cacciolati, C., Hanon, O., Dufouil, C., et al. (2013). Categories of hypertension in the elderly and their 1-year evolution. *Journal of Hypertension, 31*(4), 680–689.

Canadian Health Institute. (2013). *Health Indicators 2013*. Retrieved from https://secure.cihi.ca/free_products/HI2013_EN.pdf

Castellon, X., & Bogdanova, V. (2013). Screening for subclinical atherosclerosis by noninvasive methods in asymptomatic patients with risk factors. *Clinical Interventions in Aging, 8*, 573–580.

Colquhoun, D. M., Bunker, S. J., Clarke, D. M., et al. (2013). Screening, referral and treatment of depression in patients with coronary heart disease. *Medical Journal of Australia, 198*(9), 483–484.

Conference Board of Canada. (2010). *The Canadian heart health strategy: Risk factors and future cost implications report*. Ottawa, ON: Author.

Dalusung-Angosta, A. (2011). The impact of tai chi exercise on coronary heart disease: A systematic review. *Journal of the American Academy of Nurse Practitioners, 23*(7), 376–381.

de Boer, S. P., Serruys, P. W., Valstar, G., et al. (2013). Life-years gained by smoking cessation after percutaneous coronary intervention. *American Journal of Cardiology, 112*(9), 1311–1314. doi:10.1016/j.amjcard.2013.05.075

Doering, L. V., Chen, B., Bodan, R. C., et al. (2013). Early cognitive behavioral therapy for depression after cardiac surgery. *Journal of Cardiovascular Nursing, 28*(4), 370–379.

Eckel, R. H., Jakicic, J. M., & Ard, J. D. (2014). 2013 AHA/ACC Guideline on Lifestyle Management to Reduce Cardiovascular Risk: A report of the American College of Cardiology/American Heart Association Task Force on Practice Guidelines. *Circulation, 129*(25 Suppl. 2), S76–S99.

Ellam, S., & Williamson, G. (2013). Cocoa and human health. *Annual Review of Nutrition, 33*, 105–128.

Emerging Risk Factors Collaboration. (2012). C-reactive protein, fibrinogen, and cardiovascular disease prediction. *New England Journal of Medicine, 367*(14), 1310–1320.

Estruch, R., Ros, E., Salas-Salvado, J., et al. (2013). Primary prevention of cardiovascular disease with a Mediterranean diet. *New England Journal of Medicine, 368*(14), 1279–1290.

Felix-Redondo, F. J., Grau, M., & Fernandez-Berges, D. (2013). Cholesterol and cardiovascular disease in the elderly: Facts and gaps. *Aging and Disease, 4*(3), 154–169.

Fitzgerald, K. C., Chiuve, S. E., Buring, J. E., et al. (2012). Comparison of associations of adherence to a DASH-style diet with risks of cardiovascular disease and venous thromboembolism. *Journal of Thrombosis and Haemostasis, 10*(2), 189–198.

Frazier, L., Sanner, J., Yo, E., et al. (2014). Using a single screening question for depressive symptoms in patients with acute coronary syndrome. *Journal of Cardiovascular Nursing, 29*(4), 347–353. doi:10.1097/JCN.0b013e318291ee16

Friedmann, E., Son, H., Thomas, S., et al. (2014). Poor social support is associated with increases in depression but not anxiety over 2 years in heart failure outpatients. *Journal of Cardiovascular Nursing, 29*(1), 20–28. doi:10.1097/JCN.0b013e318276fa07

Fukushima, T., Asahina, M., Fujinuma, Y., et al. (2013). Role of intestinal peptides and the autonomic nervous system in postprandial hypotension in patients with multiple system atrophy. *Journal of Neurology, 260*(2), 475–483. doi:10.1007/s00415-012-6660-x

Gionet, L., & Roshanafshar, S. (2013). *Selected health indicators of First Nations people living off reserve, Métis and Inuit* (Statistics Canada Catalogue no. 82-624-X). Retrieved from http://www.statcan.gc.ca/pub/82-624-x/2013001/article/11763-eng.htm

Go, A. S., Mozaffarian, D., Roger, V. L., et al. (2014). Heart disease and stroke statistics: 2014 update: A report from the American Heart Association. *Circulation, 128*, e1–e267.

Goff, D. C., Lloyd-Jones, D. M., Bennett, G., et al. (2014). 2013 ACC/AHA Guideline on the assessment of cardiovascular risk: A report of the American College of Cardiology/American Heart Association Task Force on Practice Guidelines. *Journal of the American College of Cardiology, 63*(25), 2935–2959. doi:10:10.1016/j.jacc.2013.11.005

Graven, L. J., & Grant, J. (2013). The impact of social support on depressive symptoms in individuals with heart failure. *Journal of Cardiovascular Nursing, 28*(5), 429–443. doi:10.1097/JCN.0b013e3182578b9d

Hagins, M., States, R., Selfe, T., et al. (2013). Effectiveness of yoga for hypertension: Systematic review and meta-analysis. *Evidence-Based Complementary and Alternative Medicine, 2013* [Article ID 649836]. doi:10.1155.2013/649863

Hartley, L., Flowers, N., Holmes, J., et al. (2013). Green and black tea for the primary prevention of cardiovascular disease. *Cochrane Database Systematic Review.* doi:10.1002/14651858.CD009934.pub2

HealthLink BC. (2012). *Metabolic syndrome: Topic overview*. Retrieved from www.healthlinkbc.ca/healthtopics/content.asp?hwid=tm6339spec

Herdman, T. H. (Ed.). (2012). *NANDA International Nursing Diagnoses: Definitions and classification* 2012–1014. Oxford, England: Wiley-Blackwell.

Hopping, B. N., Erber, E., Mead, E., et al. (2010). High level of physical activity and obesity co-exist amongst Inuit adults in Artic Canada. *Journal of Human Nutrition and Dietetics, 23*, 110–114.

James, P. A., Oparil, S., Carter, B. L., et al. (2013). 2014 Evidence-Based Guideline for the Management of High Blood Pressure in Adults: Report from the Panel Members Appointed to the Eighth Joint National

Committee (JNC 8). *Journal of the American Medical Association.* Advance online publication. doi:10.1001/jama.2013.284427

Kariuki, J. K., Stuart-Shor, E. M., & Hayman, L. L. (2013). The concept of risk as applied to cardiovascular disease. *Journal of Cardiovascular Nursing, 28*(3), 201–203.

Kim, H. S., & Cho, K. I. (2013). Impact of chronic emotional stress on myocardial function in postmenopausal women and its relationship with endothelial dysfunction. *Korean Circulation Journal, 43,* 295–302.

Lagro, J., Meel-van den Abeelen, A., de Jong, D. L., et al. (2013). Geriatric hypotensive syndromes are not explained by cardiovascular autonomic dysfunction alone. *Journals of Gerontology: Medical Sciences, 68*(5), 581–589.

Li, J., & Siegrist, J. (2012). Physical activity and risk of cardiovascular disease: A meta-analysis of prospective cohort studies. *Indian Journal of Environmental Research and Public Health, 9,* 391–407.

Lim, L. S., Haq, N., Mahmood, S., et al. (2011). Atherosclerotic cardiovascular disease screening in adults: American College of Preventive Medicine position statement on preventive practice. *American Journal of Preventive Medicine, 40*(3), 381.e1–10. doi:10.1016/j.amepre.2010.11.021

Liu, R., So, L., Mohen, S., et al. (2010). Cardiovascular risk factors in ethnic populations within Canada: Results from national cross-sectional surveys. *Open Medicine, 4*(3). Retrieved from http://www.openmedicine.ca/article/view/372/343

Lo, H., Yeh, C. Y., Chang, S. C., et al. (2012). A tai chi exercise programme improved exercise behaviour and reduced blood pressure in outpatients with hypertension. *International Journal of Nursing Practice, 18*(6), 545–551.

Miller, M., Stone, N. J., Ballantyne, C., et al. (2011). Triglycerides and cardiovascular disease: A scientific statement from the American Heart Association. *Circulation, 123,* 2292–2333.

Miuri, K., Stamler, J., Brown, I., et al. (2013). Relationship of dietary monounsaturated fatty acids to blood pressure: The international study of macro/micronutrients and blood pressure. *Journal of Hypertension, 31*(6), 1144–1150.

Mody, P., Gupta, A., Bikdeli, B., et al. (2012). Most important articles on cardiovascular disease among racial and ethnic minorities. *Circulation Cardiovascular Quality and Outcomes, 5,* e33–e41.

Mosca, L., Benjamin, E., Berra, K., et al. (2011). Effectiveness-based guidelines for the prevention of cardiovascular disease in women—2011 update. *Circulation, 123,* 1243–1262.

Neylon, A., Canniffe, C., Anand, S., et al. (2013). A global perspective on psychosocial risk factors for cardiovascular disease. *Progress in Cardiovascular Disease, 55*(6), 574–581.

Ng, S. M., Wang, C. W., Ho, R. T., et al. (2012). Tai chi exercise for patients with heart disease: A systematic review of controlled clinical trials. *Alternative Therapies in Health and Medicine, 18*(3), 16–22.

Nilsson, P., Boutouyrie, P., Cunha, P., et al. (2013). Early vascular ageing in translation: From laboratory investigations to clinical applications in cardiovascular prevention. *Journal of Hypertension, 31,* 1517–1526.

Noguchi, Y., Asayama, K., Staessen, J. A., et al. (2013). Predictive power of home blood pressure and clinic blood pressure in hypertensive patients with impaired glucose metabolism and diabetes. *Journal of Hypertension, 31*(8), 1593–1602. doi:101097/0b013e328361732c

Okonta, N. R. (2012). Does yoga therapy reduce blood pressure in patients with hypertension? *Holistic Nursing Practice, 26*(3), 137–141.

Oliva, R. V., & Bakris, G. L. (2012). Management of hypertension in the elderly population. *Journal of Gerontology: Medical Sciences, 67*(12), 1343–1351.

Omboni, S., Gazzola, R., Carabelli, G., et al. (2013). Clinical usefulness and cost effectiveness of home blood pressure telemonitoring: Meta-analysis of randomized controlled studies. *Journal of Hypertension, 1,* 455–468.

Pearson, T. A., Palaniappan, L., Artinian, N., et al. (2013). American Heart Association guide for improving cardiovascular health at the community level, 2013 update. *Circulation, 127,* 1730–1753.

Pepersack, T., Gilles, C., Petrovic, M., et al. (2013). Prevalence of orthostatic hypotension and relationship with drug use amongst older patients. *Acta Clinic Belgium, 68*(2), 107–112.

Peterson, J. A. (2012). One theoretic framework for cardiovascular disease prevention in women. *Journal of Cardiovascular Nursing, 27*(4), 295–302.

Prata, J., Ramos, S., Martins, A., et al. (2014). Women with coronary artery disease: Do psychosocial factors contribute to a higher cardiovascular risk? *Cardiology in Review, 22*(1), 25–29.

Rabito, M. J., & Kaye, A. D. (2013). Complementary and alternative medicine and cardiovascular disease: An evidence-based review. *Evidence Based Complementary and Alternative Medicine, 2013,* 1–8. doi:10.1155/2013/672097

Rees, K., Hartley, L., Flowers, N., et al. (2013, August 12). "Mediterranean" dietary pattern for the primary prevention of cardiovascular disease. *Cochrane Database Systematic Review, 8* [Article ID] CD009824.

Salehi-Abargouei, A., Maghsoudi, Z., Shirani, F., et al. (2013). Effects of dietary approaches to stop hypertension (DASH)-style diet on fatal or non-fatal cardiovascular diseases—Incidence: A systematic review and meta-analysis on observational prospective studies. *Nutrition, 29*(4), 611–618.

Savarese, G., Gotto, A. M., Paolillo, S., et al. (2013). Benefits of statins in elderly subjects without established cardiovascular disease: A meta-analysis. *Journal of the American College of Cardiology, 62*(22), 2290–2299.

Scholl, J. (2012). Traditional dietary recommendations for the prevention of cardiovascular disease: Do they meet the needs of our patients? *Cholesterol, 2012,* 1–9 [Article ID 367898]. doi:10.1155/2012/367898

Setayeshgar, S., Whiting, S. J., & Vatanparast, H. (2013). Prevalence of 10-year risk of cardiovascular diseases and associated risks in Canadian adults: The contribution of cardiometabolic risk assessment introduction. *International Journal of Hypertension, 2013,* 1–8 [Article ID 276564]. doi:10.1155/2013/276564

Smith, S. C., Collins, A., Ferrari, R., et al. (2012). Our time: A call to save preventable death from cardiovascular disease (heart disease and stroke). *Circulation, 126,* 2769–2775.

Son, J. T., & Lee, E. (2012). Postprandial hypotension among older residents of a nursing home in Korea. *Journal of Clinical Nursing, 21*(23–24), 3565–3573.

Son, J. T., & Lee, E. (2013). Comparison of postprandial blood pressure reduction in elderly by different body position. *Geriatric Nursing, 34*(4), 282–288. doi:10.1016/j.gerinurse.2013.03.004

Statistics Canada. (2011). *Smoking and mortality.* Retrieved from http://www.hc-sc.gc.ca/hc-ps/tobac-tabac/legislation/label-etiquette/mortal-eng.php#note4

Statistics Canada. (2012). *Health indicator profile, annual estimates, by age group and sex, Canada, provinces, territories, health regions (2011 boundaries) and peer group* (CANSIM table 105-0501). Ottawa, ON: Author.

Steptoe, A., & Kivimaki, M. (2013). Stress and cardiovascular disease: An update on current knowledge. *Annual Review of Public Health, 34,* 337–254.

Stone, N. J., Robinson, J., Lichtenstein, C., et al. (2013). 2013 ACC/AHA Guideline on treatment of blood cholesterol to reduce atherosclerotic cardiovascular risk in adults: A report of the American College of Cardiology/American Heart Association Task Force on Practice Guidelines. *Circulation, 129*(29 Suppl. 2), S1–S85. Retrieved from http://circ.ahajournals.org/content/early/2013/11/11/01.cir.0000437738.63853.7a.citation

Suls, J. (2013). Anger and the heart: Perspectives on cardiac risk, mechanisms and interventions. *Progress in Cardiovascular Disease, 55*(6), 538–547.

Taylor, F., Huffman, M. D., Macedo, A. F., et al. (2013, January 31). Statins for the primary prevention of cardiovascular disease. *Cochrane Database Systematic Review, 1* [Article ID CDC004816]. doi:10.1002/14651858.CDC004816.pub5

Thurston, R. C., Rewak, M., & Kubzansky, L. D. (2013). An anxious heart: Anxiety and the onset of cardiovascular diseases. *Progress in Cardiovascular Disease, 55*(6), 524–537.

U.S. Preventive Services Task Force. (2012). *The Guide to Clinical Preventive Services 2012: Recommendations of the U.S. Preventive Services Task Force.* Agency for Health care Research and Quality, Publication no. 12-05154. Retrieved from www.ahrq.gov

van Hateren, K. J., Kleefstra, N., Blanker, M. H., et al. (2012). Orthostatic hypotension, diabetes, and falling in older patients. *British Journal of General Practice, 62*(603), e696–e702.

Veenstra, G. (2012). Expressed racial identify and hypertension in a telephone survey sample from Toronto and Vancouver, Canada: Do socioeconomic status, perceived discrimination and psychosocial stress explain the relatively high risk of hypertension for Black Canadians. *International Journal for Equity in Health, 11*, 58. doi:10.1186/1475-9276-11-58

Weber, M. A., Schiffrin, E. L, White, W. B., et al. (2014). Clinical practice guidelines for the management of hypertension in the community: A statement by the American Society of Hypertension and the International Society of Hypertension. *Journal of Hypertension, 32*(1), 3–15.

Weihua, L., Yougang, W., & Jing, W. (2013). Reduced or modified dietary fat for preventing cardiovascular disease. *Journal of Cardiovascular Nursing, 28*(3), 204–205.

Whelton, P. K., Appel, L., Sacco, R., et al. (2012). Sodium, blood pressure, and cardiovascular disease: Further evidence supporting the American Heart Association sodium reduction recommendations. *Circulation, 126*, 2880–2889.

Xin, W., Lin, Z., & Li, X. (2013). Orthostatic hypotension and the risk of congestive heart failure: A meta-analysis of prospective cohort studies. *PLoS One, 8*(5), e63169.

Ye, C., Foster, G., Kaczorowski, J., et al. (2013). The impact of a cardiovascular health awareness program (CHAP) on reducing blood pressure: A prospective cohort study. *BMC Public Health, 13*, 1230. doi:10.1186/1471-2458-13-1230

Zanasi, A., Tincani, E., Evandri, V., et al. (2012). Meal-induced blood pressure variation and cardiovascular mortality in ambulatory hypertensive elderly patients. *Journal of Hypertension, 30*(11), 2125–2132.

chapter 21

Respiratory Function

The primary functions of respiration are to supply oxygen to and remove carbon dioxide from the blood. Adequate respiratory performance is essential to life because all body organs and tissues need oxygen. Healthy, nonsmoking, older adults are able to compensate for age-related changes, but risk factors, such as smoking, anesthesia and acute or chronic diseases, can impair respiratory function in significant ways.

 AGE-RELATED CHANGES THAT AFFECT RESPIRATORY FUNCTION

As with other physiologic functions, it is difficult to distinguish the effects of age-related changes from those caused by disease processes and external influences, such as environmental factors. Although these influences occur throughout the life span, their cumulative effects become more pronounced in older adults, especially when combined with risk factors. Age-related changes of the respiratory system are summarized in this section, and effects of these changes are discussed in the section on functional consequences.

Upper Respiratory Structures

The nose and other upper respiratory structures are affected by age-related changes that can affect comfort and function in the following ways:

- Degenerative changes in connective tissue causing the nose to have a retracted columella (the lower edge of the septum) and a poorly supported, downwardly rotated tip
- Diminished blood flow to the nose, causing the nasal turbinates to become smaller
- Thicker mucus in nasopharynx due to degenerative changes in submucosal glands
- Stiffening of trachea due to calcification of cartilage
- Blunted cough and laryngeal reflexes
- Atrophy of the laryngeal nerve endings

Chest Wall and Musculoskeletal Structures

The rib cage and the vertebral musculoskeletal structures are affected by the same kind of age-related changes that affect other musculoskeletal tissue: the ribs and vertebrae become osteoporotic, the costal cartilage calcifies and the respiratory muscles weaken. Because of these age-related processes, the

Promoting Respiratory Wellness in Older Adults

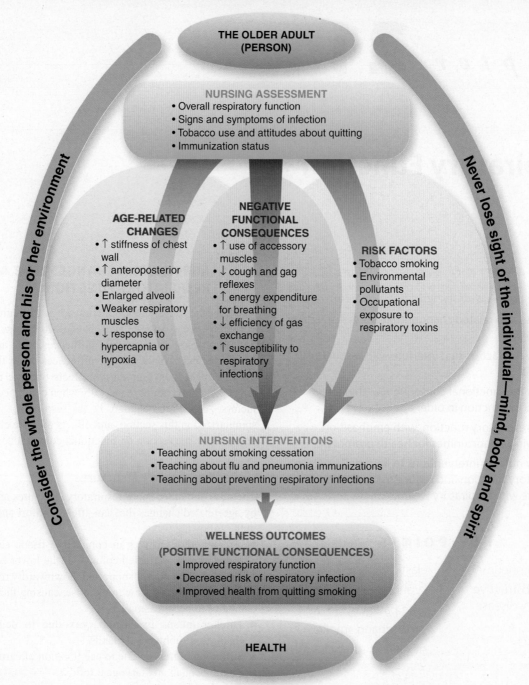

THE OLDER ADULT (PERSON)

NURSING ASSESSMENT
- Overall respiratory function
- Signs and symptoms of infection
- Tobacco use and attitudes about quitting
- Immunization status

AGE-RELATED CHANGES
- ↑ stiffness of chest wall
- ↑ anteroposterior diameter
- Enlarged alveoli
- Weaker respiratory muscles
- ↓ response to hypercapnia or hypoxia

NEGATIVE FUNCTIONAL CONSEQUENCES
- ↑ use of accessory muscles
- ↓ cough and gag reflexes
- ↑ energy expenditure for breathing
- ↓ efficiency of gas exchange
- ↑ susceptibility to respiratory infections

RISK FACTORS
- Tobacco smoking
- Environmental pollutants
- Occupational exposure to respiratory toxins

NURSING INTERVENTIONS
- Teaching about smoking cessation
- Teaching about flu and pneumonia immunizations
- Teaching about preventing respiratory infections

WELLNESS OUTCOMES
(POSITIVE FUNCTIONAL CONSEQUENCES)
- Improved respiratory function
- Decreased risk of respiratory infection
- Improved health from quitting smoking

HEALTH

Consider the whole person and his or her environment

Never lose sight of the individual—mind, body and spirit

following structural changes occur: **kyphosis** (i.e., an increased curvature of the spine), shortened thorax, chest wall stiffness and increased anteroposterior diameter of the chest. Overall, these age-related changes compromise chest wall expansion, and older adults need to expend more energy to achieve respiratory efficiency.

Lung Structure and Function

Even in healthy older adults, lungs become smaller and flabbier, and age-related changes affect the **lung parenchyma**, which is the part of the respiratory system where

gas exchange takes place. Changes that have the most effect on respiratory function are as follows:

- **Ductectasia** (i.e., the alveoli enlarge and their walls become thinner) begins around the age of 20 or 30 years and continues throughout adulthood, resulting in a gradual increase in the amount of anatomic dead space.
- The pulmonary artery becomes wider, thicker and less elastic.
- The number of capillaries diminishes.
- The pulmonary capillary blood volume decreases.
- The mucosal bed, where diffusion occurs, thickens.

Elastic recoil is the characteristic that keeps the airway open during inspiration by resisting expansion and maintaining a positive pressure across the lung surface. If the airways close prematurely, air is trapped and the lungs cannot expire to their maximum capacity. A combination of age-related changes in the parenchyma and elastic fibres interferes with elastic recoil, which results in early airway closure. Because of this and other age-related changes, gas exchange is compromised in the lower lung regions and inspired air is preferentially distributed in the upper regions. Effects of these changes include decreased arterial oxygen pressure (Pao_2) and changes in airflow rates.

Compensatory changes in respiratory rate are made under conditions of hypercapnia or hypoxia. The response to hypercapnia is initiated by a central chemoreceptor, located in the medulla, whereas the response to hypoxia is initiated by peripheral chemoreceptors, located in the carotid and aortic bodies. Age-related changes reduce the ventilatory response to both hypoxia and hypercapnia, so instead of—or in addition to—experiencing breathlessness or other respiratory symptoms when blood gases are abnormal, older adults are likely to develop mental changes.

Changes in Immune Function

Age-related alterations in the immune system affect respiratory function, even in healthy older adults. For example, studies confirm that age-related alterations of T cells (i.e., a component of the immune system that is essential for protecting against infections and malignancies) are a major factor contributing to the increased prevalence of lung diseases among older adults (Lee et al., 2012).

 ## RISK FACTORS THAT AFFECT RESPIRATORY WELLNESS

For people of any age, tobacco smoking is the single most important risk factor for lung disease and impaired respiratory function. The risks and consequences are both immediate and cumulative. Other risks are mentioned because, particularly for nonsmokers, they can be addressed through health promotion interventions to improve respiratory function. For smokers, however, it is imperative to focus attention on the serious negative consequences of smoking.

Tobacco Use

Tobacco smoking causes detrimental effects through multiple heat and chemical actions on the respiratory system. Harmful physiologic effects on the respiratory system include bronchoconstriction, impaired air flow, inflammation of the mucosa throughout the respiratory tract and inhibited ciliary action, leading to increased coughing and mucous secretions and diminished protection from harmful organisms. The most serious consequence of smoking is a significantly increased risk of developing diseases of the lungs, cardiovascular system and many other systems.

Thus, smoking-related diseases are considered the world's most preventable cause of death. Even though pipes, cigars and **smokeless tobacco** products (such as electronic cigarettes and chewing tobacco or gum) are sometimes viewed as safer than cigarettes, all forms and doses of tobacco are associated with serious health consequences, which are similar to those of cigarette smoking (Canadian Cancer Society, http://www.cancer.ca/en/cancer-information/cancer-101/what-is-a-risk-factor/tobacco/smokeless-tobacco/?region=on).

The Canadian Cancer Society (2014) has cited some evidence-based examples of the serious risks and detrimental effects as follows:

- In 2013, 25,500 Canadians were diagnosed with lung cancer.
- Smoking is responsible for 30% of all cancer deaths and is related to more than 85% of lung cancer cases.
- Each year, more than 250 Canadians die from lung cancer as a result of long-term exposure to tobacco smoked by other people (secondhand smoke) at home, at work and when they are out and about.
- Smoking increases the risk of all the following types of cancers: paranasal sinus, nasopharynx, nasal cavity, lip, oral cavity, larynx, pharynx, esophagus, lung, kidney, bladder, stomach, pancreas, colorectum, ovary, uterine, cervix and acute myeloid leukemia. There is limited evidence of the link between smoking and breast cancer in women.
- Smoking is a major cause of heart disease, cerebrovascular disease (including stroke) chronic bronchitis and emphysema; it is also associated with gastric ulcers.
- Smoking has been suggested as a risk factor for Alzheimer disease (Alzheimer Society Canada, 2014) because of its effect on blood supply to the brain.

Researchers are also identifying links between smoking and conditions that disproportionately affect older adults, including all of the following: cognitive impairment (Rincon & Wright, 2013; Okusaga et al., 2013); osteoporosis (Ní Chróinín et al., 2013); cataracts (Richter et al., 2012); age-related macular degeneration (Willeford & Rapp, 2012) and hearing loss (Yamasoba et al., 2013). Studies that are especially relevant to health promotion for older adults focus on beneficial effects of quitting during older adulthood. For example, Gellert and colleagues (2013) compared new onset of cardiovascular events in 8,807 current, never and former smokers aged 50 to 74 for a mean follow-up of 9.1 years and concluded that smoking cessation was highly and rapidly beneficial for older adults.

 DIVERSITY NOTE

Results from the Canadian Community Health Survey (CCHS) 2009/2010 identify that daily smoking rates are higher among women with low income and low levels of education. The largest number of daily and occasional smokers can be found in the Yukon, Nunavut and Northwest Territories. It has been estimated that smoking rates in the Aboriginal population may be as twice as high as in other regions of Canada.

Another potentially detrimental health effect related to smoking that has implications for care of older adults is the potential for altering the effects of medications. Interactions can occur in people who smoke or use nicotine products (including smokeless tobacco) and in people who have recently quit smoking. Interactions can be due directly to the physiologic effects of nicotine or they may be caused by the hydrocarbons in tobacco smoke, which can affect hepatic metabolism of some medications. Additional information and examples of drug–nicotine interactions are discussed in Chapter 8.

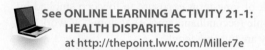

Wellness Opportunity

Be aware of opportunities to teach older adults about potential interactions between medications and nicotine products, which are often overlooked.

See **ONLINE LEARNING ACTIVITY 21-1:**
HEALTH DISPARITIES
at http://thepoint.lww.com/Miller7e

Secondhand Smoke and Other Environmental Factors

Secondhand smoke (also called passive smoke or environmental tobacco smoke) is a mixture of smoke that comes from lit tobacco products and smoke that is exhaled by the smoker. Health Canada cites the 1972 Surgeon General's Report, in which evidence indicates that there is no safe level of exposure to secondhand smoke (http://www.hc-sc.gc.ca/hc-ps/tobac-tabac/body-corps/second-eng.php). The following statistics cited by the Canadian Cancer Society (2013) substantiate the risks associated with secondhand smoke:

- Secondhand smoke contains more than 7,000 chemicals and more than 70 known carcinogens.
- There is limited evidence that secondhand smoke increases the risk for breast cancer.
- Breathing in secondhand smoke can trigger asthma attacks and increase the chances of getting chest infections like bronchitis and pneumonia.
- Effects of secondhand smoke include coughing, wheezing, chest tightness and reduced lung function.

Studies are also exploring an association between secondhand smoke and cognitive impairment in older adults, with evidence that it is an important risk factor for dementia (Chen et al., 2013; Orsitto et al., 2012).

Another environmental risk factor that can lead to negative functional consequences is the inhalation of air pollutants. Like the effects of cigarette smoking, the effects of air pollution are cumulative over many years and, therefore, have an increased impact on older adults who have been exposed to air pollutants for as many as eight or nine decades. Occupational exposure to toxic substances is another risk associated with long-term and cumulative consequences. For example, older adults who worked in occupations such

Box 21-1 Workforces With an Increased Risk for Harmful Respiratory Effects

Firefighters	Farmers, agricultural workers, grain handlers
Miners	
Traffic controllers	Construction workers
Shipyard workers	Paper mill workers
Rubber workers	Workers exposed to the following: dust, fumes, gases, nickel, arsenic, beryllium, chromium or radiation
Aluminum workers	
Iron and steel foundry workers	
Tunnel and street repair orkers	
Asbestos workers	
Quarry workers	

as mining and firefighting would not have been protected by recommendations from the Canadian Centre for Occupational Health and Safety. In addition, much of the information now available on the harmful effects of certain chemicals was not widely available when these older adults were working. Even though the exposure to harmful substances may have occurred long ago, the signs and symptoms may not manifest until later adulthood. Box 21-1 lists some job categories that are associated with an increased risk of respiratory disease.

Additional Risk Factors

Older adults are likely to have additional risks associated with conditions (e.g., obesity or chronic illness) that interfere with their usual ability to obtain adequate physical activity, which is necessary to maintain optimal respiratory function. In addition, even brief periods of bedrest during acute illnesses can increase the risk of pneumonia or exacerbate the effects of chronic lung conditions. Kyphosis is associated with poor posture and shallow breathing patterns, which can diminish respiratory function in older adults. Lack of vaccinations increases the risk for pneumonia and influenza, as discussed in the section on preventing lower respiratory infections.

Medications increase the risk for impaired respiratory function in several ways. For example, sedatives and anticholinergic medications can affect upper airway function by drying the mucus. Medications may also influence cough reflexes or cause a persistent dry cough (e.g., angiotensin-converting enzyme inhibitors).

Wellness Opportunity

Recognize the importance of encouraging and assisting patients who are in bed to change position, sit in a chair and walk as an essential intervention for promoting good respiratory function.

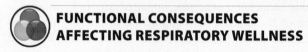

FUNCTIONAL CONSEQUENCES AFFECTING RESPIRATORY WELLNESS

Because of age-related changes, even healthy nonsmoking older adults experience diminished respiratory efficiency and reduced total pulmonary function, as measured with

TABLE 21-1 Functional Consequences of Age-Related Changes Affecting Respiratory Function

Change	Consequence
Degenerative changes affecting nose and upper airway structures	Snoring, mouth breathing, decreased efficiency of cough and gag reflexes, perception of nasal stuffiness
Increased anteroposterior diameter, chest wall stiffness, weakened muscles and diaphragm	Increased use of accessory muscles, increased energy expended for respiratory efficiency
Enlargement of alveoli, thinning of alveolar walls, diminished number of capillaries	Diminished efficiency of gas exchange, decreased arterial oxygen pressure (Pao_2)
Decreased elastic recoil and early airway closure	Changes in lung volumes, slight decrease in overall efficiency

spirometry (Ren et al., 2012). Although this functional consequence is hardly noticeable when older adults are performing their usual activities, under conditions of physiologic stress they are likely to experience dyspnea and fatigue because their respiratory system is less efficient in gas exchange. Degenerative changes of the upper airway structures cause additional minor functional consequences, as delineated in Table 21-1. In summary, healthy older adults expend more energy to achieve the same respiratory efficiency as younger adults, but the overall effects on healthy nonsmoking older people are minimal. Older adults who smoke or have other risk factors experience the same negative consequences as younger adults, but the effects are cumulative and the consequences are more serious.

Increased Susceptibility to Lower Respiratory Infections

Even for healthy nonsmoking older adults, the most important functional consequence related to respiratory wellness is due to a combination of age-related changes in the respiratory tract and the immune system. Because of this combination of age-related changes, older adults have higher rates of illness and death due to all types of lower respiratory infections, including pneumonia, influenza and West Nile viral infection (Goldstein, 2012). Pneumonia and influenza are the eighth leading cause of death among older adults 65 to 84 years of age, and the sixth leading cause of Canadians 85 years of age and older (Statistics Canada, 2012). Additional factors that commonly occur in older adults to increase their risk for lower respiratory infections, even for nonsmokers, include age-related diminished physiologic reserve and cumulative effects of exposure to toxins, including tobacco smoke, occupational dusts and indoor and outdoor air pollution (Fragoso & Gill, 2012). Additional factors that further compromise the ability of older adults to defend against respiratory infections include frailty, dysphagia, serious illness and diminished functional status.

The implications of oral health for systemic health and risk of infection are often overlooked. Poor oral care in hospitalized patients and long-term care residents in another condition that increases the risk for pneumonia (Tada & Miura, 2012). There are barriers to oral care for older patients in nursing homes, including the lack of specific designated personnel to perform oral care, resident noncompliance with care and choice of oral care itself. However, overcoming these barriers may prove to be a cost-effective use of resources. Aspiration pneumonia is a very costly illness for older residents. It seems likely that cost savings, as well as improved quality of life, would be the result of an intervention to prevent cases of pneumonia in nursing homes. Another complicating factor is the difficulty of diagnosing lower respiratory infections during early stages because the manifestations are subtle and nonspecific, as discussed in the section on nursing assessment of respiratory function.

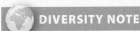

DIVERSITY NOTE

Among Canadians aged 35 to 79 years, 4% reported having been diagnosed by a health professional with COPD, chronic bronchitis or emphysema, women (5%) were significantly more likely to report a diagnosis than were men (3%) (Statistics Canada, n.d.).

Aspiration pneumonia, defined as an inflammation of the lungs caused by food or secretions entering into the bronchial tree, is a serious respiratory condition that is common in older adults with risk factors. One major risk factor for aspiration pneumonia is dysphagia, which affects 25% of independently living older adults and more than 50% of those in nursing homes (Clave et al., 2012; Serra-Prat et al., 2012). Other factors that increase the risk for aspiration pneumonia include achlorhydria, general debility, tube feeding, malnutrition and dehydration, decreased cough reflex, diminished salivary flow, compromised immune function and diminished level of consciousness.

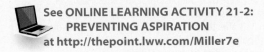

See ONLINE LEARNING ACTIVITY 21-2: PREVENTING ASPIRATION at http://thepoint.lww.com/Miller7e

Increased Susceptibility to Tuberculosis

About 1,600 new cases of tuberculosis (TB) are reported in Canada every year (Health Canada, 2013). Older adults are at increased risk for TB because of weaker immune systems. Risk factors for TB in older adults include smoking, diabetes, malnutrition and debilitating conditions. Historically, the TB rate among Aboriginal people was almost six times greater than the overall Canadian rate in 2008 and in Nunavut, it was more than 38 times the national rate (184.4 cases per 100,000 population), which suggests that older Aboriginal adults are perhaps at increased risk (CPHA, n.d.).

In recent years, the incidence of TB has been decreasing steadily across all age groups; however, rates remain high for

A Student's Perspective

I was glad to interact with someone who has emphysema and to learn about her struggles and about how care needs to be specialized for her because of her condition. Listening to E. A.'s breath sounds was frightening to me. I knew she was unable to breathe well, but I had no idea it was that obstructed. The struggle and stress her condition puts on her body to breathe is saddening. I really am amazed she is able to function as well as she does with her decreased level of oxygen.

I really enjoyed how talkative E. A. was. I had no problem getting information from her to complete her functional health assessment. It really hit me after I walked out of the nursing home on Friday that she literally talked to me for 3 hours. She was absolutely beside herself just to have someone there to listen and to interact with. I was glad I was able to give that to her. I believe this experience with E. A. will help me in the future to remember to give the emotional care as well as the physical.

In the next week, the things I would like to improve include supporting and promoting E. A. to get up and get dressed. I would like to help her with performing ADLs and help make her morning more worthwhile. I think helping E. A. become a little more productive could also help improve her social interactions. This is an area she needs a lot of help with, and I hope this week I will be able to give her support.

Jenna W.

Aboriginal, foreign-born and racial/ethnic minorities (Public Health Agency of Canada [PHAC], 2007). A higher incidence of TB in long-term care residents is associated with many risk factors, including the ease with which this disease can spread. Moreover, altered and more subtle disease manifestations interfere with identification and treatment of TB in older adults.

 DIVERSITY NOTE

The rate of TB in Canada is among the lowest in the world, with a steady decrease over the past three decades. However, certain cultural groups, including Aboriginal populations, are disproportionately affected by TB. Their rate is much higher than those of non-Aboriginal Canadian-born groups. One reason may be linked to the social determinants of health as both malnutrition and poor sanitation contribute to the spread of TB.

PATHOLOGIC CONDITION AFFECTING RESPIRATORY FUNCTION: CHRONIC OBSTRUCTIVE LUNG DISEASE

Chronic obstructive lung disease (COPD) is a term that refers to two lung diseases, emphysema and chronic bronchitis, which are characterized by chronic airflow obstruction that interferes with normal breathing. In Canada, COPD is the fourth leading cause of death for older adults, with 80% to 90% of the deaths caused by smoking (Canadian Lung Association). Conditions that increase the risk for developing COPD include smoking (the most significant factor), exposure to

Box 21-2 Evidence-Informed Nursing Practice

Background: Living with chronic obstructive pulmonary disease (COPD) has physical, psychological and social consequences for older adults. Activities of daily living become difficult because of shortness of breath, coughing and debilitating fatigue.

Question: Do people with COPD assimilate or downplay their health limitations with age?

Method: A cross-sectional survey study of 87 Albertans aged from 44 to 82. The St. George's Respiratory Questionnaire measured their health limitations

and the Attitudes to Aging Questionnaire assessed their views of aging.

Findings: Participants downplayed their symptoms and psychosocial impact and remained positive about psychosocial losses. Acknowledging activity limitations had negative outcomes for their views of the physical changes of aging.

Implications for Nursing Practice: Nurses need to consider how older adults with COPD perceive aging and how they adapt; this will influence their possible health care services.

secondary smoke and other air pollutants, increased age, genetic predisposition, low socioeconomic status and history of significant childhood respiratory disease.

The most common manifestations of COPD are cough, dyspnea, wheezing and chronic sputum production. The condition is progressive and its cumulative effects become more disabling as the person ages. Consequences of COPD for older adults include longer and more frequent hospitalizations, an increased risk for being discharged to nursing facilities and impaired health-related quality of life. Studies indicate that 80% of older adults with COPD have concurrent disease and are likely to attribute dyspnea to other conditions, including aging (Akgun et al., 2012). National data indicate that people with COPD are more likely to have several coexisting conditions, including (in order of prevalence) arthritis, depression, osteoporosis, cancer, coronary heart disease, congestive heart failure and stroke (Schnell et al., 2012) (Box 21-2).

An important health promotion implication when caring for older adults with COPD is to encourage participation in programs that support self-management, such as the ones listed in the resources related to this chapter (refer to Online Learning Activity 21-5). In addition, it is important to encourage participation in physical activity, which is an essential self-management intervention for improving symptoms in people with COPD (Thorpe & Kumar, 2012). Box 21-3 summarizes recommendations for nursing assessment and care for people with dyspnea, which is called the sixth vital sign in people with COPD (Registered Nurses Association of Ontario, 2010).

 See **ONLINE LEARNING ACTIVITY 21-3: ARTICLE ON EVIDENCE-BASED PRACTICE RELATED TO PHYSICAL ACTIVITY FOR PEOPLE WITH COPD** at http://thepoint.lww.com/Miller7e

Box 21-3 Evidence-Based Practice: Nursing Care of Patients With Dyspnea

Statement of the Problem

Dyspnea is the sixth vital sign in people with chronic obstructive pulmonary disease (COPD).

Recommendations for Nursing Assessment

- Assess all the following: vital signs, pulse oximetry, lung sounds, chest wall shape and movement, accessory muscle use, productive or nonproductive cough, peripheral edema, ability to complete a full sentence, level of consciousness.
- Assess current level of dyspnea and usual breathing pattern and level of dyspnea, using visual analogue or numeric quantitative scale.
- Assess for hypoxemia/hypoxia.
- Assess swallowing difficulties.
- Identify signs and symptoms of stable and unstable dyspnea and acute respiratory failure.
- Screen for COPD in adults older than 40 years who have a history of smoking by asking each patient these three questions: (1) Do you have progressive activity-related shortness of breath? (2) Do you have a persistent cough and sputum production? (3) Do you experience frequent respiratory tract infections?
- Advocate for spirometry testing for patients who have a history of smoking and are older than 40 years.
- If inhaler is used, assess self-administration technique.

Recommendations for Nursing Interventions

- Acknowledge and accept patient's self-report of dyspnea.
- Administer prescribed oxygen therapy, ventilation modalities and medications (e.g., bronchodilators, corticosteroids, antibiotics, psychotropics).
- Implement smoking-cessation strategies; consider nicotine replacement and other smoking-cessation modalities during hospitalization.
- Remain with patient during episodes of acute respiratory distress.

Recommendations for Teaching Older Adults and Caregivers About Dyspnea

- Prescribed medications, including correct technique for inhaler use.
- Administration of oxygen therapy if prescribed.
- Strategies for secretion clearance, energy conservation, relaxation techniques, nutrition and breathing retraining.
- Influenza and pneumococcal vaccinations.
- Pulmonary rehabilitation and exercise training as appropriate.
- Smoking-cessation strategies if appropriate.
- Disease self-management strategies: action plan, awareness of baseline symptoms and activity level, recognition of factors that worsen symptoms, early recognition of infection or acute exacerbation.

Source: Registered Nurses Association of Ontario. (2010). *Nursing care of dyspnea: The 6th vital sign in individuals with chronic obstructive pulmonary disease.* Toronto, ON: RNAO. Retrieved from www.rnao.ca

---

 DIVERSITY NOTE

Women report worse symptoms than do men for similar severity of COPD due to smaller lung capacity, and smaller airways and muscles required for breathing. At the same time, women have 20% to 60% lower mortality rates from COPD and are less likely to die during hospital admissions (Canadian Women's Health Network, n.d.).

 NURSING ASSESSMENT OF RESPIRATORY FUNCTION

Although physical examination of overall respiratory function does not differ significantly in older adults, it is imperative to be aware of variations in the manifestations of lower respiratory infections in older adults. Another difference is that older adults may have different life experiences with regard to exposure to environmental toxins and attitudes about tobacco use. From a wellness perspective, nursing assessment of respiratory function focuses on identifying opportunities for health promotion, detecting lower respiratory infections, assessing smoking behaviours and identifying other risk factors.

Identifying Opportunities for Health Promotion

Nurses interview older adults, or their caregivers, to identify the risk factors that are amenable to health promotion interventions. Because smoking is the risk factor that has the most serious detrimental effects on health, assess the potential for influencing all smokers, even older adults, to quit. Health education is based on assessment information about health-related behaviours, such as quitting smoking and avoiding secondhand smoke, as well as preventive interventions, such as influenza and pneumonia vaccinations. Nurses also assess the attitudes of older adults about these preventive measures, so they can plan appropriate educational approaches. Last, include questions about overall respiratory function to identify problems that can be addressed in the nursing care plan. Box 21-4 presents an interview format that nurses can use to assess risk factors, overall respiratory function and opportunities for health education.

Wellness Opportunity

Initiate a discussion about health-promoting behaviours by asking a question such as "What do you do to avoid secondhand smoke?"

Detecting Lower Respiratory Infections

The term *detection* is more accurate than *assessment* with regard to lower respiratory infections because these conditions commonly present atypically in older adults and treatment may be delayed, increasing the risk for serious complications, including death. Rather than presenting with a fever, cough and purulent sputum, older adults are more likely to have subtler and nonspecific disease manifestations. Even initial chest radiography may not provide accurate diagnostic information. A review of studies by Akgun and colleagues

Box 21-4 Guidelines for Assessing Respiratory Function

Questions to Identify Risk Factors for Respiratory Problems

- Have you had any respiratory problems, such as asthma, chronic lung disease, pneumonia or other infections?
- Do you have a family history of chronic lung disease?
- Have you ever had tuberculosis?
- Have you ever worked in a job where you were exposed to dust, fumes, smoke or other air pollutants (e.g., in mining, farming or any of the occupations listed in Box 21-1)?
- Have you lived in neighbourhoods where there was a lot of pollution from traffic or factories?
- Do you smoke now, or have you ever smoked? (If yes, continue with the questions in Box 21-5.)
- Are you now, or have you been, exposed to passive smoke in home, work or social environments?

Questions to Identify Opportunities for Education About Disease Prevention and Health Promotion

- Have you ever had a pneumonia vaccination? *If yes,* when was the vaccination administered and has the need for a booster been evaluated if the initial immunization was before the person was 65 years old?
- Do you get annual influenza vaccinations?

Questions to Assess Overall Respiratory Function

- Do you have any problems with breathing?
- Do you have any wheezing?
- Do you have spells of coughing? *If yes,* when do they occur? How long do they last? What brings them on? Are they dry or productive? Does the phlegm come from your throat or lungs? What does the phlegm look like?
- Do you ever have trouble getting enough air during any particular activities or when you lie down at night?
- Have you stopped doing any particular activities because of problems breathing? For example, have you stopped going up or down stairs, or have you limited the amount of walking you do? (For people with mobility limitations, this question might not be relevant.)
- Do you ever have any chest pain or feelings of heaviness or tightness in your chest?
- Do you use more than one pillow at night, or make any other adjustments, because of trouble with breathing?
- Do you wake up at night because of coughing or difficulty with breathing?
- Do you ever feel as though you can't catch your breath?
- Do you have trouble breathing when the weather is hot, cold or humid?
- Do you tire easily?

(2012) summarized the following manifestations of several types of pneumonia in older adults:

- Bacterial pneumonia: tachypnea, delirium, failure to thrive, malaise, and falls
- Viral pneumonia: bronchospasm and recent-onset dyspnea
- Aspiration pneumonia: gradual course and low-grade fevers

An important assessment consideration is to recognize that older adults do not necessarily exhibit the expected manifestations of pneumonia. The most significant finding on physical assessment of the lungs may be a diminished intensity of lung sounds or the presence of abnormal sounds, which are very nonspecific findings. In addition, a change in mental status or another alteration in functional status, such as falls or incontinence, may be a major clue to pneumonia. Thus, an important nursing responsibility is to detect nonspecific manifestations of pneumonia and collect additional information. This is essential for ensuring a timely diagnosis and preventing complications.

As with other lower respiratory infections, nonspecific assessment findings can delay and complicate the diagnosis of TB in older adults. The atypical presentation of TB in older adults can lead to delayed diagnosis and treatment and a higher rate of serious consequences, including death. The common occurrence of false-negative tuberculin skin test reactions in older adults is another reason that TB may be undetected; however, the two-step Mantoux test with tuberculin purified protein derivative (PPD) is the recommended method of assessing for previous exposure to TB. Because TB often occurs as a reactivation of dormant disease, nurses must be particularly alert for manifestations of this disease in older adults who have a history of TB.

Assessing Smoking Behaviours

Although smoking affects all people, regardless of age, some aspects of smoking behaviours differ according to age cohorts. The cohort of people born between 1910 and 1930, for example, is the first age group to be exposed to the social pressures that encouraged smoking without knowing about its detrimental effects. As a result, people who began smoking in the early 1920s, when it became a popular habit for men in Canada, may have smoked for four or five decades before finding out that smoking is harmful. For women in Canada, smoking was not socially acceptable until the mid-1940s. Although the percentage of older adults among current smokers is lower than for other age groups, older smokers may have an outlook reflected in statements such as, "If I've smoked this long and am still alive, why should I quit now?" Also assess the older adult's knowledge about health effects of smoking and benefits related to quitting and attempt to identify misconceptions.

In addition to assessing attitudes and knowledge about smoking, ask about types of nicotine product used and past and current smoking patterns. For example, older adults may be smoking cigarettes that have no filters and higher levels of tar and nicotine. Some older adults, in fact, may still roll their own cigarettes using loose tobacco. In addition, assess the older adult's perception of smoking as a manifestation of his or her rights and autonomy. For example, nursing home residents may view smoking as the one remaining indicator of their former life and the one pleasurable activity that they can control.

Personal attitudes and knowledge about smoking can influence nursing care, especially in relation to older adults. For example, ageism can lead to the view that smoking cessation would not be beneficial for older adults. Similarly,

Box 21-5 Guidelines for Nursing Assessment of Older Adults Who Smoke

Questions to Assess Smoking Behaviours

- How long have you smoked?
- How much do you smoke?
- What do you smoke?
- Have you smoked other types of tobacco in the past?

Questions to Assess Knowledge of the Risk From Smoking

- Do you think there are any harmful effects of smoking for people in general?
- Do you think you are at risk for any harmful effects from smoking?
- Do you think there are any benefits to quitting smoking?

Questions to Assess Attitudes Toward Smoking

- Have you ever thought about quitting smoking?
- Has any health professional ever talked to you about quitting smoking?
- What do you think about the idea of quitting smoking?
- Have you ever tried to quit? *If yes*, what was your experience with the attempt?
- Would you be interested in finding out about quitting smoking now?

although rights of older adults who choose to smoke need to be respected, they should not be excluded from health promotion interventions about smoking based on age alone. Use information in Box 21-5 as a guide to assessing smoking habits, knowledge and attitudes that are pertinent to developing health promotion interventions.

Wellness Opportunity

To assess smoking behaviours from a whole-person perspective, ask questions about the older adult's knowledge of the detrimental effects of smoking, as well as his or her perception of smoking as an expression of autonomy.

 See **ONLINE LEARNING ACTIVITY 21-4: THROUGH THE STOREYS OF SMOKERS WHO QUIT** at http://thepoint.lww.com/Miller7e

Identifying Other Risk Factors

In addition to assessing tobacco use as a risk factor, identify factors that affect respiratory function, including present and past exposure to secondhand smoke and other respiratory toxins. Occupational exposure to certain harmful substances is particularly important for smokers because the risk of either one of these factors is compounded when the other factor is present. Another consideration is to assess the person's level of activity and identify limitations in mobility or physical activity that can influence the potential improvement in level of activity. If, for example, people have limited mobility because of arthritis, they may not be able to engage in vigorous physical exercise, but they might benefit greatly from water exercises.

Wellness Opportunity

To set the stage for health education about preventive measures, assess the older adult's understanding of influenza and pneumonia vaccinations.

Identifying Normal Age-Related Variations

The usual assessment methods of inspection, palpation, percussion and auscultation are used for all adults, but the following minor variations are common in healthy older adults:

- Slight increase in the normal respiratory rate, which ranges from 16 to 24 respirations per minute
- Increased anteroposterior diameter
- Forward-leaning posture because of kyphosis
- Increased resonance on percussion
- Diminished intensity of lung sounds
- Increased presence of adventitious sounds in the lower lungs

Begin the assessment of respiratory function by observing the person's breathing pattern in different positions, such as walking or sitting. To facilitate auscultation, ask the older adult to sit upright, cough before auscultation and breathe with his or her mouth open. When observing respirations in a sleeping older adult, assess for brief periods of apnea, which are associated with sleep problems, as discussed in Chapter 24.

Unfolding Case Study

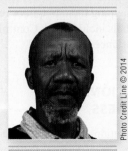
Photo Credit Line © 2014

Part 1: Mr. R. at 70 Years of Age

Mr. R. is 70 years old and comes with his wife to the senior centre where you provide weekly nursing services. Both Mr. and Mrs. R. smoke one to two packs of cigarettes a day. Mr. R. has mild COPD and Mrs. R. has hypertension and coronary artery disease. Every October, the senior centre offers influenza shots for anyone older than 65 years. As you are preparing to give influenza shots, Mr. and Mrs. R. come to you and ask, "Is this the shot that takes care of pneumonia? Our daughter said we should get a pneumonia shot every year, but we don't want a flu shot because our friend says she got the flu from one of those shots and she'll never get a shot again. Can you just give us the pneumonia shot today? We got one from the doctor last year but it's too expensive to get it from him."

THINKING POINTS

- What myths and misunderstandings do Mr. and Mrs. R. express?

- What further assessment questions would you ask?
- What health promotion teaching would you do?

QSEN APPLICATION

QSEN Competency	Knowledge/Skill/Attitude	Learning Activity Related to Mr. and Mrs. R.
Patient-centred care	(K) Integrate understanding of multiple dimensions of patient-centred care.	Identify misinformation about flu and pneumonia shots communicated by Mr. and Mrs. R.
	(K) Describe strategies to empower patients in all aspects of the health care process.	Use a nonjudgmental approach to provide correct information about flu and pneumonia shots.
	(S) Provide patient-centred care with sensitivity and respect for diversity of human experience.	
	(A) Value seeing health care situations "through patients' eyes."	
Evidence-based practice	(S) Base individualized care plan on patient values, clinical expertise and evidence.	Use simple patient-teaching handouts from a reliable source to provide accurate information about pneumonia and flu shots (e.g., www.cdc.gov).

NURSING DIAGNOSIS

The nursing diagnosis of Ineffective Breathing Pattern would be applicable when the nursing assessment identifies factors that may impair the older adult's respiratory function. If impaired respiratory function interferes with activities of daily living, a nursing diagnosis of Activity Intolerance might be appropriate. A nursing diagnosis of Risk for Infection may be appropriate for debilitated or chronically ill older adults, particularly those who live in group settings where other residents have respiratory infections. For older adults who smoke, use the nursing diagnosis of Risk-Prone Health Behaviour, which is defined as "impaired ability to modify lifestyle/behaviours in a manner that improves health status" (Herdman, 2012, p. 155).

Wellness Opportunity

Use the wellness nursing diagnosis of Readiness for Enhanced Immunization Status when administering immunizations for influenza or pneumonia.

PLANNING FOR WELLNESS OUTCOMES

Wellness-oriented care plans for all older adults address their increased vulnerability to pneumonia, influenza and TB by using NOC labels such as Immune Status, Immunization

Behaviour and Risk Control: Communicable Disease. The Nursing Outcomes Classification (NOC) label of Knowledge: Health Behaviours is applicable for older adults who would benefit from health education about quitting smoke, obtaining immunizations or preventing respiratory infections. A specific and measurable outcome of successful health education might be that older adults obtain immunizations against pneumonia and influenza.

Wellness Opportunity

Nurses promote wellness when their care plans address the immunization status of older adults.

Respiratory Status is the NOC label that is applicable in care plans related to the nursing diagnosis of Ineffective Breathing Pattern. When caring for older adults who smoke, always consider the possibility of helping them to quit or reduce smoking. Applicable NOC labels include Risk Control: Tobacco Use and Knowledge: Substance Use Control.

NURSING INTERVENTIONS FOR RESPIRATORY WELLNESS

For all older adults, nursing interventions to promote respiratory wellness focus on preventing respiratory infections, protecting from secondhand smoke and quitting smoking (if applicable). The following Nursing Interventions Classification (NIC) labels are pertinent to these goals: Environmental Risk Protection, Health Education, Immunization/Vaccination Management, Infection Control, Infection Protection, Referral and Smoking Cessation Assistance.

Promoting Respiratory Wellness

Smoking is the single most important preventable cause of disease and death in Canada and therefore should be a major target of disease prevention activities for all people who smoke tobacco. Because older smokers are likely to have smoking-related functional consequences, smoking cessation will address secondary or tertiary prevention rather than primary prevention. Smoking cessation is widely recognized as a cost-effective health promotion activity that health care professionals should routinely address (Wilkinson et al., 2012).

For all older adults, disease prevention and health promotion interventions related to respiratory function include pneumonia and influenza vaccinations and education about the importance of avoiding environmental tobacco smoke. These interventions are discussed in the following sections and summarized in Boxes 21-5 and 21-6. In addition, numerous educational materials are available for use in disease prevention and health promotion interventions, and many of these are available in languages other than English.

Wellness Opportunity

Nurses promote self-care behaviours by encouraging older adults to use patient-teaching materials, which are available from such agencies as Health Canada and the Lung Association of Canada.

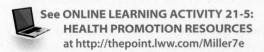

See ONLINE LEARNING ACTIVITY 21-5:
HEALTH PROMOTION RESOURCES
at http://thepoint.lww.com/Miller7e

Preventing Lower Respiratory Infections

Interventions to prevent pneumonia and influenza are particularly important because the majority of deaths due to these diseases are among people aged 65 and older (PHAC, 2012). Moreover, pneumonia and influenza are the only diseases of all the leading causes of death in older adults that can be prevented through immunizations and without major investment of time, money and motivation. Nurses also have important roles in addressing TB, particularly for medically compromised older adults in long-term and residential care facilities. The following sections discuss the role of the nurse in preventing these types of lower respiratory infections, with emphasis on health education interventions.

Box 21-6 Health Promotion Teaching About Respiratory Problems

Factors That Increase the Risk for Pneumonia and Influenza

- Diabetes or any chronic lung, heart or kidney disease
- Hospitalization within the past year for heart or lung diseases
- Severe anemia or a debilitating condition
- Confinement to bed or very limited mobility
- Residence in a long-term care facility or other group living setting
- Immunosuppressive medications

Preventing Respiratory Infection

- Wash your hands frequently with an antibacterial soap or hand sanitizer.
- Avoid hand-to-mouth and hand-to-eye contact.
- Avoid inhaling air that has been contaminated with particles from the cough or sneeze of someone with an infection.
- Avoid crowds during the influenza season.
- Be sure that influenza and pneumonia vaccinations are up to date.

Information About Influenza Vaccinations

- New vaccinations are developed every year on the basis of information about the strains of viruses that are most likely to affect people during the influenza season.
- Vaccines are made from inactivated viruses and, therefore, should have few or no side effects.
- People who are allergic to eggs and egg products should NOT receive influenza immunizations.
- Immunizations do not offer immediate protection because there is a 2- to 3-week delay in developing an antibody response.
- Every year, the manufacturers of the influenza vaccine provide recommendations as to the best time for administering the vaccine for optimal effectiveness. The best time is during the late fall, but the exact time period will vary slightly from year to year.
- Vaccines are not 100% effective, but they are helpful for most older people.
- Influenza immunizations provide protection against the most serious viruses but not against all types of respiratory infections.
- The duration of effectiveness of vaccinations may be shorter than 6 months in some older people; therefore, one vaccination might not protect the person through the entire season.
- Influenza shots are free for seniors.

Information About Pneumonia Vaccinations

- Pneumonia vaccinations are recommended for people older than 65 years of age.
- Pneumonia vaccinations were considered one-time-only immunizations, but boosters are now being recommended for older adults who received their initial immunization 5 or more years ago.
- Side effects, if they occur, are not serious and will subside within a few days.
- Common side effects include a slight fever accompanied by pain, redness or tenderness at the injection site.
- Pneumonia vaccinations are free in Canada for adults 65 years of age and older.

Nutritional Considerations

- Include foods high in zinc and vitamins A, B-complex, C and E.

The influenza and pneumococcal vaccines are safe and well tolerated in older adults, and studies indicate that these measures reduce morbidity and mortality and decrease hospitalization admission rates for respiratory infections. The PHAC (2013) recommends a single dose of pneumococcal 23-valent polysaccharide vaccine (Pneu-P-23) for all people aged 65 or older. Pneumonia vaccinations are also recommended for older adults who are uncertain about their vaccination status.

Immunization rate for influenza and pneumococcal vaccinations has been increasing gradually during the past decade. Many institutional settings have standing orders for influenza and pneumonia vaccinations, and nurses play a primary role in implementing this health promotion intervention in community, residential and institutional settings. In addition, all health care workers should receive annual influenza vaccinations to prevent transmission, thereby indirectly reducing mortality from influenza in the older population. Box 21-6 summarizes current information about influenza and pneumonia immunizations, along with information about risk factors for these illnesses.

See ONLINE LEARNING ACTIVITY 21-6:
IMMUNIZATION OF SPECIFIC POPULATIONS
at http://thepoint.lww.com/Miller7e

Interventions to prevent pneumonia and other lower respiratory tract infections are an important aspect of health promotion for older adults. For example, assuring the provision of good oral hygiene, including measures to prevent plaque accumulation, is an evidence-based nursing intervention for preventing pneumonia, especially aspiration pneumonia (Johnson, 2012). Additional nursing interventions for preventing lower respiratory infections include meticulous attention to handwashing and optimal positioning and turning of patients who have limited mobility.

Eliminating the Risk From Smoking

Educational interventions for older smokers begin by addressing attitudes that influence health-related behaviours. For example, if an older person expresses an "I'm-too-old-to-change" attitude, an initial step is to explore the older adult's understanding of his or her ability to change behavioural patterns. Even though older adults may be long-term smokers, their success rate for quitting is higher than that of younger adults. Information about models of behaviour change (discussed in Chapter 5) is applicable to helping smokers quit.

Another commonly expressed belief that nurses can address through health education is "It's too late to do any good." When nurses encounter this type of attitude, they can emphasize that the substantial health benefits derived

from quitting smoking are both immediate and long term. Benefits from smoking cessation for people of any age include improved quality of life, decreased susceptibility to smoking-related illnesses (e.g., heart disease and cancer) and a more rapid recovery from illnesses that usually are exacerbated by smoking. Health benefits of quitting smoking occur at any age, and people who quit at the age of 65 or older increase their life expectancy by 2 to 3 years (van Meijgaard & Fielding, 2012).

Wellness Opportunity

Nurses support wellness in older adults by communicating that old age is not an inevitable barrier to changing health-related behaviours: It's never too late to quit.

Evidence-based guidelines emphasize the importance of nurses and other health care providers initiating the topic of tobacco dependence and routinely identifying and intervening with all tobacco users—including light smokers and smokeless tobacco users—at every opportunity (Sarna et al., 2012; Wilkinson et al., 2012). Additional points of evidence-based guidelines are as follows:

- Tobacco dependence is a chronic disease that may require repeated interventions; however, effective treatments can significantly increase rates of long-term abstinence.
- Individual, group and telephone counselling methods are effective; problem solving and social support as part of treatment are especially effective counselling interventions.
- Nicotine-based medications that reliably increase long-term smoking abstinence are nicotine gum, inhaler, lozenge, patch and nasal spray.
- Non-nicotine medications that are effective for smoking cessation include sustained-release bupropion (Wellbutrin™) and varenicline (Chantix™); Health Canada has issued warnings about serious cardiovascular and neuropsychiatric symptoms that can occur with varenicline and continues to monitor this product.
- Counselling and medication are effective for treating tobacco dependence, but the combination of these methods is more effective than either alone.

Nonpharmacologic interventions that are effective for smoking cessation include exercise, guided imagery, breathing techniques, positive self-talk, journalling, integration of rewards and identification of habit breakers for events that trigger smoking (Jackson, 2012). Box 21-7 can be used as a guide to teaching older adults about quitting smoking.

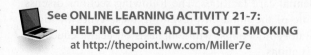

See ONLINE LEARNING ACTIVITY 21-7:
HELPING OLDER ADULTS QUIT SMOKING
at http://thepoint.lww.com/Miller7e

Unfolding Case Study

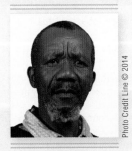

Photo Credit Line © 2014

Part 2: Mr. R. at 77 Years of Age

Mr. R. is now 77 years old and attends the senior centre with his wife three times a week for meal and social programs. During your weekly senior wellness clinic, he comes to have his blood pressure checked and says that he is thinking about quitting smoking, but that his son just quit and gained a lot of weight and had a lot of trouble sleeping. He's not sure if quitting smoking is worth the effort, especially because his son has been so miserable since he quit. Also, at his age, it probably won't do any good to quit now, he says.

THINKING POINTS

- What further questions would you ask to assess Mr. R.'s readiness to discuss quitting smoking?
- What health promotion teaching would you do?

- What would your response be if you determine that Mr. R. is not ready to consider quitting smoking?

QSEN APPLICATION

QSEN Competency	Knowledge/Skill/Attitude	Learning Activity Related to Mr. R.
Patient-Centred Care	(K) Integrate understanding of multiple dimensions of patient-centred care.	Elicit additional information about Mr. R.'s fears of quitting smoking and being too old to benefit.
	(K) Examine common barriers to active involvement in patients in their own health care processes.	Ask about previous personal experiences with quitting smoking.
	(A) Value seeing health care situations "through patients' eyes."	Using pertinent information from Box 21-7, teach Mr. R. about quitting smoking.
Teamwork and Collaboration	(K) Recognize contributions of other individuals and groups in helping patient achieve health goals.	Encourage Mr. R to use resources for quitting smoking (e.g., from Canadian Cancer Society site smokers helpline http://www.smokershelpline.ca/)
Evidence-Based Practice	(S) Locate evidence reports related to clinical practice topics and guidelines.	Read guidelines and teaching tools for health care professionals to help patients quit smoking from the Government of Canada at http://healthycanadians.gc.ca/health-sante/tobacco-tabac/index-eng.php

EVALUATING EFFECTIVENESS OF NURSING INTERVENTIONS

Measuring the effectiveness of interventions for the nursing diagnosis of Ineffective Breathing Pattern is based on a reassessment of subjective indicators such as ease of breathing and objective indicators such as lung sounds and respiratory rate and rhythm. An indicator of successful health education interventions for older adults with Ineffective Breathing Pattern is that they can accurately identify factors that can be addressed to improve their respiratory function. Interventions for the nursing diagnosis of Risk for Infection can be documented on a record of the person's history of immunizations for pneumonia and influenza. For older adults who smoke, effectiveness of interventions are measured by the person's increased knowledge about the detrimental effects of smoking and by his or her willingness to develop a plan to stop smoking. Long-term effectiveness would be evaluated by the person's successful participation in the smoking cessation program.

Box 21-7 Health Promotion Teaching About Cigarette Smoking

Attitudes About Smoking

- Stopping smoking at any age is more beneficial than continuing to smoke.
- Many of the harmful effects of smoking are reversed once the smoker quits.
- Although some of the effects of past smoking are irreversible, all of the harmful effects of future smoking can be avoided by quitting now.
- Smoking is a major risk factor for many cancers, including those of the lung, head, stomach, kidney and pancreas.
- Smoking is a major risk factor for lung and heart disease, including high blood pressure and heart attacks.
- Passive smoking (inhaling smoke from the air) is associated with an increased risk for many diseases.

Type of Tobacco

- The lower the tar and nicotine content of cigarettes, the less harmful the effects. Many cigarettes with lower tar and nicotine levels, however, have additional chemical additives that can be harmful.
- Pipe and cigar smokers are at a higher risk for chronic lung disease than nonsmokers, just as cigarette smokers are.
- The harmful effects of tobacco use on the mouth and upper respiratory tract are equal for all types of tobacco, including smokeless tobacco. All smokers have the same risk for developing cancer of the mouth and upper respiratory tract. Snuff, chewing tobacco and smokeless tobacco contain nicotine and many other harmful chemicals. The only advantage of smokeless tobacco is that it does not affect other people nearby.

Approaches to Quitting

- Any reduction in present tobacco use is better than maintaining the current level. The negative effects of smoking are directly proportional to the number of cigarettes inhaled.
- Various forms of prescription and over-the-counter nicotine substitutes (e.g., gum, skin patches, nasal sprays) are available and may be helpful, especially when used in conjunction with counselling and self-help techniques.
- Besides nicotine substitutes, some non-nicotine prescription medications and over-the-counter products may be effective as a component of a smoking-cessation program.
- People who are trying to quit smoking should discuss their goals with a health care professional to identify the methods that may be most effective.
- Many self-help programs are available for support and education regarding quitting smoking.
- Information about group programs can be obtained on the Internet or by calling the local office of any of the following organizations: Canadian Cancer Society or the Canadian Lung Association.

Nonpharmacologic Practices to Help Quit Smoking

- Exercise, music, imagery, massage, meditation, affirmations, deep breathing, stress reduction, social support, or individual or group counselling.

Unfolding Case Study

Part 3: Mr. R at 83 Years of Age

Mr. R. is now 83 years old and recently moved into an assisted living complex where you are employed as the nurse. When he comes in for his flu shot, he asks you how he can get some nicotine gum because he has heard that this is a good way to cut down on cigarettes. Now that he lives in the assisted living complex, he can't smoke in the dining room, and he'd like to chew nicotine gum before and after he eats. He admits that he smokes a pack of cigarettes every day but denies having experienced any bad effects from smoking. Mr. R. sees his doctor for COPD and takes Flovent, two puffs twice a day, and Serevent, two puffs twice a day.

Photo Credit Line © 2014

NURSING ASSESSMENT

You begin your nursing assessment by exploring Mr. R.'s attitudes about smoking and ascertaining his knowledge about the harmful effects of cigarette smoking. Mr. R. says he thought about quitting smoking many times but never actually tried to quit because his wife smoked even more than he did until she died a few months ago. He felt it would be too hard to quit as long as she was smoking two packs per day. He also states that he's heard a lot about passive smoking and he figured it wasn't worth trying to quit as long as he was around his wife's cigarette smoke. He states that he's been smoking for 40 years, and if he hasn't gotten lung cancer by now, he's not going to get it at his age. To comply with the rules in the assisted living facility, Mr. R. says he plans to chew nicotine gum when he can't smoke cigarettes, but he sees no reason to quit.

In assessing Mr. R.'s knowledge about the effects of cigarette smoking, you determine that he is aware of some of the harmful effects of passive smoking but has very little information about the detrimental effects of cigarette smoking. He relates that his wife died of lung cancer, but he attributes her death to a history of breast cancer, which she had 10 years before the lung cancer. Mr. R. has no knowledge about cigarette smoking as a risk factor for cardiovascular disease, nor does he realize that his hypertension poses an additional risk. Mr. R. reports that he has experienced no ill effects from cigarette smoking, but when you ask about his history of respiratory infections, he admits he had pneumonia 3 years ago. He says that he received a pneumonia shot, so he doesn't have to worry about getting pneumonia again, and that he has had bronchitis several times, but now that he won't be out shovelling snow, he doesn't worry about getting any lung infections either.

NURSING DIAGNOSIS

Based on the assessment findings, an appropriate nursing diagnosis would be Ineffective Health Maintenance, related to insufficient knowledge about the effects of tobacco use and self-help resources. Some of Mr. R.'s statements reflect a lack of accurate information about the harmful effects of cigarette smoking, particularly regarding risks for respiratory infections and impaired cardiovascular function. Other statements probably reflect an intellectualization of his continued smoking. Your intuition tells you that, with some education and support, he may be willing to quit smoking.

NURSING CARE PLAN FOR MR. R.

Expected Outcome	Nursing Interventions	Nursing Evaluation
Mr. R. will increase his knowledge about the harmful effects of cigarette smoking.	• Give Mr. R. brochures and illustrations provided by the Government of Canada and use them to discuss the effects of cigarette smoking. • Use brochures from the Heart & Stroke Foundation of Canada to discuss the risk factors for cardiovascular disease. • Discuss cigarette smoking as a risk factor for respiratory infections. • Give Mr. R. a copy of Box 21-7 and discuss the immediate and long-term benefits of quitting smoking.	• Mr. R. will verbalize correct information about the risks of cigarette smoking. • Mr. R. will describe the benefits derived from quitting smoking.
Mr. R. will be knowledgeable about techniques for quitting smoking.	• Using information from the Canadian Lung Association, discuss some of the strategies for quitting smoking (e.g., quitting "cold turkey," using nicotine substitutes, participating in self-help groups).	• Mr. R. will describe the advantages and disadvantages of the various methods of quitting smoking.
Mr. R. will quit smoking.	• Identify the method Mr. R. prefers for quitting smoking. • Emphasize the importance of nutrition, exercise and adequate fluid intake. • Agree on realistic goals for smoking cessation. • Discuss supportive resources. Set up weekly appointments at the senior wellness clinic for support and further discussions.	• Mr. R. will report that he has stopped or significantly reduced his smoking.

THINKING POINTS

- How would you assess Mr. R.'s readiness and motivation to quit smoking?
- What health education approach would you take with Mr. R.?
- What additional interventions or health education points would you use for Mr. R.?

QSEN APPLICATION

QSEN Competency	Knowledge/Skill/Attitude	Learning Activity Related to Mr. R.
Patient-centred care	(K) Integrate understanding of multiple dimensions of patient-centred care. (S) Elicit patient values, preferences and expressed needs. (A) Value seeing health care situations "through patients' eyes."	Explore Mr. R.'s attitudes about smoking and assess his knowledge about harmful effects of smoking. Discuss realistic goals for quitting smoking as an important intervention for promoting health.

QSEN Competency	Knowledge/Skill/Attitude	Learning Activity Related to Mr. R.
Teamwork and collaboration	(K) Recognize contributions of other individuals and groups in helping patient achieve health goals.	Use information from Box 21-7 to discuss ways of quitting smoking.
	(S) Integrate the contributions of others who play a role in helping patient achieve health goals.	Facilitate the use of Internet resources and support groups pertinent to quitting smoking.
Evidence-based practice	(S) Base individualized care plan on patient values, clinical expertise and evidence.	Use educational materials from the Heart & Stroke Foundation of Canada, the Canadian Lung Association and the Government of Canada to teach about detrimental effects of smoking and beneficial effects of quitting.

Chapter Highlights

Age-Related Changes That Affect Respiratory Wellness (Tables 21-1)

- Upper airway changes (e.g., calcification of cartilage)
- Increased anteroposterior diameter
- Chest wall stiffness, weakened muscles
- Alveoli enlarged and have thinner walls
- Alterations in lung volumes and airflow
- Decreased compensatory response to hypercapnia and hypoxia

Risks Factors That Affect Respiratory Wellness (Box 21-1)

- Tobacco smoking
- Environmental factors (e.g., pollution, dry air, second-hand smoke)
- Occupational hazards

Functional Consequences Affecting Respiratory Wellness

- Mouth breathing, diminished cough reflex, less efficient gag reflex
- Increased use of accessory muscles, increased energy expended for breathing
- Diminished efficiency of gas exchange, decreased Pao levels
- Decreased vital capacity, slight decrease in overall efficiency
- Increased susceptibility to lower respiratory infections

Pathologic Condition Affecting Respiratory Wellness: COPD

- COPD: a group of diseases, including emphysema, chronic bronchitis and a subset of asthma, characterized by chronic airflow obstruction

Nursing Assessment of Respiratory Function (Boxes 21-3 and 21-4)

- Overall respiratory function
- Detection of lower respiratory infections
- Tobacco use and attitudes regarding smoking

Nursing Diagnosis

- Health-Seeking Behaviours
- Ineffective Breathing Pattern
- Risk for Infection

Planning for Wellness Outcomes

- Vital Signs, Respiratory Status: Airway Patency and Respiratory Status: Ventilation
- Immune Status, Immunization Behaviour and Community Risk Control
- Knowledge: Health Behaviours
- Risk Control: Tobacco Use and Knowledge: Substance Use Control

Nursing Interventions to Promote Respiratory Wellness (Boxes 21-5 and 21-6)

- Prevention and detection of pneumonia and influenza
- Health education about smoking cessation

Evaluating Effectiveness of Nursing Interventions

- Ease of breathing
- Up-to-date status for pneumonia immunization
- Influenza immunization every year
- For older adults who smoke: active participation in smoking-cessation behaviours

Critical Thinking Exercises

1. What will a healthy, nonsmoking, 83-year-old person experience in his or her daily life with regard to respiratory function?
2. What would you include in a health education program, designed for older adults, on the prevention of pneumonia and influenza?
3. How would you address the following statement made by a 71-year-old person: "I've lived this long and don't have lung cancer; why should I start worrying now?"

4. Find the names, addresses and phone numbers of local agencies that would be appropriate resources for
someone interested in quitting smoking. Contact at least
one of these organizations to find out specific information about support groups, written materials and other
resources.

 **For more information about the topics discussed
in this chapter, be sure to check out the
interactive Online Learning Activities and
other helpful resources**
at http://thepoint.lww.com/Miller7e

REFERENCES

Akgun, K. M., Crothers, K., & Pisani, M. (2012). Epidemiology and management of common pulmonary diseases in older persons. *Journal of
Gerontology: Biological Sciences, 67A*(3), 276–291.

Alzheimer Society Canada. (2014). *Risk factors*. Retrieved from http://
www.alzheimer.ca/en/About-dementia/Alzheimer-s-disease/Risk-factors

Canadian Cancer Society. (2014). *Lung cancer*. Retrieved from http://www
.cancer.ca/en/cancer-information/cancer-type/lung/statistics/?region=on

Canadian Lung Association. (2014). *Chronic obstructive pulmonary disease*. Retrieved from https://www.lung.ca/copd

Canadian Women's Health Network. (n.d.). *Chronic disease: What do sex
and gender have to do with it?* Retrieved from http://www.cwhn.ca/en/
resources/primers/chronicdisease

Chen, R., Wilson, K., Chen, Y., et al. (2013). Association between environmental tobacco smoke exposure and dementia syndromes. *Occupational and Environmental Medicine, 70*(1), 63–69.

Clave, P., Rofes, L., Carrion, S., et al. (2012). Pathophysiology, relevance
and natural history of oropharyngeal dysphagia among older people.
Nestle Nutrition Institute Workshop Series, 72, 57–66.

Fragoso, C. A. V., & Gill, T. M. (2012). Respiratory impairment and the aging lung. *Journal of Gerontology: Medical Sciences, 67A*(3), 264–275.

Gellert, C., Schöttker, B., Müller, H., et al. (2013). Impact of smoking and
quitting on cardiovascular outcomes and risk advancement periods
among older adults. *European Journal of Epidemiology, 28*(8), 649–658.

Goldstein, D. R. (2012). Role of aging on innate responses to viral infections. *Journal of Gerontology: Biological Sciences, 67A*(3), 242–246.

Hall, J. E. (2011). *Guyton and Hall textbook of medical physiology* (12th
ed.). Philadelphia, PA: Elsevier.

Health Canada. (2013). *Tuberculosis*. Retrieved from http://www.hc-sc.
gc.ca/hc-ps/dc-ma/tuberculos-eng.php

Herdman, T. H. (Ed.). (2012). *NANDA International Nursing Diagnoses: Definitions and classification 2012–1014*. Oxford, England:
Wiley-Blackwell.

Jackson, C. (2012). Smoking cessation. In B. Dossey & L. Keegan (Eds.),
Holistic nursing: A handbook for practice (6th ed., pp. 513–538). Boston, MA: Jones & Bartlett.

Johnson, V. B. (2012). Evidence-based practice guideline: Oral hygiene
care for functionally dependent and cognitively impaired older adults.
Journal of Gerontological Nursing, 38(11), 11–19.

Lee, N., Shin, M. S., & Kang, I. (2012). T-Cell biology in aging, with a
focus on lung disease. *Journal of Gerontology: Biological Sciences,
67A*(3), 254–263.

Low, G., Ross, C., Stickland, M., et al. (2013). Perspectives of aging among
persons living with chronic obstructive pulmonary disease. *Western Journal
of Nursing Research, 35*(7), 884–904. doi:10.1177/0193945913478844

Ní Chróinín, D., Glavin, P., & Power, D. (2013). Awareness of osteoporosis, risk and protective factors and own diagnostic status. *Archives of
Osteoporosis, 8*(1–2), 117.

Okusaga, O., Stewart, M. C., Butcher, I., et al. (2013). Smoking, hyper-
cholesterolaemia and hypertension as risk factors for cognitive impairment in older adults. *Age and Ageing, 42*(3), 306–311.

Orsitto, G., Turi, V., Venezia, A., et al. (2012). Relation of secondhand
smoking to mild cognitive impairment in older inpatients. *Scientific
World Journal, 2012*(2012), 5.

Public Health Agency of Canada. (2007). *Life and breath: Respiratory
disease in Canada.* Retrieved from http://www.phac-aspc.gc.ca/publi-
cat/2007/lbrdc-vsmrc/index-eng.php

Public Health Agency of Canada. (2012). *Statement on seasonal influenza
vaccine for 2012–2013.* Retrieved from http://www.phac-aspc.gc.ca/
publicat/ccdr-rmtc/12vol38/acs-dcc-2/index-eng.php

Public Health Agency of Canada. (2013). *Canadian immunization guide.*
Retrieved from http://www.phac-aspc.gc.ca/publicat/cig-gci/p03-02-
eng.php

Registered Nurses Association of Ontario. (2010). *Nursing care of dyspnea: The 6th vital sign in individuals with chronic obstructive pulmonary disease.* Toronto, ON: RNAO. Retrieved from www.rnao.ca

Ren, W. Y., Li, L., Zhao, R. Y., et al. (2012). Age-associated changes in
pulmonary function: A comparison of pulmonary function parameters
in healthy young adults and the elderly living in Shanghai. *Chinese
Medical Journal, 125*(17), 3064–3068.

Richter, G. M., Choudhury, F., Torres, M., et al. (2012). Risk factors for
incident cortical, nuclear, posterior subcapsular, and mixed lens opaci-
ties. *Ophthalmology, 119*(10), 2040–2047.

Rincon, F., & Wright, C. B. (2013). Vascular cognitive impairment. *Current Opinion in Neurology, 26*(1), 29–36.

Sarna, L., Bialous, S. A., Ong, M. K., et al. (2012). Increasing nursing
referral to telephone quitlines for smoking cessation using a web-based
program. *Nursing Research, 61*(6), 433–440.

Schnell, K., Weiss, C. O., Lee, T., et al. (2012). The prevalence of
clinically-relevant comorbid conditions in patients with physician-
diagnosed COPD. *BioMed Central Pulmonary Medicine, 12*, 26.

Serra-Prat, M., Palomera, M., Gomez, C., et al. (2012). Oropharyngeal
dysphagia as a risk factor for malnutrition and lower respiratory tract
infection in independently living older persons. *Age and Ageing, 41*(3),
376–381.

Statistics Canada. (2012). *Leading causes of death in Canada* (Catalogue
no. 84-215-XWE). Ottawa, ON: Government of Canada.

Statistics Canada. (n.d.). *Chronic obstructive pulmonary disease in Canadians, 2009 to 2011.* Retrieved from http://www.statcan.gc.ca/pub/82-
625-x/2012001/article/11709-eng.htm

Tada, A., & Miura, H. (2012). Prevention of aspiration pneumonia with
oral care. *Archives of Gerontology and Geriatrics, 55*(1), 16–21.

Thorpe, O., & Kumar, S. (2012). Barriers and enables to physical activity
participation in patients with COPD: A systematic review. *Journal of
Cardiopulmonary Rehabilitation and Prevention, 32*, 359–369.

van Meijgaard, J., & Fielding, J. E. (2012). Estimating benefits of past,
current, and future reductions in smoking rates using a comprehensive
model with competing causes of death. *Preventing Chronic Disease, 9*,
E122. doi:10.5888/pcd9.110295

Wilkinson, J., Bass, C., Diem, S., et al. (2012). *Preventive services for
adults.* Bloomington, MN: Institute for Clinical Systems Improvement.
Retrieved from www.guideline.gov

Willeford, K. T., & Rapp, J. (2012). Smoking and age-related macular degeneration. *Optometry and Vision Science, 89*(11), 1662–1666.

Yamasoba, T., Lin, F. R., Someya, S., et al. (2013). Current concepts in
age-related hearing loss: Epidemiology and mechanistic pathways.
Hearing Research, 303, 30–38.

chapter 22

Mobility and Safety

LEARNING OBJECTIVES

After reading this chapter, you will be able to:

1. Delineate age-related changes that affect mobility and safety.

2. Identify risk factors that increase the risk of osteoporosis and influence the safety and mobility of older adults.

3. Discuss the following functional consequences: diminished musculoskeletal function, increased susceptibility to fractures and increased susceptibility to falls.

4. Discuss the psychosocial and long-term consequences of falls, fractures and osteoporosis.

5. Conduct a nursing assessment of musculoskeletal performance and risks for falls and osteoporosis.

6. Identify interventions directed toward safe mobility and the elimination of risks for falls and osteoporosis.

KEY POINTS

body sway

bone density

fall risk assessment tools

fear of falling

fragility fracture

osteoarthritis

osteopenia

osteoporosis

personal emergency response systems

sarcopenia

Mobility is one of the most important aspects of physiologic function because it is essential for maintaining independence and because serious consequences occur when independence is lost. For older adults, mobility is influenced by age-related changes to some extent, but risk factors play a much larger role. Because of the many risks that affect mobility, falls and fractures are an unfortunately common occurrence in old age. Older adults, then, have the dual challenge of maintaining mobility skills and avoiding falls and fractures. For these reasons, safety is an integral aspect of mobility.

AGE-RELATED CHANGES THAT AFFECT MOBILITY AND SAFETY

The bones, joints and muscles are the body structures most closely associated with mobility, but many additional functional aspects are involved in *safe* mobility. Neurologic function, for example, influences all facets of musculoskeletal performance, and visual function influences the ability to interact safely with the environment. In the musculoskeletal system, osteoporosis is the age-related change that has the most significant overall impact, has been studied the most and is most amenable to interventions aimed at prevention and management.

Bones

Bones provide the framework for the entire musculoskeletal system; they work with the muscular system to facilitate movement. Additional functions of bone in the human body include storing calcium, producing blood cells and supporting and protecting body organs and tissues. Bone is composed of a hard outer layer, called cortical or compact bone,

Promoting Musculoskeletal Wellness in Older Adults

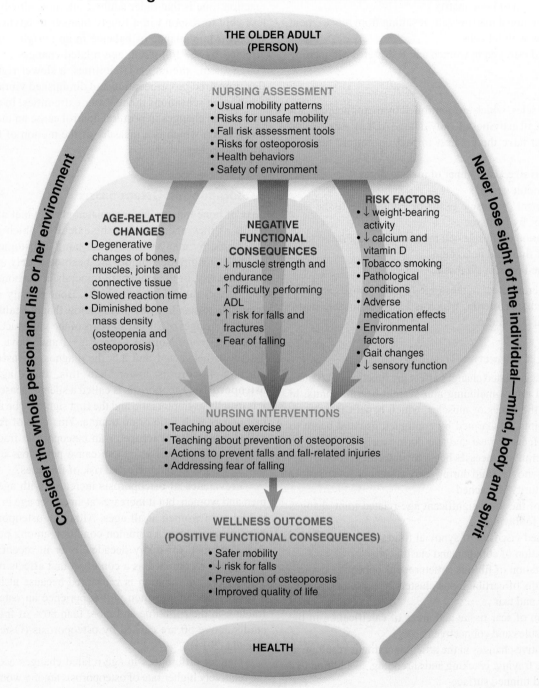

THE OLDER ADULT (PERSON)

NURSING ASSESSMENT
- Usual mobility patterns
- Risks for unsafe mobility
- Fall risk assessment tools
- Risks for osteoporosis
- Health behaviors
- Safety of environment

AGE-RELATED CHANGES
- Degenerative changes of bones, muscles, joints and connective tissue
- Slowed reaction time
- Diminished bone mass density (osteopenia and osteoporosis)

NEGATIVE FUNCTIONAL CONSEQUENCES
- ↓ muscle strength and endurance
- ↑ difficulty performing ADL
- ↑ risk for falls and fractures
- Fear of falling

RISK FACTORS
- ↓ weight-bearing activity
- ↓ calcium and vitamin D
- Tobacco smoking
- Pathological conditions
- Adverse medication effects
- Environmental factors
- Gait changes
- ↓ sensory function

NURSING INTERVENTIONS
- Teaching about exercise
- Teaching about prevention of osteoporosis
- Actions to prevent falls and fall-related injuries
- Addressing fear of falling

WELLNESS OUTCOMES (POSITIVE FUNCTIONAL CONSEQUENCES)
- Safer mobility
- ↓ risk for falls
- Prevention of osteoporosis
- Improved quality of life

HEALTH

Consider the whole person and his or her environment

Never lose sight of the individual—mind, body and spirit

and an inner, spongy meshwork, called trabecular or cancellous bone. The proportion of cortical to trabecular components varies according to bone type. Long bones, such as the radius and femur, are composed of as much as 90% cortical cells, whereas flat and vertebral bones are composed primarily of trabecular cells. Both cortical and trabecular bone components are affected by age-related changes, but the rate and impact of age-related changes differ in the two types of bone.

Bone growth reaches maturity in early adulthood, but bone remodelling continues throughout one's lifetime. The following age-related changes affect this remodelling process in all older adults:

- Increased bone resorption (i.e., breakdown of bone that is necessary for remodelling)
- Diminished calcium absorption
- Increased serum parathyroid hormone
- Impaired regulation of osteoblast activity

- Impaired bone formation secondary to reduced osteoblastic production of bone matrix
- Fewer functional marrow cells resulting from replacement of marrow with fat cells
- Decreased estrogen in women and testosterone in men

Muscles

Skeletal muscles, which are controlled by motor neurons, directly affect all activities of daily living (ADLs). Age-related changes that have the greatest impact on muscle function include

- Decreased size and number of muscle fibres
- Loss of motor neurons
- Replacement of muscle tissue by connective tissue and, eventually, by fat tissue
- Deterioration of muscle cell membranes and a subsequent escape of fluid and potassium
- Diminished protein synthesis

The overall effect of these age-related changes is a condition called **sarcopenia**, which is a loss of muscle mass, strength and endurance.

Joints and Connective Tissue

Numerous age-related changes affect the function of all musculoskeletal joints, including non–weight-bearing joints. In contrast to the bones or muscles, which benefit from exercise, the joints are harmed by continued use and begin to show the effects of wear and tear during early adulthood. In fact, degenerative processes begin to affect the tendons, ligaments and synovial fluid during early adulthood, even before skeletal maturity is reached.

Some of the most significant age-related joint changes include the following:

- Diminished viscosity of synovial fluid
- Degeneration of collagen and elastin cells
- Fragmentation of fibrous structures in connective tissue
- Outgrowths of cartilaginous clusters because of continuous wear and tear
- Formation of scar tissue and areas of calcification in the joint capsules and connective tissue
- Degenerative changes in the articular cartilage resulting in extensive fraying, cracking and shredding, in addition to a pitted and thinned surface

Consequences of these changes include impaired flexion and extension, decreased flexibility of the fibrous structures, diminished protection from forces of movement, erosion of the bones underlying the outgrowths of cartilage and diminished ability of the connective tissue to transmit the tensile forces that act on it.

Nervous System

Age-related changes in the central and peripheral nervous system may be a primary mechanism involved with diminished muscle function in older adults (Manini et al.,

2013). For example, an effect of the age-related delayed reaction time is that older adults walk more slowly and are less able to respond in a timely manner to environmental stimuli. Maintenance of balance in an upright position is affected by the following age-related changes of the nervous system: altered visual abilities, a slower righting reflex, impaired proprioception and diminished vibratory and positioning sensations in the lower extremities. In addition, age-related changes in postural control cause an increase in **body sway**, which is a measure of the motion of the body while standing.

Osteopenia and Osteoporosis

Loss of bone mass is an age-related change that affects all adults as they age; however the extent to which it occurs is affected by many variables. As bone densitometry (i.e., a simple imaging technique) has become widely available, **bone density**, or the amount of minerals in the bone, is now routinely evaluated in older adults. Bone density is scored according to standard deviations below that of healthy adults between the ages of 20 and 29 years of the same race and sex, called a *T-score*. Normal T-score is -1 and above. When a T-score is between 1 and 2.5, the diagnosis is **osteopenia**; when a T-score is lower than this, the diagnosis is **osteoporosis**. Osteoporosis is called a silent disease because it is usually asymptomatic and the first sign may be a fracture that occurs with little or no trauma. This type of fracture is called a **fragility fracture** or an osteoporotic fracture. As osteoporosis progresses, it can cause pain, loss of height, dowager's hump and increased risk of fractures.

Prevalence of osteoporosis increases with age in both men and women, but it increases at an earlier age in men and is higher in women at all ages. Although osteoporosis has been recognized as a common condition among postmenopausal women for many decades, only in recent decades has it been recognized as a condition that affects men also. This increased attention is warranted because at least 1 in 3 women and 1 in 5 men will experience an osteoporotic fracture in their lifetime and more than 80% of fractures in adults above 50 are caused by osteoporosis (Osteoporosis Canada, 2014).

Gender differences in age-related changes account for the relatively higher rate of osteoporosis among women compared with men. Both men and women reach peak bone mass in their mid-30s; then there are significant difference in rates of bone loss. Men experience about 1% annual bone loss after peak bone mass has been reached, and this bone loss is steady across their remaining lifetime. In contrast, women experience a rapid period of bone loss beginning during the transition to and early phase of menopause, which is more than they will experience in their remaining lifetime (McClung, 2012). During the first decade after the onset of menopause, the annual rate of bone loss may be as great as 7%, but after menopause, it is between 1% and 2%. In summary, osteoporosis occurs in both men and women, but women have a much greater percentage of bone loss over their lifetime and experience greater bone loss at an earlier age.

DIVERSITY NOTE

Osteoporosis affects both men and women, but the onset is about a decade earlier in women. Another difference is that men are more likely to have heterogeneous risk factors rather than age-related changes primarily (Herrera et al., 2012).

RISK FACTORS THAT AFFECT MOBILITY AND SAFETY

Risk factors affect overall musculoskeletal function and safe mobility, which is a concern for all older adults. Additional risk factors of concern are those that contribute to osteoporosis, fractures, and falls. These risks are of particular importance to nurses because health promotion interventions are appropriate for addressing many of the risk factors, and this, in turn, can prevent the serious functional consequences associated with falls and fractures.

Risk Factors That Affect Overall Musculoskeletal Function

Physical inactivity and nutritional deficits are major risk factors for diminished musculoskeletal function in older adults. Low level of physical activity (i.e., lack of exercise) is the most commonly occurring risk for poor musculoskeletal function across the full spectrum of health and functioning ranging from healthy older adults to those who are frail or seriously ill. This is particularly pertinent to health promotion because interventions to improve physical activity in older adults have extensive benefits, not only for improving overall musculoskeletal function and preventing falls and fractures, but also for many other aspects of functioning, as discussed throughout this book.

Nutritional deficits are important risk factors for diminished musculoskeletal performance. For example, researchers have focused on vitamin D deficiency because this vitamin is essential for absorption of calcium and bone health. Studies in many countries find a strong association between low serum levels of vitamin D (also call 25[OH]D) and low bone density and increased risk for fragility fractures and mobility limitations in otherwise healthy older adults (e.g., Houston et al., 2013; Mosele et al., 2013; Narula et al., 2013). Adequate dietary intake of calcium is also strongly associated with good musculoskeletal function; however, excessive calcium intake in the form of dietary supplements is associated with adverse effects, as discussed in the section on health education about osteoporosis. Other dietary factors that increase the risk for poor overall musculoskeletal function include low intake of high-quality proteins (i.e., less than 1 g/kg of body weight daily from sources such as soy and whey), and inadequate food sources of vitamin B_{12} and folic acid (Mithal et al., 2013; Reidy et al., 2013).

Risk Factors for Osteoporosis and Fragility Fractures

In addition to risks that affect overall musculoskeletal function, some conditions increase the risk for osteoporosis and osteoporotic fractures, as listed in Box 22-1. Although some risk factors, such as age, ethnicity and family history, cannot be changed, other conditions can be addressed through health promotion interventions. Current emphasis is on modifiable risk factors, including low level of weight-bearing activity, cigarette smoking, excessive alcohol consumption and inadequate intake of calcium and vitamin D. Hormonal changes also affect the risk for osteoporosis, particularly with regard to estrogen in women, which has been the focus of research

---

Box 22-1 Risk Factors for Osteoporosis and Fragility Fractures

Factors That Increase the Risk for Osteoporosis

- Age 65 or 70 years or older for women and men, respectively
- Family history of osteoporosis or osteoporotic fracture
- Low calcium intake, both past and current
- Vitamin D deficiency
- Lack of weight-bearing activity
- Hormonal deficiency from age-related changes or pathologic conditions
- Cigarette smoking
- Excessive alcohol intake
- Pathologic conditions (e.g., hypogonadism, hyperparathyroidism, thyrotoxicosis, malabsorption, low gastric acid, pre- or post-solid organ transplant, low gastric acid)
- Medications (e.g., corticosteroids, anticonvulsants, anticoagulants, aromatase inhibitors, cancer chemotherapeutic agents)

Additional Factors That Increase the Risk for Fragility Fracture

- Postmenopausal status for women, age 75 years or older for men, younger age in the presence of other risk factors
- Female sex
- Multiple risk factors for osteoporosis
- Previous fragility fracture, especially in combination with undertreatment of osteoporosis
- Family history of hip fracture
- Body mass index (BMI) less than 18.5 kg/m²
- Current or previous use of oral or systemic glucocorticoids
- Falling
- Rheumatoid arthritis

Sources: Levis, S., & Theodore, G. (2012). Summary of AHRQ's comparative effectiveness review of treatment to prevent fractures in men and women with low bone density or osteoporosis: Update of 2007 report. *Journal of Managed Care Pharmacy, 18*(Suppl. B), S1–S15; National Clinical Guideline Centre. (2012). *Guideline Summary Osteoporosis: Assessing the risk of fragility fractures.* Retrieved from www.guideline.gov/content.aspx?id=38410&search=osteoporosis; Yurgin, N., Wade, S., Satram-Hoang, S., et al. (2012). Research Article: Prevalence of fracture risk factors in postmenopausal women enrolled in the POSSIBLE US Treatment cohort. *International Journal of Endocrinology, 2013*, 1–9. doi:10.1155/2013/715025.

for many decades. For example, a 34-year longitudinal study found that menopause before 47 years is associated with increased risk of osteoporosis and fragility fractures (Svejme et al., 2013). When medications or pathologic conditions are a primary underlying cause, the condition is referred to as secondary osteoporosis.

In recent years, there is increasing attention to identifying risks for fragility fractures with emphasis on preventing hip fractures, which are strongly associated with serious and permanent negative consequences. In particular, a major focus of hospital quality and safety initiatives is the prevention of fractured hips that result from in-hospital falls in medical and postsurgical patients. Common risk factors for in-hospital hip fractures from falls include dementia, increased age, altered mental status and adverse medication effects (Zapatero et al., 2013).

Since 2012, the International Osteoporosis Foundation has been promoting the Capture the Fracture campaign with the goal of implementing best practices to reduce the incidence of fragility fractures, which occur every 3 seconds worldwide (Akesson et al., 2013). A major focus of this initiative is to prevent hip fractures in people who have already had a fracture because a history of any prior fracture almost doubles the risk for another fracture (International Osteoporosis Foundation, 2012). Osteoporosis Canada has implemented a similar campaign called Fracture Liaison Services (see http://www.osteoporosis.ca/fracture-liaison-service/?utm_source=Home+Page&utm_medium=Menu+Button&utm_campaign=FLS). Conditions that increase the risk for fragility fractures are listed in Box 22-1. It is imperative to consider that a combination of risk factors significantly increases the risk for fragility fractures. One study found that more than one half of patients who sustained a fragility fracture had low levels of serum vitamin D and nearly one third had another underlying condition (Bogoch et al., 2012).

Risk Factors for Falls

Falling is unfortunately very common among older adults, and it has been the focus of much attention in Canada and many other countries for decades. More than a half century ago, an article titled "On the Natural History of Falls in Old Age" began with the following declaration: "The liability of old people to tumble and often to injure themselves is such a commonplace of experience that it has been tacitly accepted as an inevitable aspect of aging, and thereby deprived of the exercise of curiosity" (Sheldon, 1960, p. 1685). In recent years, geriatricians and gerontologists have challenged this view that falls are a normal consequence of aging or are accidental or random events. There is now wide agreement that falls and mobility problems result from multiple, diverse and interacting risk factors. The current clinical approach is to identify the most likely causes and contributing conditions and to plan interventions to prevent falls.

Unfolding Case Study

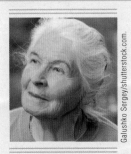

Galushko Sergey/shutterstock.com.

Part 1: Ms. M. at 58 Years of Age

Ms. M. is 58 years old and works as the secretary in the Senior Circle of Care program where you conduct health screening and educational programs. This senior wellness program is sponsored by one of the hospitals in Winnipeg, Manitoba. Ms. M.'s responsibilities include finding and organizing health education materials under the direction of the nurses. You often go to lunch with her and discuss social and health-related topics. Ms. M. has always been inquisitive about health-related concerns, and one day she asks your advice about osteoporosis. She says that both she and her mother, who is 83 years old, have been receiving fliers about getting a bone density test, and that her mother asked if she would go with her so that they could both be tested. You know from past conversations that Ms. M.'s mother fractured her wrist a long time ago, but otherwise is relatively healthy. Ms. M. is fairly healthy, although she admits that she "could stand to lose a little weight and get more exercise." You also know from previous discussions that Ms. M. has been using hormonal replacement therapy for several years as prescribed by her gynecologist. In your work as a wellness nurse, you have developed and presented several health education programs about osteoporosis, so you are familiar with recent literature on osteoporosis.

THINKING POINTS

- Based on what you know about Ms. M., what would you tell her about her risk factors for osteoporosis?
- Based on what you know about Ms. M.'s mother, what additional information would you want to know before advising her about a test for her mother?
- What suggestions would you make to help Ms. M. become more knowledgeable about osteoporosis?

Numerous studies have been published about risks for falls, with variable conclusions. Systematic reviews identify a history of falls and use of walking aids as the strongest predictors of falls in hospitals, nursing homes and community settings (Deandrea et al., 2013). Deandrea and colleagues suggest that these two conditions are not causal factors, but are indicators of an underlying problems that need to be addressed. A consistent research finding is that falls are the result of a combination of risk factors, rather than one isolated risk factor. Moreover, the risk of falls increases in proportion to the number of fall risk factors. Current emphasis is on preventing serious fall-related injuries, such as fractures and traumatic brain injury, because up to one fifth of falls in older adults results in injury, hospitalization or death (Moller et al., 2013). Risk factors for falls can be categorized according to their origin as follows: age-related changes, common pathologic conditions and functional impairments, medication effects and environmental factors (Box 22-2).

Box 22-2   Risk Factors for Falls

Pathologic Conditions and Functional Impairments

- Age-related conditions (e.g., nocturia, osteoporosis, gait changes, postural hypotension, sensory deficits)
- Cardiovascular diseases (e.g., arrhythmias or myocardial infarction)
- Respiratory diseases (e.g., chronic obstructive pulmonary disease [COPD])
- Neurologic disorders (e.g., parkinsonism, cerebrovascular accident [CVA])
- Metabolic disturbances (e.g., dehydration, electrolyte imbalances)
- Musculoskeletal problems (e.g., osteoarthritis)
- Transient ischemic attack (TIA)
- Vision impairments (e.g., cataracts, glaucoma, macular degeneration)
- Cognitive impairments (e.g., dementia, confusion)
- Psychosocial factors (e.g., depression, anxiety, agitation)

Medication Effects and Interactions

- Antiarrhythmics
- Anticholinergics, including ingredients in over-the-counter products (e.g., diphenhydramine)
- Anticonvulsants
- Diuretics
- Benzodiazepines and other hypnotics
- Antipsychotics
- Antidepressants
- Alcohol

Environmental Factors

- Inadequate lighting
- Lack of handrails on stairs
- Slippery floors
- Throw rugs
- Clutter, cords or other objects in the walking path
- Unfamiliar environments
- Highly polished floors
- Improper height of beds, chairs or toilets
- Physical restraints

Pathologic Conditions and Functional and Cognitive Impairments

Nocturia, sleep problems, gait changes, sensory changes, orthostatic hypotension, decreased muscle strength and central nervous system changes are conditions that can increase the risk of falls in older adults. In addition, vision impairment is an independent risk for falls in older adults because of its effects on mobility, balance, safety, fear of falling and ability to perform daily activities (Aartolahti et al., 2013; Reed-Jones et al., 2013). In general, commonly occurring pathologic conditions can increase the risk for falls in older adults in all of the following ways:

- Pathologic conditions can cause functional impairments that affect vision, balance or mobility.
- Pathologic conditions may be treated with medications that create risks for falling.
- Chronic conditions often interfere with optimal exercise and other health practices that are important in promoting safe mobility.

Depression and cognitive impairments can increase the risk for falls, especially in combination with other risk factors. For example, both dementia and depression diminish one's awareness of the environment and can interfere with the ability to process information about environmental stimuli. Older adults with dementia have at least a twofold fall risk, which is associated with slowed gait and executive dysfunction (Kearney et al., 2013). The following combination of factors is likely to increase the risk for falls in people with dementia: concurrent conditions, vision impairment, impaired balance and slowed psychomotor speed (Chen et al., 2012; Martin et al., 2013). Depressed older adults are at increased risk for falls secondary to gait changes, adverse medication effects and a diminished ability to concentrate on and respond to environmental factors. One study found that antidepressant medications increased the risk of outdoor falls by 70% (Quach et al., 2013). Considering all of these possible associations, it is not surprising that most falls resulting in injuries occur in people who have functional impairments and multiple, chronic medical problems.

Medication Effects

Numerous studies have identified hundreds of medications that can contribute to falls and attempts have been made to identify those medications that are associated with the highest risk of falls. Central nervous system drugs, such as hypnotics, antipsychotics and antidepressants, are medications most often identified as independent and significant risks for falls in institutional and community-based settings (Costa-Dias et al., 2013; Lamis et al., 2012; van Strien et al., 2013; Whitney et al., 2012). Central nervous system drugs with long half-lives are associated with the highest risk for falls (Obayashi et al., 2013; Olazaran et al., 2013). Diuretics also are associated with increased risk for falls and fractures, particularly during the first week after initiation of the drug

(Berry, Zhu, et al., 2013b). Use of more than four medications is another commonly identified risk for falls (Damian et al., 2013; Freeland et al., 2012).

Studies also identify medication-related factors that increase the risk of fall-related injuries. For example, anticoagulant medications, which are commonly used for stroke prevention, increase the risk for serious bleeding if a fall occurs. Dosing of medications also can affect the risk for fall-related injuries. Studies indicate that the risk for hip fractures in nursing home residents may be especially high soon after a hypnotic is initiated or when the dose of an antipsychotic is adjusted (Berry, Lee, et al., 2013a; Rigler et al., 2013).

Although most studies have focused on prescription medications, over-the-counter medications also can create risks for falls through their adverse effects on psychomotor function. Many over-the-counter preparations for pain, colds and insomnia contain alcohol or anticholinergics. These ingredients may themselves pose risks or may interact with other medications to increase the risk for falls. The adverse effects of diphenhydramine, a widely used ingredient in over-the-counter products for sleep, colds and allergies, have received much attention in the media and medical literature. Diphenhydramine has been associated with significant adverse effects on the psychomotor skills necessary for safe driving, and some provincial health bodies, such as Alberta Health Services, have drawn attention to the problems of driving while using medications containing diphenhydramine (www.albertahealthservices.ca/Researchers/if-res-policy-impaired-driving-background.pdf).

The following adverse medication effects can increase the risk for falls: confusion, depression, sedation, arrhythmias, hypovolemia, orthostatic hypotension, delayed reaction time, diminished cognitive function and changes in gait and balance (e.g., ataxia, decreased proprioception, increased body sway). Thus, any medication that has one or more of these adverse effects may increase the risk for falls. Other considerations that influence the risk of falls include medication–disease interactions, medication–medication interactions and medication–alcohol interactions.

An approach to identifying the relationship between medications and an increased risk for falls is to consider the underlying mechanism of the medication action, as well as the pathologic condition and the potential interactions among various factors. For example, orthostatic hypotension can result from pathologic conditions, age-related changes or adverse medication effects and can increase the risk for falls. If an 80-year-old person has a pathologic condition (e.g., Parkinson disease) that may cause orthostatic hypotension, and if the person is taking a medication (e.g., a vasodilator) that causes orthostatic hypotension, the risk for falls significantly increases. Therefore, rather than memorizing all of the medications known to increase the risk for falls, nurses can focus their attention on the underlying mechanisms that increase the risk for falls. Some medications that are likely to increase the risk for falls are listed in Box 22-2.

Environmental Factors

Some environmental hazards were discussed in Chapter 7 in relation to safety, but additional environmental influences must be considered specifically in relation to falls. In institutional settings, for example, falls are most likely to occur in the bedroom and bathroom. In the bedroom, most falls occur while the person is getting in or out of bed, and some falls are related to climbing over side rails or footboards. In the bathroom, falls generally occur while transferring on or off toilet seats or while hurrying to urinate or defecate. In community settings, most falls occur in the home, particularly in stairways, bedrooms and living rooms. Environmental hazards that increase the risk of falls in homes include clutter, poor lighting and lack of handrails on stairs or grab bars in bathrooms.

Physical Restraints

Physical restraints have been used since the 1960s in institutional settings with the intent of protecting impaired people from injury and reducing staff workload. Historically, the belief that using physical restraints protects vulnerable people from falls and shields the institution from liability was widespread. Since the 1990s, however, there has been increasing evidence that the use of physical restraints is not effective for fall prevention and in fact is associated with substantial risk of serious injury or fatality (Gray-Miceli & Quigley, 2012; Luo et al., 2011). Agencies that have recommended using less restrictive devices include the Canadian Patient Safety Institute, the Canadian Nurses Association and the Alzheimer Society of Canada. In addition, Canadian legislation has also limited the use of restraints; one example is the Mental Health Act in Ontario and the Criminal Code of Canada.

PATHOLOGIC CONDITION AFFECTING MUSCULOSKELETAL FUNCTION: OSTEOARTHRITIS

Osteoarthritis is a degenerative inflammatory disease affecting joints and attached muscles, tendons and ligaments; it is characterized by pain, swelling and limited movement in joints. Osteoarthritis, a leading cause of disability in Canada, affects older adults disproportionately. Although not all older adults have symptoms of osteoarthritis, the condition is often viewed as an extreme progression of age-related changes. Osteoarthritis is a complex disease process that results from the interplay of risk factors such as trauma, genetics, obesity and age-related changes.

 DIVERSITY NOTE

In Canada, men and women are equally affected (The Arthritis Society, n.d.). Using data from a large population survey in Canada, Rahman et al. (2013) identified that osteoarthritis was significantly associated with the presence of heart disease, angina and congestive heart failure in older adults.

Unfolding Case Study

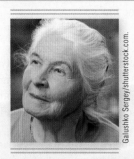

Part 2: Ms. M. at 67 Years of Age

Ms. M. is now 67 years old and has retired from her secretarial job. She attends weekly social and lunch gatherings at the local senior centre, where you are the wellness nurse. One day she comes to the centre with a cast on her left wrist and reports that she fractured her wrist when she slipped and fell on ice in her driveway. Ms. M. stopped taking hormonal therapy several years ago because she had been taking it for 10 years and was concerned about long-term effects. You also know that she takes medications for arthritis, hypertension and depression and that she self-monitors her blood pressure. In the past 10 years, she has gradually gained "a little weight every year" and her current height/weight is 1.6 m/79 kg, which is a BMI of 31. She participates in the weekly "mall walkers" exercise program but rarely exercises independently. She says that "my housework is enough exercise" and that the weekly group exercise activity is "as much as my arthritis will tolerate." She lives in a small one-floor house. Although Ms. M. says she is not really concerned about sustaining any more fractures because she views the recent fall as a "fluke of bad winter luck," she makes an appointment to talk with you. During the appointment, she reports that she is a "little concerned about osteoporosis."

THINKING POINTS

- What risk factors for osteoporosis can you identify from what you already know about Ms. M.?
- What risk factors for falls and fall-related injuries can you identify from what you already know about Ms. M.?

- Can you identify any factors that reduce her risk for falls or fractures?
- What additional information about Ms. M. would be helpful in identifying additional risks for osteoporosis?
- What additional information would be helpful in identifying additional risks for falls and fractures?

QSEN APPLICATION

QSEN Competency	Knowledge/Skill/Attitude	Application to Ms. M. at 67 Years
Patient-centred care	(K) Integrate understanding of multiple dimensions of patient-centred care.	Identify Ms. M.'s risks for fractures.
	(K) Describe strategies to empower patients in all aspects of the health care process.	Identify positive aspects of Ms. M.'s lifestyle so you can build on these when teaching about health promotion strategies.
	(K) Examine common barriers to active involvement of patients in their own health care processes.	Address Ms. M.'s lack of knowledge about osteoporosis and prevention of fragility fractures.
Evidence-based practice	(K) Describe how the strength and relevance of available evidence influence the choice of intervention.	Apply evidence-based information from Box 22-1 to assess risks for osteoporosis and fragility fractures and teach Ms. M. about prevention of fragility fractures.
	(S) Base individualized care plan on patient values, clinical expertise and evidence.	

Because self-care is an important aspect of managing osteoarthritis, nurses focus on health education interventions. Nurses can encourage participation in self-management programs, which are effective for management of pain and prevention of disability in osteoarthritis (Shelton, 2013). In addition, nurses can teach people with osteoarthritis about the following self-care practices that are recommended in evidence-based guidelines (Davies, 2011; Moskowitz, 2013):

- Participating in aerobic, resistance, land-based and aquatic exercise programs that focus on improving musculoskeletal strength, balance and endurance (e.g., yoga, aquatherapy, tai chi)

- Avoiding high-impact activities
- Wearing good shock-absorbing shoes
- Balancing weight-bearing activities with rest periods
- Losing weight if appropriate
- Using orthotics, supports, braces and shoe inserts as appropriate
- Using canes, walkers and other assistive devices as appropriate to relieve weight-bearing joints, improve balance or achieve independent functioning
- Using moist heat and analgesics for pain

Care plans for managing osteoarthritis are most effective when they are based on an interprofessional approach that

Galushko Sergey/shutterstock.com.

includes medicine, nursing, and physical and occupational therapy. Because there are many medical and surgical interventions for osteoarthritis, nurses emphasize the importance of obtaining regular medical care for ongoing evaluation and treatment as this condition changes. An important nursing role is facilitating referrals to physical and occupational therapists to improve muscle strength and promote safe and independent functioning. Online Learning Activity 22-1 provides links to reliable sources of information about physical activity and self-management interventions for people with arthritis.

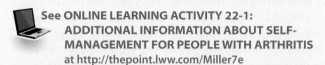

See **ONLINE LEARNING ACTIVITY 22-1: ADDITIONAL INFORMATION ABOUT SELF-MANAGEMENT FOR PEOPLE WITH ARTHRITIS** at http://thepoint.lww.com/Miller7e

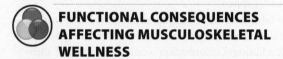

Wellness Opportunity

Older adults with osteoarthritis need to engage in self-care activities, including making responsible decisions about promoting optimal comfort and functioning.

FUNCTIONAL CONSEQUENCES AFFECTING MUSCULOSKELETAL WELLNESS

Older adults can partially compensate for age-related changes that affect overall musculoskeletal function through health promotion interventions, such as good nutrition and physical activity. The functional consequences of osteoporosis, however, are quite serious, as are the functional consequences that result from the many risk factors that contribute to falls and fractures in older adults. As with many other aspects of function in older adulthood, cumulative and interacting effects of risk factors rather than age-related changes most significantly affect function and quality of life.

Effects on Musculoskeletal Function

Muscle strength, endurance and coordination are affected to some extent by age-related changes, even in the absence of risk factors. Beginning around the age of 40 years, muscle strength declines gradually, resulting in an overall decrease of 30% to 50% by the age of 80 years, with a greater decline in muscle strength in the lower extremities than in the upper extremities. Diminished muscle strength is attributed primarily to age-related loss of muscle mass, called sarcopenia. In addition, a person's current level of activity and lifelong patterns of exercise can influence muscle strength at any age. Muscle endurance and coordination diminish as a result of age-related changes in the muscles and central nervous system. Because of these changes, older adults experience muscle fatigue after shorter periods of exercise compared with their younger counterparts.

Joint function begins to decline during early adulthood and progresses gradually to cause the following changes in range of motion:

- Decreased range of motion in the upper arms
- Decreased lower back flexion
- Decreased external rotation of the hip
- Decreased hip and knee flexion
- Decreased dorsiflexion of the foot

These changes result in slowed performance of daily activities, such as writing, eating, grooming and putting shoes and socks on; difficulty climbing stairs and curbs; and an overall diminished ability to respond to environmental stimuli.

Gait changes, which differ in men and women, are one of the more noticeable functional consequences that occur after the age of 75 years. Older women develop a narrower standing and walking gait and bowlegged-type changes that affect the lower extremities and alter the angle of the hip. Older men develop a wider walking and standing gait, characterized by less arm swing, a shorter stride, decreased steppage height, and a more flexed position of the head and trunk than when they were younger. The overall impact of these changes is that older men and women have a slower walking speed and spend more time in the support phase of gait than in the swing phase. There is substantial individual variation, but the average rate of decline in gait speed is 1% each year between the ages of 65 to 69; this rate gradually increases to 4% per year for adults older than 80 (White et al., 2013). It is important to note that any significant gait changes that occur are not due to aging alone but are consequences of other conditions, such as osteoarthritis or neurologic disorders (e.g., dementia, Parkinson disease).

Susceptibility to Falls and Fractures

The combination of age-related changes and multiple interacting risk factors doubly jeopardizes older adults by increasing the probability of both falls and fractures. Falls account for more than half of all injuries among Canadians 65 years and above. Twenty to thirty percent of community-dwelling Canadian older adults experience one fall each year, and half of those will fall more than once (Public Health Agency of Canada, 2014). Fractures are not unique to older adults, but they do differ in many respects from those that occur in younger populations. First, osteoporotic fractures occur with little or no trauma, for example, from an impact that is no more severe than that which results from falling to the floor from a standing position. Second, the risk of fractures increases in direct relation to age. Third, it is more likely that fractures in older adults, particularly hip fractures, will have serious consequences affecting independence, quality of life, and morbidity and mortality. Studies show that older adults who have had hip fractures are at increased risk for functional decline, recurrent falls, permanent admission to a nursing facility and shortened life expectancy (Frost et al., 2013; Gill et al., 2013; Tajeu et al., 2013). The likelihood of dying from a fall-related injury increases with age; among older adults, 20% of deaths related to injury can be traced back to a fall (Public Health Agency of Canada, 2014).

Fear of Falling

Since the early 1990s, there has been increasing attention to **fear of falling**, which is excessive anxiety about falling that leads to activity avoidance and decline in functioning. It is considered a major problem that affects between 40% and 75% of long-term care residents and up to 76.6% of community-dwelling older adults (Kim & So, 2013; Lach & Parsons, 2013). Rather than leading to a cautious awareness of actions to prevent falls, fear of falling increases the risk for falling and leads to additional serious negative consequences. Studies have found that fear of falling can lead to functional decline, increased dependency, significant activity restrictions, depression, social isolation and increased risk for falling (Huang et al., 2013; Lach & Parsons, 2013).

Another concern is that caregivers of older adults may be quite anxious about potential falls, and this can lead to increased caregiver burden and increased vigilance (Dow et al., 2013). In some cases, caregivers restrict the older adult's activities or decide to move the person to a setting that provides a greater level of assistance or supervision than the older person desires. Although a move to a more restrictive environment will not necessarily protect the person from falls, and may even increase the risk of falls, the caregivers may derive some peace of mind because they perceive that the older person is safer. Similarly, caregivers may begin using restraints or otherwise limiting the person's mobility; however, as already discussed, restraints do not prevent falls and are likely to contribute to more serious fall-related injuries. Nurses have important roles in addressing caregivers' fear of falls by teaching about fall-prevention interventions, as discussed in the section on promoting caregiver wellness.

Wellness Opportunity

Nurses respect older adults' autonomy and involve them in decisions by creatively finding ways to ensure safety while also allowing as much freedom of movement as possible.

NURSING ASSESSMENT OF MUSCULOSKELETAL FUNCTION

Nursing assessment of musculoskeletal function focuses on identifying risks for falls, fractures and osteoporosis, with particular attention to those factors that can be modified or alleviated through nursing interventions. Nurses can use a fall risk assessment tool to identify older adults who might benefit from appropriate preventive interventions.

Assessing Musculoskeletal Performance

Assessment of overall musculoskeletal performance begins with observation of the person's mobility and activities. In addition to watching the person walk, it is especially important to observe the person getting up from a chair. The Timed Up and Go (TUG) test is an evidence-based and simple-to-use tool for assessing gait speed and balance that has been widely used since the early 1990s in many health care and home settings. The test is a reliable measure of gait speed, as well as an indicator of fall risk and ability to safely perform ADLs. The TUG, which is illustrated in Fig. 22-1 can be administered in 5 minutes or less and it can be used repeatedly to identify declines or improvements over time. Higher scores (i.e., longer time to complete the tasks) are associated with increased risk for falls. Cut-off scores between 12 and 14 seconds are discussed in the literature, but a score of 12.47 seconds is recommended in a review of studies (Murphy & Lowe, 2013). Before administering this test, it is important to explain and demonstrate the procedure and have the person wear regular footwear and use usual assistive devices.

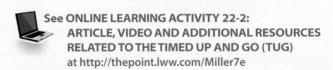

See **ONLINE LEARNING ACTIVITY 22-2:**
ARTICLE, VIDEO AND ADDITIONAL RESOURCES
RELATED TO THE TIMED UP AND GO (TUG)
at http://thepoint.lww.com/Miller7e

Assessment information is also obtained by asking questions about the person's ability to perform ADLs. When limitations are identified, it is important to find out whether the older adult is using assistive devices to improve safety, mobility, balance, independence or overall function. If the person is not using such devices—and may benefit from them—it is important to assess the person's knowledge about the availability of such devices. It is important to assess the person's attitude about using assistive devices because attitudes are likely to influence the acceptability of using recommended aids. Nurses can use the criteria for the functional assessment of all ADLs provided in Chapter 7 together with the assessment information in this chapter.

In addition to experiencing minor changes in performing ADLs, older adults experience diminished height and changes in posture. Older adults may or may not be concerned about or aware of a loss of height; however, a loss of about 2 to 4 cm per decade is normal, owing to osteoporosis and other age-related changes. Including a question about the person's usual height and any noticeable loss of height will give the nurse an opportunity to assess the older adult's awareness of this change. Although the functional consequences of decreased height are minimal, older people who never were very tall may experience increased difficulty performing activities that depend on height. In these situations, they may find that it is safer and more effective to use assistive devices, such as long-handled reachers. They may also need encouragement to rearrange cupboards so that the most frequently used items are accessible. Another assessment implication of decreased height is that the pant legs of older adults may be too long, especially if the person also has lost weight. Therefore, nurses observe whether the length of clothing increases the risk for falls because this risk can be alleviated through relatively simple interventions. Box 22-3 summarizes guidelines for assessing overall musculoskeletal performance in older adults.

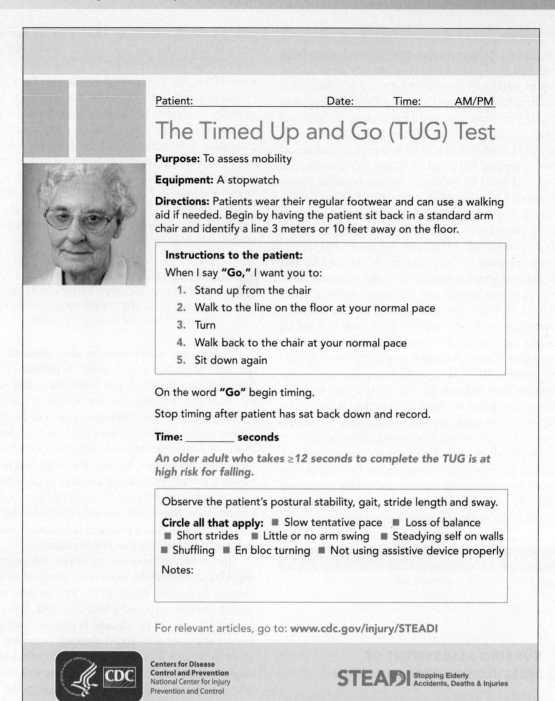

Patient: _____ Date: _____ Time: _____ AM/PM

The Timed Up and Go (TUG) Test

Purpose: To assess mobility

Equipment: A stopwatch

Directions: Patients wear their regular footwear and can use a walking aid if needed. Begin by having the patient sit back in a standard arm chair and identify a line 3 meters or 10 feet away on the floor.

> **Instructions to the patient:**
>
> When I say **"Go,"** I want you to:
>
> 1. Stand up from the chair
> 2. Walk to the line on the floor at your normal pace
> 3. Turn
> 4. Walk back to the chair at your normal pace
> 5. Sit down again

On the word **"Go"** begin timing.

Stop timing after patient has sat back down and record.

Time: _____ seconds

An older adult who takes ≥12 seconds to complete the TUG is at high risk for falling.

> Observe the patient's postural stability, gait, stride length and sway.
>
> **Circle all that apply:** ■ Slow tentative pace ■ Loss of balance ■ Short strides ■ Little or no arm swing ■ Steadying self on walls ■ Shuffling ■ En bloc turning ■ Not using assistive device properly
>
> Notes:

For relevant articles, go to: **www.cdc.gov/injury/STEADI**

CDC Centers for Disease Control and Prevention National Center for Injury Prevention and Control

STEADI Stopping Elderly Accidents, Deaths & Injuries

FIGURE 22-1 The Timed Up and Go Test (TUG). (Reprinted from the CDC; http://www.cdc.gov/homeandrecreationalsafety/pdf/steadi/timed_up_and_go_test.pdf.)

Identifying Risks for Osteoporosis

Risks for osteoporosis are assessed in all older adults because some health promotion interventions for osteoporosis—such as adequate intake of calcium and vitamin D and participation in regular weight-bearing exercise—are universally applicable. Nurses also identify modifiable risk factors, such as smoking and drinking excessive amounts of alcohol that can be alleviated through lifestyle interventions. Nurses obtain much of the information regarding risks for osteoporosis during an overall assessment or health history, and they consider this information in relation to mobility and safety. Evidence-based guidelines recommend that people at risk for osteoporotic fractures are best identified through a combination of bone density measurement and an assessment of clinical risk factors (Agency for Healthcare Research and Quality, 2012). See Box 22-3 for assessment questions and considerations relating to osteoporosis.

Box 22-3 Guidelines for Assessing Overall Musculoskeletal Function and Risks for Falls, Osteoporosis and Fragility Fractures

Questions to Assess Overall Musculoskeletal Performance

- Do you have any trouble performing your usual activities because of joint limitations?
- Do you have any pain or discomfort in your joints?
- Do you ever feel like you are losing your balance?
- Do you have any trouble walking or getting around?
- Do you use any assistive devices (e.g., a walker, quad cane, reaching devices) to help you do things?

Questions to Assess Risks for Osteoporosis and Fragility Fractures

Questions to Ask All Older Adults

- Do you know of any blood relatives who have had osteoporosis or who have sustained fractures late in life?
- Have you sustained any fractures during your adult years? (If yes, ask additional questions regarding age at the time, type, location, circumstances, treatment and so on.)
- What is your usual intake of foods high in calcium and vitamin D, and do you take any supplements?
- Have you ever had your bone density measured?
- Do you take any medications for prevention or management of osteoporosis?
- If you have osteoporosis, have you ever talked with your primary care practitioner about prevention of fractures?

Questions to Assess Risk for Falls and Fear of Falling

- Have you had any falls in the past few years? (If yes, ask additional questions about the circumstances and ask about pertinent risk factors as summarized in Box 22-2.)
- Do you have any concerns about falling? (If yes, ask additional questions about specific fears, such as, *What do you think might happen if you were to fall?*)
- Do you take any precautions to prevent falls?

- Are there any activities you would like to do, but do not do, because of any difficulty moving or getting around? (If yes, ask about specific activities, such as shopping, using public transportation and so on.)
- Are there any activities you would like to do, but do not do, because you are afraid of falling? (If yes, ask about specific activities, such as going up or down stairs, taking a bath or shower and so on.)

Observations Regarding Overall Musculoskeletal Performance

- Measure and record the person's present height and stated peak height.
- Observe the individual's walking and gait pattern.
- Use the Timed Up and Go (TUG) test (Fig. 22-1).

Information From the Overall Assessment That Is Also Useful in Assessing Musculoskeletal Function

- Observe and document a functional assessment, as described in Chapter 7.
- How much exercise does the person get on a regular basis? In particular, how much weight-bearing exercise?
- Does the person smoke cigarettes?
- How much alcohol does the person consume?
- What is the person's usual daily intake of calcium and vitamin D?
- Does the person have any medical conditions that are associated with falls or osteoporosis (as summarized in Boxes 22-1 and 22-2)?
- Is the person taking any prescription or over-the-counter medications that might create risks for falls?
- Does the person have postural hypotension?
- Is the person moderately or seriously visually impaired?
- Does the person have any cognitive impairments or other psychosocial impairments (e.g., depression) that diminish his or her attention to the environment or interfere with the ability to respond to environmental stimuli?

Wellness Opportunity

From a holistic perspective, nurses ask older adults to identify enjoyable ways of engaging in weight-bearing activities.

Identifying Risks for Falls and Injury

Identifying fall risks is an essential and multidimensional part of health care for all older adults because it is imperative to initiate preventive interventions. The best assessment information is obtained by observing the person in his or her environment and paying particular attention to the person's awareness of and attention to unsafe conditions. Observations also provide information about adaptive behaviours that otherwise might not be acknowledged. For example, a person might state that he or she has no difficulty with stair climbing, but observations might reveal that the person performs this activity in a highly unsafe manner. When nurses do not have the opportunity to observe home environments directly, they can observe the person in the immediate environment and ask the person or caregivers about the older adult's ability to function safely in that setting. They can also consider referrals to home care agencies for home assessment as part of the discharge plan.

Another important aspect of assessing the environment in any setting is identifying the factors that are likely to cause serious injury if a fall does occur. For example, stationary objects such as bathroom sinks or heavy wooden furniture or bathroom sinks can cause serious head injuries if someone falls near the object. The guidelines summarized in Chapter 7 can be used to assess the safety of any environment and can be applied to all older adults, particularly those who have intrinsic risk factors for falls.

Important assessment information can be obtained simply by asking one or two questions. For example, a nursing study found that asking hospitalized patients what they would do if they need to go to the toilet helped identify patients who were at high risk for falls (Ko et al., 2012). Similarly, the Registered Nurses Association of Ontario (RNAO, 2005) in its best practice guidelines, *Prevention of Falls and Fall Injuries in the Older Adult*, recommends that practitioners ask all older adults if they fell or experienced difficulty walking in the initial assessment. Box 22-3 includes assessment questions that are applicable to older adults who are independent or relatively independent.

Wellness Opportunity

Whenever possible, nurses actively involve the older adult and family members in identifying environmental factors that either support or create risks for safe mobility.

Many **fall risk assessment tools** are used to identify people who are at risk for falls so that preventive measures can be implemented. Two types of fall risk assessment tools are functional assessment scales and nursing fall risk tools. Functional assessment scales focus on the person's gait and balance and are used by rehabilitation therapists. Nurses can informally assess gait and balance by asking the person to sit in a firm, straight-backed chair with armrests, stand up from the chair and walk a few steps, then turn around and return to the chair. Nurses also can observe the usual walking pattern of the person, paying particular attention to any gait or balance unsteadiness or unusual patterns. If any abnormalities are noted, nurses can facilitate referrals for further evaluation by a physical therapist. Nursing fall risk assessment tools, such as the Hendrich II Fall Risk Model (Fig. 22-2), are widely used in institutional settings, as well

Hendrich II Fall Risk Model

RISK FACTOR	RISK POINTS	SCORE
Confusion/Disorientation/Impulsivity	4	
Symptomatic Depression	2	
Altered Elimination	1	
Dizziness/Vertigo	1	
Gender (Male)	1	
Any Administered Antiepileptics (Anticonvulsants): (Carbamazepine, Divalproex Sodium, Ethotoin, Ethosuximide, Felbamate, Fosphenytoin, Gabapentin, Lamotrigine, Mephenytoin, Methsuximide, Phenobarbital, Phenytoin, Primidone, Topiramate, Trimethadione, Valproic Acid)[1]	2	
Any Administered Benzodiazepines:[2] (Alprazolam, Chloridiazepoxide, Clonazepam, Clorazepate Dipotassium, Diazepam, Flurazepam, Halazepam,[3] Lorazepam, Midozolam, Oxazepam, Temazepam, Triazolam)	1	
Get-Up-and-Go Test: "Rising from a Chair" If unable to assess, monitor for change in activity level, assess other risk factors, document both on patient chart with date and time.		
Ability to Rise in Single Movement—No Loss of Balance With Steps	0	
Pushes Up, Successful in One Attempt	1	
Multiple Attempts Successful	3	
Unable to Rise Without Assistance During Test If unable to assess, document this on the patient chart with the date and time.	4	
(A Score of 5 or Greater = High Risk)	TOTAL SCORE	

On-going Medication Review Updates:

[1] Levetiracetam (Keppra) was not assessed during the original resreach conducted to create the Hendrich Fall Risk Model. As an antieptileptic, levetiracetam does have a side effect of somnolence and dizziness, which contributes to its fall risk and should be scored (effective June 2010).

[2] The study did not include the effect of benzodiazepine-like drugs since they were not on the market at the time. However, due to their similarity in drug structure, mechanism of action and drug effects, they should also be scored (effective January 2010).

[3] Halazepam was included in the study but is no longer available in the United States (effective June 2010).

FIGURE 22-2 The Hendrich II Fall Risk Model, a fall risk assessment tool recommended by the Hartford Institute for Geriatric Nursing. (Used with permission from Ann Hendrich, Inc.)

as home and community-based settings. Online Learning Activity 22-3 provides additional information and links to fall risk assessment tools that are commonly used by nurses in various settings.

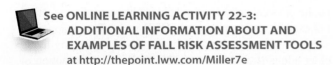

See ONLINE LEARNING ACTIVITY 22-3:
ADDITIONAL INFORMATION ABOUT AND
EXAMPLES OF FALL RISK ASSESSMENT TOOLS
at http://thepoint.lww.com/Miller7e

Although fall risk assessment tools are useful in identifying people who are at high risk for falls, they do not address the underlying causes. When older adults have several risk factors or have already had fall-related injuries, a comprehensive fall assessment should be performed in an interprofessional setting, such as a geriatric assessment program. A comprehensive fall assessment addresses all the following: mental status, nutrition, environment, medications, pathologic conditions, functional assessment, usual footwear and a complete physical examination (including visual acuity,

musculoskeletal function, neurologic function and cardiovascular status).

Because fear of falling has negative functional consequences in addition to those associated with actual falls, nurses include at least one question about fear of falling in any assessment of falls and fall risk. If the older person expresses a fear of falling, it is important to ask additional questions in relation to specific activities that may be associated with fears or falls. If the older person relies on family or other caregivers for assistance, it is important to assess caregiver concerns and observations. Assessment questions aimed at identifying fear of falling and related negative functional consequences are included in Box 22-3.

Wellness Opportunity

Nurses can use the nursing diagnosis Readiness for Enhanced Self-Health Management for healthy older adults who are willing to explore opportunities for improving musculoskeletal function and preventing falls and fractures.

Unfolding Case Study

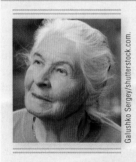

Galushko Sergey/shutterstock.com.

Part 3: Ms. M. at 74 Years of Age

Ms. M. is now 74 years old and goes to the senior centre three or four times weekly for lunch. You have been the wellness nurse at the centre for several years and are quite familiar with Ms. M. because she frequently attends your weekly healthy aging class. After your recent class on "Keeping Your Bones Healthy and Moving Well," she made an appointment to see you. She tells you that she has significantly cut down on her exercise because she experienced pain in one knee about a month ago after she took a long walk in the park with her dog. She talked with her doctor about this and was told to start taking ibuprofen, but she has not started taking it because she is not sure how much to take and her knee does not bother her except when she takes a long walk. She used to take her dog for daily walks, but now she ties him outside and stays indoors. Current prescription medications are enalapril, 5 mg twice daily, and hydrochlorothiazide, 25 mg daily. She also takes a multiple vitamin daily and acetaminophen 1,000 mg every 6 hours as needed. She continues to live in her one-floor house and is independent in doing all of her household chores. She is also responsible for all year-round outdoor maintenance activities, including mowing the lawn, raking leaves and shovelling snow.

THINKING POINTS

- What assessment questions from Box 22-3 would you ask Ms. M. at this time?
- Would you use any information from Box 22-1 or Box 22-2 at this time?

- What myths or misunderstandings related to mobility and exercise might be influencing Ms. M.?
- Would you take any steps to assess Ms. M.'s home environment for fall risks?

NURSING DIAGNOSIS

Impaired Physical Mobility is a nursing diagnosis that is applicable when the assessment identifies limitations in mobility of an older adult. This diagnosis is defined as "limitation in independent, purposeful physical movement of the body or of one or more extremities" (Herdman, 2012, p. 224). Related factors common in older adults include arthritis, depression, chronic pain, fractured hip and neurologic disorders (e.g., dementia or Parkinson disease). The nursing diagnosis of Risk for Falls is applicable for older adults who have a history of or risks for falls. Related factors common in older adults include all those factors listed in Box 22-2. If older adults have a diagnosis of osteoporosis or a history of fractures and their risks for falls and fractures are not being addressed, the nursing diagnosis of Ineffective Health Maintenance is used because the focus is on secondary prevention.

PLANNING FOR WELLNESS OUTCOMES

When planning care for older adults who are at risk for osteoporosis, nurses identify wellness outcomes that focus on primary and secondary prevention. In these situations, any of the following Nursing Outcomes Classification (NOC) terms might be pertinent: Health Promoting Behaviour, Knowledge: Health Promotion, Risk Control or Risk Detection.

Nursing goals for an older adult with a nursing diagnosis of Impaired Physical Mobility focus on restoring functional abilities, preventing further loss of function and preventing falls and injuries. NOC terminology applicable to an older adult with this nursing diagnosis include Ambulation, Balance, Endurance, Mobility or Activity Tolerance.

Care of older adults with a nursing diagnosis of Risk for Falls focuses on preventing the occurrence of falls and fall-related injuries by implementing fall-prevention programs. The following NOC terminology would be applicable with regard to safety and fall prevention: Fall-Prevention Behaviour, Falls Occurrence, Risk Control, Risk Detection, Safe Home Environment and Safe Health Care Environment.

Wellness Opportunity

Wellness outcomes that address the body–mind–spirit interrelatedness for people who are afraid of falling include Anxiety Self-Control, Coping, Fear Self-Control and Quality of Life.

NURSING INTERVENTIONS FOR MUSCULOSKELETAL WELLNESS

Nurses have numerous opportunities to promote musculoskeletal wellness because most older adults can benefit from learning about health promotion interventions for improved musculoskeletal function and prevention of osteoporosis, falls and fractures. Thus, interventions focus not only on direct actions to prevent falls but also on teaching about eliminating or addressing risks. Some Nursing Interventions Classification (NIC) terminologies that would be applicable to the interventions discussed in the following sections include Environmental Management: Safety, Exercise Promotion, Fall Prevention, Health Education, Risk Identification and Teaching: Individual.

Promoting Healthy Musculoskeletal Function

Healthy older adults experience only a slight decline in overall musculoskeletal function, but they can compensate for these minor functional consequences by maintaining an active lifestyle. Various types of exercise are beneficial in promoting healthy musculoskeletal function, and nurses can encourage older adults to incorporate several exercise strategies into their regular health behaviour routines. Positive musculoskeletal effects of exercise include improved functioning, increased bone strength and prevention of falls and disability. Flexibility exercises can improve range of motion, and weight-bearing

exercise is an essential intervention for osteoporosis. Moderate aerobic exercise can prevent loss of muscle mass in older adults and is especially important for those who are intentionally trying to lose weight. Thus, an important nursing intervention is to help older adults identify ways in which they can incorporate physical activity as a daily health promoting practice. For example, using an exercise DVD is an effective approach to improving musculoskeletal function in community-living older adults (McAuley et al., 2013). Because promotion of physical activity is a wellness outcome that affects many aspects of functioning, this topic is addressed in Chapter 5.

In recent years, there has been increasing attention to holistic types of exercise that address balance, mobility and the mind–body connection. Tai chi, which is a traditional Chinese martial art and a mind–body exercise that involves focused attention and a series of fluid and continuous movements, has been used in Asian countries for centuries and is now widely available in Western countries. Many studies and systematic reviews have confirmed the following beneficial effects of tai chi related to musculoskeletal function (Huang et al., 2011; Tousignant et al., 2013; Wei et al., 2013):

- Improved balance and neuromuscular coordination
- Increased muscle strength, flexibility and endurance
- Improved postural stability
- Decreased risk of falls and fractures
- Reduced fear of falling

Studies also found that long-term participation in tai chi has beneficial effects, including fall prevention, for older adults with chronic conditions that affect musculoskeletal function, such as osteoarthritis, Parkinson disease and peripheral neuropathy (Lauche et al., 2013; Manor et al., 2013; Tsang, 2013; Yan et al., 2013) (see Box 22-4 for research on the importance of recognizing cultural preferences in recommending exercise to older adults). .

Yoga is another body–mind therapy that is effective for improving balance and mobility in older adults (Tiedemann et al., 2013). Recent studies identify positive outcomes of dancing as an intervention for improving balance and preventing falls in older adults, including those age 85 and

Box 22-4 Evidence-Informed Nursing Practice

Background: Canada is a multicultural country with a diversity of cultural practices. Western and Eastern biomedical beliefs about exercise and health practices can differ.

Question: How do Western beliefs compare and contrast with traditional Chinese medicine conceptions of health and exercise?

Method: In-depth interviews were conducted with 15 immigrant Chinese older adults who participated in fitness activities.

Findings: Many of the participants used traditional Chinese practices to promote their health.

Implications for Nursing Practice: Recognition of cultural practices by nurses will potentially facilitate health education of the older adult. Exercise was done by participants because it improved their level of happiness.

Source: Jette, S., & Vertinsky, P. (2011). "Exercise is medicine": Understanding the exercise beliefs and practices of older Chinese immigrant in British Columbia, Canada. *Journal of Aging Studies, 25*, 272–284.

older and those with dementia (e.g., Abreu & Hartley, 2013; Hackney et al., 2013). Advantages of dance-type exercises is that they are safe, feasible, enjoyable and have a high adherence rate (Granacher et al., 2012). The Feldenkrais method is another holistic form of exercise that has been found to improve balance and mobility and to decrease fear of falling in older adults (Connors et al., 2011).

> ### Wellness Opportunity
>
> Walking, dancing, swimming, tai chi and bicycle riding are examples of wellness interventions that are enjoyable and have positive effects on the body, mind and spirit.

Teaching About Osteoporosis

Interventions for prevention and treatment of osteoporosis need to be an integral part of fracture-prevention regimens for older adults, particularly in health care settings where a major focus of care is on chronic conditions (e.g., home care and long-term care settings). Although primary care practitioners are responsible for diagnosing and treating osteoporosis, nurses are responsible for health education about osteoporosis interventions and prevention of fractures. Because awareness about osteoporosis in men is just beginning to develop, nurses have a particular responsibility for teaching older men about screening for osteoporosis. It is also important to focus health education on older adults who already have had fractures because secondary prevention measures are often overlooked. See Online Learning Activity 22-4 for additional information about prevention and treatment of osteoporosis, including health education materials for multicultural communities.

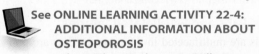

See ONLINE LEARNING ACTIVITY 22-4: ADDITIONAL INFORMATION ABOUT OSTEOPOROSIS at http://thepoint.lww.com/Miller7e

> ### Wellness Opportunity
>
> Promoting self-care practices to prevent osteoporosis is particularly important when teaching older adults who have a history of falls or fractures.

Health education includes information about risk factors with emphasis on developing a plan to address the modifiable risk factors. Nurses can encourage older adults with risk factors to ask their primary care practitioner about screening tests and interventions. All adults can benefit from lifestyle interventions for osteoporosis, and teaching about these self-care activities is well within the realm of nursing responsibilities. Important self-care interventions for osteoporosis include daily weight-bearing activities, quitting smoking and limiting alcohol intake.

Nurses can also teach older adults and their caregivers about the importance of adequate intake of calcium and

A Student's Perspective

This past week, I chose to do the water aerobics with the older adults at the health and fitness centre. I was encouraged by the vitality and general zest for life that these older women showed. I was enlightened by their sense of pride in their health and level of activity. I left with the impression that this group activity was something that each of them attributed her good health to. I also noted that they got more out of this activity than just physical exercise. The social connection that these women had was truly admirable. They were constantly encouraging each other and me during the class. They also used the time just to connect with each other and discuss normal life events.

My take-away lesson from this experience was the importance of having opportunities like this for older adults to exercise their muscles as well as their social personalities. Older adults are often portrayed as socially inferior in today's popular culture, but I felt these older women were living truly balanced lives, maybe more so than me in some respects. I think that often I find myself so busy that I do not take time to invest myself in more meaningful relationships—something that these people are obviously benefiting from.

Clint H.

vitamin D. The new guidelines for vitamin D recommend daily supplements of 400 to 1,000 IU for adults below age 50 without osteoporosis or conditions affecting vitamin D absorption. For adults above 50, supplements of between 800 and 2,000 IU are recommended (Health Canada, 2012). A registered dietitian, if available, can evaluate a food journal to determine the usual intake of calcium and vitamin D. If intake does not provide at least 1,000 to 1,200 mg of calcium and 800 to 2,000 international units of vitamin D, then health teaching focuses either on increasing dietary intake to the recommended amount or on taking a daily supplement. In long-term care facilities, all care plans should include a review of nutritional interventions for osteoporosis, particularly in relation to preventing fractures. Nurses can take the lead in involving dietitians and primary care providers in developing and implementing appropriate preventive interventions. Box 22-5 summarizes health promotion information that can be used as a guide for teaching older adults about osteoporosis.

A major goal of pharmacologic interventions for osteoporosis is prevention of osteoporotic fractures, which are associated with serious consequences, including chronic pain, decreased quality of life and significant morbidity and mortality. In recent years, many types of medications have been approved for prevention of fragility fractures, which are in addition to the menopausal hormonal therapy that was widely used until the mid-1990s. A systematic review of 567 clinical studies published between 2005 and 2011 identified the following pharmaceutical agents as effective for preventing fragility fractures in postmenopausal women with

Box 22-5 Health Promotion Teaching About Osteoporosis

Health Promotion Interventions for Early Detection and Treatment

- Review risk factors for osteoporosis as summarized in Box 22-1.
- Plan interventions for modifiable risk factors using Boxes 22-1 and 22-3 as guides.
- Encourage discussion with the primary care provider about bone density tests.
- Encourage discussion with the primary care provider about medical interventions for osteoporosis if risk factors are present.
- Encourage discussion with the primary care provider about prevention of fractures if osteoporosis is diagnosed.

Lifestyle Interventions

- Implement weight-bearing exercise regimen for one-half hour daily.
- Engage in activities such as yoga, swimming, massage, acupressure and tai chi.
- Wear supportive shoes.
- Discontinue cigarette smoking.
- Maintain ideal body weight.
- Avoid excessive alcohol intake.

Nutritional Interventions

- A daily intake of at least 1,000 mg of calcium from food sources is recommended, rather than using calcium supplements that may have adverse effects.
- Foods that are high in calcium include milk, cheese, yogurt, custard, ice cream, raisins, tofu, canned salmon or sardines, and broccoli and other dark green vegetables.
- If a higher dose of calcium is required, for example for osteoporosis, this should be under the direction of a primary care practitioner.
- Provide adequate dietary intake of vitamin D and use supplement if needed to assure daily intake of at least 800 to 1,000 IU vitamin D.
- People with low serum vitamin D levels may require higher daily doses, which should be taken under the direction of a primary care practitioner.

osteoporosis (Agency for Health care Research and Quality Effective Health Care Program, 2012):

- Biphosphonates: alendronate (Fosamax), risedronate (Actonel), zoledronic acid (Zometa), ibandronate (Boniva)
- Denosumab (Xgeva, Prolia)
- Menopausal hormone therapy (e.g., Premarin)
- Raloxifene (Evista)
- Parathyroid hormone (e.g., Teriparatide)

It is important to note that all these medications reduced incidence of vertebral fractures; however, the only ones that reduced the risk for hip fracture were alendronate, risedronate, zoledronic acid and denosumab. Because all these medications are associated with various adverse effects, including serious ones, such as thromboembolic events and increased risk for breast cancer, it is imperative to advise older women to discuss the benefits and risks with their primary care practitioners so they can make informed decisions about this important preventive intervention.

Because most clinical trials of medical interventions for osteoporosis focus primarily on women, much less evidence is available about safe and effective pharmacologic treatments for men with the disease. On the basis of a systematic review of studies, the Endocrine Society Task Force on Osteoporosis in Men (Watts et al., 2012) recommended that men at high risk for fracture be treated with one of the following medications: alendronate, risedronate, zoledronic acid or parathyroid hormone. The Task Force emphasized that selection of a pharmaceutical agent should be individualized on the basis of factors such as fracture history, severity of osteoporosis and risk for hip fracture.

In summary, there is sound evidence that pharmacologic treatment of osteoporosis can improve bone density, reduce the rate of bone loss and decrease the risk for fragility fractures, including hip fracture. Evidence is less clear about pharmacologic interventions for older adults who do not have osteoporosis, but have risks for it. Decisions about preventive pharmacologic interventions for people at risk for osteoporosis and fractures must be based on an appraisal of the relative risks and benefits of any particular intervention. Pharmacologic treatment is just one component of a comprehensive management plan that must also include nutritional intake of calcium and vitamin D, physical activity to maintain musculoskeletal function and reduce the risk of falls, and patient education regarding osteoporosis and fall prevention. Use Online Learning Activity 22-5 for current evidence-based information related to osteoporosis and other aspects of musculoskeletal wellness.

See ONLINE LEARNING ACTIVITY 22-5: RESOURCES FOR HEALTH PROMOTION MATERIALS RELATED TO MUSCULOSKELETAL WELLNESS
at http://thepoint.lww.com/Miller7e

Preventing Falls and Fall-Related Injuries

Because falls are multifaceted in their causes, they are best addressed through interprofessional fall-preventions programs that address conditions in a particular setting and those factors that are unique to each at-risk person. Comprehensive programs focus not only on reducing fall episodes but also on preventing fall-related injuries if a fall does occur. Key aspects of fall-prevention programs in institutional settings are the identification of people who are at risk for falls and the consistent implementation of preventive actions by all staff. Thus, an important part of these programs is the education of all professional and nonprofessional staff members who have contact with the person who is at risk for falls. Education may involve strategies to heighten staff awareness of the importance of reducing fall risks. For example, posters and brochures may be used initially and periodically as reminders. Also, some form of patient/resident or chart identification can be used to draw attention to those people who have an increased risk for falls. Box 22-6 describes a fall-prevention program that could be adapted for use in institutional settings, and Box 22-7 summarizes evidence-based recommendations related to preventing falls in community-dwelling older adults.

Unfolding Case Study

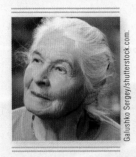

Galushko Sergey/shutterstock.com.

Part 4: Ms. M. at 79 Years of Age

Recall that you are the nurse at the wellness program where Ms. M., now 79 years old, regularly attends your health education programs. On the basis of additional assessment information, you know that Ms. M. does not take any calcium or vitamin D supplements because she drinks milk twice daily and believes that this should be sufficient. She stopped having menstrual periods when she was 50 years old and began hormonal therapy a few years later. She stopped taking estrogen when she was in her mid-60s because she began "hearing too many bad things about estrogen." Ms. M. fractured her wrist 4 years ago when she reached her arms out to diminish the impact of a fall. At that time, orthopedic surgeon said that her x-rays showed that her "bones were a little thin but not bad for her age." She has not had any further x-rays or any bone density tests and says her primary care practitioner has never brought up the subject of osteoporosis because "I guess he's too worried about my heart problems to be concerned about my bones." Although she fell once when she was raking leaves last fall and tripped over a small tree stump, she has had no serious fall-related injuries since she fractured her wrist. She does not smoke and drinks alcohol only on major social occasions. When you assessed her blood pressure, you found that her blood pressure while standing was 146/86 mm Hg and while reclining was 128/78 mm Hg. Her record of self-monitored blood pressure readings indicates that her usual blood pressure is around 134/82 mm Hg. Her vision is adequate, but she has stopped driving at night and is being monitored by her ophthalmologist for progression of bilateral cataracts. Her eye doctor told her that she is likely to need cataract surgery sometime during the next 2 to 3 years.

THINKING POINTS

- What further assessment information would you want to have?
- What health promotion interventions would you advise for Ms. M.? Specifically, what health teaching would you do with regard to further assessment, lifestyle interventions, nutrition and nutritional supplements and pharmacologic interventions?
- What educational materials would you use for Ms. M.?
- What follow-up health promotion would you consider for Ms. M.? Specifically, how would you work with Ms. M. to develop lifelong health promotion interventions?

QSEN APPLICATION

QSEN Competency	Knowledge/Skill/Attitude	Application to Ms. M. at 79 Years
Patient-centred care	(K) Integrate understanding of multiple dimensions of patient-centred care.	Use information in Boxes 22-2 and 22-3 to identify conditions that increase the risk for falls and fractures.
	(K) Describe strategies to empower patients in all aspects of the health care process.	Use effective communication skills to explore Ms. M.'s willingness to address risks.
	(S) Elicit patient values, preferences and expressed needs.	
Evidence-based practice	(K) Describe how the strength and relevance of available evidence influence the choice of intervention.	Use Online Learning Activities 22-4 and 22-5 to find additional evidence-based information related to management of osteoporosis and prevention of fractures.
	(S) Read original research and evidence reports related to clinical practice.	Teach Ms. M. about evidence-based interventions for osteoporosis as summarized in Box 22-5.
	(A)Value evidence-based practice as integral to determining the best clinical practice.	

Box 22-6 A Fall-Prevention Program for Older Adults Being Cared for in Hospitals or Nursing Homes

Identification of Patients/Residents Who Are at Risk for Falling

- Use a nursing judgment and a fall risk assessment tool to identify any risks for falling and fall-related injuries (e.g., medications, osteoporosis, medical conditions, history of falls, impaired cognition, diminished alertness, impaired mobility, age 75 years or older).
- Document the risk factors on the designated fall assessment guide.
- Use an interprofessional approach to address any risk factors for falls, osteoporosis or fall-related injuries.
- Frequently reassess the risks for falls and fall-related injuries at predetermined times (e.g., every shift, every day, whenever there is a change in the patient's/resident's functional status).
- Use colour-coded items (e.g., brightly coloured stickers for the chart, a brightly coloured wrist band, signs near the person's bed and outside the room) to identify those who are included in the fall-prevention program.

Education of the Staff, Patient/Resident and Family

- Instruct the patient or resident and family about the fall-prevention program and provide written information about preventing falls and obtaining help if falls occur.
- Provide staff education about the fall-prevention program and the risk factors for falls, especially those factors that the staff influences (e.g., use of restraints, selection of footwear).

- Use posters and fliers to heighten staff awareness of the fall-prevention program.

Interventions to Be Implemented for All High-Risk Patients/Residents

- Keep the call light within reach at all times.
- Respond quickly to calls for assistance.
- Assess toileting needs at frequent intervals.
- Make sure that ambulatory patients wear sturdy, nonslip footwear when out of bed.
- Offer assistance with activities of daily living (ADLs) and try to anticipate the person's needs before help is needed.
- Encourage the person to call for help when needed.
- Assure close monitoring and frequently checks for all patients/residents who cannot be relied on to call for help.
- Make sure the bed is in the lowest position possible and the wheels are locked.
- Carefully and frequently assess the environment for factors that increase the risk for either falls or fall-related injuries; address all modifiable risk factors.
- Consider the use of a movement-detection device.
- Adhere to institutional policies about use of physical restraints, including bedrails.
- If appropriate, orient the person to person, place and time every shift and as needed.
- Document fall-prevention interventions on the person's chart.

Box 22-7 Evidence-Based Practice: Preventing Falls in Older Adults in Community Settings

Statement of the Problem

- About 30% of community-dwelling older adults fall each year.
- Many studies in recent years have identified evidence-based interventions that are effective for reducing falls, risks for falls and fall-related injuries.

Recommendations for Screening and Assessment

- Ask older adults if they have had a fall during the past year.
- Find out details about circumstances of each fall.
- Ask about gait and balance problems.
- Perform simple test for gait and balance (e.g., Timed Get Up and Go).
- Arrange for multifactorial fall risk assessment including comprehensive physical examination, functional assessment, environmental assessment, medical history and medication review.

Evidence-Based Fall-Prevention Interventions

- Implementation of interventions for individual fall risks identified during multifactorial assessment
- Participation in a multiple component group or home-based exercise program that includes balance, strength and gait-training exercises
- Optimal management of all medical conditions, especially cardiac arrhythmias and postural hypotension
- Modification of prescription medication regimens, including gradual withdrawal of psychotropic medication
- Treatment of vision impairment: cataract surgery as needed, not using multifocal lenses while walking

- Management of foot problems and footwear
- Vitamin D supplementation for people with lower serum vitamin D levels
- Home safety assessment and modification, which is particularly effective for people who are visually impaired and when delivered by an occupational therapist

Recommendations for Nursing Interventions

- Facilitate implementation of applicable evidence-based interventions.
- Teach about recommended level of physical activity for older adults: 2.5 hours of moderate-intensity or 1.25 hours of vigorous-intensity aerobic physical activity every week, plus muscle-strengthening activities twice weekly and balance training 3 or more days per week for those with risks for falls.
- Teach about self-care actions, including using appropriate assistive devices and safety measures (e.g., antislip shoe devices in icy conditions).

Source: American Geriatrics Society and British Geriatrics Society. (2010). *AGS/BGS Clinical Practice Guideline: Prevention of falls in older persons* (guidelines summary NGC-9165). Retrieved from www.ahrq.gov; Gillespie, L. D., Robertson, M. C., Gillespie, W. J., et al. (2012). Interventions for preventing falls in older people living in the community (Review). *Cochrane Database of Systematic Reviews* (9) [Article number CD007614. doi:10.1002/14651858.CD007146.pub3; Public Health Agency of Canada. (2011). *You CAN prevent falls!* Retrieved from http://www.phac-aspc.gc.ca/seniors-aines/publications/public/injury-blessure/prevent-eviter/index-eng.php; U.S. Preventive Services Task Force. (2012). Prevention of falls in community-dwelling older adults: U.S. Preventive Services Task Force recommendation statement. *Annals of Internal Medicine, 157*(3), 197–204.

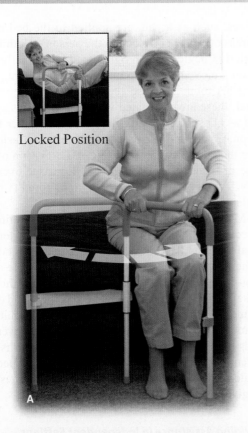

Locked Position

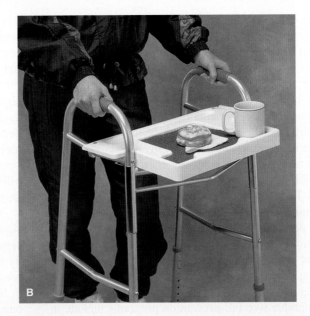

FIGURE 22-3 The use of assistive devices can help reduce the risk of falls. **(A)** Transfer assistive devices are used to facilitate safer transfer in and out of beds. **(B)** Walkers are available in various styles with wheels, brakes, baskets, seats and other features to improve safety and mobility. (Photographs reprinted with permission from ActiveForever.com.)

Addressing Intrinsic Risk Factors

Because any gait and balance impairment increases the risk for falls, interventions that improve mobility are likely to be beneficial in preventing falls. Interventions for improving mobility are implemented primarily by therapists, nurses and nursing staff, often through an interprofessional approach. Teaching about the proper use of mobility aids and other assistive devices (Fig. 22-3) is an important part of fall-prevention programs. Nurses are responsible for raising questions about whether an older adult may benefit from the use of mobility aids or assistive devices and facilitating a referral to a physical therapist for evaluation and teaching. In community settings, nurses can teach older adults and their caregivers about the availability of various mobility aids, transfer assistance devices and other aids that might improve safety. Nurses can suggest that older adults seek professional help with selecting appropriate mobility aids and assistive devices. Home health care equipment supplies have therapists or staff members who can provide advice and assist with processing insurance claims. When mobility aids are prescribed, nursing responsibilities include making sure that the aids are accessible, encouraging the person to use the aids, and facilitating referrals for reassessment if questions arise about the safety or effectiveness of the mobility aids.

Because proper footwear is essential to prevent slips and falls, nurses can advise older adults about wearing nonslip footwear for safety. Walking outdoors can be particularly

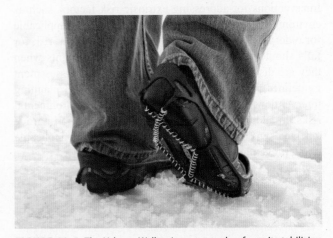

FIGURE 22-4 The Yaktrax Walker is an example of a gait-stabilizing device that can be used to prevent falls on slippery outdoor surfaces. (Photograph reprinted with permission from Yaktrax, LLC.)

hazardous, especially when winter conditions create a dangerous environment for older people who have a predisposition for falls. Nurses can emphasize the importance of removing ice and snow from walkways and help older adults explore resources for assistance with this. For example, a local organization may provide snow removal or outdoor maintenance services at little or no cost. In addition, a simple gait-stabilizing device, such as the Yaktrax Walker (Fig. 22-4), may help prevent outdoor falls when it is applied and worn properly.

In recent years, fall-prevention literature has emphasized the effectiveness of various exercise routines as an intervention for reducing intrinsic fall risk. An important role for nurses is to identify those older adults who may benefit from gait and balance training programs and to facilitate referrals for physical therapy when appropriate. Nurses are also responsible for encouraging adequate and consistent follow-through with recommended exercise programs. In long-term care settings, nurses generally oversee restorative nursing programs in which nursing assistants help residents with walking and other exercise regimens established by physical therapists. These restorative nursing routines are essential aspects of fall-prevention programs. Group exercise programs are also widely used as fall-prevention interventions that are beneficial to all at-risk people. Many programs incorporate exercises aimed specifically at improving gait, balance, ankle strength or other aspects of fall prevention.

Comprehensive fall-prevention programs include interprofessional interventions for specific risks, including pharmacists for addressing medication effects or neurologists for addressing pathologic conditions. If an interprofessional team is not available for a comprehensive approach, nurses have essential roles in identifying appropriate professional resources and facilitating referrals for these services.

Addressing Extrinsic Risk Factors

Interventions for addressing extrinsic risk factors, such as environmental conditions and use of restraints, are applicable for older adults in any setting. Patients who are at risk for falls should receive referrals for home assessments when they are discharged from hospitals. The safety assessment guidelines provided in Chapter 7 can help with planning interventions that may eliminate or reduce environmental risks. In addition, environmental modifications to improve a person's vision, as discussed in Chapter 17, are applicable to fall prevention.

> **Wellness Opportunity**
>
> Fall-prevention interventions that address the person–environment relationship can be as simple and effective as involving older adults in decisions about removing or replacing slippery throw rugs.

Using Monitoring Devices in Institutional Settings

Monitoring devices can be useful in alerting staff to potentially unsafe patient/resident movement; however, concerns have been raised about the overuse and negative consequences of some types of devices. All monitoring devices contain a mechanism for transmitting a signal to a remote location (e.g., a nursing station) when activated by certain levels of patient/resident movement. Some devices, such as a pad, are applied to the bed or chair, whereas others are attached to the person's clothing. Less restrictive devices are programmed specifically for the person's movement in a confined environment, such as his or her room. Because alarm-type devices emit a loud signal, these are associated with negative consequences, such as (1) staff responding to the alarm rather than the person, (2) disruptive noise, which can be confusing when more than one alarm is sounding, (3) provision of a false sense of security for staff and (4) decreased overall mobility for the person who is being monitored (Crogan & Dupler, 2014).

Most movement-detection devices were originally designed for institutional use, but simplified monitoring and signal systems have now been developed for home use by family caregivers. In home settings, a simple auditory room-monitoring device (i.e., a "baby room monitor") may be useful when caregivers need to detect the sound of someone moving around in another room. A major limitation of any movement-detection device is that its effectiveness depends on the timely response of someone who is able to prevent the fall. These devices are not useful for people living alone or for people without responsible and responsive caregivers.

Providing Assistance in Independent Settings

For people living alone and at risk for falls, it is important to consider interventions for summoning help in a timely manner if falls occur. Many types of **personal emergency response systems** are available, and these involve the use of a small portable transmitter that is worn on the person's body or clothing. Fig. 22-5 illustrates one example of a commonly used personal emergency response system. When the person falls, he or she can summon help by using the transmitter to signal a receiver unit attached to the telephone. In turn, a call is automatically made to the personal emergency response system provider, who then checks in with the person on a speaker-phone system and calls the local emergency response team or a contact person, such as a neighbour or family member if the person needs help. Some of these devices are set up so that a monitoring call is made to the person once a day if the person does not push a reset button or otherwise notify the company that he or she is well.

The effectiveness of personal emergency response system depends on the ability of the fallen person to signal for help and on the availability of a helping person. A major limitation of such devices is that cognitively impaired people may not be able to learn to use them. Hospitals, home care agencies and local senior organizations provide information about local personal emergency response system programs, and information about national programs is available on the Internet. Cordless phones, especially if preprogrammed for emergency help and placed within

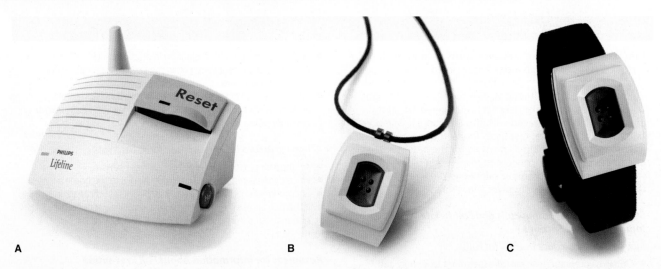

A   **B**   **C**

FIGURE 22-5 Example of a personal emergency response system receiver with **(A)** white "box," **(B)** necklace and **(C)** bracelet. (Used with permission from Philips Respironics.)

reach where someone might fall, can also be used for obtaining help.

Preventing Fall-Related Injuries

When falls cannot be prevented, interventions are directed toward reducing the risk of fractures and other serious fall-related injuries. Two interventions for preventing fall-related injuries that should be used for people who are at risk for falls are (1) to implement evidence-based measures for osteoporosis (discussed previously) and (2) to adapt the environment as much as possible to reduce the risk for fall-related injuries. Heavy furniture that is in a pathway where a fall is likely to occur can be moved out of the way or replaced with items that would move easily if the person falls into them. Also, hard edges of sinks and built-in cabinets can be padded. Particular attention should be paid to padding hard edges of bathroom cabinets and either padding or removing swinging shower doors. Using a bed that can be adjusted to a very low position can reduce risk of injury from falling out of bed. Soft mats can be placed near beds and in other locations where people are likely to fall, but caution must be used so that these pads do not become fall risks.

External hip protectors have been available since the 1990s, and studies conducted during the first decade of their use indicated statistically significant reductions in hip fracture rates; however, conclusions from more recent studies are not as positive. A review of studies published since 2001 concluded that effectiveness of hip protectors in institutional settings remains "obscure," and there is no evidence of clinically significant effectiveness for older adults in community settings (Skorga & Young, 2012).

Finally, it is imperative to recognize that restraints do not necessarily reduce the risk of falls and are associated with more serious fall-related injuries, as already discussed. In recent years, federal regulations have mandated that health care institutions develop policies for restraint reduction or restraint-free care. Evidence-based guidelines emphasize the need for individualized care plans to prevent falls and for education of patients, family members and all caregiving staff members about the concept of restraint-free care as well as fall-prevention measures. Nurses play important roles in decisions about using restraints, as discussed in Chapter 9. Evidence-based practices for prevention of falls in institutional settings are summarized in Box 22-6.

Wellness Opportunity

Health promotion interventions need to be broad and include precautions to minimize the risk of injury if falls do occur.

Addressing Fear of Falling

Any interventions that reduce the risk of falls are also likely to reduce a person's fear of falling, but some people may need additional interventions to address this problem. For example, nurses can address fear of falling in the same way they address other fears: encourage the expression of feelings and provide education and reassurance about interventions that are being implemented as part of an individualized fall-prevention care plan. Family members and caregivers should be included in nursing interventions and health education to address fear of falling. For people living alone, a personal emergency response system may be very reassuring and at least alleviate the fear of being helpless if a fall occurs.

Box 22-8 Caregiver Wellness

Family caregivers often experience stress because their older relative desires to remain independent even though he or she is at risk for falls, has already had a fall or even is a "frequent faller." In these situations, caregivers weigh the right of the older adult to take risks versus the need for safety and protection. When faced with this situation, it is important to use professional resources for promoting as safe and independent functioning as possible for the older person and peace of mind for concerned relatives. Implementing some strategies that promote safety and prevent injuries and thereby help to relieve caregiver stress follow.

Strategies for Preventing Falls and Fall-Related Injuries in Home Settings

Interventions to Reduce the Risk for Falls

- Obtain a comprehensive fall risk assessment to identify and address risks related to medical conditions, medication effects and functional limitations.
- Obtain ophthalmologic evaluation to assure optimal visual function (e.g., cataract surgery may improve safety).
- Arrange for a home visit by a physical therapist or other qualified professional to identify and address environmental risks.
- Modify the home for safety by installing grab bars, handrails, good lighting and other appropriate modifications for safe and independent mobility.

Actions to Promote Safe and Independent Functioning

- Arrange for occupational and physical therapy evaluations and recommendations for assistive devices, home modification for safety and therapeutic exercises.

- Encourage frequent participation in enjoyable and beneficial physical activity programs, such as dancing, tai chi and water exercises.
- Encourage the person to engage in home-based physical activity by using videos, Wii Fit and simple exercise equipment; consider doing these activities with them.

Actions to Assure Timely Response for Assistance

- Arrange for personal emergency response system.
- Place cordless phones in strategic locations in the home.
- Encourage the person to keep a cell phone handy at all times.
- If the person has memory problems, frequently remind him or her about the importance of calling for help when needed.

Resources for Information About Fall Prevention in Home Settings

- Centre for Hip Health and Mobility, http://www.hiphealth .ca/en/Canada Mortgage and Housing Corporation, http:// www.cmhc-schl.gc.ca/en/co/acho/acho_012.cfm
- National Center for Patient Safety Falls Toolkit, www.patientsafety. va.gov/Safey/Topics/fallstoolkit/index.html
- Simon Fraser University Technology for Injury Prevention in Seniors (TIPS) program, http://www.sfu.ca/tips
- For resources in Chinese and Punjabi, access http://www2.gov .bc.ca/gov/topic.page?id=7025C57E37BD4C038EB01C92D81 B3F27

Promoting Caregiver Wellness

In home and community settings, preventing falls and fall-related injuries are major responsibilities for caregivers of people who have risks for falls or a history of falls. This responsibility can significantly increase the stress for families as they try to balance the desire of the older adult to have privacy and independence against the risk of the person falling and incurring significant, or even fatal, injuries. Nurses working in home care settings often address this issue and weigh the responsibility to respect autonomy versus the responsibility to assure safety. Information in Chapters 9 and 10 is applicable to ethical issues when working with caregivers to address these questions.

On the practical side, nurses can address caregiver stress related to their concerns about falls by arranging for an interprofessional approach to risk assessment and interventions for preventing falls and fall-related injuries. These assessments are available at outpatient geriatric assessment programs and through skilled home care agencies for people

who are homebound. Nurses also can teach caregivers about fall-prevention strategies and resources for additional information, as described in Box 22-8.

EVALUATING EFFECTIVENESS OF NURSING INTERVENTIONS

Nursing care for older adults with impaired musculoskeletal function is evaluated by the degree to which the person achieves and maintains the highest possible level of independence and safe mobility. Nursing care of older adults who are at high risk for osteoporosis is evaluated according to the degree to which the older adult incorporates preventive measures in his or her daily life. For example, older adults might begin a regimen of three half-hour periods of weight-bearing exercise weekly. The nursing care of older adults who are at high risk for falls and fall-related injuries is evaluated according to the extent to which falls and serious injuries are prevented. Nurses cannot, of course, measure the number of falls that do not occur, but they can measure the risk factors that have been addressed in the care plan. Evaluation of these risk factors is facilitated by careful documentation of interventions, such as environmental modifications and fall-prevention programs.

Unfolding Case Study

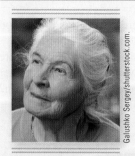

Galushko Sergey/shutterstock.com.

Part 5: Ms. M. at 89 Years of Age

Ms. M. is now 89 years old and has been admitted to the hospital for heart failure. Additional diagnoses include arthritis, osteoporosis, recurrent depression, early-stage dementia and history of fractured wrist at age 75 and fractured hip 3 years ago. Current medications include furosemide (Lasix), 40 mg twice daily; enalapril (Vasotec), 10 mg twice daily; alendronate (Fosamax), 70 mg; Os-Cal with D; and sertraline (Zoloft), 50 mg at bedtime. Ms. M. lives alone in an assisted-living facility, where she receives help with her medications and goes to the dining room for meals. You are the nurse on the acute care floor assigned to her care on the day of admission.

NURSING ASSESSMENT

During your initial nursing assessment, Ms. M. is quiet and withdrawn. When you ask about her living situation, she says she moved to the assisted-living facility after the hospitalization and rehabilitation for her fractured hip. At the time of the injury, she had been living alone. She had fallen while making her way to the bathroom at night and remained lying on the floor until her daughter came to visit her the next morning. During the past year, Ms. M. reports that she has fallen twice in the assisted-living facility, but that she has been able to call for help and has not had any serious injuries. You determine that Ms. M. will need help in ambulating to the bathroom and that she should be supervised whenever she gets out of bed.

Ms. M. confides that she is worried that she will have to move to the nursing home section of her facility if she falls again. She is very depressed about her lack of energy and her hospitalization for heart failure. A mental status assessment indicates that Ms. M. is alert and oriented but that her short-term memory is impaired. She has a great deal of difficulty with abstract ideas, such as learning to use the call button. You check her vital signs, which are within normal range, with no evidence of postural hypotension.

NURSING DIAGNOSIS

In addition to the nursing diagnoses related to Ms. M.'s medical condition, you identify a nursing diagnosis of Risk for Falls. Related factors include a history of falls and fractures, weakness, diuretic and cardiovascular medications, depression and impaired cognition. You are concerned about preventing falls during her hospitalization.

Nursing Care Plan for Ms. M.

Nursing Evaluation	Expected Outcome	Nursing Interventions
Ms. M. will ambulate safely and avoid falls during her hospitalization.	• Identify Ms. M. as a participant in the fall-prevention program by using an orange wrist bracelet, posting a Fall Alert sign near her bed and placing an orange Fall Alert sticker on her chart. • Provide Ms. M. with a brochure that explains the fall-prevention program. • Reassess fall risks every shift and document these on the Fall Assessment form included in Ms. M.'s chart. • Talk with Ms. M.'s physician about a referral for physical therapy. • Keep the call light button within her reach and review instructions for its use every shift. • Assess benefits and risks of using bedrails, and discuss these with Ms. M. and her family. • Make sure that the bed is in the lowest possible position with the wheels locked. • Use a movement-detection bed pad and explain to Ms. M. that the purpose of the pad is to ensure that the staff knows when she needs to get out of bed. • Every 2 hours, when Ms. M. is awake, the nursing staff will ask her if she needs to go to the bathroom.	• Ms. M. will receive assistance with ambulation every time she is out of bed. • Ms. M. will not fall during her hospitalization.

THINKING POINTS

- If you were the nurse on the acute care floor where Ms. M. was a patient, what concerns would you address in a discharge plan? Would you identify any additional nursing diagnoses related to safe mobility and musculoskeletal function? What additional nursing interventions would you plan to supplement this care plan that is focused on preventing falls during Ms. M.'s hospitalization?

- If you were a nurse in the assisted-living facility where Ms. M. lives, what concerns would you have about her care? How would you address these concerns in a care plan?

QSEN APPLICATION

QSEN Competency	Knowledge/Skill/Attitude	Application to Ms. M. at 89 Years
Patient-centred care	(K) Integrate understanding of multiple dimensions of patient-centred care. (K) Examine common barriers to active involvement of patients in their own health care processes. (S) Elicit patient values, preferences and expressed needs. (S) Provide patient-centred care with sensitivity and respect for diversity of the human experience. (S) Communicate care provided and needed at each transition in care. (A) Value seeing health care situations "through patients' eyes."	Use fall risk assessment tool and additional assessment information from Box 22-3 to develop fall-prevention interventions on the basis of identified needs. Use effective communication skills to explore psychosocial factors that influence Ms. M.'s current health situation. Identify interventions to assure continuity of care when Ms. M. is discharged.
Teamwork and collaboration	(K) Describe scopes of practice and role of health care team members. (K) Recognize contributions of other individuals and groups in helping patient achieve health goals. (S) Integrate the contributions of others who play a role in helping patient achieve health goals.	Facilitate referral for physical therapy to address fall risks. Facilitate referral for social worker to address psychosocial needs. Talk with primary care practitioner and social worker about a referral for comprehensive geriatric assessment services for assessing fall risk and mental status, either during hospitalization or after Ms. M. is discharged.

Chapter Highlights

Age-Related Changes That Affect Mobility and Safety

- Degenerative changes in bones, muscles, joints and connective tissue
- Central nervous system changes: slowed reactions time, body sway
- Diminished bone density (i.e., osteopenia and osteoporosis)

Risk Factors That Affect Mobility and Safety

- Risk factors for impaired musculoskeletal function: physical inactivity, nutritional deficits (e.g., low intake of foods high in calcium and vitamin D)
- Risk factors for osteoporosis and fractures: lack of weight-bearing activity, increased age, tobacco smoking, excessive alcohol consumption, certain medications (e.g., corticosteroids) (Box 22-1)
- Risk factors for falls: pathologic conditions and functional and cognitive impairments, medication effects, environmental factors, physical restraints (Box 22-2)

Pathologic Condition Affecting Musculoskeletal Wellness: Osteoarthritis

- Osteoarthritis

Functional Consequences Affecting Musculoskeletal Wellness

- Diminished muscle strength, endurance and coordination
- Increased difficulty performing ADLs
- Increased susceptibility to falls

- Increased susceptibility to fractures and other fall-related injuries
- Fear of falling

Nursing Assessment of Musculoskeletal Function (Box 22-3)

- Assessing overall musculoskeletal performance (Fig. 22-1)
- Identifying risks for osteoporosis
- Assessing for safety of the environment
- Using fall risk assessment tools (Fig. 22-2)

Nursing Diagnosis

- Wellness nursing diagnosis: Readiness for Enhanced Self-Health Management
- Related to fall risks: Impaired Physical Mobility, Risk for Falls, Ineffective Health Maintenance

Planning for Wellness Outcomes

- Balance, Endurance, Mobility, Activity Tolerance
- Risk Control, Risk Detection
- Fall-Prevention Behaviour
- Safe Home Environment, Safe Health Care Environment

Nursing Interventions for Musculoskeletal Wellness

- Promoting healthy musculoskeletal function
- Teaching about osteoporosis (e.g., early detection and treatment, lifestyle interventions, nutritional interventions, medications) (Box 22-5)
- Preventing falls and fall-related injuries by addressing intrinsic and extrinsic risk factors in institutional and community settings (Boxes 22-6 and 22-7, Figs. 22-3 and 22-4)
- Using monitoring devices in institutional settings and personal emergency response systems in home settings (Fig. 22-5)
- Addressing fear of falling
- Promoting caregiver wellness (Box 22-8)

Evaluating Effectiveness of Nursing Interventions

- Maintenance of highest level of safe mobility
- Incorporation of preventive measures in daily life to ensure safety and prevent osteoporosis
- Expressed feelings of safety and improved quality of life

Critical Thinking Exercises

1. Identify factors that increase or reduce the risk for osteoporosis.
2. Describe how each of the following age-related changes or risk factors might increase an older person's risk for falls and fractures: nocturia, osteoporosis, medications, altered gait, pathologic conditions, sensory impairments, cognitive impairments, functional impairments, slowed reaction time.
3. Describe the environmental factors that you would assess, in both home and institutional settings, to identify potential risks for falls.
4. Describe how you would design and implement a fall-prevention program in a long-term care facility.
5. How would you deal with a daughter who demanded that restraints be used whenever her 84-year-old mother, who is a patient on your acute care floor, is sitting in a chair?
6. What information would you include in health education about osteoporosis?
7. Use the Internet to find information about fall-prevention products that you might use in clinical practice.

 For more information about topics discussed in this chapter, be sure to check out the interactive Online Learning Activities and other helpful resources at http://thepoint.lww.com/Miller7e

REFERENCES

Aartolahti, E., Hakkinen, A., Lonnroos, E., et al. (2013, September 4). Relationship between functional vision and balance and mobility performance in community-dwelling older adults. *Aging Clinical and Experimental Research, 25,* 545–552.

Abreu, M., & Hartley, G. (2013). The effects of salsa dance on balance, gait, and fall risk in a sedentary patient with Alzheimer's dementia, multiple comorbidities, and recurrent falls. *Journal of Geriatric Physical Therapy, 36*(2), 100–107.

Agency for Healthcare Research and Quality. (2012). *Guideline synthesis: Screening and risk assessment for osteoporosis.* Retrieved from www.guideline.gov/syntheses/printView.aspx?id=38658

Agency for Healthcare Research and Quality Effective Health Care Program. (2012). *Clinical research summary: Muscle, bone, and joint conditions: Osteoporosis* (Publication no. 12-EHC023-3). Retrieved from www.effectivehealthcare.ahrq.gov/lbd.cfm

Akesson, K., Marsh, D., Mitchell, P. J., et al. (2013). Capture the fracture: A Best Practice Framework and global campaign to break the fragility fracture cycle. *Osteoporosis International, 24,* 2135–2152.

Berry, S. D., Lee, Y., Cai, S., et al. (2013a). Non-benzodiazepine sleep medications and hip fractures in nursing home residents. *Journal of the American Medical Association Internal Medicine, 173*(9), 754–761.

Berry, S. D., Zhu, Y., Choi, H., et al. (2013b). Diuretic initiation and the acute risk of hip fracture. *Osteoporosis International, 24*(2), 689–695.

Bogoch, E. R., Elliot-Gibson, V., Wang, R. Y., et al. (2012). Secondary causes of osteoporosis in fracture patients. *Journal of Orthopedic Trauma, 26*(9), e145–e152.

Chen, T. Y., Peronto, C. L., & Edwards, J. D. (2012). Cognitive function as a prospective predictor of falls. *Journals of Gerontology: Psychological Sciences and Social Sciences, 67*(6), 720–728.

Connors, K. A., Galea, M. P., & Said, C. M. (2011). Feldenkrais method balance classes improve balance in older adults: A controlled trial. *Evidence-Based Complementary and Alternative Medicine, 2011,* 1–9. doi:10.1093/ecam/nep055

Costa-Dias, M. J., Oliveira, A. S., Martins, T., et al. (2013). Medication fall risk in old hospitalized patients: A retrospective study. *Nurse Education Today, 34*(2), 171–176. doi:10.1016/j.nedt.2013.05.016

Crogan, N. L., & Dupler, A. E. (2014). Quality improvement in nursing homes. *Journal of Nursing Care Quality, 29*(1), 60–65.

Damian, J., Pastor-Barriuso, R., Valderrama-Gama, E., et al. (2013). Factors associated with falls among older adults living in institutions. *BioMed Central Geriatrics, 13*(1), 6. doi:10.1186/1471-2318-13-6

Davies, P. S. (2011). New developments in the treatment of osteoarthritis: A focus on women. *Pain Management Nursing, 12*(1), S17–S22.

Deandrea, S., Bravi, F., Turati, F., et al. (2013). Risk factors for falls in older people in nursing homes and hospitals: A systematic review and meta-analysis. *Archives of Gerontology and Geriatrics, 56*(3), 407–415. doi:10.1016/j.archger.2012.12.006

Dow, B., Meyer, C., Moore, K. J., et al. (2013). The impact of care recipient falls on caregivers. *Australian Health Review, 37*(2), 162–157.

Freeland, K. N., Thompson, A. N., Zhao, Y., et al. (2012). Medication use and associated risk of falling in geriatric outpatient population. *Annals of Pharmacotherapeutics, 46*(9), 1188–1192.

Frost, S. A., Nguyen, N. D., Center, J. R., et al. (2013). Excess mortality attributable to hip-fracture: A relative survival analysis. *Bone, 56*(1), 23–29.

Gill, T. M., Murphy, T. E., Gahbauer, E. A., et al. (2013). Association of injurious falls with disability outcomes and nursing home admission in community-living older persons. *American Journal of Epidemiology, 178*(3), 418–425.

Granacher, U., Muehlbauer, T., Bridenbaugh, S. A., et al. (2012). Effects of salsa dance training on balance and strength performance in older adults. *Gerontology, 58*(4), 305–312.

Gray-Miceli, D., & Quigley, P. A. (2012). Fall prevention: Assessment, diagnoses, and intervention strategies. In M. Boltz, E. Capezuti, T. Fulmer, et al. (Eds.), *Evidence-based practice protocols for best practice* (4th ed., pp. 268–297). New York, NY: Springer.

Hackney, M. E., Hall, C. D., Echt, K. V., et al. (2013) Dancing for balance: Feasibility and efficacy in oldest-old adults with visual impairment. *Nursing Research, 62*(2), 138–143.

Health Canada. (2012). *Vitamin D and calcium: Updated dietary reference intakes*. Retrieved from http://www.hc-sc.gc.ca/fn-an/nutrition/vitamin/vita-d-eng.php

Herdman, T. H. (Ed.). (2012). *NANDA International Nursing Diagnoses: Definitions and classification 2012–1014*. Oxford, England: Wiley-Blackwell.

Herrera, A., Lobo-Escolar, A., Mateo, J., et al. (2012). Male osteoporosis: A review. *World Journal of Orthopedics, 3*(12), 223–234.

Houston, D. K., Neiberg, R. H., Tooze, J. A., et al. (2013). Low 25-hydroxyvitamin D predicts onset of mobility limitation and disability in community-dwelling older adults: The Health ABC Study. *Journals of Gerontology: Biological Sciences and Medical Sciences, 68*(2), 181–187.

Huang, W.-N., Chi, W.-C., Hu, L.-J., (2013). Associations between fear of falling and functional balance in older adults. *International Journal of Therapy and Rehabilitation, 20*(2), 101–106.

Huang, T. T., Yang, L. H., & Liu, C. Y. (2011). Reducing the fear of falling among community-dwelling elderly adults through cognitive-behavioural strategies and intense tai chi exercise: A randomized controlled trial. *Journal of Advances in Nursing, 67*(5), 961–971.

International Osteoporosis Foundation. (2012). *Capture the fracture*. Retrieved from www.iofbonehealth.org

Kearney, F. C., Harwood, R. H., Gladman, J. R., et al. (2013). The relationship between executive function and falls and gait abnormalities in older adults: A systematic review. *Dementia, Geriatrics, and Cognitive Disorders, 36*(1–2), 20–35.

Kim, S., & So, W. Y. (2013). Prevalence and correlates of fear of falling in Korean community-dwelling elderly subjects. *Experimental Gerontology, 48*(11), 1323–1328. doi:10.1016/j.exger.2013.08.015

Ko, A., Van Nguyen, H., Chan, L., et al. (2012). Developing a self-reported tool on fall risk based on toileting responses on in-hospital falls. *Geriatric Nursing, 33*(1), 9–16.

Lach, H. W., & Parsons, J. L. (2013). Impact of fear of falling in long-term care: An integrative review. *Journal of the American Medical Directors Association, 14*(8), 573–577.

Lauche, R., Langhorst, J., Dobos, G., et al. (2013). A systematic review and meta-analysis of tai chi for osteoarthritis of the knee. *Complementary Therapies in Medicine, 21*(4), 396–406.

Lamis, R. L., Kramer, J. S., Hale, L. S., et al. (2012). Fall risk associated with inpatient medications. *American Journal of Health Systems Pharmacy, 69*(1), 1888–1894.

Luo, H., Lin, M., & Castle, N. (2011). Physical restraint use and falls in nursing homes: A comparison between residents with and without dementia. *American Journal of Alzheimer's Disease and Other Dementias, 26*(1), 44–50.

Manini, T. M., Hong, S. L., & Clark, B. C. (2013). Aging and muscle: A neuron's perspective. *Current Opinion in Clinical Nutrition, 16*, 21–26.

Manor, B., Lipsitz, L. A., Wayne, P. M., et al. (2013). Complexity-based measures inform tai chi's impact on standing postural control in older adults with peripheral neuropathy. *BioMed Central Complementary and Alternative Medicine, 13*(1), 87. doi:10.1186/1472-6882-13-87

Martin, K. L., Blizzard, V. K., Srikanth, V. K., et al. (2013). Cognitive function modifies the effects of physiological function on the risk of multiple falls: A population-based study. *Journals of Gerontology: Biological Sciences and Medical Sciences, 68*(9), 1091–1097.

McAuley, E., Wojcicki, T. R., Gothe, N. P., et al. (2013). Effects of a DVD-delivered exercise intervention on physical function in older adults. *Journals of Gerontology: Biological Sciences and Medical Sciences, 68*(9), 1076–1082.

McClung, M. R. (2012). Revisiting the prevention of bone loss at menopause. *Menopause: The Journal of the North American Menopause Society, 19*(11), 1173–1175.

Mithal, A., Bonjour, J. P., Boonen, S., et al. (2013). Impact of nutrition on muscle mass, strength, and performance in older adults. *Osteoporosis International, 24*(5), 1555–1566.

Moskowitz, R. W. (2013). The 2012 ACR guidelines for osteoarthritis: Not a cookbook. *Cleveland Clinic Journal of Medicine, 80*(1), 26–32.

Moller, U. O., Midlov, P., Kristensson, J., et al. (2013). Prevalence and predictors of falls and dizziness in people younger and older than 80 years of age—A longitudinal cohort study. *Archives of Gerontology and Geriatrics, 56*, 160–168.

Mosele, M., Coin, A., Manzato, E., et al. (2013). Association between serum 25-hydroxyvitamin D levels, bone geometry, and bone mineral density in healthy older adults. *Journals of Gerontology: Biological Sciences and Medical Sciences, 68*(8), 992–998.

Murphy, K., & Lowe, S. (2013). Improving fall risk assessment in home care: Interdisciplinary use of the Timed Up and Go (TUG). *Home Health care Nurse, 31*(7), 389–396.

Narula, R., Tauseef, M., Ahmad, I. A., et al. (2013). Vitamin D deficiency among postmenopausal women with osteoporosis. *Journal of Clinical and Diagnostic Research, 7*(2), 336–338.

Obayashi, K., Araki, T., Nakamura, K., et al. (2013). Risk of falling and hypnotic drugs: Retrospective study of inpatients. *Drugs in Research and Development, 13*, 159–164.

Olazaran, J., Valle, D., Serra, J. A., et al. (2013). Psychotropic medications and falls in nursing homes: A cross-sectional study. *Journal of the American Medical Directors Association, 14*, 213–217.

Osteoporosis Canada. (2014). *Osteoporosis facts & statistics*. Retrieved from http://www.osteoporosis.ca/osteoporosis-and-you/osteoporosis-facts-and-statistics/

Public Health Agency of Canada. (2014). *Seniors' falls in Canada: Second report*. Retrieved from www.phac-aspc.gc.ca/...falls.../seniors_falls-chutes_aines-eng.pdf

Quach, L., Yang, F. M., Berry, S. D., et al. (2013, July 1). Depression, antidepressants, and falls among community-dwelling elderly people: The MOBILIZE Study. *Journals of Gerontology: Biological Sciences and Medical Sciences, 68*(12), 1575–1581. doi:10.1093/gerona/glt084

Rahman, M. M., Kopec, J. A., Cibere, J., et al. (2013). The relationship between osteoarthritis and cardiovascular disease in a population health survey: A cross-sectional study. *British Medical Journal Open, 3*, e002624. doi:10.1136/bmjopen-2013-002624

Reed-Jones, R. J., Solis, G. R., Lawson, K. A., et al. (2013). Vision and falls: A multidisciplinary review of the contributions of visual impairment to falls among older adults. *Maturitas, 75*(1), 22–28.

Registered Nurses Association of Ontario. (2005). *Prevention of falls and fall injuries in the older adult.* Retrieved from http://rnao.ca/sites/rnao-ca/files/Prevention_of_Falls_and_Fall_Injuries_in_the_Older_Adult.pdf

Reidy, P. T., Walker, D. K., Dickinson, J. M., et al. (2013). Protein blend ingestion following resistance exercise promotes human muscle protein synthesis. *Journal of Nutrition, 143*(4), 410–416.

Rigler, S. K., Shireman, T. I., Cook-Wiens, G. J., et al. (2013). Fracture risk in nursing home residents initiating antipsychotic medications. *Journal of the American Geriatrics Society, 61*(5), 715–722.

Sheldon, J. H. (1960). On the natural history of falls in old age. *British Medical Journal, 2,* 1685–1690.

Shelton, L. R. (2013). A closer look at osteoarthritis. *The Nurse Practitioner, 38*(7), 30–36.

Skorga, P., & Young, C. F. (2012). Hip protectors for preventing hip fractures in older people: A review summary. *Clinical Nurse Specialist, 26*(6), 308–309.

Svejme, O., Ahlborg, H. G., Nilsson, J.-A., et al. (2013). Low BMD is an independent predictor of fracture and early menopause of mortality in post-menopausal women: A 34-year prospective study. *Maturitas, 74,* 341–345.

The Arthritis Society. (n.d.). *Osteoarthritis.* Retrieved from www.arthritis.ca/page.aspx?pid=941

Tajeu, G. S., Delzell, E., Smith, W., et al. (2013). Death, debility, and destitution following hip fracture. *Journals of Gerontology: Biological Sciences and Medical Sciences.* Advance online publication. doi:10.1093/gerona/glt.105

Tiedemann, A., O'Rourke, S., Sesto, R., et al. (2013). A 12-week Iyengar Yoga program improved balance and mobility in older community-dwelling people: A pilot randomized controlled trial. *Journals of Gerontology: Biological Sciences and Medical Sciences, 68*(9), 1068–1075.

Tousignant, M., Corriveau, H., Roy, P. M., et al. (2013). Efficacy of supervised tai chi exercises versus conventional physical therapy exercises in fall prevention for frail older adults: A randomized controlled trial. *Disability and Rehabilitation, 35*(17), 1429–1435.

Tsang, W. W. (2013). Tai chi is effective in reducing balance impairments and falls in patients with Parkinson's disease. *Journal of Physiotherapy, 59*(1), 55.

van Strien, A. M., Koek, H. L., van Marum, R. J., et al. (2013). Psychotropic medications, including short acting benzodiazepines, strongly increase the frequency of falls in elderly. *Maturitas, 74*(4), 357–362.

Watts, N. B., Adler, R. A., Bilezikian, J. P., et al. (2012). Osteoporosis in men: An Endocrine Society clinical practice guideline. *Journal of Endocrinology and Metabolism, 97*(6), 1802–1822.

Wei, G.-X., Xu, T., Fan, F.-M., et al. (2013). Can tai chi reshape the brain? A brain morphometry study. *PLoS ONE, 8*(4), e61038. Retrieved from www.plosone.org

White, D. K., Neogi, T., Nevitt, M. C., et al. (2013). Trajectories of gain speed predict mortality in well-functioning older adults: The Health, Aging, and Body Composition Study. *Journals of Gerontology: Biological Sciences and Medical Sciences, 68*(4), 456–464.

Whitney, J., Close, J. C., Lord, S. R., et al. (2012). Identification of high risk fallers among older people living in residential care facilities: A simple screen based on easily collectable measures. *Archives of Gerontology and Geriatrics, 55*(3), 690–695.

Yan, J. H., Gu, W. J., Sun, J., et al. (2013). Efficacy of tai chi on pain, stiffness and function in patients with osteoarthritis: A meta-analysis. *PLoS ONE, 8*(4), e61672. Retrieved from www.plosone.org

Zapatero, A., Barba, R., Canora, J., et al. (2013). Hip fracture in hospitalized medical patients. *BioMed Central Musculoskeletal Disorders, 14*(15). Retrieved from www.biomedcentral.com/1471-2474/14/15

chapter 23

Integumentary Function

LEARNING OBJECTIVES

After reading this chapter, you will be able to:

1. Delineate age-related changes that affect the skin, hair, nails and glands.
2. Describe risk factors that can affect skin wellness for older adults.
3. Discuss the functional consequences of age-related changes and risk factors that affect the skin, hair, nails and glands.
4. Assess skin in older adults, and recognize normal and pathologic skin changes.
5. Describe the assessment, prevention and management of pressure ulcers.
6. Implement nursing interventions to address the following aspects of skin care: maintenance of healthy skin, prevention of xerosis and referrals for the treatment of pathologic skin lesions.

KEY POINTS

basal cell carcinoma

melanoma

photoaging

photosensitivity

pressure ulcer

squamous cell carcinoma

staging system

xerosis

For many people, and particularly for older adults, skin is the most visible indicator of the combined effects of biologic aging, lifestyle and environment. Thus, the skin, hair and nails have not only physiologic functions but also many social functions. Physiologically, the skin directly affects all of the following processes:

- Thermoregulation
- Excretion of metabolic wastes
- Protection of underlying structures
- Synthesis of vitamin D
- Maintenance of fluid and electrolyte balance
- Sensation of pain, touch, pressure, temperature and vibration

The social functions of the skin include facilitating communication and serving as an indicator of race, gender, work status and other personal characteristics.

Hair serves to protect underlying organs, primarily the skin, from injury and adverse temperatures. In addition, in social contexts, the length and style of one's hair can reflect certain characteristics such as age, gender and personality. Although hair is one of the most visible manifestations of aging, hair colour can easily be altered if grey is viewed as an undesirable indicator of age. Like the skin and hair, nails have both a physiologic and social capacity. Physiologically, nails protect the underlying tissue from injury. In social contexts, nails can reflect personal characteristics such as grooming and occupational activities.

AGE-RELATED CHANGES THAT AFFECT THE INTEGUMENTARY SYSTEM

The skin is the largest, as well as the most visible, body organ. Structurally, the skin comprises three layers: the epidermis, the dermis and the subcutaneous tissue. Hair, nails and sweat glands are also parts of the integumentary system. As with many other aspects of functionality, it is difficult to distinguish between changes that are strictly attributable to aging and those that occur because of risk factors. Genetics, lifestyle and environmental factors exert a significant effect on skin throughout the life span and have a cumulative effect in older adults.

Promoting Skin Wellness in Older Adults

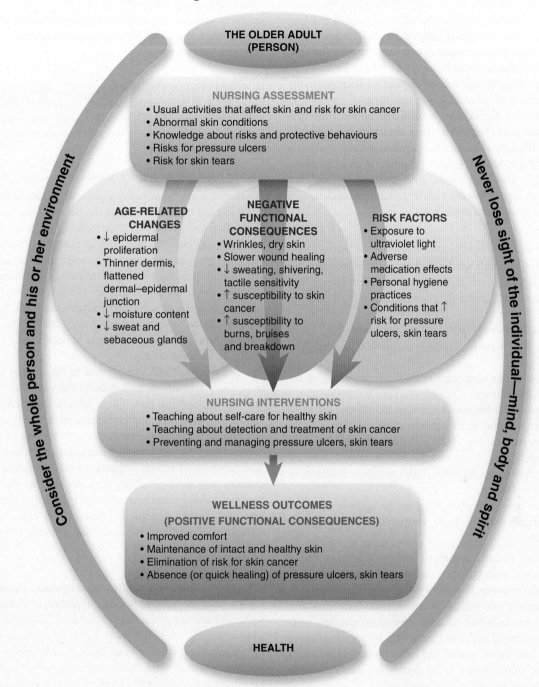

THE OLDER ADULT (PERSON)

Consider the whole person and his or her environment

Never lose sight of the individual—mind, body and spirit

NURSING ASSESSMENT
- Usual activities that affect skin and risk for skin cancer
- Abnormal skin conditions
- Knowledge about risks and protective behaviours
- Risks for pressure ulcers
- Risk for skin tears

AGE-RELATED CHANGES
- ↓ epidermal proliferation
- Thinner dermis, flattened dermal–epidermal junction
- ↓ moisture content
- ↓ sweat and sebaceous glands

NEGATIVE FUNCTIONAL CONSEQUENCES
- Wrinkles, dry skin
- Slower wound healing
- ↓ sweating, shivering, tactile sensitivity
- ↑ susceptibility to skin cancer
- ↑ susceptibility to burns, bruises and breakdown

RISK FACTORS
- Exposure to ultraviolet light
- Adverse medication effects
- Personal hygiene practices
- Conditions that ↑ risk for pressure ulcers, skin tears

NURSING INTERVENTIONS
- Teaching about self-care for healthy skin
- Teaching about detection and treatment of skin cancer
- Preventing and managing pressure ulcers, skin tears

WELLNESS OUTCOMES (POSITIVE FUNCTIONAL CONSEQUENCES)
- Improved comfort
- Maintenance of intact and healthy skin
- Elimination of risk for skin cancer
- Absence (or quick healing) of pressure ulcers, skin tears

HEALTH

Epidermis

The epidermis is the relatively impermeable outer layer of skin that serves as a barrier, preventing both the loss of body fluids and the entry of substances from the environment. The density of the epidermis varies depending on the part of the body it covers. The epidermis comprises layers of cells that undergo a continual cycle of regeneration, cornification and shedding. Epidermal cells develop in the innermost layer of the epidermis and continually migrate to the surface of the skin where they are shed. With increasing age, these cells become larger and more variable in shape, and the rate of epidermal turnover gradually decreases.

Melanocytes are epidermal cells that give the skin its colour and provide a protective barrier against ultraviolet radiation. Beginning around the age of 25 years, the number of active melanocytes decreases by 18% to 20% each decade. Although this decline occurs in both sun-exposed and sun-protected skin, the density of melanocytes in exposed skin is double or triple that in unexposed skin. With increased age, the number of Langerhans cells, which serve as macrophages, also decreases in both sun-exposed and sun-protected skin; the decrease ranges from 50% to 70% in sun-exposed skin. Another age-related change is a decrease in the moisture content of the outer epidermal layer.

Papillae give the skin its texture and connect the epidermis to the underlying dermis at the dermal–epidermal junction. With increased age, the papillae retract, causing a flattening of the dermal–epidermal junction and diminishing the surface area between the epidermis and dermis. This age-related change slows the transfer of nutrients and oxygen between the dermis and epidermis.

Dermis

The primary functions of the dermis include temperature regulation, sensory perception and nourishment for all skin layers. Components of the dermis function in the following ways:

- *Collagen* constitutes 80% of the dermis and provides elasticity and tensile strength to prevent tearing and overstretching.
- *Elastin* maintains skin tension to allow stretching in response to movement.
- *Dermal ground substance* determines skin turgor and elastic properties owing to its water-binding capacity.
- *Blood vessels in the deep plexus* facilitate efficient thermoregulation.
- *Blood vessels in the superficial plexus* supply nutrients to the epidermal layer.
- *Cutaneous nerves* receive and transmit sensory information regarding pain, pressure, temperature, and deep and light touch.

Beginning in early adulthood, dermal thickness gradually diminishes, with collagen thinning at a rate of 1% per year. Elastin increases in quantity and decreases in quality because of age-related and environmentally induced changes. The dermal vascular bed decreases by approximately one-third with increased age; this contributes to the atrophy and fibrosis of hair bulbs, sweat and sebaceous glands. Additional age-related changes in the dermis include a decrease in the number of fibroblasts and mast cells.

Subcutaneous Tissue and Cutaneous Nerves

The subcutis is the inner layer of fat tissue that protects the underlying tissues from trauma. Additional functions include the storage of calories, insulation of the body and regulation of heat loss. With increased age, some areas of subcutaneous tissue atrophy, particularly in the plantar foot surface and in sun-exposed areas of the hands, face and lower legs. Other areas of subcutaneous tissue hypertrophy, however, with the overall effect being a gradual age-related increase in the proportion of body fat during older adulthood. This increased body fat is more pronounced in women than in men and is most noticeable in the waists of men and the thighs of women. Age-related changes also affect the cutaneous nerves responsible for sensations of pressure, vibration and light touch.

 DIVERSITY NOTE

In adult humans, the dermis is thicker in men but the epidermis and subcutaneous tissue are thicker in women (Makrantonaki et al., 2012).

Sweat and Sebaceous Glands

Eccrine and apocrine sweat glands originate in the dermal layer and are most abundant in the palms of the hands, soles of the feet and axillae. Eccrine glands, which are important for thermoregulation, open directly onto the skin surface and are most abundant on the palms, soles and forehead. Apocrine glands are larger than eccrine glands and open into hair follicles, primarily in the axillae and genital area. The sole function of these glands is to produce secretions, which create a distinctive body odour when they decompose. Both eccrine and apocrine glands decrease in number and functional ability with increased age.

Sebaceous glands are present in the dermal skin layer over every part of the body except the palms of the hands and the soles of the feet. These glands continually secrete sebum—a substance that combines with sweat to form an emulsion. Functionally, sebum prevents the loss of water and serves as a mild retardant of bacterial and fungal growth. The secretion of sebum begins to diminish during the third decade, with women having a greater decline than men. In younger adults, sebum production is closely related to the size of the sebaceous glands; however, in older adults, the sebaceous glands increase in size but produce less sebum.

Nails

The rate of nail growth is influenced by many factors including age, climate, state of health, circulation to and around the nails, and activity of the fingers and toes. Nail growth begins to slow in early adulthood, with a gradual decrease of 30% to 50% during a normal life span. Nails of older adults gradually become thinner, fragile, brittle and more prone to splitting. In appearance, the older nail is dull, opaque, longitudinally striated, and yellow or grey, with decreased lunula size.

Hair

Hair colour and distribution change to some degree in all older adults, with the most noticeable changes being baldness and grey hair. About half of adults at the age of 50 years have greying hair, which occurs owing to decreased production of melanin and a gradual replacement of pigmented hairs by nonpigmented ones. Also at the age of 50 years, about 60% of men have a noticeable degree of baldness, which is attributable to a change in production from coarse terminal hair to fine vellus hair. Hair distribution is also affected by age-related changes, with patches of coarse terminal hair developing over the upper lip and lower face in older women and in the ears, nares and eyebrows of older men. Another age-related change is a progressive loss of body hair, initially in the trunk, then in the pubic area and axillae.

> **DIVERSITY NOTE**
>
> Caucasians have earlier onset and greater skin wrinkling than other groups; whereas, Asians and Africans experience more problems related to skin pigmentation (Vierkotter & Krutmann, 2012).

RISK FACTORS THAT AFFECT SKIN WELLNESS

The risk factors that influence the skin and hair of older adults include heredity, lifestyle and environmental factors, and adverse medication effects. Lifestyle and environmental factors have a cumulative effect that manifests more fully during later adulthood, but it is important to identify the risk factors that nurses can address through health education. Risk factors associated with pressure ulcers and skin cancer are addressed in the section on *Pathologic Conditions Affecting Skin*.

Genetic Influences

Heredity plays an important role in the development of skin and hair changes. People with fair skin, light hair and light eyes are more sensitive to the effects of ultraviolet radiation than people with dark skin, as evidenced by the fact that skin cancers are common in light-skinned people of northern European ancestry but rare in African Canadians.

Health Behaviours and Environmental Influences

Smoking, sun exposure, emotional stress, and substance or alcohol abuse are the health behaviours and environmental factors that significantly affect skin wellness. Exposure to ultraviolet radiation is the most significant environmental factor, but adverse climate conditions can also cause negative functional consequences. For example, because the water content of the stratum corneum is influenced by relative humidity, **xerosis** (dry skin) is exacerbated when the relative humidity is below 30%.

Cigarette smoking is another factor that has been associated with detrimental skin changes, as well as with faster rates of developing baldness and grey hair (Gatherwright et al., 2012, 2013). Effects of smoking on the skin include all of the following:

- More wrinkles
- Greyish discolouration
- Diminished ability to protect against ultraviolet radiation damage
- Increased risk of skin cancer

Sociocultural Influences

Cultural factors, societal attitudes and advertising trends influence hygiene and skin care practices. People in industrialized societies place a high value on frequent bathing and the use of commercial products for hygienic and cosmetic purposes. Although most of the personal practices associated with these values are desirable or harmless in younger adults, they may adversely affect older adults. For example, frequent bathing with harsh deodorant soaps may cause or exacerbate dry skin problems in an older person.

> **Wellness Opportunity**
>
> From a holistic nursing perspective, nonjudgmentally consider the influence of cultural and societal attitudes on personal care practices and address any factors that negatively affect self-esteem. An example is the practice of Inuit people who used lemming (small rodents) skins as bandages, which acted as an antiseptic agent. Caribou, seal, or bear fat were used for the same purpose. This might be viewed negatively by southern living Canadians.

Medication Effects

Common adverse medication effects involving the skin include pruritus, dermatoses and photosensitivity reactions. Less common adverse medication effects on the skin and hair include alopecia and pigmentation changes of the skin or hair. Cytotoxic agents are the type of drug most commonly associated with hair loss, but other drugs that can cause alopecia include anticoagulants, nonsteroidal anti-inflammatory agents and cardiovascular medications.

Dermatoses, or rashes, are the most frequently cited adverse medication effect, and they can be caused by virtually any medication. Medication-related skin eruptions vary widely in their manifestations, including their onset. Drug rashes can occur from 1 day to 4 weeks after initiating or discontinuing the causative medication; the most common type of drug-related skin reaction is maculopapular eruptions. Antibiotics are the type of medication most often associated with skin eruptions; however, any medication can cause skin reactions. Medications that commonly cause dermatitis include antibiotics, nonsteroidal anti-inflammatory drugs, anticonvulsants, and antihypertensive agents (Turk et al., 2013).

Photosensitivity is an adverse medication effect that causes an intensified response to ultraviolet radiation. The inflammatory reaction is initially distributed over sun-exposed areas, but it may spread to nonexposed areas and persist even after the medication is discontinued. Photosensitivity may begin during a seasonal exposure to bright sunlight or during a vacation in an unusually hot climate. Amiodarone, furosemide, naproxen, phenothiazines, sulfonamides, tetracyclines, and thiazides are examples of medications that can cause photosensitivity reactions. St. John's wort and other herbal preparations may also increase the risk of photosensitivity.

In addition to causing adverse effects, medications can indirectly cause skin problems by exacerbating age-related changes. For example, fluid loss from diuretics can exacerbate xerosis and cause further discomfort or skin problems for the older adult. Another example of the combined effects of aging and medications is that older adults taking anticoagulants are likely to bruise easily, and bruising may become extensive.

 ## FUNCTIONAL CONSEQUENCES AFFECTING SKIN WELLNESS

Age-related changes and risk factors negatively affect many functions of the skin including thermoregulation, tactile sensitivity and wound healing. Age-related changes do not interfere with the protective function of the nails; however, the nails in older persons are brittle and more likely to split. People who hold negative attitudes about aging may experience psychosocial consequences when changes in the appearance of the skin and hair become visible indicators of aging.

Delayed Wound Healing and Increased Susceptibility to Skin Problems

The regeneration of healthy skin takes twice as long for an 80-year-old as for a 30-year-old person. In perfectly intact skin, this slowed regeneration has no noticeable effects. When skin integrity is compromised, however, this age-related change contributes to delayed wound healing, even for superficial wounds. The consequences of age-related changes that affect the healing of deep wounds include an increased risk for postoperative wound disruption, decreased tensile strength of healing wounds and increased risk of secondary infections.

Age-related changes in all layers of the skin combine with the effects of long-term exposure to the sun and other risk factors to increase the susceptibility of older adults to many types of problems (e.g., skin tears, pressure ulcers, stasis dermatitis), as delineated in Table 23-1 and described in the section on *Pathologic Conditions Affecting Skin*. In addition, the age-related diminished immune function increases older adults' susceptibility to skin cancers, cutaneous fungal infectionsand herpes zoster (commonly called *shingles*) (Chang et al., 2013).

Photoaging

Photoaging is the term used to describe skin changes that occur because of exposure to ultraviolet radiation, even at levels that do not cause any detectable sunburn. These changes are sometimes viewed as premature aging; however, they are biologically distinct processes that occur independently and are superimposed on normal aging changes. One reason for the misconception that photoaging is an age-related change is that the cumulative effects of ultraviolet radiation may not be evident until later adulthood. Common characteristics of photoaging are as follows:

- Coarse, leathery, and ruddy or yellowed appearance
- Deep wrinkles, particularly on the face and neck
- Pathologic lesions and seborrheic and actinic keratoses
- Thickened epidermis
- Enlarged sebaceous glands
- Marked loss of elasticity
- Dilated and tortuous blood vessels
- Numerous freckles

Smoking is another condition that contributes to the development of photoaging (Durai et al., 2012). Recent studies are focusing on factors that counteract the effects of sun exposure and reduce the risk for photoaging. For example, a survey of dietary intake of 2,920 adults in France found that healthy dietary habits and higher consumption of olive oil were associated with reduced evidence of facial photoaging (Latreille et al., 2012).

Comfort and Sensation

Dry skin is one of the most universal complaints of older adults; indeed, it has been observed in up to 85% of non-institutionalized older people. Age-related changes, such as diminished output of sebum and eccrine sweat, contribute to

---

TABLE 23-1 Functional Consequences Affecting Skin and Appendages

Age-Related Change	Consequence
Decreased rate of epidermal proliferation	Delayed wound healing; increased susceptibility to infection
Flattened dermal–epidermal junction; thinning of dermis; degenerative changes of collagen; increased quantity, but decreased quality, of elastin	Decreased resiliency; increased susceptibility to injury, bruising, mechanical stress, ultraviolet radiation and blister formation
Reductions in dermal blood supply and the number of melanocytes and Langerhans cells	Decreased intensity of tanning; irregular pigmentation; increased susceptibility to skin cancer; diminished dermal clearance, absorption and immunologic response
Reductions in eccrine sweat, subcutaneous fat and dermal blood supply	Decreased sweating and shivering; increased susceptibility to hypothermia or hyperthermia
Decreased moisture content	Dry skin; discomfort
Decreased number of Meissner's and Pacinian corpuscles	Diminished tactile sensitivity; increased susceptibility to burns
Slowed nail growth	Increased susceptibility to cracking and injury; delayed healing
Changes in hair colour, quantity and distribution	Negative impact on self-esteem in proportion to negative attitudes

a decrease in the moisture content of the skin. Risk factors that may contribute to dry skin include stress, smoking, sun exposure, dry environments, excessive perspiration, adverse medication reactions, excessive use of soap and certain medical conditions (e.g., hypothyroidism).

Tactile sensitivity begins to decline around the age of 20 years, eventually causing older adults to have a diminished and less intense response to cutaneous sensations. This decline is attributable, at least in part, to age-related changes in Pacinian and Meissner's corpuscles, which are the skin receptors that respond to vibration. Other contributing factors include lower body temperature and functional alterations in the central nervous system. Functionally, older adults are more susceptible to scald burns because of their diminished ability to feel dangerously hot water temperatures.

Thermoregulation is also affected by age-related reductions in eccrine sweat, subcutaneous fat and dermal blood supply. These age-related changes interfere with sweating, shivering, peripheral vasoconstriction and vasodilation, and insulation against adverse environmental temperatures. Thus, older adults are more at risk for the development of hypothermia and heat-related illnesses, as discussed in Chapter 25.

Cosmetic Effects

The overall cosmetic effect of age-related skin changes is that the skin looks paler, thinner and more translucent, and is irregularly pigmented. Age-related changes that cause these cosmetic effects include decreased melanocytes and diminished dermal circulation. Additional indicators of age-related skin changes include sagging and wrinkling, which are caused by age-related changes in the epidermis and dermis, particularly those affecting collagen. Decreased subcutaneous tissue contributes to sagging skin, particularly over the upper arms, by allowing gravity to pull the skin downward. Various skin growths and lesions that are common in older adults are described in the section on *Nursing Assessment*.

Although these changes in appearance are gradual and do not interfere significantly with physiologic function, the psychosocial consequences of these changes can be significant because of the social value placed on personal appearance and negative attitudes that may be held about growing old. Regardless of age, one's physical appearance has been shown to be an important determinant of self-perception, and modern societies associate attractiveness with young-looking skin.

> **Wellness Opportunity**
>
> Nurses can promote positive attitudes about aging by challenging societal perspectives that associate beauty only with youth.

Because of the high visibility of the face and neck, any signs of increased age that are prominent around the eyes and mouth may be particularly bothersome to the person who wants to avoid visible indications of age. Characteristic signs of advanced age that are evident around the eyes include increased pigmentation, crow's-feet wrinkles, and fat and fluid accumulation in the upper lid and under the eye. Also, because of diminished skin elasticity and the loss and shifting of subcutaneous fat, the neck skin sags, and a double chin may develop. Table 23-1 summarizes the functional consequences resulting from age-related changes of the skin, hair, nails and glands.

PATHOLOGIC CONDITIONS AFFECTING SKIN: SKIN CANCER AND PRESSURE ULCERS

Skin Cancer

A serious functional consequence of the age-related skin changes and long-term sun exposure is the increased incidence of skin cancers in older adults. Skin cancer, defined as an abnormal growth of skin cells, is the most common—as well as the most preventable—type of cancer. Older adults are highly vulnerable to the two most common types of skin cancer, primarily because of the cumulative effects of sun exposure. **Basal cell carcinoma**, the most common type accounting for 90% of all skin cancers in this country, occurs most often on the head and neck (Fig. 23-1A). It affects 50 to 60,000 Canadians each year (Canadian Skin Cancer Foundation, 2012). If diagnosed and treated during its early stage, the cure rate for basal cell carcinoma is close to 100%; however, if left untreated, it invades the surrounding tissue. **Squamous cell carcinoma**, the second most common type, occurs most commonly on the head, neck, forearms and dorsal hands (Fig. 23-1B). However, exact rates of nonmelanoma skin cancer (basal and squamous) are difficult to accurately identify since most cancer registries in this country do not collect information on them. Read more: http://www.cancer.ca/en/cancer-information/cancer-type/skin-non-melanoma/statistics/?region=on#ixzz30TMIckkX.

Melanoma, which originates in the melanocytes, is the most serious type of skin cancer and the one most likely to be fatal (see Fig. 23-1C). The incidence and mortality rates of melanoma have been gradually increasing throughout most of the developed world during the past 25 years (Geller et al., 2011). The Melanoma Network of Canada (n.d.) states that approximately 1 in 63 men will develop melanoma during his lifetime and 1 in 79 women.

> **DIVERSITY NOTE**
>
> Melanoma is more common in men, light-skinned people and older adults; however, the incidence in younger women is increasing rapidly, due in part to trends in indoor tanning (i.e., tanning beds) (Little & Eide, 2012). Nonwhites and older adults are likely to have more advanced disease when diagnosed and lower survival rates (Pollack et al., 2011; Wu et al., 2011).

Early detection and treatment are imperative for improving the outcomes of all types of skin cancer, and nurses have an essential role in assessing and teaching older adults about skin cancer, as discussed in the sections on *Nursing Assessment and Nursing Interventions*. Nurses also need to

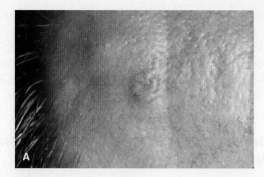

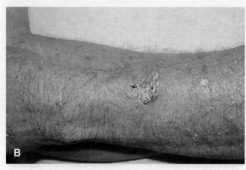

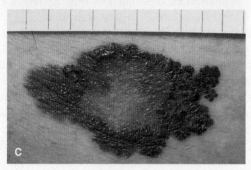

FIGURE 23-1 Common types of skin cancer. (**A**) Basal cell carcinoma. (**B**) Squamous cell carcinoma. (**C**) Melanoma. (**A** & **B**, Reprinted with permission from Rosenthal, T. C., Williams, M. E., & Naughton, B. J. [2007]. *Office care geriatrics*. Philadelphia, PA: Lippincott Williams & Wilkins; **C**, From Goodheart, H. P. [2003]. *Goodheart's photoguide of common skin disorders*. Philadelphia, PA: Lippincott Williams & Wilkins.)

be alert to risk factors, so they consider these in their assessments and address them in health promotion. Advanced age increases the risk for all types of skin lesions including skin cancers. Exposure to ultraviolet rays, including those from tanning booths, is a risk factor that is highly associated with skin cancers and that is most amenable to protective measures. Other risks for melanoma include family history, fair skin, light hair colour, sunburn susceptibility, number of severe sunburns and multiple nevi on extremities (Walls et al., 2013). Recent studies are also exploring stress as a risk factor, based on the higher incidence of melanoma in people who are immunosuppressed and those with highly stressful occupations (Sinnya & DeAmbrosis, 2013).

Wellness Opportunity

Nurses promote self-care for wellness by teaching older adults to examine their skin for suspicious changes once a month.

Box 23-1 Evidence-Informed Nursing Practice

Background: Skin tears occur in those with fragile skin and are more frequently seen in older adults than in other age groups. Some skin tears are unavoidable but many are preventable.

Question: What is the prevalence of skin tears in the Canadian population residing in long-term care facilities?

Method: The setting was a 114-bed long-term care facility in Eastern Ontario. One hundred and thirteen residents were assessed for presence of skin tears, the number of skin tears and location. Skin tears were categorized according to the Payne Martin Classification system.

Findings: Twenty-five (22%) of the participating residents had skin tears. Category I accounted for 51% of skin tears, 16% were Category II, and 33% were Category III. Individuals who had more than 1 skin tear had at least 1 Category III skin tear. The most common locations were arms (48%), lower legs (40%) and hands (12%). Etiologic factors included blunt trauma such as banging into objects (44%), trauma associated with activities of daily living (20%), and falls (12%); 24% were categorized as idiopathic.

Implications: Nurses need to place greater emphasis upon the assessment of risk factors contributing to the presence of skin tears.

Source: LeBlanc, K., Christensen, D., Cook, D., et al. (2013). Prevalence of skin tears in a long-term care facility. *Journal of Wound, Ostomy & Continence Nursing, 40,* 580–584.

Skin Tears

Skin tears are traumatic wounds involving the dermis and/or epidermis layers of the skin and usually caused by friction, rubbing, or a shearing force (see Box 23-1). Skin tears commonly occur in older adults because of a combination of age-related skin changes and risk factors, such as frailty, limited mobility and poor nutrition. In December 2011, the International Skin Tear Advisory Panel proposed a Skin Tear Classification System to establish a common language for documenting skin tears and to facilitate research and development of best practices (LeBlanc et al., 2013). Skin tears are classified as follows:

1. No skin loss, with an average of 10 days to heal
2. Partial thickness (i.e., epidermis separated from the dermis), with an average of 14 days to heal
3. Full thickness (i.e., both epidermis and dermis separated from underlying tissue), with an average of 21 days to heal (Holmes et al., 2013; LeBlanc et al., 2013)

Online Learning Activity 23-1 illustrates a case study and provides comprehensive information about care and management of skin tears for older adults in home settings.

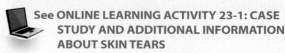

See **ONLINE LEARNING ACTIVITY 23-1: CASE STUDY AND ADDITIONAL INFORMATION ABOUT SKIN TEARS** at http://thepoint.lww.com/Miller7e

Pressure Ulcers

In recent years, the focus on the development, prevention and management of pressure ulcers has increased significantly. Although pressure ulcers have been a topic of concern since the 1970s, it is now being addressed as an essential aspect of patient safety in Canada and many other countries.

Definition and Overview

A **pressure ulcer** is "any lesion caused by unrelieved pressure that results in damage to underlying tissue. Pressure ulcers usually occur over a bony prominence and are staged to classify the degree of tissue damage observed" (Registered Nurses Association of Ontario [RNAO], 2011, p. 19). Many factors contribute to the development of pressure ulcers, but the immediate determinant is the degree to which tissues can tolerate the intensity and duration of pressure. People who are unable to move around independently, even for short periods (e.g., during surgery) are most vulnerable. Figure 23-2 illustrates areas of the body that are most susceptible to development of pressure ulcers, with sacrum/coccyx and heel being the first and second most common sites.

Medical devices can also be a source of pressure to cause *medical device–related pressure ulcers*. Device-related pressure ulcers account for 9.1% of ulcers, with the ears being the most common location (Ayello & Sibbald, 2012). Medical devices that are commonly associated with increased risk for pressure ulcers include masks, orthotics, tubing, immobilizers, stockings or boots, nasogastric tubes, cervical collars or braces, and tracheostomy tubes and ties (Apold & Rydrych, 2012; Coyer et al., 2014).

Since the early 2000s, there has been increasing attention to incidence, prevalence and serious consequences of pressure ulcers. This increased attention is due to the steadily growing awareness of safety issues in hospitalized patients, with pressure ulcers being identified as one of the top three concerns (Gadd, 2012). In 2002, the RNAO published the first version of its *Best Practice Guidelines on Risk Assessment and Prevention of Pressure Ulcers*, which was last revised in 2011. The guideline emphasizes a comprehensive approach to assessment of risks and implementation of evidence-based interventions to address risks. Nurses have consistently provided strong leadership in addressing this important issue through organizations such as the Canadian Association for Enterostomal Therapy, the Canadian Association of Wound Care, and the RNAO.

In addition to concerns about quality of care, long-term care facilities have incentives to initiate comprehensive pressure ulcer prevention programs because their accreditation status might be reduced. Efforts are also being made to develop evidence-based guidelines for home health care agencies, with emphasis on addressing the unique needs of home care patients. For example, in home health care settings, options for interventions may be limited by economic and insurance status, and care plans rely almost entirely on caregiving resources, which may also be limited (Bergquist-Beringer & Daley, 2011).

Health care practitioners in acute care settings are mandated to document the presence of any skin breakdown on admission and during the hospitalization. In addition, all acute care settings have increased their efforts to prevent pressure ulcers in all their patients as a major focus of quality improvement programs. Currently, goals for hospital-acquired

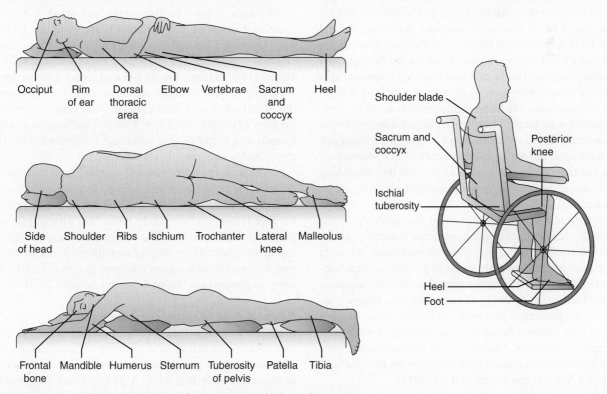

FIGURE 23-2 The risk for the development of pressure ulcers is higher at these points.

pressure ulcer (HAPU) prevention are based on evidence that most pressure ulcers are preventable and have been re-framed from "reduction in number" to "zero HAPU" (Stotts et al., 2013).

 DIVERSITY NOTE

Analysis of data related to pressure ulcers across the skin pigmentation spectrum shows that persons with darkly pigmented skin have a higher incidence of serious pressure ulcers. Clinicians need to pay particular attention to a variety of indicators for detection of early-stage pressure ulcers (Ayello & Sibbald, 2012).

Functional Consequences

Pressure ulcers are associated with many serious functional consequences, including pain, loss of function and decreased quality of life. The RNAO guidelines emphasize the important role of nurses in assessing and intervening for pain in patients with pressure ulcers. This emphasis is warranted because patients with pressure ulcers report that pain is their most distressing symptom and pressure-related pain is often experienced even before skin breakdown is evident (Briggs et al., 2013). Studies have identified HAPUs as a major risk for all the following: doubling the length of stay, increased rates of mortality during the hospitalization or within 30 days of discharge, and increased rates of bacteremia with multi-drug resistant organisms with a poor outcome (Braga et al., 2013; Lyder et al., 2012; Theisen et al., 2012).

Risk Identification

Evidence-based tools are used to identify and rate risk factors for pressure ulcer development. In Canada, the Braden Scale (Fig. 23-3) is commonly used as a screening tool and the RNAO recommends this tool as the best practice for identifying older adults who are at risk for the development of pressure ulcers. The Norton and Waterloo scales are also commonly used, with reviews of studies indicating that all three of these scales can help identify patients at risk for pressure ulcers who might benefit from targeted interventions (Chou et al., 2013). It is important to recognize, however, that these tools are not necessarily predictive of pressure ulcers, but their major purpose is to provide the initial step in pressure ulcer prevention programs (Kelechi et al., 2013; Kelleher et al., 2012).

A current focus of research is on the reliability of the Braden Scale in predicting pressure ulcers in specific groups of hospitalized patients. These studies emphasize the need to focus on specific subscale scores (e.g., friction/shear subscale) to implement preventive plans that address individual needs (Tescher et al., 2012). A comprehensive research review of the predictive power of the Braden Scale in adult critical care patients found that the subscales for Sensory Perception, Mobility, Moisture, and Friction/Shear were more predictive of pressure ulcer development than the subscales for Activity and Nutrition (Cox, 2012).

Current research is focusing on critically ill patients who develop HAPU and have multiple risk factors, including ones that are not identified on risk assessment tools. For example, Bry and colleagues (2012) reported a study of 82 patients who had at least 1 HAPU and found that all patients had multiple risk factors, yet almost one-quarter of the Braden scores were graded as low risk. Similarly, Black and colleagues (2012) found that critically ill patients shared a unique pattern of pressure ulcer risk with the following characteristics: elderly, immobile, inactive, dehydrated, undernourished, anemic, moist skin, sedated or unconscious, and mechanically ventilated and requiring head-of-the-bed elevation. Studies of HAPU in postsurgical patients have identified the following risk factors: diabetes, longer operative time, recurrent surgeries, and low body mass index (Liu et al., 2012; Tschannen et al., 2012). Studies such as these underscore the importance of using evidence-based tools in conjunction with clinical judgment as one component of a comprehensive assessment of all factors that increase the risk for pressure ulcers.

Staging Classifications

Since 1975, the National Pressure Ulcer Advisory Panel (NPUAP) (in the United States) has promoted the use of a **staging system**, which is an assessment system that classifies pressure ulcers according to anatomic depth of soft-tissue damage. This staging system is widely used in Canada. In 2009, the NPUAP and the European Pressure Ulcer Advisory Panel (EPUAP) jointly issued a revised classification system, as described, illustrated and summarized in Table 23-2.

Once a pressure ulcer is identified according to the defined stages, it must be frequently reassessed to evaluate the effectiveness of interventions. Since 1996, the NPUAP has encouraged the use of a standardized tool for assessing changes in pressure ulcers called the Pressure Ulcer Scale for Healing (PUSH) tool. The PUSH tool scores pressure ulcers according to size, exudates and tissue type, with changes in the PUSH score over time indicating the progression or regression of the pressure ulcer. This tool has been assessed in Canada and found to be a valid and appropriate tool (Hon et al., 2010).

Although the term "reverse staging" has been used to describe the progression of a later-stage pressure stage to a healed stage, the NPUAP has advised against this practice because it does not accurately reflect the pathophysiologic processes that occur. The NPUAP provides many educational resources related to the staging classification and the PUSH tool. The tool includes quick reference guides in English and other languages (see Online Learning Activity 23-2).

Evidence-Based Practice for Pressure Ulcers

Financial and quality-of-care implications related to pressure ulcers have led to an abundance of information about interventions for preventing and healing pressure ulcers, as summarized in Box 23-2. Although much progress has

BRADEN SCALE FOR PREDICTING PRESSURE SORE RISK

Patient's Name _____ Evaluator's Name _____ Date of Assessment

SENSORY PERCEPTION Ability to respond meaningfully to pressure-related discomfort	**1. Completely Limited** Unresponsive (does not moan, flinch or grasp) to painful stimuli, due to diminished level of consciousness or sedation. OR limited ability to feel pain over most of body.	**2. Very Limited** Responds only to painful stimuli. Cannot communicate discomfort except by moaning or restlessness. OR Has a sensory impairment which limits the ability to feel pain or discomfort over 1/2 of body.	**3. Slightly Limited** Responds to verbal commands, but cannot always communicate discomfort or the need to be turned. OR Has some sensory impairment which limits ability to feel pain or discomfort in 1 or 2 extremities.	**4. No Impairment** Responds to verbal commands. Has no sensory deficit which would limit ability to feel or voice pain or discomfort.			
MOISTURE Degree to which skin is exposed to moisture	**1. Constantly Moist** Skin is kept moist almost constantly by perspiration, urine, etc. Dampness is detected every time patient is moved or turned.	**2. Very Moist** Skin is often, but not always moist. Linen must be changed at least once a shift.	**3. Occasionally Moist:** Skin is occasionally moist, requiring an extra linen change approximately once a day.	**4. Rarely Moist** Skin is usually dry, linen only requires changing at routine intervals.			
ACTIVITY Degree of physical activity	**1. Bedfast** Confined to bed.	**2. Chairfast** Ability to walk severely limited or nonexistent. Cannot bear own weight and/or must be assisted into chair or wheelchair.	**3. Walks Occasionally** Walks occasionally during day, but for very short distances, with or without assistance. Spends majority of each shift in bed or chair.	**4. Walks Frequently** Walks outside room at least twice a day and inside room at least once every two hours during waking hours.			
MOBILITY Ability to change and control body position	**1. Completely Immobile** Does not make even slight changes in body or extremity position without assistance.	**2. Very Limited** Makes occasional slight changes in body or extremity position but unable to make frequent or significant changes independently.	**3. Slightly Limited** Makes frequent though slight changes in body or extremity position independently.	**4. No Limitation** Makes major and frequent changes in position without assistance.			
NUTRITION Usual food intake pattern	**1. Very Poor** Never eats a complete meal. Rarely eats more than 1/2 of any food offered. Eats 2 servings or less of protein (meat or dairy products) per day. Takes fluids poorly. Does not take a liquid dietary supplement. OR Is NPO and/or maintained on clear liquids or IV's for more than 5 days.	**2. Probably Inadequate** Rarely eats a complete meal and generally eats only about 1/2 of any food offered. Protein intake includes only 3 servings of meat or dairy products per day. Occasionally will take a dietary supplement. OR Receives less than optimum amount of liquid diet or tube feeding.	**3. Adequate** Eats over half of most meals. Eats a total of 4 servings of protein (meat, dairy products) per day. Occasionally will refuse a meal, but will usually take a supplement when offered. OR Is on a tube feeding or TPN regimen which probably meets most of nutritional needs.	**4. Excellent** Eats most of every meal. Never refuses a meal. Usually eats a total of 4 or more servings of meat and dairy products. Occasionally eats between meals. Does not require supplementation.			
FRICTION & SHEAR	**1. Problem** Requires moderate to maximum assistance in moving. Complete lifting without sliding against sheets is impossible. Frequently slides down in bed or chair, requiring frequent repositioning with maximum assistance. Spasticity, contractures or agitation leads to almost constant friction.	**2. Potential Problem** Moves feebly or requires minimum assistance. During a move skin probably slides to some extent against sheets, chair, restraints or other devices. Maintains relatively good position in chair or bed most of the time but occasionally slides down.	**3. No Apparent Problem** Moves in bed and in chair independently and has sufficient muscle strength to lift up completely during move. Maintains good position in bed or chair.				

Total Score

FIGURE 23-3 The Braden Scale is a widely used screening tool to identify people at risk for pressure ulcers. Scores: 15–18, at risk; 13–14, moderate risk; 10–12, high risk; less than 9, very high risk. (From Braden B., & Bergstrom, N. [1988]. Reprinted with permission. Permission to use this tool should be sought at www.bradenscale.com.)

been made in identifying interventions for preventing and healing pressure ulcers, research is ongoing and recommendations continue to develop. For example, repositioning is consistently identified as an effective measure; however, the long-standing criterion of turning patients every 2 hours has been replaced with the recommendation to individualize repositioning schedules based on the patient's condition, care goals, vulnerable skin areas and type of support surface being used (Accreditation Canada, 2013; Chou et al., 2013).

Because research is ongoing and plentiful, nurses can keep up-to-date on evidence-based recommendations by exploring information in the resources described in Online Learning Activity 23-2.

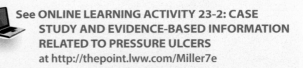

See **ONLINE LEARNING ACTIVITY 23-2: CASE STUDY AND EVIDENCE-BASED INFORMATION RELATED TO PRESSURE ULCERS** at http://thepoint.lww.com/Miller7e

TABLE 23-2 Stages of Pressure Ulcer Development

Stage	Description		
0	Normal skin	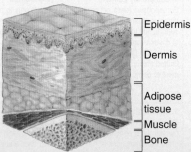 Epidermis Dermis Adipose tissue Muscle Bone	
I	**Non-blanchable erythema.** Intact skin with non-blanchable redness of a localized area usually over a bony prominence. Darkly pigmented skin may not have visible blanching; its colour may differ from the surrounding area. The area may be painful, firm, soft, warmer or cooler as compared to adjacent tissue. Category I may be difficult to detect in individuals with dark skin tones. May indicate "at risk" persons.	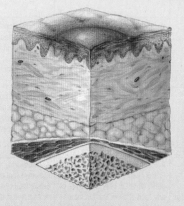	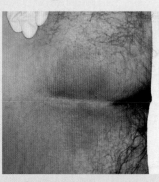
II	**Partial thickness.** Partial thickness loss of dermis presenting as a shallow open ulcer with a red pink wound bed, without slough. May also present as an intact or open/ruptured serum-filled or sero-sanginous filled blister. Presents as a shiny or dry shallow ulcer without slough or bruising*. This category should not be used to describe skin tears, tape burns, incontinence associated dermatitis, maceration or excoriation. *Bruising indicates deep tissue injury.	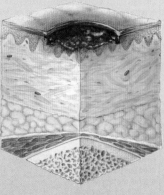	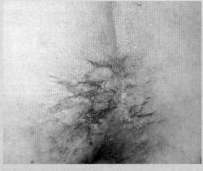
III	**Full thickness skin loss.** Full thickness tissue loss. Subcutaneous fat may be visible but bone, tendon or muscle is not exposed. Slough may be present but does not obscure the depth of tissue loss. May include undermining and tunneling. The depth of a Category/Stage III pressure ulcer varies by anatomical location. The bridge of the nose, ear, occiput and malleolus do not have (adipose) subcutaneous tissue and Category/Stage III ulcers can be shallow. In contrast, areas of significant adiposity can develop extremely deep Category/Stage III pressure ulcers. Bone/tendon is not visible or directly palpable.	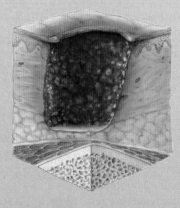	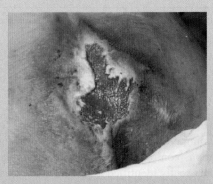

Stage	Description
IV	**Full thickness tissue loss.** Full thickness tissue loss with exposed bone, tendon or muscle. Slough or eschar may be present. Often includes undermining and tunneling. The depth of a Category/Stage IV pressure ulcer varies by anatomical location. The bridge of the nose, ear, occiput and malleolus do not have (adipose) subcutaneous tissue and these ulcers can be shallow. Category/Stage IV ulcers can extend into muscle and/or supporting structures (e.g., fascia, tendon or joint capsule) making osteomyelitis or osteitis likely to occur. Exposed bone/muscle is visible or directly palpable. 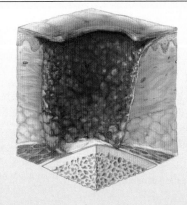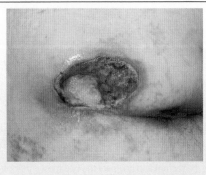
Unstageable	**Full thickness skin or tissue loss—depth unknown.** Full thickness tissue loss in which actual depth of the ulcer is completely obscured by slough (yellow, tan, gray, green or brown) and/or eschar (tan, brown or black) in the wound bed. Until enough slough and/or eschar are removed to expose the base of the wound, the true depth cannot be determined; but it will be either a Category/Stage III or IV. Stable (dry, adherent, intact without erythema or fluctuance) eschar on the heels serves as "the body's natural (biological) cover" and should not be removed. 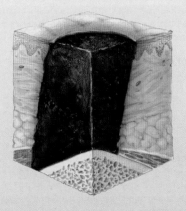
Suspected deep tissue injury	**Depth unknown.** Purple or maroon localized area of discoloured intact skin or blood-filled blister due to damage of underlying soft tissue from pressure and/or shear. The area may be preceded by tissue that is painful, firm, mushy, boggy, warmer or cooler as compared to adjacent tissue. Deep tissue injury may be difficult to detect in individuals with dark skin tones. Evolution may include a thin blister over a dark wound bed. The wound may further evolve and become covered by thin eschar. Evolution may be rapid exposing additional layers of tissue even with optimal treatment. 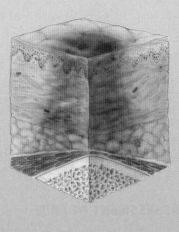

Text reprinted from National Pressure Ulcer Advisory Panel and European Pressure Ulcer Advisory Panel. (2009). *Prevention and treatment of pressure ulcers: Clinical practice guideline.* Washington, DC: National Pressure Ulcer Advisory Panel. Retrieved from www.npuap.org. Used with permission of the National Pressure Ulcer Advisory Panel.

Box 23-2 Evidence-Based Practice: Pressure Ulcers

Statement of the Problem

- Pressure ulcers, defined as a localized injury to the skin and/or underlying tissue as a result of pressure or pressure in combination with shear, are a major focus of quality-of-care initiatives in all health care settings.
- Underlying causative factors are a combination of pressure intensity and duration and tissue tolerance.
- Risk factors include immobility, surgery, frailty, older age, friable skin, incontinence, compromised nutritional status, cognitive impairment, comorbid conditions and dependence in activities of daily living.
- The sacrum and heels are the two most common sites for the development of pressure ulcers; other common sites are the ears, elbows, coccyx and ischium.
- Pressure ulcers differ physiologically from moisture-associated dermatitis or surface injury caused by moisture or friction.
- Complications of pressure ulcers include sepsis, cellulitis, osteomyelitis, increased length of stay, and financial and emotional cost.
- Detection of Stage I pressure ulcers is particularly challenging in patients with darkly pigmented skin, and these patients are more likely to die from pressure ulcers.

Recommendations for Nursing Assessment

- Identify risk factors using a valid and reliable tool (e.g., Braden Scale).
- Perform a head-to-toe skin assessment on admission to a facility, on discharge, whenever the patient's condition changes, and at appropriate intervals.
- Additional components of a comprehensive assessment for pressure ulcer risk include a history and physical examination.
- Assess and reassess pressure ulcers according to the most recent NPUAP Pressure Ulcer Staging System.
- During assessments, use natural or halogen lighting rather than fluorescent lighting.
- Because patients with darkly pigmented skin may not meet the normal criteria for Stage I pressure ulcers, consider additional parameters (e.g., differences in skin over bony prominences compared with surrounding skin, alterations in pain or local sensation, deviations from the usual colour for that person).
- If available, use technologic devices to improve the detection of Stage I pressure ulcers in patients with darkly pigmented skin.

Recommendations for Nursing Interventions

- Pressure redistribution interventions: individualize repositioning schedules, and use pressure redistribution surfaces (e.g., static mattresses and overlays, alternating pressure mattress, gel cushions).

- Positioning interventions: raise heels to eliminate pressure, keep head of bed in lowest height, maintain 30° tilted side-lying position, avoid positioning directly on the trochanter and avoid doughnut-shaped devices.
- Use protective methods, such as heel protection boots.
- Decrease the risk of friction and shear: have patient use trapeze to lift self off bed; staff can use transfer or lifting devices.
- Nutritional interventions: assessment of nutritional status and appropriate referrals for the services of registered dieticians; provision of adequate calories, nutrients, hydration; and appropriate use of supplements.
- Daily nutrient needs for prevention and treatment of pressure ulcers: 30 to 35 calories/kg body weight, 1.25 to 1.5 g/kg protein, 1 mL fluid intake per kilocalorie, vitamin and mineral supplements to compensate for deficiencies, with less than 40 mg elemental zinc.
- Protect skin from moisture: manage incontinence, keep skin clean and dry, use absorbent products, change linens frequently and use moisture barrier skin protectant.
- Skin care: individualize bathing frequency; avoid hot water and excessive rubbing; use moisturizer lotion; protect skin from urine, stool, and other sources of moisture; and do not massage bony prominences.
- Manage treatment measures including wound cleansing, moist wound dressings, debridement, pain management, and referral to wound care specialists.
- Education of professionals, patients, caregivers.

Cultural Considerations for Interventions

- Dressings for pressure ulcers may contain animal-derived collagen that conflicts with the patient's ideology or cultural background as in the following examples: porcine products for Jewish or Muslim patients, bovine products for Hindu patients, and honey-based products for patients who follow a vegan diet.
- Obtain information about products with animal-based collagen and discuss with patients who may have cultural conflicts.

Sources: Ayello, E. A., & Sibbald, R. G. (2012). Preventing pressure ulcers and skin tears. In M. Boltz, E. Capezuti, T. Fulmer, et al. (Eds.), *Evidence-based geriatric nursing protocols for best practice* (4th ed., pp. 298–323). New York, NY: Springer; Boyer, D. (2013). Cultural considerations in advanced wound care. *Advances in Skin and Wound Care, 26*(3), 110–111; Chou, R., Dana, T., Bougatsos, C., et al. (2013). *Pressure ulcer risk assessment and prevention: Comparative effectiveness*. Rockville, MD: Agency for Healthcare Quality and Research, Publication No. 12(13)-EHC148-EF2013; Institute for Clinical Systems Improvement. (2012). *Guideline summary NGC-8962: Pressure ulcer prevention and treatment protocol*. Available at National Guideline Clearinghouse, Retrieved from www.guideline.gov; Posthauer, M. E., Collins, N., Dorner, B., et al. (2013). Nutritional strategies for frail older adults. *Advances in Skin and Wound Care, 26*(3), 128–140.

NURSING ASSESSMENT OF SKIN

Because the skin is the largest and most visible organ of the body, it is relatively easy to identify problems that affect it. In addition, the integumentary system provides clues to other areas of physiologic and psychosocial function, such as nutrition, hydration and personal care. Nurses collect information about the skin, hair and nails during an assessment interview and through physical examination procedures. Opportunities for direct examination also arise during routine nursing care activities, such as assisting with personal care or listening to the lung and heart sounds. Assessment of the skin, hair and nails can also provide information to validate or raise questions about other areas of function. For example, the observation that an older man has a beard of several days' growth, when combined with assessment information about his overall function, may support conclusions about the need for assistance with personal care activities.

Identifying Opportunities for Health Promotion

Assessment questions identify the person's perception of problems, risk factors that may contribute to skin problems,

Box 23-3 Interview Questions for Assessing the Integument

Questions to Assess Risk Factors and Skin Problems

- Do you have any concerns about or trouble with your skin?
- Do you have any problems with rashes, itching, swelling or dry skin?
- Do you have any sores that will not heal?
- Do you bruise easily?
- Have you been treated for skin cancer or any other skin problems?
- How much time do you spend in the sun?
- Do you spend time in tanning booths?
- Do you do anything to protect yourself from the effects of the sun?

Questions to Assess Personal Care Practices

- How do you manage your bathing?
- How often do you take a bath or shower?
- What temperature water do you use?
- Do you use soap every time you bathe?
- What kind of soap do you use?
- Do you use any kind of skin lotion, creams or ointments? What kind do you use and how frequently do you use it? Where do you apply it?
- Do you have any problems with your fingernails or toenails?
- Do you get or need any help with nail care?

and any personal care behaviours that influence hair and skin status. Assessing these aspects of skin care can help identify opportunities for health education about risk factors and healthy skin care practices. Older adults may initiate a discussion about age spots or other noticeable skin changes, and they are usually very receptive to information about skin and hair care. Information about medications and other risk factors, which is obtained as part of the overall assessment, is incorporated into the skin assessment. Likewise, other pertinent information obtained during a comprehensive assessment, such as information about fluid intake, nutritional status, and mobility and safety, is applicable to the assessment of the skin. Box 23-3 summarizes assessment questions related to the skin and nails.

Observing Skin, Hair and Nails

Close inspection of the skin in a warm, private and well-lit environment is an essential component of skin assessment. Examination of the skin is particularly important because older adults may focus on cosmetic conditions, such as skin tags, instead of questioning more serious conditions such as skin cancer. Assessment observations of skin include all the following: colour, turgor, dryness, overall condition, bruises, and any growths or pathologic conditions. Cultural variations are also noted. For example, skin changes may be difficult to assess in people with dark pigmentation.

The common occurrence of various skin lesions complicates the assessment of skin in older adults. Although most of these changes are harmless, some are cancerous or precancerous. An important aspect of health promotion is to reassure the older adult about the harmless changes and to encourage medical evaluation of the questionable ones. In general, the following characteristics of a skin lesion warrant medical evaluation:

- Redness
- Swelling
- Dark pigmentation
- Moisture or drainage
- Pain or discomfort
- Raised or irregular edges around a flat centre

In addition, any lesion that undergoes change, or any sore that does not heal within a reasonable time, requires further evaluation. Evaluation is also indicated when, because of its location, a mole or other skin lesion is subject to frequent rubbing or irritation.

Document all the following characteristics of any skin lesions: size, shape, colour, location, macular (flat) versus papular (raised), superficial versus penetrating, discrete versus diffuse borders, and the presence or absence of inflammation, redness or discharge. Terminology related to various skin lesions in older adults is confusing, and many terms are used interchangeably. Table 23-3 describes some of the terms used for skin lesions that are common in older adults; some of these lesions are shown in Figure 23-4.

Nursing assessment of the skin, hair and nails can provide clues to a broad spectrum of physiologic functioning, particularly in combination with additional assessment information. For example, brown-stained fingertips are an indication of cigarette use, and feces under the fingernails and around the cuticle may be a clue to constipation. In some circumstances, toenails provide clues to mobility difficulties, particularly when extremely long nails curl under the toes. Observations of the skin may provide the only objective evidence of serious functional problems that the older person might not otherwise acknowledge. For example, multiple bruises, particularly in various stages of healing, may be a significant clue to falls, alcoholism, self-neglect, or physical abuse. Observation and documentation of these signs are particularly important when neglect or abuse is suspected as described in detail in Chapter 10 (see Chapter 10 for a detailed description of elder abuse).

In assessing the skin for clues to the broader aspects of function, keep in mind that some of the usual manifestations may be altered in older adults. For example, skin turgor on the hands or arms is an indication of hydration status; however, this is not necessarily a reliable indicator in frail older adults. Also, age-related changes make it difficult to assess patterns of wound healing using the same standards that are applied to younger adults.

Observations of the hair, skin and nails can also provide clues to self-care abilities and aspects of psychosocial function. For example, poor personal grooming may be indicative

TABLE 23-3 Common Skin Lesions in Older Adults

Common Term(s)	Description
Age spots, liver spots, senile freckles	Pale to dark brown macules, occurring most frequently on exposed areas
Actinic keratosis, solar keratosis	Red, yellow, brown, or flesh-coloured papules or plaques; gritty texture; surrounded by erythema; *premalignant*
Senile purpura	Areas of brown or bluish discolouration that look like bruising
Seborrheic keratosis	Brown or black papules or plaques with sharp edges and a waxy or wartlike texture; appearing most frequently on trunk and face
Sebaceous hyperplasia	Yellowish, doughnut-shaped elevations; common on face, particularly in men
Senile angiomas, cherry or ruby angiomas, telangiectasia	Bright, ruby–red, pinpoint, superficial elevations of small blood vessels
Spider angiomas	Tiny, red papules with radiating arms; *may indicate a pathologic condition*
Venous stars	Bluish, irregular, sometimes spider-shaped lesions, appearing mainly on the legs or the chest
Venous lakes, benign venous angiomas	Bluish papules with sharp borders, appearing mainly on the lips or the ears
Acrochordons, skin tags	Flesh-coloured, pedunculated, or stalklike lesions
Corns, calluses	Hard masses of keratin caused by repeated pressure or irritation
Xanthelasma	Fatty deposits, usually around the eyes; *may be related to a pathologic condition*, particularly if large or numerous

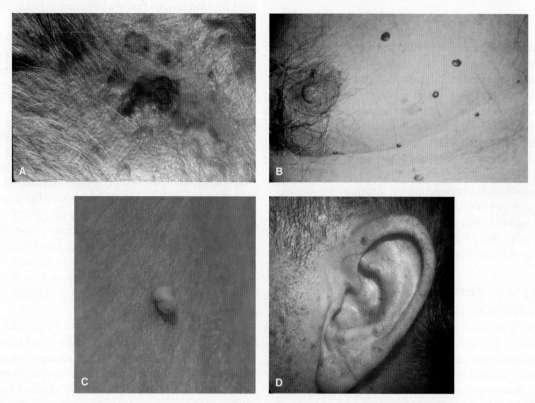

FIGURE 23-4 Common skin lesions in older adults. **(A)** Seborrheic keratosis. **(B)** Cherry angioma. **(C)** Skin tag. **(D)** Venous lakes or benign venous angiomas. (**A** & **D**, Reprinted with permission from Rosenthal, T. C., Williams, M. E., & Naughton, B. J. [2007]. *Office care geriatrics*. Philadelphia, PA: Lippincott Williams & Wilkins; **B**, Reprinted with permission from Weber, J., & Kelley, J. [2002]. *Health assessment in nursing* [2nd ed.]. Philadelphia, PA: Lippincott Williams & Wilkins; **C**, Courtesy of Stiefel Laboratories)

of functional limitations or psychosocial influences such as lack of motivation or awareness due to depression or dementia. The use of unusually deep hues of hair colouring or facial cosmetics may indicate impaired colour perception. Box 23-4 summarizes nursing observations pertaining to the integumentary system.

Box 23-4 Observations Regarding the Integument

Examination of the Skin

- What is the colour?
- Are there any areas of irregular pigmentation?
- Are there any areas of sunburn or tan?
- Are there areas that are discoloured in any way?
- Are there any indications of poor circulation, particularly in the extremities (e.g., varicosities, or areas of red, blue, or brown discolouration indicative of chronic stasis problems in the lower extremities)?
- What is the skin temperature?
- Is there a marked difference between the temperature of the extremities and that of the rest of the body?
- How does the skin feel in terms of moisture? Is it dry? Clammy? Oily?
- What is the skin's texture? Is it smooth or rough?
- Does the skin look tissue-paper thin?
- What is the turgor of the abdominal skin?
- Are scars present? (If so, describe their location and appearance.) Are there any signs of falling or physical abuse?
- Are any of the lesions described in Table 23-3 present?

Examination of the Hair and Nails

- What are the colour, texture and general condition of the hair?
- What is the distribution pattern of the hair?

- Is there any evidence of dandruff, scaling or other problems with the hair?
- What are the colour, length, cleanliness and general condition of the toenails and fingernails?
- What are the colour and general condition of the nail beds of the toes and fingers?

Personal Care Practices

- What is the person's overall appearance with regard to grooming and attention to personal attractiveness?
- If grooming is poor, does the person express concern about this or provide an explanation?
- Are there any psychosocial factors that influence personal care practices (e.g., is the person socially isolated or overburdened with caregiving responsibilities and, therefore, inattentive to personal care)?
- Are any of the following signs of neglect evident: presence of a body odour; unkempt, uncut, or matted hair; unusually long and unkempt fingernails or toenails; patches of brown crust on the skin; bruises; or any pathologic skin conditions?

Unfolding Case Study

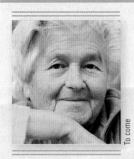

To come

Part 1: Ms. S. at 84 Years of Age

Ms. S. is an 84-year-old white woman who lives in her own home on the coast of New Brunswick. She is quite active and healthy and enjoys golfing and "beachcombing." She attends the local senior centre, where you are the wellness nurse. The local chapter of the Canadian Cancer Society is co-sponsoring a skin cancer screening day at the senior centre, and you have been asked to prepare a health education program titled "Checking Your Skin for Serious Changes." You are also assisting the dermatologist with the screening examinations. Ms. S. attends the health education part of your program and says she is not sure if she can stay for the screening. She has just one "age spot," and she knows it is not serious because she has "had a couple skin cancers removed, and this one looks different." You look at the questionable spot, and you assess it as a brown, raised plaque with a gritty texture, about 1 cm in diameter.

THINKING POINTS

- What additional assessment information would you want to obtain from Ms. S.?
- How would you use Table 23-3 and Boxes 23-3 and 23-4 in your assessment?

- What advice would you give to Ms. S. about her skin?

(continued)

Unfolding Case Study (continued)

QSEN APPLICATION

QSEN Competency	Knowledge/Skill/Attitude	Application to Ms. S. When She Is 84 Years of Age
Evidence-based practice	(K) Describe how the strength and relevance of available evidence influence the choice of intervention. (S) Base individualized care plan on patient values, clinical expertise and evidence. (A) Value evidence-based practice as integral to determining the best clinical practice.	Apply evidence-based information in Table 23-3 and Boxes 23-3 and 23-4 when you assess Ms. S. and teach her about the importance of participating in the health education program that includes a screening performed by a dermatologist.
Teamwork and collaboration	(K) Recognize contributions of other individuals and groups in helping patient achieve health goals. (S) Integrate the contributions of others who play a role in helping patient achieve health goals.	Assume leadership role in coordinating plans for dermatologist to provide screenings for skin cancer during health education program.

NURSING DIAGNOSIS

When older adults have any skin breakdown, nurses can use the nursing diagnosis of Impaired Skin Integrity, defined as "altered epidermis and/or dermis" (Herdman, 2012, p. 436). When older adults have any risk factors for skin tears or pressure ulcers, nurses can use the nursing diagnosis of Risk for Impaired Skin Integrity, which is defined as "at risk for alteration in epidermis and/or dermis" (Herdman, 2012, p. 437). Related factors that commonly affect older adults include medications, incontinence, dehydration, limited mobility, nutritional deficits or a combination of these factors.

If the older adult has any skin lesion that requires medical evaluation, the nursing diagnosis of Ineffective Health Maintenance might be applicable. This is defined as the "inability to identify, manage and/or seek out help to maintain health" (Herdman, 2012, p. 157). This nursing diagnosis might also be pertinent for older adults who do not use protective measures when they are exposed to ultraviolet radiation from sunlight or tanning beds.

Wellness Opportunity

Nurses can use the wellness nursing diagnosis of Readiness for Enhanced Knowledge: Skin Care for older adults who are interested in learning how to address risks for conditions such as dry skin and skin cancer.

PLANNING FOR WELLNESS OUTCOMES

When older adults have conditions that affect skin comfort or integrity, nurses identify wellness outcomes as an essential part of the nursing process. Similarly, when they have risks for conditions that can cause skin problems (e.g., skin cancer or pressure ulcers), nursing goals focus on prevention.

Wellness Opportunity

Nurses promote wellness when they plan outcomes to address skin comfort and the prevention of skin cancer.

For healthy older adults with risk factors (e.g., history of skin cancer) or minor skin problems (e.g., xerosis), applicable Nursing Outcomes Classification (NOC) terminology includes Comfort Level, Tissue Integrity: Skin and Mucous Membranes, Knowledge: Health Behaviour, Health Seeking Behaviour, Nutritional Status, Risk Control: Cancer, and Risk Control: Sun Exposure.

For older adults with pressure ulcers or other types of wounds or skin breakdown, NOC terms include Impaired Skin Integrity, Wound Healing: Primary Intention, and Wound Healing: Secondary Intention. Outcomes are achieved through interventions discussed in the following section.

NURSING INTERVENTIONS FOR SKIN WELLNESS

Nurses have many opportunities for promoting wellness with regard to comfort, self-esteem and maintenance of a healthy integumentary system. Nursing interventions for healthy older adults focus on promoting self-responsibility for identifying and seeking further evaluation for harmful or precancerous lesions. Interventions for physically compromised older adults focus on maintaining intact skin and managing pressure ulcers. The following Nursing Interventions

Classification (NIC) terminologies can be used to document interventions: Hair Care, Health Education, Health Screening, Nutrition Therapy, Positioning, Pressure Management, Pressure Ulcer Prevention, Pruritus Management, Risk Identification, Self-Esteem Enhancement, Skin Surveillance and Wound Care.

Promoting Healthy Skin

Because one's overall health significantly affects the condition of the skin, maintenance of optimal nutrition and hydration is an important intervention in the skin care of older adults. Health promotion interventions also address environmental factors and personal care practices that influence the condition of the skin. Box 23-5 can be used as a guide to teaching older adults, or caregivers of dependent older adults, about skin health. Although much of the gerontologic nursing literature advocates limiting baths or showers to one to three times weekly, it is not clear that there is a cause–effect relationship between bathing or showers and dry skin. Other factors, including smoking, dehydration, sun exposure, low environmental humidity and the use of harsh cleansing products, are likely to contribute to skin problems in older adults.

Currently, there is controversy about health promotion recommendations related to exposure to sunlight because sunlight is required for vitamin D synthesis in humans and it is beneficial in treating seasonal affective disorder and many skin conditions, including psoriasis and fungal mycosis (Wilson et al., 2012). In contrast, it is a well-recognized cause of wrinkles, photoaging, all types of skin cancer and other skin conditions, as well as increased risk for diseases of other systems (e.g., cataracts, immunosuppression) (Al-Mutairi et al., 2012). Concerns about vitamin D deficiency from lack of exposure to sunlight include increased incidence of or poor outcome for autoimmune conditions, infectious diseases, cardiovascular disease and various types of cancers (e.g., skin, breast, colon) (Mason & Reichrath, 2013). Current recommendations emphasize the importance of a balanced approach that encourages small amounts of sun exposure each day for adequate vitamin D synthesis, but not so much that would lead to increased skin cancer risk (Bonevski et al., 2013).

Although questions have been raised about the safety and efficacy of sunscreens, recent Food and Drug Agency (FDA) regulatory guidelines emphasize the following (Jou et al., 2012; Latha et al., 2013):

- All sunscreening agents must be tested and meet requirements for claims about effectiveness.
- Claims for broad-spectrum agents must protect from both ultraviolet A and ultraviolet B rays.
- Claims for reduction of skin cancer and skin aging can be made only with a SPF between 15 and 50.
- Claims of "waterproof," "sweatproof," or "sunblocks" are not permitted because they overemphasize the product's efficacy.
- Claims of "water resistant" need to be substantiated by tests for 40 or 80 minutes.

- Acceptable forms of sunscreen include oils, gels, sprays, creams, pastes, butters and ointment; forms that are *not* acceptable include wipes, powders, shampoos, towelettes and body washes.

> **Box 23-5 Health Promotion Teaching About Skin Care for Older Adults**
>
> *Maintaining Healthy Skin*
> - Include adequate amounts of fluid in the daily diet.
> - Use humidifiers to maintain environmental humidity levels of 40% to 60%.
> - Apply moisturizing lotions twice daily or as needed.
> - Use moisturizing lotions immediately after bathing, when the skin is still moist.
> - Avoid massaging over bony prominences when applying lotions.
> - Avoid skin care products that contain perfumes or isopropyl alcohol.
> - Avoid multiple-ingredient preparations because unnecessary additives may cause allergic responses.
> - Inspect skin monthly for suspicious-looking changes.
>
> *Personal Care Practices*
> - When bathing or showering, use soap sparingly or use a mild, unscented soap (e.g., Dove, Tone, Basis, Aveeno).
> - Maintain water temperatures for bathing at about 32°C to 37°C.
> - Rinse well after using soap. Whirlpool baths stimulate circulation, but moderate temperatures should be maintained.
> - Apply moisturizing products after bathing, rather than using them in the bath water, to minimize the risk for falls on oily surfaces and to maximize the benefits of the emollient.
> - Use emollient products containing petrolatum or mineral oil (e.g., Keri, Eucerin, Aquaphor, Vanicream, Vaseline).
> - If you use bath oils, take extra safety precautions to prevent slipping.
> - If moisturizing products are applied to the feet, wear nonskid slippers or socks before walking.
> - Dry your skin thoroughly, particularly between your toes and in other areas where your skin rubs together.
> - When drying your skin, use gentle, patting motions rather than harsh, rubbing motions.
> - Obtain regular podiatric care.
>
> *Preventing Sun Damage and Skin Cancers*
> - Wear wide-brimmed hats, sun visors, sunglasses and light-coloured clothing when exposed to the sun.
> - Wear clothing made of cotton, rather than polyester fabrics, because ultraviolet rays can penetrate polyester.
> - Apply sunscreen products liberally beginning 1 hour before sun exposure and reapplying at frequent intervals.
> - Use sunscreen lotions with an SPF of 30. Avoid exposure to the sun between 10:00 AM and 4:00 PM.
> - Protect yourself from ultraviolet rays even on cloudy days and when you are in the water (lake, pool, ocean).
> - Artificial tanning booths use ultraviolet type A rays, which have been found to cause damage and increase the risk for skin cancers.
>
> *Preventing Injury From Abrasive Forces*
> - Do not use starch, bleach or strong detergents when laundering clothing or linens.
> - Use soft terry or cotton washcloths.
> - If waterproof pads are necessary, make sure that an adequate amount of soft, absorbent material is placed near the body.

Studies suggest that use of sunscreens can prevent skin aging and this is not a contributing factor for vitamin D deficiency (Hughes et al., 2013; Lin et al., 2011). This information can be incorporated in health education about use of sunscreens to protect older adults from skin cancer and other skin changes. Online Learning Activity 23-3 lists resources for teaching older adults about prevention of skin cancer.

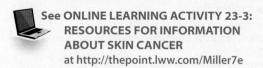

See **ONLINE LEARNING ACTIVITY 23-3:**
RESOURCES FOR INFORMATION
ABOUT SKIN CANCER
at http://thepoint.lww.com/Miller7e

Preventing Skin Wrinkles

The best methods of preventing skin lesions and wrinkles are avoiding too much exposure to sunlight and using a sunscreen and other protective measures (as summarized in Box 23-5) when exposure to sunlight is unavoidable. Topical products containing α- or β-hydroxy acids may be beneficial in reversing wrinkles and promoting the regression of solar keratoses. Be alert to the possibility that older adults might develop an allergic or sensitivity reaction to some of the ingredients in topical products. Information about the harmful effects of sunlight should be included in health education about the maintenance of healthy skin and prevention of undesirable cosmetic and pathologic skin changes. Also, encourage people who are concerned about wrinkles and dry skin to discuss medical interventions with their primary care provider.

Wellness Opportunity

Nurses promote wellness by teaching that exposure to ultraviolet light—by sunlight or tanning lights—is a major factor in the occurrence of skin wrinkles, skin cancer and other skin changes.

Preventing Dry Skin

Petrolatum and other emollients are effective in alleviating dry skin discomfort, because they moisturize and lubricate the skin. The effectiveness of an emollient is based on its ability to prevent water evaporation, so the beneficial effects will be enhanced when it is applied to skin that already has some degree of moisture. Thus, an emollient agent is most effective when it is applied to moist skin immediately after bathing. See Box 23-5 for information on the use of emollients and other interventions designed to prevent or care for dry skin in older adults.

Detecting and Treating Harmful Skin Lesions

Early detection and treatment of cancerous or precancerous skin lesions are key factors in preventing serious functional consequences, because the cure rate for most skin cancers approaches 100% with early excision. The nurse's role is to detect any suspicious-looking lesions and to encourage or facilitate further evaluation. Encourage all older adults to use the following guide to identify any skin changes that require further evaluation:

- **A**symmetric shape: irregular or different-looking sides
- **B**order that is irregular: ragged, notched, blurred, irregular
- **C**olour change: different shades, uneven distribution
- **D**iameter: larger than a quarter of an inch (6 mm), increasing

If older adults or their caregivers have avoided medical evaluation because of fears about cancer, provide reassurance about the high cure rate and the minimal chance of long-term problems if early treatment is initiated. Similarly, if they have ignored suspicious changes because they attribute them to "normal aging," teach about the importance of further evaluation. Box 23-5 includes health promotion information about the prevention and early detection of skin cancer.

Unfolding Case Study

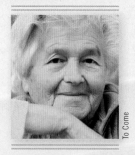

To Come

Part 2: Ms. S. at 86 Years of Age

Ms. S. is 86 years old and continues to attend the senior centre in New Brunswick where you are responsible for presenting a health education program titled "Maintaining Healthy Skin." You plan to emphasize the importance of self-care techniques such as checking for skin changes. Ms. S. is very interested in attending the program and tells you she will be bringing her 80-year-old sister, who also lives in New Brunswick. Ms. S. worries about her sister because she uses a wheelchair and is very frail. You know that several of the participants at the senior program use wheelchairs, and you plan to include health education about preventing pressure ulcers.

THINKING POINTS

- Outline your health education points for a half-hour program including specific points about preventing pressure ulcers.
- How would you use Table 23-2 and Box 23-5 in your program?

- Find additional information that you would consider using as educational materials for this program.

QSEN APPLICATION

QSEN Competency	Knowledge/Skill/Attitude	Application to Ms. S. When She Is 86 Years of Age
Evidence-based practice	(K) Describe how the strength and relevance of available evidence influence the choice of intervention.	Use Table 23-2 and Box 23-5 for evidence-based information in the health education program.
	(S) Base individualized care plan on patient values, clinical expertise and evidence.	
	(A) Value evidence-based practice as integral to determining the best clinical practice.	

Wellness Opportunity

Nurses address the body–mind–spirit interrelationship by allaying unreasonable fears about skin cancer.

EVALUATING EFFECTIVENESS OF NURSING INTERVENTIONS

Nursing care for older adults with dry or itching skin is evaluated by determining the degree to which the interventions alleviate the person's complaints. It may take several weeks for older adults to feel the full effects of skin care interventions because of an age-related delay in dermal response to external stimuli. Also, there is a great deal of individual variation among older adults in their response to interventions. Thus, it may be necessary to evaluate the effects of one type of soap or lotion for several weeks before trying a different brand if the problem does not resolve. Because environmental humidity affects skin comfort, environmental conditions may also influence the evaluation of interventions.

The effectiveness of interventions for older adults at risk for skin breakdown is measured by the absence of skin tears or pressure ulcers. The effectiveness of interventions for pressure ulcers is determined by the rate of healing and prevention of complications such as osteomyelitis. Because significant cost and quality-of-life issues are associated with pressure ulcers, preventing skin breakdown can have far-reaching positive consequences for older adults who are at risk for developing pressure ulcers.

Unfolding Case Study

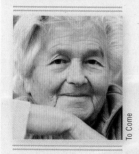

Part 3: Ms. S. at 92 Years of Age

Ms. S. is now 92 years old and lives in an assisted-living facility in New Brunswick. She ambulates with a walker and needs assistance with meals, medications and personal care. Three months ago, her doctor prescribed hydrochlorothiazide 25 mg every morning for isolated systolic hypertension. She has a history of arthritis but does not take any medication for it. Ms. S. attends your monthly nursing clinic for health education and blood pressure monitoring. When she comes to see you in January, she complains of dry skin and discomfort.

NURSING ASSESSMENT

You interview Ms. S. about her personal care practices and find out that she soaks in the tub in lukewarm water three times weekly and enjoys using bath salts and perfumed skin lotions. She spends much of her leisure time outdoors on the patio or in the air-conditioned solarium. She does not use sunscreens because she thinks they are unnecessary and too oily. She states that she has not had sunburn for several years, and that she has built up a good tolerance to the sun. She does not wear sunglasses or sun hats. She reports that she has had three skin cancers removed in the past 10 years, one from her cheek, one from her arm and one from her ear lobe. She says she does not worry about recurrent skin cancer because she no longer swims outside or sits by the swimming pool. Also, because she does not get sunburned, she believes she is not at risk for skin cancer.

Inspection of Ms. S.'s skin reveals dry, wrinkled skin on her face and arms, and unevenly tanned skin on her face, neck and extremities. She has many age spots over the exposed skin areas but no suspicious-looking lesions. Ms. S. has blue eyes and fair skin.

(continued)

Unfolding Case Study (continued)

NURSING DIAGNOSIS

Your nursing diagnosis is Ineffective Health Maintenance related to excessive sunlight exposure and insufficient knowledge of the effects of ultraviolet light. Evidence for this diagnosis comes from her misconceptions about risk factors for skin cancer and other skin problems. Also, you identify her lack of knowledge about the potential photosensitivity reactions associated with use of hydrochlorothiazide as a factor that contributes to Ineffective Health Maintenance.

NURSING CARE PLAN FOR Ms. S.

Expected Outcome	Nursing Interventions	Nursing Evaluation
Ms. S.'s discomfort from dry skin will be alleviated.	• Discuss and describe age-related skin changes. • Discuss risk factors that contribute to skin discomfort (e.g., bath salts, perfumed lotions, unprotected exposure to sunlight). • Use Box 23-5 to teach Ms. S. about skin care practices directed toward alleviating dry skin.	• Ms. S. will report that she no longer experiences skin discomfort and dryness.
Ms. S.'s knowledge about risk factors for skin cancer will increase.	• Discuss the relationship between skin cancer and exposure to ultraviolet rays. • Explain that any exposure to ultraviolet rays is a risk factor for skin cancer. • Emphasize that a history of skin cancer increases the chance of recurrent skin cancer.	• Ms. S. will verbalize an awareness of the risk factors for skin cancer.
The factors that increase Ms. S.'s risk of skin problems and skin cancer will be eliminated.	• Inform Ms. S. that hydrochlorothiazide may increase the risk for photosensitivity, making protective measures increasingly important. • Use Box 23-5 as a guide for discussing measures to avoid sun damage. • Emphasize the importance of using sunscreens and wearing wide-brimmed hats when in the solarium or outside.	• Ms. S. will use measures to reduce the risk for skin cancer and sun damage.

THINKING POINTS

- What risk factors would you address in your care plan?
- How would you promote Ms. S.'s personal responsibility for skin care, including addressing risks for skin cancer?

QSEN APPLICATION

QSEN Competency	Knowledge/Skill/Attitude	Application to Ms. S. When She Is 92 Years of Age
Patient-centred care	(K) Integrate understanding of multiple dimensions of patient-centred care.	Identify the conditions that are likely to cause dry skin and increase the risk for skin problems.
	(K) Describe strategies to empower patients in all aspects of the health care process.	Provide accurate information to dispel myths and misunderstanding and improve Ms. S.'s knowledge about risks for skin cancer.
	(K) Examine nursing roles in assuring coordination, integration and continuity of care.	Recognize the important health promotion role of nurses in teaching about self-care actions to prevent skin dryness and cancer.
Evidence-based practice	(S) Base individualized care plan on patient values, clinical expertise and evidence. (A) Value evidence-based practice as integral to determining the best clinical practice.	Apply evidence-based guidelines summarized in Box 23-5 to teach about measures to prevent sun damage.

Chapter Highlights

Age-Related Changes That Affect Skin Wellness (Table 23-1)

- Thinner dermis, flattened dermal–epidermal junction
- Diminished moisture content
- Decreased dermal blood supply
- Fewer sweat and sebaceous glands
- Nails become thinner, fragile, brittle, prone to splitting
- Changes in patterns of hair distribution

Risks Factors That Affect Skin Wellness

- Genetic factors (hair colour and distribution, skin colour, skin cancer)
- Smoking, sun exposure, stress
- Personal hygiene practices
- Adverse medication effects
- Factors that increase the risk for skin breakdown

Functional Consequences Affecting Skin Wellness (Table 23-1)

- Delayed wound healing
- Increased susceptibility to skin problems (skin cancer, breakdown, pressure ulcers)
- Xerosis (dry skin), discomfort
- Irregular pigmentation and other cosmetic changes
- Decreased tactile sensitivity, increased susceptibility to burns
- Diminished sweating and shivering, increased susceptibility to hypothermia and heat-related conditions

Pathologic Conditions Affecting Skin Wellness (Fig. 23-1, Table 23-2)

- Skin cancer: basal cell carcinoma, squamous cell carcinoma, melanoma
- Skin tears
- Pressure ulcers (Box 23-2)
- Risk for pressure ulcers (Figs. 23-2 and 23-3)

Nursing Assessment of Skin (Table 23-3, Boxes 23-3 and 23-4)

- Abnormal skin conditions
- Personal care practices
- Skin lesions common in older adults (Table 23-3, Fig. 23-4)

Nursing Diagnosis

- Readiness for Enhanced Knowledge: Skin
- Impaired Skin Integrity (or Risk for)
- Ineffective Health Maintenance

Planning for Wellness Outcomes

- Comfort Level
- Tissue Integrity: Skin and Mucous Membranes
- Nutritional Status
- Risk Control: Cancer
- Wound Healing

Nursing Interventions for Skin Wellness (Box 23-5)

- Health promotion teaching about healthy skin
- Preventing skin wrinkles
- Preventing dry skin
- Detecting and treating suspect skin changes

Evaluating Effectiveness of Nursing Interventions

- Alleviation of complaints (e.g., dryness)
- Evaluation of suspect skin changes
- Absence of pressure ulcers in high-risk older adults
- Wound healing

Critical Thinking Exercises

1. What changes would a healthy 85-year-old person notice with regard to his or her skin, hair and nails?
2. Describe the questions you would ask and the observations you would make to assess the skin, hair and nails of an 82-year-old person.
3. Describe at least eight skin lesions that are normal and three skin lesions that require further evaluation.
4. You are asked to give a 20-minute presentation on "Maintaining Healthy Skin" at a senior centre. Outline the content of your health education program.
5. What would you teach the family caregivers of a 74-year-old woman who sits in a wheelchair for 14 hours a day with regard to the prevention of pressure ulcers?

 For more information about the topics discussed in this chapter, be sure to check out the interactive Online Learning Activities and other helpful resources at http://thepoint.lww.com/Miller7e

REFERENCES

Accreditation Canada. (2013). *Implementation of turning clocks for pressure ulcer prevention and management*. Retrieved from http://www.accreditation.ca/implementation-turning-clocks-pressure-ulcer-prevention-and-management

Al-Mutairi, N., Issa, B. I., & Nair, V. (2012). Photoprotection and vitamin D status. *Indian Journal of Dermatology, Venerology and Leprology, 78*(3), 342–349.

Apold, J., & Rydrych, D. (2012). Preventing device-related pressure ulcers. *Journal of Nursing Care Quality, 27*(1), 28–34.

Ayello, E. A., & Sibbald, R. G. (2012). Preventing pressure ulcers and skin tears. In M. Boltz, E. Capezuti, T. Fulmer et al. (Eds.), *Evidence-based geriatric nursing protocols for best practice* (4th ed., pp. 298–323). New York, NY: Springer.

Bergquist-Beringer, S., & Daley, C. M. (2011). Adapting pressure ulcer prevention for use in home health care. *Journal of Wound Ostomy and Continence Nursing, 38*(2), 145–154.

Black, J., Berke, C., & Urzendowski, G. (2012). Pressure ulcer incidence and progression in critically ill subjects. *Journal of Wound Ostomy and Continence Nursing, 39*(3), 267–273.

Bonevski, B., Bryant, J., Lambert, S., et al. (2013). The ABC of vitamin D: A qualitative study of the knowledge and attitudes regarding vitamin D deficiency amongst selected population groups. *Nutrients, 5,* 915–927. doi:10.3390/nu5030915

Braga, I. A., Pirett, C. C., Ribas, R. M., et al. (2013). Bacterial colonization of pressure ulcers: Assessment of risk for bloodstream infection and impact on patient outcomes. *Journal of Hospital Infections, 83*(4), 314–320.

Briggs, M., Collinson, M., Wilson, L., et al. (2013). The prevalence of pain at pressure areas and pressure ulcers in hospitalized patients. *BioMed Central Nursing, 12*(1), 19.

Bry, K. E., Buescher, D., & Sandrik, M. (2012). Never say never: A descriptive study of hospital-acquired pressure ulcers in a hospital setting. *Journal of Wound Ostomy and Continence Nursing, 39*(3), 274–280.

Canadian Skin Cancer Foundation. (2012). *Basal cell carcinoma.* Retrieved from http://www.canadianskincancerfoundation.com/basal-cell-carcinoma.html

Chang, A. L., Wong, J. W., Endo, J. O., et al. (2013). Geriatric dermatology review: Major changes in skin function in older patients and their contribution to common clinical challenges. *Journal of the American Medical Directors Association, 14*(10), 724–730.

Chou, R., Dana, T., Bougatsos, C., et al. (2013). *Pressure ulcer risk assessment and prevention: Comparative effectiveness.* Rockville, MD: Agency for Healthcare Quality and Research, Publication No. 12(13)-EHC148-EF.

Cox, J. (2012). Predictive power of the Braden Scale for Pressure Sore Risk in adult critical care patients. *Journal of Wound Ostomy and Continence Nursing, 39*(6), 613–621.

Coyer, F. M., Stotts, N. A., & Blackman, V. S. (2014). A prospective window into medical device-related pressure ulcers in intensive care. *International Wound Journal, 11*(6), 656–664. doi:10.1111/wj.12026

Durai, P. C., Thappa, D. M., Kumari, R., et al. (2012). Aging in elderly: Chronological versus photoaging. *Indian Journal of Dermatology, 57*(5), 343–352.

Gadd, M. M. (2012). Preventing hospital-acquired pressure ulcers. *Journal of Wound Ostomy and Continence Nursing, 39*(3), 292–294.

Gatherwright, J., Liu, M. T., Amirlak, B., et al. (2013). The contribution of endogenous and exogenous factors to male alopecia: A study of identical twins. *Plastic and Reconstructive Surgery, 131*(5), 794e–801e.

Gatherwright, J., Liu, M. T., Gliniak, C., et al. (2012). The contribution of endogenous and exogenous factors to female alopecia: A study of identical twins. *Plastic and Reconstructive Surgery, 130*(6), 1219–1226.

Geller, A. C., Swetter, S. M., Oliveria, S., et al. (2011). Reducing mortality in individuals at high risk for advanced melanoma through education and screening. *Journal of the American Academy of Dermatology, 65*(5 Suppl. 1), S87–S94.

Herdman, T. H. (Ed.). (2012). *NANDA International Nursing Diagnoses: Definitions and classification 2012–1014.* Oxford, England: Wiley-Blackwell.

Holmes, R. F., Davidson, M. W., Thompson, B. J., et al. (2013). Skin tears: Care and management of the older adult at home. *Home Healthcare Nurse, 31*(2), 90–101.

Hon, J., Lagden, K., McLaren, A.-M., et al. (2010). A prospective, multicenter study to validate use of the pressure ulcer scale for healing (PUSH) in patients with diabetic, venous, and pressure ulcers. *Ostomy Wound Management, 56,* 26–36.

Hughes, M. C., Williams, G. M., Baker, P., et al. (2013). Sunscreen and prevention of skin aging: A randomized trial. *Annals of Internal Medicine, 158*(11), 781–790.

Jou, P. C., Feldman, R. J., & Tomecki, K. J. (2012). UV protection and sunscreens: What to tell patients. *Cleveland Clinic Journal of Medicine, 79*(6), 427–435.

Kelechi, T. J., Arndt, J V., & Dove, A. (2013). Review of pressure ulcer risk assessment scales. *Journal of Wound, Ostomy and Continence Nurses Society, 40*(3), 232–236.

Kelleher, A. D., Moorer, A., & Makic, M. F. (2012). Peer-to-peer nursing rounds and hospital-acquired pressure ulcer prevalence in a surgical intensive care unit. *Journal of Wound, Ostomy and Continence Nurses Society, 39*(2), 152–157.

Latha, M. S., Martis, J., Shobha, V., et al. (2013). Sunscreening agents: A review. *Journal of Clinical and Asthetic Dermatology, 6*(11), 16–24.

Latreille, J., Kesse-Guyot, E., Malvy, D., et al. (2012). Dietary monounsaturated fatty acids intake and risk of skin photoaging. *PLOS One, 7*(9), e44490. Retrieved from www.plosone.org

LeBlanc, K., Baranoski, S., Holloway, S., et al. (2013). Validation of a new classification system for skin tears. *Advances in Skin & Wound Care, 26*(6), 263–266.

Lin, J. S., Eder, M., Weinmann, S., et al. (2011). *Evidence Synthesis Number 82: Behavioral counseling to prevent skin cancer: Systematic evidence review to update the 2003 U. S. Preventive Services Task Force recommendation.* Rockville, MD: Agency for Healthcare Research and Quality. Retrieved from www.ahrq.gov

Little, E. G., & Eide, M. J. (2012). Update on the current state of melanoma incidence. *Dermatology Clinics, 30*(3). doi.016/det.2012.04.001

Liu, P., He, W., & Chen, H.-L. (2012). Diabetes mellitus as a risk factor for surgery-related pressure ulcers. *Journal of Wound, Ostomy and Continence Nurses Society, 39*(5), 495–499.

Lyder, C. H., Wang, Y., Metersky, M., et al. (2012). Hospital-acquired pressure ulcers: Results from the national Medicare Patient Safety Monitoring System study. *Journal of the American Geriatrics Society, 60*(9), 1603–1608.

Makrantonaki, E., Bekou, V., & Zouboulis, C. C. (2012). Genetics and skin aging. *Dermato Endocrinology, 4*(3), 280–284.

Mason, R. S., & Reichrath, J. (2013). Sunlight vitamin D and skin cancer. *Anticancer Agents in Medical Chemistry, 13*(1), 83–97.

Melanoma Network of Canada. (n.d.). *Melanoma facts.* Retrieved from http://www.melanomanetwork.ca/facts-summary/

Pollack, L. A., Berkowitz, Z., Weir, H. K., et al. (2011). Melanoma survival in the United States, 1992 to 2005. *Journal of the American Academy of Dermatology, 65*(5 Suppl. 1), S78–S86.

Registered Nurses Association of Ontario. (2011). *Risk assessment and prevention of pressure ulcers.* Toronto, ON: Author. Retrieved from http://rnao.ca/bpg/guidelines/risk-assessment-andprevention-pressure-ulcers

Sinnya, S., & DeAmbrosis, B. (2013, June 6). Stress and melanoma: Increasing evidence towards a causal basis. *Archives of Dermatology Research, 305*(9), 851–856.

Stotts, N. A., Brown, D. S., Donaldson, N. E., et al. (2013). Eliminating hospital-acquired pressure ulcers: Within our reach. *Advances in Skin and Wound Care, 26*(1), 13–18.

Tescher, A., Branda, M., Bryne, T., et al. (2012). All at-risk patients are not created equal. *Journal of Wound, Ostomy and Continence Nursing, 39*(3), 282–291.

Theisen, S., Drabik, A., & Stock, S. (2012). Pressure ulcers in older hospitalised patients and its impact on length of stay: A retrospective observational study. *Journal of Clinical Nursing, 21*(3–4), 380–387.

Tschannen, D., Bates, O., Talsma, A., et al. (2012). Patient-specific and surgical characteristics in the development of pressure ulcers. *American Journal of Critical Care, 21,* 116–125.

Turk, B. G., Gunaydin, A., Ertam, I., et al. (2013). Adverse cutaneous drug reactions among hospitalized patients: Five year surveillance. *Cutaneous Ocular Toxicology, 32*(1), 41–45. doi:10.3109/15569527.2012.702837

Vierkotter, A., & Krutmann, J. (2012). Environmental influences on skin aging and ethnic-specific manifestations. *DermatoEndocrinology, 4*(3), 227–231.

Walls, A. C., Han, J., Li, T., et al. (2013, April 13). Host risk factors, ultraviolet index of residence, and incident malignant melanoma in situ among US women and men. *American Journal of Epidemiology, 177*(9), 997–1005.

Wilson, B. D., Moon, S., & Armstrong, F. (2012). Comprehensive review of ultraviolet radiation and the current status on sunscreens. *Journal of Clinical and Aesthetic Dermatology, 5*(9), 18–22.

Wu, X. C., Eide, M. J., King, J., et al. (2011). Racial and ethnic variations in incidence and survival of cutaneous melanoma in the United States, 1999–2006. *Journal of American Academy of Dermatology, 65*(5 Suppl. 1), S26–S37.

chapter 24

Sleep and Rest

LEARNING OBJECTIVES

After reading this chapter, you will be able to:

1. Delineate age-related changes that affect sleep and rest patterns in older adults.

2. Identify psychosocial, environmental and physiologic risk factors that influence sleep and rest in older adults.

3. Discuss sleep changes and problems common in older adults.

4. Assess sleep patterns in older adults to identify opportunities for health promotion to improve sleep.

5. Identify nursing interventions to promote optimal sleep and to address risks that interfere with sleep in older adults.

KEY POINTS

advanced sleep phase

circadian rhythm

Epworth Sleepiness Scale (ESS)

excessive daytime sleepiness

insomnia

obstructive sleep apnea (OSA)

periodic limb movements during sleep (PLMS)

Pittsburgh Sleep Quality Index (PSQI)

restless legs syndrome (RLS)

sleep latency

protein synthesis accelerate, and cognitive and emotional information is processed. Recent studies increasingly emphasize the major role of sleep in modulating metabolic, endocrine and cardiovascular systems (Rizzi et al., 2011). Thus, the quantity and quality of sleep affect many aspects of wellness.

Before the 1930s, research on sleep was nonexistent, and nocturnal sleep was viewed as the absence of daytime activity, rather than as an activity in its own right. In the 1950s, our understanding of sleep patterns improved significantly on the basis of polygraphic measurements that identified distinct sleep cycles. During the 1970s, sleep disorder centres were established to conduct research on sleep and offer comprehensive evaluation and treatment programs for persons suffering from sleep disorders. Now, sleep-related concerns are widely recognized as a major health issue and a major focus of research. In addition, health care practitioners have increasingly recognized the importance of addressing sleep as an essential aspect of health promotion (Canadian Sleep Society, http://www.canadiansleepsociety.ca). Because older adults are as likely as younger adults to benefit from newer information and technology, it is important to understand the commonly occurring sleep problems of older adults so that they too can benefit from evidence-based approaches to addressing this important health-related quality-of-life concern.

AGE-RELATED CHANGES THAT AFFECT SLEEP AND REST

A half century of sleep research has provided a strong base of information about age-related changes in sleep patterns, as well as the many sleep disorders that affect older adults. Sleep patterns of older adults are affected by complex relationships among a wide range of physiologic, environmental and psychosocial factors. This section describes age-related changes in sleep characteristics according to the quantity of time spent in bed and the depth and quality of sleep.

Approximately one-third of a person's lifetime is spent in sleep and rest activities, yet little attention is paid to the essential physiologic and psychosocial functions accomplished through these activities. During sleep and rest, many metabolic processes decelerate, production of growth hormone increases, and tissue repair and

Promoting Sleep Wellness in Older Adults

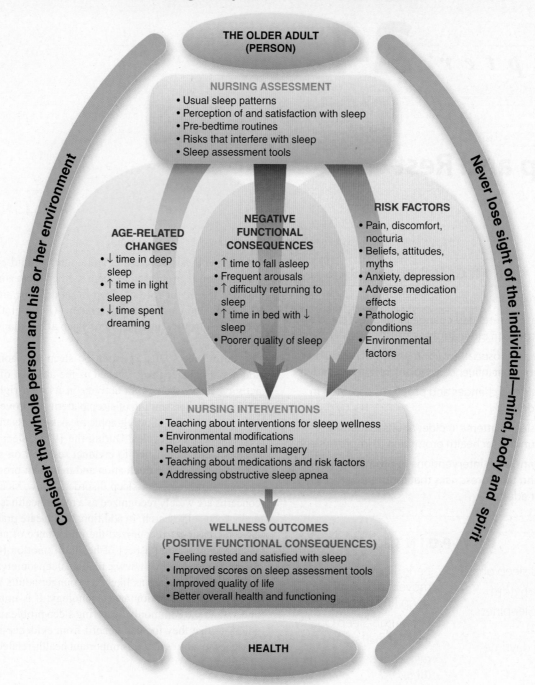

THE OLDER ADULT (PERSON)

NURSING ASSESSMENT
- Usual sleep patterns
- Perception of and satisfaction with sleep
- Pre-bedtime routines
- Risks that interfere with sleep
- Sleep assessment tools

AGE-RELATED CHANGES
- ↓ time in deep sleep
- ↑ time in light sleep
- ↓ time spent dreaming

NEGATIVE FUNCTIONAL CONSEQUENCES
- ↑ time to fall asleep
- Frequent arousals
- ↑ difficulty returning to sleep
- ↑ time in bed with ↓ sleep
- Poorer quality of sleep

RISK FACTORS
- Pain, discomfort, nocturia
- Beliefs, attitudes, myths
- Anxiety, depression
- Adverse medication effects
- Pathologic conditions
- Environmental factors

NURSING INTERVENTIONS
- Teaching about interventions for sleep wellness
- Environmental modifications
- Relaxation and mental imagery
- Teaching about medications and risk factors
- Addressing obstructive sleep apnea

WELLNESS OUTCOMES
(POSITIVE FUNCTIONAL CONSEQUENCES)
- Feeling rested and satisfied with sleep
- Improved scores on sleep assessment tools
- Improved quality of life
- Better overall health and functioning

HEALTH

Consider the whole person and his or her environment

Never lose sight of the individual—mind, body and spirit

Sleep Quantity

Sleep efficiency, which is the percentage of time asleep during the time in bed, ranges from 80% to 90% for younger people and diminishes to 50% to 70% for older people (Misra & Malow, 2008). This diminished sleep efficiency is attributed both to prolonged **sleep latency**, which is the time required to fall asleep, and to an increased number of awakenings during the night. Older adults are likely to take daytime naps, which can be beneficial in compensating for less nighttime sleep (Cohen-Mansfield & Perach, 2012).

Sleep Quality

Nocturnal sleep patterns are described in terms of sleep cycles and sleep stages. Each sleep cycle, which lasts between

70 and 120 minutes, is a combination of sleep stages. Sleep stages are classified according to the presence of rapid eye movement (REM) or the absence of this characteristic (non-REM). In adults, a cycle typically begins with Stage I non-REM (lightest sleep), progresses through Stage IV (deepest sleep), recurs in reverse order, and is followed by REM sleep (dream stage). As the cycle repeats during the night, non-REM length decreases and REM increases, so more time is spent in dream stage. During the non-REM stages, hormones are released, muscles relax, body systems slow and essential restorative functions take place.

In addition to the presence of rapid eye movements, REM sleep is characterized by the following physiologic changes: flaccid muscles, increased gastric acid secretions, increased cerebral blood flow, fluctuating blood pressure and thermoregulation, increased rate and irregular rhythm of pulse and respirations. These physiologic alterations can exacerbate some medical problems. For example, increased gastric acid secretion during REM sleep may precipitate gastrointestinal pain for people with peptic ulcer disease. Likewise, people with chronic obstructive pulmonary disease (COPD) may experience dyspnea or even a respiratory crisis because of decreased oxygen saturation during REM periods.

Because the length of the lightest sleep stage increases gradually throughout adulthood, older adults experience longer periods of drowsiness without actual sleep during the early part of the night. In addition, older adults shift more frequently in and out of lighter sleep stages. Between the ages of 20 and 40 years old, the proportion of deep sleep (Stages III and IV) decreases gradually until the age of 70 years, when it levels off. In both younger and older adults, Stage IV sleep increases significantly during the night after sleep loss. The number of episodes of REM sleep does not change significantly in older adults, but episodes are shorter, resulting in proportionately less time spent in REM. Also, REM sleep stages shift toward the earlier part of the night in older adults. Table 24-1 summarizes the usual adult sleep cycle and typical age-related changes in sleep patterns.

Circadian Rhythm

Sleep patterns are determined, in part, by an individual's **circadian rhythm**, also known as a *biologic clock*. Body functions that have a circadian pattern include thermoregulation, sleep–wake cycles, and secretion of many hormones, including cortisol and melatonin. The sleep–wake circadian rhythm generally causes adults to become sleepy between 10 PM and midnight and to awaken feeling rested between 6 AM and 8 AM. With increasing age, **advanced sleep phase** occurs, causing older adults to become sleepy earlier in the evening and to awaken earlier in the morning. Age-related alterations in circadian rhythm affect sleep quantity and quality, and these disturbances are likely to be exacerbated by lack of exposure to bright light.

TABLE 24-1 Age-Related Changes in Sleep

Sleep Characteristics	Healthy Older Adults (vs. Healthy Younger Adults)
Non-REM	Gradual increase in length of light sleep stages with less time in deep sleep More frequent shifts in and out of light sleep
REM (dream stage)	Shorter episodes Begins earlier in the night Less intense
Sleep initiation	Longer time to fall asleep
Sleep maintenance	More frequent arousals
Sleep efficiency	Reduced amount of sleep during time in bed, more time in napping to compensate
Sleep schedule	Shift in nocturnal sleep phase to earlier bedtime and wakening

Non-REM, non–rapid eye movement; REM, rapid eye movement.

RISK FACTORS THAT CAN AFFECT SLEEP

This section provides an overview of risk factors that commonly occur in older adults and lead to the common complaint of sleep problems, which are discussed in the section on *Functional Consequences*. Pain, dementia and delirium are risk factors that are common in older adults and are discussed in Chapters 28 and 14.

Psychosocial Factors

Anxiety and boredom are psychosocial factors that nurses can address through health promotion interventions to improve sleep in older adults. For example, lack of information about age-related sleep changes can cause anxiety and excessive worry about sleep. Anxiety is associated with difficulty falling asleep, frequent arousals during the night and difficulty returning to sleep. Health education interventions discussed later in this chapter can be used to teach about actions to improve sleep. When anxiety and worry is associated with other causes, nurses can teach about stress-reduction interventions, as discussed in the section on *Nursing Interventions for Sleep Wellness*.

Older adults with few or no interesting activities, work demands, social responsibilities or environmental stimuli may find it particularly difficult to establish healthy sleeping patterns. Socially isolated older adults may stay in bed for long periods because of boredom, lack of motivation, difficulty concentrating or a desire to withdraw from stressful situations. Similarly, if an older adult spends all of his or her time in the same room, the lack of differentiation between space for waking and sleeping activities may interfere with sleep patterns. Interventions discussed in Chapter 12 can be used to address this risk.

Environmental Conditions

Noise and many other environmental conditions can significantly influence sleep patterns, particularly for patients in acute care settings. Studies confirm that noise in general and staff conversations in particular are a major source of disrupted sleep and contribute significantly to diminished sleep quantity and quality in hospitalized (Adachi et al., 2013; Little et al., 2012; Yoder et al., 2012). Studies also show a positive relationship between improved sleep and the implementation of nursing interventions to reduce nighttime noise and care-related activities (Li et al., 2011).

Environmental conditions can be problematic for people who live in institutional settings or with other people as in the following examples:

- Lack of privacy and sleeping in close proximity to others
- Uncomfortably low or high temperatures (often due to inadequate heating or cooling systems)
- Excessive light in bedrooms, patient/resident rooms and hallways
- Insufficient exposure to bright light during the day, leading to diminished production of melatonin
- Hot and humid conditions, especially for menopausal women who experience more nighttime hot flashes when the air is hot and humid

Needs and schedules of others in long-term care facilities or home settings can influence sleep of older adults. For example, in institutional settings, the time for awakening patients/residents is often based on the most efficient use of nursing and dietary time, and patients/residents are expected to adjust their sleep routines accordingly. Similarly, dependent older adults in home settings may have to adjust their sleep routines to the schedule of family caregivers who have work responsibilities. In home settings, older adults who are caregivers may have their sleep interrupted by dependent family members who require care during the night.

Pathologic Conditions and Functional Impairments

Pathologic conditions interfere with sleep and increase the risk for sleep-related disorders for many different reasons, as delineated in Table 24-2. In addition to these conditions that directly interfere with sleep, many pathologic conditions are strongly associated with sleep problems, but the cause–effect relationship is unclear. For example, conditions that impair physical or cognitive function (e.g., dementia, Parkinson disease) have underlying pathophysiologic mechanisms that are similar to those involved with sleep disorders (e.g., restless legs syndrome, circadian rhythm sleep disorders) (Watson & Viola-Saltzman, 2013). There is a strong correlation between lower level of functioning and poor sleep in residents of nursing homes and assisted-living facilities, but the relationship between these variables is unclear (Fung et al., 2012; Valenza et al., 2013). Nocturia (discussed in Chapter 19), a common occurrence in older adults, is significantly associated with decreased quantity and quality of sleep (Zeitzer et al., 2013).

Obstructive sleep apnea is a specific sleep disorder that affects many older adults and is discussed in the section on *Pathologic Conditions Affecting Sleep*. In recent years, researchers and clinicians have focused on two sleep-related movement disorders: restless legs syndrome and periodic limb movements during sleep, which are strongly associated with sleep disturbances. Increased age is a risk factor for both RLS and PLMS, and symptoms may increase over time. Researchers currently are exploring potential causative relationship between dopamine deficiency and RLS and PLMS (Bliwise et al., 2012; Silber, 2013).

Restless legs syndrome (RLS), also known as *Willis–Ekbom disease*, is characterized by an almost irresistible urge to move the legs, which is often accompanied by unpleasant leg sensations. Symptoms of RLS occur in a circadian rhythm, with peak severity during the evening and night, which can interfere both with initiating and maintaining sleep. During waking hours, RLS disrupts periods of rest and relaxation. An additional characteristic is that the symptoms are not due to another condition, such as leg cramps, fibromyalgia, arthritis or positional discomfort. Risk factors for

TABLE 24-2 Pathophysiologic Factors Affecting Sleep	
Risk Factor	**Sleep Alteration**
Arthritis	Chronic pain and discomfort that interfere with sleep
COPD	Awakening as a result of apnea and respiratory distress
Nocturia	Sleep disruptions due to needing to void
Diabetes mellitus	Awakening secondary to nocturia or poorly controlled blood glucose levels; increased incidence of OSA
Gastrointestinal disorders, ulcers	Nocturnal pain secondary to increased gastric secretions during REM sleep
Hypertension	Early-morning awakening
Hyperthyroidism	Increased difficulty falling asleep
Nocturnal angina	Awakening without perception of pain, especially during REM sleep
PLMS, RLS	Awakening caused by recurrent involuntary leg movements
Malignancies	Increased incidence of RLS
Chronic kidney disease	Increase incidence of PLMS, RLS and OSA
Parkinsonism	Increased time awake; decreased amount of sleep
Dementia	Alterations of all sleep stages
Delirium	Increased somnolence *or* inability to sleep

COPD, chronic obstructive pulmonary disease; OSA, obstructive sleep apnea; PLMS, periodic limb movements in sleep; REM, rapid eye movement; RLS, restless legs syndrome.

RLS include genetic predisposition, iron deficiency, chronic renal failure, peripheral neuropathy and adverse effects of medications (e.g., most antidepressants, antipsychotic agents and possibly antihistamines) (Silber, 2013). In addition to causing major sleep problems, RLS is associated with increased risk for anxiety, depression and hypertension (Gupta et al., 2013; Salas & Kwan, 2012).

Periodic limb movements during sleep (PLMS), also known as *nocturnal myoclonus*, is the occurrence of brief muscle contractions, spaced at intervals of about 20 to 40 seconds, which cause leg jerks, or rhythmic movements of muscles in the foot or leg. They may occur several times to more than 200 times nightly, with increased occurrence during the first half of the night. PLMS can contribute to complaints of insomnia, frequent arousals and increased daytime sleepiness. They are also associated with increased risk for cardiovascular disease (Koo et al., 2011). In addition to increased age as a risk factor, PLMS is more common in people with RLS, diabetes, Parkinson disease, Lewy body dementia and sleep disorders (Hibi et al., 2012; Roux, 2013; Silber, 2013).

Wellness Opportunity

Nurses promote wellness by identifying subtle risk factors, such as chronic pain and discomfort, that are often overlooked and that can be addressed through many types of holistic interventions.

Effects of Bioactive Substances

Adverse effects of medications and other bioactive substances can interfere with sleep in a number of ways. Prescription medications that can cause disturbed sleep include steroids, antidepressants, aminophylline preparations, thyroid extracts, antiarrhythmic medications and centrally acting antihypertensives. These effects are not unique to older adults; however, adverse effects of medication are more likely to occur in older adults, as discussed in detail in Chapter 8.

Caffeine is a central nervous system stimulant that lengthens the sleep latency period and causes awakening during the night. Although low doses of nicotine can have relaxing and sedative effects, higher doses interfere with sleep because of nicotine's stimulant effect as well as its effects on respiration. Alcoholic beverages initially induce drowsiness but also suppress REM sleep and cause frequent awakenings, resulting in less total sleep and more daytime sleepiness. People who abstain from alcohol after long-term abuse may experience insomnia for a few years after withdrawing from it. Alcohol and other central nervous system depressants can exacerbate sleep disorders and lead to additional detrimental effects. Table 24-3 summarizes the effects of various medications and chemicals on sleep in older adults.

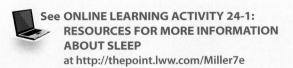

See ONLINE LEARNING ACTIVITY 24-1: RESOURCES FOR MORE INFORMATION ABOUT SLEEP
at http://thepoint.lww.com/Miller7e

TABLE 24-3 The Effect of Various Medications and Chemicals on Sleep

Medication or Chemical	Sleep Alteration
Alcohol	Suppression of REM sleep; early-morning awakening
Alcohol or hypnotic withdrawal	Sleep disturbances; nightmares
Anticholinergics	Hyperreflexia; overactivity; muscle twitching
Barbiturates	Suppression of REM sleep; nightmares; hallucinations; paradoxical responses
Benzodiazepines	Awakening secondary to apnea
β-Blockers	Nightmares
Corticosteroids	Restlessness; sleep disturbances
Diuretics	Awakening for nocturia; sleep apnea secondary to alkalosis
Theophylline, levodopa, isoproterenol, phenytoin	Interference with sleep onset and sleep stages
Antidepressants	PLMS; suppression of REM sleep

PLMS, periodic limb movements in sleep; REM, rapid eye movement.

FUNCTIONAL CONSEQUENCES AFFECTING SLEEP WELLNESS

The overall functional consequences of age-related changes in sleep are insufficient, inefficient and poor quality sleep, as summarized in Table 24-1. In addition, the high prevalence of risk factors that can interfere with sleep increases the vulnerability of older adults to sleep disorders and complaints. Common sleep complaints of older adults include daytime sleepiness, difficulty falling asleep and frequent arousals during the night. Within Canada, the first ever survey on sleep apnea was conducted in 2009 as part of the Canadian Community Health Survey. The results of this survey revealed that an estimated 858,900 Canadians reported having sleep apnea, and of these individuals, three-quarters were over the age of 45 years (Public Health Agency of Canada, 2010). Health consequences of poor sleep include impaired cognitive functions and increased risk for stroke, cancer, obesity, diabetes, depression, metabolic syndrome, substance abuse and all-cause mortality (Harand et al., 2012; Hung et al., 2013; Mander et al., 2013; National Center on Sleep Disorders Research, 2011).

Depression is a condition that is strongly associated with sleep problems, but it is difficult to determine if it is a risk for or functional consequence (i.e., cause or effect) of sleep problems. People who are depressed take longer to fall asleep, have less deep sleep and more light sleep, awaken more frequently during the night and earlier in the morning, and feel less rested in the morning. Although these sleep problems are commonly viewed as symptoms of depression, recent studies suggest that depression in older adults is a consequence of sleep disorders, particularly insomnia and excessive daytime sleepiness (EDS) (Baglioni & Riemann, 2012; Jaussent et al., 2011).

PATHOLOGIC CONDITIONS AFFECTING SLEEP: SLEEP DISORDERS

In the late 1970s, sleep disorders were classified systematically, and standards were established to diagnose these disorders. **Insomnia** is a chronic or acute sleep disorder characterized by a complaint of poor sleep quality or difficulty initiating or maintaining sleep that causes daytime impairment. Because people with chronic insomnia experience symptoms during the night and day, it is considered a 24-hour condition (Neubauer, 2013). Prevalence of insomnia is 10% to 20% with about half of those having a chronic course (Buysse, 2013).

Excessive daytime sleepiness, defined as the inability to maintain alertness, is characterized by hypersomnolence (i.e., falling asleep at periodic intervals during a 24-hour period). Excessive daytime sleepiness differs from fatigue, which manifests as difficulty sustaining a high level of functioning. An evidence-based geriatric nursing protocol for best practice states that daytime sleepiness should not be dismissed as an insignificant condition; rather, it should be evaluated by health care providers because it can have significant health effects (Chasens & Umlauf, 2012). Box 24-1 summarizes guidelines for nursing assessment and interventions related to excessive daytime sleepiness.

Obstructive sleep apnea (OSA) is a sleep disorder that has been the focus of much research and clinical attention in the past several decades. Primary manifestation of OSA are (1) the involuntary cessation of airflow for 10 seconds or longer (i.e., apnea) and (2) the occurrence of more than five to eight of these episodes per hour. This condition occurs because the muscles responsible for holding the throat open relax during sleep and block the passage of air. Symptoms of OSA include daytime fatigue, morning headaches, diminished mental acuity and loud snoring punctuated by brief periods of silence.

E B P   Box 24-1 Evidence-Based Practice: Excessive Sleepiness

Statement of the Problem

- Healthy older adults experience the following changes in sleep: an increase in transient arousals, longer time until sleep onset and Stage I sleep, and decrease in quantity and quality of restorative slow-wave sleep.
- Excessive sleepiness—defined as the inability to maintain alertness or vigilance because of hypersomnolence—is common in older adults.
- Primary causes of excessive sleepiness include OSA, insomnia and restless legs syndrome.
- Secondary causes include medications, psychiatric illnesses (e.g., depression and anxiety) and medical conditions (e.g., respiratory illness, heart failure, neurologic conditions, painful chronic conditions).
- Lifestyle factors and pre-bedtime behaviours are contributing factors that can be addressed through health promotion.
- Because 22% to 61% of hospitalized patients experience sleep disturbances, routine care should include interventions to assess and improve sleep.
- Daytime sleepiness is often viewed falsely as normal or unpreventable in older adults; this misperception reduces the likelihood that this condition will be appropriately evaluated and treated.
- Consequences of sleepiness include decreased alertness, delayed reaction time and diminished cognitive performance.

Recommendations for Nursing Assessment

- Obtain a sleep history, based on information from both the patient and family members, including information about sleep patterns and sleep-related behaviours.
- Use the Epworth Sleepiness Scale as a valid and reliable tool for identifying excessive sleepiness.
- Use the STOP-BANG tool for identifying risks for OSA: Snoring, Tired, Observed gaps in breathing, blood Pressure high, BMI more than 35, Age over 50, Neck circumference greater than 40 cm, and Gender male.
- Assess sleep history and identify primary and secondary causes of excessive sleepiness.

- When possible, observe patients for snoring, apnea during sleep, excessive leg movements during sleep, and difficulty staying awake during normal daytime activities.

Recommendations for Patient Teaching

Teach older adults and caregivers about the following sleep-promoting measures:
- Use the bed only for sleeping or sex.
- Develop consistent and rest-promoting bedtime routines and maintain the same schedule daily.
- If awakened during the night, avoid looking at the clock.
- Avoid or limit naps to 10 to 15 minutes.
- Sleep in a cool, quiet environment.
- Avoid the following before bedtime: caffeine, nicotine, alcohol, large meals, exercise and emotionally charged activities.
- If you cannot fall asleep after 15 or 20 minutes, go to another room and engage in a quiet activity until you are sleepy again.

Recommendations for Care

- Work with primary care practitioners to ensure optimal management of medical conditions, psychological disorders and symptoms that interfere with sleep.
- Teach patients and families about lifestyle measures for improving sleep among all family members.
- Incorporate sleep-hygiene measures and ongoing treatment of existing sleep disorders into the plan of care for older adults in all settings.
- Work with prescribing practitioners to review and, if appropriate, adjust medications that can cause drowsiness or sleep impairment.
- Suggest referral to a sleep specialist for moderate or severe sleepiness or a clinical profile consistent with major sleep disorders.

Sources: Chasens, E. R., & Umlauf, M. G. (2012). Excessive sleepiness. In M. Boltz, E. Capezuti, T. Fulmer, et al. (Eds.), *Evidence-based geriatric nursing protocols for best practice* (4th ed., pp. 74–88). New York, NY: Springer; Slater, G., & Steier, J. (2012). Review article: Excessive daytime sleepiness in sleep disorders. *Journal of Thoracic Disease, 4*(6), 608–616.

OSA is not exclusively a condition of older adults, but the prevalence of apnea increases with advancing age, beginning around the fifth decade, and is higher in men than in women. Prevalence rates for adults older than 60 years range from 32% to 62% (Sforza & Roche, 2012) (see Box 24-2). Additional factors associated with increased risk for OSA include obesity, diabetes, stroke, Parkinson disease, congestive heart failure, genetic predisposition, craniofacial anatomic features, and the use of alcohol or medications that depress the respiratory centre (Panossian & Daley, 2013).

 DIVERSITY NOTE

OSA is 1.5 to 4 times more common in men than in women (Panossian & Daley, 2013).

OSA is a major focus of researchers and clinicians because of the increasing evidence that it causes serious consequences, and even death, when it is untreated. Studies confirm a strong link between OSA and all the following medical conditions: stroke, hypertension, cerebral ischemia and many types of cardiovascular disease (e.g., arrhythmias, coronary heart disease) (Cho et al., 2013; Das & Khan, 2012; Levy et al., 2012; Winklewski & Frydrychowski, 2013). Moreover, effective treatment of OSA results in improved cardiac function, reduced cardiovascular disease and decrease in mortality rates (Baquet et al., 2012; Kasai, 2012; Vijayan, 2012; Yang et al., 2013). In addition, OSA interferes with quality of life because it causes excessive daytime sleepiness and other cognitive effects. Studies are also investigating a potential causative relationship between OSA and cognitive impairment (Grigg-Damberger & Ralls, 2012; Sforza & Roche, 2012).

 See **ONLINE LEARNING ACTIVITY CHECKPOINT 24-2: LEARNING MORE ABOUT OBSTRUCTIVE SLEEP APNEA** at http://thepoint.lww.com/Miller7e

 NURSING ASSESSMENT OF SLEEP

Identifying Opportunities for Health Promotion

In recent years, nurses and other health care professionals have recognized the importance of assessing sleep as an essential aspect of wellness and quality of life. Nurses assess sleep patterns to determine the adequacy of the person's usual sleep and rest patterns and to identify factors that either contribute to or interfere with the quality and quantity of sleep. Goals of nursing assessment are (1) to identify health-promoting behaviours that can be encouraged and (2) to identify conditions that interfere with sleep so that these can be addressed. Many of the contributing factors are addressed through educational interventions, such as correction of misinformation or lack of knowledge. Box 24-3 provides guidelines for interviewing

Box 24-2 Evidence-Informed Nursing Practice

Background: As part of the Canadian Community Health Survey conducted by Statistics Canada (2009), the Public Health Agency of Canada developed the Sleep Apnea Rapid Response Survey to evaluate the prevalence of sleep apnea among Canadian adults.
Question: What is the prevalence of sleep apnea in Canadians 18 years of age and older?
Method: A representative sample of 8,647 Canadian adults were surveyed about whether or not they have been informed by a health care professional that they have sleep apnea.
Findings: While the prevalence of self-reported sleep apnea was 3% among individuals 18 years of age and older, the rate rose to 5% among those 45 years of age or older. Three-quarters of those reporting sleep apnea were 45 years of age and older. Of the individuals who had risk factors or symptoms of sleep apnea (e.g., loud snoring, having someone else report a stoppage of breathing when sleeping, high blood pressure, being very overweight), 73% were men and 76% were older than 50 years of age. Additionally, those who indicated being diagnosed with sleep apnea were more likely (than the general population) to be diagnosed with diabetes, heart disease, and depression or other forms of mood disorders.
Implications for Nursing Practice: Nurses should assess their older clients for sleep problems, as well as assess for risk factors and symptoms of sleep apnea. Interventions found in Boxes 24-4 and 24-5 can be offered to clients to enhance their sleep. Further, nurses can recommend that older adults be referred to a sleep clinic if they suspect they have sleep apnea or are experiencing significant problems sleeping.

Source: Public Health Agency of Canada. (2010). *Fast facts from the 2009 Canadian Community Health Survey—Sleep apnea rapid response* [Cat. HP35-19/1-2010E]. Ottawa, ON: Author.

 Box 24-3 Guidelines for Assessing Sleep and Rest

Questions to Assess the Perception of Quality and Adequacy of Sleep

- On a scale of 1 to 10, with 10 as the highest, how would you rate your sleep?
- When you awaken in the morning, do you feel like you are rested?
- Do you feel drowsy or sleepy during the day or early evening?
- Does fatigue interfere with your desired daytime activity level?

Questions to Identify Opportunities for Health Education

- What is your usual time for getting into bed?
- Describe your usual activities during the daytime and evening.
- What factors help you fall asleep (e.g., food or drink, relaxation strategies, environmental influences)?
- What conditions interfere with good sleep (e.g., pain, discomfort, anxiety, depression)?
- Do you take any medicines to help you sleep?
- Do you take medicines to help you stay awake during the day?
- Do you drink alcoholic or caffeinated beverages, or take medicines that contain alcohol or caffeine during the late afternoon or evening? (If yes, how much and what kind?)
- Do you smoke or use nicotine products? (If yes, what kind and how much?)
- Are you aware, or has anyone told you, that you snore or stop breathing during your sleep?
- Do your legs kick or jump involuntarily while you sleep?

(continued)

Box 24-3 *(continued)*

Questions to Assess Nighttime Sleep Pattern

- Where do you sleep at night (e.g., bed, couch, recliner chair)?
- How long does it usually take to fall asleep after you get into bed?
- Do you think you lie awake too long before falling asleep?
- After you fall asleep, how many times do you wake up during the night?
- What kinds of things disturb your sleep during the night (e.g., getting up to urinate; activities of roommates or other people in the setting; environmental factors, such as noise or lighting)?
- If changes in living arrangements have occurred in the past few months, has your sleep pattern changed since (e.g., since you came to this nursing home; since your spouse passed away)?

independent older adults and caregivers of dependent older adults about sleep and rest patterns.

In addition to obtaining information from older adults and their caregivers, nurses observe behavioural indicators of sleep and rest patterns. This is especially important when objective observations are contrary to subjective complaints. For example, older adults may complain of not sleeping at all, but when observed by caregivers, they may appear to be sleeping during the entire night. By contrast, older adults who deny any problems sleeping may nap frequently and readily fall asleep during daytime activities.

Wellness Opportunity

Be aware of opportunities to help older adults identify self-care measures to improve sleep quantity and quality, rather than view this as an inevitable consequence of aging.

Evidence-Based Assessment Tools

Older adults can use evidence-based sleep assessment tools for self-assessment or for self-reporting to health care professionals. Two easy-to-use and readily available tools that have been tested for validity and reliability are the **Pittsburgh Sleep Quality Index (PSQI)** and the **Epworth Sleepiness Scale (ESS)**. The PSQI assesses sleep quality and patterns over the past month, and the ESS focuses on daytime sleepiness over the past week. Additionally, the Quebec Sleep Questionnaire (QSQ) assesses the quality of life for individuals with OSA. This tool was initially developed and validated in French (French Canadian), but an English version has been provided (Lacasse et al., 2004). Online Learning Activity 24-3 provides links to additional information about and illustration of these tools.

 See **ONLINE LEARNING ACTIVITY 24-3: TOOLS FOR ASSESSING SLEEP IN OLDER ADULTS** at http://thepoint.lww.com/Miller7e

NURSING DIAGNOSIS

When healthy older adults are interested in learning self-care activities to improve their sleep pattern, the nursing diagnosis of Readiness for Enhanced Sleep is applicable. This wellness nursing diagnosis is defined as "a pattern of natural, periodic suspension of consciousness that provides adequate rest, sustains a desired lifestyle, and can be strengthened" (Herdman, 2012, p. 220). Nursing diagnoses pertinent to older adults who have sleep problems include Insomnia, Disturbed Sleep Pattern and Sleep Deprivation.

Unfolding Case Study

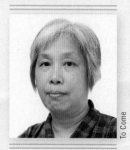

Part 1: Mrs. Z. at 66 Years of Age

Mrs. Z. is 66 years old and recently retired from her job as office manager for a law firm. She considers herself to be in good health, although she has had hypertension for 20 years and osteoarthritis for the past several years. She self-monitors her blood pressure and takes atenolol, 50 mg daily. She occasionally takes an over-the-counter analgesic medication when her arthritis pain bothers her. She just started going to the local senior centre once a week for lunch and social and educational activities. During one of your weekly senior wellness clinics, Mrs. Z. comes to talk with you about her difficulty sleeping. She reports that since she has retired, she often wakes up several times during the night and has difficulty returning to sleep. She used to sleep an average of 7 to 8 hours nightly and could easily return to sleep if she woke up during the night. Now she is lucky if she gets 6 hours of sleep because she lies in bed for several hours. She used to go to bed between 10 PM and 11 PM and get up promptly between 6:30 AM and 7 AM. Now that she is retired, she goes to bed around 11 PM, but stays in bed until 10 AM if she wakes up during the night and does not get a full night's sleep.

THINKING POINTS

- What age-related changes may be contributing to Mrs. Z.'s dissatisfaction with her sleep?
- What risk factors might be contributing to Mrs. Z.'s dissatisfaction with her sleep?

- What further assessment information would you need to obtain, and how would you obtain it?

PLANNING FOR WELLNESS OUTCOMES

When older adults experience sleep disturbances or have risk factors that affect sleep patterns, nurses identify wellness outcomes as an essential part of the nursing process. Nursing Outcomes Classification (NOC) terms that most directly relate to interventions to enhance sleep or address sleep problems in older adults are Sleep, Rest, Health Promoting Behaviour, Fatigue Level, Comfort Status: Environment, Personal Well-Being, Anxiety Level, Knowledge: Health Behaviour, and Pain: Disruptive Effects. Sleep–Rest Pattern is an appropriate NOC when the focus is on risk factors, such as noise, family schedules and patterns of relaxation (Moorhead et al., 2013).

NURSING INTERVENTIONS FOR SLEEP WELLNESS

Nursing interventions to promote sleep wellness for older adults include health education and direct interventions, such as environmental modifications and comfort and relaxation strategies. It is important to adapt these interventions to the individual needs of older adults in various settings. For example, in community settings, the focus is on teaching older adults and their caregivers about self-care interventions that can improve sleep patterns. In long-term care settings, the focus is on interventions that can be implemented routinely to improve sleep patterns of residents. In hospital settings, the focus of care is primarily on acute medical problems, but sleep disturbances should not be overlooked as an important health concern. The following pertinent Nursing Interventions Classification (NIC) terminologies are appropriate for documentation of interventions: Sleep Enhancement, Anxiety Reduction, Exercise Promotion, Music Therapy, Risk Identification, Environmental Management, Pain Management, Relaxation Therapy and Autogenic Training.

Teaching Older Adults About Interventions for Sleep Wellness

Increasing attention is paid to nonpharmacologic interventions for improving sleep and alleviating insomnia, with emphasis on safe and effective alternatives to medications, which can have many adverse effects (see the section on *Educating Older Adults About Medications and Sleep*). Box 24-4 summarizes current research conclusions about nonpharmacologic interventions for improving sleep.

See ONLINE LEARNING ACTIVITY 24-4: JOURNAL ARTICLE AND ADDITIONAL RESOURCES FOR EVIDENCE-BASED INTERVENTIONS at http://thepoint.lww.com/Miller7e

An important aspect of health promotion is to teach older adults about normal age-related changes and help them identify risk factors that can affect their sleep, as described in Tables 24-1 and 24-2. When contributing factors

---

EBP **Box 24-4 Evidence-Based Practice: Research Conclusions About Nonpharmacologic Interventions to Improve Sleep**

- Meditation, mindfulness and mindfulness-based stress reduction are consistently identified as effective interventions for improving sleep (Gross et al., 2011; Nagendra et al., 2012; Ong et al., 2012).
- Daily moderate physical activity improves sleep for older adults (Guimaraes et al., 2008; King et al., 2008; Kline et al., 2012; Uchida et al., 2012).
- Muscle relaxation techniques (e.g., progressive muscle relaxation, autogenic training) improve sleep, particularly when stress is a contributing condition (Sharma & Andrade, 2012).
- Many studies find strong support for cognitive behavioural treatment for insomnia (e.g., Katofsky et al., 2012; Troxel et al., 2012; Williams et al., 2013).
- Studies find good support for the use of yoga and tai chi (body–mind interventions) in improving sleep (Sarris & Byrne, 2011; Sobana et al., 2013).
- Acupuncture and acupressure may be effective for sleep disorders, based on their effects on serotonin, dopamine and endogenous opioids, with stronger evidence in support of acupressure (Lu et al., 2013; Sarris & Byrne, 2011).

- Listening to soothing music is effective for improving sleep quality (Su et al., 2012).
- Melatonin, a sleep-regulating hormone produced by the pineal gland, can be effective in managing circadian sleep disorders and jet lag (Kostoglou-Athanassiou, 2013).
- L-Tryptophan (an exogenous amino acid that is converted into serotonin) may increase sleepiness and decrease length of time for sleep onset, particularly in healthy adults (Sarris & Byrne, 2011).
- A systematic review of studies found that lavender oil may be helpful for promoting sleep (Fismer & Pilkington, 2012).
- Some, but not all studies, have found that valerian (an herbal product), alone or in combination with hops or kava, may improve sleep (Sarris & Byrne, 2011).
- Earplugs and eye masks can improve sleep in critical care patients (Jones & Dawson, 2012).
- Massage therapy is beneficial for improving sleep, for example, for menopausal symptoms (Oliveira et al., 2012) and for people with dementia in nursing homes (Harris et al., 2012).

are identified, help older adults plan interventions to address risks such as stress and chronic pain or discomfort. In addition, use information in Box 24-5 to teach about self-care actions (sometimes called *sleep hygiene*) for promoting sleep wellness. If older adults are not familiar with relaxation techniques, give them a copy of Box 24-6 and teach them about deep breathing, progressive relaxation and mental imagery.

Box 24-5 Health Promotion Teaching About Sleep

Actions to Take

- Establish a bedtime ritual that is effective for you, and try to follow it every night.
- Maintain the same daily schedule for waking, resting and sleeping.
- Take a warm, relaxing bath in the afternoon or early evening.
- After 1:00 PM, avoid foods, beverages and medications that contain caffeine or stimulants (e.g., tea, cocoa, coffee, chocolate, sugar, refined carbohydrates, and some over-the-counter pain relievers and cold preparations).
- Pre-bedtime foods that promote sleep include milk (warm), chamomile tea and a light snack of complex carbohydrates (e.g., whole grains).
- Use one or more of the following relaxation methods: imagery, meditation, deep breathing, progressive relaxation, soothing music, body or foot massage, rocking in a chair, reading nonstimulating materials or watching nonstimulating television.
- Perform daily moderate aerobic exercise, preferably before the late afternoon, but avoid vigorous exercise in the evening.
- Ensure adequate intake of the following nutrients: zinc, calcium, magnesium, manganese, vitamin C and vitamin B complex.

Actions to Avoid

- Do not drink alcohol before bedtime because it may cause early-morning awakening. If you use alcohol, use only in small amounts.
- Do not smoke cigarettes in the evening because nicotine is a stimulant.
- If your bedtime is temporarily changed, try to keep your waking time as close to the usual time as possible, and avoid staying in bed beyond your usual waking time.
- Do not use your bed for reading or other activities not associated with sleeping.
- If you awaken during the night and cannot return to sleep, get out of bed after 30 minutes and engage in a nonstimulating activity, such as reading, in another room.
- Arise at your usual time, even if you have not slept well.

Complementary and Alternative Care Practices

- Yoga, tai chi, meditation, imagery, aromatherapy, massage, soothing music, relaxation techniques, and a warm bath or warm footbath may be effective in promoting sleep.
- Melatonin, a sleep-regulating hormone, can be effective in improving sleep, but it can interact with other medications and also can cause daytime sleepiness.

Special Precautions

- Although widely promoted as sleep aids, herbs should be used with caution in older adults because of their possible adverse effects.
- Inform your health care professionals about any use of herbs, aromatherapy, or other complementary and alternative care practices.

Box 24-6 Relaxation and Mental Imagery Techniques That Promote Sleep

Deep Breathing

- Focus your attention on your breathing; extend your belly and draw in a deep breath as you count.
- Hold your breath for three or four counts.
- Exhale completely.
- Repeat this pattern, focusing your total attention on breathing.
- Phrases, such as "I am sleepy," or counting may be repeated during each exhalation to help keep your attention focused on breathing.

Progressive Relaxation

- Start by focusing your attention on the muscles in your toes.
- Flex or tense these muscles, and then relax them.
- Repeat two or three times.
- Focus your attention on the muscles in your foot.
- Flex or tense, then relax these muscles, two or three times.
- Repeat this process, progressively focusing on different muscle groups and proceeding from your feet to your head.

Mental Imagery

- Begin with deep breathing exercises to relax yourself.
- Focus your attention on a serene and peaceful scene, visualize the setting, and imagine the sounds (e.g., a beach with waves gently washing ashore).
- Imagine yourself in the setting, lying relaxed, enjoying the environment.
- Keep your attention focused on the scene.
- Imagine repetitive motions, such as waves on the beach or sheep jumping over a fence.

Encourage older adults to use CD players with automatic shutoffs or other devices to listen to soothing music or provide instructions for deep breathing, guided imagery or relaxation exercises.

Wellness Opportunity

Health education about sleep is particularly important in community and long-term care settings because nurses have more opportunities to focus on quality-of-life issues.

Improving Sleep for Older Adults in Institutional Settings

Older adults in acute and long-term care settings have a high prevalence of sleep disturbances, and these disturbances can lead to serious and detrimental health consequences, as already delineated. Nurses who work evening or night shifts have many opportunities to engage in direct care activities that promote good nighttime sleep, which are in addition to environmental interventions discussed in the next section.

For older adults in any setting, nursing responsibilities include addressing factors that interfere with sleep, ensuring the most comfortable environment possible, and individualizing care plans so that they incorporate personal preferences for optimal sleep conditions. The following relatively simple nursing actions can improve sleep in hospitalized patients:

supporting the person's usual sleeping schedule and routines, providing assistance with personal care and comfortable positioning, providing comfort measures (e.g., warm beverage, a brief massage) and maintaining a quiet environment with minimal lighting.

If dementia or depression interferes with sleep onset, a helpful intervention is to simply stay with the older person to provide reassurance until the person is able to fall asleep. In addition, relief of pain, anxiety and physical discomfort are nursing responsibilities that can affect the sleep of older adults. Older adults who are cognitively impaired may not request analgesics but may give nonverbal cues that pain is interfering with sleep, as discussed in Chapter 28. Be alert to this possibility and assess for chronic or acute pain, and recognize that an analgesic taken 30 minutes before bedtime may help induce sleep in people with chronic pain or discomfort.

Because daytime activities influence sleep patterns, care plans in long-term care settings should incorporate appropriate types and amounts of activities in each older adult's daily routine. Also, residents should be exposed to adequate bright lights during the day. Evening and nighttime routines need to be based on a comprehensive assessment of the needs of the older adult and consider any conflicting needs. For example, for some older adults, the need for an uninterrupted night's sleep may outweigh the potential benefits of being awakened for nighttime care tasks. In many situations, the needs can be addressed during the person's usual waking time, rather than performing the tasks on a rigid schedule designed for the convenience of staff.

Modifying the Environment to Promote Sleep

Environmental modifications are among the simplest and most effective interventions to improve sleep, especially in institutional settings. Actions, such as closing bedroom doors and adjusting bedroom lighting, can improve sleep. Elimination of unnecessary staff-initiated noise, especially conversations at the nursing station, is another helpful intervention for patients/residents located near the centre of nursing activity. In long-term care settings, nurses can document preferences for bedtime routines that promote sleep on each resident's care plan and ensure that these measures are carried out by nursing staff. In long-term care settings where residents share rooms, decisions about room assignments should take into consideration the compatibility of individual needs. Once room assignments have been made, roommate behaviours that interfere with sleep can be addressed by a room change, if necessary.

If a noisy environment contributes to sleeping difficulties, and the noise cannot be controlled or eliminated, the older person may wish to use earplugs. People who live alone, however, should be cautioned about the danger of blocking out protective noises, such as that of a smoke alarm. If environmental noise cannot be eliminated, it can be masked by white noise (e.g., using a fan, air conditioner, soft music or recordings of white noise). In addition to addressing noise in the environment, temperature should be adjusted in the sleeping area. The nighttime room temperature should be comfortable, and is usually slightly lower than during the day. In cooler environments, the older adult should wear a nightcap to prevent loss of heat through the head.

Educating Older Adults About Medications and Sleep

Hypnotics may be effective for short-term management of sleep disorders, especially in temporary circumstances, such as in acute care settings; however, the adverse effects of some hypnotics can outweigh their advantages. Guidelines for evidence-based practice emphasize that sedative-hypnotic medications should not be used for treatment of insomnia in older adults, particularly in nursing home residents (Brandt & Piechocki, 2013).

Benzodiazepines (e.g., flurazepam [Dalmane], triazolam [Halcion], temazepam [Restoril]) were the most commonly prescribed sleep medication for older adults until the early 1990s. However, recent guidelines emphasize that this class of drugs should not be used as hypnotics because they are associated with serious adverse effects, including falls, fractures, cognitive and functional impairments, and increased risk of infections, dementia and coronary artery disease (American Geriatrics Society, 2012; deGage et al., 2012; Huang et al., 2012).

Nonbenzodiazepine agents (e.g., zolpidem [Ambien], zaleplon [Sonata], eszopiclone [Lunesta] and ramelteon [Rozerem]) have been available since 1993 but recent studies indicate that these drugs are associated with serious adverse effects, including increased risk of fractures (Kang et al., 2012). In addition, older adults often use over-the-counter medications, such as diphenhydramine and other antihistamines, for their sedating effects; however, there is little evidence that they are effective for improving sleep when used for more than several days and they are associated with serious adverse effects because of their strong anticholinergic actions, such as drowsiness, tachycardia, urinary retention and confusion. Box 24-7 summarizes pertinent teaching points that nurses can use to educate older adults and their caregivers about the effects of alcohol, medications and certain chemicals on sleep.

Wellness Opportunity

Nurses have important roles in correcting misperceptions about sleep and teaching older adults about nonpharmacologic ways of improving sleep.

Teaching About Management of Sleep Disorders

Evidence-based guidelines emphasize the important role that nurses have in identifying and referring patients for sleep disorders because they see patients sleep more than any other health care professionals. Thus, when older adults have sleep disturbances that do not respond to health promotion interventions, it is important to teach them about many safe and effective interventions for addressing sleep problems. Nurses

Box 24-7 Health Promotion Teaching About Medications and Sleep

- Older adults are more susceptible than younger adults to the adverse effects of many prescription sleeping medications, including benzodiazepines (e.g., flurazepam, triazolam and temazepam).
- Over-the-counter sleeping preparations usually contain diphenhydramine and can have adverse effects, such as confusion, constipation or blurred vision, either alone or in combination with other medications.
- Sleeping medications, even over-the-counter ones, are likely to have adverse effects that interfere with daytime function and with the quality of nighttime sleep.
- Many hypnotic medications are not effective for long-term use because of increasing tolerance, which may develop within the first week and usually develops after a month of regular use.
- Sleep medications can interfere with the dream stage of sleep and cause a rebound effect, characterized by nightmares and excessive dreaming, after they are discontinued.
- Alcohol is likely to cause nightmares and awakenings during the latter part of the night.
- Medications that can interfere with sleep include steroids, diuretics, theophylline, anticonvulsants, decongestants and thyroid hormone.
- Combining a sleeping medication with any other medication can be harmful or even fatal.

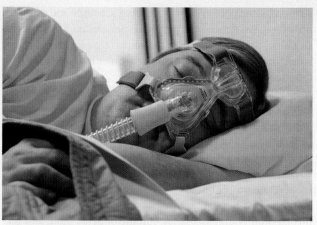

FIGURE 24-1 A CPAP machine. (Used with permission from Philips Healthcare.)

can also emphasize the importance of addressing sleep disorders as a health issue and encourage older adults to talk with their primary care practitioner about a referral for a comprehensive sleep evaluation.

Teaching about interventions for OSA is an important nursing responsibility because of the serious health consequences that develop when the condition is not adequately treated. This is especially important as the disorder affects so many older adults and is associated with serious health consequences, as discussed earlier in this chapter.

Many types of interventions are available for treating OSA, so obtaining a comprehensive evaluation and treatment at a sleep disorders clinic should be considered. The "gold standard" for treating OSA is continuous positive airway pressure (CPAP) therapy, which is effective in improving symptoms and preventing serious complications. Although CPAP adherence is an essential first-line treatment for OSA, there is a high rate of nonadherence, which nurses can address through health education (Carlucci et al., 2013). Although most people who use CPAP equipment do so independently in their homes, older adults in hospitals and long-term care settings may need assistance with managing their nightly treatments. Figure 24-1 illustrates an older adult using a CPAP machine.

 DIVERSITY NOTE

Men require higher pressures of CPAP than women for effective management of symptoms (Ralls & Grigg-Damberger, 2012).

Wellness Opportunity

Nurses promote sleep wellness for older adults who experience sleep problems by teaching about the importance of having any sleep disorder evaluated by a knowledgeable professional.

Unfolding Case Study

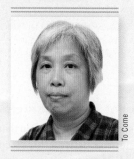

Part 1: Mrs. Z. at 66 Years of Age (continued)

Mrs. Z. returns for further discussion of her sleep problem after filling out the Pittsburgh Sleep Quality Index based on her experiences during the past month. In addition, she has followed your instructions to keep a "sleep log" describing her daily activities, including exercise, and the effect of these activities on her sleep. Per your request, she has documented the types of foods and beverages she consumes regularly. You review the assessment information with her and find out that when she is home she spends most of her time reading or doing crossword puzzles. She attends the senior centre weekly, plays bridge two evenings a week, and goes to lunch with friends a few times every week. She enjoys gardening during the summer but has no other interest in physical activities. She avoids exercise because she is afraid that physical activity "will get the old arthritis all stirred up." On further questioning, she estimates that when she worked, she walked about one-half mile daily. She drinks about "a pot" of coffee daily and has coffee and cookies at bridge games. She enjoys a glass of wine in the evenings. When she wakes up during the night, she usually gets up and goes to the bathroom, then returns to bed and lies there "thinking" until she returns to sleep. Her sleep log reflects that she often stays awake for as long as 2 hours before returning to sleep. She says she's heard that melatonin is good for insomnia and asks your opinion about trying it.

THINKING POINTS

- What myths and misunderstandings about sleep would you address?
- What risk factors might you address through health education?
- Because you can see Mrs. Z. weekly at the wellness clinic, you can develop a long-term teaching plan. How

would you establish priorities for immediate and long-term goals?
- What information from Boxes 24-4 to 24-7 would you use for health education with Mrs. Z.?

EVALUATING EFFECTIVENESS OF NURSING INTERVENTIONS

The effectiveness of interventions for the nursing diagnosis of Disturbed Sleep Pattern or for the wellness diagnosis of Readiness for Enhanced Sleep can be measured subjectively or objectively. A subjective measurement would be that the

older adult reports that he or she feels rested and refreshed upon awakening in the morning. If a sleep assessment tool is used during the initial assessment, it can be used again for a reassessment after interventions have been implemented. An example of an objective measurement would be that the older adult can sleep for 6 to 8 hours at night with only brief interruptions, and that the person looks and acts rested during the day.

Unfolding Case Study

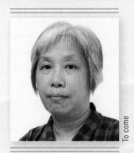

Part 2: Mrs. Z. at 79 Years of Age

Mrs. Z. is now 79 years old and is being admitted to a rehabilitation unit after a total hip replacement. Her diagnoses include osteoarthritis and osteoporosis. After a few weeks on the unit, she plans to return to her ranch-style home where she lives with her husband. Before surgery, she was independent in her activities of daily living, and she expects to regain her independence and walk with a walker. The hospital transfer form has orders for acetaminophen 1,000 mg every 8 hours and zolpidem tartrate 5 mg at bedtime as needed.

NURSING ASSESSMENT

During the admission interview, you ask Mrs. Z. about her sleep patterns. She states that for the past few years, she has been awakened frequently at night by her hip pain and other arthritic discomforts. In addition, she reports that she would usually get up three or four times during the night to go to the bathroom. When questioned further, she explains that the pain and discomfort would wake her, and so she would go to the bathroom because she wanted to move around, not because she felt an urge to urinate that often. Although her doctor had prescribed medications for pain, she did not take them regularly because

she was concerned about adverse effects. During her 1-week hospitalization, she had taken a sleeping pill several times as well as Tylenol with codeine. Mrs. Z. expresses anxiety about sleeping in the rehabilitation unit because she says that the noise in the hospital was very disruptive to her sleep. She reports that she feels rested in the morning if she gets at least 6 hours of sleep during the 8 hours she spends in bed. During her hospitalization, she never felt rested in the morning and was unable to sleep for 6 hours except when she took sleeping pills. Mrs. Z. says that listening to relaxing music helps her to fall asleep.

NURSING DIAGNOSIS

In addition to nursing diagnoses related to Mrs. Z.'s osteoarthritis and hip surgery, you identify a nursing diagnosis of

Disturbed Sleep Pattern. Related factors are pain, age-related changes and environmental conditions. You decide that you

(continued)

Unfolding Case Study

will not list nocturia as an associated factor because Mrs. Z. does not feel an urge to void during the night. Rather, she wakes up with pain and then goes to the bathroom. You decide to list age-related changes as a related factor because it is important for Mrs. Z. to understand that even though she may not awaken with pain, she may awaken because of age-related changes.

NURSING CARE PLAN FOR Mrs. Z.

Expected Outcome	Nursing Interventions	Nursing Evaluation
Mrs. Z. will identify factors that influence her sleep pattern.	• Describe age-related changes in sleep patterns. • Discuss the important role of pain-relieving measures in promoting good sleep.	• Mrs. Z. will be able to describe the age-related changes and other conditions that affect her sleeping patterns.
Mrs. Z. will consistently obtain 6 hours of sleep nightly without the aid of sleeping medications.	• Administer Tylenol as ordered and evaluate its effectiveness in controlling Mrs. Z.'s pain. • Explain that sleeping medications should be avoided, except for periodic use in short-term situations. See Online Learning Activity 24-4 for instructions: Canadian Sleep Society Insomnia Rounds for physicians. • Assign Mrs. Z. to a room that is not close to the nursing station. • Make sure Mrs. Z.'s door is closed at night. • Encourage Mrs. Z. to play quiet music at bedtime. • Give Mrs. Z. a copy of Boxes 24-5 and 24-6 and discuss additional nonpharmacologic methods for promoting sleep.	• Mrs. Z. will report that she is not awakened by pain. • Mrs. Z. will report that she feels rested upon awakening in the morning.

THINKING POINTS

- What additional assessment information pertinent to Mrs. Z.'s sleep patterns would you like to have, and how would you obtain this information?
- What additional nursing interventions would you include in the care plan to address Mrs. Z.'s Disturbed Sleep Pattern? Would you use any of the information in Box 24-5 or give her a copy of it?

- What concerns specifically related to sleep would you have about Mrs. Z. after she is discharged from the rehabilitation unit to her own home? How would you address these concerns in your health promotion interventions?

QSEN APPLICATION

QSEN Competency	Knowledge/Skill/Attitude	Application to Mrs. Z When She Is 79 Years of Age
Patient-centred care	(K) Integrate understanding of multiple dimensions of patient-centred care.	Identify preexisting conditions as well as immediate risks that can affect Mrs. Z.'s sleep.
	(K) Describe strategies to empower patients in all aspects of the health care process.	Teach Mrs. Z. about normal sleep changes and risk factors so that she feels more control over her sleep.
	(K) Examine nursing roles in ensuring coordination, integration, and continuity of care.	Recognize that it is important to address sleep concerns as part of a comprehensive care plan in long-term care settings.
	(S) Communicate care provided and needed at each transition in care.	Teach Mrs. Z. about interventions she can use at home after being discharged.
	(A) Value seeing health care situations "through patients' eyes."	

Chapter Highlights

Age-Related Changes That Affect Sleep and Rest Patterns (Table 24-1)

- Diminished sleep efficiency
- Alterations in sleep cycles and stages
- Shifts in circadian rhythm

Risks Factors That Affect Sleep Wellness (Tables 24-2 and 24-3)

- Psychosocial factors: beliefs, attitudes, anxiety, depression, boredom
- Environmental factors: noise, light, lack of privacy
- Pathologic conditions and functional impairment (e.g., pain and discomfort, medication effects, physiologic disorders)
- Restless legs syndrome and periodic limb movements during sleep

Functional Consequences Affecting Sleep Wellness

- Longer time needed to fall asleep
- Frequent arousals during the night
- More time in bed to achieve same quantity of sleep
- Diminished quality of sleep (less dreaming and deep sleep)

Pathologic Condition Affecting Sleep Wellness

- Insomnia
- Excessive daytime sleepiness (Box 24-1)
- Obstructive sleep apnea (OSA)

Nursing Assessment of Sleep (Box 24-3)

- Perception of quantity and quality of sleep
- Factors that affect sleep
- Usual sleep patterns and behaviours that affect it
- Actual sleep pattern (observed in institutional settings)
- Evidence-based assessment tools: Pittsburgh Sleep Quality Index (PSQI) and Epworth Sleepiness Scale (ESS)

Nursing Diagnosis

- Readiness for Enhanced Sleep
- Disturbed Sleep Pattern

Planning for Wellness Outcomes

- Sleep
- Rest
- Comfort level
- Personal well-being

Nursing Interventions for Sleep Wellness (Boxes 24-3 through 24-7)

- Teaching about interventions to promote healthy sleep patterns
- Modifying the environment
- Individualizing care in institutional settings
- Explaining relaxation and mental imagery techniques
- Teaching about medications that affect sleep
- Addressing OSA

Evaluating Effectiveness of Nursing Interventions

- Expressed feelings of being rested upon awakening
- Improved score on sleep assessment tool
- Observations that the person is sleeping at night

Critical Thinking Exercises

1. What is an older adult likely to experience with regard to sleep and rest patterns? How would you explain these changes to an older adult?
2. Identify three specific factors in each of the following categories that might interfere with sleep: environmental influences, physiologic disturbances and psychosocial factors.
3. How would you assess an 82-year-old person who comes to the nursing clinic at the senior wellness centre complaining of feeling tired all the time and not getting enough sleep?
4. What would you include in a half-hour presentation on "Tips for Good Sleep" for participants in a senior wellness program at a community-based centre?
5. What information about sleep and rest would you include in an in-service program for evening and night-shift nursing assistants employed in a long-term care facility?

 For more information about the topics discussed in this chapter, be sure to check out the interactive Online Learning Activities and other helpful resources at http://thepoint.lww.com/Miller7e

REFERENCES

Adachi, M., Staisiunas, P. G., Knutson, K. L., et al. (2013). Perceived control and sleep in hospitalized older adults. *Journal of Hospital Medicine, 8*(4), 184–190. doi:10.1002/jhm.2023

American Geriatrics Society. (2012). American Geriatrics Society updated Beers Criteria for potentially inappropriate medication use in older adults. *Journal of the American Geriatrics Society, 60*, 616–631.

Baglioni, C., & Riemann, D. (2012). Is chronic insomnia a precursor to major depression? Epidemiological and biological findings. *Current Psychiatry Reports, 14*(5), 511–518.

Baquet, J. P., Barone-Rochette, G., Tamisier, R., et al. (2012). Mechanisms of cardiac dysfunction in obstructive sleep apnea. *National Review of Cardiology, 9*(12), 879–688.

Bliwise, D. L., Trotti, L. M., Yesavage, J. A., et al. (2012). Periodic leg movements in sleep in elderly patients with Parkinsonism and Alzheimer's disease. *European Journal of Neurology, 19*(6), 18–23.

Brandt, N. J., & Piechocki, J. M. (2013). Treatment of insomnia in older adults. *Journal of Gerontological Nursing, 39*(4), 48–54.

Buysse, D. J. (2013). Insomnia. *Journal of the American Medical Association, 309*(7), 706–716.

Carlucci, M., Smith, M., & Corbridge, S. J. (2013). Poor sleep, hazardous breathing: An overview of obstructive sleep apnea. *The Nurse Practitioner, 38*(3), 20–27.

Chasens, E. R., & Umlauf, M. G. (2012). Excessive sleepiness. In E. Capezuti, D. Zwicker, M. Mezey, et al. (Eds.), *Evidence-based geriatric nursing protocols for best practice* (4th ed., pp. 74–88). New York, NY: Springer.

Cho, E. R., Kim, H., Seo, H. S., et al. (2013, February 1). Obstructive sleep apnea as a risk factor for silent cerebral infarction. *Journal of Sleep Research, 22*(4), 452–458. doi:10.1111/jsr.12034

Cohen-Mansfield, J., & Perach, R. (2012). Sleep duration, nap habits, and mortality in older persons. *Sleep, 35*(7), 1003–1009.

Das, A. M., & Khan, M. (2012). Obstructive sleep apnea and stroke. *Expert Review of Cardiovascular Therapies, 10*(4), 525–535.

deGage, S. B., Begaud, B., Bazin, F., et al. (2012, September 27). Benzodiazepine use and risk of dementia. *British Medical Journal, 345*, e6231. doi:10.1136/bmj.e6231

Fismer, K. L., & Pilkington, K. (2012). Lavender and sleep: A systematic review of the evidence. *European Journal of Integrative Medicine, 4*(4), e436–e447.

Fung, C. H., Martin, J. L., Chung, C., et al. (2012). Sleep durations among older adults in assisted living facilities. *American Journal of Geriatric Psychiatry, 20*(6), 485–493.

Grigg-Damberger, M., & Ralls, F. (2012). Cognitive dysfunction and obstructive sleep apnea: From cradle to tomb. *Current Opinion in Pulmonary Medicine, 18*(6), 580–587.

Gross, C. R., Kreitzer, M. J., Reilly-Spong, M., et al. (2011). Mindfulness-based stress reduction vs. pharmacotherapy for primary chronic insomnia. *Explore, 7*(2), 76–87.

Guimaraes, L. H., de Carvalho, L. B., Yanaguibashi, G., & do Prado, G. (2008). Physically active women sleep more and better than sedentary women. *Sleep Medicine, 9*, 488–493.

Gupta, R., Lahan, V., & Goel, D. (2013). Prevalence of restless legs syndrome in subjects with depressive disorder. *Indian Journal of Psychiatry, 55*(1), 70–73.

Harand, C., Bertran, F., Doidy, F., et al. (2012). How aging affects sleep-dependent memory consolidation? *Frontiers in Neurology, 3*, 8. doi:10.3389.fneuro.2012.00008

Harris, M., Richards, K. C., & Grando, V. T. (2012). The effects of slow-stroke back massage on minutes of nighttime sleep in persons with dementia and sleep disturbances in the nursing home: A pilot study. *Journal of Holistic Nursing, 30*(4), 255–263.

Herdman, T. H. (Ed.). (2012). *NANDA International Nursing Diagnoses: Definitions and classification 2012-1014.* Oxford, England: Wiley-Blackwell.

Hibi, S., Yamaguchi, Y., Umeda-Kameyama, Y., et al. (2012). The high frequency of periodic limb movements in patients with Lewy body dementia. *Journal of Psychiatry Research, 46*(12), 1590–1594.

Huang, A. R., Mallet, L., Rochefort, C. M., et al. (2012). Medication-related falls in the elderly. *Drugs and Aging, 29*(5), 359–376.

Hung, H. C., Yang, Y. C., Ou, H. Y., et al. (2013). The association between self-reported sleep quality and metabolic sndrome. *PLoS One, 8*(1), e53404. doi:10.1371/jounal.pone.0054304

Jaussent, I., Bouyer, J., Ancelin, M.-L., et al. (2011). Insomnia and daytime sleepiness are risk factors for depressive symptoms in the elderly. *Sleep, 34*(8), 1103–1110.

Jones, C., & Dawson, D. (2012). Eye masks and earplugs improve patient's perception of sleep. *Nursing in Critical Care, 17*(5), 247–254.

Kang, D. Y., Park, S., Rhee, C. W., et al. (2012). Zolpidem use and risk of fracture in elderly insomnia patients. *Journal of Prevention and Public Health, 45*(4), 2219–2226.

Kasai, T. (2012). Sleep apnea and heart failure. *Journal of Cardiology, 60*(2), 78–85.

Katofsky, I., Backhaus, J., Junghanns, K., et al. (2012). Effectiveness of a cognitive behavioral self-help program for patients with primary insomnia in general practice. *Sleep Medicine, 13*(5), 463–468.

King, A. C., Pruitt, L. A., Woo, S., et al. (2008). Effects of moderate-intensity exercise on polysomnographic and subjective sleep quality with mild to moderate sleep complaints. *The Journals of Gerontology. Series A, Biological Sciences and Medical Sciences, 63*(9), 997–1004.

Kline, C. E., Sui, X., Hall, M. H., et al. (2012). Dose-response effects of exercise training on the subjective sleep quality of postmenopausal women: Exploratory analysis of a randomised control trial. *British Medical Journal Open, 2012*(2), e001044. doi:10.1136/bmjopen.2012.001044

Koo, B. B., Blackwell, T., Ancoli-Israel, S., et al. (2011). Association of incident cardiovascular disease with periodic limb movements during sleep in older men. *Circulation, 124*(11), 1223–1231.

Kostoglou-Anthanassiou, I. (2013). Therapeutic applications of melatonin. *Therapeutic Advances in Endocrinology and Metabolism, 4*(1), 13–24.

Lacasse, Y., Bureau, M.-P., & Series, F. (2004). A new standardized and self-administered quality of life questionnaire specific to obstructive sleep apnoea. *Thorax, 59*, 494–499. doi:10.1136/thx.2003.011205

Levy, P., Tamisier, R., Arnaud, C., et al. (2012). Sleep deprivation, sleep apnea and cardiovascular diseases. *Frontiers in Bioscience, 4*, 2007–2021.

Li, S. Y., Wang, T. J., Vivienne Wu, S. F., et al. (2011). Efficacy of controlling night-time noise and activities to improve patients' sleep quality in a surgical intensive care unit. *Journal of Clinical Nursing, 20*(3–4), 396–407.

Little, A., Ethier, C., Ayas, N., et al. (2012). A patient survey of sleep quality in the intensive care unit. *Minerva Anestesilogica, 78*(4), 406–414.

Lu, M.-J., Lin, S.-T., Chen, K.-M., et al. (2013). Acupressure improves sleep quality of psychogeriatric inpatients. *Nursing Research, 62*(2), 130–137.

Mander, B. A., Rao, V., Lu, B., et al. (2013). Prefrontal atrophy, disrupted NREM slow waves and impaired hippocampal-dependent memory in aging. *Nature Neuroscience, 16*(3), 357–364.

Misra, S., & Malow, B. A. (2008). Evaluation of sleep disturbances in older adults. *Clinics in Geriatric Medicine, 24*, 15–26.

Moorhead, S., Johnson, M., Maas, M. L., et al. (Eds.). (2013). *Nursing outcomes classification (NOC)*. Philadelphia, PA: Elsevier.

Nagendra, R. P., Maruthai, N., & Kutty, B. M. (2012). Meditation and its regulatory role on sleep. *Frontiers in Neurology, 3*. doi:10.3389/fneur.2012.00054

National Center on Sleep Disorders Research. (2011). *National Institutes of Health Sleep Disorders Research Plan* [NIH Publication No. 11-7820]. Washington, DC: U.S. Department of Health and Human Services.

Neubauer, D. N. (2013). Chronic insomnia. *Continuum, 19*(1), 50–66.

Oliveira, D. S., Hachul, H., Goto, V., et al. (2012). Effect of therapeutic massage on insomnia and climateric symptoms in postmenopausal women. *Climacteric, 15*(1), 21–29.

Ong, J. C., Ulmer, C. S., & Manber, R. (2012). Improving sleep with mindfulness and acceptance. *Behaviour Research and Therapy, 50*, 651–660.

Panossian, L., & Daley, J. (2013). Sleep-disordered breathing. *Continuum, 19*(1), 86–103.

Public Health Agency of Canada. (2010). *Fast facts from the 2009 Canadian Community Health Survey—Sleep apnea rapid response* [Cat. HP35-19/1-2010E]. Ottawa, ON: Author.

Ralls, F. M., & Grigg-Damberger, M. (2012). Roles of gender, age, race/ethnicity, and residential socioeconomics in obstructive sleep apnea syndromes. *Current Opinion in Pulmonary Medicine, 18*(6), 568–573.

Rizzi, M., Barrella, M., Kotzalidis, G. D., et al. (2011). Periodic limbic movement disorder during sleep as diabetes-related syndrome? *International Scholarly Research Network,* 1–5. doi:1-.5402/2011/246157

Roux, F. J. (2013). Restless legs syndrome: Impact on sleep-related breathing disorders. *Respirology, 18*(2), 236–245.

Salas, R. E., & Kwan, A. B. (2012). The real burden of restless legs syndrome. *American Journal of Managed Care, 18*(9 Suppl.), S207–S212.

Sarris, J., & Byrne, G. J. (2011). A systematic review of insomnia and complementary medicine. *Sleep Medicine Reviews, 15*, 99–106.

Sforza, E., & Roche, F. (2012, May 29). Sleep apnea syndrome and cognition. *Frontiers in Neurology, 3*, 87. doi:10.3389/fneur.2012.00087

Sharma, M. P., & Andrade, C. (2012). Behavioural interventions for insomnia: Theory and practice. *Indian Journal of Psychiatry, 54*(4), 359–366.

Silber, M. (2013). Sleep-related movement disorders. *Continuum, 19*(1), 170–184.

Sobana, R., Parthasarathy, S., & Duraisamy, et al. (2013). The effect of yoga therapy on selected psychological variables among male patients with insomnia. *Journal of Clinical & Diagnostic Research, 7*(1), 55–57.

Su, C. P., Lai, H. L., Chang, E. T., et al. (2013). A randomized controlled trial of the effects of listening to non-commercial music on quality of nocturnal sleep and relaxation indices in patients in medical intensive care unit. *Journal of Advanced Nursing, 69*(6), 1377–1389. doi:10.1111/j.1365-2648

Troxel, W. M., Germain, A., & Buysse, D. J. (2012). Clinical management of insomnia with brief behavioral treatment. *Behavioral Sleep Medicine, 10*(4), 266–279.

Uchida, S., Shioda, K., Morita, Y., et al. (2012, April 2). Exercise effects on sleep physiology. *Frontiers in Neurology, 3*, 48. doi:10.3389/jneur.2012.00048

Valenza, M. C., Cabrera-Martos, I., Martin-Martin, L., et al. (2013). Nursing homes: Impact of sleep disturbances on functionality. *Archives of Gerontology and Geriatrics, 56*(3), 432–436.

Vijayan, V. K. (2012). Morbidities associated with obstructive sleep apnea. *Expert Review of Respiratory Medicine, 6*(5), 557–566.

Watson, N. F., & Viola-Saltzman, M. (2013). Sleep and comorbid neurologic disorders. *Continuum, 19*(1), 148–169.

Williams, J., Roth, A., Vatthauer, K., et al. (2013). Cognitive behavioral treatment of insomnia. *Chest, 143*(2), 554–565.

Winklewski, P. J., & Frydrychowski, A. F. (2013). Cerebral blood flow, sympathetic nerve activity and stroke risk in obstructive sleep apnoea. *Blood Pressure, 22*(1), 27–33.

Yang, M.-C., Lin, C.-Y., Lai, C.-C., et al. (2013). Factors affecting positive airway pressure therapy acceptance in elderly patients with obstructive sleep apnea in Taiwan. *Respiratory Care, 58*(9), 1504–1513. doi:10.4187/respcare.02176

Yoder, J. C., Staisiunas, P. G., Meltzer, D. O., et al. (2012). Noise and sleep among adult medical inpatients. *Archives of Internal Medicine, 172*(1), 68–70.

Zeitzer, J. M., Bliwise, D. L., Hernandez, B., et al. (2013). Nocturia compounds nocturnal wakefulness in older individuals with insomnia. *Journal of Clinical Sleep Medicine, 9*(3), 259–262.

chapter 25

Thermoregulation

LEARNING OBJECTIVES

After reading this chapter, you will be able to:

1. Describe age-related changes that affect an older adult's normal body temperature, febrile response to illness, and response to hot and cold environmental temperatures.

2. Identify risk factors that affect thermoregulation in older adults and increase the potential for hypothermia or heat-related illness.

3. Assess the following aspects of thermoregulation: baseline temperature, risks for altered thermoregulation, hypothermia, heat-related illness and febrile response to illness.

4. Discuss the functional consequences of altered thermoregulation in older adults.

5. Implement health promotion interventions for preventing hypothermia and heat-related illness in older adults.

KEY POINTS

accidental hypothermia   heat-related illness

acclimatize   hypothermia

heat exhaustion   thermoregulation

heat stroke

The primary function of thermoregulation is to maintain a stable core body temperature in a wide range of environmental temperatures. In the presence of infections, thermoregulation also assists in maintaining homeostasis. Under normal circumstances, the core body temperature is maintained at 36.1°C to 37.2°C through complex physiologic mechanisms governing heat production and dissipation.

Because older adults experience age-related changes and additional risk factors that affect thermoregulation, they are vulnerable to **hypothermia,** an abnormally low body temperature, and **hyperthermia**, an abnormally elevated body temperature, for example from heat stroke, fever or similar conditions. The term **heat-related illness** is used in this chapter when hyperthermia occurs in response to hot environmental temperatures, in contrast to when it is related to pathophysiologic causes. This chapter focuses on nursing assessment and interventions related to altered thermoregulation in older adults.

AGE-RELATED CHANGES THAT AFFECT THERMOREGULATION

With increased age, subtle alterations in thermoregulation occur, and these become important considerations in caring for healthy, as well as frail, older adults. **Thermoregulation** is a complex adaptive response that involves many internal and external influences. Internal conditions that affect thermoregulation include metabolic rate, pathologic processes, muscle activity, peripheral blood flow, amount of subcutaneous fat, central nervous system function, temperature of the blood flowing through the hypothalamus, and effects of medications and other bioactive substances. External influences on thermoregulation include environmental temperature, humidity level, airflow, and the type and amount of clothing and covering used. The following sections address these factors in relation to the ability of older adults to respond to environmental temperatures and in relation to normal body temperature.

Response to Cold Temperatures

In cold environmental temperatures, the body normally initiates physiologic mechanisms to prevent loss of body heat and increase heat production. At the same time, individuals usually initiate protective behaviours to warm the body and protect themselves from adversely cold temperatures.

Promoting Healthy Thermoregulation in Older Adults

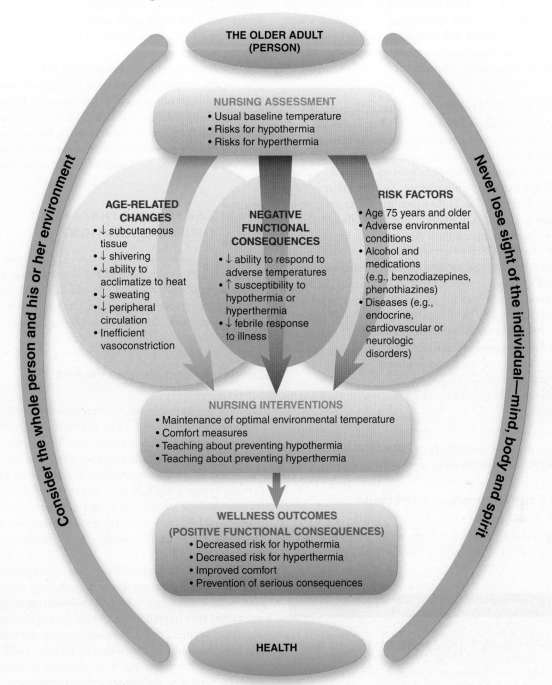

THE OLDER ADULT (PERSON)

NURSING ASSESSMENT
• Usual baseline temperature
• Risks for hypothermia
• Risks for hyperthermia

AGE-RELATED CHANGES
• ↓ subcutaneous tissue
• ↓ shivering
• ↓ ability to acclimatize to heat
• ↓ sweating
• ↓ peripheral circulation
• Inefficient vasoconstriction

NEGATIVE FUNCTIONAL CONSEQUENCES
• ↓ ability to respond to adverse temperatures
• ↑ susceptibility to hypothermia or hyperthermia
• ↓ febrile response to illness

RISK FACTORS
• Age 75 years and older
• Adverse environmental conditions
• Alcohol and medications (e.g., benzodiazepines, phenothiazines)
• Diseases (e.g., endocrine, cardiovascular or neurologic disorders)

NURSING INTERVENTIONS
• Maintenance of optimal environmental temperature
• Comfort measures
• Teaching about preventing hypothermia
• Teaching about preventing hyperthermia

WELLNESS OUTCOMES
(POSITIVE FUNCTIONAL CONSEQUENCES)
• Decreased risk for hypothermia
• Decreased risk for hyperthermia
• Improved comfort
• Prevention of serious consequences

HEALTH

Consider the whole person and his or her environment

Never lose sight of the individual—mind, body and spirit

Physiologic mechanisms that prevent heat loss and increase heat production include shivering, muscle contraction, increased heart rate, peripheral vasoconstriction, dilation of the blood vessels in the muscles, insulation of deeper tissues by subcutaneous fat, and release of thyroxine and corticosteroid by the pituitary gland. Protective actions that people commonly initiate in cold temperatures include seeking shelter, ingesting warm fluids, wearing warm clothing or covering, and increasing activity to stimulate circulation.

The following age-related changes, which can affect processes involved with heat loss or production, are likely to interfere with an older person's ability to respond to cold temperatures:
● Inefficient vasoconstriction
● Decreased cardiac output
● Decreased muscle mass
● Diminished peripheral circulation
● Decreased subcutaneous tissue
● Delayed and diminished shivering

These changes begin during the fifth decade, but their cumulative effects are experienced during the seventh or eighth decade. The overall outcome of these changes is a dulled perception of cold and a concomitant lack of stimulus to initiate protective actions, such as adding more clothing or raising the environmental temperature.

Response to Hot Temperatures

In hot environmental temperatures, or when metabolic heat production is high, the normal mechanisms for heat dissipation are the production of sweat to facilitate evaporation and the dilation of peripheral blood vessels to facilitate heat radiation. When exposed to hot climates or engaged in strenuous activity daily for 7 to 14 days, healthy adults are able to **acclimatize** (i.e., gradually increase their metabolic efficiency to adapt to higher temperatures). See box 25-1 for evidence to inform practice. Delayed acclimatization may explain the phenomenon of increased incidence of heat exhaustion during the third or fourth days of heat waves (Hansen et al., 2011).

The older person's ability to acclimatize and respond to heat stress is altered by the following age-related changes:

- Higher threshold for the onset of sweating
- Diminished response when sweating occurs
- Dulled sensation of warm environments
- Renal and cardiovascular changes
- Diminished thirst sensation, which can lead to inadequate fluid intake

The overall effect of these changes is that even healthy older adults are more susceptible to heat-related illnesses because they are less able to adapt to hot environments.

Normal Body Temperature and Febrile Response to Illness

The long-standing norm for body temperature has been 37°C; however, a systematic review of studies related to body temperature norms and a study of 18,630 healthy adults concluded that normal body temperature for healthy adults is lower than 37°C, with older adults having an oral temperature range of 36.1°C to 36.3°C (Lu et al., 2010; Waalen & Buxbaum, 2011).

An elevated temperature, or fever, is the body's protective response to pathologic conditions, such as cancer, infection, dehydration or connective tissue disease. This protective response is blunted in older adults because of age-related changes involving thermoregulation and the immune system. Implications for nursing care are discussed in the sections on *Functional Consequences* and *Nursing Assessment*.

 RISK FACTORS THAT AFFECT THERMOREGULATION

Increased age is a risk factor for both hypothermia and heat-related illnesses, which are likely to occur even in moderately cold or hot environments. In addition, pathophysiologic disorders, adverse medication reactions and socioeconomic conditions increase the risk for serious consequences related to altered thermoregulation.

Conditions That Increase the Risk for Hypothermia

The risk for hypothermia is increased by conditions that decrease heat production (e.g., inactivity, malnutrition, endocrine disorders, neuromuscular conditions), increase heat loss (e.g., burns, vasodilation) or affect the normal thermoregulatory process (pathologic conditions of the central nervous system). Medical disorders that predispose to hypothermia include stroke, sepsis, malnutrition, multiple sclerosis, renal insufficiency, Parkinson disease and endocrine disorders (e.g., hypothyroidism, hypoglycemia, hypoadrenalism) (Davis, 2012).

Medications and alcohol can predispose a person to hypothermia by suppressing shivering, inducing vasodilation or affecting the central nervous system. Medications most often associated with hypothermia include antipsychotics (including newer atypical ones), benzodiazepines, tricyclic antidepressants, opioids and barbiturates (Davis, 2012; Kreuzer et al., 2012). Excessive use of alcohol can increase the risk for hypothermia by dulling sensory perceptions and interfering with cognitive skills necessary for initiating protective behaviours.

Conditions That Increase the Risk for Heat-Related Illness

The risk for heat-related illness is increased by physiologic alterations that increase internal heat production (e.g., hyperthyroidism, diabetic ketoacidosis) or interfere with the ability to respond to heat stress (e.g., cardiovascular disease, fluid or electrolyte imbalance). In addition, medical disorders, such as cardiovascular disease and Parkinson disease, can

---

Box 25-1 Evidence-Informed Nursing Practice

Background: While daily physical activity is important for maintaining functional capacity and independence, most older Canadians do not engage in enough activities.

Question: What influence does summer time weather variations in Canada have upon the physical activity of older adults?

Method: Forty-eight randomly selected members of a local community centre wore an accelerometer for a single 7-day period over the late spring and early summer period and completed a physical activity logbook. Local weather conditions were collected from the national weather service.

Findings: Age and air quality were found to have a significant influence upon activity levels.

Implications for Nursing Practice: Older adults should be encouraged to engage in indoor activities on a daily basis. Well-ventilated places for such activities are important.

Source: Brandon, C. A., Gill, D. P., Speechley, M., et al. (2009). Physical activity levels of older community-dwelling older adults are influenced by summer weather variations. *Applied Physiology, Nutrition & Metabolism, 34*(2), 182–190.

worsen the severity of heat-related illness and decrease the chance of full recovery. For example, case studies of heat-stroke in patients with Parkinson disease reported multiorgan dysfunction and permanent neurologic damage (Yamashita et al., 2012).

Medications can predispose to heat-related illness by increasing diuresis (e.g., diuretics), increasing heat production (e.g., salicylate intoxication), or interfering with sweating (e.g., anticholinergics) or peripheral vasodilation (e.g., β-adrenergic blocking agents). A study comparing adverse medication reactions in older adults during heat waves and normal summers implicated the following medications: diuretics, serotonic antidepressants, angiotensin-converting enzyme inhibitors, and proton pump inhibitors (Sommet et al., 2012). Alcohol increases the risk for heat-related illness by inducing diuresis, and excessive alcohol can increase the risk by increasing heat production.

Environmental and Socioeconomic Influences

Environmental temperatures—especially in combination with low socioeconomic indicators—can increase the vulnerability of older adults, particularly those older than 75 years, to hypothermia or heat-related illness (Hansen et al., 2011; Romero-Ortuno et al., 2013). Although people who live in geographic areas with extreme temperature variations are especially vulnerable, frail older adults often develop hypothermia or heat-related conditions even in moderately hot or cold climates because of additional interacting conditions. For example, heat-related illness can be precipitated in older adults by moderate exercise in hot and humid weather, especially if fluid intake is not adequate. Insufficient fluid intake is another contributing condition, and this is likely to occur if older adults rely solely on their sensation of thirst, which is decreased owing to age-related changes.

In addition to the obvious influence of hot or cold temperatures, homelessness, substandard living conditions, and diets deficient in protein and calories are conditions associated with both hypothermia and heat-related illness. Heat waves are especially hazardous for older adults living in environments with poor ventilation, lack of air-conditioning, and high levels of humidity and air pollutants. Older adults who live in urban areas with high crime rates may keep windows closed for safety considerations. In Great Britain, the term *urban hypothermia* has been used with reference to older adults living alone in poorly heated dwellings.

Social isolation is a factor that increases the risk for progression of heat-related illness or hypothermia because people rarely are able to self-report these conditions. Thus, they may not receive help in a timely manner. Older adults who live alone and have dementia may be at increased risk if they do not have the cognitive skills to adjust the thermostat and wear proper clothing or the ability to recognize the symptoms and call for help in a timely manner. Additional risk factors are summarized in Box 25-2.

Box 25-2 Risk Factors for Hypothermia or Heat-Related Illness in Older Adults

Risks for Hypothermia and Heat-Related Illness

- Age 75+ years
- Adverse environmental temperatures
- Pathophysiologic alterations
- Socioeconomic conditions related to poor housing

Risks for Hypothermia

- Alcohol, especially excessive amounts
- Stroke
- Diabetes or hypoglycemia
- Endocrine disorders (e.g., hypothyroidism, hypoadrenalism)
- Malnutrition
- Parkinson disease
- Peripheral neuropathy
- Medications: opioids, antipsychotics, barbiturates, benzodiazepines and tricyclic antidepressants

Risks for Heat-Related Illness

- Alcohol and alcohol withdrawal
- Dehydration
- Diabetic ketoacidosis
- Hyperthyroidism
- Excessive exercise or even moderate exercise in hot and humid environments
- Medications: diuretics, cardiovascular agents and anticholinergic agents (including antihistamines, phenothiazines, tricyclic antidepressants)

Wellness Opportunity

Although the weather cannot be controlled, it is important to identify the environmental factors that affect thermoregulation and that can be addressed through health education about protective actions.

Behaviours Based on Lack of Knowledge

Lack of knowledge about age-related vulnerability to hypothermia and heat-related illness may create risks secondary to inadequate protective measures. For example, when the use of air-conditioning or heating is curtailed as a cost-saving measure, younger adults may be able to adjust to the moderately hot or cool temperature, whereas an older adult may develop hypothermia or a heat-related illness under the same circumstances. If older adults and their caregivers are not aware of the age-related decrease in the perception of environmental temperatures, they may not take appropriate protective measures, such as removing or adding clothing.

In the presence of infection or other pathophysiologic alterations, lack of knowledge about normal temperature in older adults may result in undetected illnesses. For example, caregivers and health care professionals may falsely assume that no infection is present if there is no fever. Similarly, if they believe that the baseline temperature for all adults is 37°C, they may not recognize an elevated temperature in someone whose baseline temperature is lower than this.

FUNCTIONAL CONSEQUENCES ASSOCIATED WITH THERMOREGULATION IN OLDER ADULTS

A healthy older adult in a comfortable environment will experience few, if any, functional consequences of altered thermoregulation. In the presence of any risk factor, however, hypothermia or heat-related illness may develop in an older adult. Even moderately adverse environmental temperatures can precipitate hypothermia or heat-related illness in an older adult, especially in the presence of additional predisposing factors, such as certain medications or pathologic conditions. For older adults in whom hypothermia or heat-related illness develops, the risk of subsequent morbidity or mortality from this condition is greater than that for their younger counterparts.

In Canada, hypothermia and heat-related illness usually are seasonal hazards that occur during cold spells and heat waves. Compared to other countries, there have been few quantitative studies of the adverse effects of heat waves in Canada. An exception is the work of Alberini et al. (2011), who in 2010 surveyed five Canadian cities to identify how individuals perceived the heat, what was their experience with heat-related illness and how they protected themselves from excessive heat. About 21% of participants reported feeling unwell during a recent heat spell. The rate which participants reported a heat-related illness was higher among those with cardiovascular or respiratory illnesses. Extreme heat events were estimated to cause an average of 120 deaths in the city of Toronto alone per year (Cheng & Campbell, 2005).

Altered Response to Cold Environments

Increased age is associated with an increased vulnerability to hypothermia because most older adults are less aware of a low core body temperature, less efficient in their physiologic response to cold and less apt to take corrective actions when necessary. A low environmental temperature usually contributes to hypothermia, and the term **accidental hypothermia** is used when low environmental temperature is the primary cause of the condition. Even in normal environmental temperatures, however, the condition can result from serious alterations in homeostasis, such as can occur with anesthesia or endocrine or neurologic disorders. Accidental hypothermia can occur in older adults as a consequence of exposure to moderately cool temperatures, and may affect as many as 10% of older adults living in winter climates (e.g., Canada, Great Britain and parts of the United States).

In the early stages of hypothermia, the older adult probably will not shiver or complain of feeling cold. In the absence of any protective measures, hypothermia will progress, clouding mental function. The effects of impaired thermoregulation are cumulative, and hypothermia progresses rapidly after the core body temperature falls to 33.9°C. The age-related diminished ability of the kidney to conserve water and the common occurrence of inadequate fluid intake in older adults exacerbate the effects of hypothermia. If the process is not reversed, death from hypothermia will result from the myocardial effects of seriously impaired thermoregulation. Figure 25-1 illustrates physiologic effects of hypothermia according to stages from mild to severe.

Altered Response to Hot Environments

Functional consequences that affect an older adult's ability to respond to hot environments include delayed and diminished sweating and inaccurate perception of environmental temperatures. Because of these functional consequences, the older adult is more likely to have heat-related illnesses, including heat exhaustion and heat stroke. **Heat exhaustion** is a condition that develops gradually from depletion of fluid, sodium or both. It can occur in active or immobilized older people who are dehydrated or underhydrated and exposed to hot environments. **Heat stroke** is an even more serious condition that is likely to occur in active older adults because of a combination of age-related thermoregulatory changes and risk factors, such as overexertion and warm environments. Heat stroke can also occur in immobilized older adults in hot environments, either as a progression of untreated heat exhaustion or as a result of a combination of risk factors. The underlying mechanism in heat stroke is an inability to balance the rates of heat production and dissipation. This balance depends primarily on sweating and cardiac output.

In hot environments, the effects of altered thermoregulation are cumulative, and heat-related illnesses progress rapidly after the body temperature reaches 40.6°C. If fluid volume is not adequate to meet the requirements for effective sweating, then heat-related illness will progress even more rapidly. If heat-related illness is not reversed, death will result from respiratory depression. One study found that heat waves were associated with statistically significant increases in cardiovascular and diabetes mortality and higher emergency room admissions for renal disease (Wang et al., 2012).

Altered Thermoregulatory Response to Illness

Age-related changes in the thermoregulatory centres of the hypothalamus diminish the older adult's febrile response to illness and infections. Thus, infections are likely to be undetected until they progress and manifest as a functional decline or change in mental status. Older adults with infections may have a normal or even lower than normal temperature, but when their temperature is compared with their baseline temperature, at least a slight elevation is evident. An implication of this is that impaired temperature regulation can have deleterious results in older adults and a subtle temperature change may be a significant indicator of an underlying disease that requires medical attention (Chester & Rudolph, 2011).

Altered Perception of Environmental Temperatures

Older adults often report feeling cool or cold, even in very warm environments, and they generally prefer environmental

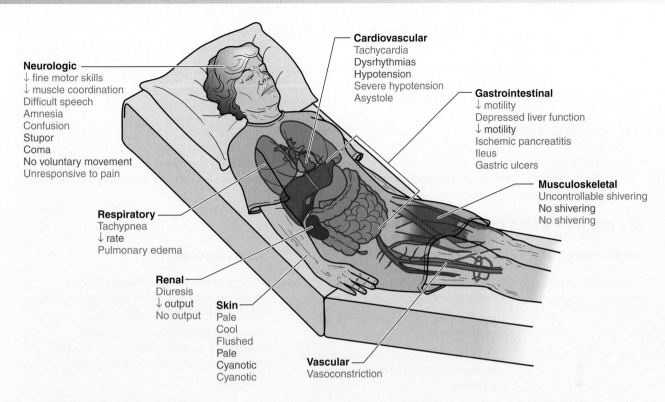

Red = mild (91.4°F–95°F [33°C–35°C]); Green = moderate (85.2°F–89.6°F [29°C–32°C]); Blue = severe (<85.2°F [<29°C]).

FIGURE 25-1 Physiologic effects of hypothermia according to stages from mild to severe. (From Davis, R. A. [2012]. The big chill: Accidental hypothermia. *American Journal of Nursing, 112*[1], 41.)

temperatures that are at least 23.9°C. Inaccurate perceptions of environmental temperatures are associated with pathophysiologic conditions, such as dementia, thyroid disorders, or cardiovascular inefficiency, rather than with age-related changes alone.

Psychosocial Consequences of Altered Thermoregulation

Psychosocial consequences are associated with hypothermia, heat-related illness or diminished fever response. If hypothermia or heat-related illness is overlooked, or if interventions are not initiated at an early stage, the condition may progress to the point of impairing cognitive function. Likewise, if a diminished or delayed febrile response to an infection is not recognized, a treatable condition may be overlooked and treatment may unintentionally be delayed or denied. Untreated infections are likely to progress in severity and, in older adults, may manifest primarily as a functional decline, such as impaired cognition.

Unfolding Case Study

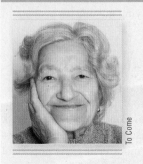

Part 1: Mrs. T. at 76 Years of Age

Mrs. T. is 76 years old and lives alone in a large farmhouse in a rural area in central Saskatchewan. She has lived on this 20-acre farm for 49 years and has been a widow for 2 years. She has four children and eight grandchildren, but they all live in other provinces. Mrs. T. has been able to manage her farm with a part-time farmhand who comes a couple of times a week to help feed the several dozen chickens and collect eggs. When her farmhand doesn't come, she manages the chores by herself. She has hypertension and type 2 diabetes, and manages reasonably well medically. She adheres to her diabetic diet and takes her medications daily. She sends her farmhand to the city once weekly for groceries and drives to the nearby church on Sundays. Once a month she attends the senior centre, where you are the nurse. It is the middle of July, and summer in Saskatchewan this year has been unusually hot and humid. A drought and heat wave are predicted for central

(continued)

Unfolding Case Study (continued)

Saskatchewan and you are planning to present a health education program called "Hot Tips for Surviving the Summer." You are particularly concerned about Mrs. T. and several other participants who live in isolated areas and have little contact with others.

THINKING POINTS

- What factors increase the risk of Mrs. T. developing a heat-related illness? Which ones would you discuss in your health education program?

- In your health education program, how would you explain heat-related illnesses and the associated signs and symptoms?

QSEN APPLICATION

QSEN Competency	Knowledge/Skill/Attitude	Application to Mrs. T.
Patient-centred care	(K) Describe how diverse backgrounds function as a source of values.	When planning the educational program, identify aspects of rural living that increase the risks for heat-related illnesses.
	(S) Elicit patient values, preferences and expressed needs.	During the educational program, elicit information from Mrs. T. about ways in which she can reduce the risks for heat-related illnesses.
	(S) Provide patient-centred care with sensitivity and respect for diversity of the human experience.	
	(A) Value seeing health care situations "through patients' eyes."	

NURSING ASSESSMENT OF THERMOREGULATION

Nursing assessment of thermoregulation addresses the older person's baseline body temperature, any risk factors for altered thermoregulation, manifestations of hypothermia or heat-related illness, and febrile response to illness. This information is essential for planning health education interventions to prevent hypothermia and heat-related illness. Assessment information is also crucial for detecting hypothermia or heat-related illnesses as quickly as possible so that appropriate interventions can be initiated before serious or irreversible effects occur. Assessment information is also important in detecting infections at an early stage. Nurses obtain much of the pertinent information about risk factors as part of the overall assessment; they also obtain information by observing the environment, measuring the person's body temperature, and interviewing the older adult and the caregivers of dependent older adults.

Assessing Baseline Temperature

Body temperature measurements show a diurnal fluctuation of 1°C to 1.3°C, with lower temperatures during sleeping and greater fluctuations during periods of fever-inducing illness. Because older adults normally have a lower body temperature and may have a diminished febrile response to infection, it is especially important to determine the person's usual temperature, as well as to characterize the usual pattern

of diurnal variation. Because many types of thermometers are now available (e.g., oral, rectal, tympanic and bladder probes), it is important to document the method used for assessing temperature. Also, when assessing for hypothermia, it is advisable to use several methods and to make sure that the thermometers are able to detect low body temperatures.

Nurses can encourage older adults in home settings to determine their usual temperature by recording their temperature at different times of the day for several days when they are feeling well. Doing this seasonally by people who live in fluctuating climates and annually by those who live in stable climates provides a baseline for comparison when symptoms of illness or functional decline occur. In long-term care settings, baseline temperature data, including normal fluctuations, should be documented on the chart. Box 25-3 summarizes the principles underlying nursing assessment of thermoregulation in older adults.

Identifying Risk Factors for Altered Thermoregulation

Anyone older than 75 years is at risk for altered thermoregulation, as are older adults who have one or more of the risk factors listed in Box 25-2. Because many of the risk factors for altered thermoregulation are modifiable, it is important to identify those that can be addressed through health promotion interventions. Information about medications and pathologic disorders is obtained during the overall assessment, and it is important to identify any conditions that predispose the

Box 25-3 Guidelines for Assessing Thermoregulation

Principles of Temperature Assessment

- Document the person's baseline body temperature and its diurnal and seasonal variations.
- Assume that even a small elevation above the baseline temperature is a clue to the presence of a pathologic process.
- Document actual temperature and deviations from the baseline, rather than using such terminology as "afebrile."
- Carefully follow all the standard procedures for accurate temperature measurement. Use a thermometer that registers temperatures lower than 35°C.
- Consider the influence of temperature-altering medications when evaluating a temperature reading (e.g., medications that mask a fever).
- Do not assume that an infection will necessarily be accompanied by an elevated temperature.
- Remember that, in the presence of an infection, a decline in function or change in mental status may be an earlier and more accurate indicator of illness than an alteration in temperature.
- Do not assume that an older adult will initiate compensatory behaviours or complain of discomfort when exposed to adverse environmental temperatures.

Questions to Assess Risk Factors for Hypothermia or Heat-Related Illness

- Do you have any particular health problems that occur in hot or cold weather?
- Are you able to keep your house or room at a comfortable temperature in both summer and winter months?
- What do you do to cope with hot temperatures in the summer?
- Do you have any difficulty paying your utility bills?
- What forms of protection against the cold do you use in the winter months (e.g., electric blanket, supplemental sources of heat)?
- Have you ever received medical care for exposure to heat or cold?
- Have you ever fallen and not been able to get up or get help?

Observations to Assess Risk Factors for Hypothermia or Heat-Related Illness

- Does the older person live in a house where the temperature is kept below 21.1°C during the winter?
- Does the person drink alcohol or take temperature-altering medications (see Box 25-2)?
- Does the person live alone? If so, what is the frequency of outside contacts?
- Does the person have any pathologic conditions that predispose him or her to hypothermia (e.g., endocrine, neurologic or cardiovascular disorders)?
- Is the person's fluid and nutritional intake adequate?
- Does the person have postural hypotension? (See Chapter 20, Table 20-2 and Boxes 20-1 and 20-2 for assessment criteria relating to postural hypotension.)
- Is the person immobilized or sedentary? Is the person's judgment impaired because of dementia, depression or other psychosocial disorders?
- Does the person live in a poorly ventilated dwelling without air-conditioning?
- Are atmospheric conditions very hot, humid or polluted?
- Does the person engage in active exercise during hot weather?
- Does the person have any chronic illness that predisposes him or her to heat-related illness?
- Is the person at risk for hyponatremia or hypokalemia because of medications or chronic illnesses?

person to hypothermia or heat-related illness. In addition to assessing for risks for hypothermia or heat-related illnesses, recognize that a low baseline body temperature is a risk for undetected fever. It is important to document the person's baseline temperature and note this as a risk factor for both hypothermia and undetected febrile conditions if temperature is below 36.7°C.

Most nurses do not have the opportunity to observe and assess the older adult's home environment, but they can ask pertinent questions and listen for clues to detect environmental risk factors. For example, older adults who live alone and express concern about keeping the house warm in winter should be considered to be at risk for hypothermia. Likewise, older adults who live in poor housing conditions, or with family members who keep the house at low temperatures during winter months, should be considered to be at risk for hypothermia. Older adults who live in poorly ventilated houses without air-conditioning should be considered to be at risk for heat-related illness during heat waves. Interview questions aimed at identifying risk factors for altered thermoregulation are listed in Box 25-3.

Wellness Opportunity

From a holistic perspective, nurses consider that fears about paying utility bills in the winter or about personal safety when windows are open can increase the risk for hypothermia or heat-related conditions.

Assessing for Hypothermia

Hypothermia is best detected by measuring core body temperature with a thermometer that registers below 35°C. Cool skin in unexposed areas, such as the abdomen and buttocks, is a distinguishing characteristic of hypothermia. The environmental temperature may be only moderately cool and the older person will not necessarily shiver or complain of feeling cold. Even in environmental temperatures of 20°C or 20.6°C, an older person may become hypothermic, especially if other risk factors such as immobility or hypothermia-inducing medications are present. Early signs of hypothermia are subtle, and the most objective assessment tool is a comparison of the person's body temperature with their usual baseline temperature. As untreated hypothermia progresses, additional signs may include lethargy, slurred speech, mental changes, impaired gait, puffiness of the face, slowed or irregular pulse, low blood pressure, slowed tendon reflexes and slow, shallow respirations. Severe stages of hypothermia are characterized by muscular rigidity, diminished urinary function and a progression of all other manifestations to the point of stupor and coma. The skin will feel very cool, and, contrary to what might be expected, the colour of the skin will be pink. Also contrary to what might be expected, a hypothermic person may not shiver, particularly if the body temperature is below 32.2°C.

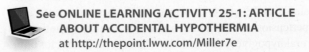

See ONLINE LEARNING ACTIVITY 25-1: ARTICLE ABOUT ACCIDENTAL HYPOTHERMIA at http://thepoint.lww.com/Miller7e

Assessing for Heat-Related Illness

Manifestations of heat-related illnesses range from mild headache to life-threatening respiratory and cardiovascular disturbances. In the early stages of heat-related illness, the person will feel weak and lethargic and may complain of headache, nausea and loss of appetite. The skin will be warm and dry, and the sweating response may be absent, especially if the person's fluid intake is low. As the heat-related condition progresses, these manifestations will be exacerbated, and the following signs will become evident: dizziness, dyspnea, tachycardia, vomiting, diarrhea, muscle cramps, chest pain, mental impairment and a wide pulse pressure.

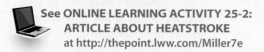

See ONLINE LEARNING ACTIVITY 25-2:
ARTICLE ABOUT HEATSTROKE
at http://thepoint.lww.com/Miller7e

Assessing the Older Adult's Febrile Response to Illness

Because the manifestations of delayed or diminished febrile response to infections are likely to be very subtle, nurses assess for any temperature changes from the person's baseline as well as for additional signs of illness, such as a decline in function or change in mental status. Nurses should also examine assumptions about thermoregulation that may apply to younger adults but not to older adults. For example, the expectation that pneumonia is accompanied by an elevated temperature is not necessarily applicable to older adults, as discussed in Chapter 21. Thus, nurses in long-term care facilities need to be particularly vigilant about subtle temperature changes and other manifestations of fever. A more reliable indicator of elevated temperature in older adults would be an increase of 1°C above the person's baseline. See Box 25-3 for a summary of some of these considerations.

Wellness Opportunity

A holistic assessment for febrile conditions requires that nurses identify subtle manifestations, such as behaviour changes and slight elevations above the person's baseline temperature, even if the temperature is within the so-called normal range.

NURSING DIAGNOSIS

Pertinent nursing diagnoses in the class of Thermoregulation are Hypothermia (i.e., body temperature below normal range), Hyperthermia (i.e., body temperature elevated above normal range) and Ineffective Thermoregulation (i.e., temperature fluctuation between hypothermia and hyperthermia). In addition, the nursing diagnosis of Risk for Imbalanced Body Temperature is applicable when the person has risk factors for hypothermia or heat-related illness. For example, an 83-year-old woman with diabetes, dementia and hypertension who is taking a diuretic, an antipsychotic and an oral hypoglycemic would have many risk factors for both

hypothermia and heat-related illness. Related factors that are common in older adults include immobility, advanced age, medication effects, adverse environmental conditions, and acute and chronic illnesses. For older adults living alone, social isolation may be a related factor that increases the risk for experiencing more serious consequences if hypothermia or heat-related illness occurs.

Wellness Opportunity

Nurses can use the nursing diagnosis of Readiness for Enhanced Knowledge: Prevention of Hypothermia (or Hyperthermia) for older adults and their caregivers who are interested in learning to address risks for these conditions.

PLANNING FOR WELLNESS OUTCOMES

When caring for older adults with risks for hypothermia or heat-related illness, nurses identify wellness outcomes as an essential component of the nursing process. Nurses can use the following Nursing Outcomes Classification (NOC) terminologies in their care plans addressing risks for altered thermoregulation: Health Promoting Behaviour, Hydration, Knowledge: Health Behaviour, Knowledge: Personal Safety, Risk Detection, Risk Control, Safe Home Environment, Thermoregulation, and Vital Signs: Body Temperature.

Outcomes vary depending on the setting. In acute care settings, nurses are more likely to focus on outcomes that pertain to the patient's immediate physical condition (e.g., Hydration, Thermoregulation, and Vital Signs: Body Temperature). A focus of nursing care in long-term care settings is early detection of infections. In home and other community settings, nurses might be able to provide group or individual health education for older adults who are at risk for development of hypothermia or heat-related illness, especially during times of extreme weather conditions. In these situations, nurses focus more on teaching about self-care and environmental modifications to prevent hypothermia or heat-related illness.

Wellness Opportunity

Nurses promote wellness when their care plans include health-promoting behaviours to prevent hypothermia and heat-related illness.

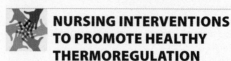

NURSING INTERVENTIONS TO PROMOTE HEALTHY THERMOREGULATION

Health promotion interventions to address altered thermoregulation are directed toward primary prevention of hypothermia and heat-related illness. Health promotion interventions also address early detection of altered thermoregulation and prompt initiation of interventions to restore thermal balance and to prevent detrimental effects. Comfort interventions are initiated to promote well-being in older adults. Nurses can use the following Nursing Interventions Classification (NIC) terminologies to document interventions: Temperature Regulation, Hypothermia Treatment, Hyperthermia Treatment, Environmental Management, Health Education, Risk Identification, Surveillance, and Teaching: Individual (or Group).

Addressing Risk Factors

Maintenance of an environmental temperature of around 23.9°C is the single most important intervention to prevent hypothermia or heat-related illness. In addition, relative humidity can be altered to minimize the discomfort and detrimental effects associated with extremely warm or cool environments. With comfortable indoor temperatures, the ideal humidity is between 40% and 50%, although an acceptable range is between 20% and 70%. Older adults can be encouraged to humidify the air in their homes during the dry winter months by using humidifiers, either alone or with their heating systems. Simpler measures, such as keeping pans of water on heating vents or using a vaporizer near the bed at night, may be appropriate if a humidifier is unavailable.

An intervention for older adults at risk for hypothermia or heat-related illnesses is to teach about government- and community-sponsored programs that provide assistance for addressing needs related to weather-related risks. For example, the Government of Canada supports Canada Mortgage and Housing (CMHC) programs that help older adults to adapt their home to meet their changing needs through *home adaptations*, *modification strategies*, and *financial assistance* programs.

Other government-sponsored programs provide financial assistance, such as low-interest loans and the Emergency Repair Program (for rural seniors) for home winterization and modernization measures to protect against adverse weather conditions. There are also programs specific to meet the needs of those living in harsher weather parts of Canada, for example, the *Home Adaptations for Seniors' Independence* for older adults living in the Yukon. Older people and their family caregivers can be encouraged to take advantage of these programs.

Wellness Opportunity

Nurses promote wellness for socially isolated older adults by identifying ways of developing a system of social contact, such as a friendly phone call program, that ensures daily contact during periods of adversely hot or cold weather.

Promoting Healthy Thermoregulation

In cool environmental temperatures, interventions to prevent hypothermia include using adequate clothing and covering, especially for the hands, feet and head because these areas of the body have the heaviest concentration of nerve endings that are sensitive to heat loss. Nurses can encourage older adults to wear caps, thermal socks and several layers of warm clothing when appropriate. Electric blankets used during the night are a relatively inexpensive form of protection in cool environments, but proper safety precautions must be taken. Space heaters often are used to provide intense heat in a small area, but they can create serious fire and safety hazards. In addition to environmental considerations, special attention must be directed toward ensuring adequate nutrition, including fluid intake, and treating any pathologic conditions.

During heat waves, heat-related illness can affect older adults living in their own homes or in long-term care settings that are not air-conditioned. In long-term care facilities without air-conditioning, nurses need to ensure that all residents have adequate fluid intakes. Nurses must also observe for early signs of heat-related illness, especially in residents who are immobile or who have medical problems, such as endocrine or circulatory disorders, that predispose them to heat-related illness. If only parts of the facility are air-conditioned, nurses can encourage residents to spend time in those areas and can provide assistance for residents who have mobility limitations.

Nurses can teach older adults living in community settings about measures to cool the environment, such as those summarized in Box 25-4. Older adults may be reluctant to use fans or air-conditioners because of a desire to save money on utility bills; however, if they understand the health risks associated with heat-related illness, they may use these appliances judiciously. If the home setting cannot be cooled adequately during heat waves, encourage older adults to

---

 Box 25-4 Health Promotion Teaching About Hypothermia and Heat-Related Illness

Environmental and Personal Protection Considerations for Preventing Hypothermia

- Maintain a constant room temperature as close to 23.9°C as possible, with a minimum temperature of 21.1°C.
- Use a reliable, clearly marked thermometer to measure room temperature.
- Wear close-knit, but not tight, undergarments to prevent heat loss; wear several layers of clothing.
- Wear a hat and gloves when outdoors; wear a nightcap and socks for sleeping.
- Wear extra clothing in the early morning when your body metabolism is at its lowest point.
- Use flannel bed sheets or sheet blankets.
- Use an electric blanket set on a low temperature.
- Take advantage of programs that offer assistance with utility bills and home weatherization.

(continued)

Box 25-4 *(continued)*

Environmental and Personal Protection Action to Prevent Heat-Related Illnesses

- Maintain room temperatures below 29.4°C.
- If your residence is not air-conditioned, use fans to circulate the air and cool the environment.
- During hot weather, spend time in public air-conditioned settings, such as libraries or shopping malls.
- Drink extra noncaffeinated, nonalcoholic liquids, even if you don't feel thirsty.
- Wear loose-fitting, lightweight, light-coloured, cotton clothing.
- Wear a hat or use an umbrella to protect yourself against sun and heat when you are outside.
- Avoid outdoor activities during the hottest time of the day (i.e., between 10:00 AM and 2:00 PM); perform them during the cooler hours of the morning or evening.
- Place an ice pack or cold, wet towels on your body, especially on the head, the groin area and armpits. Take cool (about 75°F [23.9°C]) baths or showers several times daily during heat waves, but do not use soap every time.

Health Promotion Actions for Maintaining Optimal Body Temperature

- Maintain adequate fluid intake by drinking 8 to 10 glasses of noncaffeinated, nonalcoholic liquid daily.
- Do not rely on your thirst sensation as an indicator of the need for fluid.
- Eat small, frequent meals rather than heavy meals.
- Avoid drinking caffeinated beverages, such as cola and coffee.
- Avoid drinking alcohol.
- In cold weather, engage in moderate physical exercise and indoor activities to increase circulation and heat production.

Nutritional Considerations

- Maintain good nutrition, especially zinc, selenium, and vitamins A, C and E.

Preventive Measures and Additional Approaches

- Know your normal temperature in the morning and in the evening.
- Know the difference in your temperature in the winter and the summer.
- Obtain pneumonia and influenza immunizations (as discussed in Chapter 21).
- Obtain tetanus and diphtheria vaccinations every 10 years.
- Be aware that melatonin and other bioactive substances (see Box 25-2) might alter thermoregulation; use these substances only under the advice of a health care professional.

spend time in air-conditioned public places. Additional self-care actions to prevent heat-related illness during heat waves include the provision of adequate fluids and the avoidance of heavy meals and strenuous exercise. Box 25-4, which summarizes interventions for the prevention of heat-related illness, can be used as a patient education tool for older adults.

Unfolding Case Study

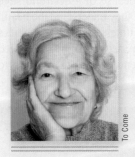

Part 1: Mrs. T. at 76 Years of Age (continued)

Recall that Mrs. T. is 76 years old and a participant at the senior centre where you will be presenting a health education program.

THINKING POINTS

- How would you incorporate assessment information into your health education program?
- How would you use information from Box 25-4 to teach about preventing heat-related illnesses?
- What specific suggestions would you make about early detection of heat-related illnesses to the participants at this rural senior centre?
- How would you find health education materials to use for your program?

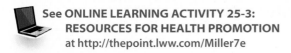

See ONLINE LEARNING ACTIVITY 25-3:
RESOURCES FOR HEALTH PROMOTION
at http://thepoint.lww.com/Miller7e

Promoting Caregiver Wellness

Caregivers of older adults who have risks for hypothermia or heat-related illness may benefit from the health promotion resources that are listed in the Online Learning Activity 25-3. For example, caregivers may be interested in finding out about programs for assistance with utility bills or home modifications for improved energy efficiency and comfort. Use the information in Box 25-4 to teach about strategies for preventing hypothermia and heat-related illnesses. In addition, it is important to encourage caregivers to establish a plan for at least daily communication with socially isolated older adults, especially during heat waves or cold spells.

EVALUATING EFFECTIVENESS OF NURSING INTERVENTIONS

Nurses evaluate care of older adults diagnosed with risk for hypothermia/heat-related illness or imbalanced body temperature according to the extent to which the risks are eliminated. It is not always possible to know whether risk factors were eliminated, but nurses can evaluate the effectiveness of their teaching by asking for feedback from older adults and their caregivers. Nurses can also suggest referrals for resources and ask the older adult about his or her intent to follow through. For example, if housing and financial factors increase the risk of hypothermia and heat-related illnesses, nurses can refer the older adult to a program such as those provided by Canada Mortgage and Housing and document the person's response to this information. When nurses teach about preventing hypothermia and heat-related illnesses, effectiveness is evaluated on the basis of the person's ability to describe ways of decreasing the risk factors for hypothermia or heat-related illnesses.

Unfolding Case Study

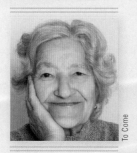

Part 2: Mrs. T. at 87 Years of Age

Mrs. T. is now 87 years old and continues to live alone in her own home in a rural area of central Saskatchewan. She has a history of hypertension and diabetic retinopathy, and was recently hospitalized for uncontrolled diabetes. Upon discharge from the hospital in November, she was referred to Home Care for teaching about insulin administration and monitoring of her diabetic care.

NURSING ASSESSMENT

During your initial visit, you observe that Mrs. T.'s house is poorly maintained and has no insulation or other weatherization. Mrs. T. tells you that she has lived in this house for 60 years and that, in recent years, she has had difficulty keeping up with maintenance because of her poor eyesight and limited income. She has few social contacts, but her daughter visits her every other week and a neighbour visits weekly and brings her groceries. About once a month, friends pick her up and take her to church. Your assessment reveals that although Mrs. T. has difficulty preparing meals because of her poor eyesight, she is independent in all other activities of daily living.

During your initial visit, you identify several risk factors for hypothermia, so during subsequent visits you follow up with further assessment. You learn that Mrs. T. was taken to the emergency department in January, 2 years ago, to be treated for hypothermia. She recalls that her daughter had come for her usual visit and had found her in a very weak and confused state. Her description of the situation is that "they just warmed me up at the hospital and sent me home again. I could have done that myself if my daughter would have just let me be." It is apparent that she did not consider her condition to be of particular concern. In the winter, she keeps her utility bills low by using a small, portable heater in the living room during the day and moving it into the bedroom at night. Mrs. T. keeps her thermostat at 18.3°C during the day and 15.6°C at night. A neighbour told her that the county office on aging had a program to assist with utility bills, but she is embarrassed to ask her daughter to drive her to the office to apply for this "welfare help."

NURSING DIAGNOSIS

In addition to addressing the nursing diagnoses related to Mrs. T.'s diabetes, you identify a nursing diagnosis of Hypothermia. Related factors include advanced age, diabetes, social isolation, poor housing conditions, low environmental temperatures and a history of hypothermia.

(continued)

Unfolding Case Study (continued)

NURSING CARE PLAN FOR Mrs. T.

Expected Outcome	Nursing Interventions	Nursing Evaluation
Mrs. T.'s knowledge about risk factors for hypothermia will be increased.	• Discuss risk factors for hypothermia, with emphasis on Mrs. T.'s diabetes, social isolation, environmental conditions and history of hypothermia.	• Mrs. T. will be able to state at least four factors that place her at risk for hypothermia.
Mrs. T.'s knowledge about ways of preventing hypothermia will be increased.	• Use Box 25-3 to discuss interventions to prevent hypothermia and to explore ways of applying these interventions to Mrs. T.'s situation.	• Mrs. T. will implement strategies aimed at reducing her risk for hypothermia.
The risk factor of low temperatures in Mrs. T.'s house will be eliminated.	• Inform Mrs. T. about CMHC programs and explain that she may qualify for assistance with utility bills as well as help with weatherization. • Emphasize that CMHC is an important housing agency which may help to prevent hypothermia in older adults. • Ask Mrs. T.'s permission to contact CMHC.	• Mrs. T. will accept assistance from CMHC. • Mrs. T. will have her house weatherized. • Mrs. T. will keep her thermostat at 21.1°C during the winter.
The risk factor of social isolation will be eliminated.	• Suggest home-delivered meals to Mrs. T. as a means of providing prepared meals and daily contact. • Emphasize that one of the purposes of such programs is to ensure that socially isolated older adults have daily contact with someone who can monitor their well-being. • Ask Mrs. T. for permission to contact her daughter to suggest that she call her mother daily during cold spells to make sure she is okay.	• Mrs. T. will accept home-delivered meals. • Mrs. T.'s daughter will phone daily during cold spells.

THINKING POINTS

- How would you address Mrs. T.'s perception that hypothermia does not have serious health-related implications?

- What additional interventions might you consider to address Mrs. T.'s risk for hypothermia?

QSEN APPLICATION

QSEN Competency	Knowledge/Skill/Attitude	Application to Mrs. T. When She Is 87 Years Old
Patient-centred care	(K) Describe strategies to empower patients in all aspects of the health care process.	Identify misinformation and lack of information that interfere with the use of available resources.
	(K) Examine common barriers to active involvement in patients.	Recognize that Mrs. T values her independence, and emphasize that prevention of hypothermia is an important way to maintain health and autonomy.
	(S) Elicit patient values, preferences and expressed needs.	
	(A) Value seeing health care situations "through patients' eyes."	
Teamwork and collaboration	(K) Recognize contributions of other individuals and groups in helping patient achieve health goals.	Provide information about community resources and obtain permission to facilitate a referral for CMHC assistance.
	(S) Integrate the contributions of others who play a role in helping patient achieve health goals.	Obtain permission to involve Mrs. T's daughter in the care plan.

Chapter Highlights

Age-Related Changes That Affect Thermoregulation

- Inefficient vasoconstriction
- Decreased cardiac output
- Diminished subcutaneous tissue and muscle mass
- Decreased peripheral circulation
- Delayed and diminished shivering
- Diminished ability to acclimatize to heat

Risks Factors That Affect Thermoregulation (Box 25-2)

- Environmental factors (e.g., temperatures, humidity)
- Socioeconomic and housing factors (e.g., poor ventilation, inadequate heat, lack of air-conditioning)
- Insufficient knowledge about altered thermoregulation
- Medications and alcohol
- Chronic and acute conditions (e.g., infections; cardiovascular, endocrine and neurologic conditions)
- Inactivity
- Social isolation

Functional Consequences Affecting Thermoregulation

- Compromised ability to respond to hot or cold environments
- Increased susceptibility to hypothermia and heat-related illness
- Lower baseline temperature
- Diminished febrile response to infections
- Dulled perception of environmental temperatures

Nursing Assessment of Thermoregulation (Box 25-3)

- Establish baseline temperature, including diurnal variations
- Identify risks for hypothermia or heat-related illness
- Observe for additional manifestations of infections

Nursing Diagnosis

- Hypothermia
- Hyperthermia
- Ineffective Thermoregulation
- Risk for Imbalanced Body Temperature
- Readiness for Enhanced Knowledge: Prevention of Hypothermia (or Hyperthermia)

Planning for Wellness Outcomes

- Health Promoting Behaviour
- Knowledge: Personal Safety
- Risk Detection
- Risk Control
- Safe Home Environment
- Thermoregulation

Nursing Interventions to Promote Healthy Thermoregulation (Box 25-4)

- Maintaining healthy environmental conditions
- Teaching about measures to protect from hypothermia
- Teaching about measures to prevent heat-related illness
- Promoting caregiver wellness

Evaluating Effectiveness of Nursing Interventions

- Evidence that risk factors are eliminated
- Feedback about improved knowledge regarding prevention of hypothermia and heat-related illness
- Feedback about referrals for community resources

Critical Thinking Exercises

1. Describe four major functional consequences that an older adult is likely to experience with regard to thermoregulation. How would you explain these changes to an older adult?
2. Explain how each of the following factors might affect an older person's thermoregulation: medications, pathologic conditions, environmental conditions, socioeconomic factors and lack of knowledge.
3. What would you include in an assessment of thermoregulation in an older adult?
4. What would you teach older adults about hypothermia and its prevention?
5. What would you teach older adults about heat-related illnesses and their prevention?
6. Find appropriate health education materials on the Internet to use in teaching older adults about hypothermia and heat-related illnesses.

 For more information about the topics discussed in this chapter, be sure to check out the interactive Online Learning Activities and other helpful resources at http://thepoint.lww.com/Miller7e

REFERENCES

Alberini, A., Gans, W., & Alhassan, M. (2011). Individual and public-program adaptation: Coping with heat waves in five cities in Canada. *International Journal of Environmental Research and Public Health, 8*, 4679–4701.

Cheng, C. S., & Campbell, M. (2005). *Differential and combined impacts of winter and summer weather and air pollution due to global warming on human mortality in south-central Canada* (Technical Report Health Policy Research Program, Health Canada). Retrieved from http://www.toronto.ca/health/hphe/pdf/weather_air_pollution_impacts.pdf

Chester, J. G., & Rudolph, J. L. (2011). Vital signs in older patients: Age-related changes. *Journal of the American Medical Directors Association, 12*(5), 337–343.

Davis, R. A. (2012). The big chill: Accidental hypothermia. *American Journal of Nursing, 112*(1), 38–46.

Hansen, A., Bi, P., Nitschke, M., et al. (2011). Perceptions of heat-susceptibility in older persons: Barriers to adaptation. *International Journal of Environmental Research and Public Health, 8*(12), 4714–4728.

Kreuzer, P., Landgrebe, M., Wittmann, M., et al. (2012). Hypothermia associated with antipsychotic drug use: A clinical case series and review of current literature. *Journal of Clinical Pharmacology, 52*(7), 1090–1097.

Lu, S. H., Leasure, A. R., & Dai, Y. T. (2010). A systematic review of body temperature variations in older people. *Journal of Clinical Nursing, 19*(1–2), 4–16.

Romero-Ortuno, R., Tempany, M., Dennis, L., et al. (2013). Deprivation in cold weather increases the risk of hospital admission with hypothermia in older people. *Irish Journal of Medical Sciences, 182*(3), 513–518.

Sommet, A., Durrieu, B., Lapeyre-Mestre, M., et al. (2012). A comparative study of adverse drug reactions during two heat waves that occurred in France in 2003 and 2006. *Pharmacoepidemiologic and Drug Safety, 21*(3), 285–288.

Waalen, J., & Buxbaum, J. N. (2011). Is older colder or colder older? The association of age with body temperature in 18,630 individuals. *Journal of Gerontology: Biological Sciences, 66A*(5), 487–492.

Wang, X. Y., Barnett, A. G., Yu, W., et al. (2012). The impact of heatwaves on mortality and emergency hospital admissions from non-external causes in Brisbane, Australia. *Occupational and Environmental Medicine, 69*(3), 163–169.

Yamashita, S., Uchida, Y., Kojima, S., et al. (2012). Heatstroke in patients with Parkinson's disease. *Neurological Sciences, 33*(3), 685–687.

chapter 26

Sexual Function

LEARNING OBJECTIVES

After reading this chapter, you will be able to:

1. Describe age-related changes that affect sexual function in older adults.

2. Discuss risk factors that influence older adults' interest in, opportunities for and performance of sexual activities.

3. Discuss the functional consequences affecting sexual wellness in older adults.

4. Assess your own attitudes about sexual function in older adults.

5. Apply assessment guidelines in clinical settings when it is appropriate to address sexual wellness.

6. Teach older adults about interventions to promote sexual wellness.

KEY POINTS

andropause	menopausal hormonal therapy (MHT)
erectile dysfunction	
female sexual dysfunction	menopause
	perimenopause
hot flashes	postmenopause
human immunodeficiency virus (HIV)	prostatic hyperplasia
	urethritis
	vaginitis

Because sexual function in older adults encompasses many physiologic and psychosocial aspects of sexuality and intimate relationships, this chapter's perspective is broad. Although sexual function is not a dominant focus of gerontological nursing care in most situations, it is a very important component of quality of life for older adults. Thus, in long-term care settings and other situations in which quality of life is a focus of nursing care, an essential nursing responsibility is assessing sexual function and implementing interventions to promote sexual wellness.

 AGE-RELATED CHANGES THAT AFFECT SEXUAL FUNCTION

Loss of reproductive ability at the onset of menopause in women is an age-related change in sexual function that is clearly delineated. Additional and more subtle age-related changes in sexual function include diminished reproductive abilities in older men and alterations in both male and female responses to sexual stimulation. Older adults generally can compensate for any age-related changes in their response to sexual stimulation; however, when risk factors are present, they may experience additional changes in sexual function. This section focuses on age-related changes affecting physiologic aspects of sexual function. The wide range of commonly occurring risk factors are discussed in the Risk Factors and Pathologic Conditions sections.

Changes Affecting Older Women

Hormonally regulated cycles, called *menses*, begin during adolescence and control female reproductive abilities. Beginning around the fifth decade of life, the frequency of ovulation diminishes and menstrual cycles become shorter and irregular. **Menopause** (i.e., the cessation of menses), which typically occurs around the age of 49 to 51 years, is a clear indicator that reproduction is no longer possible. **Perimenopause** refers to the several years before menopause when women begin experiencing manifestations of approaching menopause (e.g., changes in menstrual cycles, vasomotor symptoms, vaginal dryness). **Postmenopause** begins 12 months after a woman's last menstrual cycle.

Promoting Sexual Wellness in Older Adults

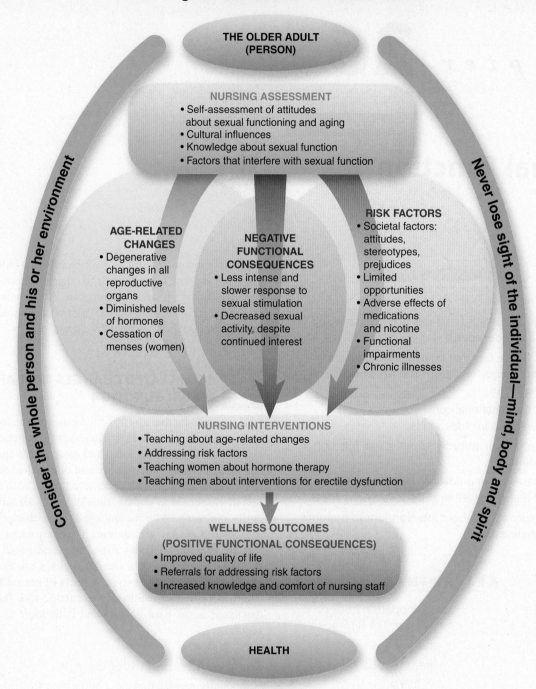

THE OLDER ADULT (PERSON)

NURSING ASSESSMENT
- Self-assessment of attitudes about sexual functioning and aging
- Cultural influences
- Knowledge about sexual function
- Factors that interfere with sexual function

AGE-RELATED CHANGES
- Degenerative changes in all reproductive organs
- Diminished levels of hormones
- Cessation of menses (women)

NEGATIVE FUNCTIONAL CONSEQUENCES
- Less intense and slower response to sexual stimulation
- Decreased sexual activity, despite continued interest

RISK FACTORS
- Societal factors: attitudes, stereotypes, prejudices
- Limited opportunities
- Adverse effects of medications and nicotine
- Functional impairments
- Chronic illnesses

NURSING INTERVENTIONS
- Teaching about age-related changes
- Addressing risk factors
- Teaching women about hormone therapy
- Teaching men about interventions for erectile dysfunction

WELLNESS OUTCOMES (POSITIVE FUNCTIONAL CONSEQUENCES)
- Improved quality of life
- Referrals for addressing risk factors
- Increased knowledge and comfort of nursing staff

HEALTH

Consider the whole person and his or her environment

Never lose sight of the individual—mind, body and spirit

In addition to affecting reproductive ability, menopause influences other aspects of sexual function, predominantly because of the accompanying decline in endogenous estrogen levels. Production of estradiol by the ovaries is the primary source of estrogen before menopause, but after menopause, the primary source is estrone, which is converted from androstenedione in skin and fat tissue. Although endogenous estrogen levels decline in all postmenopausal women, the extent and manifestations are influenced by factors such as the following: length of time since onset of menopause, production of hormones by the adrenal cortex, clearance rates of androgens and estrogens, and body weight, with higher body fat being positively correlated with higher levels of estrogen.

About 75% to 80% of all menopausal women experience hot flashes (also called *hot flushes*) with 20% requesting treatment for severe symptoms (Elkins et al., 2013; Okeke et al., 2013). **Hot flashes** are a vasomotor symptom characterized by the sudden onset of heat, perspiration and flushing that spreads from the head to trunk. Symptoms last from 1 to 5 minutes, and may be accompanied by chills, nausea, anxiety, palpitations and clamminess. Although severity of symptoms varies significantly, hot flashes can cause embarrassment, sleep disruptions, significant discomfort and interruptions in activities, including sexual activities. Hot flashes gradually subside in most women after 1 to 7 years, but as many as 40% experience them for more than 7 years (Whiteley et al., 2013).

Diminished estrogen levels can directly affect sexual function for older women in several ways. One of the more obvious effects is that breasts become more pendulous and have more fat and less mammary tissue. Vaginal dryness from diminished secretions is another noticeable effect that can affect sexual pleasure unless compensatory interventions, such as a lubricant, are used. Less obvious changes include loss of fullness of the labia, diminished quantity of pubic hair and atrophy of sexual organs.

In addition to these effects on sexual function and quality of life, estrogen deficiency affects many nonreproductive tissues, including brain, bone, heart, liver and muscle, and is associated with increased risk for osteoporosis, cardiovascular disease, Alzheimer disease and metabolic dysfunction (Cui et al., 2013; Mauvais-Jarvis et al., 2013; Nedergaard et al., 2013). Menopausal hormonal changes have been identified as a risk factor for depression, but some studies suggest that the relationship is complex and may be more strongly associated with psychosocial factors, such as coping skills and social support (Gibbs et al., 2012; Lin et al., 2013; Pimenta et al., 2012).

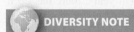
DIVERSITY NOTE

Women in China, Korea and Japan have a lower prevalence of menopausal symptoms, and this may be associated with higher dietary intake of soy products (Im et al., 2012).

Changes Affecting Older Men

Male reproductive function depends on the secretion of testosterone and other hormones, the production and release of sperm, and the motility of sperm through the urethra. All male reproductive organs undergo age-related degenerative changes, and production of viable sperm gradually diminishes; however, some men never lose their reproductive abilities.

The term **andropause** (or *male menopause*) has been used to describe the age-related decline in testosterone in men that begins around the age of 30 years and is analogous to the age-related decline in estrogen in women. Cross-sectional and longitudinal data vary widely, with some studies indicating that up to 20% of men older than 60 years and 50% of those older than 80 have serum testosterone levels below the lower limits of young adults (Horstman et al., 2012; Surampudi et al., 2012). Researchers emphasize that much of the variation is associated with comorbid conditions, such as metabolic syndrome, type 2 diabetes and cardiovascular disease (Pantalone & Faiman, 2012). In recent years, the term

androgen deficiency in the older male (also called *late-onset hypogonadism, testosterone deficiency syndrome*) has been used to describe a condition in which the serum testosterone level is abnormally low and is associated with symptoms such as low libido, **erectile dysfunction**, decreased vitality and depressed mood (McGill et al., 2012). Recent studies suggest that low serum testosterone levels are associated not only with diminished sexual function but also with increased risk for pathologic conditions, such as anemia, diabetes and osteoporosis (Spitzer et al., 2013).

 RISK FACTORS THAT AFFECT SEXUAL FUNCTION

Many types of risk factors can affect sexual function and expressions of sexuality, ranging from individual, physical, functional and psychosocial factors to broader societal and cultural influences. Although many of these risks affect people at any age, older adults are likely to experience several or more risks and some risks are unique to older adults. This section provides an overview of risk factors that occur most commonly in older adults.

Myths and Attitudes in Society

Because personal attitudes about sexuality are shaped by societal influences, it is important to consider the societal context of attitudes about sexuality, particularly with regard to women and older adults. Strict Victorian standards of morality in Europe and North America strongly influenced many generations, beginning in the 1800s and including those who are older adults today. According to Victorian standards, masturbation, homosexual activity, public displays of affection, and sex with anyone except a marital partner were totally taboo. Women's sexuality was a particular target of negative attitudes, and medical practitioners removed a woman's sexual organs as a usual treatment.

Victorian perspectives were dominant until 1953 when Kinsey and colleagues published their study of *Sexual Behaviors in the Human Female*. This "Kinsey report" brought public attention to previously taboo topics, such as orgasm, masturbation, premarital sex and marital infidelity, and was a major turning point in perspectives on female sexuality. Although attitudes about sexuality have changed significantly, older adults may lack accurate information about sexuality and may resist attempts to discuss topics that they consider taboo. This is particularly true for women born in 1925 or before (Farrell & Belza, 2011).

Another factor that influences perspectives on sexuality and aging is the strong association in Western societies between sexual attractiveness and physical attributes in very gender-specific and stereotypical ways. For example, male sexuality is associated with the image of a tanned, muscular and youthful man and female sexuality is associated with the image of a thin, but adequately endowed, young woman. Because these images contrast sharply with typical portrayals of older adults as physically unattractive, they foster a stereotype of "sexless seniors."

DIVERSITY NOTE

Ethnicity may influence sexual desire. Euro-Canadian women report greater sexual desire and less sexual guilt than Chinese Canadian women (Woo et al., 2012).

These societal influences promote the false perception that older adults have lost the interest in or capacity for sexual activity. This can become a self-fulfilling prophecy if older adults believe this stereotype. Even if older adults do not believe these stereotypes, they may be embarrassed to acknowledge their sexual desires and activities for fear of being considered abnormal.

Wellness Opportunity

Nurses need to avoid reinforcing, or even buying into, the pervasive societal attitudes about "sexless seniors."

In addition to being affected by myths and stereotypes, older people who are gay, lesbian, bisexual and transgender (LBGT) usually have long-term experiences of prejudice and misinformation related to their sexual orientation and identity. Even though attitudes have changed in recent years, these diverse groups of sexual minorities have experienced decades of stigma and discrimination and they are more likely than younger generations to be "closeted" and secretive about their sexual orientation. In addition, the disproportionately high death rate among gay men in Canada between the ages of 25 and 44 when HIV/AIDS was at its peak (1987–1996) had a strong influence on social networks and personal lives of those who are now reaching older adulthood (Schanzer, 2003). A review of studies identified many health disparities among LGBT older adults; however, studies also identified many areas of strength and resiliency among these groups (Van Wagenen et al., 2013).

Wellness Opportunity

Nurses can holistically address sexual wellness by being nonjudgmental about choices of close personal relationships.

Social Circumstances

Availability of a satisfactory partner is a major factor that influences opportunities for sexual activities during older adulthood, and this is especially true for older heterosexual women (Wood et al., 2012). Although higher levels of sexual interest and activity are reported by men at any age compared with women at a similar age, this gender difference widens during older adulthood. This is partly attributable to fact that women outnumber men among persons aged 65 to 79, wherein there were estimated to be 90 males per 100 females in late 2012, and in those aged 80 and above, there were an estimated 61 males per 100 females (Statistics Canada, 2013).

Similarly, the proportion of married women also decreases with increasing age, as illustrated in Figures 26-1 and 26-2. Another contributing factor for women is the common occurrence of poor health in their male partners (Syme et al., 2013).

Privacy is generally considered a requisite for sexual activity, and adults who live in their own homes are usually able to arrange for this. However, older adults who live in institutions, group settings, or family homes may find it difficult or impossible to arrange for privacy, especially if their sexual needs are ignored or considered abnormal or even morally deviant. Even if some privacy is possible in institutional settings, additional environmental constraints include the inability to lock doors and ensure total privacy and the unavailability of anything larger than a single bed.

Wellness Opportunity

Nurses in long-term care settings need to create opportunities for privacy if a resident desires this.

Adverse Effects of Medication, Alcohol and Nicotine

Almost three decades ago, a study published in the *Journal of the American Medical Association* (Slag et al., 1983) identified adverse effects of medication as the single largest cause of erectile dysfunction in men. Slag and colleagues found that 34% of 1,180 male patients in a medical clinic were impotent, and 25% of the 188 subjects who subsequently underwent further evaluation were found to have medication-induced erectile dysfunction. In recent years, there has been increasing attention to sexual adverse effects of medications as a major factor that influences quality of life and adherence to prescribed regimens. Although most studies have focused on men, medications are a common cause of sexual dysfunction in both men and women (Wood et al., 2012).

Medications adversely affect sexual function through a variety of mechanisms, including their influence on the release of hormones and their actions on the autonomic and central nervous systems. Specific adverse medication effects that interfere with sexual function in men include a decreased or absent libido; difficulty obtaining or maintaining an erection; dry, premature or retrograde ejaculation; and inability to achieve orgasm. Women may experience the following medication-induced limitations in sexual function: diminished vaginal lubrication, decreased or absent libido, and inability to achieve orgasm. Box 26-1 lists some of the medications that are commonly associated with sexual dysfunction. These effects usually disappear when the medication is discontinued, and occasionally the effects will disappear if the dose is decreased.

Because alcohol depresses the central nervous system, it can interfere with sexual function. Although alcohol can decrease inhibitions and heighten sensual and sexual interest in social settings, excessive amounts can depress the central nervous system and interfere with sexual performance. Moderate amounts of alcohol normally do not interfere with

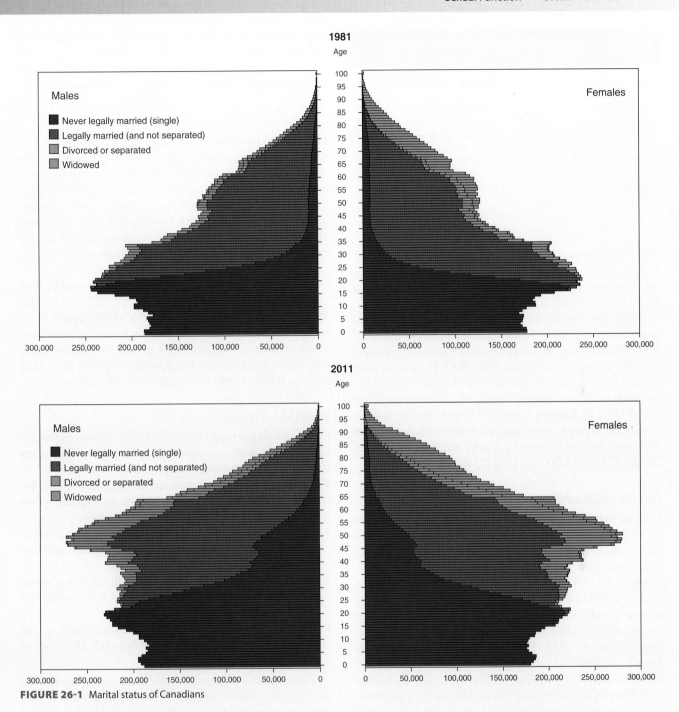

FIGURE 26-1 Marital status of Canadians

Category	65+	85+
Total—legal marital status	24,726,815	276,305
Single (never legally married)	7,816,050	16,085
Married (and not separated)	12,941,965	49,425
Separated but still legally married	698,245	2,215
Divorced	1,686,035	9,595
Widowed	1,584,530	198,980

FIGURE 26-2 Canadian Women 65+ and 85+, Marital Status, 2011. (Calculated from Statistics Canada. [2012]. *2011 Census of population Catalogue no. 98-XCB2011041*. Ottawa ON: Author. Data do not include common law relationships.)

Box 26-1 Medications that can Interfere with Sexual Function

ACE inhibitors	Calcium-channel blockers
α-Adrenergic blockers or agonists	Diuretics
Antidepressants	Dopamine agonists
Antiepileptics	Histamine H$_2$ antagonists
Antihistamines	Monoamine oxidase inhibitors (MAOIs)
Antiparkinson agents	Nonsteroidal anti-inflammatory drugs (NSAIDs)
Antipsychotics	
Benzodiazepines	Alcohol, nicotine and recreational drugs
β-Blockers	

---

sexual performance; however, in combination with other risk factors, such as medications or pathologic conditions, even small amounts of alcohol may be detrimental to the sexual performance of older adults.

Cigarette smoking was first identified as a cause of erectile dysfunction in the mid-1980s, and recent studies have confirmed that smoking increases the risk for sexual dysfunction in both men and women (Glina et al., 2013; Harte & Meston, 2012; Kim et al., 2011). Nicotine interferes with circulation to the sexual organs and accentuates the effects of other risk factors, such as diabetes, hypertension and vascular disease. In addition, cigarette smoking is associated with earlier onset of menopause and increased intensity and frequency of hot flashes (Hayatbakhsh et al., 2012; La Marca et al., 2013).

Effects of Chronic Conditions

Chronic conditions that have consistently been identified as having detrimental effects on sexual wellness include pain, cancer, diabetes, cardiovascular disease and obstructive sleep apnea (Ryan & Gajraj, 2012; Santos et al., 2012; Syme et al., 2013). Prevalence of erectile dysfunction in men with diabetes is 50% or more, with higher rates being associated with obesity, older age, physical inactivity and taking calcium-channel blockers (Sharifi et al., 2012, Shamloul & Ghanem, 2013; Thorve et al., 2011). In addition to erectile dysfunction, men with diabetes are likely to experience retrograde ejaculation (Fedder et al., 2013). Women with diabetes or metabolic syndrome also have a high prevalence of sexual dysfunction, such as problems with orgasm or lubrication, with increased age being an independent risk factor (Copeland et al., 2012; Martelli et al., 2012; Pontiroli et al., 2013). Depression is another chronic condition that is strongly associated with sexual dysfunction in men and women (Pastuszak et al., 2013; Wood et al., 2012).

Cardiovascular disease (e.g., heart failure) is strongly associated with many aspects of sexual dysfunction, including decreased libido, inhibited performance and pleasure, and decreased frequency of sexual activities (Hoekstra et al., 2012). Sexual function is affected not only by the physical manifestations of coronary heart disease (e.g., angina and reduced levels of activity) and adverse effects of medications, but also by psychological factors that commonly occur in people with cardiovascular disease. For example, even when no physiologic basis exists for abstaining from sexual intercourse after a myocardial infarction, sexual activity is often limited or absent because of fatigue, depression, diminished sexual desire, and fears and anxiety of the person or the sexual partner.

Gender-Specific Conditions

Prostatic hyperplasia (also called *benign prostatic hypertrophy*) is a common pathologic condition in which the prostate gland gradually enlarges and affects the urinary tract and sexual function. Men with prostatic hyperplasia often experience erectile dysfunction, ejaculatory dysfunction and urinary incontinence, which can interfere with enjoyment of sexual activities. Estimates of the prevalence of erectile dysfunction in men who have had prostatectomy for prostate cancer ranges from 25% to 90% (Tutolo et al., 2012).

Sexual function in older women can be affected by their increased susceptibility to inflammations, such as **urethritis** and **vaginitis** because of the thinning of the vaginal tissue and the decreased acidity and quantity of vaginal secretions. These conditions can occur after intercourse and cause urinary urgency and burning that persists for several days. They also can interfere with enjoyment of sexual intercourse.

Functional Impairments

Functional impairments associated with chronic conditions can interfere with enjoyment of sexual activity in many ways, as in the following examples:

- Chronic obstructive pulmonary disease may cause hypoxia and severe shortness of breath in response to the high physiologic demands of sexual activity.
- Arthritis and other musculoskeletal disorders are likely to be associated with pain, stiffness, muscle spasms and limited flexibility.
- Urinary incontinence can interfere with satisfying sexual relationships in people of any age, but this condition is more common in older adults.
- Medical conditions and adverse medication effects can have physiologic effects that interfere with all phases of sexual function.

Functional limitations increase with advancing age and are likely to combine with other risk factors to interfere with sexual function. In addition to direct effects of functional limitations, people with visible disabilities are often misperceived as unable to engage in sexual activities. This stigma and cultural bias can distort one's overall sexual self-concept and have a negative impact on sexual function and relationships (Esmail et al., 2010). This is particularly relevant to older adults who live in institutional settings because attitudes of the staff members can affect the residents' expressions of sexuality.

Sensory impairments can also interfere with sexual function because sensory stimulation is an important part of sexual pleasure and intimate communication. For example, an older adult with impaired hearing may find it difficult or impossible to carry on the intimate conversations that are often a part of sexual interactions. Similarly, hearing impairments can interfere with professional efforts to assess and counsel older adults on this sensitive topic. Likewise, impairments affecting vision, smell or touch can interfere with some of the usual sensual stimulation associated with sexual activities.

Attitudes and Behaviours of Families and Caregivers

In addition to societal influences, the attitudes and behaviours of family members and caregivers can affect sexual wellness of older adults, particularly for those who are dependent on others for their care. In institutional settings, attitudes of staff members can significantly affect the way in which residents express or repress their sexual needs. Staff members in long-term care facilities are generally unprepared to address issues related to sexuality and aging. Moreover, studies have found a notable lack of policies to guide staff responses to residents' sexual expressions or romantic behaviours (Cornelison & Doll, 2012; Elias & Ryan, 2011).

In general, sexual needs of older adults are ignored unless they are expressed in private and not brought to the attention of staff. When staff in long-term care facilities observe sexual expressions of residents, they are likely to view these behaviours as a problem rather than an expression of unmet need (Cornelison & Doll, 2012). Another concern in institutional settings is that family members are often involved with decisions about a resident's sexual expressions, even when the person is competent. This occurs either because the staff initiate the contact with the family or the family requests assistance from the facility in setting boundaries on the resident's expressions of sexuality.

Effects of Dementia on Sexual Expressions

When older adults are cognitively impaired, issues related to sexual expression are compounded by concerns about competency, decision making, the personal meaning of behaviours and whether the behaviour arises from dementia. Loss of sexual desire is the most common effect of dementia on sexual function; however, some people with dementia experience hypersexuality and demand frequent sexual intercourse. People with dementia may exhibit behaviours that are considered sexually inappropriate, such as exposing oneself, sexual talk, physically intimate touch or getting into bed with someone. However, these behaviours are usually caused by cognitive impairments rather than sexual impulses. For example, hypersexual behaviours and increased sexual desire are common manifestations of cognitive impairment due to frontal lobe disorders (e.g., fronto-temporal dementia) (Mendez & Shapira, 2013).

Prevalence of inappropriate sexual behaviours in people with dementia ranges from 2% to 17%, with higher rates reported in men (Lochlainn & Kenny, 2013). It is important to consider that behaviours associated with sexuality may be expressions of unmet needs related to touch, intimacy and interpersonal relationships. Sometimes, the behaviours are normal but they become problematic because of the context or the environment. For example, masturbating or disrobing in public places are considered sexually inappropriate

behaviours, but these actions may be due to dementia-related disinhibition.

For people in institutional settings, questions may arise about the ability of the person with dementia to make decisions about intimate relationships and sexual expressions. This is particularly problematic with regard to nonmarital relationships and behaviours involving spousal infidelity. These decisions are complex and should consider not only the effect on the spouse, but also whether sexual interactions could be beneficial or positive for the person with dementia.

 See **ONLINE LEARNING ACTIVITY 26-1: EVIDENCE-BASED INFORMATION ABOUT ISSUES REGARDING SEXUALITY** at http://thepoint.lww.com/Miller7e

 FUNCTIONAL CONSEQUENCES AFFECTING SEXUAL WELLNESS

Sexual function involves reproduction, response to sexual stimulation and interest and participation in sexual activity. With increased age, reproductive aspects become less significant, but many studies verify that sexual well-being is an important component of overall quality of life throughout older adulthood (Syme et al., 2013). Although age-related changes directly affect reproduction, other aspects of sexuality are affected more directly by risk factors. In addition, because sexual dysfunctions commonly occur in older men and women as a consequence of risk factors, these are discussed in this section.

Reproductive Ability

For women, loss of reproductive ability is a functional consequence of menopause, caused by the cessation of ova production within 1 year of the last menstrual cycle. Another functional consequence affecting reproduction in women is the increased risk that a fetus will be defective if ova are fertilized during the premenopausal years. On the positive side, older women frequently experience fewer constraints and inhibitions when they no longer are concerned about pregnancy (Gray & Garcia, 2012). The reproductive ability of men, by contrast, gradually declines with age but does not cease completely.

Response to Sexual Stimulation

The Masters and Johnson (1966) investigation has been widely recognized as the landmark study of human physiologic response to sexual stimulation. This classic study of 694 adults in a laboratory setting identified four phases of physiologic response to sexual stimulation in men and women. An analysis of data on older subjects led to the following conclusions:

- Older adults maintain their ability to respond to sexual stimulation, but their response is slower and less intense.
- Regularly engaging in sexual activity helps older adults respond to sexual stimulation.
- Any major changes in response to sexual stimulation are associated with risk factors rather than aging, per se.

TABLE 26-1 Functional Consequences for Response to Sexual Stimulation

Phase	Changes in Female Response	Changes in Male Response
Excitement phase	Breasts not as engorged Sexual flush diminished Delayed or diminished vaginal lubrication Decreased expansion of vaginal wall Decreased vasocongestion of labia	Longer time required to attain erection Less firm erection Longer maintenance of erection before ejaculation Increased difficulty regaining an erection if lost Reduced scrotal and testicular vasocongestion
Plateau phase	Decreased areolar engorgement Less intense sexual flush Less intense myotonia Decreased vasocongestion of labia Reduced Bartholin gland secretions Slower/less marked uterine elevation	Diminished nipple turgidity and sexual flush Less intense muscle tension Slower penile erectile response Delayed and diminished testicular elevation Fewer rectal sphincter contractions Diminution of ejaculatory expulsion force by about 50%
Orgasmic phase	Fewer rectal sphincter contractions Decreased number and intensity of orgasmic contractions	Absent or diminished sense of ejaculatory inevitability Fewer and less intense ejaculatory contractions
Resolution phase	Slower loss of nipple erection Quicker return to preexcitement stage	Slower loss of nipple erection Longer refractory period Rapid penile detumescence and testicular descent

Although older adults were greatly underrepresented in this study, the findings of Masters and Johnson have been widely accepted as the knowledge base about age-related changes in physiologic response to sexual stimulation. Normal age-related changes in male and female responses to sexual stimulation and the associated consequences are discussed in the following sections and summarized in Table 26.1. In recent years, there has been increasing emphasis on multifactorial factors that influence all aspects of sexuality, with emphasis on sexual wellness as a component of quality of life for older adults.

Sexual Interest and Activity

During the 1940s and 1950s, the Kinsey surveys first brought information about sexual behaviours of older adults to public attention by concluding that the frequency of sexual activity gradually declines with increasing age, but sexual interest and competence do not necessarily decline. Sexual interest, attitudes, activity and satisfaction are a continuation of lifelong patterns, and they remain stable in older adulthood unless risk factors interfere with sexual function. As discussed in the Risk Factors section, conditions that commonly affect sexual interest and activity in older adults include social circumstances, poor health, pathologic conditions, adverse medication effects and influences of family and caregivers. The sexual needs and interest of older adults, including residents of long-term care facilities, do not necessarily decrease, but their opportunities for sexual activity are often limited.

In recent decades, studies of sexuality and aging have focused on broader aspects, such as affection, friendships and intimacy. For older adults, these aspects of sexual function may become more important as the number of opportunities for sexual activities diminishes. For example, one of the first studies addressing sexual behaviours found that the most common sexual activities in a sample of 202 adults aged 80 to 102 years were touching and caressing without sexual intercourse (Bretschneider & McCoy, 1988). More recent studies have confirmed that older men and women who engage in more frequent sexual touching report higher levels of satisfaction (Galinsky, 2012). Additional components of sexuality that are especially important for older adults include kissing, hugging, intimacy, fantasy, masturbation, oral sex, loving words, physical closeness and expressions of affection (Lochlainn & Kenny, 2013; Muzacz & Akinsulure-Smith, 2013). A study of healthy community-dwelling older women (median age 67) found that one third reported low libido, but half were sexually active and maintained arousal, lubrication and orgasm (Trompeter et al., 2012).

In summary, older adults do not lose their interest in or capacity for sexual activity because of age-related changes, but risk factors such as misinformation, social circumstances, pathologic conditions, environmental constraints and adverse medication effects commonly interfere with sexual function. Many studies confirm that healthy older adults remain sexually active, particularly if they have positive attitudes, accurate information and access to a healthy partner (DeLamater, 2012; Trompeter et al., 2012; Van Wagenen et al., 2013). A normal consequence of aging, however, is that the response of older men and women to sexual stimulation is slower, less intense and of shorter duration. As one 79-year-old man reported, "It's like sparklers, not fireworks."

Sexual Dysfunction in Men and Women

Erectile dysfunction, defined as the inability to achieve or maintain an erection sufficient for satisfactory sexual function, is the most common sexual dysfunction affecting older men. Until the early 1990s, this condition was called *impotence*, but the National Institutes of Health in the United States proposed this change in terminology to reflect the broader understanding of erectile dysfunction as a complex condition associated with many interacting factors. This same term is advocated by the Canadian Urological Association, the Canadian Male Sexual Health Council and other leading health care associations in this country. Although erectile dysfunction is not the only type of male sexual dysfunction, it is the one that has been studied the most and has received the most public attention since 1998 because of the availability of medications, such as sildenafil (Viagra), and the widespread publicity about these medications that continues today. Other types of male sexual dysfunction include problems with ejaculation and diminished desire. Men at any age are likely to experience erectile dysfunction, but the incidence increases gradually with increasing age. It is currently viewed as a complex disease associated with multiple interacting factors, as discussed in the Risk Factors section.

In recent years, health care practitioners and pharmaceutical companies have started addressing **female sexual dysfunction**, similar to the way in which erectile dysfunction has been addressed since the early 1990s. Female sexual dysfunction includes disorders that affect sexual desire (including motivation and physical drive), sexual arousal, orgasm or pain during sexual activities (i.e., dyspareunia or vaginismus). Many of the same risk factors associated with erectile dysfunction are also associated with female sexual dysfunction: diabetes, cardiovascular disease, cigarette smoking, pelvic surgeries and adverse medication effects. An additional risk factor for women is diminished estrogen levels.

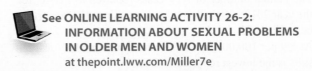

See **ONLINE LEARNING ACTIVITY 26-2: INFORMATION ABOUT SEXUAL PROBLEMS IN OLDER MEN AND WOMEN** at thepoint.lww.com/Miller7e

PATHOLOGIC CONDITION AFFECTING SEXUAL WELLNESS: HUMAN IMMUNODEFICIENCY VIRUS

Health care practitioners who provide care to older adults are increasingly aware of the need to address **human immunodeficiency virus (HIV)** as a sexually transmitted infection that is becoming more common among older adults. Studies identify one in four reported AIDS cases (26%) were among older Canadians in 2011. Among all reported AIDS cases since 1979, more than half of reported cases among older Canadians (52%) were among gay men and other men who have sex with men; one in five were among people who acquired HIV through heterosexual contact (20%) (Canadian AIDS Society, 2013). The effectiveness of antiretroviral therapy since the late 1980s has enabled many HIV-infected people to live longer with this condition, which is now considered a chronic disease, before it progresses to acquired immunodeficiency syndrome (AIDS). As a result of the use of highly effective antiretroviral

Unfolding Case Study

Part 1: Mr. and Mrs. J. at 73 and 71 Years of Age

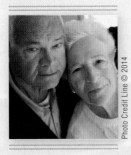

Photo Credit Line © 2014

You are the "wellness nurse" at the senior centre where Mr. and Mrs. J. come for the meal program and social interaction. Mr. J. is 73 years old and has hypertension and a history of a heart attack. He takes diltiazem (Cardizem), 300 mg daily; furosemide (Lasix), 20 mg daily; and propranolol (Inderal), 80 mg three times daily. Mrs. J., who is 71 years old, describes herself as generally healthy, but with a history of depression and some arthritis. She takes ibuprofen (Motrin), 400 mg four times daily, and sertraline (Zoloft), 50 mg daily. During your nursing clinics, Mr. J. and several other men have asked you about the drug that is advertised on television for men who have trouble satisfying their partners. The senior centre director also has noticed an increased interest in this topic and has asked that you plan a group health information session called "Sexuality and Aging."

THINKING POINTS

- Develop a plan for teaching older adults about the normal changes in sexual function that they are likely to experience.
- What risk factors would you discuss in relation to sexuality and aging?

- What educational materials would you use?
- What teaching would you do about interventions?

treatments during the past two decades, fewer than one third of the people who have been diagnosed and treated will die from conditions traditionally associated with HIV/AIDS. By 2015, 50% of HIV-infected individuals will be age 50 and older (Adekeye et al., 2012; Cahill & Valadéz, 2013).

Within *Estimates of HIV prevalence and incidence in Canada* (Public Health Agency of Canada [PHAC], 2013), the following data (from 2012) were identified:

- The annual number of HIV cases reported to PHAC for the year 2012 was the lowest reported since HIV reporting began in 1985.
- At 5.9 per 100,000, the 2012 rate of positive HIV test results is the lowest reported to date.
- Of the 534 at birth HIV-positive diagnoses in 2012, 312 (58.4%) were born in Africa and the Middle East, 139 (26.0%) in the Americas, 58 (10.9%) in Asia and Oceania and 25 (4.7%) in Europe.
- Of the HIV case reports indicating race/ethnicity information, 52.7% were attributed to Whites and 23.3% to Aboriginals. This was followed by the Blacks (13.1%), Asian (4.3%), Latin American (3.1%) and South Asian/West Asian/Arab (2.5%) categories.
- At the national level, distinct differences were observed between the sexes in terms of age at diagnosis of HIV and of AIDS, whereby diagnosis tended to be made at a younger age in females than in males.
- The proportion of HIV cases among older Canadians (50 years and older) has been gradually increasing since reporting began in 1985, and males outnumber females in the older age groups, particularly in the 30-to-39-year and the 40-to-49-year age groups.

 DIVERSITY NOTE

Aboriginal people in Canada are overrepresented in the HIV epidemic (PHAC, 2012).

The diagnosis of HIV/AIDS for people at any age is always accompanied by major health-related issues, but some issues are more unique to older adults, as summarized in Box 26-2. Although nurses in gerontological care settings are not expected to be experts in all aspects of HIV/AIDS, they are expected to holistically assess and address the complex needs of older adults with this condition. And, perhaps first and foremost, they should be able to communicate a nonjudgmental approach in all interactions with people who have risks for, or a diagnosis of, HIV/AIDS.

An important assessment consideration is that HIV may initially manifest as a nonspecific viral illness with signs and symptoms similar to seasonal flu or mononucleosis. These early manifestations may subside after several weeks, and HIV antibodies will appear in the blood between 3 and 6 weeks after the initial infection. If appropriate treatment is initiated in a timely manner, people with HIV can expect to live well into older adulthood, although they are likely to experience additional health issues, as summarized in Box 26-2.

Box 26-2   Issues Associated With HIV/AIDS in Older Adults

Issues Related to Diagnosis and Progression

- Older adults are likely to be diagnosed at a later stage, due to lack of screening, poor awareness of risk factors and failure of health care professionals to recognize and treat HIV/AIDS.
- Older adults have a shorter interval before progression to AIDS, particularly if HIV was diagnosed after the age of 60 years.
- HIV-positive older adults are at increased risk for dying due to AIDS or other conditions.

Associated Medical Concerns

- Older adults with HIV/AIDS are likely to be dealing with commonly occurring comorbidities, such as cardiovascular disease and some cancers (e.g., lung, leukemia, melanoma, all areas of the gastrointestinal tract).
- Dementia and cognitive impairment occurs more frequently in older HIV patients.
- Older adults have a diminished and delayed immune response to treatments.
- Metabolism of antiretroviral medications is altered in older adults, and this may lead to liver toxicity and other adverse effects.
- Common adverse effects of antiretroviral therapy include osteoporosis, pancreatitis, lipid disorders, peripheral neuropathy and high serum levels of lactic acid.

Associated Psychosocial Issues

- Older adults with HIV/AIDS have high rates of depression.
- Older adults are more likely to have less social support due to ageism, living alone, perceived stigma and nondisclosure of HIV status.
- Caregivers of people with HIV/AIDS experience significant levels of stress, which is exacerbated by associated factors such as stigma, uncertainty, depression, social isolation and impaired cognitive function.

Treatment of HIV generally includes a combination of antiretroviral agents and other types of medications to control disease progression. The pharmacologic regimen requires close monitoring for therapeutic and adverse effects. Adherence is a common problem for people with HIV/AIDS, for various reasons including cost of medications and adverse effects, making these issues important aspects of assessing older adults with HIV/AIDS.

Nurses have important responsibilities with regard to promoting wellness for older adults with HIV/AIDS, including addressing related psychosocial needs. For example, older gay men with HIV/AIDS are particularly susceptible to depression related to stigma, rejection and social isolation (Jang et al., 2011). Assessment and intervention guidelines for depression discussed in Chapter 15, including those related to suicide, are applicable for older adults with HIV/AIDS. In addition to addressing medical conditions related to HIV/AIDS, nursing interventions address psychosocial aspects for the person with HIV/AIDS and his or her caregivers. In addition, consider the cultural needs by suggesting resources specific for people who identify as LGBT or other minorities (e.g., black) (Box 26-3).

Box 26-3   Evidence-Informed Nursing Practice

Background: The deleterious effects of HIV stigma are well documented. However, little is known about what factors exacerbate or lessen the effects of HIV stigma.

Question: What are the predictors of overall HIV stigma?

Method: Adults above the age of 50 who were living with HIV in Ontario completed a questionnaire. Multiple linear regression analysis was conducted on 378 completed responses.

Findings: Being female, heterosexual, engaging in maladaptive coping and having poor self-rated health were associated with overall greater stigma. Whereas, being older, having greater mastery, increased emotional-informational social support and having experienced a longer time span since HIV diagnosis were associated with lower levels of stigma.

Implications for Nursing Practice: Nurses may need to initiate psychosocial interventions to promote the mental well-being of older adults living with HIV.

Source: Emlet, C. A., Brennan, D. J., Brennenstuhl, S., et al. (2013). Protective and risk factors associated with stigma in a population of older adults living with HIV in Ontario. *AIDS Care, 25*(10), 1330–1339.

Teaching about safe sex is a nursing responsibility that is often overlooked when caring for older adults, but it is particularly important with regard to preventing and managing HIV. Older adults need to recognize that safe sex practices are imperative for anyone who has sex with someone other than a long-term partner who is 100% monogamous. Nurses also need to teach about early detection of HIV and other sexually transmitted infections and encourage appropriate testing for anyone with risk factors. Recognize that even though health professionals are reluctant to initiate discussions with older adults about sexually transmitted infections, older adults themselves are receptive to this information (Slinkard & Kazer, 2011). Nurses can incorporate information about safe sex in their health education about sexual activity for older adults, as discussed in the section on nursing interventions and summarized in Box 26-6 later in this chapter.

See ONLINE LEARNING ACTIVITY 26-3: INFORMATION ABOUT OLDER ADULTS AND HIV/AIDS at http://thepoint.lww.com/Miller7e

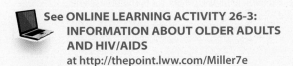

NURSING ASSESSMENT OF SEXUAL FUNCTION

Nurses do not necessarily include sexual function in every assessment, but it is an essential aspect when addressing quality-of-life issues that affect day-to-day function. Thus, assessment of sexual function is especially important in home care and long-term care settings (e.g., nursing facilities, group homes, assisted-living facilities). Sexual function is often neglected in nursing assessments because of the high degree of privacy associated with sexual function and the stereotype of the "sexless senior" that is prevalent in Canadian society. In addition, gender or generational differences between the health professional and the older person may interfere with an assessment of sexual function. Although all of these factors may explain why sexual function in older adults is so often overlooked, they do not justify its exclusion.

Self-Assessment of Attitudes About Sexual Function and Aging

Because of the private nature of sexual function and associated emotional responses and cultural factors, nurses are often uncomfortable discussing it. Additional discomfort occurs because nurses are not confident in dealing with concerns about human sexuality as an integral part of their nursing practice. They are even less comfortable initiating this topic with older adults or with people who are not in a traditional marital relationship. Thus, an assessment of personal attitudes about sexuality and aging is a prerequisite to addressing sexual wellness. Box 26-4 lists some of the questions nurses can use to examine their own attitudes toward the sexual function of older adults. Some questions are specific to adults in long-term care facilities because of the dominant role of nurses in addressing sexual function as a quality-of-life issue for residents.

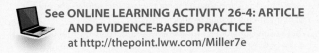

See ONLINE LEARNING ACTIVITY 26-4: ARTICLE AND EVIDENCE-BASED PRACTICE at http://thepoint.lww.com/Miller7e

Wellness Opportunity

Nurses should take time for self-assessment to increase their comfort with, openness to and sensitivity about issues related to sexual wellness for older adults.

Significant cultural differences between the nurse and the older adult may increase the difficulty of discussing sexual function. Box 26-5 summarizes some cultural aspects of sexual function that may be applicable to nursing assessment. Nurses may also be uncomfortable discussing sexual function with older adults who are LGBT or in any nontraditional relationship. Thus, an important aspect of self-assessment is to identify attitudes toward nontraditional sexual activities because these attitudes can influence the assessment and care of people who do not conform to the nurse's expectations. When assessing sexual function, establish a trusting relationship, have an awareness of gay and lesbian culture and other nontraditional sexual relationships, and communicate a nonjudgmental attitude by using appropriate or gender-neutral terminology. For example, the word *partner* includes a spouse, as well as a same-sex relationship, and asking about someone who is a *confidant* is broader than asking about marital status. Terminology related to people who identify as LGBT is delineated in Box 26-5.

Box 26-4 Assessing Personal Attitudes Toward Sexuality and Aging

What Do I Believe About Sexuality and Aging?

- Do I hold the misconception that older people, especially unmarried ones, are no longer interested in or capable of sexual activities?
- Do I believe the subtle messages that inaccurately associate sexual activities only with youth and attractiveness?
- Do I hold age-specific standards regarding sexual activity and romantic relationships? (e.g., Do I think it is okay for young adults to kiss or hold hands, but inappropriate or "cute" for older people to do this?)

What Do I Believe About the Nurse's Role With Regard to the Sexual Function of Older Adults?

- Do I base my nursing practice on the misconception that sexual function is strictly a private matter that health professionals should not address?
- Do I view sexual function as an activity of daily living that should be included in a comprehensive assessment of long-term care needs of older adults?
- Do I feel more comfortable discussing sexual function with people who are of the same gender and age range as myself, but very uncomfortable in discussing this matter with people who are old enough to be my parents or grandparents?
- Do I avoid discussion of sexual function with older adults because I believe they are not interested in sexual activity or are uncomfortable discussing this topic?
- Do I avoid discussing sexual function with older adults who are not in traditional marital relationships?
- What beliefs do I hold about the assessment of sexual function on the basis of the age of the person? For example, do I think sexual function should be assessed in sexually active teenagers who are at risk for unwanted pregnancy, but not older people?
- Am I comfortable incorporating health education about safe sex practices with older adults?

What Is My Attitude About Various Expressions of Sexual Activity?

- How do I view sexual activity and romantic relationships between unmarried people, or between people of the same gender?
- How do I view masturbation?
- Do my views about masturbation or sexual activity between unmarried or same-gender people influence my assessment of and interventions for people who engage in these activities?
- Am I tolerant and nonjudgmental toward people whose views and practices are nontraditional or different from mine?

For Nurses in Settings Where Long-Term Needs Are Addressed

- How do I feel about the rights of residents to engage in sexual activity in private, either with themselves or people of their own choosing?
- Do I try to ensure privacy for those residents who desire it?
- If I am aware of the sexual activities of a resident, do I think that I should inform the administrator, a family member or another "responsible adult?"

Box 26-5 Cultural Considerations: Cultural Aspects of Sexual Function

Expressions of Sexuality and Intimacy

- In some cultures, direct eye contact, especially between a man and woman, is interpreted as an expression of intimacy.
- In some cultures, it is taboo for a man to be alone with a woman other than his wife.
- Touching another person (particularly of the opposite sex) is considered taboo in many cultures.
- In some cultures, heterosexual men and women commonly hold hands with another person of the same gender.
- Only a few cultures value sexual equality between men and women.
- Homosexuality is accepted in some cultures but is considered taboo or is kept secret among family members in others.

Assessment Considerations

- In some cultures, it is considered taboo for postmenopausal women to have their breasts or vagina examined, even by a health care provider.
- Menopausal manifestations may vary in different cultural groups (e.g., most Japanese women do not experience hot flashes).

Terms Describing Sexual Orientation (i.e., one's sexual and romantic attraction)

- *Heterosexual:* sexual attraction to people of the opposite sex
- *Bisexual:* sexual attraction to both men and women
- *Homosexual:* sexual attraction to people of the same sex; the term applies to both men and women and is associated more with biologic aspects rather than with lifestyle characteristics.
- *Gay:* the term that is associated with lifestyle characteristics of men who feel romantically attracted to other men
- *Lesbian:* the term that is associated with lifestyle characteristics of women who feel romantically attracted to other women

Terms Describing Sexual Orientation (i.e., a combination of biologic characteristics and social roles)

- *Transgender:* people whose gender identity, gender expression or behaviour do not conform to that typically associated with the sex to which they were assigned at birth
- *Female-to-male* or *male-to-female transgenders* may be preparing for or recovering from sexual reassignment surgery, or they may be using long-term hormonal therapy as a nonsurgical option.

Assessing Sexual Function in Older Adults

Two goals of assessing sexual function in older adults are to provide an opportunity for the older adult to discuss any concerns related to sexual function and to identify risk factors, including lack of information, that affect the person's sexual wellness. Although the extent of the assessment varies according to individual circumstances, it minimally includes questions about the gynecologic aspects for women and genitourinary aspects for men. Incorporate these questions into a routine assessment of overall function and then ask an additional open-ended question about sexual interest and activities. When problems or risk factors are identified, obtain enough additional information to suggest appropriate resources for further evaluation. Box 26-6 summarizes guidelines for assessing sexual function in older adults. In addition, nurses have important roles in teaching about screening for HIV/AIDS (Slinkard & Kazer, 2011).

The Hartford Institute for Geriatric Nursing recommends that nurses use the PLISSIT assessment model as a

Box 26-6 Guidelines for Assessing Sexual Function in Older Adults

Interview Atmosphere and Communication Techniques

- Ensure both privacy and comfort.
- Be nonjudgmental and matter-of-fact in verbal and nonverbal communication.
- If feasible, sit face-to-face in chairs, rather than conducting the interview while the person being interviewed is in bed.
- If feasible, allow the person being interviewed to wear usual daytime clothing, rather than a hospital gown.

Initiation and Discussion of the Topic

- Begin by acknowledging feelings of discomfort and by stating the reason for discussing this topic. (e.g., "I know that sexuality is a private matter and people are often uncomfortable discussing this topic. However, as a nurse, I consider sexuality to be an aspect of health and well-being, and it may have a significant bearing on your overall care.")
- Include statements that address stereotypes and require a response from the older adult. (e.g., "Our society tends to view old people as being uninterested in sex, but for most older people, this is not true. Many older people are less sexually active than when they were younger, but this is not because of age-related changes. Have you experienced any changes in your sexual activities in the past few years?")
- Initiate the topic near the end of a comprehensive assessment interview, and begin with questions about the physiologic aspects of male or female function, such as those that follow.
- Incorporate at least one question to assess the appropriateness of including information about safe sex practices in your health teaching. (e.g., "If you have sex with partners other than someone who is in a long-term monogamous relationship with you, what precautions do you take?")

Interview Questions to Assess Male Sexual Function

- Have you ever had prostate problems or related surgery? Have you ever been told that you have or had an enlarged prostate?
- How often do you undergo a complete medical examination? When was your last complete physical examination done?
- Do you ever experience dribbling of urine or have problems holding your water?
- Do you have any trouble initiating the stream of urine?
- After you have urinated (passed water), do you still feel like you haven't emptied your bladder completely?
- Do you have to get up during the night to empty your bladder? If so, how many times?
- Have you ever noticed any blood in your urine?
- Do you ever have any discharge from your penis?
- Do you have any sores, lumps, ulcers, irritations or areas of inflammation on your penis or scrotum?
- Do you have any trouble with erection or ejaculation?

Interview Questions to Assess Female Sexual Function

- How many children, if any, have you had? How many pregnancies?
- At what ages did your menstrual periods begin and end?
- Have you ever had a Pap (Papanicolaou) test? When was your most recent Pap test and gynecologic examination?
- Have you ever had a mammogram? When was the most recent one?
- Have you ever been taught to examine your breasts for lumps?
- Do you examine your breasts for lumps? How often?
- Have you noticed any changes in your breasts? Do you ever have any discharge from your nipples?

- Do you have any burning, itching or irritation in the vaginal area?
- Do you ever have any vaginal discharge or bleeding?
- Do you have any difficulties with sexual intercourse?

Principles for Assessing Sexual Interest and Activities

- If the older adult makes a clear statement that this topic is irrelevant, do not insist on further questions. If the older adult responds to questions, however, do not discontinue the interview because of your own discomfort.
- Do not assume that an assessment of sexual function is irrelevant to unmarried people.
- For both married and unmarried older adults, use open-ended questions to elicit information about intimate relationships (e.g., "Is there anything you would like to ask or discuss about intimate relationships?").
- For a married person, open-ended questions may be asked about the partner's influence on sexual activities (e.g., "Has your husband experienced any changes in his health that have affected your sexual activities?").
- Listen for statements that reflect myths, a negative self-image or self-fulfilling prophecies, such as "Of course I stopped being interested in sex after menopause," or "I can't have an erection because I have prostate trouble."
- If risk factors, such as certain medications or pathologic conditions, have been identified earlier in the interview, ask additional questions, such as "Have you had any difficulties with sexual activities since your heart attack?" or "Do you have any questions about the possible effects of diabetes on sexual activity?"
- Emphasize the clinical reason for the questions. ("Sometimes certain illnesses or medications interfere with sexual function, and we want to identify any problems you might be having in this area.")
- Use open-ended questions that allow for either closure of the topic or a further discussion of issues. ("Is there anything you would like to discuss with regard to your sexual relationships?")

---

routine nursing assessment for older adults. The four components of this model are as follows:

- Obtaining *Permission* from the client to initiate sexual discussion
- Providing *Limited Information* about sexual function
- Giving *Specific Suggestions* for the individual to proceed with sexual relations
- Providing *Intensive Therapy* surrounding the issues of sexuality for the client

Online Learning Activity 26-5 provides additional information demonstrating the application of this tool in a clinical setting.

 See **ONLINE LEARNING ACTIVITY 26-5: EVIDENCE-BASED TOOL FOR ASSESSING SEXUALITY FOR OLDER ADULTS** at http://thepoint.lww.com/Miller7e

NURSING DIAGNOSIS

When nurses identify risks that interfere with sexual function, or when older adults express an interest in discussing sexual function, the appropriate nursing diagnosis is Ineffective Sexuality Pattern, defined as "expressions of concern regarding own sexuality" (Herdman, 2012, p. 325). Related factors commonly identified in older adults include medication effects, endocrine diseases (e.g., diabetes), cardiovascular diseases, genitourinary conditions, functional impairments secondary to chronic conditions (e.g., limited range of motion as a result of arthritis), psychosocial circumstances (e.g., lack of a partner) and myths and misunderstandings about age-related changes. The case example at the end of this chapter addresses this nursing diagnosis.

Wellness Opportunity

The nursing diagnosis of Readiness for Enhanced Knowledge: Sexual Function would be applicable to older adults who express an interest in learning about the effects of aging or risk factors on sexual wellness.

PLANNING FOR WELLNESS OUTCOMES

Increased knowledge about sexual functioning is an expected outcome for older adults who lack accurate information about age-related changes and risk factors. An outcome for residents of long-term care facilities would be Client Satisfaction: Protection of Rights. For a long-term care resident who is LGBT, an applicable outcome would be Client Satisfaction: Cultural Needs Fulfillment. Nurses can use the following additional Nursing Outcomes Classification (NOC) terminologies in care plans to promote sexual wellness for older adults: Body Image, Health Beliefs, Knowledge: Sexual Functioning, Personal Well-Being, Self-Esteem and Sexual Functioning.

Wellness Opportunity

Quality of Life is a wellness outcome for older adults who achieve more satisfying relationships through a variety of expressions of intimacy.

 ## NURSING INTERVENTIONS TO PROMOTE HEALTHY SEXUAL FUNCTION

Nurses have many opportunities to teach older adults about healthy sexual function as an important aspect of quality of life, particularly in community and long-term care settings. Teaching about age-related changes and risk factors is especially important for gerontological nurses because many older adults, as well as family and caregivers, hold stereotypes or have little accurate information about sexuality and aging. For documentation in care plans, use the following Nursing Interventions Classification (NIC) terminologies: Body Image Enhancement, Energy Management, Health Education, Patient Rights Protection, Risk Identification, Role Enhancement, Self-Awareness Enhancement, Self-Esteem Enhancement and Teaching: Sexuality.

Teaching Older Adults About Sexual Wellness

Unlike sex therapists or primary health care providers, nurses are not expected to provide sex education or direct interventions; however, nurses are expected to address sexual function as a quality-of-life concern. Nursing responsibilities also include teaching about safe sex practices for older adults who are sexually active with anyone other than their long-term monogamous partner. Health education about sexual wellness for older adults includes the following information:

- Acknowledgment that sexual function is within the usual realm of health promotion for older adults, especially in long-term care settings
- Effects of age-related changes on sexual function
- Risk factors that cause or contribute to problems with sexual function
- Resources for addressing identified problems and risk factors
- Protection from sexually transmitted infections

In addition, nurses in long-term care settings often need to address attitudes of the staff members, families and residents by providing accurate information and modelling nonjudgmental behaviours.

It is important to use excellent communication skills and ensure privacy and confidentiality when teaching older adults or caregivers about age-related changes and risk factors that affect sexual function. Use an approach that is open, respectful, nonjudgmental and gender neutral. Box 26-7 is a teaching tool written in nontechnical terms that can be used for health education of older adults. As with many other aspects of health education, emphasize that major changes in sexual function are not due to age-related changes alone, which are summarized in Table 26.1. Use Online Learning Activity 26-6 to explore resources for reliable information about sexuality and aging.

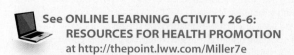 See **ONLINE LEARNING ACTIVITY 26-6: RESOURCES FOR HEALTH PROMOTION** at http://thepoint.lww.com/Miller7e

Wellness Opportunity

Nurses promote personal responsibility for sexual wellness by suggesting sources of accurate information that older adults can use.

Addressing Risk Factors

If an older adult with significant changes in sexual function also has a pathologic condition, takes a medication or uses any substance that might be a contributing factor, provide information about the potential influence of these risk factors. This is particularly important when the older person inaccurately attributes sexual problems to aging rather than to a manageable and reversible risk factor. For example, an older man may attribute a problem with attaining an erection to age-related changes, when, in fact, he has diabetes and takes an antihypertensive

Box 26-7 Health Education About Sexual Activity for Older People

- Older people remain fully capable of enjoying orgasm, but their response to sexual stimulation usually is slower, less intense and of shorter duration. Increasing the amount and diversity of sexual stimulation and experimenting with different positions can compensate for these changes and increase sexual enjoyment.
- The "use it or lose it" principle applies to sexual activity.
- Sexual problems in older people occur for the same reasons they occur in younger people. That is, they may be related to illness or disability, medications or alcohol, or psychological and relationship factors. A cause of sexual problems that is unique to older people is the self-fulfilling prophecy of the "sexless senior" stereotype.
- The following habits enhance sexual enjoyment: exercising regularly, avoiding or limiting consumption of alcohol, maintaining optimal health and nutrition, using hearing aids and corrective lenses as needed and engaging in sexual activities when you are relaxed and your energy level is at its peak.
- If you experience problems with sexual function, seek advice from a professional who is skilled in working with older people. Medical help can be obtained from a urologist, gynecologist or other medical specialist. If there is no medical basis for the problem, a sex therapist or marriage counsellor might be helpful.
- If you engage in sexual activity with anyone other than your long-term monogamous partner, protect yourself from sexually transmitted infections and talk with your health care practitioner about being tested periodically.

Facts Specific to Older Men

- Periodic difficulties with erection and ejaculation do not necessarily indicate that you are impotent.
- After you've reached orgasm, it may be 1 or 2 days before you are able to reach full orgasm again.
- Many new treatment options are available for treating erectile dysfunction (impotence). If your health care provider cannot provide up-to-date information about these options, ask for a referral for an appropriate evaluation and discussion of various options.

Facts Specific to Older Women

- Using a water-soluble lubricant will compensate for decreased vaginal lubrication. Do ***not*** use petroleum jelly because it is not a very effective lubricant for this purpose and can predispose you to infection.
- Estrogen is beneficial in preventing some problems with sexual function, but the relative risks and benefits of such therapy should be considered and discussed thoroughly with your primary care provider.
- You may have vaginal irritation or urinary tract infections, especially after sexual intercourse, because of age-related thinning of the vaginal wall. Such problems may be avoided by the following interventions:
- Drink plenty of fluids.
- Use an estrogen cream or vaginal lubricant.
- Maintain good hygiene in the vaginal area.
- If you have a male partner, have him thrust his penis downward, toward the back of your vagina.
- Empty your bladder before and after intercourse.

medication that is associated with erectile dysfunction. Use Box 26-1 to identify some of the medications that can interfere with sexual function. When a potential relationship between a risk factor and sexual problems is identified, suggest that the older adult seek professional advice. A complete medical evaluation by a primary care provider who is knowledgeable about the sexual problems of older adults is a good starting point. When a review of medications identifies adverse effects that contribute to sexual dysfunction, alternative drugs or reduced doses may resolve the problem. For example, people with hypertension are less likely to have sexual dysfunction when treated with calcium-channel blockers, angiotensin-converting enzyme inhibitors or peripheral α-adrenergic receptor blockers. After medical problems are addressed, a mental health professional may be an appropriate resource if problems with sexual function persist.

Arthritis is one of the most common pathologic conditions affecting older adults, and, in many cases, it is self-managed with little or no medical supervision. Often, the symptoms are not severe enough to motivate the older adult to seek medical evaluation and treatment, but they may interfere with sexual activities. In such cases, nurses can use Box 26-8 to teach about self-care interventions that may be effective in improving the quality of sexual activities for the older adult with arthritis. Nurses can also suggest that older adults who have arthritis obtain pamphlets from local chapters of The Arthritis Society.

Another pathologic condition often associated with sexual dysfunction is coronary artery disease, particularly in those who have had myocardial infarctions or who have undergone coronary artery bypass surgery. Nurses have important—but often overlooked—roles in providing information about sexual concerns for male and female patients and their partners not only immediately after a myocardial infarction but also for a prolonged period after initial recovery (Byrne et al., 2013; Steinke et al., 2011). Nurses can encourage older adults to discuss these concerns with their

Box 26-8 Health Education About Sexual Activity for People With Arthritis

The pain, fatigue and joint limitations of arthritis may interfere with, but do not have to curtail, your enjoyment of sexual activity. In fact, sexual activity can be beneficial to you because it stimulates the release of cortisone, adrenalin and other chemicals that are natural pain relievers. The following actions may enhance your sexual enjoyment and minimize the effects of arthritis:

- Engage in sexual activity when you feel least fatigued and most relaxed.
- Use analgesic medications and other methods of pain relief before engaging in sexual activity.
- Use relaxation techniques before engaging in sexual activity. Relaxation techniques that may be helpful for arthritis include warm baths or showers and the application of hot packs to the affected joints.
- Maintain optimal health through good nutrition and a proper balance of rest and activity.
- Experiment with different sexual positions and use pillows for comfort and support.
- Increase the time spent in foreplay.
- Use a vibrator if your ability to massage is limited by arthritis.
- Use a water-soluble jelly for vaginal lubrication.

Box 26-9 Health Education About Sexual Activity for People With Cardiovascular Disease

- Participation in a medically supervised exercise program can reduce oxygen requirements during sexual activity and improve the quality of your sex life.
- The typical energy expenditure for sexual intercourse is equivalent to that used for climbing two flights of steps.
- Do not engage in sexual activity in extremely hot and humid environments.
- Wait 3 hours after consuming alcohol or a large meal before initiating sexual activity.
- Engage in sexual activity when your energy is at its peak and you are feeling rested and relaxed.
- Avoid sexual activity during times of intense emotional stress.
- Avoid engaging in sexual activity with a partner with whom you are uncomfortable (e.g., an extramarital partner).
- Experiment with different positions to find one that is least demanding of your energy.
- Consider using nitroglycerin, if ordered by your primary care provider, as needed before sexual activity.
- Know that many types of oral medications for erectile dysfunction can cause serious (even fatal) interactions with nitrates.
- Consult your primary care provider if you experience chest pain during or after sexual activity, or breathlessness or heart palpitations persisting for 15 minutes after orgasm.

primary care practitioner and can provide health education using the general guidelines outlined in Box 26-9.

Promoting Sexual Wellness in Long-Term Care Settings

Responsibilities of nurses in long-term care settings to address sexual needs differ from those responsibilities of nurses in acute care or home settings in the following ways:

- Intense medical needs of patients in acute care settings take precedence over sexual needs.
- The short duration of stay in acute care settings is not conducive to addressing long-term sexual needs of patients.
- Because of the high degree of privacy and autonomy for people in their own homes, home care nurses are not routinely concerned about sexual needs.

Residents in long-term care facilities, however, usually are not acutely ill, are planning to stay in the facility for a long time and do depend on the nursing staff to ensure the privacy necessary to meet their personal needs. Thus, the nurse in long-term care facilities must address the sexual needs of residents as an integral part of the overall care plan.

Staff education is an important part of addressing the sexual needs of older adults in long-term care facilities because staff members need to know about all aspects of sexuality and aging, including the lifelong interest in and need for sexual activity and intimate relationships. Audiovisual materials can be used to stimulate discussion about the unique aspects of meeting sexual needs in institutional settings and about the responsibilities and limitations of staff members. Nurses generally participate in such in-services as

part of the interprofessional team, which also includes social service and administrative staff. Presenters and discussion leaders should be nonjudgmental and matter-of-fact so that they model the most effective approach for addressing this sensitive topic.

When the ability of a cognitively impaired resident to give informed consent is questionable, an interprofessional team can assess competence to participate in an intimate relationship. Emphasis should be placed on the Residents' Rights bill, as defined by the federal government in the 1987 Nursing Home Reform Law. Sexual needs of residents of long-term care facilities are protected through the rights to:

- Self-determination
- Participation in their own care
- Independence in making personal decisions
- Reasonable accommodation of their needs and preferences
- Privacy and unrestricted communication with any person of their choice
- Immediate access by their relatives and others, subject to reasonable restriction with the resident's permission

In addition to educating staff members about the sexual needs and rights of residents, nurses are responsible for ensuring privacy for those residents who desire it. If a resident does not have a private room, staff members try to provide privacy, while still respecting the rights of any roommates. Sometimes, the role of the nurse will be that of a negotiator, assisting residents in reaching mutually acceptable agreements about privacy and shared space.

Wellness Opportunity

Nurses respect autonomy by working with other staff members to assess the ability of someone with dementia to make decisions about expressions of sexuality.

Teaching Women About Interventions

Hormonal therapy refers to the use of estrogen alone or with progestogen for symptoms of natural or surgically induced menopause. Use of **menopausal hormonal therapy (MHT)** (also called hormonal replacement therapy) has a long and controversial history, beginning in the 1940s when it was a common medical intervention to alleviate vasomotor symptoms associated with menopause. During the early 2000s, results of large longitudinal studies, such as the Women's Health Initiative, raised questions about the safety of MHT, including the increased risk for serious diseases, such as cancers and cardiovascular events. As a result of these studies, many women who had been taking MHT for years discontinued these medications and fewer women initiated this intervention.

Currently, researchers continue to investigate the safety and efficacy of MHT and longitudinal data provide information about women who had previously used MHT, as well as those who currently or never used MHT. On the basis of continually evolving evidence, major organizations such as the North American Menopause Society and international consensus groups update their recommendations at least every 2 years. Increasingly, emphasis is placed on the importance of basing decisions about MHT on an individualized assessment of the person's risks and benefits by a knowledgeable health care practitioner (de Villiers et al., 2013; North American Menopause Society, 2012). Because these recommendations change frequently on the basis of evolving evidence, it is important to keep up to date on current recommendations through reliable resources listed in Online Learning Activity 26-6.

Because of the controversy surrounding MHT, there is an increasing need for evidence-based recommendations about nonprescription therapies for menopausal symptoms. Reviews of well-controlled studies have found little support for phytoestrogens (e.g., red clover and soya extracts) or herbal products (e.g., black cohosh); these reviews also raise concerns about adverse effects (Leach & Moore, 2012; Pitkin, 2012; Villaseca, 2012). Interventions that are highly recommended and without controversy are those that emphasize a healthy lifestyle (e.g., regular exercise, stress management, nutritious food, healthy weight, no smoking). In addition, recent studies indicate that some body–mind interventions (e.g., yoga, hypnosis, relaxation, cognitive-behavioural group treatment) have potential for improving quality of life for menopausal women (Cramer et al., 2012; Elkins et al., 2013; Green et al., 2013; Lindh-Åstrand & Nedstrand, 2012). Women can be encouraged to use water-soluble lubricants or prescription estrogen cream for vaginal dryness.

Teaching Men About Interventions

Interventions for erectile dysfunction have been available for several decades, but until recently, these interventions were not widely used, in part, because men did not seek help for this condition. Since 1998, extensive publicity about oral agents that are safe and easy-to-use interventions has brought much attention to this topic and it is now commonly recognized as a treatable condition. Sildenafil (Viagra) is the most commonly used drug of this type, called oral phosphodiesterase-5 inhibitors, and additional drugs in this class are vardenafil (Levitra), tadalafil (Cialis) and the most recently approved one, avandavil (Stendra). These drugs are widely used as first-line therapies for erectile dysfunction in older adults, with 60% to 80% response rates compared with placebos (Kedia et al., 2013). Common adverse effects of these drugs include headache, flushing, indigestion, dizziness and nasal congestion. Some recent studies are finding "emerging evidence" that these drugs are associated with hearing impairments (Thakur et al., 2013). These drugs are contraindicated for men taking nitrate medications because they can cause serious and even fatal adverse effects.

Testosterone replacement therapy has gained increasing attention in recent years, with many questions being raised about the safety and efficacy of this intervention. Current guidelines emphasize that testosterone therapy can improve sexual function in hypogonadal men, but decisions about treatment need to be individualized because information about long-term effects, including adverse effects, is lacking (Baer, 2012). Some herbal preparations (e.g., yohimbine) are promoted for enhancing sexual function in men; however, evidence-based information is unavailable to support these so-called interventions.

In addition to the oral agents that are widely publicized, several types of penile prostheses, such as the vacuum erection device, are used as safe and effective treatments for erectile dysfunction. Some of these devices require a surgical procedure, but some can be self-administered. Another pharmacologic approach is the administration of a vasoactive drug, such as alprostadil, as either an intracavernosal injection or a transurethral suppository. Nurses do not need to be familiar with the details of these procedures, but they need to know enough about interventions to suggest that men discuss their options with a physician.

It is also important to discuss interventions to address risk factors that cause or contribute to sexual dysfunction. For example, teach about smoking cessation, healthy practices, and optimal management of chronic conditions as interventions for sexual wellness. Psychotherapy and behavioural therapy are primary or adjunctive treatment options to address the psychosocial issues that may be contributing to erectile dysfunction. Decisions about appropriate treatment options must be based on a comprehensive evaluation by a urologist or a primary care provider who is knowledgeable about erectile dysfunction. The primary responsibility of nurses is to keep current on the types of interventions that are available and to teach about the importance of seeking help for erectile dysfunction.

EVALUATING EFFECTIVENESS OF NURSING INTERVENTIONS

Nursing care for older adults with the diagnosis of Ineffective Sexuality Pattern is evaluated by the degree to which risk factors are eliminated, particularly through the provision of accurate information. For example, older adults may verbalize an improved understanding of the age-related changes that affect their response to sexual stimulation. In turn, this information can alleviate anxiety about sexual performance and improve quality of life. Interventions to alleviate risk factors, such as medical conditions or adverse medication/chemical effects, would be considered successful if the older adult follows through with a referral to an appropriate resource. One measure of successful intervention in long-term care settings would be that staff members increase their understanding of the sexual needs of older adults and are more comfortable allowing appropriate sexual expressions by the residents.

Unfolding Case Study

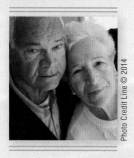

Photo Credit Line © 2014

Part 2: Mr. and Mrs. J. at 73 and 71 Years of Age

Mr. and Mrs. J. are now 75 and 73 years old, respectively, and they have moved to an assisted-living facility where you are the nurse. Their health conditions have not changed significantly in the past 2 years, with the exception of Mrs. J. having more difficulty walking because of her arthritis. Mr. and Mrs. J. recently moved to the facility because they needed help with transportation and wanted to live in a place where they had fewer responsibilities and more time to enjoy life. During one of their appointments, Mrs. J. becomes tearful and says she has been disappointed in their move from their own home. She says, "Now we have the time to enjoy our life together, but we seem to be in each other's way all the time. When we lived in our own home, we were so busy with the yard and the housekeeping and all the daily chores, we never had time to think about what we enjoy together. Now I don't have to cook meals and worry about getting to the grocery store, but we aren't enjoying the time we have together."

NURSING ASSESSMENT

On further discussion, Mrs. J. acknowledges that she talked with her husband about having more "intimate time and resuming sexual activities that have decreased in the past few years because we were always so tired and never seemed to have much time." In reply, Mr. J. stated that "We're probably too old to do those things, and old people shouldn't expect to have the fun in bed that we used to have." Mrs. J. says she used to believe that, but recently she's been talking with some of the other women in the assisted-living facility who seem to be enjoying sexual activities. Mr. and Mrs. J. relate that they had a good sexual relationship until Mr. J.'s heart attack 5 years ago. After that, he lost interest in sexual activities, even though he was told he could resume all his usual activities except for very strenuous activity, such as shovelling snow. Mrs. J. says she masturbates occasionally, but she doesn't find that very satisfying. Mrs. J. expresses concern about being comfortable in the sexual position they used previously because her arthritis has gotten worse in the past few years.

NURSING DIAGNOSIS

You address Ineffective Sexuality Patterns as your nursing diagnosis for Mr. and Mrs. J. Related factors include myths and lack of information about the age-related changes and risk factors that influence sexual function. Potential risk factors that you identify are Mr. J.'s medications and his lack of information about sexual function after a heart attack.

NURSING CARE PLAN FOR MR. AND MRS. J.

Expected Outcome	Nursing Interventions	Nursing Evaluation
Mr. and Mrs. J.'s knowledge about age-related changes and risk factors that affect sexual function will be increased.	• Use Box 26-7 as a basis for discussion of sexual function in later adulthood.	• Mr. and Mrs. J. will verbalize correct information about sexual function in older adulthood.
The risk factors associated with Mr. J.'s heart attack and medication regimen will be addressed.	• Explain that many medications for heart problems and high blood pressure are associated with problems with sexual function. • Use Box 26-8 as a basis for discussing sexual activity as it relates to people with heart problems. • Encourage Mr. J. to talk with his primary care provider about his medication regimen and about his heart condition. Suggest that he inquire whether a different medication would effectively treat his high blood pressure without interfering with sexual function.	• Mr. J. will agree to talk with his primary care provider about the potential relationship between his medications and heart condition and his lack of sexual activity.
The risk factors associated with Mrs. J.'s arthritis will be addressed.	• Use Box 26-7 to discuss sexual activity as it relates to people with arthritis.	• Mrs. J. will identify ways to increase her comfort during sexual activities.

THINKING POINTS

- What risk factors are likely to influence Mrs. J.'s enjoyment of sexual activity?
- What risk factors are likely to affect Mr. J.'s enjoyment of sexual activity?
- What health education would you provide for Mrs. J., and what patient teaching tools would you use?
- What health education would you provide for Mr. J., and what patient teaching tools would you use?

QSEN APPLICATION

QSEN Competency	Knowledge/Skill/Attitude	Application to Mr. & Mrs. J. When They Are 75 and 73 Years Old
Patient-centred care	(K) Integrate understanding of multiple dimensions of patient-centred care.	Base care plan on an assessment of individual needs of both Mr. J. and Mrs. J.
	(K) Describe strategies to empower patients in all aspects of the health care process.	Provide information about age-related changes and risk factors that affect sexual function is an intervention for empowering Mr. and Mrs. J. toward resolution of their sexual issues.
	(K) Discuss principles of effective communication.	
	(S) Elicit patient values, preferences and expressed needs.	
	(S) Provide patient-centred care with sensitivity and respect for diversity of the human experience.	Assess your own attitudes related to sexuality in older adults, so you can effectively discuss this topic with Mr. and Mrs. J.
	(S) Assess own level of communication skill in encounters with patients and families.	Communicate a nonjudgmental and open attitude when discussing this sensitive topic.
Evidence-based practice	(S) Base individualized care plan on patient values, clinical expertise and evidence.	Stay current on the topic of sexual function in older adults by exploring the resources listed in Online Learning Activities 26-1 and 26-6.
	(S) Read original research and evidence reports related to clinical practice.	
	(A) Value evidence-based practice as integral to determining the best clinical practice.	

Chapter Highlights

Age-Related Changes That Affect Sexual Wellness

- Diminished levels of hormones and degenerative changes of reproductive organs in both men and women
- Women: cessation of menses, onset of menopause, loss of reproductive ability
- Men: low testosterone (i.e., andropause), gradual decline, but not total loss of reproductive ability

Risk Factors That Affect Sexual Wellness

- Societal influences, especially on attitudes, stereotypes and prejudices
- Effects of attitudes and behaviours of families and caregivers, especially on dependent older adults
- Limited opportunities for sexual activity (lower ratio of men to women, health conditions)
- Adverse effects of medication, alcohol and nicotine (Box 26-1)
- Chronic conditions
- Gender-specific conditions
- Functional impairments and dementia

Functional Consequences Affecting Sexual Wellness

- Reproductive ability: ceases in women, diminishes in men
- Response to sexual stimulation: slower and less intense (Table 26.1)
- Sexual interest and activity: maintenance of interest and capacity in most older adults, but diminished sexual activity due to risk factors
- Male and female sexual dysfunction

Pathologic Condition Affecting Sexual Wellness: Human Immunodeficiency Virus

- Increasing numbers of adults aged 50 years and older have HIV/AIDS.
- Health-related concerns associated with HIV/AIDS in older adults (Box 26-2)
- Risk factors differ for older adults (less likely to be tested or to practice safe sex).
- Nurses have important roles in identifying new cases of HIV, assessing risks for sexually transmitted infections and assessing treatment issues (i.e., adverse effects, drug interactions).
- Nurses need to teach about safe sex practices.

Nursing Assessment of Sexual Function

- Self-assessment of attitudes about sexual function and aging (Box 26-4)
- Assessment of cultural influences (Box 26-5)
- General principles of and specific interview questions for nursing assessment (Box 26-6)
- Using the PLISSIT assessment model

Nursing Diagnosis

- Readiness for Enhanced Knowledge: Sexual Functioning
- Ineffective Sexuality Pattern

Planning for Wellness Outcomes

- For residents in long-term care facilities: Client Satisfaction, Protection of Rights, Cultural Needs Fulfillment
- Body Image
- Personal Well-Being
- Self-Esteem
- Sexual Functioning

Nursing Interventions to Promote Sexual Wellness (Boxes 26-6 through 26-8)

- Teaching older adults about sexual wellness: age-related changes and risk factors
- Addressing risk factors: teaching about sexual activity for people with arthritis or cardiovascular disease
- Promoting sexual wellness in long-term care facilities: staff education, protection of rights, ensuring privacy
- Teaching women about interventions for the effects of menopause and men about interventions for erectile dysfunction

Evaluating Effectiveness of Nursing Interventions

- Provision of accurate information to dispel myths and misconceptions
- Improved quality of life
- Referrals to health care professionals for addressing risk factors
- Increased knowledge and comfort of staff in long-term care facilities

Critical Thinking Exercises

1. Describe the attitudinal risk factors on the parts of society, older adults and health care providers that can interfere with healthy sexual function in older adults.
2. Summarize the functional consequences that are likely to affect sexual function in healthy older men and women.
3. What are the responsibilities of nurses in each of the following settings related to assessment of sexual function in older adults: community setting, acute care facility and long-term care facility?

4. Describe the assessment and health education approaches you might use for a 73-year-old married man who confides that he has difficulty making his wife "happy in bed."
5. Spend a few minutes answering all the questions included in Box 26-4, Assessing Personal Attitudes Toward Sexuality and Aging. What did you learn about yourself?

 For more information about the topics discussed in this chapter, be sure to check out the interactive Online Learning Activities and other helpful resources at http://thepoint.lww.com/Miller7e

REFERENCES

Adekeye, O. A., Heiman, H. J., Onyeabor, O. S., et al. (2012). The new invincibles: HIV screening among older adults in the U.S. *PLoS ONE, 7*(8), e43618. doi:10.1371/journal.pone.0043618

Baer, J. T. (2012). Testosterone replacement therapy to improve health in older males. *The Nurse Practitioner, 37*(8), 39–44.

Bretschneider, J. G., & McCoy, N. L. (1988). Sexual interest and behavior in healthy 80- to 100-year olds. *Archives of Sexual Behavior, 17,* 109–129.

Byrne, M., Doherty, S., Murphy, A. W., et al. (2013). The CHARMS Study: Cardiac patients' experiences of sexual problems following cardiac rehabilitation. *European Journal of Cardiovascular Nursing, 12*(6), 558–566.

Cahill, S., & Valadéz, M. S. W. (2013). Growing older with HIV/AIDS: New public health challenges. *American Journal of Public Health, 103*(3), e7–e15.

Canadian AIDS Society. (2013). *HIV and aging in Canada*. Retrieved from http://www.cdnaids.ca/files.nsf/pages/hiv_aging_1-introduction-factsheet/$file/HIV_aging_1-Introduction-FactSheet.pdf

Copeland, K. L., Brown, J. S., Creasman, J. M., et al. (2012). Diabetes mellitus and sexual function in middle-aged and older women. *Obstetrics and Gynecology, 120*(2), 331–340.

Cornelison, L. J., & Doll, G. M. (2012). Management of sexual expression in long-term care: Ombudsmen's perspectives. *The Gerontologist, 53*(5), 780–789. doi:10.1093/geront/gns162

Cramer, H., Lauche, R., Langhorst, J., et al. (2012). Effectiveness of yoga for menopausal symptoms: A systematic review and meta-analysis of randomized controlled trials, *Evidence Based Complementary and Alternative Medicine,* 2012, 1–11. doi:1155/2012/863905

Cui, J., Shen, Y., & Li, R. (2013). Estrogen synthesis and signaling pathways during ageing. *Trends in Molecular Medicine, 19*(3), 197–209.

DeLamater, J. (2012). Sexual expression in later life: A review and synthesis. *Journal of Sex Research, 49*(2–3), 125–141.

de Villiers, T. J., Gass, M. L. S., Haines, C. J., et al. (2013). Global consensus statement on menopausal hormone therapy. *Maturitas, 74,* 391–392.

Elias, J., & Ryan, A. (2011). A review and commentary on the factors that influence expressions of sexuality by older people in care homes. *Journal of Clinical Nursing, 20*(11–12), 1668–1676.

Elkins, G. R., Fisher, W. I., Johnson, A. K., et al. (2013). Clinical hypnosis in the treatment of postmenopausal hot flashes. *Menopause, 20*(3), 291–298.

Esmail, S., Darry, K., Walter, A., et al. (2010). Attitudes and perceptions towards disability and sexuality. *Disability Rehabilitation, 32*(14), 1148–1155.

Farrell, J., & Belza, B. (2011). Are older patients comfortable discussing sexual health with nurses? *Nursing Research, 61*(1), 51–57.

Fedder, J., Kaspersen, M. D., Brandslund, I., et al. (2013). Retrograde ejaculation and sexual dysfunction in men with diabetes mellitus. *Andrology, 1*(4), 602–606. doi:10.1111/j.2047-2927.2013.00083.x

Galinsky, A. M. (2012). Sexual touching and difficulties with sexual arousal and orgasm among U.S. older adults. *Archives of Sexual Behavior, 41*(4), 875–890.

Gibbs, A., Lee, S., & Kulkarni, J. (2012). What factors determine whether a women becomes depressed during perimenopause? *Archives of Women's Mental Health, 15*(5), 323–332.

Glina, S., Sharlip, I. D., & Hellstrom, W. J. (2013). Modifying risk factors to prevent and treat erectile dysfunction. *Journal of Sex Medicine, 10*(1), 115–119.

Gray, P. B., & Garcia, J. R. (2012). Aging and human sexual behavior. *Gerontology, 58*, 446–452.

Green, S. M., Haber, E., McCabe, R. E., et al. (2013). Cognitive-behavioral group treatment for menopausal symptoms. *Archives of Women's Mental Health, 16*(4), 325–332.

Harte, C. B., & Meston, C. M. (2012). Association between smoking cessation and sexual health in men. *British Journal of Urology International, 109*(6), 888–896.

Hayatbakhsh, M. R., Clavarino, A., Williams, G. M., et al. (2012). Cigarette smoking and age of menopause. *Maturitas, 72*(4), 346–352.

Herdman, T. H. (Ed.). (2012). *NANDA International Nursing Diagnoses: Definitions and classification* 2012-1014. Oxford, England: Wiley-Blackwell.

Hoekstra, T., Lesman-Leegle, I., Luttik, M. L., et al. (2012). Sexual problems in elderly male and female patients with heart failure. *Heart, 98*(22), 1647–1652.

Horstman, A. M., Dillon, E. L., Urban, R. J., et al. (2012). The role of androgens and estrogens in healthy aging and longevity. *Journals of Gerontology: Biological Sciences and Medical Sciences, 67*(11), 1140–1152.

Im, E.-O., Ko, Y., Hwang, H., et al. (2012). "Symptom-specific or holistic": Menopausal symptom management. *Health Care Women International, 33*(6), 575–592.

Jang, H., Anderson, P. G., & Mentes, J. C. (2011). Aging and living with HIV/AIDS. *Journal of Gerontological Nursing, 37*(12), 4–7.

Kedia, G. T., Ückert, S., Assadi-Pour, F., et al. (2013). Avanafil for the treatment of erectile dysfunction. *Therapeutic Advances in Urology, 5*(1), 35–41.

Kim, T. H., Kim, S. M., Kim, J. J., et al. (2011). Does metabolic syndrome impair sexual function in middle- to old-aged women? *Journal of Sex Medicine, 8*(4), 1123–1130.

La Marca, A., Sighinolfi, G., Papaleo, E., et al. (2013). Prediction of age at menopause from assessment of ovarian reserve may be improved by using body mass index and smoking status. *PLoS ONE, 8*(3), e57005.

Leach, M. J., & Moore, V. (2012). Black cohosh for menopausal symptoms. *Cochrane Database Systematic Review, 2012*(9) [CD007244]. doi:10.1002/14651858.CD007244.pub2

Lin, H. L., Hsiao, M. C., Liu, Y. T., et al. (2013). Perimenopause and incidence of depression in midlife women. *Climacteric, 16*(3), 381–386.

Lindh-Åstrand, L., & Nedstrand, E. (2012). Effects of applied relaxation on vasomotor symptoms in postmenopausal women: A randomized controlled trial. *Menopause: The Journal of the North American Menopause Society, 20*(4), 401–408.

Lochlainn, M. N., & Kenny, R. A. (2013). Sexual activity and aging. *Journal of the American Medical Directors Association, 14*(8), 565–572.

Martelli, V., Valisella, S., Moscatiello, S., et al. (2012). Prevalence of sexual dysfunction among postmenopausal women with and without metabolic syndrome. *Journal of Sex Medicine, 9*(2), 4334–441.

Masters, W. H., & Johnson, V. E. (1966). *Human sexual response*. Boston, MA: Little Brown.

Mauvais-Jarvis, F., Clegg, D. J., & Hevener, A. L. (2013). The role of estrogens in control of energy balance and glucose homeostasis. *Endocrinology Review, 34*(3), 309–338.

McGill, J. J., Shoskes, D. A., & Sabanegh, E. S. (2012). Androgen deficiency in older men. *Cleveland Clinic Journal of Medicine, 79*(11), 797–806.

Mendez, M. F., & Shapira, J. S. (2013). Hypersexual behavior in frontotemporal dementia. *Archives of Sex and Behavior, 42*(3), 501–509.

Muzacz, A. K., & Akinsulure-Smith, A. M. (2013). Older adults and sexuality. *Journal of Mental Health Counseling, 35*(1), 1–14.

Nedergaard, A., Henriksen, K., Karsdal, A. M., et al. (2013). Menopause, estrogens and frailty. *Gynecological Endocrinology, 29*(5), 418–423.

North American Menopause Society. (2012). The 2012 hormone therapy position statement of the North American Menopause Society. *Menopause: The Journal of the North American Menopause Society, 19*(3), 257–271.

Okeke, T. C., Ezenyeaku, C. C., Ikeako, L. C., et al. (2013). An overview of menopause associated vasomotor symptoms and options available in its management. *Nigerian Journal of Medicine, 22*(1), 7–14.

Pantalone, K. M., & Faiman, C. (2012). Male hypogonadism. *Cleveland Clinic Journal of Medicine, 79*(10), 717–725.

Pastuszak, A. W., Badhiwala, N., Lipshultz, L. I., et al. (2013). Depression is correlated with the psychological and physical aspects of sexual dysfunction in men. *International Journal of Impotence Research, 25*(5), 194–199. doi:10.1038/ijir.2013.4

Pimenta, F., Leal, I., Moroco, J., et al. (2012). Menopausal symptoms. *Maturitas, 73*(4), 324–331.

Pitkin, J. (2012). Alternative and complementary therapies for menopause. *Menopause International, 18*(1), 20–27.

Pontiroli, A. E., Cortelazzi, D., & Morabito, A. (2013). Female sexual dysfunction and diabetes: A systematic review and meta-analysis. *Journal of Sex Medicine, 10*(4), 1044–1051. doi:10.1111/jsm.12065

Public Health Agency of Canada. (2012). *At a glance: HIV and AIDs in Canada: Surveillance Report to December 31st, 2012.* Retrieved from http://www.phac-aspc.gc.ca/aids-sida/publication/survreport/2012/dec/index-eng.php

Public Health Agency of Canada. (2013). *HIV and AIDS in Canada: Surveillance Report to December 31,* 2012. Retrieved from http://www.phac-aspc.gc.ca/aids-sida/publication/survreport/2012/dec/index-eng.php

Ryan, J. G., & Gajraj, J. (2012). Erectile dysfunction and its association with metabolic syndrome and endothelial function among patients with type 2 diabetes mellitus. *Journal of Diabetes Complications, 26*(2), 141–147.

Santos, T., Drummond, M., & Botelho, F. (2012). Erectile dysfunction in obstructive sleep apnea syndrome. *Review of Portuguese Pneumologica, 18*(2), 64–71.

Schanzer, D. L. (2003). Trends in HIV/AID|S mortality in Canada, 1987–1998. *Canadian Journal of Public Health, 94*(2), 135–139.

Shamloul, R., & Ghanem, H. (2013). Erectile dysfunction. *Lancet, 381*(9861), 153–165.

Sharifi, F., Asghari, M., Jaberi, Y., et al. (2012). Independent predictors of erectile dysfunction in type 2 diabetes mellitus. *ISRN Endocrinology, 2012*(2012), 1–5 [Art. ID 502353]. doi:10.5402/2012/5023553

Slag, M., Morley, J. E., Elson, M. K., et al. (1983). Impotence in medical clinic patients. *Journal of the American Medical Association, 249*, 1736–1740.

Slinkard, M. S., & Kazer, M. W. (2011). Older adults and HIV and STI screening. *Geriatric Nursing, 32*(5), 341–349.

Spitzer, M., Huang, G., Basaria, S., et al. (2013). Risks and benefits of testosterone therapy in older men. *Nature Reviews of Endocrinology, 9*(7), 414–424. doi:10.1038/nrendo.2013.73

Statistics Canada. (2013). *Annual demographic estimates: Canada, provinces and territories.* Retrieved from http://www5.statcan.gc.ca/bsolc/olc-cel/olc-cel?lang=eng&catno=91-215-XWE

Steinke, E. E., Mosack, V., Barnason, S., et al. (2011). Progress in sexual counseling by cardiac nurses, 1994 to 2009. *Heart & Lung, 40*(3), e15–e24. doi:10.1016/j.hrtlng.2010.10.001

Surampudi, P. N., Wang, C., & Swerdloff, R. (2012). Hypogonadism in the aging male: Diagnosis, potential benefits and risks of testosterone replacement therapy. *International Journal of Endocrinology, 2012,* 1–20 [Art. ID 625434]. doi:10.1155/2012/625434

Syme, M. L., Klonoff, E. A., Macera, C. A., et al. (2013). Predicting sexual decline and dissatisfaction among older adults. *Journals of Gerontology: Psychological Sciences and Social Sciences, 68*(3), 323–332.

Thakur, J. S., Thakur, S., Sharma, D. R., et al. (2013). Hearing loss with phosphodiesterase-5 inhibitors. *Laryngoscope, 123*(6), 1527–1530. doi:10.1002/lary.23865

Thorve, V. S., Kshirsagar, A. D., Vyawahare, N. S., et al. (2011). Diabetes-induced erectile dysfunction. *Journal of Diabetes Complications, 25*(2), 129–136.

Trompeter, S. E., Bettencourt, R., & Barrett-Connor, E. (2012). Sexual activity and satisfaction in healthy community-dwelling older women. *The American Journal of Medicine, 125*, 37–43.

Tutolo, M., Briganti, A., Suardi, N., et al. (2012). Optimizing postoperative sexual function after radical prostatectomy. *Therapeutic Advances in Urology, 4*(6), 347–365.

Van Wagenen, A., Driskell, J., & Bradford, J. (2013). "I'm still raring to go": Successful aging among lesbian, gay, bisexual, and transgender older adults. *Journal of Aging Studies, 27*, 1–14.

Villaseca, P. (2012). Non-estrogen conventional and phytochemical treatments for vasomotor symptoms. *Climacteric, 19*(2), 115–124.

Whiteley, J., Wagner, J.-S., Bushmakin, A., et al. (2013). Impact of the severity of vasomotor symptoms on health status, resource use, and productivity. *Menopause: The Journal of the North American Menopause Society, 20*(5), 518–524.

Woo, J. S. T., Brotto, L. A., & Gorzalka, B. B. (2012). The relationship between sex guilt and sexual desire in a community sample of Chinese and Euro-Canadian Women. *Journal of Sex Research, 49*(3), 290–298.

Wood, A., Runciman, R., Wylie, K. R., et al. (2012). An update on female sexual function and dysfunction in old age and its relevance to old age psychiatry. *Aging and Disease, 3*(5), 373–384.

part **5**

Promoting Wellness in All Stages of Health and Illness

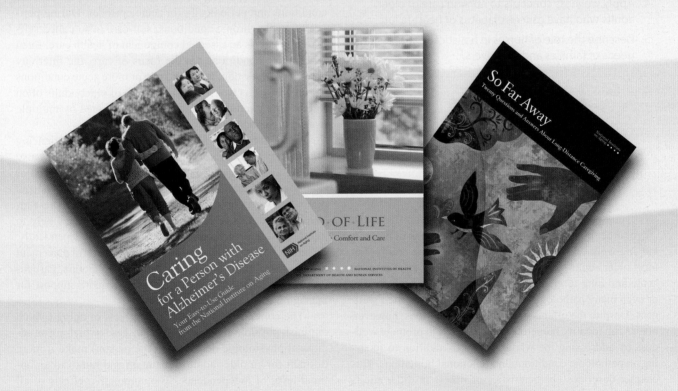

Caring for Older Adults During Illness

S everal factors differentiate care of older adults from that of other populations and add to the challenge of promoting wellness. Foremost among these is the reality that most older adults—and all of those whom nurses care for in acute and long-term care settings—are coping with several or even many pathologic conditions that threaten their wellness. Despite the effects of pathologic conditions, however, nurses can identify numerous opportunities to promote wellness by addressing the whole person in addition to focusing on pathologic conditions and functional limitations. This chapter describes characteristics of illness in older adults and discusses an approach to holistic care that is applicable for older adults who have chronic or progressively declining conditions. Concepts are applied to nursing care for older adults who have cancer, diabetes and heart failure. Needs of caregivers of older adults are also addressed in this chapter.

CHARACTERISTICS OF ILLNESS IN OLDER ADULTS

Older adults commonly have one or more chronic conditions that gradually accumulate and affect their daily functioning and quality of life. In fact, in 2009, one quarter of Canadians aged 65 to 79 and 37% of those 80 years of age and older reported having four or more chronic conditions (Public Health Agency of Canada, 2010). Consequently, they typically receive health care on a continuing basis for chronic conditions and periodically for acute episodes. During periods of stable chronic conditions, self-care (also called self-management) is an essential component of health care. Even when acute conditions are the focus of care, the interplay between chronic conditions and one or more acute conditions is likely to affect care. Thus, the health of older adults often fluctuates unpredictably and is usually affected by multiple interacting conditions.

When nurses care for older adults who are experiencing illness, they address not only the acute conditions but also the interaction among acute and chronic conditions. For example, older adults with heart failure may be hospitalized off and on when their condition becomes unstable. These intermittent periods of care in hospital settings are likely to interfere with the person's ability to function independently. Eventually, these conditions can lead to long-term placement in an assisted living or other type of nursing facility, particularly if the older adult does not have adequate support for managing care at home.

The combined and cumulative effects of aging (which diminish physiologic reserves) and disease (which place additional physiologic demands on the person) make it more difficult for an older adult to maintain and return to an optimal level of independence. The cumulative effects of all these intermittent and interacting forces can lead to a "yo-yoing" effect: the person experiences a cycle of ups and downs in health, with the "yo-yo" failing to return to the height of its previous cycle. With diminishing resiliency during subsequent cycles, the yo-yo eventually loses its ability to bounce back. Promoting wellness involves holistically addressing the changing needs of older adults as they progress through these cycles of ups and downs. Wellness nursing care also involves implementing interventions directed toward "rewinding the yo-yo" by building on the person's strengths and supporting health-promoting self-care actions.

> ### Wellness Opportunity
>
> By attending to the body–mind–spirit interconnectedness of older adults, nurses can identify opportunities to provide physical comfort and support emotional and spiritual growth even in situations involving inevitable physical decline.

Multimorbidity

In recent years, there has been increasing recognition of the complexity of providing medical care for older adults who have combinations of chronic conditions and intermittent acute conditions. In 2012, the Canadian Institutes of Health Research (CIHR)–Institute of Aging published "Living Longer, Living Better," its 2013–2018 strategic plan. Within this plan, one priority is to address the importance of interventions appropriate for older adults with multiple chronic conditions, or **multimorbidity**. Multimorbidity is associated with poorer quality of life and greater use of health care resources (CIHR Institute of Aging, 2012). In relation to the priority focused upon developing interventions that address the complexity of older adults' health, this report suggests the following:

- Interventions should be holistic and based upon an understanding of the impact conditions have upon older adults' physical and mental health and overall wellness.
- It is important to establish a continuum of integrated services that begins with preventative support and moves through to medical care.
- Interventions should be tailored toward the diversity of caregivers and their needs.
- Services and interventions need to improve the quality of life for individuals and families living with neurodegenerative diseases, such as Alzheimer disease.

Although this priority and its related foci are developed for primary care practitioners, they are pertinent to the provision of nursing care for older adults. This is especially important in relation to the roles of nurses as advocates, coordinators of care and communicators with patients, families, caregivers, physicians and other professionals.

Atypical Presentation

Atypical presentation (i.e., signs and symptoms of a disease differ from what is expected because they are altered, subtle, absent or nonspecific) is common in older adults. For example, falls, changes in behaviour or functioning and vague physical manifestations (e.g., increased fatigue or loss of appetite) are common atypical presentations of infection (e.g., pneumonia or urinary tract infection). In addition, the expected manifestations of an infection, such as elevated temperature or specific complaints of pain or discomfort, may be absent. Atypical presentation of disease is especially common in those who are cognitively impaired or older than 85 years. Adverse effects of medication may also present atypically, and this can interfere with timely recognition and management (Petrovic et al., 2012). A major nursing responsibility is to maintain a heightened awareness of the potential for atypical presentation of disease and explore all potential underlying causes of signs and symptoms of illness in older adults.

Geriatric Syndromes

The term **geriatric syndromes** refers to conditions that do not fit a specific disease category but have a significant negative effect on the older person's level of functioning and quality of life. The most commonly cited geriatric syndromes are falls, frailty, malnutrition, urinary incontinence, functional decline, pressure ulcers and cognitive impairment (including delirium). Although definitions of geriatric syndromes vary, experts agree that these conditions are highly prevalent and caused by the interplay among several risk factors and underlying conditions. Another characteristic of geriatric syndromes is that they diminish the person's ability to adapt to stressors and are associated with substantial morbidity and poor outcomes (Kane et al., 2012; Wang et al., 2013). Current emphasis is on addressing specific risks and causative factors so that interventions can be initiated to prevent geriatric syndromes or minimize the serious consequences. For example, much attention focuses on addressing adverse effects of the psychoactive drugs that are strongly associated with falls, delirium and hospitalization (Wierenga et al., 2012).

Since the early 2000s, **frailty** has been discussed in geriatric literature as a syndrome arising from the "physiologic triad" of sarcopenia (i.e., loss of muscle mass) and immune and neuroendocrine dysregulation (Fried et al., 2001). Frailty is now widely recognized as a complex geriatric syndrome and patients are considered frail when they have three or more of the following conditions: low level of physical activity, slow walking speed, unintentional weight loss (i.e., 4.5 kg or more during the past year), weakness (measured by diminished handgrip strength) and self-reported exhaustion (Koller & Rockwood, 2013).

Experts agree that frailty is multifactorial and that a comprehensive definition should include assessment of six domains: cognition, mental health, nutrition, physical functioning, mobility, and gait speed (Rodríquez-Mañas et al., 2013). Many studies find that frailty leads to many serious negative consequences, including increased mortality and admissions to hospitals and long-term care facilities and decreased functioning and quality of life (e.g., Drubbel et al., 2013; Shamliyan et al., 2013). Studies also emphasize that identification of frailty in hospitalized older adults should be an important first step in preventing adverse events in this group of patients who are at increased risk for serious outcomes (Bagshaw & McDermid, 2013). An international consensus group of experts recommends frailty screening for all persons above 70 years and those with significant weight loss related to chronic disease because this condition can potentially be prevented or treated with specific modalities, including exercise, nutritional interventions, vitamin D and reduction of polypharmacy (Morley et al., 2013).

See **ONLINE LEARNING ACTIVITY 27-1: ADDITIONAL INFORMATION ABOUT CHARACTERISTICS OF ILLNESS IN OLDER ADULTS** at http://thepoint.lww.com/Miller7e

CONNECTING THE CONCEPTS OF WELLNESS, AGING AND ILLNESS

Although the concepts of wellness and aging may seem contradictory when caring for older adults who are acutely and chronically ill, it is relatively easy to apply wellness to older adults in their 70s who are healthy, functional and satisfied with their lives. The greater challenge is to apply the concept of wellness to the nursing care of people who not only are in their 80s, 90s, or even older, but also have several chronic condition or are seriously ill or dying. It is necessary in these circumstances to emphasize that wellness applies to the broader context of the body–mind–spirit interrelationship as well as one's relationships with self, others and all that is sacred to the individual.

When caring for older adults who are ill, nurses have unique opportunities to promote wellness by addressing needs related not only to physical comfort, health and function but also to emotional welfare and spiritual well-being, as in the following examples:

- Helping older adults identify personal strengths that are not dependent on their physical health and functioning (e.g., emotional, interpersonal and spiritual qualities), then identifying strategies that build on or improve these personal characteristics
- Supporting and promoting interpersonal relationships, including the development of new relationships and support resources, that can improve the older adult's health, functioning and quality of life
- Helping older adults identify realistic goals for quality of life, which can be identified in any situation when wellness is conceptualized in the context of the body–mind–spirit interrelationship
- Facilitating the use of new resources and strengthening the support resources that already are in place for older adults, their families and caregivers
- Identifying ways of supporting wellness for families and caregivers of dependent older adults

Health promotion is an essential part of nursing care for *all* older adults, including those who have serious chronic or acute illnesses and even those with life-limiting conditions.

Unfortunately, ageist attitudes of health professionals, older adults and family members can create barriers to health promotion. Although health care professionals may believe that there is little or no benefit from improving health behaviours in later life, this belief is not supported by evidence (Pascucci et al., 2012). Nurses and other health care professionals must be careful not to be influenced by ageist attitudes suggesting that older adults are too old—or too sick or impaired—to learn or change behaviours and to benefit from improved health behaviours.

Personal responsibility for health is an important aspect of wellness for older adults because self-care is essential for achieving optimal health in people who have chronic illnesses. Nurses can help identify ways to assume personal responsibility for health, even when the older adult must depend on others for care. Because personal responsibility for health—with regard to both overall wellness and specific chronic conditions—often requires that a person address health-related behaviours, nurses can apply principles of behaviour change as discussed in Chapter 5.

Self-efficacy is another aspect of health promotion that nurses can influence through health promotion interventions. This may be particularly important for older adults who live alone and need to self-manage care for one or more chronic conditions (Melchior et al., 2013). Nurses have numerous opportunities to address self-efficacy, for example by providing positive feedback about progress older adults are making toward managing a complex medication routine. Challenging ageist attitudes and communicating confidence in an older adult's ability to learn and apply new information is another intervention for improving self-efficacy.

Even when illnesses compromise the health, functioning and quality of life of older adults, nurses can usually identify wellness-oriented outcomes and interventions if they use a holistic perspective. For example, nurses can suggest that older adults who have difficulty engaging in outdoor walking or exercises that require good balance and mobility explore other options in group settings, such as aquatic exercise or tai chi programs. Programs such as these are available in most communities, and they can provide additional positive outcomes, such as increased socialization. Table 27-1 lists examples of Nursing Outcomes Classification (NOC) and Nursing Interventions Classification (NIC) labels that apply to psychosocial, comfort, health promotion and spiritual needs. Nurses can incorporate these outcomes and interventions into care plans in conjunction with addressing the needs that are directly related to the primary health conditions.

HOLISTICALLY CARING FOR OLDER ADULTS WHO ARE ILL: FOCUSING ON CARE AND COMFORT

Care and comfort are core components of all nursing, but they become even more important when a cure is not feasible. Equating aging with inability to cure is not only inaccurate and

TABLE 27-1 Nursing Outcomes and Nursing Interventions Classifications for Promoting Wellness in Older Adults During Illness

Type of Needs	Nursing Outcomes Classification (NOC)	Nursing Interventions Classification (NIC)
Psychosocial needs	Anxiety Level, Coping, Decision Making, Fear Level, Participation in Health Care Decisions, Personal Autonomy, Personal Well-Being, Self-Direction of Care, Self-Esteem, Social Involvement, Stress Level, Suffering Severity	Anxiety Reduction, Counselling, Coping Enhancement, Decision-Making Support, Emotional Support, Patient Rights Protection, Resiliency Promotion, Support Group, Simple Guided Imagery, Touch
Comfort needs	Comfort Level, Pain Control, Pain: Disruptive Effects, Sleep, Symptom Control, Thermoregulation	Pain Management, Positioning, Simple Massage, Temperature Regulation
Health promotion needs	Fall Prevention Behaviour, Health-Promoting Behaviour, Immunization Behaviour, Knowledge: Diet, Disease Process, Health Behaviour, Health Resources, Illness Care, Medication, Nutritional Status, Physical Fitness, Risk Control, Risk Detection, Self-Care Status, Safe Home Environment	Anticipatory Guidance, Environmental Management: Comfort/Safety, Exercise Promotion, Fall Prevention, Health Education, Immunization Management, Nutrition Management, Risk Identification, Self-Responsibility Facilitation, Simple Relaxation Therapy, Skin Surveillance, Sleep Enhancement, Surveillance: Safety
Spiritual needs	Hope, Spiritual Health	Active Listening, Forgiveness Facilitation, Guilt Work Facilitation, Hope Instillation, Presence, Reminiscence Therapy, Religious Ritual Enhancement, Self-Awareness Enhancement, Spiritual Growth Facilitation, Spiritual Support
Quality-of-life needs	Leisure Participation, Personal Well-Being, Quality of Life	Animal-Assisted Therapy, Aromatherapy, Family Involvement Promotion, Humour, Music Therapy

A Student's Perspective

I learned a lot from my interview this past week. The woman I spoke with has gone through a lot of hardships in her life—and is still going through hardships—but she continues to move forward despite setbacks. She is suffering from physical ailments, but her faith in God keeps her head above water. This woman was open to questioning and insightful with her answers. For being a quiet woman, she has a lot of inner strength she pulls on.

For a while after she was diagnosed with multiple sclerosis, she suffered depression and lost five dress sizes unintentionally. She also became fatigued and withdrawn. This was in line with how it has been shown that physical ailments can cause stress in a person and that this in turn can cause other physical ailments. She was fortunate (if it can be called so) to be able to lose the amount of weight that she did and not have severe consequences. If this were to happen to someone of lesser weight, the results may have been more serious. This is a firsthand experience of how depression can cause more than just sad feelings as effects. Once she accepted her fate, she gained back two dress sizes and is holding there, which she is content with.

Her daughter has also been diagnosed with multiple sclerosis, which is a blessing and burden at the same time. Her daughter has been diagnosed at a much younger age and has more serious problems with it, causing her to be periodically hospitalized. It is difficult for a mother to watch her daughter go through this, but it's a blessing that she has someone to share the experience with.

As stated earlier, her faith in God keeps her head above water. She still has her bouts with frustration, but she believes that God only gives what we can handle and that He is always there for her. Her strength is encouraging to the people around her. I know it has given me strength.

Anita M.

potentially damaging to older adults but also a disservice to older adults to focus only on curing disease when treatments are more detrimental or risky than the underlying conditions. Caring for older adults often involves a combination of caring and curing, with the emphasis shifting away from curing and more toward caring as disease conditions progress and accumulate. Moreover, because of the complexity of illness in older adults, rarely is there a clearly defined "turning point" when the focus changes from cure to care. Thus, goals of care may fluctuate or include a combination of curing one condition while simultaneously providing care and comfort for other conditions. Increasingly, geriatricians, gerontologists, ethicists and gerontological nurses are challenged to identify ways to improve *quality* of life for people whose *quantity* of life is limited.

The emergence and expansion of **palliative care** programs in recent years provides a framework for promoting wellness during serious illness, and this model is increasingly used to address the complex and cumulative effects of conditions for which there is no cure. Palliative care is characterized by all the following (Canadian Hospice Palliative Care Association, 2013; Meier, 2011):

- Palliative care is both a philosophy of care and an organized system for achieving best possible quality of life for patients and their family caregivers.
- Recipients of care are patients and their families facing problems associated with a broad range of persistent, life-threatening or recurring conditions that adversely affect their daily functioning or will predictably reduce life expectancy (e.g., frailty, acute stroke, malignancies, dementia and other neurodegenerative conditions).
- Goals are to prevent and relieve suffering, enhance quality of life, optimize function, assist with decision making and provide opportunities for personal growth.

- Ideally, palliative care is initiated early in the course of an illness and at the same time as curative or disease-modifying treatments.

Palliative care services were initially developed as an integral aspect of hospice services, but in Canada, these programs are also now available independently of hospice programs. Currently, palliative care programs are available both within and outside hospice programs and in some Canadian urban hospitals (Canadian Hospice Palliative Care Association, n.d.).

Despite the progress made in implementing palliative care services, only 16% to 30% of Canadians have access to hospice palliative care services (Canadian Hospice Palliative Care Association, 2012). These services are not available in many rural areas within Canada. Furthermore, it is estimated that for those who use palliative care services, they incur about 25% of the costs due to accessing home-based services (such as nurses) and personal services (Canadian Hospice Palliative Care Association, 2012).

In many countries, like Canada, the terms palliative care and hospice are used interchangeably. Within Canada, the term hospice is often used to describe care given in the community, such as a hospice situated within its own building, rather than within a hospital (Canadian Hospice Palliative Care Association, n.d.). Generally, recipients of hospice services must have a prognosis of living for 3 months or less and they agree to forego curative therapies. In contrast, palliative care can be provided at any point during the course of a chronic declining condition and concurrently with life-prolonging therapies or as a main focus of care for as long as the person has the serious illness. Because health care literature commonly associates palliative care with end-of-life care, palliative care is discussed in this chapter in its broader context (i.e., outside of hospice) and it is discussed in Chapter 29 as an integral aspect of hospice care. Figure 27-1 illustrates the continuum of palliative care as described by Passmore (2013) as an ongoing approach to preserving comfort, dignity, autonomy and quality of life for people with dementia.

Palliative care models are based on an interprofessional team approach, with nurses assuming essential roles. They are particularly applicable to holistically addressing the needs of older adults because of the emphasis on quality of life during serious illness. Palliative care emphasizes respect for the individual, sharing caring moments, allowing older adults to direct their own care and honouring the intrinsic worth and uniqueness of each person. Some characteristics of palliative care programs that are particularly pertinent to promoting wellness in older adults include the following:

- A primary focus on ensuring physical comfort and psychosocial and spiritual well-being
- Comprehensive management of distressing symptoms
- Education and support of families and all support people (e.g., friends, volunteers, significant others)
- Consultation, education and support of professional caregivers (e.g., nurses, nursing assistants, primary care providers)

Palliative care also includes nursing care directed toward optimizing function and encouraging physical activity and other healthy lifestyle activities (Canadian Hospice Palliative Care Association, 2013).

Nurses have an important responsibility to recognize the appropriateness of a referral for palliative care and to initiate discussion of this option with older adults and their families. This is particularly important with regard to teaching about the difference between hospice care and palliative

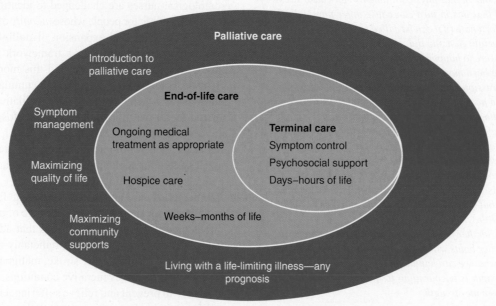

FIGURE 27-1 The palliative care continuum. (Copyright © 2013. Michael J. Passmore. Neuropsychiatric symptoms of dementia: Consent, quality of life, and dignity. *BioMed Research International.* doi:10/1155/2013/230234)

care because this is beginning to change in Canada. When discussing palliative care services with older adults or their families, emphasize that although these services are provided within all hospice programs, they are also available outside of hospice programs, and they have a broader range of admission criteria. For example, the World Health Organization (WHO) suggests that palliative care is applicable early in the course of a life-threatening illness (http://www.who.int/cancer/palliative/definition/en/), and not just at the end of life. When discussing palliative care, the term "supportive care" may be more acceptable and can be used interchangeably with palliative care (Maciasz et al., 2013).

Nurses can use Table 27-2 as a guide to conditions that may prompt the initiation of palliative care discussions, as listed by the Institute for Clinical Systems Improvement (2013) (http://www.icsi.org/asset/K056ab/PalliativeCare.pdf). Many of the indicators, including unintentional weight loss, unstable medical conditions and frequent hospitalizations are readily identified and can serve as "red flags" for initiating a discussion of palliative care services. Because these programs are multidimensional and holistically address needs of older adults, families and caregivers, they are an important component of wellness nursing care in many situations.

It is also important to provide information about palliative care programs that are available independently of hospice programs. A number of Canadian hospitals have nursing and medical staff trained in palliative care. Some hospitals have specialized palliative care units where individuals can have their symptoms managed. Additionally, outpatient palliative care programs may be run through hospitals or through home care (Canadian Virtual Hospice, 2011). Recognize that palliative care services are generally more available in urban areas; individuals living in rural Canada may not have the same palliative care options. Older adults should be counselled to contact the palliative care association within their province (Canadian Virtual Hospice, 2011). For a list of provincial/territorial palliative care associations, please see Online Learning Activity 27-2.

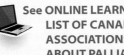

See **ONLINE LEARNING ACTIVITY 27-2: LIST OF CANADIAN PALLIATIVE CARE ASSOCIATIONS FOR INFORMATION ABOUT PALLIATIVE CARE IN SPECIFIC PROVINCES AND TERRITORIES** at http://thepoint.lww.com/Miller7e

APPLYING WELLNESS CONCEPTS IN SPECIFIC PATHOLOGIC OR CHRONIC CONDITIONS

All clinically oriented chapters in this book discuss ways in which nurses promote wellness in relation to usual aspects of functioning and some common chronic conditions of older adults. Although it is beyond the scope of this book to address pathophysiologic conditions in depth, the following sections present information specific to promoting wellness in older adults who have cancer, diabetes or heart failure. These three conditions are discussed within the framework of the Functional Consequences Theory to illustrate the application of wellness concepts within the context of health promotion.

TABLE 27-2 Examples of Conditions and Symptoms That Indicate a Need for Palliative Care

Condition	Indicators of the Need for Palliative Care
Cancer	• Pain, dyspnea, anorexia and any other symptom that is not well controlled • When condition is likely incurable, even while person is undergoing treatment (e.g., radiation, chemotherapy) • When disease progresses even with treatment • When significant care is required to meet basic needs
Dementia	• Significant behavioural problems that are distressful to the person with dementia or to caregivers • Nutritional concerns (e.g., weight loss, eating/feeding limitations, risk for choking) • Frequent hospitalizations and/or unstable medical conditions • Concomitant medical conditions (e.g., heart failure, pneumonia) • When decisions about medical care need to be made • Progression to late-stage dementia
Heart failure	• Progression to late-stage heart failure despite optimal medical management • Dyspnea, pain or other symptoms that are unresponsive to treatment • The need for frequent medical care or hospitalizations • Significant decline in functioning
Chronic obstructive pulmonary disease (COPD)	• Orthopnea, dyspnea, difficulty managing symptoms related to breathing • Substantial weight loss • Anxiety, fear of death
Parkinson disease	• Significant decline in functioning • Nutritional concerns, especially involving swallowing difficulties and weight loss

Sources: Brown, M. A., Sampson, E. L., Jones, L., et al. (2013). Prognostic indicators of 6-month mortality in elderly people with advanced dementia: A systematic review. *Palliative Medicine, 27*(5), 389–400; Miyasaki, J. M. (2013). Palliative care in Parkinson's disease. *Current Neurology and Neuroscience Reports, 13*(8), 367–372; Parikh, R. B., Kirch, R. A., Smith, T. J., et al. (2013). Early specialty palliative care: Translating data in oncology into practice. *New England Journal of Medicine, 369*(24), 2347–2351; Passmore, 2013; Thoonsen, B., Engels, Y., van Rijswijk, E., et al. (2012). Early identification of palliative care patients in general practice. *British Journal of General Practice, 62*(602), e625–e631.

Promoting Wellness for Older Adults With Cancer

Because cancer requires the passage of time before it reaches the stage of being a diagnosable disease, the increasing incidence of cancer is associated with increased age. Eighty-eight percent of Canadians who develop cancer are above 50 years of age (Canadian Cancer Society's Advisory Committee on Cancer Statistics, 2013). Twenty-eight percent of new diagnoses of cancer occur in individuals 60 to 69 years of age and 43% of new diagnoses occur in seniors 70 years of age and older. The overall 5-year survival rate for those diagnosed with cancer is 63%; however, this varies greatly depending upon the type of cancer. For instance, thyroid cancer has a 98% 5-year survival rate, but pancreatic cancer has only an 8% 5-year survival rate. Breast, colon and prostate cancers are the most common diagnoses among cancer survivors (Canadian Cancer Society's Advisory Committee on Cancer Statistics, 2013). Studies indicate that older cancer patients are diagnosed at a later stage and are at risk for inadequate treatment (Cataldo et al., 2013; Clough-Gorr et al., 2013).

Decisions about screening and treatment of cancer in older adults can be complicated for several reasons. First, older adults have been underrepresented in clinical trials, so there are fewer evidence-based guidelines about recommendations. Second, they are likely to have coexisting conditions that increase their susceptibility to adverse effects of treatments. Third, decisions about screening and treatment may be influenced by ageism. Current emphasis is on basing decisions not on chronologic age alone but on a multidimensional assessment that considers all the following: effects of normal age-related changes, physical and psychosocial health and functioning, effects of accumulated chronic conditions, life expectancy, potential benefits versus harms, and the individual's values and preferences (Eckstrom et al., 2013; Overcash, 2012).

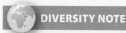 **DIVERSITY NOTE**

Survival rates following a breast cancer diagnosis are lower among First Nations women in Ontario than their white counterparts. This is believed to be due to breast cancer being diagnosed at a later stage in First Nations women (Ontario Cancer Facts, 2010).

Nursing Assessment

From a health promotion perspective, nurses assess older adults to identify their knowledge and attitudes about screening for the types of cancer most likely to develop. For example, skin cancer is one of the most commonly occurring types and it can be readily detected through self-examination. Thus, it is important to assess the older adult's knowledge about skin changes, as discussed in Chapter 23. Nurses also assess older adult's knowledge about interventions for preventing cancer because this provides a base for identifying health promotion goals. When caring for an older adult who has cancer, nurses promote wellness by identifying psychosocial aspects, such as the meaning of cancer for the individual, coping strengths and supports and the person's ability to participate in decisions about screening and care.

Wellness Nursing Diagnoses and Wellness Outcomes

Readiness for Enhanced Knowledge is a wellness nursing diagnosis applicable for older adults who are interested in learning about screening and prevention of cancer. For older adults who have been diagnosed with cancer, this diagnosis would be applicable for those who are interested in learning more about holistically oriented resources such as palliative care or hospice services.

Two Nursing Outcomes Classifications (NOC) applicable to prevention and early detection of cancer are Health-Promoting Behaviour and Knowledge: Health Behaviour. Outcomes that are pertinent to holistically caring for older adults with cancer include Comfort, Coping and Quality of Life.

Nursing Interventions

Cancer is an important focus of health promotion efforts because about one third of the cases could be prevented through healthy lifestyle choices, such as exercise, eating healthy and not smoking (Canadian Cancer Society's Advisory Committee on Cancer Statistics, 2013). Health promotion interventions focus on teaching older adults about primary prevention and early detection of cancer, as summarized in Box 27-1. Nurses can encourage older adults and surrogate decision makers to discuss cancer detection and treatment options with their primary care providers with an emphasis on quality of life.

 Box 27-1 Health Promotion Interventions Related to Cancer and Older Adults

Teaching About Primary Prevention

- Stop smoking (if applicable).
- Avoid secondhand smoke.
- Maintain ideal body weight.
- Consume at least five servings of fresh fruit and vegetables and 26 to 35 g of fibre daily (Canadian Diabetes Association).
- Limit intake of fats, red meats and fried foods.
- Avoid excessive exposure to sunlight.
- Avoid excessive alcohol consumption.

Screening Recommendations in Canada by the Canadian Task Force on Preventative Health Care (http://canadataskforce.ca/2011/11)

- Annual or biennial fecal occult blood test or fecal immuno-chemical test (FIT) for those who do not have increased risk of colorectal cancer.
- Flexible sigmoidoscopy may or may not be included with the fecal occult blood test or the fecal immunochemical test.
- Guidelines for prostate-specific antigen and rectal digital examination for men not provided by Canadian Task Force on Preventative Health Care, but men are encouraged to discuss these tests with their physicians.
- Annual or biennial mammogram for women between the ages of 50 and 74 years, and Pap test every 3 years for women up to age 69 if they have had three prior normal Pap tests.
- Screening for hypertension when visiting primary health care provider.

For older adults already diagnosed with cancer, nurses address all aspects of pain and comfort (see Chapter 28). Also, because people with cancer sometimes use complementary and alternative therapies, nurses can encourage them to discuss these therapies with their primary care practitioner and obtain information from reliable sources (e.g., the Canadian Cancer Society). It is important to discuss the use of complementary or alternative medicines as some are not recommended when undergoing treatment (Canadian Cancer Society, 2014). In addition, encourage the use of self-care practices, such as yoga, prayer and meditation, to alleviate symptoms associated with cancer and cancer treatments. Additional wellness-oriented nursing interventions include offering hope, support and encouragement and considering referrals for hospice and palliative care. Online Learning Activity 27-3 provides additional information about nursing assessment and interventions related to cancer in older adults.

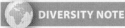

> **See ONLINE LEARNING ACTIVITY 27-3:**
> **RESOURCES FOR ADDITIONAL INFORMATION**
> **ABOUT NURSING ASSESSMENT AND**
> **INTERVENTIONS RELATED TO CANCER**
> at http://thepoint.lww.com/Miller7e

> **Wellness Opportunity**
>
> Nurses can promote personal responsibility for wellness by teaching older adults about screening and preventive actions they can take.

Promoting Wellness for Older Adults With Diabetes Mellitus

Diabetes mellitus is one of the most common chronic conditions in older adults, with a prevalence of 24.1% in seniors between 70 and 74 years of age, and just above 25% in those between the ages of 75 and 79 years of age (Public Health Agency of Canada, 2011). Age-related changes that increase the risk for developing diabetes include declining beta cell function and increased insulin resistance (glucose intolerance). In addition to age-related changes, risk factors for diabetes include obesity, hypertension, family history, physical inactivity, high levels of triglycerides and low levels of high-density lipoproteins. Serious consequences of diabetes include renal failure, retinopathy, neuropathy, cognitive decline, lower extremity amputations and cardiovascular diseases, including stroke, hypertension, myocardial infarction and coronary artery disease. Additional serious consequences in older adults include higher mortality, decreased functional status and increased risk of residing in a long-term care facility (Kirkman et al., 2012).

> **DIVERSITY NOTE**
>
> Between 2008 and 2010, age-adjusted rates of diagnosed diabetes among First Nations individuals was 17.2% for those living on a reserve, 10.3% for First Nations persons living off reserve and 7.3% for Metis. These rates are significantly higher than the 5% rate of diabetes among non-Aboriginal individuals (Public Health Agency of Canada, 2011).

Disease management and nursing care related to diabetes are complicated by the common occurrence of concomitant conditions in older adults. For example, infections can affect the optimal doses of insulin and hypoglycemic agents, and chronic arthritis or periodic flare-ups of gout are likely to affect the older adult's level of activity. Another complicating factor is that older adults are likely to be taking medications (e.g., prednisone) that can lead to disease instability. Self-management of diabetes is affected by conditions that occur more commonly in older adults (e.g., dementia, functional limitations) and by situational circumstances, such as dependence on others or financial constraints that affect ability to purchase medications and appropriate foods.

Nursing Assessment

Although nurses are not expected to diagnose diabetes, they are expected to know about variations in diagnostic indicators that are specific to older adults. For example, the renal threshold for glucose increases in older adults, so glycosuria may not be an accurate indicator. The Canadian Diabetes Association (2013) states that any one of the following conditions is a diagnostic indicator for diabetes:

- Glycoated hemoglobin (HbA_{1c}) of 6.5% or more
- Fasting plasma glucose of 7.0 mmol/L or greater (8-hour fast)
- 2-hour blood glucose value during oral glucose tolerance test greater than or equal to 11.1 mmol/L with a glucose load of 75 g

The HbA_{1c} is routinely used to monitor glucose control in people with diabetes over the previous months, with the target goal being a level less than 7% to reduce microvascular and neuropathic complications. Although a target goal of 7% to 7.5% is appropriate for healthy older adults, the Canadian Diabetes Association (2013) recommends that less stringent targets may be safer and more appropriate for older adults who are frail or who have dementia. The recommended glycemic target is less than 8.5% for frail older adults (Canadian Diabetes Association, 2013).

In addition to the usual nursing assessment parameters for diabetes, a holistic nursing approach for older adults addresses related issues, such as the meaning of the condition, the influence of ageist attitudes that affect management and socioeconomic and cultural influences. Box 27-2 summarizes some questions that are more specific to assessment of diabetes in older adults from a wellness perspective.

Wellness Nursing Diagnoses and Wellness Outcomes

Readiness for Enhanced Knowledge is a wellness nursing diagnosis applicable for older adults who are interested in learning about diabetes, particularly with regard to improved understanding of how this condition affects their health. Nurses can use the wellness nursing diagnosis of Readiness for Enhanced Self-care when they care for older adults who are interested in improving personal responsibility for management of their condition, including preventing complications.

Box 27-2 Assessment Guidelines for Older Adults With Diabetes

Considerations About the Meaning of Diabetes

- What terminology is appropriate for discussing the condition (e.g., older adults may refer to diabetes as "sugar")?
- What is the person's understanding of diabetes?

Considerations for Disease Management

- What is the person's understanding of personal responsibility for managing diabetes?
- Socioeconomic influences: Who does grocery shopping and meal preparation? What foods are included in the usual meal pattern? What is the usual "budget" for food? Where does the person eat meals?
- What cultural factors affect health beliefs, disease management, food preparation, eating patterns and health-related behaviours, such as exercise?
- What concomitant conditions affect the older adult's self-care abilities?

Considerations Regarding the Influence of Ageist Attitudes

- Do ageist attitudes (of the older adult, caregiver or health care professionals) interfere with setting wellness-oriented goals? (e.g., "I've been eating doughnuts for breakfast all my life, why should I worry about that now at my age?")
- Does the older adult (or do others) inaccurately associate a sense of hopelessness with his or her condition because of advanced age? (e.g., "At my age, I can't do anything about my sugar levels.")

Nursing Outcomes Classification (NOC) terms that would be pertinent to promoting wellness in older adults with diabetes include Diabetes Self-management, Blood Glucose Level, Health-Promoting Behaviour, Knowledge: Diabetes Management and Self-care Status.

Nursing Interventions

Teaching about self-management is the cornerstone of diabetes care, and group programs are particularly effective for older adults (Tshiananga et al., 2012). Benefits of group interventions for older adults with diabetes include improvements in glycemic control, self-efficacy, emotional coping, quality of life, and decreased levels of distress and depressive symptoms (Beverly et al., 2013). Thus, in addition to individual teaching about diabetes, a primary nursing responsibility is facilitating referrals for group educational programs.

When caring for older adults with diabetes, nurses often need to address conditions that make self-management more difficult, such as involving and teaching caregivers and compensating for memory deficits. Older adults with diabetes may benefit from referrals for community-based services, including home-delivered meals, assistance with grocery shopping or meal preparation, participation in group meal programs, transportation to appointments, and assistance with medication management or glucose monitoring. An intervention for older adults with limited mobility is to consider referrals for aquatherapy classes as a way of engaging

in safe and enjoyable physical activity. Online Learning Activity 27-4 provides links to health promotion information about diabetes self-management, including materials for culturally diverse groups.

See **ONLINE LEARNING ACTIVITY 27-4: RESOURCES FOR ADDITIONAL INFORMATION ABOUT HEALTH PROMOTION FOR OLDER ADULTS WITH DIABETES** at http://thepoint.lww.com/Miller7e

Wellness Opportunity

Nurses can teach all older adults about actions they can take to lessen the likelihood of developing diabetes, as well as what they can do to reduce complications from this disease by accessing the Canadian Diabetes Association website (www.diabetes.ca).

Promoting Wellness for Older Adults With Heart Failure

Heart failure is the most common reason for hospitalization in Canadians above the age of 65 years (Canadian Heart Failure Network, n.d.). In addition to recurrent hospitalizations, other common consequences of heart failure in older adults include the following:

- Increased likelihood for developing arrhythmias, which can threaten life or cause syncopal episodes
- Increased risk for hypotension and falls because of compromised cardiovascular function and adverse medication effects
- Increased risk for hospital-acquired iatrogenic conditions, such as *Clostridium difficile* infection
- Increased risk for drug interactions and adverse medication effects, especially if the older adult has concomitant conditions and requires several types of medications
- High incidence of sleep disorders
- Shorter life expectancy

Because of consequences such as these—which make it a major source of chronic disability, increased mortality and impaired quality of life—heart failure in older adults has emerged as a major focus of health promotion interventions.

DIVERSITY NOTE

Canadian men are more likely to be referred to heart failure clinics than are Canadian women. Also, younger adults are more likely to be referred than their older counterparts (Feldman et al., 2013).

Nursing Assessment

Nurses assess for signs and symptoms of heart failure in older adults using the same assessment techniques that apply to adults of any age. However, older adults are more likely to have concomitant conditions that can affect the assessment. For example, because older adults with mobility limitations may not exert themselves enough to experience dyspnea, nurses need to consider other limiting factors when they assess the effects of heart failure on respirations. It is important to ask very direct questions about specific symptoms because early symptoms may be attributed to aging or chronic conditions.

Another assessment consideration is that older adults with heart failure are likely to have some degree of chronic renal failure, which often fluctuates within an abnormal range. Thus, nurses need to identify and document the older adult's usual indicators of renal function (i.e., ranges of blood urea nitrogen and creatinine that are typical for that individual). It is also important to assess for electrolyte imbalances and adverse medication effects, which are commonly associated with diminished renal function, as discussed in Chapter 8. This is especially important with regard to medications, such as digoxin that have a narrow therapeutic range.

In addition to assessing signs and symptoms of heart failure, nurses assess risk factors, paying particular attention to those that can be addressed through health promotion interventions. Factors that increase the risk for heart failure include hypertension, coronary artery disease, myocardial infarction, family history of heart failure, hyperthyroidism, diabetes, smoking and obesity. Even though older adults may have long-term patterns of behaviour that affect disease management (e.g., smoking, inadequate physical activity, high-sodium diets), nurses need to assess attitudes about changing these behaviours so that they can address this in health promotion teaching. Additional wellness-focused assessment considerations that are important for older adults who have heart failure are outlined in Box 27-3.

Box 27-3 Assessment Guidelines for Older Adults With Heart Failure

Considerations About the Meaning of Heart Failure

- What is the older adult's understanding of heart failure?
- What terminology is appropriate for discussing the condition? Does the term failure cause anxiety or fear?
- What personal experiences or those of significant others are influencing the older adult's response to cardiovascular disease? (e.g., How life-threatening does the person perceive this to be?)

Considerations Regarding the Influence of Ageist Attitudes

- Do ageist attitudes interfere with health promotion interventions? (e.g., Do health care providers avoid teaching about smoking cessation because they think the person is too old to quit or to benefit from quitting?)

Considerations Regarding Disease Management

- Does the older adult have questions or fears about engaging in therapeutic or enjoyable activities (e.g., exercise, swimming, sexual relationships)? If so, would he or she benefit from health education about this?
- Do socioeconomic factors affect disease management (e.g., limited income that interferes with ability to purchase needed medications or healthy foods)?

Wellness Nursing Diagnoses and Wellness Outcomes

Nurses can use the wellness nursing diagnosis of Readiness for Enhanced Therapeutic Regimen Management to promote increased personal responsibility for management of heart failure and prevention of hospitalizations and other complications. The wellness nursing diagnosis of Readiness for Enhanced Fluid Balance might be applicable when older adults with heart failure are interested in learning about actions they can take to improve and maintain fluid and electrolyte balance.

Outcomes that are pertinent to promoting wellness in older adults with heart failure include Cardiac Disease Self-Management, Energy Conservation, Health-Promoting Behaviour and Knowledge: Cardiac Disease Management.

Nursing Interventions

Wellness-oriented care plans for older adults with heart failure focus on teaching about actions the person can take to achieve the best possible level of functioning and quality of life despite the chronic condition. For example, nurses can teach older adults about planning appropriate rest and energy-management techniques to achieve optimum quality of life with limited energy. Teaching about symptom recognition is an important aspect of self-care because older adults may not associate signs and symptoms with heart failure and this may be a factor in unnecessary hospital admissions (Lam & Smeltzer, 2013). From a holistic perspective, nurses also need to address psychosocial consequences associated with heart failure, such as fear, anxiety, loneliness and depression (discussed in Chapters 12, 13 and 15). Another consideration is that people with heart failure often experience pain, dyspnea and other distressing symptoms (Light-McGroary & Goodlin, 2013; Wilson & McMillan, 2013). In these situations, a referral for palliative care may be appropriate (Pastor & Moore, 2013). Online Learning Activity 27-5 provides links to an article about palliative care for heart failure and other additional resources about nursing interventions for heart failure.

See ONLINE LEARNING ACTIVITY 27-5: ARTICLE ABOUT PALLIATIVE CARE FOR HEART FAILURE AND ADDITIONAL RESOURCES RELATED TO NURSING ASSESSMENT AND MANAGEMENT OF OLDER ADULTS WITH HEART FAILURE at http://thepoint.lww.com/Miller7e

Wellness Opportunity

Because stress-reduction activities are especially important when older adults have chronic conditions, such as heart failure, nurses can suggest relaxation and health promotion activities such as deep breathing, meditation, prayer and guided imagery.

ADDRESSING NEEDS OF FAMILIES AND CAREGIVERS

During periods of illness—whether acute, chronic or declining—importance of relationships increases in proportion to the need not only for physical care but also for emotional and spiritual care. Thus, when nurses care for older adults during illness, families and caregivers are an integral focus of care because the multifaceted needs of dependent older adults cannot be met without a strong support system. Despite the increasing availability of formal services for older adults in Canada, family caregivers still provide a significant number of hours of care every week to older adults with limitations in their activities of daily living. In fact, one in ten caregivers in Canada spends 30 hours a week or more in providing supportive care (Sinha, 2013). Providing support for older adults can be stressful for caregivers (see Box 27-4).

In most health care settings, the extent to which nurses can address caregiver needs is limited by time constraints and the need to focus on the immediate and complex needs of the older adult. Despite these limitations, however, nurses can use the Modified Caregiver Strain Index (Fig. 27-2) to identify families who may benefit from more in-depth assessment and follow-up. Box 27-5 summarizes evidence-based information about nursing assessment and interventions related to family caregiving. Table 27-3 lists NOC and NIC terms that are pertinent to promoting wellness for caregivers. Supplemental materials related to this topic, including resources for family caregivers, are provided in Online Learning Activity 27-6.

Box 27-4 Evidence-Informed Nursing Practice

Background: Canadians spend significant effort and time in caring for family members, whether they be children, spouses, grandparents or parents.

Question: What are the consequences of caregiving upon family members caring for a loved one?

Method: As part of the General Social Survey, Canadians were asked about whether they provide caregiving to a family member, who that family member is and what the psychological, physical and financial effects of caregiving are.

Findings: Of the individuals (15 years of age and older) who reported to be caregivers, 27% provided care to their mothers, 11% to their fathers, 13% to a grandparent and 8% to their spouses. For caregivers who were 45 to 65 years of age, almost 50% provided care to a parent. Among those caring for a parent, 30% reported "aging" or "frailty" as reasons for caregiving. Others noted cardiovascular disease (12%), cancer (11%) and dementia (7%). Although those caring for a parent reported less psychological distress than those caring for a child, 21% of caregivers supporting a parent admitted to feeling depressed and 34% caring for spouses experienced depression.

Implications for Nursing Practice: Nurses need to be aware that the stress of caregiving is partly related to the relationship between those needing care and those providing support (e.g., adult child providing care to an aging parent or aging adult supporting ailing spouse). Depression among caregivers is common; nurses should be aware of the supports for caregivers within their communities.

Source: Turcotte, M. (2013). *Statistics Canada—Family caregiving: What are the consequences?* (Catalogue no. 75-006-X). Ottawa, ON: Statistics Canada.

See ONLINE LEARNING ACTIVITY 27-6: **ADDITIONAL INFORMATION ABOUT FAMILY CAREGIVING AND LINKS TO RESOURCES FOR CAREGIVERS** at http://thepoint.lww.com/Miller7e

Box 27-5 Evidence-Based Practice: Family Caregiving

Statement of the Problem

- More than 80% of the care for dependent older adults is provided by family.
- Family caregivers are a key link in providing safe and effective transitional care as older adults move across care settings.
- Caregiving activities include assistance with daily activities, illness-related care (medication management, assessing and addressing symptoms, carrying out treatments) and care management activities (advocacy, accessing and coordinating services, navigating health care and social service systems).
- Caregivers typically experience higher levels of stress and depression and lower levels of physical health and subjective well-being.
- Increased caregiver strain is associated with lack of preparedness for the role, caring for someone with dementia and poor quality relationships between caregiver and care recipient.

Parameters of Nursing Assessment

- Caregiving context: roles and responsibilities, duration of caregiving, physical environment, financial status, potential resources, cultural factors
- Caregiver's perception of health and functional status of care recipient, including functional and cognitive limitations

- Caregiver preparedness: skills, knowledge
- Quality of relationship between caregiver and care recipient
- Indicators of problems with care: unhealthy environment, inappropriate financial management
- Caregiver's health status: self-rated health, physical and mental health, rewards of caregiving

Recommended Assessment Tool

- Modified Caregiver Strain Index (see Fig. 27-2)

Recommendations for Interventions

- Form a partnership with caregivers and use an interprofessional approach when working with caregivers.
- Identify caregivers' needs, issues and concerns and assist caregivers in developing a plan to address these.
- During hospitalizations, invite family caregivers to participate in care, on the basis of an assessment of family preference.
- Help the caregiver identify strengths in the caregiving situation.
- Assist the caregiver in finding and using resources.

Source: Messecar, D. C. (2012). Family caregiving. In E. Capezuti, D. Zwicker, M. Mezey, et al. (Eds.), *Evidence-based geriatric nursing protocols for best practice* (4th ed., pp. 469–499). New York, NY: Springer.

Directions: Here is a list of things that other caregivers have found to be difficult. Please put a checkmark in the columns that apply to you. We have included some examples that are common caregiver experiences to help you think about each item. Your situation may be slightly different, but the item could still apply.

	Yes, On a Regular Basis = 2	Yes, Sometimes = 1	No = 0
My sleep is disturbed (For example: the person I care for is in and out of bed or wanders around at night)			
Caregiving is inconvenient (For example: helping takes so much time or it's a long drive over to help)			
Caregiving is a physical strain (For example: lifting in or out of a chair; effort or concentration is required)			
Caregiving is confining (For example: helping restricts free time or I cannot go visiting)			
There have been family adjustments (For example: helping has disrupted my routine; there is no privacy)			
There have been changes in personal plans (For example: I had to turn down a job; I could not go on a vacation)			
There have been other demands on my time (For example: other family members need me)			
There have been emotional adjustments (For example: severe arguments about caregiving)			
Some behavior is upsetting (For example: incontinence; the person cared for has trouble remembering things; or the person I care for accuses people of taking things)			
It is upsetting to find the person I care for has changed so much from his/her former self (For example: he/she is a different person than he/she used to be)			
There have been work adjustments (For example: I have to take time off for caregiving duties)			
Caregiving is a financial strain			
I feel completely overwhelmed (For example: I worry about the person I care for; I have concerns about how I will manage)			

[Sum responses for "Yes, on a regular basis" (2 pts each) and "yes, sometimes" (1 pt each)]   Total Score =

FIGURE 27-2 Modified Caregiver Strain Index. (From Thornton, M., & Travis, S. S. [2003]. Analysis of the reliability of the Modified Caregiver Strain Index. *The Journal of Gerontology, Series B, Psychological Sciences and Social Sciences, 58*[2], p. S129. Copyright © The Gerontological Society of America. Reproduced by permission of the publisher.)

TABLE 27-3 Nursing Outcomes and Nursing Interventions Classifications for Promoting Wellness in Caregivers

Type of Needs	Nursing Outcomes Classification (NOC)	Nursing Interventions Classification (NIC)
Needs related to caregiver role	Caregiver Adaptation to Patient Institutionalization, Caregiver Emotional Health, Caregiver Endurance Potential, Caregiver Home Care Readiness, Caregiver Lifestyle Disruption, Caregiver–Patient Relationship, Caregiver Performance: Direct/Indirect Care, Caregiver Physical Health, Caregiver Stressors, Caregiver Well-Being	Caregiver Support, Case Management, Counselling, Energy Management, Family Support, Family Integrity Promotion, Resiliency Promotion, Role Enhancement, Self-Awareness Enhancement, Support Group
Needs related to using resources and managing care	Information Processing, Knowledge: Health Resources, Participation in Health Care Decisions, Role Performance	Decision-Making Support, Health Education, Health System Guidance, Referral, Respite Care, Support System Enhancement, Teaching: Individual, Telephone Consultation
Psychosocial needs	Anxiety Level, Coping, Decision Making, Depression Level, Family Coping, Family Resiliency, Fear Level, Grief Resolution, Loneliness Severity, Self-Esteem, Stress Level	Active Listening, Anticipatory Guidance, Anxiety Reduction, Cognitive Restructuring, Coping Enhancement, Emotional Support, Grief Work Facilitation, Mood Management, Presence, Simple Guided Imagery
Spiritual and quality-of-life needs	Hope, Leisure Participation, Quality of Life, Sleep, Social Involvement, Social Support, Spiritual Health	Forgiveness Facilitation, Guilt Work Facilitation, Hope Instillation, Humour, Sleep Enhancement, Spiritual Support

Chapter Highlights

Characteristics of Illness in Older Adults

- Presence of many interacting conditions and factors (e.g., acute illness, chronic conditions, psychosocial factors, environmental conditions, age-related changes, medication effects)
- Complexity of interpreting signs and symptoms (e.g., vague or atypical manifestations)
- Far-reaching consequences (e.g., loss of independence due to fractured hip)
- Cumulative effects of aging and illness making adaptation difficult
- Older adults likely experiencing a "yo-yoing" pattern of health, with gradually diminishing resiliency

Connecting the Concepts of Wellness, Aging and Illness

- A holistic perspective enables nurses to identify ways of promoting wellness by addressing needs related to physical health and functioning and emotional and spiritual well-being.
- An important aspect of wellness is promoting personal responsibility for health through self-care measures and management of chronic conditions.
- Nurses challenge ageist attitudes and provide health education to foster behaviour change when appropriate.
- Many NIC and NOC terms are applicable in care plans that address psychosocial, comfort, health promotion and spiritual needs (Table 27-1).

Holistically Caring for Older Adults Who Are Ill: Focusing on Caring and Comforting

- Palliative care is a holistic approach to caring for patients with advanced progressive illnesses through prevention,

assessment and treatment of pain and other physical, psychosocial and spiritual problems.
- Nurses have important roles in suggesting referrals for palliative care and talking with older adults and their families about the scope of these services.

Applying Wellness Concepts in Specific Pathologic or Chronic Conditions

Promoting Wellness for Older Adults With Cancer

- Older adults are disproportionately affected by cancer, less likely to be screened for cancer and diagnosed at a later stage.
- From a health promotion perspective, nurses assess older adults to identify their knowledge and attitudes about screening for the types of cancer that they are most likely to develop.
- Nurses holistically address the needs of older adults already diagnosed with cancer.
- Nurses can teach older adults about primary prevention interventions and about screening recommendations (Box 27-1).

Promoting Wellness for Older Adults With Diabetes

- Diabetes is common among older adults, with the highest prevalence among First Nations peoples and individuals from South and Southeast Asia.
- Disease management and nursing care related to diabetes are complicated by the common occurrence of concomitant conditions and by the increased vulnerability of older adults to complications.
- In addition to usual assessment parameters, nurses identify ageist attitudes and the meaning of diabetes (Box 27-2).
- Care plans for older adults with diabetes include all the usual interventions and additional teaching points (e.g., teaching caregivers, referring for community-based

services, appropriate ways of engaging in physical activity).

Promoting Wellness for Older Adults With Heart Failure

- Heart failure is the most common reason for hospitalization among Canadians 65 years of age and older. However, there are wellness behaviours that older adults can engage in to improve their health and thus decrease the number of hospitalizations.
- In addition to assessing all the usual signs and symptoms of heart failure, nurses assess effects of other conditions, risk factors that can be addressed through health promotion and other aspects that are specific to older adults (e.g., the effects of ageist attitudes).
- In addition to all the usual teaching points, wellness-oriented care plans focus on teaching about actions the person can take to achieve the best possible level of functioning and quality of life, despite the effects of heart failure.

Addressing Needs of Families and Caregivers

- Nurses promote caregiver well-being by identifying and addressing issues related to **caregiver burden** (Box 27-5).
- Many NIC and NOC terms are applicable in care plans that address caregivers with regard to role performance, use of resources and management of care, and psychosocial, spiritual and quality-of-life needs (Table 27-2).

Critical Thinking Exercises

1. Identify an older person (in your personal life or clinical experience) who has recently been hospitalized and address the following in relation to that person:
   - How many different conditions (e.g., acute and chronic illness, functional limitations, support resources, psychosocial factors, environmental factors) affected how the person was able to adapt to the hospitalization?
   - How did these factors affect the outcome for the person (e.g., longer hospitalization, increased dependency on others, discharge plans)?
   - Select two NOC and NIC terms from Table 27-1 that you could apply to a care plan to promote wellness for this person.

2. Think about your expectations for older adults who are affected by multiple interacting conditions and identify any ageist attitudes or assumptions that are likely to affect your care.

3. Find information about local resources for palliative care and prepare yourself to teach older adults and their families about this service.

4. Identify a situation in your personal life or clinical experience that requires caregiving assistance from a family member at least once weekly and address the following in relation to this situation:
   - What benefits (rewards) and stresses are caregivers likely to experience?

- Select two NOC and NIC terms from Table 27-2 that you could apply to a care plan to address the needs of the caregiver.

 For more information about topics discussed in this chapter, be sure to check out the interactive Online Learning Activities and other helpful resources at http://thepoint.lww.com/Miller7e

REFERENCES

American Geriatrics Society. (2012). Guiding principles for care of older adults with multimorbidity: An approach for clinicians. *Journal of the American Geriatrics Society, 60*(10), E1–E25. doi:10.1111/j.1532-5415.2012.04188.x

Bagshaw, S. M., & McDermid, R. C. (2013). The role of frailty in outcomes from critical illness. *Current Opinions in Critical Care, 19*(5), 496–503.

Beverly, E. A., Fitzgerald, S., Sitnikov, L., et al. (2013). Do older adults aged 60–75 years benefit from diabetes behavioral interventions? *Diabetes Care, 36*(6), 1501–1506.

Canadian Cancer Society. (2014). *Complementary and alternative therapies.* Retrieved from http://www.cancer.ca/en/cancer-information/diagnosis-and-treatment/complementary-therapies/?region=on

Canadian Cancer Society's Advisory Committee on Cancer Statistics. (2013). *Canadian cancer statistics 2013.* Toronto, ON: Canadian Cancer Society.

Canadian Diabetes Association. (2013). 2013 *Clinical practice guidelines for the prevention and management of diabetes in Canada.* Retrieved from https://www.diabetes.ca/for-professionals

Canadian Heart Failure Network. (n.d.). *Rationale for heart failure clinics.* Retrieved from http://www.chfn.ca/clinic-resource-manual/rationale-for-hf-clinics

Canadian Hospice Palliative Care Association. (2012). *Fact sheet: Hospice palliative care in Canada.* Retrieved from http://www.chpca.net/media/7622/fact_sheet_hpc_in_canada_may_2012_final.pdf

Canadian Hospice Palliative Care Association. (2013). *A model to guide hospice palliative care:* Based on national principles and norms of practice. Ottawa, Ontario: Author.

Canadian Hospice Palliative Care Association. (n.d.). *FAQS: What is palliative care?* Retrieved from http://www.chpca.net/family-caregivers/faqs.aspx

Canadian Virtual Hospice. (2011). *What is palliative care?* Retrieved from http://www.virtualhospice.ca

Cataldo, J. K., Paul, S., Cooper, B., et al. (2013). Differences in the symptom experience of older versus younger oncology outpatients: A cross-sectional study. *BioMed Central Cancer, 13*, 6. Retrieved from www.biomedcentral.com/1471-2407/13/6

CIHR Institute of Aging. (2012). *Living longer, living better: Canadian Institutes of Health Research Institute of Aging 2013–2018 strategic plan.* Retrieved from http://www.cihr-irsc.gc.ca/e/documents/IA_Strategic_Plan_En_v5jul13.pdf

Clough-Gorr, K. M., Noti, L., Brauchli, P., et al. (2013). The SAKK cancer-specific geriatric assessment (C-SGA): A pilot study of a brief tool for clinical decision-making in older cancer patients. *BioMed Central Medical Informatics & Decision Making, 13*, 93. Retrieved from www.biomedcentral.com/1472-6947/14/93

Drubbel, I., de Wit, N. J., Bleijenberg, N., et al. (2013). Predictions of adverse health outcomes in older people using a frailty index based on routine primary care data. *Journals of Gerontology: Medical Sciences, 68*(5), 301–308.

Eckstrom, E., Feeny, D. H., Walter, L. C., et al. (2013). Individualizing cancer screening in older adults: A narrative review and framework for future research. *Journal of General Internal Medicine, 28*(2), 292–298.

Feldman, D. E., Huynh, T., Des Lauriers, J., et al. (2013). Gender and other disparities in referral to specialized heart failure clinics following emergency department visits. *Journal of Women's Health, 22*(6), 526–531. doi:10.1089/jwh.2012.4107

Fried, L. P., Tangen, C. M., Walston, J., et al. (2001). Frailty in older adults: Evidence for a phenotype. *Journals of Gerontology: Medical Sciences, 56*(3), M146–M156.

Kane, R. L., Shamliyan, T., Talley, K., et al. (2012). The association between geriatric syndromes and survival. *Journal of the American Geriatrics Society, 60*(5), 896–906.

Kirkman, M. S., Briscoe, V. J., Clark, N., et al. (2012). Diabetes in older adults: A consensus report. *Journal of the American Geriatrics Society, 60*(12), 2342–2356. doi:10.1111/jgs.12035

Koller, K., & Rockwood, K. (2013). Frailty in older adults: Implications for end-of-life care. *Cleveland Clinic Journal of Medicine, 80*(3), 168–174.

Lam, C., & Smeltzer, S. C. (2013). Patterns of symptoms recognition, interpretation, and response in heart failure patients. *Journal of Cardiovascular Nursing, 28*(4), 348–459.

Light-McGroary, K., & Goodlin, S. J. (2013). The challenges of understanding and managing pain in the heart failure patient. *Current Opinion in Supportive and Palliative Care, 7*(1), 14–20.

Maciasz, R. M., Arnold, R. M., Chu, E., et al. (2013). Does it matter what you call it: A randomized trial of language used to describe palliative care services. *Supportive Care for Cancer, 21*(12), 3411–3419.

Meier, D. E. (2011). Increased access to palliative care and hospice services: Opportunities to improve value in health care. *The Milbank Quarterly, 89*(3), 343–380.

Melchior, M. A., Seff, L. R., Bastida, E., et al. (2013). Intermediate outcomes of chronic disease self-management program for spanish-speaking older adults in south Florida, 2008–2010. *Preventing Chronic Disease, 10.* doi:10:5888/pcd10.130016

Morley, J. E., Vellas, B., van Kan, G. A., et al. (2013). Frailty consensus: A call to action. *Journal of the American Medical Directors Association, 14*(6), 392–397.

Ontario Cancer Facts. (2010). *Diagnosis of breast cancer occurs at a later stage among First Nations women in Ontario.* Retrieved from http://www.cancercare.on.ca/common/pages/UserFile.aspx?fileId=74610

Overcash, J. (2012). Cancer assessment and intervention strategies. In M. Boltz, E. Capezuti, T. Fulmer, et al. (Eds.), *Evidence-based practice protocols for best practice* (4th ed., pp. 658–669). New York, NY: Springer.

Pascucci, M. A., Chu, N., & Leasure, A. R. (2012). Health promotion for the oldest of old people. *Nursing Older People, 24*(3), 22–28.

Passmore, M. J. (2013). Neuropsychiatric symptoms of dementia: Consent, quality of life, and dignity. *BioMed Research International.* Advance online publication. doi:10/1155/2013/230234

Pastor, D. K., & Moore, G. (2013). Uncertainties of the heart: Palliative care and adult heart failure. *Home Healthcare Nurse, 31*(1), 29–36.

Petrovic, M., van der Cammen, T., & Onder, G. (2012). Adverse drug reactions in older people: Detection and prevention. *Drugs and Aging, 29*(6), 453–462.

Public Health Agency of Canada. (2010). *The Chief Public Health Officer's report on the state of public health in Canada.* Retrieved from http://www.phac-aspc.gc.ca/cphorsphc-respcacsp/2010/fr-rc/index-eng.php

Public Health Agency of Canada. (2011). *Diabetes in Canada: Facts and figures from a public health perspective.* Retrieved from http://www.phac-aspc.gc.ca/cd-mc/publications/diabetes-diabete/facts-figures-faits-chiffres-2011/highlights-saillants-eng.php#chp6

Rodríquez-Mañas, L., Féart, C., Mann, G., et al. (2013). Searching for an operational definition of frailty: A Delphi Method based consensus statement. *Journals of Gerontology: Medical Sciences, 68*(1), 62–67.

Shamliyan, T., Talley, K. M., Ramakrishnan, R., et al. (2013). Association of frailty with survival: A systematic literature review. *Ageing Research Review, 12*(2), 719–736.

Sinha, M. (2013). *Statistics Canada—Portraits of caregivers, 2012* [Catalogue no. 89-652-X]. Ottawa, Ontario: Statistics Canada.

Tshiananga, J. K., Kocher, S., Weber, C., et al. (2012). The effect of nurse-led diabetes self-management education on glycosylated hemoglobin and cardiovascular risk factors: A meta-analysis. *Diabetes Education, 38*(1), 108–123.

Wang, S.-Y., Shamliyan, T. A., Talley, K. M. C., et al. (2013). Not just specific disease: Systematic review of the association of geriatric syndromes with hospitalization or nursing home admission. *Archives of Gerontology and Geriatrics, 57*, 16–26.

Wierenga, P. C., Buurman, B. M., Parlevliet, J. L., et al. (2012). Association between acute geriatric syndromes and medication-related hospital admissions. *Drugs and Aging, 29*(8), 691–699.

Wilson, J., & McMillan, S. (2013). Symptoms experienced by heart failure patients in hospice care. *Journal of Hospice and Palliative Nursing, 15*(1), 13–21.

chapter 28

Caring for Older Adults Experiencing Pain

LEARNING OBJECTIVES

After reading this chapter, you will be able to:

1. Differentiate between types of pain: nociceptive, acute, chronic and cancer pain.

2. Discuss unique aspects of pain in older adults, including prevalence, causes and complexities of assessment and management.

3. Examine and dispel commonly held myths and beliefs about pain in older adults.

4. Discuss cultural aspects of pain.

5. Apply evidence-based guidelines for assessment and management of pain in older adults who are cognitively impaired.

6. Describe principles of analgesic medication use in older adults.

7. Discuss evidence-based nonpharmacologic and other additional nursing interventions that are effective in managing pain in older adults.

KEY POINTS

acute pain	nociception
addiction	nonopioid analgesics
adjuvant analgesics	opioid analgesics
cancer pain	pain
chronic (persistent) pain	pain intensity
dependence	tolerance
neuropathic pain	

Pain is a biopsychosocial phenomenon with multiple dimensions, including sensory, cognitive, emotional, developmental, behavioural, spiritual and cultural influences. Pain is very common among older adults, and nursing assessment and management is further complicated by additional factors, such as age-related changes, impaired mental status and other concomitant conditions. In addition, knowledge and attitudes of care providers can enhance or interfere with accurate assessment and effective management of pain, particularly with regard to older adults. This chapter provides an overview of pain and discusses assessment and management of pain, emphasizing aspects that are most pertinent to care of older adults.

DEFINITIONS AND TYPES OF PAIN

Pain is an unpleasant sensory and subjective experience associated with actual or potential injury. The subjective quality of pain is defined as whatever the experiencing person says it is, existing whenever she or he says it does (McCaffery, 1968). Objectively, pain occurs within the context of a physiologic process that is a response to a noxious stimulus. Because pain is a very complex phenomenon, there are many ways of classifying it. The following sections describe commonly used classifications according to underlying mechanisms (i.e., nociceptive and neuropathic) and duration (i.e., acute and chronic/persistent). Cancer pain is also described because of its unique characteristics and its common occurrence in older adults.

Nociceptive and Neuropathic Pain

Nociception, which is the physiologic process that leads to the perception of a noxious stimulus as being painful,

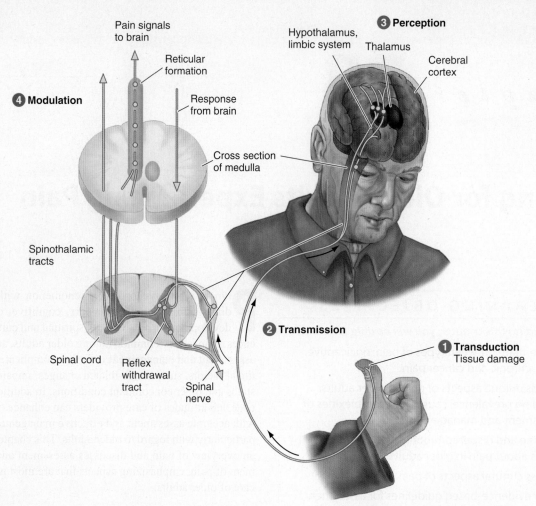

FIGURE 28-1 Processes involved in the physiology of pain. (Adapted with permission from Karch, A. M. [2011]. *Focus on nursing pharmacology* [5th ed.]. Philadelphia, PA: Lippincott Williams & Wilkins.)

involves four processes: transduction, transmission, perception and modulation (Fig. 28-1). *Transduction* involves the activation of primary nociceptive fibres (i.e., the primary afferent neurons throughout the body) when tissue damage occurs from any of the following sources: mechanical (e.g., surgery, trauma, tumour), thermal (e.g., burn, extreme cold) or chemical (e.g., toxin, chemotherapy). Excitatory compounds are released through local tissues, immune cells or nerve endings and include serotonin, bradykinin, histamine, substance P and prostaglandins. These physiologic processes set off an action potential, which is the second phase of nociception, called *transmission*. During transmission, the afferent information passes through the dorsal root ganglia to the spinal cord, where it continues to pass through multiple ascending pathways to the brainstem. Effectiveness of analgesic medications is based on their ability to modify specific aspects of transduction and transmission.

Perception, the third process of nociception, is the point at which pain becomes a conscious experience. Sensory, emotional and cognitive areas of the brain are involved in the perception of pain. Effectiveness of cognitive-behavioural

therapies and other body–mind modalities is associated with evidence that brain processes can strongly influence pain perception. The final process of nociception, *modulation*, refers to the body's responses to painful stimuli, which involves both the central and peripheral nervous systems and many neurochemicals, including serotonin, norepinephrine and endogenous opioids. Effectiveness of antidepressants for relief of pain is associated with their effects on serotonin and norepinephrine.

Neuropathic pain originates from an abnormal processing of sensory stimuli by the central or peripheral nervous system (i.e., damage to or dysfunction that affects any part of the central or autonomic nervous systems). In contrast to nociceptive pain, which is triggered by an immediate noxious stimulus, neuropathic pain can occur in the absence of immediate tissue damage or inflammation. Also in contrast to nociceptive pain, which serves to warn and protect from further injury, neuropathic pain serves no useful purpose (Pasero & Portenoy, 2011).

Neuropathic pain involves complex responses of many peripheral and central mechanisms. Peripheral mechanisms

TABLE 28-1 Comparison of Nociceptive and Neuropathic Pain

Characteristic	Nociceptive Pain	Neuropathic Pain
Underlying mechanism	*Normal* processing of noxious stimuli in response to actual or potential tissue injury or inflammation	*Abnormal* processing of sensory input sustained by damage to or dysfunction of the nervous system
Physiologic processes	Transduction, transmission, perception, modulation	Sensitization due to abnormal peripheral and central processing of noxious stimuli
Subtypes and examples according to origin	Somatic: skin, bone, joint, connective tissue, mucous membranes, subcutaneous tissue (e.g., burn, bruise, arthritis, tendonitis, fibromyalgia, myofascial pain) Visceral: gastrointestinal, urinary tract or other internal organs due to blockage, pressure or infection (e.g., tumours, cholecystitis, kidney stones)	Central pain from injury to or dysfunction of the central nervous system (e.g., poststroke pain, multiple sclerosis, spinal cord injury) Peripheral mononeuropathy results in pain along nerve pathway (e.g., nerve root compression or trigeminal neuralgia) Peripheral polyneuropathy results in pain along the distribution of many peripheral nerves (e.g., trigeminal neuropathy, postherpetic neuralgia, phantom limb, diabetic neuropathy, chronic postsurgical pain)
Common descriptors	Somatic: aching, deep, throbbing, dull, sharp, tender, gnawing, pressure Visceral: cramping, squeezing, shooting, pressure	Burning, shooting, knife-like, tingling, pins and needles
Sensory symptoms	Not common except hypersensitivity in immediate area of injury	Numbness, tingling, pricking, hypersensitive to touch
Distribution	Proximal radiation common	Distal radiation common
Motor symptoms	Weakness due to pain experience	Neurologic-associated weakness if motor nerves are involved

are activated by actual or potential tissue damage due to mechanical, thermal or chemical stimuli, as described earlier. In addition, viruses, infections, ischemia, metabolic disease (e.g., diabetes), nutritional deficiencies and neurologic diseases can activate peripheral pain mechanisms. Abnormalities in processing information during transduction and transmission combine with dysfunctions in central mechanisms to cause sensitization, which leads to increasingly stronger responses in the pain transmission pathway. When this occurs, pain is experienced with little or no stimulus. Table 28-1 compares characteristics of nociceptive and neuropathic pain and lists examples of types.

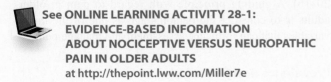

See **ONLINE LEARNING ACTIVITY 28-1: EVIDENCE-BASED INFORMATION ABOUT NOCICEPTIVE VERSUS NEUROPATHIC PAIN IN OLDER ADULTS** at http://thepoint.lww.com/Miller7e

Acute and Chronic Pain

Although the term chronic (also called persistent) pain describes the length of time the pain is experienced, there is increasing evidence that this type of pain has additional unique characteristics. Whereas acute pain has a sudden onset and is linked to a specific event, injury or illness, chronic pain develops when the central nervous system continues to process pain signals as though new injuries were occurring. Researchers are focusing on identifying the many factors that affect the transition from acute to chronic pain, which is sometimes referred to as "pain chronification." Risk factors

currently under investigation include genetic predisposition, enhanced pain perception, presence of preexisting pain and psychological factors (e.g., distress, catastrophizing) (Pergolizzi et al., 2014).

Acute pain is sharp, immediate pain from an injury to tissue, and it can also be triggered by physiologic malfunction or severe illness. It is the normal, predictable physiologic response to an adverse chemical, thermal or mechanical stimulus, and its purpose is to lead to resolution of the causative agent or event. Common causes of acute pain include burns, trauma, medical or surgical procedures, or chronic medical problems, such as cancer or postherpetic neuralgia. Acute pain is generally time limited and responds effectively to anti-inflammatory and opioid medications as well as other approaches.

Chronic (persistent) pain lasts longer than 3 to 6 months or beyond the expected time of healing from the initial causative event. National statistics reveal that the incidence of chronic pain increases with age, with Canadian women 65 years and older reporting the highest rates of pain (Reitsma et al., 2011). Physiologically, the perception of chronic pain involves many neurotransmitters and receptors involved with peripheral sensitization, central sensitization and modulation at many sites of the autonomic and central nervous system. Although the phenomenon is not well understood, there is increasing evidence that the pathophysiology of persistent pain begins with an acute nociceptive process that at some point combines with neuropathic characteristics (Taverner et al., 2014). Because this is a complex pathophysiologic process, effective management includes a pharmacologic approach with drugs that target several pain pathways in combination with nonpharmacologic interventions.

Research has led to the following conclusions about persistent pain, which have been summarized by the Institute of Medicine (IOM, 2011) in the United States and identified by the Canadian Pain Coalition and the Canadian Institute for the Relief of Pain and Disability.

- Chronic pain represents a pathologic transition from acute pain.
- Causes of chronic pain include underlying pathologic process, injury, medical treatment, surgical interventions, inflammations and neuropathic pain.
- The cause of chronic pain is not always identifiable.
- In most cases, chronic pain should be considered a disease in its own right.
- Chronic pain can affect every aspect of a person's life.
- Management of persistent pain requires a biopsychosocial approach that addresses physiologic, psychological, social, emotional and spiritual aspects of the person.

Recent studies have focused on the complex mechanisms involved with the development of chronic postsurgical pain, finding that its incidence can be reduced with the use of aggressive and early analgesic therapy (Deumens et al., 2013; Van de Ven & John Hsia, 2012). This is particularly pertinent to care of older adults recovering from surgical procedures in acute care settings, nursing facilities and independent settings. Similarly, studies of postherpetic neuralgia emphasize the early treatment with antiviral medication (McGreevy et al., 2011).

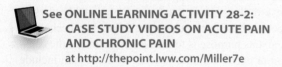

See ONLINE LEARNING ACTIVITY 28-2:
CASE STUDY VIDEOS ON ACUTE PAIN AND CHRONIC PAIN
at http://thepoint.lww.com/Miller7e

Cancer Pain

Cancer pain is a complex phenomenon caused by the cancer itself, concomitant disease or adverse effects of treatments. Cancer pain can be acute, chronic, nociceptive, neuropathic or—as is most often the case—a combination of these types. Pain is caused directly by the cancer and indirectly by effects of the cancer, such as compression due to tumour infiltration and neuropathy from chemotherapy. Studies have documented high prevalence rates of cancer pain as in the following examples (IOM, 2011):

- Multiple myeloma (100%)
- Metastatic or advanced-stage disease (64%)
- During anticancer treatment (59%)
- Breast cancer (58%)
- Lung cancer (56%), colorectal cancer (41%)

Because half of all cancers occur in people aged 65 or older, addressing cancer pain is particularly pertinent when caring for older adults.

UNIQUE ASPECTS OF PAIN IN OLDER ADULTS

Although many aspects of pain differ in older adults, research on pain in older adults lags behind other areas of pain research. There is widespread agreement, however, that pain is under-detected and poorly managed among older adults (Lynch, 2011). Nursing assessment and management of pain is challenging not only because of age-related changes but also because of coexisting conditions, such as dementia, delirium, surgery, or acute or chronic illness that affect many—if not most—older adults. Additional complicating factors include lack of evidence-based information, misconceptions and misinformation, and the presence of several types of pain (e.g., neuropathic pain plus acute pain, pain at more than one site, acute pain superimposed on chronic pain, cancer pain combined with chronic pain). This section provides an overview of unique aspects of pain in older adults, and the assessment and interventions sections address specific aspects of pain in older adults who are cognitively impaired as a result of delirium or dementia.

Age-Related Changes

Although many processes involved with pain perception can be altered by age-related changes in neurochemical, neuro-anatomic and neurophysiologic mechanisms, little is known about the functional consequences of these changes in older adults. Whereas some studies indicate that older adults have a diminished response to noxious stimuli, numerous studies also find that they are more vulnerable to experiencing severe or chronic pain and have diminished ability to tolerate severe pain (IOM, 2011).

Age-related changes in pharmacokinetics and pharmacodynamics, as discussed in Chapter 8, can affect analgesic medications in older adults and increase the risk for adverse effects. Even this aspect, however, is variable, because studies have found no age-related difference in appropriate doses of postoperative morphine, particularly when doses were normalized according to body weight (Pasero & McCaffery, 2011b). A guiding principle with regard to pain in older adults is to consider the person's age as one of the many variables that can influence assessment and management.

Prevalence and Causes

Pain, especially chronic pain, is common in older adults. Depending upon the study, between 25% and 65% of older Canadians living in independent settings report experiencing chronic pain. For those living in long-term care facilities, up to 80% acknowledge living with continuous pain (Canadian Pain Society, 2013; Hadjistavropoulos et al., 2009). Moreover, between 28% and 59% of older adults report pain at more than one site, which is due to a high prevalence of pain-causing conditions associated with more than one type of pain (e.g., nociceptive, neuropathic, inflammatory) (Reid et al., 2011).

Musculoskeletal pain is the most common type of chronic pain, and it often occurs in multiple sites, particularly the joints and back. National statistics indicate that the prevalence of arthritis, which causes chronic pain, is approximately 34% for men 65 years and older and just over 50% for senior women (Statistics Canada, 2010). Cancer is another condition that disproportionately affects aging adults and is a common cause of acute and chronic pain (Canadian Cancer Society's Advisory Committee on Cancer Statistics, 2013).

 ## FUNCTIONAL CONSEQUENCES OF PAIN IN OLDER ADULTS

Pain is associated with numerous immediate and long-term consequences, and older adults are particularly vulnerable because pain is often superimposed on other undesirable conditions. An important functional consequence of acute pain, especially if it is undertreated, is the increased risk of developing chronic pain. Additional functional consequences commonly experienced by older adults include:

- Diminished physical function to the point of disability
- Psychosocial effects: fatigue, anxiety and depression (Hawker et al., 2011)
- Increased risk of falls
- Sleep disturbances
- Weight loss
- Increased dependency
- Decreased quality of life
- Social isolation and negative effects on relationships (Lane, Hirst, & Reed, 2015).

One study of community-living older adults identified that pain negatively impacted the following: walking (38%), general activity (23%), mood (19%), enjoyment of life (16%), sleeping (15%), concentration (10%) and relationships (8%) (Brown et al., 2011) (see Box 28-1). Similarly, studies of long-term care residents found that pain had significant negative effects on both physical and psychological health, including mobility, activities of daily living, depression and life satisfaction (Tse et al., 2013). Studies also found that chronic pain is an independent risk factor for falls (Eggermont et al., 2012). Overall, any degree of pain diminishes one's quality of life and causes suffering not only for the person who experiences pain but also for all those who live with and care about that person.

CULTURAL ASPECTS OF PAIN

Cultural factors can significantly influence the way people experience, express and manage their pain, as illustrated by the examples and associated nursing implications in Box 28-2. As with all aspects of culturally appropriate care, it is imperative to be aware of different expressions of pain commonly used by cultural groups, while at the same time avoiding stereotypes and basing care on the unique characteristics of each person.

Box 28-1 Evidence-Informed Nursing Practice

Background: There is substantive evidence that race and ethnicity influence the experience of pain.
Question: What is the epidemiology of pain and what factors may influence its assessment and treatment in Aboriginal peoples of Canada?
Method: A systematic search for peer-reviewed articles was conducted in five databases. A thematic analysis was then completed.
Findings: Aboriginal people have a higher prevalence of pain symptoms than the general population. There was also evidence that this population group frequently used alternative modalities to manage pain.
Implications for Nursing Practice: Nurses need to ask Aboriginal seniors about both their pain experiences and what strategies they use to relieve their pain.

Source: Jimenez, N., Garroutte, E., Kundu, A. et al. (2012). A review of the experience, epidemiology, and management of pain among American Indian, Alaska native, and Aboriginal Canadian peoples. *Journal of Pain, 12*, 511–522. Retrieved from http://dx.doi.org/10.1016/j.jpain.2010.12.002

It is also important to recognize disparities and diversities in pain prevalence and management, as in the following examples, which are particularly relevant to care of older adults:

- Patients aged 65 or older receive inadequate doses—or even no doses—of analgesic medications for cancer or postoperative pain.
- Racial and ethnic minorities are at high risk for receiving inadequate pain relief.
- Women are more likely than men to be undertreated for pain.
- People with low health literacy or low-English proficiency, particularly recent immigrants, report greater pain.
- Higher pain rates are strongly associated with lower income and level of education.
- Across all groups, women consistently report a higher prevalence of chronic pain than men (Schopflocher et al., 2011).
- Fears, concerns and misconceptions about analgesic types and doses affect prescribing behaviours and therapeutic adherence by older adults and their caregivers.
- Older adults commonly fear negative consequences of analgesics. A common, but misconceived fear, is that of addiction (IOM, 2011; Pasero & McCaffery, 2011c; Reid et al., 2011).

A first step in assessing and managing pain in older adults is to recognize the actual and potential influences of personal biases, attitudes, experiences, misconceptions and lack of information with regard to assessing and managing pain. For example, studies using vignettes found that assessment and management of pain by nurses is influenced by their personal experiences of pain and also by their perceived acceptability of the patient's lifestyle (Pasero & McCaffery, 2011c). These factors can be addressed by self-assessment and by keeping up-to-date on evidence-based guidelines, as reviewed in the following sections.

Box 28-2 Cultural Considerations: Expressions of Pain Associated With Selected Cultural Groups

Group	Assessment and Intervention Considerations	Nursing Implications
First Nations (Aboriginal) Canadians	Depending upon the location in Canada, may have higher rates of arthritis than non-First Nations (predisposing them to chronic pain). First Nations believe that health is holistic and involves a balance in all areas of life (physical, mental, emotional, spiritual).	May use traditional approaches to wellness including sacred herbs/plants (such as sweet grass, cedar or sage) and traditional healers. However, many First Nations individuals also use "western" medicine.
African Canadians	May believe as part of their spiritual and religious foundation that pain and suffering are inevitable and must be endured; this belief may contribute to a higher pain tolerance. May believe that pain and suffering can be relieved by prayers and by a person or spiritual leader placing their hands on the person during prayer, a practice known as "the laying on of hands"; if pain persists, it may be due to lack of faith.	Teach about effectiveness of analgesics as an intervention for pain. Encourage the use of religious practices (often from a Christian tradition) as an additional intervention rather than a solitary intervention.
Arabs	Pain is regarded as unpleasant and something to be controlled; however, they may be reluctant to express pain with professionals.	Recognize that family members may request analgesics on behalf of the patient.
Chinese	Tend to describe pain in terms of diverse body symptoms rather than specific or localized. May explain pain as imbalance between yin and yang. Interventions include oils, massage, warmth, relaxation, aspirin and sleeping on the affected area.	Recognize the variation in reports of pain. Support interventions as adjuvants to analgesic medications.
Filipinos	May appear stoic owing to their belief that pain is part of living an honourable life and part of the process of spiritual purification while still on earth. May be viewed as an opportunity to reach fuller spiritual life or to atone for past transgressions. May rely on religious or spiritual practices for pain management.	Observe for signs of pain and discomfort.
Hindu	A fatalistic attitude about illness is common, and is associated with their religious beliefs of *karma*. Thus, they may be stoic and not express pain. Pain is attributed to God's will, the wrath of God, or a punishment from God that is to be borne with courage. Asian Indian Hindus may prefer herbal remedies.	Pay particular attention to nonverbal indicators of pain and ask about the meaning of their pain.
Japanese	Bearing pain is considered a virtue and a matter of family honour. *Itami* is the word for pain. Because addiction is a strong taboo, patients may be reluctant to accept pain medication.	Encourage the expression of pain as an important component of accurate assessment. Consider the use of regularly scheduled medications rather than a patient-controlled approach.
Jewish	Verbalization of pain is acceptable and common. Individuals want to know the cause of the pain, which is just as important as obtaining relief.	Talk with patients about causes of pain.

Sources: Alberta Health Services. (2009). *Health care and religious beliefs.* Retrieved from http://www.albertahealthservices.ca/ps-1026227-health-care-religious-beliefs.pdf; Purnell, L. D. (2013). *Transcultural health care* (4th ed.). Philadelphia, PA: F.A. Davis; Reading, J. (n.d.). *The crisis of chronic disease among Aboriginal peoples: A challenge for public health, population health and social policy.* Retrieved from http://www.cahr.uvic.ca/docs/ChronicDisease%20Final.pdf

NURSING ASSESSMENT OF PAIN IN OLDER ADULTS

An accurate assessment of pain is based on recognizing the unique way in which each individual experiences and expresses pain, as described in the classic definition of pain as being whatever the person experiencing it says it is (McCaffery, 1968). Despite the simplicity of this classic definition, assessment of pain is very complex, even when people can describe their pain. When a person's level of cognition is altered—for example by delirium or dementia—or when other communication barriers exist, assessment of pain is even more challenging (as discussed in the next section). Additional complications are associated with the common occurrence of concomitant conditions in older adults. For example, studies

indicate that nurses in acute care settings often overlook issues related to preexisting chronic pain (Siedlecki et al., 2014).

Identifying Common Misconceptions

Despite the common occurrence of pain in older adults, it is a major mistake to view pain as a "normal part of aging." This false belief is one of many misconceptions that can affect assessment and management of pain in older adults. Although the study of pain is an evolving and inexact science—with many unanswered questions—evidence-based information is available to dispel many of the long-held beliefs that can affect pain assessment and management (Pasero & McCaffery, 2011c). For example, a misconception that is commonly incorporated in pain assessments is that changes in vital signs

Box 28-3 Misconceptions that can Affect Assessment and Management of Pain

Misconceptions Commonly Held by Health Care Professionals

- Older adults have a high pain tolerance.
- People with dementia do not experience pain.
- People who are sleeping are not experiencing pain.
- Chronic pain is not as painful as cancer pain or acute pain.
- Changes in vital signs are an important indicator of pain.
- Behavioural manifestations are more reliable than patients' self-reports.
- Anxiety and depression directly cause pain.
- Opioids should not be used for chronic pain.

Misconceptions Commonly Held by Older Adults

- Desire to avoid a diagnosis that is serious, untreatable or life-threatening
- Fears related to addiction to or adverse effects of analgesics
- Concern about being perceived as a complainer
- Desire to maintain stoicism or avoid expression of feelings that may be perceived as a weakness
- Perceptions about pain being an atonement or punishment that should not be addressed by analgesics or other medical interventions
- Belief that morphine and strong analgesics are used only for terminal situations
- Stigma associated with prescription analgesics

are a good indicator of pain in nonverbal patients. Evidence-based guidelines emphasize that although changes in vital signs may occur concomitantly with acute pain, these indicators are not necessarily related to the presence or absence of pain (Wysong, 2014). Thus, an initial step in assessing pain is to identify misconceptions, such as the ones delineated in Box 28-3. An associated step is to keep up-to-date on evidence-based guidelines related to pain in older adults.

See ONLINE LEARNING ACTIVITY 28-3: EVIDENCE-BASED INFORMATION ABOUT NURSING ASSESSMENT AND MANAGEMENT OF PAIN IN OLDER ADULTS
at http://thepoint.lww.com/Miller7e

Obtaining Information About Pain

An important guiding principle is to assess for pain during initial contacts with patients, at frequent intervals, whenever the person's condition changes, and as an essential component of pain management interventions. During an initial contact and whenever pain is of recent onset, a comprehensive assessment, as described in this section, is imperative. A less comprehensive but comparative assessment needs to be conducted at appropriate intervals after analgesics and other pain management interventions have been administered and whenever pain management interventions are changed. For example, in acute care settings, effectiveness of analgesics should be assessed 30 to 60 minutes after administration. A comparative reassessment typically includes questions about pain intensity and length of time the intervention was effective.

Because a patient's self-report about pain is considered the "gold standard" for pain assessment, begin by asking about the person's experience of pain. Allow older adults enough time to process the information and respond, and recognize that they may refer to pain by words such as *burning, discomfort, aching, soreness* or *hurting*. Another good communication strategy is to "contextualize the older adult's pain experience" by asking older adults to describe how chronic pain affects their daily life (Clarke et al., 2012, p. 2).

Essential assessment information is also obtained by observing for nonverbal indicators of pain, such as grimacing, muscle tension, rubbing or protecting body parts, rapid or excessive eye blinking, or a sad or frightened facial expression. Information can also be elicited from family members and caregivers when additional input would be helpful, particularly if the older adult is not a reliable reporter for any reason. If the person's level of functioning has changed recently, find out if pain or discomfort is a contributing factor.

Pain rating scales are used to assess **pain intensity**, which is the subjective determination of the strength, concentration or force of the pain. Because pain intensity is an easily measured indicator that can be used to assess changes at different times, it is often referred to as the "fifth vital sign." The Numerical Rating Scale (NRS) is widely used; however, the Verbal Descriptor Scale (VDS) is the one recommended for use with older adults (see Fig. 28-2). The VDS is a reliable

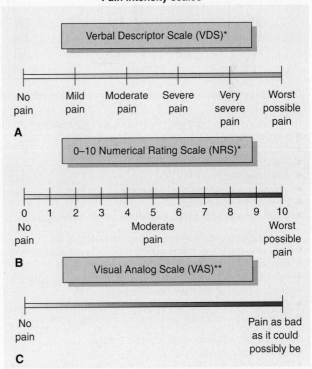

Pain intensity scales

Verbal Descriptor Scale (VDS)*

No pain | Mild pain | Moderate pain | Severe pain | Very severe pain | Worst possible pain

A

0–10 Numerical Rating Scale (NRS)*

0 1 2 3 4 5 6 7 8 9 10
No pain | Moderate pain | Worst possible pain

B

Visual Analog Scale (VAS)**

No pain | Pain as bad as it could possibly be

C

* If used as a graphic rating scale, a 10-cm baseline is recommended.

** A 10-cm baseline is recommended for VAS scales.

FIGURE 28-2 Examples of pain rating scales: **(A)** Verbal Description Scale, **(B)** Numerical Rating Scale and **(C)** Visual Analogue Scale.

and valid measure of pain intensity; moreover, studies identify it as the easiest to use for older adults and most preferred by them (Horgas et al., 2012). This scale, which can be used with the NRS, uses a continuum of verbal cues ranging from no pain to the worst pain possible. Pain rating scales provide a standardized and relatively simple measure of pain, and it is important to use the same tool at appropriate intervals and to document the findings. These tools, however, provide only one piece of information, so they need to be supplemented with self-reports and nursing observations.

Nursing assessment of pain focuses on information about the older adult's experience of acute, chronic and intermittent pain, including characteristics of different types. If the assessment addresses more than one type or location of pain, use letters for distinguishing sites and descriptors. Pain assessment also addresses the person's experiences with and concerns about analgesics. Box 28-4 can be used as a guide for assessing these components of pain. An important aspect of documenting patient experiences of pain is avoiding the use of phrases such as "complains of pain" because this is

Box 28-4   Questions to Assess Pain in Older Adults

Initial questions to ascertain need for further assessment:
- Are you experiencing pain, discomfort, aching, right now?
- Do you have more than one type of pain?
- Have you had this before or is this new? (If pain has been present before, ask about how it differs, what makes it better or worse, and other questions.)
- Describe the pain in your own words.

If the person acknowledges having pain, use a pain rating scale and document location(s) on this figure.

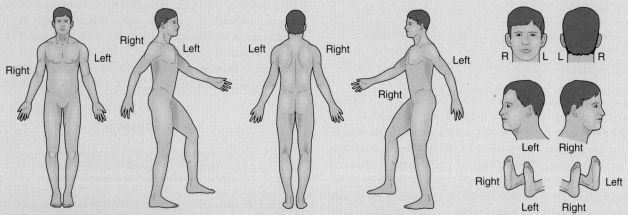

Document pain location and pain rating on relevant figure and/or body part.

Ask about the following characteristics for each type of pain reported:
- Frequency
- Duration
- Precipitating factors
- Alleviating factors
- Variations, such as changes in intensity
- Previous medical evaluation
- Usual management strategies (pharmacologic and nonpharmacologic)

Ask about effects of pain on functioning and quality of life:
- Daily activities (sleep, eating, appetite, ability to get around, level of independence, driving, and so forth)
- Level of physical activity for functioning or enjoyment
- Relationships with other (e.g., social interactions, family activities)
- Emotions (e.g., anger, happiness, irritability, mood)
- Cognitive abilities (e.g., concentration, thinking)
- Participation in enjoyable activities (e.g., hobbies, travel)

Assess the following aspects of analgesic history:
- Current and past use of analgesics
- Names, doses, and effectiveness of prescription and nonprescription analgesics
- Experiences with adverse effects
- Analgesics taken on set schedule or as needed
- Use of analgesics during previous 24 hours and influence of these on pain rating scale and other assessment information

Assess concerns about, or fear of, adverse effects, including addiction.

associated with a negative attitude toward patients and may reflect a desire that patients cope better or talk less about their pain. Rather, it is more appropriate and objective to state that patients "report pain" when documenting information about a patient's experience of pain (Pasero & McCaffery, 2011c).

Another aspect of pain assessment is using open-ended questions to identify the person's expectations for relief, as well as the meaning he or she associates with the pain. Personal goals for pain management may be based on the degree to which pain affects daily functioning and quality of life. Nurses can ask questions such as the following to assess pain management goals and potential interventions, which are particularly applicable with regard to persistent pain:

- Does the person expect to be free of pain or is a certain level of pain acceptable?
- What level of functioning is the person expecting to attain?
- Is the person interested in self-management interventions, such as a physical activity program?
- Would a referral to a pain management practitioner be helpful?
- Is it appropriate to consider a referral for physical or occupational therapy?
- Is the person interested in information about complementary and alternative medicine practices or practitioners (e.g., relaxation, guided imagery, acupuncture)?

In addition to asking assessment questions, observe and document pertinent physical assessment findings, such as skin colour, temperature, and integrity and overall appearance and level of function of the person. In addition, observe the person's verbal and nonverbal expressions of emotional responses to pain and incorporate pertinent information in the assessment.

Assessment in Older Adults Who Are Cognitively Impaired

Many studies confirm that the pain transmission process is unaltered in older adults who have dementia; however, the cognitive processing and interpretation of the pain stimulus may be impaired (Pasero & McCaffery, 2011a). Despite this evidence, many caregivers and health care professionals falsely believe that people with dementia do not experience pain. Consequently, there is a high prevalence of unrecognized and undertreated pain in older adults with dementia.

As with all aspects of pain assessment, it is essential—and challenging—to identify individual differences in the way people communicate their experience. This becomes even more challenging when assessing older adults who are cognitively impaired because dementia affects communication abilities to varying degrees. It is imperative to recognize that many older adults with mild-to-moderate dementia can verbally communicate about pain (Shega et al., 2010), and in these situations, it is appropriate to use the nursing assessment guidelines already discussed. It is also imperative to supplement the information with input from family and all caregivers, including nursing assistant staff in long-term care facilities.

In people with moderate or advanced dementia, disruptive behaviours may be the key indicator of pain, and assessment focuses on nonverbal indicators and reports from reliable observers (e.g., family and caregivers). A recent analysis of assessment data for nursing home residents found that disruptive behaviours (e.g., aggression and agitation) that do not involve locomotion were more strongly correlated with pain in comparison to behaviours (e.g., wandering) that involved locomotion (Ahn & Horgas, 2013). In all situations when caring for older adults who are cognitively impaired, keep in mind that dementia does not directly affect individuals' experience of pain, but it does alter the ability to express pain, as well as other needs.

Pain assessment in older adults who are cognitively impaired involves all the following actions:

- Elicit as much verbal and nonverbal information directly from the person as possible (Shega et al., 2010).
- Assess for indicators of underlying causes of pain, such as chronic conditions (e.g., arthritis, gout, neuralgia) or recent falls or surgical procedures.
- Use astute observations to identify behavioural indicators of pain, such as aggression, agitation, verbalizations and resistance to care activities.
- Obtain information from family members, caregivers and other reliable sources who are familiar with the person.
- Compare current assessment findings with the person's baseline function, but recognize that the person's usual level of functioning may be affected by undiagnosed and undertreated pain.

Box 28-5 summarizes specific actions nurses can take to assess pain in older adults who are cognitively impaired.

Box 28-5 Assessing Pain in Older Adults Who Have Dementia

General Principles

- Know the person and recognize that the person's ability to communicate may fluctuate.
- For people with mild-to-moderate dementia, use numerical rating scales as appropriate.
- Base assessment conclusions on multiple sources of information.
- Assess the person under several types of conditions: for example, resting, active, different times of day, during activities of daily living.

Identify Verbal Indicators of Pain

- Vocalizations such as sighing, moaning and chanting
- Repeated calling out "Help"
- Response to touching: "Ow," "Ouch," swearing or cursing
- Response to care-related activities: "Stop" or "Don't do that"
- Facial expressions, such as grimacing or furrowed brows
- Rubbing or protecting an extremity

Observe for Nonverbal Indicators

- Changes in behaviour
- Increased confusion, disorientation
- Diminished appetite

(continued)

Box 28-5 *(continued)*

- Resistance to or combativeness during care activities
- Withdrawal from social activities
- Decreased participation in physical activities
- Spending more time in bed (with or without sleep)

Look for Clues to Potential Causes of Pain (as in the following examples)

- *Skin infection:* swelling, inflammation, breakdown
- *Arthritis:* joint swelling, guarding, limited use, diminished mobility
- *Gout:* joint inflammations
- *Oral problems:* check mouth for sores, redness, open areas
- *Low back pain:* gait changes, diminished level of activity, abnormal posture
- *Urinary tract infection:* changes in behaviour, urinary frequency or incontinence

Obtain Pertinent Information From Family, Caregivers and Reliable Sources

- Identify history of chronic conditions associated with pain (e.g., gout, arthritis, peripheral or postherpetic neuropathy).
- Observe for exacerbations of previously controlled chronic conditions.
- Ask about usual manifestations of pain (e.g., wandering, agitation, withdrawal from activities).
- Find out about previous use of analgesics and nonpharmacologic interventions.
- Ask about recent falls or acute problems that could cause pain (e.g., urinary tract infections, skin tears or injuries, or bacterial infections [e.g., pneumonia]), as well as chronic conditions.

Many pain assessment tools have been developed specifically for older adults with dementia. The Pain Assessment in Advanced Dementia (PAINAD) and the Pain Assessment Checklist for Seniors with Limited Ability to Communicate (PACSLAC) are two commonly used tools. Both of these tools provide a checklist of observations that may be indicative of pain in people who cannot self-report, with each tool having different characteristics, as summarized in Table 28-2. The PACSLAC is more detailed, with 60 specific indicators listed (see Fig. 28-3). Online Learning Activity 28-4 provides additional information about the PAINAD and links to evidence-based information about commonly used tools for pain assessment in people with dementia. Any positive score on these tools should trigger further assessment and plans for interventions, for example consideration of using an analgesic medication on a trial basis (Monroe & Mion, 2012; Zwakhalen et al., 2012).

All tools for assessing pain in people with dementia focus on observation and documentation of behaviours that are indicative of pain, but false positive results on assessment tools may be associated with psychosocial distress or delirium (Jordan et al., 2011; Lints-Martindale, et al., 2012). A review of six tools concluded that the measurements most strongly associated with pain were facial expression, vocalizations and body movements (Lints-Martindale et al., 2012). Keep in mind, however, that these tools can only be used when the person is able to self-report (Monroe & Mion, 2012) and that numerical values do not capture the complexity and intensity of experienced pain.

If assessment findings indicate that the person with dementia is likely to be experiencing pain, it is important to do all of the following: assume pain is present, initiate a trial of analgesic medication, and observe changes in the person's behaviour in response to the analgesic (Pasero & McCaffery, 2011a). An analgesic trial is an integral part of the assessment, and it can also be an intervention for promoting comfort and for addressing dementia-related behaviours.

TABLE 28-2 Characteristics of PAINAD and PACSLAC

Tool Characteristic	PAINAD	PACSLAC
Indicators	Breathing independent of vocalization Negative vocalization Facial Expression Body language Consolability	Activity/body movement Negative vocalizations Facial expression Social/personality/mood Physiologic changes (e.g., sleeping, appetite)
Scoring	0 to 2 for each of 5 indicators (total 0 to 10), with higher score related to degree of pain	Checkmarks for 60 specific indicators in 4 sub-scale groups, with more checkmarks indicating pain
Recommended use	Best for daily use in acute care or frequent intervals	Best for comparisons at longer intervals for chronic pain or in long-term care settings
Validity and reliability	Supported by research	Supported by research
Original reference	Warden, V., Hurley, A. C., & Volicer, L. (2003). Development and psychometric evaluation of the Pain Assessment in Advanced Dementia (PAINAD) scale. *Journal of the American Medical Directors Association, 4,* 9–15.	Fuchs-Lacelle, S., & Hadjistavropoulos, T. (2004). Development and preliminary validation of the Pain Assessment Checklist for Seniors with Limited Ability to Communicate (PASSLAC). *Pain Management Nursing, 5,* 37–49.
Recent reference	Monroe, T. B., & Mion, L. C. (2012). Patients with advanced dementia: How do we know if they are in pain? *Geriatric Nursing, 33*(3), 226–228.	Lints-Martindale, Hadjistavropoulos, T., Lix, L., & Thorpe, L. (2012). A comparative investigation of observational pain assessment tools for older adults with dementia. *Clinical Journal of Pain, 28,* 226–237.

Pain Assessment Checklist for Seniors with Limited Ability to Communicate (PACSLAC)

Indicate with a checkmark, which of the items on the PACSLAC occurred during the period of interest. Scoring the subscales is derived by counting the checkmarks in each column. To generate a total pain, sum all subscale totals.

Facial Expression	Present
Grimacing	
Sad Look	
Tighter Face	
Dirty Look	
Change in Eyes (Squinting, dull, bright, increased eye movements)	
Frowning	
Pain Expression	
Grim Face	
Clenching Teeth	
Wincing	
Open Mouth	
Creasing Forehead	
Screwing Up Nose	

Activity/Body Movement	Present
Fidgeting	
Pulling Away	
Flinching	
Restless	
Pacing	
Wandering	
Trying to Leave	
Refusing to Move	
Thrashing	
Decreased Activity	
Refusing Medications	
Moving Slow	
Impulsive Behaviors (Repeat movements)	
Uncooperative/Resistance to Care	
Gaurding Sore Area	
Touching/Holding Sore Area	
Limping	
Clenching Fist	
Going into Fetal Position	
Stiff/Rigid	

Social/Personality/Mood	Present
Physical Aggression (e.g., pushing people and/or objects, scratching others, hitting others, striking, kicking).	
Verbal Aggression	
Not Wanting to Be Touched	
Not Allowing People Near	
Angry/Mad	
Throwing Things	
Increased Confusion	
Anxious	
Upset	
Agitated	
Cranky/Irritable	
Frustrated	

Other (Physiological Changes/Eating Sleeping Changes/Vocal Behaviors)	Present
Pale Face	
Flushed, Red Face	
Teary Eyed	
Sweating	
Shaking/Trembling	
Cold Clammy	
Changes in Sleep Routine (Please circle 1 or 2) (1) Decreased Sleep ----------------------------- (2) Increased Sleep During the Day	
Changes in Appetite (Please circle 1 or 2) (1) Decreased Appetite ----------------------------- (2) Increased Appetite	
Screaming/Yelling	
Calling Out (i.e., for help)	
Crying	
A Specific Sound of Vocalization for Pain ("ow," "ouch")	
Moaning and groaning	
Mumbling	
Grunting	
Total Checklist Score	

FIGURE 28-3 Pain Assessment Checklist for Seniors with Limited Ability to Communicate. (Reprinted with permission from Fuchs-Lacelle, S., & Hadjistavropoulos, T. [2004]. Development and preliminary validation of the Pain Assessment Checklist for Seniors with Limited Ability to Communicate (PACSLAC). *Pain Management Nursing, 5*[1], 37–49. Copyright © Shannon Fuchs-Lacelle and Thomas Hadjistavropoulos.)

In recent years, pain management is increasingly viewed as an evidence-based but underused strategy that can be incorporated with other behavioural interventions for older adults with dementia who are at risk for developing aggressive actions (Bradford et al., 2012). Recommended doses of acetaminophen for an analgesic trial are 325 to 500 mg every 4 hours or 500 to 1,000 mg every 6 hours initially with titration to stronger analgesics if pain continues to be suspected and there is no change in behaviour (Herr et al., 2011). In addition, nonpharmacologic comfort interventions (e.g., touch, communication, music, massage and environmental modifications) are essential components of assessment and management of pain in people with dementia (Lu & Herr, 2012).

In addition to considering an analgesic trial, consider initiating appropriate nonpharmacologic interventions, as described in the section *Nonpharmacologic Interventions for Managing Pain*. Because many of these interventions require active participation by the person experiencing pain, assess the individual's ability to engage in the intervention. For people with advanced dementia, consider nonpharmacologic interventions, such as music therapy, that are safe and can be used in almost any situation.

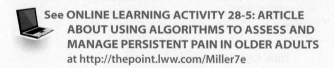

See **ONLINE LEARNING ACTIVITY 28-4:** **EVIDENCE-BASED INFORMATION ABOUT PAIN IN PEOPLE WITH DEMENTIA** at http://thepoint.lww.com/Miller7e

PHARMACOLOGIC INTERVENTIONS FOR MANAGING PAIN

Analgesic medications are the foundation of effective pain management and are the first intervention for acute and serious pain. Selection of type and dose of analgesic is based on careful evaluation of many patient variables, including age, weight, concomitant conditions and medications, and concerns about actual and potential adverse effects (including drug interactions). Keep in mind that with careful analgesic selection and monitoring there is less risk of adverse effects from medications as compared with the serious risks associated with undertreatment of pain in older adults. Nurses have major responsibilities in preventing the undertreatment of pain and at the same time providing astute assessment and management of both therapeutic and adverse effects. This is particularly important when caring for older adults who are in long-term care facilities and those who have dementia. Algorithms can be used for assessment and management of chronic pain in older adults, as described in Online Learning Activity 28-5.

See **ONLINE LEARNING ACTIVITY 28-5: ARTICLE ABOUT USING ALGORITHMS TO ASSESS AND MANAGE PERSISTENT PAIN IN OLDER ADULTS** at http://thepoint.lww.com/Miller7e

Classifications of Analgesics

Three groups of analgesics are nonopioids, opioids and adjuvants. Avoid using the term *narcotic* because this term is associated with substances that have the potential for abuse, such as cocaine, which actually have no analgesic properties. Instead, use the terms *nonopioid* and *opioid* analgesics rather than *nonnarcotics* and *narcotics*.

Nonopioid analgesics include acetaminophen; non-aspirin, nonsteroidal anti-inflammatory drugs (NSAIDs);

and aspirin. Nonopioids act at the site of the injury to decrease pain; NSAIDs, for example, inhibit the release of prostaglandin from damaged cells. **Opioid analgesics** are natural, semisynthetic or synthetic drugs that relieve pain by binding to multiple types of opioid receptors in the central nervous system. Because of this action, the release of neurotransmitters is blocked and the pain impulse cannot cross the synapse into the dorsal horn during transmission over the pain pathway. Examples of opioids are codeine, morphine, tramadol, fentanyl and methadone. **Adjuvant analgesics** are medications that have a primary indication other than the treatment of pain, such as antidepressants or anticonvulsants, but relieve pain in some conditions. Adjuvants most often act on the modulation phase along the pain pathway by interfering with the reuptake of serotonin and norepinephrine, thereby inhibiting the transmission of nociceptive impulses. All three groups are effective in the perception phase, acting in different ways to decrease the conscious experience of pain perception.

Misconceptions and Realities About Analgesics

The many misconceptions about different analgesics may affect selection of medications for pain management. Table 28-3 identifies misconceptions and realities about analgesics that are most relevant to pain management for older adults.

Because misconceptions and lack of information can lead to fears and reluctance to take appropriate medications, it is important to teach older adults and their families about tolerance, dependence and addiction. Medication **tolerance** is a physiologic protective mechanism that helps the body become accustomed to the medication so that adverse effects (except for constipation) gradually diminish. Tolerance is characterized by a decrease in one or more therapeutic effects of the medication (e.g., less analgesia) or its adverse effects (e.g., nausea, sedation or respiratory depression). Tolerance to analgesia usually occurs during the first several days to 2 weeks of therapy.

Dependence is a normal physiologic response manifested by the development of withdrawal symptoms when an opioid is suddenly discontinued after being administered repeatedly for more than 2 weeks. Tapering (i.e., gradually reducing) the dose of an opioid as pain resolves usually prevents withdrawal symptoms. Dependence is not necessarily an indicator of addiction; rather, it indicates that the medication is medically necessary for managing symptoms.

In contrast to dependence and tolerance, **addiction** is a chronic disease with biologic, neurologic and psychological characteristics, including one or more of the following in relation to a drug: craving, compulsive use, inability to control its use and continued use even when harm occurs. In reality, addiction rarely occurs in relation to analgesic medications; whereas, tolerance and dependence are normal responses that should be expected when opioids are taken for 2 to 4 weeks or longer (Pasero & McCaffery, 2011c).

TABLE 28-3 Misconceptions and Realities About Analgesics

Misconception	Evidence-Based Reality
Daily use of nonopioids is safer than long-term use of opioids.	Long-term use of NSAIDs is associated with more severe and life-threatening adverse effects; whereas the most common adverse effect of opioids is constipation, which can be addressed.
Nonopioids are not effective for severe pain.	Nonopioids alone rarely relieve severe pain, but they have an important role as adjuvants.
Polypharmacy with different types of analgesics is unacceptable.	Because different types of analgesics have unique mechanisms, it is acceptable and often recommended to use different types for specific purposes.
Rectal or parenteral administration of NSAIDs reduces the risks of GI adverse effects.	NSAIDS administered by any route inhibit prostaglandins, which are necessary to maintain the protective barrier in the GI tract.
Administering NSAIDs with an antacid reduces the risk of GI adverse effects.	Antacids may decrease the risk of GI effects, but they also decrease effectiveness of NSAIDs because they cause the drug to be released in the stomach instead of the small intestine.
Taking opioids for pain relief leads to addiction.	Addiction as a result of taking opioids for analgesia occurs less than 1% of the time.
Opioids are not effective for all types of pain.	All pain responds to opioids, but they are more effective in relieving visceral and somatic pain and less effective for neuropathic pain.
Opioids should be avoided during early stages of progressive conditions to prevent the development of tolerance.	Tolerance to opioids does not necessarily develop, and the dose usually stabilizes if the pain is stable. There is no ceiling to opioid doses and patients develop tolerance to respiratory depression.
Opioids commonly cause clinically significant respiratory depression.	If opioid doses are titrated slowly and decreased when sedation occurs, respiratory depression is rare. Tolerance to respiratory effects develops within 72 hours of regular daily doses.

Sources: Pasero, C., Portenoy, R. K., & McCaffery, M. (2011). Nonopiod analgesics. In C. Pasero & M. McCaffery (Eds.), *Pain assessment and pharmacologic management* (pp. 177–180). St. Louis, MO: Mosby Elsevier; Pasero, C., Quinn, T. W., Portenoy, R. K., et al. (2011). Opioids analgesics. In C. Pasero & M. McCaffery (Eds.), *Pain assessment and pharmacologic management* (pp. 277–282). St. Louis, MO: Mosby Elsevier.

The Canadian Guideline for Safe and Effective Use of Opioids for Chronic Non-Cancer Pain

While non-opioids are given as a first line of treatment for pain, they are not without side effects. For instance, acetaminophen (Tylenol) is the first-line treatment for mild-to-moderate pain because it is a very effective analgesic with few side effects. However, taken in large dosages, acetaminophen can be damaging to the liver. Hepatotoxicity, which is the most serious adverse effect, can occur when the recommended maximum dose of 4 g/day is exceeded.

Similarly, NSAIDS—although non-opioids—can cause significant risks to older adults. These risks include gastrointestinal bleeding, renal insufficiency or failure, decreased platelet aggregations and even death. In 2007, the National Opioid Use Guideline Group (NOUGG) was formed for the purpose of developing guidelines for the use of opioids for chronic pain not related to cancer. They released the Canadian Guideline for Safe and Effective Use of Opioids for Chronic Non-Cancer Pain in 2010 (See http://nationalpain-centre.mcmaster.ca/opioid/). The guideline was developed to assist those who prescribe opioids, but not as the standard practice to follow. Updates to the guideline may be offered in 2015 (Furlan et al., 2010).

Within the guideline offered by the NOUGG, special populations such as older adults are included. The group suggested that opioids are usually safe for older adults. They noted that while opioid abuse is much lower in aged adults than their younger counterparts, opioids should be carefully titrated and monitored to avoid deleterious effects (National Pain Centre, 2010).

Opioids can be an effective treatment option for individuals experiencing chronic, noncancer pain. Unfortunately, this option tends to be under-utilized for older adults (Kahan et al., 2011). They can also be safer than NSAIDS and cause less cognitive impairment than benzodiazepines (National Pain Centre, 2010). Often, older adults respond very well to low dosages of opioids for conditions such as rheumatoid or osteoarthritis (Kahan et al., 2011). However, dosages need to be lower than younger adults (half the dosage of their younger counterparts) and should be increased slowly if starting doses are ineffective.

There are some considerations about older adults taking opioids for pain, however. First, older adults may be at higher risk for overdose than younger adults. If they are taking benzodiazepines concurrently, they have a greater chance of becoming over sedated (National Pain Centre, 2010). Older adults can also have greater risk of falling with opioids and resultant fractures, or can experience delirium. Further, older adults with cognitive impairment who live alone at home should not take opioids, unless receiving some supervision (Kahan et al., 2011). Another adverse effect is constipation, and this is the one effect that does not subside over time. Conditions that increase the risk of developing constipation include increased age, diminished mobility, gastrointestinal conditions and medication interactions. Additional adverse effects of opioids include nausea and vomiting. Interventions for preventing and addressing constipation and altered mental state are discussed in Chapters 18 and 14, respectively.

Nurses should provide teaching to older adults and family members to seek medical help immediately if there are signs of overdose (such as over sedation or slurred speech). They should regularly assess for signs of sedation in their older patients (Kahan et al., 2011) and monitor the effectiveness of pain relief. Finally, in managing chronic pain in older individuals, good communication between health care providers (across professions), as well as between older adults, family member and professionals is crucial in helping those with chronic non-cancer-related pain (Furlan et al., 2010).

A Student's Perspective

My aging client complains periodically about pain in her shoulder. She has stated that she does not want to take anything besides aspirin when she has pain and that aspirin seems to take care of her pain. She does not take the aspirin every day. She's afraid of taking pain medications because she does not want to rely on strong medications, and she is afraid of becoming addicted. I explained to her the consequences of untreated pain and also tried to ease her fears of pain medication. She assured me that she will see her physician if the pain becomes severe when aspirin does not help her.

Thelma M.

NONPHARMACOLOGIC INTERVENTIONS FOR MANAGING PAIN

Although analgesics are the mainstay of pain management, nonpharmacologic interventions are an essential component of a comprehensive approach for all types of pain. A wellness-oriented approach to pain management for older adults involves the use of a wide variety of interventions to supplement, enhance or diminish the need for pharmacologic interventions. One major advantage of nonpharmacologic interventions is that they rarely have adverse effects. In addition, nonpharmacologic approaches often have broader benefits, such as improved comfort, reduced anxiety and improved quality of life. Lu and Herr (2012) suggest that nurses consider the following nonpharmacologic interventions listed in Box 28-6 as a part of pain management. When considering nonpharmacologic pain modalities for older adults, nurses should take into account the preferences of their clients. Based upon their upbringing, experiences and belief systems, older adults may be more comfortable with some nonpharmacologic treatments than others.

- Physical strategies: massage, reflexology, heat and cold, mild exercise, physical therapy and transcutaneous electrical nerve stimulation (TENS units).
- Cognitive-behavioural approaches: relaxation, distraction, hypnosis, biofeedback, guided imagery, music therapy, and spiritual and religious coping strategies (e.g., prayer).
- Biofield therapies and energy medicine techniques: Reiki, healing touch, therapeutic touch, acupressure and qi therapy.
- Patient and family education: addressing fears and misbeliefs by teaching about nature of pain, signs of its

---

E·B·P **Box 28-6 Evidence-Based Practice: Nonpharmacologic Interventions for Chronic Pain**

Systematic Reviews

- Low back pain: evidence in support of yoga, massage, acupuncture, spinal manipulation, progressive relaxation (Cramer et al., 2013; National Center on Complementary and Alternative Medicine, 2014).
- Acupressure is effective for relieving chronic pain of various types, including chronic headache and low back pain (Chen & Hsiu-Hung, 2014).
- Acupuncture is effective for many types of chronic pain, including osteoarthritis and back, neck, and shoulder pain (Vickers et al., 2012).
- Music is a safe, inexpensive and independent nursing function that can be used as an adjuvant approach to pain control in hospitalized patients (Cole & LoBiondo-Wood, 2014).

Individual Studies

- Healing touch may be beneficial for some older adults in long-term care settings as an adjunct for chronic pain (Wardell et al., 2012).
- Listening to personal choice of music may be a simple, safe and effective method of reducing pain in patients after open heart surgery (Özer et al., 2013).
- Using music as a routine part of nursing care is an effective practice for reducing pain intensity in patients with neuropathic pain (Korhan et al., 2014).
- Relaxation exercises are effective in reducing postoperative pain following upper abdominal surgery (Topcu & Findik, 2012).

Osteoarthritis

(National Center on Complementary and Alternative Medicine, 2012; Shengelia et al., 2013)

- Acupuncture is the complementary and alternative medicine (CAM) with the most promising evidence of potential benefit in reducing pain and improving joint mobility.
- Some research supports the use of massage and tai chi for reducing pain and improving mobility.
- Yoga may be beneficial for symptoms associated with osteoarthritis (e.g., stress and anxiety), but people with osteoarthritis need to be cautious about overstretching of affected joints and ligaments.
- A few studies, but not all, have found that a combination of glucosamine and chondroitin has potentially beneficial effects for knee osteoarthritis.
- A few, but not all studies, have found that S-Adenosyl-L-methionine (SAMe) was effective for small improvements in pain and function.
- There is some evidence to support the use of dietary supplements of devil's claw and avocado–soybean unsaponifiables (ASUs).
- Modalities with little or no evidence of benefits: homeopathy, magnets, topical dimethyl sulfoxide (DMSO), oral methylsulfonylmethane (MSM).

presence, and management goals related to comfort and function, and use of pharmacologic and nonpharmacologic approaches. (Box 28-6 summarizes recent research related to nonpharmacologic approaches to pain management.)

Another major role of nurses in pain management is making referrals for specialized services when pain does not respond to usual analgesic approaches, or when people experience chronic pain. For example, palliative care professionals are available in most hospitals and through many hospice programs. These programs, which include nurses, physicians, psychologists and sometimes other professionals such as chaplains, use an interprofessional approach to assess and manage pain. Nurses who are interested in learning more about pain management may take courses through the Canadian Pain Society. Other educational options include the certificate in Pain Management through the University of Alberta or the Western (university) pain management program. Outcomes of participation in educational programs include improved knowledge and attitudes, increased skill in pain assessment, improved confidence with administration of opioids and ability to use nonpharmacologic interventions such as relaxation (Grant et al., 2011; Williams et al., 2012).

Teaching about rehabilitation and self-management strategies is another important aspect of wellness-oriented care for older adults with chronic pain. For example, rehabilitation programs, which include exercise, physical modalities, manual techniques and assistive devices, have been found to provide pain relief, reduce disability and improve function in people with osteoarthritis of the knee and hip (Iversen, 2012). Online Learning Activity 28-6 provides information about resources for patient and caregiver teaching related to all aspects of pain management.

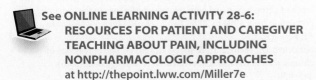

See ONLINE LEARNING ACTIVITY 28-6: RESOURCES FOR PATIENT AND CAREGIVER TEACHING ABOUT PAIN, INCLUDING NONPHARMACOLOGIC APPROACHES at http://thepoint.lww.com/Miller7e

Chapter Highlights

Definitions and Types of Pain
- Nociceptive and neuropathic pain (Fig. 28-1, Table 28-1)
- Acute and chronic (persistent) pain
- Cancer pain

Unique Aspects of Pain in Older Adults
- Age-related changes
- Prevalence and causes

Functional Consequences of Pain in Older Adults

Cultural Aspects of Pain (Box 28-2)

Nursing Assessment of Pain in Older Adults
- Identifying common misconceptions (Box 28-3)
- Obtaining information about pain (Fig. 28-2, Box 28-4)
- Assessment in older adults who are cognitively impaired (Table 28-2, Box 28-5, Fig. 28-3)

Pharmacologic Interventions for Managing Pain
- Classification of analgesics
- Misconceptions and realities about analgesics (Table 28-3)

Nonpharmacologic Interventions for Managing Pain
- Nonpharmacologic interventions (Box 28-6)
- Referrals for specialized services
- Teaching about self-management strategies

Critical Thinking Exercises

1. Identify an older person in your recent clinical experience who has talked with you about chronic pain, and address the following in relation to that person:
   - Which factors listed in Box 28-3 affect the person's experience of pain?
   - What assumptions from Box 28-4 are applicable to assessing pain in that person?
2. Review Box 28-5 and the section *Nonpharmacologic Interventions for Managing Pain*. Develop a patient-teaching strategy to improve comfort levels in a 78-year-old woman with chronic low-back pain and mild cognitive impairment.
3. Review the information about tolerance, dependence and addiction and write a sentence for each of these concepts in terms that you could use for teaching older adults and their caregivers about medication therapy.

For more information about the topics discussed in this chapter, be sure to check out the interactive Online Learning Activities and other helpful resources at http://thepoint.lww.com/Miller7e

REFERENCES

Ahn, D., & Horgas, A. (2013). The relationship between pain and disruptive behaviors in nursing home residents with dementia. *BioMed Central Geriatrics, 13*, 14. Retrieved from www.biomedcentral.com/1471-2318/13/14

Bradford, A., Shrestha, S., Snow, A. L., et al. (2012). Managing pain to prevent aggression in people with dementia: A nonpharmacologic intervention. *American Journal of Alzheimers Disease and Other Dementias, 27*(1), 41–47.

Brown, S. T., Kirkpatrick, M. K., Swanson, M. S., et al. (2011). Pain experience of the elderly. *Pain Management Nursing, 12*(4), 190–196.

Canadian Cancer Society's Advisory Committee on Cancer Statistics. (2013). *Canadian cancer statistics.* Toronto, ON: Canadian Cancer Society.

Canadian Pain Society. (2013). *Pain in Canada fact sheet*. Retrieved from http://www.canadianpainsociety.ca/pdf/pain_fact_sheet_en.pdf

Chen, Y.-W., & Hsiu-Hung, W. (2014). The effectiveness of acupressure on relieving pain: A systematic review. *Pain Management Nursing, 15*(2), 539–550. doi:10.1016/j.pmn.2012.12.005

Clarke, A., Anthony, C., Gray, D., et al. (2012). "I feel so stupid because I can't give a proper answer…" How older adults describe chronic pain: A qualitative study. *Biomed Central Geriatrics, 12*, 78. Retrieve from www.biomedcentral.com/1471-2318/12/78

Cole, L. C., & LoBiondo-Wood, G. (2014). Music as an adjuvant therapy in control of pain and symptoms in hospitalized older adults: A systematic review. *Pain Management Nursing, 15*(1), 406–425. doi:1.1016/j.pmn.2012.08.010

Cramer, H., Lauche, R., Haller, H., et al. (2013). A systematic review and meta-analysis of yoga for low back pain. *Clinical Journal of Pain, 29*(5), 450–460.

Deumens, P., Steyaert, A., Forget, P., et al. (2013). Prevention of chronic postoperative pain. *Progress in Neurobiology, 104*, 1–37. doi:10.1016/j.pneurobio.2013.01.002

Eggermont, L., Penninx, B., Jones, R., et al. (2012). Depressive symptoms, chronic pain, and falls in older community-dwelling adults: The MOBILIZE Boston Study. *Journal of the American Geriatrics Society, 60*, 230–237.

Furlan, A. D., Reardon, R., & Weppler, C. (2010). Opioids for chronic non-cancer pain: A new Canadian practice guideline. *Canadian Medical Association Journal, 182*(9), 923–930.

Grant, M., Ferrell, B., Hanson, J., et al. (2011). The enduring need for the pain resource nurse (PRN) training program. *Journal of Cancer Education, 26*(4), 5598–5603.

Hadjistavropoulos, T., Marchildon, G. P., Fine, P. G., et al. (2009). Transforming long-term care pain management in North America: The policy-clinical interface. *Pain Medicine, 10*(3), 506–520. doi:10.1111/j.1526-4637.2009.00566.x

Hawker, G. A., Gignac, M. A., Badley, E., et al. (2011). A longitudinal study to explain the pain-depression link in older adults with osteoarthritis. *Arthritis Care & Research, 63*(10), 1382–1390. doi:10.1002/acr.20298

Herr, K., Coyne, P., McCaffery, M., et al. (2011). Pain assessment in the patients unable to self-report: Position statement with clinical practice recommendations. *Pain Management Nursing, 12*(4), 230–250.

Horgas, A. L., Yoon, S. L., & Grall, M. (2012). Pain Management. In M. Boltz, E. Capezuti, T. Fulmer, et al. (Eds.), *Evidence-based practice protocols for best practice* (4th ed., pp. 246–267). New York, NY: Springer.

Institute of Medicine. (2011). *Relieving pain in America: A blueprint for transforming prevention, care, education, and research*. Washington, DC: National Academies Press.

Iversen, M. D. (2012). Rehabilitation interventions for pain and disability in osteoarthritis. *American Journal of Nursing, 112*(3 Suppl. 1), S32–S37.

Jordan, A., Hughes, J., Pakresi, M., et al. (2011). The utility of PAINAD in assessing pain in a UK population with severe dementia. *International Journal of Geriatric Psychiatry, 26*(2), 118–126.

Kahan, M., Wilson, L., Mailis-Gagnon, A., & Srivastava, A. (2011). Canadian guideline for safe and effective use of opioids for chronic non-cancer pain: Clinical summary for family physicians. Part 2: Special populations. *Canadian Family Physician, 57*, 1269–1276.

Korhan, E. A., Uyar, M., Eyigör, C., et al. (2014). The effects of music therapy on pain in patients with neuropathic pain. *Pain Management Nursing, 15*(1), 306–314. doi:1-/1-16/j.mpmn.2012.10.006

Lane, A. M., Hirst, S. P., & Reed, M. B. (2015). *Older adults: Understanding and facilitating transitions*. Dubuque, IA: Kendall Hunt.

Lints-Martindale, A. C., Hadjistavropoulos, T., Lix, L. M., et al. (2012). A comparative investigation of observational pain assessment tools for older adults with dementia. *Clinical Journal of Pain, 28*(3), 226–237.

Lu, D. F., & Herr, K. (2012). Pain in dementia: Recognition and treatment. *Journal of Gerontological Nursing, 38*(2), 8–13.

Lynch, M. E. (2011). The need for a Canadian pain strategy. *Pain Research & Management, 16*(2), 77–79.

McCaffery, M. (1968). *Nursing practice theories related to cognition, bodily pain and man-environmental interactions*. Los Angeles, CA: UCLA Students Store.

McGreevy, K., Bottros, M. M., & Raja, S. N. (2011). Preventing chronic pain following acute pain. *European Journal of Pain, 5*(2), 365–372.

Monroe, T. B., & Mion, L. C. (2012). Patients with advanced dementia: How do we know if they are in pain? *Geriatric Nursing, 33*(3), 226–228.

National Center on Complementary and Alternative Medicine. (2014). *Chronic pain and complementary health approaches: What you need to know*. Retrieved from http://nccam.nih.gov.health/pain/chronic.htm

National Center on Complementary and Alternative Medicine. (2012). *Get the facts: Osteoarthritis and complementary health approaches*. Retrieved from http://nccam.nkg/gov

National Pain Centre. (2010). *Canadian guideline for safe and effective use of opioids for chronic non-cancer pain*. Retrieved from http://nationalpaincentre.mcmaster.ca/opioid/cgop_b04_r17.html

Özer, M., Karaman Özlü, Z., Arslan, S., et al. (2013). Effect of music on postoperative pain and physiologic parameters of patients after open heart surgery. *Pain Management Nursing, 14*(1), 20–28.

Pasero, C., & McCaffery, M. (2011a). Assessment tools. In C. Pasero & M. McCaffery (Eds.), *Pain assessment and pharmacologic management* (pp. 49–142). St. Louis, MO: Mosby Elsevier.

Pasero, C., & McCaffery, M. (2011b). Initiating opioid therapy. In C. Pasero & M. McCaffery (Eds.), *Pain assessment and pharmacologic management* (pp. 442–461). St. Louis, MO: Mosby Elsevier.

Pasero, C., & McCaffery, M. (2011c). Misconceptions that hamper assessment and treatment of patients who report pain. In C. Pasero & M. McCaffery (Eds.), *Pain assessment and pharmacologic management* (pp. 20–48). St. Louis, MO: Mosby Elsevier.

Pasero, C., & Portenoy, R. K. (2011). Neurophysiology of pain and analgesia and the pathophysiology of neuropathic pain. In C. Pasero & M. McCaffery (Eds.), *Pain assessment and pharmacologic management* (pp. 1–12). St. Louis, MO: Mosby Elsevier.

Pergolizzi, J. V., Raffa, R. B., & Taylor, R. (2014). Treating acute pain in light of the chronification of pain. *Pain Management Nursing, 15*(1), 380–390. doi:10.1016/j/pmn.2012/2.07.004

Reid, M. C., Bennett, D. A., Chen, W. G., et al. (2011). Improving the pharmacologic management of pain in older adults. *Pain Medicine, 12*(9), 1336–1357.

Reitsma, M. L., Tranmer, J. E., Buchanan, D. M., et al. (2011). The prevalence of chronic pain and pain-related interference in the Canadian population from 1994 to 2008. *Public Health Agency of Canada, 31*(4), 1–13.

Schopflocher, D., Taenzer, P., & Jovey, R. (2011). The prevalence of chronic pain in Canada. *Pain Research & Management, 16*(6), 445–450.

Shega, J. W., Ersek, M., Herr, K., et al. (2010). The multidimensional experience of noncancer pain: Does cognitive status matter? *Pain Medicine, 11*, 1680–1687.

Shengelia, R., Parker, S. J., Ballin, M., et al. (2013). Complementary therapies of osteoarthritis: Are they effective? *Pain Management Nursing, 14*(4), e274–e288. doi:10.1016/j.pmn/2012.01.001

Siedlecki, S. L., Modic, M. B., Bernhofer, E., et al. (2014). Exploring how bedside nurses care for patients with chronic pain: A grounded theory study. *Pain Management Nursing, 15*(3), 565–573. doi:10.1016/j/pmn.2013.12.007

Statistics Canada. (2010). *Healthy people, healthy places – Arthritis* [82-229-X]. Ottawa, ON: Government of Canada.

Taverner, T., Closs, S. J., & Briggs, M. (2014). The journey to chronic pain: A grounded theory of older adults' experiences of pain associated with leg ulceration. *Pain Management Nursing, 15*(1), 186–198. doi:10.1016/j/pmn.2012.08.002

Topcu, S. Y., & Findik, U. Y. (2012). Effect of relaxation exercises on controlling postoperative pain. *Pain Management Nursing, 13*(1), 11–17.

Tse, M. M. Y., Wan, V. T. C., & Vong, S. K. S. (2013). Health-related profile and quality of life among nursing home residents: Does pain matter? *Pain Management Nursing, 14*(4), 173–184. doi:10.1016/j.pmn.2011.10.006

Van de Ven, T. J., & John Hsia, H. L. (2012). Causes and prevention of chronic postsurgical pain. *Current Opinion in Critical Care, 18*(4), 366–371.

Vickers, A. J., Cronin, A. M., Maschino, A. C., et al. (2012). Acupuncture for chronic pain: Individual patient data meta-analysis. *Archives of Internal Medicine, 172*(19), 1444–1453. doi:10.1001/archinternmed.2012.3654

Wardell, D. W., Decker, S. A., & Engebretson, J. C. (2012). Healing touch for older adults with persistent pain. *Holistic Nursing Practice, 26*(4), 194–202.

Williams, A. M., Toye, C., Deas, K., et al. (2012). Evaluating the feasibility and effect of using a hospital-wide coordinated approach to introduce evidence-based changes for pain management. *Pain Management Nursing, 13*(4), 202–214.

Wysong, P. R. (2014). Nurses' beliefs and self-reported practices related to pain assessment in nonverbal patients. *Pain Management Nursing, 15*(1), 176–185. doi:10.1016/j/pmn.2012.08.003

Zwakhalen, S. M. G., van der Steen, J. T., & Najim, M. D. (2012). Which score most likely represents pain on the observational PAINAD pain scale for patients with dementia? *Journal of the American Medical Directors Association, 13*(4), 384–389.

chapter 29

Caring for Older Adults at the End of Life

Written by Marlette B. Reed

Because of the dramatic increases in both life expectancy and the length of time living with chronic conditions, there has been increasing emphasis on providing supportive care during chronic and life-limiting illness and at the end of life. Many illnesses that once were fatal have become chronic conditions; as a result, much of the health care focus is on helping older adults achieve quality of life while living with disabilities and chronic conditions and at some point experience a dignified death. Major emphasis also is on addressing complex and diverse needs of family and all those people who assume caregiving roles for older adults during times of illness and at end of life. Chapter 27 discussed care of older adults during progressive chronic conditions, and this chapter addresses care at the end of life.

PERSPECTIVES ON END-OF-LIFE CARE

Concepts related to death, dying and end of life have changed since the early 1900s in Canada, when the average life expectancy at birth averaged 60.6 years for females and 58.8 years for males in 1921 (Statistics Canada, 2010a).[1] At that time, death was a common occurrence in infants, children, youth and young adults, and it often occurred unexpectedly and in homes or community settings. Families provided care during brief illnesses—which most commonly were due to communicable diseases—and there was little or no prolonged end-of-life period. Accidental deaths were common, and death was accepted as an inevitable and normal part of life (Arnup, 2013).

Many factors have contributed to major shifts in the perceptions of death and dying and the ways in which end-of-life care is provided in Canada. By the 1950s, improved health care (vaccinations, more hospitals, greater public health education) led to longer life expectancies; it also led to the medicalization of end-of-life care (Arnup, 2013). By 1950, more than half of Canadians died in hospital (Smith & Nickel, 2003). The term **medicalization of end-of-life care** will be defined and discussed further in Trends in End-of-life Care.

---

[1]Canadian Aboriginal peoples are understood to have had a much shorter life expectancy in the early 1900s than the population as a whole. Comparable statistics for this time period are not available, but the high mortality rates for children in residential schools (some reports of close to 50%) are indicative of this understanding. See Bryce (1922). By the 1930s and 1940s, death rates were estimated to be greater than 700 deaths per 100,000 persons, "among the highest ever reported in a human population" (Arnup, 2013, p. 11).

When Does End-of-Life Care Begin?

Death has traditionally been defined as the cessation of all biologic functions. In many situations, however, major medical and technological developments have changed the perception of death from a clearly defined event to an evolving process. This is especially common in acute care settings, where, for example, a patient can be considered legally dead resulting from the absence of brain function, but not be clinically dead if medical technology has sustained heart and lung functioning. For many older adults, the **end of life** may be a gradual process that is associated with the cumulative effects of chronic illness and many interacting conditions, rather than a single cause. In many cases, a major medical event, such as sepsis or a fractured hip, becomes the "tipping point" that causes the older adult to transition from a state of chronic illness to an end-of-life state in which death occurs.

Nurse researchers at the Pennsylvania State University (Penrod et al., 2011) described the course and duration of three end-of-life trajectories as follows:

- Expected death trajectory: steep progressive decline, often measured in clinical benchmarks, with prolonged terminal phase
- Mixed death trajectory: initial successful treatment and period of stability, followed by steep decline and short terminal phase
- Unexpected death trajectory: slow decline (i.e., periodic exacerbations with recovery never reaching former level of health), followed by extremely short terminal phase

Penrod and colleagues (2012) applied this concept to caregiving through the end of life, with emphasis on the need for caregivers to "seek normal" during each phase of the trajectory, as illustrated in Figure 29-1. Although this model is applied to caregiving, it illustrates the different experiences of older adults and their caregivers across three end-of-life trajectories. It is important to recognize that the early phase of these trajectories may be subtle and recognized only in retrospect, as is often the case with dementia.

Views of Death and Dying in Western Culture

Western culture tends to deny or ignore the universality of death (Arnup, 2013; Lane, Hirst, & Reed, 2013) and this influences the type of health care services provided to people who are dying. Social gerontology studies have identified the following four contemporary values or beliefs that shape perceptions about aging and death in Western societies (Markson, 2003):

1. Work and activity are intertwined with self-worth, and chronic illness or disability is associated with the end of productivity and loss of purpose. Consequently, people may not acknowledge illness and aging because they are viewed as predecessors to death.
2. Through self-determination and individual responsibility, anyone can do anything if he or she tries hard enough. Because human life has inherent limitations, this false mentality is a major underpinning to the denial of aging and death in the 21st century.

3. Medical advances of the last several decades foster the belief that aging, illness and even death can be manipulated, managed and controlled.
4. Authority over and responsibility for death has subtly transferred from religious leaders to physicians. Consequently, the ability to cure illness and prolong life has imbued life and death with qualities that are more humanistic and less overtly spiritual.

Despite these prevalent attitudes and beliefs, acknowledgement and acceptance of death has been increasing, along with a focus on a more holistic view of end-of-life care. This change is due largely to the baby boom generation facing its own aging process while simultaneously dealing with their parents' aging and health issues. In addition, people living with serious and progressive conditions that significantly limit quality of life are increasingly expressing a desire to control their destiny.

Older Adults' Perspectives on Death and Dying

Although younger generations may feel they are invincible and immune to disease or death, older adults tend to be more aware and accepting of the inevitability of death, in part because they have experienced the deaths of family and friends, often including those who are younger than they are. Even though illness and functional limitations are common during older adulthood, older adults who develop a holistic perspective recognize that old age can present opportunities for fulfillment and self-actualization (Lane et al., 2013). As such, a "good death" is viewed as part of the process of "aging well," and both processes are individualized. Defining a "good death" for older adults is extremely personal and strongly influenced by one's level of function, independence and quality of life. Also, although older adults may have an increased awareness of the inevitability of death, true acceptance of death is not a clearly defined process and even at the end of life, humans "rhythmically oscillate between acceptance and nonacceptance of death" (McLeod-Sordjan, 2013, p. 391). And for some older adults, the term "good death" is an oxymoron; they, or their family members, may never come to accept that a death can be "good" (Lane et al., 2013).

A Student's Perspective

This week, I learned that it is okay to accept that an elderly patient is ready to die and that is his/her wish. I had a patient who requested that we not perform any measures—just give him his beer with lunch, wine with dinner and some pain medicine to make him comfortable. He stated that he has led a good life and is ready to go see God. That is really hard for me because it's my job to help people and save lives. The other aspect of that is helping people die a dignified death—it's just a really TOUGH aspect!!!

Sarah E.

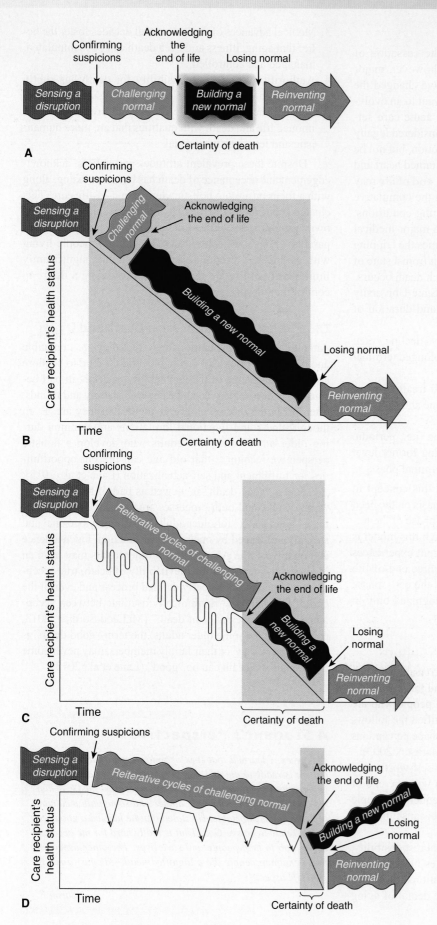

FIGURE 29-1 A model of caregiving through the end of life illustrating variations in the course and duration of phases. **(A)** Basic model, **(B)** caregiving across the expected death trajectory, **(C)** caregiving across the mixed death trajectory, **(D)** caregiving across the unexpected death trajectory. (Adapted with permission from SAGE Publications, Penrod, J., Hupcey, J. E., Shipley, P. Z., et al. [2012]. A model of caregiving through the end of life: Seeking normal. *Western Journal of Nursing Research, 34*[2], 175–193.)

Culturally Diverse Perspectives on Death and Dying

Because cultural perspectives exert a strong influence on end-of-life experiences, all health care professionals need to be aware of their own culturally based perceptions as well as those that influence older adults. Cultural influences can affect all the following aspects of end-of-life care:

- Perceptions of a good death
- Acceptance of hospice palliative care services
- Lines of communication about pending death and end-of-life decisions
- Expectations about medical interventions (e.g., decisions about resuscitation)
- Place where death occurs
- Practices and rituals near the end of the dying process and immediately following death
- Decisions about autopsy or organ donations

An important step in providing culturally appropriate nursing care is to explore one's own beliefs about death, dying and the end of life. Some questions to ponder for self-awareness and insight include the following (Ohio State University Health Sciences Center, Office of Geriatrics & Gerontology, 2003):

- When you hear the word "death," what comes to your mind? What do you personally fear the most? What are you most curious about?
- How old were you the first time someone close to you died? How was grief handled in your family? What do you believe happens to you when you die?
- Have you ever seen anyone die? What was that like for you?
- How do your own attitudes and previous experiences affect the way you work with dying patients now?

These types of questions elucidate a nurse's "lens" through which she processes loss and death. That paradigm is vital in working with the dying over the long term, as not having a way to deal with ongoing loss quickly burns a nurse out. She may experience physical and emotional symptoms that keep her from her work, or keep her from doing it effectively. A recent study in Great Britain showed that 10% of nurses missed more than 6 days due to illness in a 3-month period; 20% indicated that they have come to work when they were too ill to do their job (Van Stolk et al., 2009).[2] Being aware of one's own culturally based beliefs and attitudes is essential for a nurse's self-care.

Nurses also need to identify the culturally based beliefs and attitudes held by each person for whom they provide care. Religion and spirituality are two aspects of culture that are particularly powerful in relation to beliefs about death, dying and end-of-life decisions. Although it may be easy to ask about a person's religious affiliation as part of a nursing assessment, the more challenging aspect of providing

culturally appropriate care is identifying *the particular person's* beliefs and values that affect *his or her* care; within cultural and religious groups, there can be significantly differing needs. Nurses accomplish this by asking exploratory questions with a nonjudgmental approach about customs, beliefs and concerns about death, dying, afterlife and end of life, as described in the section on communication.

In clinical settings, nurses are integrally involved with one of the most concrete aspects of end-of-life care: postmortem care. This care is directed by institutional policies and standards of care and is a routine aspect of nursing care. What is not routine, however, is the incorporation of end-of-life rituals, which are often culturally based and are an essential aspect of supporting families and caregivers. An American study of long-term care nurses found that those who were foreign born stressed the need for end-of-life rituals whereas those born in the United States did not see this as important (Periyakoil et al., 2013). Though this study was limited in that its data came from a single health care system, it illustrates a universal principle in caregiving: caregivers bring with them cultural and religious beliefs and practices

A Student's Perspective

I found myself in a situation today in which I quickly recognized the importance of the lesson on cultural sensitivity in nursing. My aging client unfortunately had a significant change over the weekend, and her husband requested for her to be transported to the palliative care unit within the hospital. As she and I sat on her bed, she verbalized her acceptance that her disease is terminal. She wept as she voiced her heartache in telling her family of her "disappointment." Even though she is Catholic, because of her Chinese heritage and her family's Buddhist belief in "saving face," she worries that she has let her family down. While she expressed her thoughts, I listened and provided emotional support, which seemed to ease some of her grief. We transported her to the palliative care unit, and I assisted in making her comfortable with the new environment. When I went out to the nurses' station to give my report, the receiving nurse's first comment to me was, "I see she is Asian and you have her religious preference documented as Catholic. Are you sure that is correct?" Because of our recent discussions and reading on cultural sensitivity, I quickly realized how we as nurses can make incorrect assumptions in categorizing individuals on the basis of their ethnicity. I reported about my client's childhood history, her parents' belief in Buddhism, the Catholicism she was taught in school, and her long and strong Catholic faith. I found myself really understanding the importance of educating ourselves as nurses about different cultures and the effect of cultural belief systems on individualized health care. As difficult as it was for me to leave my client in a strange environment, I felt that the information I had learned and shared would enable the staff to be respectful of her beliefs, which in turn would be a positive experience for my client during her stay.

Deborah L.

[2]As a result of this study, the National Health Service in Great Britain formulated a response to address these issues. See Nash (2011).

Box 29-1 Cultural Considerations: Death Rituals Commonly Associated With Specific Groups

Group	Death Ritual	Intervention
African Canadians	May respond to news of death of a loved one by *falling out* (i.e., sudden collapse, paralysis and inability to see or speak). There may be wailing present. Loved ones may cover their heads with a blanket or covering.	Recognize that this is a culturally based response; that the physical responses are not medical emergencies can be evidenced by a number of the community present experiencing these symptoms, as well as by others in the community who have come to provide support who can provide you with assurances (especially if those evidencing these symptoms do not speak English). As a nurse, provide support.
European Canadians	Believe that the dying person should not be left alone.	Make accommodations for family members to be present at all times.
Hindus	Priest and eldest son may perform death rites, with all male relatives assisting; women may respond with loud wailing.	Provide a supportive and private environment; offer understanding of death rituals and grief behaviours.
Japanese	Family members gather at the bedside at the time of death, with the eldest son having particular responsibilities at the time (as determined by the family).	Notify eldest son of pending death, identify lines of communication if eldest son is not available.
Jewish	Dying person should not be left alone in their dying; also, family will often remain with the body of their loved one who has just passed away. Death rituals vary and some are not performed on the Sabbath or holy days.	Ask the closest relative specifically about postmortem practices.
Koreans	Family members are expected to stay with the person who is dying and assist with care. If the family are Christian, there will be a number of the community who come at a passing; singing and praying is common.	Support family in caring for the person. Provide the family and their community with the time and space, if possible, to pray and sing.
Ismailis (Muslims)	There will be reading from the Qur'an, as well as prayers. Family members will ask for their loved one's eyes to be closed. Particularly in larger urban centres, members of the mosque bereavement committee will come to provide support to the grieving family after death. They will also call the funeral home and assist the family with funeral preparations.	Provide privacy for the readings and prayers. Also, if possible, close the deceased person's eyes.
Buddhists	Many Buddhists desire that the body of their loved one not be touched for a certain period of time (1–12 hours post-mortem). This is to allow the spirit to leave the body. Also, the family may request quietness; overt displays of emotion may be reserved for outside of the room.	Discuss with the family *ahead of time* what their desires are post-mortem. As much as possible, accommodate their desire to have the body not touched after passing. (Sometimes families will be accommodating of nursing needs to take out sites, etc.)
Vietnamese	Flowers are avoided during illness because they are usually reserved for rites of the dead.	Ask permission from the patient or family before placing flowers in a room.

Sources: Purnell, L. D. (2013). *Transcultural health care* (4th ed.). Philadelphia, PA: F. A. Davis; Cloutier, K. (2012). *Customs and traditions: In times of death and bereavement* (3rd ed.). Calgary, AB: McInnis and Holloway.

that impact how they do care[3] (see Box 29-1). As with other aspects of culturally appropriate care, it is important for caregivers entrusted with postmortem care to be cognizant of their own cultural and religious lenses, as well as to be aware of the different practices associated with particular groups represented by their patients. An effective way of

[3]An international study involving foreign-born health care workers in Canada, the United States, the United Kingdom and Ireland addressed the demands of caring for aging populations and diminishing work forces. In these four nations, a lack of funding for the care of older adults (and hence low-paying jobs), with a resistance on the part of native-born workers to enter this profession, has resulted and is predicted to continue to result in a significant number of foreign-born caregivers for older adults. See Spencer et al. (2010).

addressing this issue with patients is to inquire ahead of time about preferences of older adults, families and caregivers and incorporate pertinent information in the care plan. In an end-of-life situation, it is not uncommon for families to change their minds over time on postmortem care/rituals. Here, an evolving care plan, with communication between nurses occurring both interpersonally and on this plan, can ensure that family wishes are carried out.

Trends in Providing End-of-life Care

Just as medical and technological advances, such as control of communicable diseases and medical and surgical treatments for serious illnesses, changed perspectives on death,

major medical advances that began during the 20th century shifted the approach to end-of-life care. By the middle of the 20th century, health care facilities had become centres for curing disease and health care professionals viewed death as something to be avoided because it symbolized failure. Prolonging life, even at the expense of quality, was viewed as the ultimate accomplishment: a symbol of success for patients, families and the health care teams involved. The term **medicalization of end-of-life care** describes care that focuses on prolonging life through the use of medical technology rather than on interventions for comfort and quality of life. As a result of the medicalization of end-of-life care, patients often suffered through treatments that did not cure. And sadly, death was understood to be a "medical failure" (Arnup, 2013, p. 8). This affected the quality of care. "Nurses often did a poor job in caring for the dying because they were neither emotionally prepared nor practically trained in what to do. The curriculum taught them how to save lives, not how to care for the dying" (Smith & Nickel, 2003, p. 336).

A shift away from the medicalization of end-of-life care began in Canada with the hospice palliative care movement in the 1960s and 1970s. However, nurses and other health care professionals have continued to raise concerns about the need to improve end-of-life care in hospitals because studies confirm that despite the increased attention to this issue, patients continue to experience pain, indignity, social isolation and uncomfortable symptoms related to ineffective and unwanted life-sustaining treatments, particularly in intensive care units (Seaman, 2013). Much of this concern is associated with poor communication between professionals and families about end-of-life decision-making (Wiegand et al., 2013). The Canadian Association of Critical Care Nurses (CACCN) has issued a comprehensive position statement about end-of-life care in intensive care units addressing the need for effective communication between professionals and patients/families, as well as between interprofessional team members. It also advocates further training in end-of-life issues for those working in critical care environments (CACCN, 2011). An expected outcome of the increasing use of hospice palliative care services is that the care of the dying, in whatever setting they reside, will continue to improve (see the section on hospice palliative care).

In Canada, the 1990s saw a significant reduction in funding for universal health care, which affected the number of hospitalizations and length of stays in hospital (Canadian Institute for Health Information, 2005). This too contributed to the deinstitutionalization of many health and life issues, including death. In Canada, the number of deaths that occur within hospital settings sits at about 66% (Statistics Canada, 2012). With renewed emphasis upon palliative care, as mentioned previously, this has opened the door for more home care palliative care and residential hospices. However, funding was, and continues to be, a major issue.

This does not mean, however, that Canadians are all receiving adequate end-of-life care. Only 16% to 30% of dying Canadians have access to hospice palliative care; access is highly dependent upon region in Canada (CHPCA Fact Sheet, 2013). Canadian families often shoulder about a quarter of the cost of care, and almost two thirds indicated that they could not provide the necessary number of hours required to care for loved ones at home (CHPCA Fact Sheet, 2013). And it is a reality that many Canadian deaths will occur in hospital; Dr. Sharon Baker, a palliative care specialist with the London Health Sciences Centre (ON), said, "The most important thing is to recognize that people will die in hospital and we need to provide a good, humane environment for those people. The biggest problem right now isn't that people are dying in hospital. It's that people aren't dying well in hospital" (Cairns & Ahmad, 2011, n.p.).

As the Canadian population continues to age, it is estimated that toward the end of this decade, there will be more seniors than children (The Canadian Press, 2012) and that by 2036, seniors could account for between 23% and 25% of the population (Statistics Canada, 2010b). Currently, 92.1% live independently, with the rest of the above-65 population living in residences for seniors or in nursing homes.

It should be stated that the term "nursing home" does not refer to all collective living arrangements for seniors (Statistics Canada, 2010b). Within Canadian society has come, in the past several decades, a proliferation of options for seniors in terms of living arrangements. "Independent living" incorporates the +55 population living within their own homes, as well as seniors' apartments and complexes.[4] Within collective arrangements, seniors may live in "assisted living" that provides some aids to daily living (such as meal preparation and rides to appointments). Independent living and assisted living arrangements do not fall under the jurisdiction of our health care system; hence health care dollars are not spent here. Another collective arrangement is a nursing home or "continuing care facility" (Lane et al., 2013).[5] Nursing homes are facilities for the disabled and/or elderly who need nursing/medical care (and hence have coverage under our universal health care system), and, with the deinstitutionalization of Canadian health care, the criterion for placement is quite rigorous. One source estimated that about 10% of Canadians die in nursing homes (Cairns & Ahmad, 2011).

There is much discussion in our country about how we will cope with fewer adults working (due to low birth rates) and many more seniors to look after. "Often described as the 'crisis' of the aging baby boomers, this population shift poses a number of major social and health care policy challenges" (Arnup, 2013, p. 4). Our aging population will die later, having coped with (and received care for) a number of chronic health conditions. From an end-of-life perspective, hospital deaths are costly to our health care system. The pressure to

[4]The term "senior" can be applied to those 55 years and older, as well as those 65 years and above. Particularly in housing arrangements that are designed for the "mature" population, the definition of *senior* tends to be the 55-year mark.

[5]For a fuller discussion of housing arrangements available for seniors in Canada (both conventional and unconventional), see Lane et al. (2013).

care for aging family members within the home is increasing. Members of the "sandwich generation" are caring for their children and their aging parents simultaneously (Lane et al., 2013).

Whether a Canadian senior dies in hospital, in a nursing home or at home, the emphasis now in the health care system is upon greater palliative care in each setting. Hospitals have palliative care units, and some hospitals house "hospices" within their walls; residential hospices exist typically within urban settings, residents within nursing homes are receiving palliative care coming into them, and palliative care teams within the community provide care within homes for dying older adults. The call is for an "integrated palliative care approach" for Canada, where clinicians in all setting will be able to recognize when an older adult and his family could benefit from palliative care and would be able to connect them with the resources that are both available and appropriate for their needs (Hodgson, 2012, p. 4).

From a financial perspective, palliative care makes sense: it is estimated that hospital-based palliative care may save the health care system up to $8,000 per patient (Hodgson, 2012) and reduces the cost of end-of-life care by 50% or more, mainly through reducing the number of intensive care unit admissions, diagnostic tests, medical interventions and the length of hospital stay (Hodgson, 2012). While it is widely accepted that there is much room for improvement within Canadian health care regarding palliative care, we are learning. Greater emphasis is being put into medical and nursing education, public awareness campaigns are being run, and the social and spiritual benefits of palliative care are enormous. The increased emphasis on the "rehumanizing" of end-of-life care, which recognizes and respects the process of death and dying as an important and meaningful stage of the continuum of human life, is reconnecting dying individuals with their own souls, with their loved ones and (sometimes) with the Transcendent. Lynn Keegan and Carole Ann Drick (2011) are two nurses who are leading a movement to implement the "Golden Room" concept for providing end-of-life care for a dignified death. They propose a model that changes the consciousness around death and dying to one of acceptance and reverence. In this model, rather than being an ending, death is "a sacred passage, a time of honouring, a time for goodness, a time for compassion, a time for peace, dignity, and most of all gentle release" (Keegan & Drick, 2011, p. 154).

As end-of-life care is becoming a more integral part of the medical mainstream, the issue of quality of life versus quantity of life at all costs has broadened the professional perspective. Nurses and other health care professionals increasingly realize that they can find meaning, rewards and satisfaction in caring for people at the end of life and for families and others who are an integral part of the dying person's support network. Hospice palliative care professionals play a key role in promoting awareness and understanding of holistic end-of-life care, both as direct providers of care and as consultants for those who are less skilled in this area, as discussed in the section on hospice palliative care.

Current Legal and Ethical Concerns

Ethical and legal questions and challenges are escalating as citizens, governments, institutions and health care professionals express concerns about care and policies that directly affect end-of-life care.

In three countries in the western world, physician-assisted suicide and euthanasia have been made legal: The Netherlands, Belgium and Luxembourg. In the United States, the state of Oregon passed the Death With Dignity Act in 1997. This bill was passed by the majority of voters, allowing terminally ill and competent adults to request a lethal injection for the purpose of ending their lives (Death With Dignity National Center, 2013). Since that time, physician-assisted suicide has been legalized in three other states: Montana, Vermont and Washington.

There are significant structures put around the right to die in the United States. Jablonski and colleagues (2012) described the following requirements that are built into the Death With Dignity Act to control its use:

- The person must make several requests for assisted suicide, with at least 15 days between first and last request.
- Two physicians must determine that the person is competent.
- Information must be provided about hospice, but there is no requirement that the person enrol in hospice.
- Physicians and institutions are not required to provide physician-assisted death.

In Canada, at this time, physician-assisted suicide and euthanasia are illegal. But the "right to die" is being discussed vigorously. In 2013, the Quebec National Assembly proposed **Bill 52**: *An Act Respecting End-of-Life Care* (Bill 52, 2013). It allows for the euthanasia of adults with capacity (mentally competent) who are dying. In this legislation, doctors are allowed to give lethal injection (as opposed to the patients themselves), "making it the first jurisdiction in North America to allow physicians to deliberately end patients' lives" (Hamilton, 2014, n.p.). At the time of this writing, the bill was blocked in the provincial legislature, but the debate within the province and within the country is expected to continue. Though health care is under provincial jurisdiction, the Criminal Code is federal. So a provincial bill allowing euthanasia would contravene the Criminal Code, which does not permit it: provincial jurisdiction (medical issues) opposes federal jurisdiction (legal issues) (Reichel, 2014). The debate is expected to go to the Supreme Court of Canada. There is much dispute, and this issue is value-laden.

For example, note the terminology used in this heated discussion; those who believe in "the right to die" will use the term "medical aid in dying" (e.g., Bill 52, 2013, p. 10) as opposed to "physician-assisted suicide." The debate comes down to fundamental beliefs about life, autonomy (the right to one's own values and, if possible, decision-making), beneficence (doing what is good) and about the role of health care and health care providers in dying.

In the midst of this ethical debate resides much misinformation in the Canadian public. Difficult experiences of dying elderly relatives years ago will result in some Canadians' approving of euthanasia, without the knowledge of all the advances in pain control, as well as the legal latitude of palliative care. Particular to the debate in Quebec, retired lawyer Michel Racicot of Living With Dignity made allusion to this: "Quebecers already have the right to refuse or to discontinue treatment. They already have the right to say 'no' to overtreatment and to receive effective painkillers and, if necessary, sedation to reduce their pain. These actions have nothing to do with euthanasia" (Physicians' Alliance for Total Refusal of Euthanasia, 2013, n.p.). Regarding difficult dying experiences, a number of studies have shown that when issues such as pain—physical, emotional or psychological—are alleviated, patients who had been thinking about euthanasia no longer wish to die in that way (Materstvedt et al., 2003; Segers, 1988; Teno et al., 2011; von Gunten, 2012).

At the heart of impassioned discussion in the public is the phrase "dying with dignity." This phrase has increasingly become associated with the "right to die" movement (particularly in the United States). But it is used by parties on both sides of the debate. Those who favour physician-assisted suicide and/or euthanasia speak of not wanting disability, lack of continence and the existential angst of facing into death; to them, dying with dignity means not having to experience these things. Those against physician-assisted suicide and euthanasia speak of the human dignity and sense of the sacred that can be present in the midst of this experience, for the dying individual, family members and caregivers. There is also the recognition that the dying experience can be a time of significant emotional and spiritual growth for the dying individual and his or her family members (Lane et al., 2013).

Carleton University professor Dr. Katherine Arnup (2013) stated, as one who volunteers in a hospice and supported her father through his terminal illness, that "there is nothing inherently undignified in the care that is required at the end of life. Rather, dignity resides in the quality and nature of the care provided and in the attitudes of both the caregiver and the recipient of care" (p. 16). Fenigsen (2012) agreed and stated, "We are told that to be assisted by medical technology entails loss of dignity, as if the dignity of honest, caring, courageous people, our parents and spouses, could somehow be drained out of them through medical devices" (p. 73).

Whether euthanasia becomes legal in Canada has huge professional implications. Health care providers are wary. In a 2013 Canadian Medical Association survey, only 1 in 5 Canadian physicians would be willing to carry out a request from one of their patients for euthanasia (Kirkey, 2014, n.p.). In a very gentle article about this subject from a physician's perspective, Dr. Manual Borod, a palliative care physician at the Montreal General Hospital and head of the division of supportive and palliative care programs at Montreal's McGill University, spoke of his practice and his philosophy. He indicated that his discomfort with Bill 52 is not because of religious or "right to life" reasons, but rather because the parameters of the legislation are too broad. He noted that for intractable physical or psychological suffering, he can

(without Bill 52) prescribe palliative sedation. And he spoke of the value that palliative care can add to individual patients' and their families lives. Summing up his position, he states,

> *I can't say that I would never—under any circumstance— consider hastening death. That is too extreme. But, I just don't see the need for it . . . I feel very strongly about not forcing treatment, about letting people die and not getting in the way. But we don't have to kill them.* (Kirkey, 2013, n.p.)

The aged are particularly affected by the outcome of end-of-life decisions within our land, as they are, as a demographic, most close to the end of life. Chapter 9 discusses issues related to decision-making and advance directives, and Online Learning Activity 29-1 provides additional information pertinent to nursing roles and responsibilities for end-of-life care.

 See **ONLINE LEARNING ACTIVITY 29-1: RESOURCES FOR ADDITIONAL INFORMATION ABOUT LEGAL AND ETHICAL ISSUES RELATED TO END-OF-LIFE NURSING CARE** at http://thepoint.lww.com/Miller7e

HOSPICE PALLIATIVE CARE

The terms *hospice* and *palliative care* both refer to an interprofessional approach to care that holistically addresses the needs of people with life-limiting conditions, as well the needs of their families and others who care for and care about them. In Canada, these two terms are used interchangeably, and, as evidenced in this chapter, as often used in combination: **hospice palliative care** (Arnup, 2013).[6] "End-of-life care" is also used interchangeably with hospice palliative care. The definition for palliative care in Canada is as follows: "[A] type of health care for patients and families facing life-threatening illness. (It) helps patients to achieve the best quality of life right up until the end of life" (Canadian Virtual Hospice, 2003–2014). Hospice care will be focused upon separately now, as "hospice" is not just a philosophy of care and resulting practice, but it also has a history as an international movement.

Hospice Care

Hospice care refers to a philosophy of care that seeks to support dignified dying or a good death experience for people with terminal illnesses and for their families and caregivers. The term *hospice* (from the same linguistic root as "hospitality") was first applied to specialized care for dying patients in the 1960s by physician and nurse Dame Cicely Saunders, who founded the first modern hospice—St. Christopher's— in a residential suburb of London. During a guest lecture

---

[6]In the United States, these terms are closely associated, but differ in that palliative care refers to the alleviating of suffering throughout a serious illness, whereas hospice care is limited to end-of-life care (the dying individual has a life expectancy of 6 months or less).

for medical students, nurses, social workers and chaplains at Yale University, Saunders introduced the idea of hospice care and emphasized holistic services and symptom control. This lecture sparked interest, which led to the development of hospice care as it is known today.

Another influencing factor was the publication of the book *On Death and Dying* by psychiatrist Elisabeth Kübler-Ross in 1969. This book, based on interviews with dying patients, identified five stages through which many terminally ill patients progress: denial, anger, bargaining, depression and acceptance (Kübler-Ross, 1969). This book was well received by the public and health care professionals and drew attention to the needs of dying people. In 1972, Kübler-Ross testified at the U.S. Senate Special Committee on Aging, pleading for federal legislation to provide resources for supporting end-of-life care at home.

In Canada, the founder of our hospice palliative care movement is Dr. Balfour Mount. In the 1970s, he utilized the model of Cicely Saunders' hospice, but sought to enact that within Montreal's Royal Victoria Hospital (Comeau, 2014). Since that time, palliative care units within hospitals and hospices, as well as palliative home care, have grown throughout the country.

The value of hospice services is great. Hospice treats the person, not just the disease. It focuses on the family, not simply the patient; and it emphasizes the quality of life, not just the duration. Hospice services are provided by interprofessional teams and include the following services: physicians, nurses, health care aides, social workers, spiritual counsellors, volunteers, bereavement counsellors, and speech, physical and occupational therapists. Some programs offer additional services such as music, art, reiki and pet therapy. These services are provided by public and private agencies in any setting, including homes, hospitals, short- or long-term residential facilities or freestanding hospice centres. And, as mentioned earlier, hospice services are much more cost-effective than hospitalization.

Eligibility criteria for hospice include physician referral and, generally, a patient prognosis of 6 months or less (the prognosis may vary according to facility). As well, the patient has decided to focus upon comfort measures, rather than a cure; additionally, there is agreement that resuscitation will not be used when symptoms bring about death (Canadian Virtual Hospice, 2003–2014). An important role for nurses in all settings is to encourage older adults and their families to find information about hospice even in the absence of a clearly defined "terminal" phase. Hospice programs usually arrange for exploratory meetings to discuss services, and they can suggest other resources in the community if the person is not immediately eligible.

There is, within our nation, widespread recognition on the part of government and the health care system that hospice palliative care is not accessible to many Canadians (see Box 29-2). In 2000, a Canadian Senate report—*Quality End-of-Life Care: The Right of Every Canadian*—called for the federal government, in conjunction with the provinces and

---

Box 29-2 Evidence-Informed Nursing Practice

Background: Research has shown that there are significant regional differences in palliative care availability within Canada. As well, there are significant differences in terms of who has access and who accesses that care. Canada's Aboriginal population (First Nations, Metis and Inuit peoples) experience both: while almost 60% of Aboriginal peoples now live within urban settings, many do not choose to access palliative care, due to lack of cultural sensitivity within the system. In rural settings, there is often less available palliative care, and if no reserves are within that area, the Aboriginal peoples may have "blended in" with the population, not identifying themselves as Aboriginal for fear of prejudice; as a result, cultural practices may have been lost or set aside. The researchers of this article identified that currently there is no national standard for Aboriginal palliative care.

Question: From the standpoint of formal and informal palliative care providers, what are the issues for rural Aboriginal peoples in receiving quality palliative care in their dying?

Method: Researchers chose an area of rural British Columbia in which there is a small Aboriginal population living, with no reserves: the West Kootenay-Boundary region of British Columbia. In this qualitative study, 31 formal (paid) and informal (volunteers, pastors, family caregivers) palliative care providers were interviewed; there was a semistructure guide used, and the majority of questions were open ended.

Findings: Some of the challenges of WKB region's Aboriginal population were clear: the Aboriginal people in this area of British Columbia are understood to be "invisible" in that they are a small minority in this region, and prejudice against them keeps some from identifying their Aboriginal heritage. Other findings were not clear: Some of the interviewees felt that there was a denial to access of palliative care services through existing prejudices; others felt that the Aboriginal peoples in the area chose not to access services available to them because they were not interested in them.

Nursing Practice Implications: In order to provide culturally safe palliative care for Aboriginal peoples in the region, there needs to be training for palliative care workers in cultural sensitivity, death needs to occur in the place of the patient's choice and a patient must be able to carry out meaningful cultural practices, such as smudging. There is a large gap in the palliative care literature regarding the Canadian Aboriginal people's experience with receiving care, and, as such, more research needs to be conducted.

Source: Castleden, H., Crooks, V., Hanlon, N., et al. (2010). Providers' perceptions of Aboriginal palliative care in British Columbia's rural interior. *Health and Social Care in the Community, 18*(5), 483–491. doi:10.1111/j.1365-2524.2010.00922.x

---

territories, to develop a strategy for quality end-of-life care available to all in our nation. The Quality End-of-Life Care Coalition of Canada (QECCC, 2014) came together as what was then 24 health care agencies (it now is more than 36) to seek to develop such a strategy, guided by the mission statement: ". . . all Canadians have the right to quality end-of-life care that allows them to die with dignity, free of pain, surrounded by their loved ones, in a setting of their choice" (n.p.). This coalition, made up by more than 36 Canadian health care organizations, is seeking to develop a comprehensive strategy for end-of-life care. It has developed a "Blueprint for Action: 2010–2020." With the demographic pressure of increased numbers of older adults, fewer adult children to care for them, as well as the stresses of an overburdened health care system, concerted efforts are being made to address current needs and prepare for the future. The comprehensive plan involves a number of facets, including the education of the public *about* the benefits of hospice palliative care and the education of health care professionals *in* hospice palliative care; the need of greater funds directed to this area of health care; government benefits for caregivers (such as the Compassionate Care Benefit); providing quality hospice palliative care in regions which do not yet have it; and encouraging Canadians to have end-of-life conversations before the reality is upon them. For example, Canadians are encouraged to complete Advanced Care Planning[7] (QECCC, 2010).

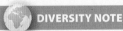

DIVERSITY NOTE

Studies show that ethnicity, cultural and religious beliefs impact many end-of-life decisions, including the use of hospice palliative care. Patients of North American and Northern European descent are more likely to favour end-of-life options with less technology (such as hospice care). Physicians of similar descent are likely to recommend such options. Also, patients from East Asian communities are less likely to speak openly about death, including to the family member who is dying; hence these families may utilize hospice palliative care less frequently (Fowler & Hammer, 2013). While there is diversity among aboriginal Canadians, many would prefer to die at home with family and friends (as opposed to being transported to major cities to die in hospital) and some older aboriginals believe that telling the truth about the diagnosis may jeopardize an individual's health (The Royal Society of Canada, 2011).

PROMOTING WELLNESS AT THE END OF LIFE

Wellness at the end of life is closely connected to the concept of a "good death." Because the phrase "death with dignity" is increasingly associated with physician-assisted suicide and euthanasia, terms such as **dignified death** or dignified care are more appropriate for describing a good death. The degree to which hospital care is perceived as dignified is influenced by many variables, such as the following ones that are directly related to nurses: attitude and behaviours, promotion of patient independence, professional commitment and competency, and verbal and nonverbal communication, including compassionate behaviour and taking enough time (Lin et al., 2013; Manookian et al., 2013).

Some characteristics of dignified care identified by older adults in studies (Cairns et al., 2013; van Gennip et al., 2013) that are most pertinent to maintaining their personhood (Hirst et al., 2013), as well as promoting wellness at the end of life, are as follows:

- Being treated as an individual and with respect, including the proper use of his/her name
- Maintaining independence, while having basic care needs met

- Being involved in decision-making
- Having privacy and a safe environment
- Being listened to (including some socialization with caregiving staff) and having needs and wishes respected
- Experiencing good communication
- Feeling peaceful and ready to die
- Absence of anxiety and depressive mood

These characteristics are in accord with the "Dying Patient's Bill of Rights," a document created at a workshop on "The Terminally Ill Patient and the Helping Person" by Linda Austin (1975) to identify concretely the dignified care that dying people deserve (Box 29-3). This document continues to be helpful as a guide for defining goals and interventions for individualized end-of-life care.

In the Nursing Outcomes Classification (NOC), a Dignified Death (now called Dignified Life Closure, to reflect American discourse on end-of-life) is defined as "personal actions to maintain control when approaching end of life"; it includes the following specific outcomes that are within the realm of nursing care: maintains physical independence, participates in decisions related to care, shares feelings about dying, maintains sense of control of remaining time, completes meaningful goals, shares feelings about dying, discusses spiritual concerns and experiences, exchanges affection with others and controls treatment choices, including food and drink intake (Moorhead et al., 2013, p. 201). Nursing interventions to achieve these outcomes are discussed in the next section.

Box 29-3   The Dying Person's Bill of Rights

I have the right to be treated as a living human being until I die.
I have the right to maintain a sense of hopefulness, however changing its focus may be.
I have the right to express my feelings and emotions about my approaching death in my own way.
I have the right to participate in decisions concerning my care.
I have the right to expect continuing medical and nursing attention even though cure goals must be changed to comfort goals.
I have the right not to die alone.
I have the right to be free from pain.
I have the right to have my questions answered honestly.
I have the right not to be deceived.
I have the right to have help from and for my family in accepting my death.
I have the right to die in peace and with dignity.
I have the right to retain my individuality and not be judged for my decisions, which may be contrary to the beliefs of others.
I have the right to be cared for by caring, sensitive, knowledgeable people who will attempt to understand my needs and will be able to gain some satisfaction in helping me face my death.
I have the right to be cared for by those who can maintain a sense of hopefulness, however changing this might be.
I have the right to expect that the sanctity of the human body will be respected after death.
I have the right to discuss and enlarge my religious and/or spiritual experiences, whatever these may mean to others.

Source: Austin, L. (1975). *Dying patient's bill of rights*. Created at The Terminally Ill Patient and the Helping Person Workshops. Sponsored by the Southwest Michigan Inservice Education Council in Lansing, MI.

---

[7]Fowler and Hammer (2013) indicated that while the majority of Canadians do not wish to have aggressive treatment in their dying, relatively few have spoken to family members and their physicians about what their wishes are. This is indicative of our reluctance in Canada to speak about dying.

Perceptions of dignity at the end of life are influenced by religious teachings. For example, the dignity and value of life in the Christian faith is rooted in Jesus, who was human and gave respect to all human life, as created in "the image of God" (Gen. 1:25–26). In the Jewish faith, dignity of life is based in the belief that life and death are in God's hands, and humans have the responsibility to live life to the fullest and have life last as long as possible (Zamer & Volker, 2013). In Buddhism, the dignity of human life is rooted in the belief that each individual life is a manifestation of a universal life force (Soka Gakkai International, 2014).

A Student's Perspective

When I left the nursing home today I felt better about working with people facing the certain end of their lives. Mr. F. had a really positive attitude about his inoperable brain tumour and it made me understand that I am the one who feels uncomfortable with death. He expressed that his life has meaning and that he is here for a reason. He told me about some of his goals in life: he plans to get out of the nursing home so that he can travel around the country in an RV with his wife. He seemed to imply that even if that goal never occurred, it was OK, that it was mostly something to look forward to. All of the communication with Mr. F. had a huge impact on me. It gave me a whole new perspective on how people view their lives. This man is suffering from this terrible disease, yet he still finds hope and has goals in life.

Erin H.

NURSING SKILLS AND INTERVENTIONS FOR END-OF-LIFE CARE

Caring for people at the end of life is one of the most challenging aspects of nursing, and, when it is done well, it can be rewarding for all involved. For hospice palliative care nursing certification (2008), much is required in terms of knowledge and skills understood to be essential for quality end-of-life care. The following is a broad summary of the requirements:

- Effective symptom management
- Advocating for patient's quality of life
- Effective communication with patient and his or her family about prognosis, treatment, goals of care, the dying process and death
- Assisting the patient with maintaining and promoting functional capacity, as is possible
- Comprehensive, compassionate whole-person care, including psychological and spiritual support for patients and their families
- Knowledge of grief and of bereavement services

The next sections discuss nursing skills in relation to communication and management of symptoms, and Box 29-4 summarizes some nursing interventions that are pertinent to end-of-life care.

Box 29-4 Supportive Interventions for Relationship Building

Presence	A core nursing intervention, presence can be described as a "gift of self" in which the nurse is available and open to the situation.
	Presence can be demonstrated through verbal communication, valuing what the patient says, accepting the patient's meaning for things and remembering or reflecting.
Compassion	The nurse strives to be totally and compassionately *with* the patient and family, allowing the most positive experience.
Touch	A powerful therapeutic intervention, touch communicates an offer of unconditional acceptance. It can be both healing and life affirming, a means of communicating genuine care and compassion.
Recognition of Autonomy	The nurse realizes and respects the individual's right to make end-of-life decisions.
Honesty	The nurse is often in a frontline position to communicate/explain what can be expected. Compassionate honesty builds trust with the older adult facing death and his or her family.
Expert Communication	At any given moment, nurses need to be able to assess the patient and family, implement a plan to comfort them and communicate clearly and supportively throughout.
Assisting in Transcendence	At the highest level of care, nurses provide emotional support that facilitates the experience of self-transcendence and a sense of triumph over death.

Source: Saunderson, C. A., & Brener, T. H. (Eds.). (2007). *End of life: A nurse's guide to compassionate care* (p. 6). Philadelphia, PA: Lippincott Williams & Wilkins.

It is beyond the scope of this book to offer comprehensive information about this topic, but links to resources for more in-depth information are provided in Online Learning Activity 29-2.

See **ONLINE LEARNING ACTIVITY 29-2:**
ADDITIONAL RESOURCES ABOUT PROVIDING
NURSING CARE AT THE END OF LIFE
at http://thepoint.lww.com/Miller7e

Communication

When caring for people at the end of life, communication is critically important to all involved, and its importance is magnified by the complexity and uncertainty of the circumstances. In these situations, nurses can help people who are dying and their caregivers express their needs by using open, honest, direct and empathetic communication, even when they may be unsure about what to say. See Box 29-5

Box 29-5 Communicating With Dying Patients and Their Families

What to Say

Tell me more about ….
What questions do you have about your condition?
What are you most concerned about right now?
How are you feeling right now?
I hear your concern [worry, frustration].
How can I be helpful?
I'm here to listen and I'll do my best to help [support, alleviate discomfort].
Take your time.
Is there someone I can call to help with this? [e.g., family, religious person, medical professional]
It's okay to cry. This is very sad for you.
Would you prefer to be left alone?
Would you like to share some memories?

Nonverbal Communication

Maintain active presence.
Use touch purposefully.
Communicate patience and respectful waiting.
Learn to be comfortable with silence.
Allow yourself to cry and express emotions in an appropriate and supportive way.

for examples of verbal and nonverbal communication techniques that are appropriate for end-of-life care. It is essential to base all communication on the assumption that people who are dying are able to hear what is being said either to or about them, even if they appear to be unresponsive. An important aspect of communication is to create and support an environment that is appropriate for the needs of the person who is dying as well as his or her family. Sensory components of a supportive environment include music, silence, sounds of nature, pleasant scents, conversations with loved ones, warm blankets and other comfort items. At times the needs of the person dying and his or her family members will conflict; when this occurs, the needs of the *patient* take precedence.

Offering Spiritual Support

Spiritual care is as an essential aspect of nursing care at all times and it becomes even more important at the end of life. Specific ways in which nurses can address spiritual needs at the end of life are described by the (American) Hospice and Palliative Nurses Association (2010) as follows:

- Listening reflectively to the patient's and family's story with a compassionate presence
- Demonstrating empathy and the ability to journey with others in their suffering
- Recognizing and responding to spiritual distress and facilitating the discovery of meaning in the experience of illness, suffering, grief and loss
- Eliciting key concerns with respect, including feelings of hopelessness, loss, brokenness and other unmet spiritual and religious needs

- Identifying and responding to ethical issues and conflicts and assisting and supporting others in the application of their own values in decision-making
- Willingness to create therapeutic and healing spaces in which spiritual expression can occur
- Facilitating the use of symbol and ritual according to the needs and values of the patient and family
- Offering sensitivity, prayer, music, scripture or other readings that are meaningful to the patient and family
- Supporting spiritual strengths of the patient and family
- Seeking additional resources as needed by the patient and family including chaplaincy or other spiritual providers

Chapters 12 and 13 in this book provide additional information about nursing assessment and intervention related to spiritual care for older adults.

Nursing diagnoses pertinent to spiritual care during the end of life are Risk for Spiritual Distress, Spiritual Distress and Readiness for Enhanced Spiritual Well-Being. The following nursing interventions relevant to spiritual care at the end of life are as follows: Active Listening, Coping Enhancement, Emotional Support, Guilt Work Facilitation, Hope Instillation, Presence, Religious Ritual Enhancement, Spiritual Support and Touch. This skill set of both diagnoses and interventions is a tall order, and the interprofessional team is invaluable! When a nurse feels out of her depth in the area of spiritual care, he or she can make a referral for pastoral care, in the form of a hospital chaplain, a parish nurse or another form of spiritual support (in accordance with the dying person's desires). Hospice programs provide spiritual support for both patients and their families.

Managing Physical Symptoms

Although the end-of-life process is individualized and unpredictable, some symptoms occur commonly and require

A Student's Perspective

I had a special experience with a man at the rehab centre. "Mort" and I had great conversations, and he quickly became a friend. Mort was suffering from cardiovascular failure, and I knew he did not have long to live. I interviewed Mort and then wrote a paper about his life. I wrote the paper early so that I could read it to Mort before his health declined any more. I read my paper to Mort one morning, and he listened with a seeming sense of sacredness about the words being read. This was his life, and I could tell that it meant a lot to him that I wrote it all down. When I finished, Mort simply said, "I thank you . . . I thank you." He asked me to put the paper in a safe place so it would not get ruined. Mort and I had a special connection; he was a hero to me. The following week, I went to the centre and found out that Mort had passed away. I am grateful that I had the opportunity to know Mort and to grow and learn from his good life. I am glad that I could serve him at this final time and help him reflect on his life.

Amy C.

expert and timely nursing care. A systematic review of the prevalence of symptoms during the last 2 weeks of life identified the following as the most commonly occurring ones: dyspnea (56.7%), pain (52.4%), respiratory secretions (51.4%) and confusion (50.1%) (Kehl & Kowalkowski, 2012). Additional symptoms that are often addressed at the end of life include fatigue and weakness, constipation, nausea and vomiting, dehydration and decreased appetite. Because these symptoms usually occur in combination, management is challenging and it is not always possible to control every symptom completely.

Nurses can use information in Table 29-1 and the following sections as a guide to nursing assessment and interventions for some of the commonly occurring symptoms. In

TABLE 29-1 Guide to Nursing Assessment and Interventions for Common Symptoms at the End of Life

Symptom	Nursing Assessment	Nursing Interventions	Pharmacologic Interventions
Fatigue (asthenia)	Assess for associated conditions, including infection, fever, pain, depression, insomnia, anxiety, dehydration, hypoxia, medication effects.	Inform older adult and family of the normality of fatigue at end of life. Pace activities and care according to tolerance. Encourage exercise if tolerated. Promote optimal sleep, with regular times of rest, sleep and waking.	Corticosteroids, although generally contraindicated in older adults, may decrease fatigue in patients with cancer. Treat associated conditions (e.g., with antibiotics, antidepressants) if patients desire it.
Constipation	Identify risks (e.g., chronic laxative users, medications). Perform abdominal assessment, including palpation for distention, tenderness or masses and auscultation of bowel sounds and pitch. Assess patients taking pain medications daily. Monitor the character of the bowel movements. Check the rectum if the older adult has not had a bowel movement in more than 3 days or is leaking liquid stool (which can occur with an impaction).	Anticipate and prevent constipation with emphasis on fibre, fluid intake and activity, but recognize that patients may have difficulty tolerating the optimal interventions. Promote regular routine. Strongest propulsive contractions occur after breakfast; provide patient privacy at this time.	Individualize laxative regimen on the basis of the cause(s) of constipation, history and preferences. Use bulk-forming and stool-softening agents for patients with normal peristalsis. A laxative regimen (with stimulant laxative) may be ordered for patients taking a pain medication known to cause constipation. Stimulant laxatives are the most appropriate for opioid-induced constipation.
Dyspnea	*Respiratory:* Assess vital signs, including oxygen saturation, breathing pattern and use of accessory muscles. Auscultate breath sounds. Assess cough (type, if present). Check for tachypnea and cyanosis. *General:* Assess for restlessness, anxiety and activity tolerance.	Pace activities and rest. Provide oxygen, usually at 2–4 L per cannula (avoid using face mask because of discomfort and sensation of smothering). Provide calm reassurance. Use a fan to circulate air and help reduce the feeling of breathlessness. Position for optimal respiratory function (e.g., leaning forward over a table with a pillow on top is helpful for chronic obstructive pulmonary disease [COPD]; on the side with head slightly elevated for unresponsive patient). Teach patient to use pursed-lip breathing, and encourage relaxation techniques to reduce muscle tightness and associated sensation of breathlessness.	Treat causes. Treat symptoms with morphine or hydromorphone, which relieves the breathless sensation in almost all cases. Use antianxiety agents or antidepressants if appropriate (and if perception of breathlessness is exaggerated because of anxiety or depression). Corticosteroids can be used for their anti-inflammatory effects in certain conditions (e.g., COPD, radiation pneumonitis).
Nausea and vomiting	Assess for potential cause (e.g., constipation, bowel obstruction). Palpate abdomen and check for distention. Assess vomitus for fecal odour. Assess heartburn and nausea, which may occur after meals in squashed stomach syndrome. Assess pain (e.g., pain on swallowing may indicate oral thrush; pain on standing may be caused by mesenteric traction). Hiccups occur with uremia.	Offer frequent, small meals; serve foods cold or at room temperature. Apply damp, cool cloth to face when nauseated. Provide oral care after vomiting.	Medications need to be specific to the cause: • Squashed stomach syndrome, gastritis and functional bowel obstruction: metoclopramide (contraindicated in full bowel obstruction) • Chemical causes, such as morphine, hypercalcemia or renal failure: haloperidol • If caused by dysfunction of vomiting centre (e.g., associated with mechanical bowel obstruction, increased intracranial pressure, motion sickness): meclizine or diphenhydramine

Symptom	Nursing Assessment	Nursing Interventions	Pharmacologic Interventions
Dehydration	Assess for clinical signs of hydration (e.g., skin turgor over the upper chest or forehead). Assess buccal membranes for moisture. Assess vital signs: pulse, orthostatic blood pressure.	Encourage fluids as tolerated; offer ice chips and popsicles if swallowing. Provide frequent oral care; use swabs or moistened toothettes.	Give intravenous fluids or administer clysis per advance directives. Discuss continued diuretic use with physician.
Anorexia and cachexia	Assess for weight loss. Assess for levels of weakness and fatigue. Conduct physical examination for decreased fat, muscle wasting, decreased strength. Assess mental status, including depression.	Remove unpleasant odours. Provide frequent oral care. Treat pain optimally. Provide frequent, small meals. Provide companionship. Serve meals in a place that is separate from the bed area. Involve patient with meal planning. Collaborate with dietician for nutritional analysis and meal planning. Encourage culturally appropriate foods. Consider using an alcoholic beverage before meals.	Medications that are used to stimulate appetite, promote weight gain and provide a sense of well-being: megestrol acetate, corticosteroids, and mirtazapine. Metoclopramide is used to improve gastric motility and appetite.

addition, nurses can use information in Chapter 28 to address pain, which is a symptom that occurs frequently at the end of life and is one of the most feared symptoms associated with death. This chapter addresses the symptoms only in relation to the end of life; other pertinent topics are discussed more comprehensively in other chapters: confusion or delirium (Chapter 14), depression (Chapter 15), constipation (Chapter 18) and sleep problems (Chapter 24).

Fatigue (Asthenia)

Fatigue is one of the most commonly reported symptoms at the end of life. Fatigue is often described as tiredness, or lack of physical strength and endurance, or decreased mental concentration. Older adults may have reduced energy or activity tolerance caused by chronic conditions, so it is important for the nurse to establish a baseline for comparison and meaningful interpretation. Fatigue is generally a symptom with underlying causes related to disease processes or conditions, such as anemia, malnutrition, infection, drug therapy or depression. Other concurrent end-of-life symptoms, such as pain and dyspnea, may exacerbate fatigue.

Constipation

Constipation, a reduced frequency of bowel movements, can include passing hard stools, straining to pass a stool or impaction (hard stool that is blocked). Constipation may be accompanied by pain, abdominal fullness and reduced bowel sounds. In general, older adults are at increased risk for constipation because of medications, dietary patterns and decreased physical activity. Factors that increase the risk for constipation at the end of life include pain medications (discussed in Chapter 28), dehydration, kidney failure, elevated calcium levels and disease effects (e.g., ascites, spinal cord damage, colon or pelvic cancers).

Dyspnea

Dyspnea occurs commonly in conditions involving cardiorespiratory function (e.g., heart failure, lung cancer, chronic obstructive pulmonary disease), and it also occurs during advanced stages of other conditions. Studies have identified dyspnea as one of the most distressing symptoms experienced by many people with advanced progressive diseases, and it often evokes feelings of fear, anxiety and panic (Campbell, 2012; Yates & Zhao, 2012). Descriptive terms include shortness of breath, breathlessness, suffocation and being smothered. A recent nursing review of literature by Lowey et al. (2013) recommended the following framework, called the ADRA (Assess, Document, Re-Assess, Advocate) as an integral part of care for patients with end-stage illnesses:

- Assess all patients for dyspnea intensity and severity, using a standardized and validated tool.
- Document comprehensive information about assessment, pharmacologic and nonpharmacologic interventions, and patient's responses.
- Reassess dyspnea and response to interventions.
- Advocate for patients by discussing wishes and preferences for care.

Nausea and Vomiting

Nausea and vomiting are common symptoms associated with terminal illness. Causes of nausea and vomiting at the end of life include the following:

- Irritation/obstruction of gastrointestinal tract (bowel obstruction, constipation, cancer tumour, delayed emptying of stomach from ascites, tumour pressure [often called *squashed stomach syndrome*])
- Medication side effect (particularly opioids such as morphine)
- Ear infection or labyrinthitis

- Electrolyte imbalance, sepsis
- Kidney failure, liver failure
- Increased intracranial pressure (brain tumour, cerebral edema, intracranial bleeding, metastasis)
- Foul odours
- Anxiety, fear

Dehydration

Because older adults normally have an age-related decrease in body water, they become dehydrated more easily. Causes of dehydration at the end of life include reduced or inadequate oral intake, medications such as diuretics, vomiting, diarrhea and fever. Symptoms of dehydration can interfere with comfort by causing dry mouth, constipation, confusion and skin impairment.

Anorexia and Cachexia

Additional symptoms include anorexia, a lack of appetite that progresses to the inability to eat and cachexia, which is a general state of malnutrition in which there is loss of fat, muscle and bone mineral content. Even before the terminal illness, older adults often have less lean tissue, so there is less reserve and malnutrition can progress quickly. Factors that contribute to anorexia and cachexia include nausea and vomiting, constipation, dehydration, weakness, depression, pain, oral candidiasis or dry mouth, gastritis and medication side effects.

Symptoms During the Active Dying Process

When it becomes apparent that a dying person has only a few days to live, it is especially important that the nurse work closely with the individual and his or her family to help them understand the dying process and anticipate changes. Guidance about what to expect helps reduce fear and anxiety.

Characteristic physical signs indicate the **active dying** process. In most situations, the individual has become totally dependent on others for all aspects of care, with less wakeful or alert time. Levels of consciousness may change or fluctuate. The person has little or no interest in the oral intake of food or fluids. Physiologic changes occur in breathing patterns, circulation slows down, sensory awareness decreases and muscle weakness occurs as a result of decreased tone. In addition to these physiologic manifestations, delirium and restlessness are common during the last weeks of life. Table 29-2 summarizes some signs and symptoms that occur within days of death. The overall focus of nursing care at this point is to continue to promote physiologic and psychological comfort, while assisting the older adult in achieving a peaceful, dignified death.

Providing Emotional Support and Caring for Oneself

Two aspects of end-of-life care that are particularly challenging are providing emotional support for the patient and family and caring for oneself. The Supportive Care Department at the City of Hope National Medical Center have developed a pocket-sized CARES tool for guiding nursing care of hospitalized patients who are dying (Freeman, 2013). Online Learning Activity 29-3 provides a link to complete information about CARES, which is an acronym for Comfort, Airway, Restlessness, Emotional, Support and Self-Care. Box 29-6 illustrates the guides for providing emotional support and self-care.

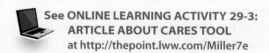

See **ONLINE LEARNING ACTIVITY 29-3: ARTICLE ABOUT CARES TOOL** at http://thepoint.lww.com/Miller7e

---

TABLE 29-2 Signs and Symptoms of Death Within Days

Physiologic Change	Signs and Symptoms
Altered breathing patterns	• Breathing initially becomes more shallow. • Cheyne-Stokes respirations • Noisy breathing (death rattle)
Changing circulation	• Limbs, ears and nose become cold to touch or mottled in appearance. • Decreased blood pressure • Pulse may weaken and become irregular. • Diaphoresis • Possible increase in dependent edema • No urine output or small amount of very dark urine (anuria or oliguria)
Decreased muscle tone	• Relaxed facial muscles, lower jaw drops, mouth opens • Decreased/loss of gag reflex • Difficulty swallowing • Abdominal distention due to decreased gastrointestinal activity • Possible urinary and fecal incontinence due to relaxation of sphincter muscles
Decreased senses	• Reduced level of consciousness • Blurred or distorted vision • Decreased taste and smell (probable continued sense of hearing)

Source: Saunderson, C. A., & Brener, T. H. (Eds.). (2007). *End of life: A nurse's guide to compassionate care.* Philadelphia, PA: Lippincott Williams & Wilkins.

Box 29-6 Implementing CARES Emotional Support

The CARES tool addresses Comfort, Airway, Restlessness and delirium, Emotional and spiritual support, and Self-care for dying patients and their caregivers. CARES was developed by Bonnie Freeman, RN, DNP, ANP, Department of Supportive Care Medicine, City of Hope National Medical Centre, in Duarte, California.

Emotional, Spiritual, Psychosocial and Cultural Support

Providing emotional, spiritual, psychosocial and cultural support to the patient and family allows nurses to care for the soul. This is the very foundation of caring for the dying. It is important to implement various resources. For example:

- Notify supportive care team members for assistance and specify whether the resources are for patient, staff or both.
- Always work to retain the patient's dignity and feelings of value.
- Remember every family is unique and grieves differently.

Good Communication Is Essential

- Make sure that communication exists with the family and interprofessionally.
- Take your cues from family members. Do not assume you know what they are thinking or feeling.
- Clarify how much the family wants to know.
- Clarify goals of care.
- Clarify privacy needs.
- Just be with patient and family and sit in silence.
- Work with family to provide favourite activities, smells, sounds, etc.
- Support rituals and assist with obtaining desired clergy or equipment.

Other Activities and Methods of Support

- Your humanity is needed the most now. Always be available. Your very presence is reassuring to the family.
- The family is an important part of your patient care and becomes your focus as the patient becomes more unresponsive.

- — Be sure families are getting rest and breaks.
- — Provide coffee, water, etc.
- — Continue to be available to answer questions.
- — You cannot take away their pain. Acknowledge their emotions and be present.
- Play patient's favourite music.
- Position bed so patient can see out a window.
- Encourage family to provide patient's favourite hat, clothing, etc.
- Lower or mute lighting in the patient's room.
- Consider bringing in a favourite pet.

Self-Care

Health care providers must allow themselves to be human and expect some personal emotional response to the death of their patient and for the grieving family. Care providers may need supportive services. Often a review and debriefing can assist with professional grieving and promote emotional health by:

- Recognizing the stressful event and thanking supportive team members.
- Reviewing what went well and what challenges need to be addressed.
- Sharing bereaved family comments.
- Addressing moral distress issues.
- Expressing issues of death anxiety and obtaining support.
- Exploring challenges and privileges of assisting a fellow human being through the dying process.
- Acknowledging the spiritual impact of witnessing death.
- Exploring how your care made a difference to the grieving family.
- Reviewing effective communication techniques, available resources and support.

Adapted with permission from Freeman, B. (2013). CARES: An acronym organized tool for the care of the dying. *Journal of Hospice & Palliative Nursing, 15*(3), 147–153. Used with permission from B. Freeman, RN, DNP, ANP and Journal of Hospice & Palliative Nursing.

Unfolding Case Study

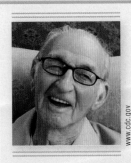

www.cdc.gov

Part 1: Mr. B. at 91 Years of Age

Mr. B. is a 91-year-old man with medical diagnoses including hypertension, type 2 diabetes mellitus, history of cerebrovascular accident and benign prostatic hyperplasia. He was taking the following medications: lisinopril (Prinivil), 20 mg daily; aspirin, 81 mg daily; furosemide (Lasix), 40 mg daily; potassium, 20 mEq daily; and acetaminophen (Tylenol) as needed for arthritis pain. He has lived at home by himself for the past 15 years since the death of his wife. He has three adult children, all living out of state, who visit on average once monthly. He is very well known in his neighbourhood as the older man who helps everyone. He loves his home and spends his days "keeping house." His favourite chores include mowing the grass in the summer and blowing the snow in the winter. He owns and drives a car to the local supermarket and barbershop and to the cemetery to visit his wife's grave. In late summer, he had an accident with his lawn mower that drew his family's attention to the fact that he was losing his strength. While mowing his grass, he fell over the lawn mower, scraping his face on the sidewalk. He required emergency department (ER) evaluation and treatment, including stitches for facial lacerations. He later admitted that, before his fall, he had been experiencing dizziness, especially when getting out of his easy chair.

Three weeks after his ER evaluation, Mr. B.'s daughter came to visit. She was shocked to see her father looking so "thin and gaunt." Mr. B. admitted that he had lost a few pounds over the summer

(continued)

Unfolding Case Study (continued)

and still didn't have much energy. He stated that he wasn't sleeping well at night, with his sleep disrupted every 30 to 45 minutes because of the need to urinate. To control his urination, he had decided to limit his drinking fluids to less than 240 cc daily. Mr. B.'s daughter noticed that in spite of his weight loss, his abdomen was very large and distended. "Do you have any aches?" she asked her father. He nodded yes and grabbed his lower abdomen.

THINKING POINTS

- On the basis of symptoms and history, what points would you address in your nursing assessment?
- What nursing problems would you address in Mr. B.'s nursing care plan?

- What are some probable causes of Mr. B.'s abdominal discomfort?
- What would the appropriate nursing interventions be?
- What health teaching would you provide?

Unfolding Case Study

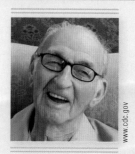
www.cdc.gov

Part 2: Mr. B. at Follow-up

Mr. B. and his daughter have a follow-up office visit with his primary care physician. On arrival, his vital signs are as follows: temperature, 36.7 PO; apical pulse, 82 beats per minute and irregularly irregular; respirations, 24 per minute; and blood pressure sitting, 98/50. When standing to walk to the scale for his weight measurement, he swayed a bit, grabbed the wall and then steadied himself. "I just got a little dizzy," he admitted. As the office nurse, you immediately grabbed the blood pressure cuff and took his blood pressure in the standing position. It was 70/40. Mr. B.'s pulse at that time was 90 and irregular. Noting the vital sign changes, the physician ordered some laboratory tests. Blood samples for testing were drawn in the office. With results pending, no changes were made in his medical care at that time.

THINKING POINTS

- What are your immediate nursing concerns for Mr. B. based on information about his decline during the past 6 months?

- What risk factors are likely to be contributing to Mr. B.'s dizziness?
- What patient teaching is indicated at this time?

Unfolding Case Study

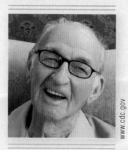
www.cdc.gov

Part 3: Mr. B. the Next Week

Mr. B.'s blood test results come back the next day, confirming dehydration and malnutrition:

- Sodium: 150
- Potassium: 3.7
- Serum albumin: 3.0
- Prealbumin: 14
- Blood urea nitrogen: 35
- Serum creatinine: 1.7

The physician discontinued Mr. B.'s furosemide and lisinopril and suggested a follow-up visit in 2 weeks. Two days before his next appointment, Mr. B.'s daughter called the office to relay that her father had fallen and was taken to the hospital for evaluation. A workup revealed that he had had a transient ischemic attack and was now too weak to eat and was experiencing difficulty swallowing. The family declined a feeding tube, and a hospice referral was made.

THINKING POINTS

- Identify two priority nursing diagnoses appropriate for Mr. B. at this time.
- For each diagnosis, list two to three nursing interventions.

- Mr. B. died in the hospital 1 week after his fall, on the day he was scheduled for discharge.

Chapter Highlights

Perspectives on End-of-Life Care (Fig. 29-1, Box 29-1)

- The end-of-life time for older adults is often a gradual process associated with cumulative effects of chronic illness and many interacting conditions.
- Views of death and dying in Western societies have shifted as a result of demographic and health care trends (e.g., increased life expectancy, medical and technical advances).
- Cultural perspectives—of society, patients and health care providers—exert a strong influence on all aspects of end-of-life care.
- Current emphasis is on "rehumanizing" end-of-life care and addressing issues concerning both cost and quality of care.

Current Legal and Ethical Concerns

- Within Canada, physician-assisted suicide and euthanasia are not legal. There is much debate about this issue, and Bill 52 was introduced in the Quebec Legislature, in favour of euthanasia. It was not passed. It is expected that the debate will continue and that it may reach the Supreme Court of Canada.
- A national strategy has been created through the Quality End-of-Life Care Coalition to make quality end-of-life care available to all Canadians.

Hospice Palliative Care

- Hospice palliative care is an interprofessional approach to care that holistically addresses needs of people with life-limiting conditions, as well as the needs of their families and caregivers. The care focuses on comfort, rather than cure.
- To qualify for hospice services, patients must have a life expectancy of 6 months or less.

Promoting Wellness at the End of Life

- Wellness at the end of life is achieved through a dignified death, as described in the Dying Patient's Bill of Rights (Box 29-3).
- The Nursing Outcomes Classification (NOC) of Dignified Life Closure is applicable to promoting wellness for patients at the end of life.

Nursing Skills and Interventions for End-of-Life Care (Boxes 29-3 through 29-5, Tables 29-1 and 29-2)

- Nurses use verbal and nonverbal communication skills that are appropriate for addressing the complexity of end-of-life situations.
- Nurses have numerous opportunities to provide spiritual care for patients and families as an integral part of end-of-life care.
- Nurses are responsible for managing physical symptoms that occur during the end of life: fatigue, constipation, dyspnea, nausea and vomiting, dehydration and anorexia.
- Interventions for emotional support for patients and families, as well as self-care for nurses, are essential aspects of end-of-life care.

Critical Thinking Exercises

1. Review the section on culturally diverse perspectives on death and dying and spend a few minutes answering the questions for self-reflection.
2. Review the information in Box 29-6 and reflect on how you would apply this information to the care of a dying patient and to the care of yourself.

 For more information about the topics discussed in this chapter, be sure to check out the interactive Online Learning Activities and other helpful resources at http://thepoint.lww.com/Miller7e

REFERENCES

Arnup, K. (2013). *Death, dying and Canadian families*. Ottawa, ON, Canada: Vanier Institute.

Austin, L. (1975). *Dying patient's bill of rights*. Created at The Terminally Ill Patient and the Helping Person Workshops. Sponsored by the Southwest Michigan Inservice Education Council in Lansing, MI.

Bill 52: An act respecting end-of-life care. (2013). Quebec, IA: Quebec Official Publisher. Retrieved from http://www.assnat.qc.ca/en/travaux-parlementaires/projets-loi/projet-loi-52-40-1.html

Bryce, P. H. (1922). *The story of a national crime*. Ottawa, ON, Canada: James Hope and Sons.

Cairns, B., & Ahmad, M. (2011, May 17). Choosing where to die: Allowing for choices: Dying at home, in a hospice or in palliative care. *CBC News*. Retrieved from http://www.cbc.ca/news/health/choosing-where-to-die-1.1002383

Cairns, D., Williams, V., Victor, C., et al. (2013). The meaning and importance of dignified care: Findings from a survey of health and social care professionals. *BioMed Central Geriatrics, 13*, 28. Retrieved from www.biomedcentral.com/1471-2318/13/28

Campbell, M. L. (2012). Dyspnea prevalence, trajectories, and measurement in critical care and at life's end. *Current Opinion in Supportive and Palliative Care, 6*(2), 168–171.

Canadian Association of Critical Care Nurses. (2011). *Providing end of life care in the Intensive Care Unit.* Retrieved from http://www.caccn.ca/en/publications/position_statements/providing_end_of_life_care_in_the_icu.html

Canadian Hospice Palliative Care Association. (2008). *Nursing Certification Examination: List of assumptions and competencies.* Retrieved from www.chpca.net

Canadian Institute for Health Information. (2005). *Hospital trends in Canada: Results of a project to create a historical series of statistical and financial data for Canadian hospitals over twenty-seven years.* Ottawa, ON: Author. Retrieved from https://secure.cihi.ca/free_products/Hospital_Trends_in_Canada_e.pdf

Canadian Virtual Hospice Team. (2003–2014). *Palliative care.* Retrieved from http://www.virtualhospice.ca

Comeau, S. (2014, April 10). A doctor for the dying. *McGill News.* Retrieved from http://publications.mcgill.ca/mcgillnews/2011/10/13/a-doctor-for-the-dying/

Death With Dignity National Center. (2013). *Death with Dignity acts.* Retrieved from www.deathwithdignity.org/acts

Fenigsen, R. (2012). Other people's lives: Reflections on medicine, ethics and euthanasia. *Issues in Law and Medicine, 28*(1), 73–87.

Fowler, R., & Hammer, M. (2013). End-of-life care in Canada. *Clinical and Investigative Medicine, 36*(3), E127–E129.

Freeman, B. (2013). CARES: An acronym organized tool for the care of the dying. *Journal of Hospice and Palliative Nursing, 15*(3), 147–153.

Hamilton, G. (2014, February 13). As Quebec set to legalize euthanasia, doctors already looking to expand who qualifies for lethal injections. *The National Post.* Retrieved from http://news.nationalpost.com/2014/02/13/as-quebec-set-to-legalize-euthanasia-doctors-already-looking-to-expand-who-qualifies-for-lethal-injections/

Hirst, S. P., Lane, A. M., & Reed, M. B. (2013). Personhood in nursing homes: An ethnographic study. *Indian Journal of Gerontology, 27*(1), 69–87.

Hodgson, C. (2012). *Cost-effectiveness of palliative care: A review of the literature.* Ottawa, ON: Canadian Hospice and Palliative Care Association.

Hospice and Palliative Nurses Association. (2010). *HPNA position statement: Spiritual care.* Retrieved from www.hpna.org

Jablonski, A, Clymin, J., Jacobson, D., et al. (2012). The Washington state Death With Dignity Act. *Journal of Hospice and Palliative Nursing, 14*(1), 45–52.

Keegan, L., & Drick, C. (2011). *End of life: Nursing solutions to death with dignity.* New York, NY: Springer.

Kehl, K. A., & Kowalkowski, J. A. (2012). A systematic review of the prevalence of signs of impending death and symptoms in the last 2 weeks of life. *American Journal of Hospice and Palliative Care, 30*(6), 601–616.

Kirkey, S. (2013, December 13). Should this doctor help people die? *The Vancouver Sun.* Retrieved from http://www.vancouversun.com/health/seniors/FINAL+EXIT+This+doctor+sees+death+daily+should+help+suffering/9284582/story.html

Kirkey, S. (2014, April 7). 'Physician-assisted death is going to become legal': Canada's right-to-die debate almost over, doctors say. *The National Post.* Retrieved from http://news.nationalpost.com/2014/04/07/physician-assisted-death-is-going-to-become-legal-canadas-right-to-die-debate-almost-over-doctors-say/

Kübler-Ross, E. (1969). *On death and dying.* New York, NY: Macmillan.

Lane, A. M., Hirst, S. P., & Reed, M. B. (2013). *Older adults: Understanding and facilitating transitions.* Dubuque, IA: Kendall Hunt.

Lin, Y. P., Watson, R., & Tsai, Y. F. (2013). Dignity in care in the clinical setting: A narrative review. *Nursing Ethics, 20*(2), 168–177.

Lowey, S. E., Powers, B. A., & Xue, Y. (2013). Short of breath and dying: State of science on opioid agents for the palliation of refractory dyspnea in older adults. *Journal of Gerontological Nursing, 39*(2), 43–52.

Manookian, A., Cheraghi, M. A., & Nasrabadi, A. N. (2013). Factors influencing patients' dignity: A qualitative study. *Nursing Ethics, 21*(3), 323–334.

Markson, E. (2003). *Social gerontology today.* Los Angeles, CA: Roxbury.

Materstvedt, L. J., Clark, D., Ellershaw, J., et al. (2003). Euthanasia and physician-assisted suicide: A view from an EAPC ethics task force. *Palliative Medicine, 17*(2), 97–101. doi:10.1191/0269216303pm673oa

McLeod-Sordjan, R. (2013). Human becoming: Death acceptance: Facilitated communication with low-English proficiency patients at end of life. *Journal of Hospice and Palliative Nursing, 15*(7), 390–395.

Moorhead, S., Johnson, M., Maas, M. L., & Swanson, E. (Eds.). (2012). *Nursing Outcomes Classification (NOC).* Philadelphia, PA: Elsevier.

Nash, S. (2011). Health and wellbeing part 1: Helping ourselves and others. *Nursing Times, 107*(22), 19, 20.

Ohio State University Health Sciences Center, Office of Geriatrics & Gerontology. (2003). *Series to understand, nurture and support end-of-life transitions (SUNSET).* Retrieved from http://sunset.osu.edu

Penrod, J., Hupcey, J. E., Baney, B., et al. (2011). End-of-life caregiving trajectories. *Clinical Nursing Research, 20*(1), 7–24.

Penrod, J., Hupcey, J. E., Shipley, P. Z., et al. (2012). A model of caregiving through the end of life: Seeking normal. *Western Journal of Nursing Research, 34*(2), 174–193.

Periyakoil, V. S., Stevens, M., & Kraemer, H. (2013). Multicultural long-term care nurses' perceptions of factors influencing patient dignity at the end of life. *Journal of the American Geriatrics Society, 61*(3), 440–446.

Physicians' Alliance for Total Refusal of Euthanasia. (2013, June 12). *Bill 52: A dangerous and discriminatory bill.* Retrieved from http://www.newswire.ca/en/story/1182723/bill-52-a-dangerous-and-discriminatory-bill

Quality End-of-Life Care Coalition of Canada. (2010). *Blueprint for action 2010–2020.* Retrieved from http://www.qelccc.ca/media/3743/blueprint_for_action_2010_to_2020_april_2010.pdf

Quality End-of-Life Care Coalition of Canada. (2014). *Canadian Hospice Palliative Care Association.* Retrieved from http://www.qelccc.ca/

Reichel, J. (2014, February 12). 'Father of palliative care' slams Quebec euthanasia bill. *The Epoch Times.* Retrieved from http://www.theepochtimes.com/n3/504138-father-of-palliative-care-slams-quebec-euthanasia-bill/?photo=2

Royal Society of Canada. (2011). *The Royal Society of Canada Expert Panel: End-of-life decision making.* Retrieved from https://rsc-src.ca/sites/default/files/pdf/RSCEndofLifeReport2011_EN_Formatted_FINAL.pdf

Seaman, J. B. (2013). Improving care at end of life in the ICU. *Journal of Gerontological Nursing, 39*(3), 52–58.

Segers, J. H. (1988). Persons on the subject of euthanasia. *Issues in Law & Medicine, 3*, 407–424.

Smith, S. L., & Nickel, D. D. (2003). Nursing the dying in Post-Second World War Canada and the United States. In G. Feldberg (Ed.), *Women, health, and nation: Canada and the United States since 1945* (pp. 330–354). Canada: McGill-Queen's University Press.

Soka Gakkai International. (2014). *Buddhism and human dignity.* Retrieved from http://www.sgi.org/buddhism/buddhist-concepts/buddhism-and-human-dignity.html

Spencer, S., Martin, S., Bourgeault, I. L., & O'Shea, E. (2010). *The role of migrant care workers in ageing societies: Report on research findings in the United Kingdom, Ireland, Canada and the United States.* Geneva, Switzerland: International Organization for Migration.

Statistics Canada. (2010a). *Life expectancy.* Retrieved from http://www.statcan.gc.ca/pub/82-229-x/2009001/demo/lif-eng.htm

Statistics Canada. (2010b). *Population projections for Canada, provinces and territories – 2009–2036.* Retrieved from www.statcan.gc.ca/pub/91-520-x/91-520-x2010001-eng.pdf

Statistics Canada. (2012). *Deaths: 2009.* Ottawa, ON: Government of Canada, Health Statistics Division.

Teno, J. M., Gozalo, P. L., Lee, I. C., et al. (2011). Does hospice improve quality of care for persons dying of dementia? *Journal of the American Geriatrics Society, 59*(8), 1531–1536. doi:10.1111/j.1532-5415.2011.03505.x

The Canadian Press. (2012). *Canada has higher proportion of seniors than ever before.* Retrieved from http://www.cbc.ca/news/canada/canada-has-higher-proportion-of-seniors-than-ever-before-1.1151526

van Gennip, I. E., Roeline, H., Pasman, W., et al. (2013). Death with dignity from the perspective of the surviving family: A survey study among family caregivers of deceased older adults. *Palliative Medicine, 27*(7), 616–624.

Van Stolk, C., Hassan, E., Austin, C., et al. (2009). *The NHS workforce health and wellbeing review.* London, England: Department of Health.

von Gunten, C. F. (2012). Evolution and effectiveness of palliative care. *American Journal of Geriatric Psychiatry, 20*(4), 291–297. doi:10.1097/JGP.0b013e3182436219

Wiegand, D. L., Grant, M. S., Cheon, J., et al. (2013). Family-centered end-of-life care in the ICU. *Journal of Gerontological Nursing, 39*(8), 60–68.

Yates, P., & Zhao, I. (2012). Update on complex nonpharmacological interventions for breathlessness. *Current Opinion in Supportive and Palliative Care, 6*(2), 144–151.

Zamer, J. A., & Volker, D. L. (2013). Religious leaders' perspectives of ethical concerns at the end of life. *Journal of Hospice and Palliative Nursing, 15*(7), 396–402.

Index

Note: Page numbers followed by the letter *b* denoted boxes, those followed by *f* denote figures, and those followed by *t* denote tables.